2

Spine Trauma

AAOS

American Academy of Orthopaedic Surgeons

2

Spine Trauma

Editors
Jack E. Zigler, MD
Frank J. Eismont, MD
Steven R. Garfin, MD
Alexander R. Vaccaro, MD, PhD

AAOS
American Academy of Orthopaedic Surgeons

AAOS
AMERICAN ACADEMY OF
ORTHOPAEDIC SURGEONS

Staff

Mark W. Wieting, *Chief Education Officer*

Marilyn L. Fox, PhD, *Director, Department of Publications*

Mary Steermann Bishop, *Senior Manager, Production and Archives*

Courtney Astle, *Editorial Production Manager*

Suzanne O'Reilly, *Graphic Designer*

Karen Danca, *Permissions Coordinator*

Charlie Baldwin, *Production Database Associate*

Abram Fassler, *Production Database Associate*

Hollie Benedik, *Page Production Assistant*

Michelle Bruno, *Publications Assistant*

Published 2011 by the

American Academy of Orthopaedic Surgeons
6300 North River Road
Rosemont, IL 60018

ISBN 978-0-89203-753-7

Printed in the USA

Bone and Joint DECADE 2002-USA-2011

Editorial Board, Spine Trauma, ed 2

Contributors

Todd Albert, MD
Richard H. Rothman Professor and Chair
Department of Orthopaedics
Rothman Institute
Thomas Jefferson University
Philadelphia, Pennsylvania

Paul A. Anderson, MD
Professor of Orthopedic Surgery
Department of Orthopedic Surgery and Rehabilitation
University of Wisconsin
Madison, Wisconsin

Alana J. Arnold, BS
Medical Student
Tufts University School of Medicine
Boston, Massachusetts

Michal Atkins, MA, OTR/L
Occupational Therapy Clinical Instructor
Department of Occupational and Recreational Therapy
Rancho Los Amigos National Rehabilitation Center
Downey, California

Eli M. Baron, MD
Neurosurgeon and Spine Surgeon
Cedars Sinai Spine Center
Cedars Sinai Medical Center
Los Angeles, California

David M. Benglis, Jr, MD
Neurosurgery PG-Y-7 Resident
Department of Neurosurgery
University of Miami
Miami, Florida

Edward C. Benzel, MD
Chairman
Department of Neurosurgery
Neurological Institute
Cleveland Clinic
Cleveland, Ohio

Christopher M. Bono, MD
Associate Professor of Orthopaedic Surgery and Chief of Spine Service
Department of Orthopaedic Surgery
Harvard Medical School
Brigham and Women's Hospital
Boston, Massachusetts

Michael J. Botte, MD
Co-Director of Hand and Microvascular Surgery
Division of Orthopaedic Surgery
Scripps Clinic
La Jolla, California

Ted Brindle, MD
Neurosurgeon
Sutter Neuroscience Medical Group
Sutter Roseville Medical Center
Roseville, California

Patrick J. Cahill, MD
Physician
Shriners Hospital for Children
Philadelphia, Pennsylvania

Terrence Cahill, MD
Department of Physical Medicine and Rehabilitation
Billings Clinic
Billings, Montana

Frank P. Cammisa, Jr, MD, FACS
Chief, Spinal Surgical Service
Spine Care Institute
The Hospital for Special Surgery
Associate Professor of Clinical Orthopaedic Surgery
Weill Medical College of Cornell University
New York, New York

Lisa Carroll, PT
Clinical Manager
Department of Physical Therapy
Rancho Los Amigos National Rehabilitation Center
Downey, California

Contributors (cont.)

Douglas G. Chang, MD, PhD
Clinical Associate Professor and Chief of Physical Medicine and Rehabilitation
Department of Orthopaedic Surgery
University of California San Diego
San Diego, California

Esteban Cuartas, MD
Department of Orthopedics
St. Luke's Cornwall Hospital
Newburgh, New York

Bradford L. Currier, MD
Professor of Orthopedics and Director of the Mayo Clinic Spine Fellowship
Department of Orthopedics
Mayo Clinic
Rochester, Minnesota

Lawrence Delasotta, MD, MPH
Research Fellow
Department of Orthopaedic Spine Surgery
Rothman Institute
Thomas Jefferson University Hospital
Philadelphia, Pennsylvania

Timothy DiIorio, MD
Research Fellow
Rothman Institute
Thomas Jefferson University
Philadelphia, Pennsylvania

Rob D. Dickerman, DO, PhD
Neurosurgeon
Plano Presbyterian Hospital
Plano, Texas

Frank J. Eismont, MD
Chairman
Department of Orthopedic Surgery
University of Miami Miller School of Medicine
Miami, Florida

Ahmad Faizan, PhD
Research Assistant
Department of Bioengineering
University of Toledo
Toledo, Ohio

Steven Falcone, MD, MBA
Associate Professor of Radiology, Neurosurgery, and Ophthalmology
University of Miami
Miami, Florida

Amir Fayyazi
VSAS Orthopaedics
Allentown, Pennsylvania

Michael G. Fehlings, MD, PhD, FRCSC, FACS
Professor of Neurosurgery
Department of Neurosurgery
University of Toronto
Toronto, Ontario, Canada

Joseph L. Ferguson, DPT, BS, MD (candidate)
Medical Student
Jefferson Medical College
Philadelphia, Pennsylvania

Daveed D. Frazier, MD
Assistant Clinical Professor of Orthopaedic Surgery
Department of Orthopaedic Surgery
Columbia University
St. Luke's Roosevelt Hospital
New York, New York

Steven R. Garfin, MD
Professor and Chair
Department of Orthopaedic Surgery
University of California San Diego
San Diego, California

Kevin D. Gerhart, MD, PhD
Chief
Spinal Cord Injury Service
VA San Diego Healthcare System
San Diego, California

Contributors (cont.)

Vijay K. Goel, PhD
Endowed Professor
Department of Bioengineering
University of Toledo
Toledo, Ohio

Jonathan N. Grauer, MD
Associate Professor
Department of Orthopaedics and Rehabilitation
Yale University School of Medicine
New Haven, Connecticut

Barth A. Green, MD, FACS
Professor and Chairman
Department of Neurosurgery
University of Miami
Miami, Florida

Jordan Gruskay, BA
Spine Research Fellow
Rothman Institute
Thomas Jefferson University Hospital
Philadelphia, Pennsylvania

Richard D. Guyer, MD
Chairman
Texas back Institute Research Foundation
Texas Back Institute
Plano, Texas
Associate Clinical Professor of Orthopedics
University of Texas Southwestern School of Medicine
Dallas, Texas

Mitchel B. Harris, MD, FACS
Chief of Orthopaedic Trauma
Brigham and Women's Hospital
Harvard Medical School
Boston, Massachusetts

James Harrop, MD
Neurosurgeon
Department of Neurological Surgery
Thomas Jefferson University Hospital
Philadelphia, Pennsylvania

Harry N. Herkowitz, MD
Chairman
Department of Orthopaedic Surgery
William Beaumont Hospital
Royal Oak, Michigan

Martin J. Herman, MD
Associate Professor
Drexel University College of Medicine
Orthopedic Center for Children
St. Christopher's Hospital for Children
Philadelphia, Pennsylvania

Joseph Hong, BS
Research Fellow
Rothman Institute
Thomas Jefferson University Hospital
Philadelphia, Pennsylvania

Steven Hwang, MD
Fellow
Department of Orthopedics
Shriners Hospital
Philadelphia, Pennsylvania

Andrew Jea, MD
Assistant Professor
Department of Neurosurgery
Baylor College of Medicine
Houston, Texas

S. Babak Kalantar, MD
Assistant Professor of Spine Surgery
Department of Orthopedics
Georgetown University Hospital
Washington, DC

Mara Karamitopoulos, MD
Resident
Department of Orthopedic Surgery
Thomas Jefferson University Hospital
Philadelphia, Pennsylvania

Contributors (cont.)

Choll W. Kim, MD, PhD
Associate Clinical Professor
Spine Institute of San Diego
Center for Minimally Invasive Spine Surgery
Alvarado Hospital and University of California San Diego
San Diego, California

Scott H. Kitchel, MD
Orthopedic Spine Surgeon
Orthopedic Spine Associates
Eugene, Oregon

Mark A. Knaub, MD
Director of Orthopaedic Spine Service
Department of Orthopaedic Surgery
Penn State Hershey Medical Center
Hershey, Pennsylvania

Lawrence T. Kurz, MD
Attending Spine Surgeon
Department of Orthopaedic Surgery
William Beaumont Hospital
Royal Oak, Michigan

Brian K. Kwon, MD, PhD, FRCSC
Associate Professor
Combined Neurosurgical and Orthopaedic Spine Program
Department of Orthopaedics
University of British Columbia
Vancouver, British Columbia, Canada

Sebastian Lattuga, MD
Chief of Spine Division North Shore
Department of Orthopaedics
North Shore Franklin Hospital
Valley Stream, New York

Darren R. Lebl, MD
Chief Resident
Department of Orthopaedic Surgery
Harvard Combined Orthopaedics
Boston, Massachusetts

Yu-Po Lee, MD
Assistant Clinical Professor
Department of Orthopaedic Surgery
University of California San Diego Medical Center
San Diego, California

Alan M. Levine, MD
Deceased

Allan Levi, MD, PhD, FRCSC, FACS
Professor of Neurological Surgery
Department of Neurological Surgery
University of Miami
Miami, Florida

Worawat Limthongkul, MD
Clinical Instructor
Department of Orthopaedics
King Chulalongkorn Memorial Hospital
Bangkok, Thailand

Michael Linn, MD
Resident
Department of Orthopaedics
University of California San Diego
San Diego, California

Travis G. Maak, MD
Chief Resident
Department of Orthopedics
Hospital for Special Surgery
New York, New York

Lauren R. Maher, BA
New Jersey Medical School
University of Medicine and Dentistry of New Jersey
Newark, New Jersey

Alberto Martinez-Arizala, MD
Associate Professor of Clinical Neurology
Miami VA Medical Center
University of Miami
Miami, Florida

Gregory S. McDowell, MD
Ortho Montana, PSC
St. Vincent's Hospital
Billings, Montana

Robert McGuire, MD
Professor and Chairman
Department of Orthopedics
University of Mississippi Medical Center
Jackson, Mississippi

Contributors (cont.)

Nancy McLaughlin, MD, PhD, FRCSC
Neurosurgeon and Fellow
Brain Tumor Center at St. John's Health Center
John Wayne Cancer Institute
Santa Monica, California

Luciano Miller Reis Rodrigues, MD
Assistant Professor
Department of Orthopaedic Surgery
FM-ABC University
São Paulo, Brazil

Sohail K. Mirza, MD, MPH
Professor and Chair
Department of Orthopaedics
Dartmouth Hitchcock Medical Center
Lebanon, New Hampshire

Jeffrey Moore, BS
Medical Student
Department of Orthopaedics
The New Jersey School of Medicine
Newark, New Jersey

Elizabeth Morrison, MD
Resident
Rothman Institute
Thomas Jefferson University Hospital
Philadelphia, Pennsylvania

Michelle Ng, BSc
Graduate Student
ICORD
University of British Columbia
Vancouver, British Columbia, Canada

Robert P. Norton, MD
Orthopaedic Surgery Resident
Department of Orthopaedics
University of Miami Miller School of Medicine
Miami, Florida

Alvin Ong, MD
Orthopaedic Surgeon
Rothman Institute
Egg Harbor Township, New Jersey

Nathaniel R. Ordway, MS, PE
Assistant Professor
Department of Orthopedic Surgery
SUNY Upstate Medical University
Syracuse, New York

Lorenzo L. Pacelli, MD
Co-Director and Orthopedic Surgeon of the Hand
Department of Orthopedics
Scripps Health
La Jolla, California

Wesley W. Parke, PhD
Deceased

William J. Peace, MD
Department of Orthopaedic Surgery
University of California San Diego
San Diego, California

Christopher H. Perkins, MD
Chief Orthopedic Resident
Department of Orthopedic Surgery
Baylor College of Medicine
Houston, Texas

Jamie Purzner, MD
Resident
Department of Neurosurgery
University of Toronto
Toronto, Ontario, Canada

Teresa Purzner, MD
Resident
Department of Neurosurgery
University of Toronto
Toronto, Ontario, Canada

Kris Radcliff, MD
Assistant Professor
Department of Orthopedic Surgery
Thomas Jefferson University
Philadelphia, Pennsylvania

Contributors (cont.)

Adriana N. Ramirez, OTR/L, BS
Spinal Injury Clinical Instructor
Department of Occupational Therapy
Rancho Los Amigos National Rehabilitation Center
Downey, California

Juan M. Raposo, MD
Orthopaedic Spine Surgeon
Miami Neck and Back Institute
Miami, Florida

Mohammad Reza Rasouli, MD
Research Fellow
Department of Orthopaedic Surgery
Rothman Institute
Thomas Jefferson University
Philadelphia, Pennsylvania

Charles A. Reitman, MD
Associate Professor
Department of Orthopedic Surgery
Baylor College of Medicine
Houston, Texas

Cheryl Resnik, MS, DPT
Associate Professor of Clinical Physical Therapy
Division of Biokinesiology and Physical Therapy
University of Southern California
Los Angeles, California

Jeffrey A. Rihn, MD
Assistant Professor
Department of Orthopaedic Surgery
Thomas Jefferson University Hospital
The Rothman Institute
Philadelphia, Pennsylvania

Reynold Rimoldi, MD
Partner
Nevada Orthopedic and Spine Center
Las Vegas, Nevada

Jonathan G. Roper, MD
Spinal Surgeon
Department of Orthopaedic Surgery
Kaiser San Diego Medical Center
San Diego, California

Stephen L. Gabriel Rothman, MD
Department of Radiology
Keck University School of Medicine
Los Angeles, California

Todd Rubin, BS
MS IV
Department of Orthopaedic Surgery
Jefferson Medical College
Philadelphia, Pennsylvania

Amer Samdani, MD
Director of Pediatric Spine Surgery
Department of Orthopedic Surgery
Shriners Hospital for Children
Philadelphia, Pennsylvania

Rajiv K. Sethi, MD
Spinal Surgeon
Group Health Neurosurgery
Virginia Mason Medical Center
Seattle, Washington

Daniel Shedid, MD, MSc, FRCSC, FABN
Neurological Surgeon
Department of Neurosurgery
University of Montreal
Notre Dame Hospital
Montreal, Quebec, Canada

Nina Singh, MD
Assistant Clinical Professor
Department of Anesthesiology and Critical Care
University of Pennsylvania
Philadelphia, Pennsylvania

Marcos Andre Sonagli, MD
Master Sciences Student
Spine Surgery Department of Clinical Surgery
Federal University of Paraná
Guritiba, Brazil

Rebecca Stinsman, BS
Editor
Department of Orthopaedics
Rothman Institute Orthopaedics
Philadelphia, Pennsylvania

Contributors (cont.)

Lilli Thompson, PT, NCS, ATP
Director, Physical Therapy Department
Chief, Rehabilitation Therapy Division
Rancho Los Amigos National Rehabilitation Center
Downey, California

Alexander R. Vaccaro, MD, PhD
The Everrett J. and Marion Gordon Professor of Orthopaedic Surgery
Professor of Neurosurgery
Co-Director of the Delaware Valley Spinal Cord Injury Center
Co-Chief of Spine Surgery
Co-Director of Spine Surgery
Department of Orthopaedics
Thomas Jefferson University and the Rothman Institute
Philadelphia, Pennsylvania

Mark Valente, DO
Spine Surgeon
Minimally Invasive Spine Institute, PA
Dallas, Texas

Michael Vives, MD
Associate Professor
Department of Orthopaedics
University of Medicine and Dentistry of New Jersey
Newark, New Jersey

Christopher Frank Wagener, MD
Spine Surgeon
Department of Coordinated Health
Center for Advanced Spine Solutions
Bethlehem, Pennsylvania

Hansen A. Yuan, MD
Professor Emeritus
Department of Orthopedic and Neurological Surgery
SUNY Upstate Medical University
Syracuse, New York

Jack E. Zigler, MD
Spine Surgeon
Medical Director
Texas Back Institute
Plano, Texas

Dedications

The current four editors would like to dedicate this second edition of *Spine Trauma* to Alan M. Levine, MD, who was the driving force behind publication of the first edition in 1998. Alan's unfortunate and untimely death in 2009 during the active phase of writing this second edition saddened all of us at the loss of our colleague and a leader in the field of spine trauma. As a tribute to Dr. Levine, the current editors have pledged all royalty interests arising from sales of this second edition to the AAOS Alan M. Levine, MD, Education Fund in Alan's memory. We hope our contributions will enhance the work of this fund in furthering the educational interests of orthopaedic surgeons.

The Editors

I would like to thank my wife Emily and my children Austin, Adam, April, Allison and Andy for not only allowing, but actually encouraging me to continue to pursue an academic career. I would like to thank my mentors Dr. Richard Rothman and the late Dr. Henry Bohlman for teaching me how medicine and spine surgery should be practiced. I want to thank my co-editors for their longstanding friendship, which has always made it fun to work together. I would also like to acknowledge the key role that Dr. Alan Levine played in the conceptualization and development of *Spine Trauma*, both the first and the second editions.

Frank J. Eismont, MD

As with any major text book, each editor is indebted and thankful to the innumerable people who participated in its creation or provided the time and support to its creators. For me, for the second edition of this book, as with all my other texts, it still certainly remains my family, secretary, nurse practitioner, mentors, and former and current fellows and residents (the latter groups as inspiration to continue to teach). However, this text in particular was created out of respect, friendship, and loyalty, to honor the memory of Dr. Alan Levine, who had a passion for patients with serious spinal disorders and cancer, a dedication to education at all levels, and a commitment to family and friends.

Steven R. Garfin, MD

I am honored to be associated with the giants of spine surgery as my co-editors. These are the physicians who taught me the principles and tenets of spinal care. May they continue to inspire and lead future generations of spine surgeons.

Alexander R. Vaccaro, MD, PhD

As in the first edition of *Spine Trauma,* I would like to dedicate this work to Dr. Henry Bohlman, who was my mentor, as well as mentor to dozens of spine surgeons around the world. Dr. Bohlman died in May 2010, leaving a legacy in his fellows that will survive for many generations. I would also like to dedicate this book to my wife Wendy, my children Jeffrey and Jennifer, and to my parents, who will display this second edition in their home as proudly as they do the first.

Jack E. Zigler, MD

Acknowledgments

All four of the editors of this text are not only surgeons who have extensive clinical involvement caring for patients with spine trauma, but are also educators who have devoted their careers to training residents and fellows. We each owe debts of tremendous gratitude to our mentors, who instilled in us an interest in spine surgery, as well as an interest in paying it forward to become teachers of new generations of spine surgeons.

We have all enjoyed the rewards of helping patients through difficult times by sharing with them our knowledge and technical skills. Each patient encounter has made us better clinicians and made us better equipped to help the next patient. Each of the physicians and surgeons we have trained has also challenged us and made us better teachers for the next group of trainees.

We would also like to acknowledge the outstanding staff in the AAOS publications department, who agreed to work with us to bring this second edition project to fruition. We are grateful to the efforts of Marilyn Fox, PhD, whose confidence in our abilities as well as those of our authors is greatly appreciated. We are especially grateful to Sharon O'Brien, our manuscript editor and project manager, whose very focused and accelerated work resulted in the timely publication of this text.

Preface

The prefaces of many texts dealing with spinal injury have commonly emphasized the importance of the team approach in the treatment of patients with this devastating problem. Beginning with George Bedbrook in his text *The Care and Management of Spinal Cord Injuries,* the emphasis has been on including the perspectives of all the health professionals involved in the complex care of spinal injury patients, from admission through the completion of rehabilitation. "My purpose in writing this book is to describe the practical, day to day care and medical management of individuals with spinal paralysis. Emphasis is placed on the team approach."[1] However, as the care of the spine-injured patient has evolved through the last several decades, many elements of this care have become more and more complex. Therefore, the editors and authors of the second edition of *Spine Trauma* have, in this text, included more up-to-date treatment algorithms for the care of these patients. Improved surgical techniques and instrumentation have evolved since the publication of the first edition in 1998, and more up-to-date information is provided for today's reader.

The team approach continues to remain the major hallmark of spinal injury care, modeled after the experience gained in the first half of the twentieth century from the rehabilitation of patients with polio. If anything, the team approach has grown even more important than it was with the establishment of spinal cord injury centers in the 1950s. The field of spinal cord injury was one of the first to recognize the value of super-specialized care with establishment of the Model Systems, developing a nationwide network of specialty centers that have been federally funded since 1973. The National Spinal Cord Injury Database was also established in 1973 and currently contains prospectively collected data on nearly 30,000 patients. This is one of the longest ongoing outcomes data collections of any field in medicine!

The first edition of this text was planned to address many of the elements of spinal injury care, such as epidemiology, emergency evaluation, and diagnosis of spine injury in the polytrauma patient. In addition, significant attention was directed to discussing the rehabilitation of the neurologically injured patient. It was evident, even in 1998 that the evolution of the acute care of the spine injured patient had progressed rapidly in the decades of the '80s and '90s, and the current editors and authors have introduced further advancements that have occurred in the past 13 years. We describe more options for radiologic imaging, for pharmacologic management of spinal cord injury, and for the surgical treatment of spinal trauma.

The first edition of this text was conceived as a departure from many of the previous works on spinal injury in that it delved more intensively and specifically into the acute management of specific types of spinal trauma in both the non-cord injured and cord-injured patient. Of all patients sustaining injuries to the spine, only 10% have significant neurologic deficit; even in injuries to the cervical region, only 40% of patients sustaining trauma to the spine have neural deficit. A large proportion of the patients are therefore not spinal cord injury patients, but rather are spinal trauma patients without neurologic injury. We thought then, and continue to think now that it is important to address the management of spinal column trauma in this population.

Both spine trauma and spinal cord injury patients can sustain either isolated injuries or multiple injuries. With the increasing prevalence of both trauma centers and spinal injury centers, more patients with significant polytrauma (spinal column injury along with other musculoskeletal and visceral injuries) are surviving. These patients may require modification of the approach to the sequencing and timing of surgical intervention, with coordination among services as the patient is initially assessed. The presence of an incomplete spinal cord injury demands that it receive primary focus in the handling of the patient to maximize potential for recovery.

A broad spectrum of professionals attends to these patients. The second edition of the text is targeted to serve the needs of those initially involved in evaluating and treating the spine trauma victim by providing a background on the etiology of spinal injury and the rationale for the remaining specific treatment pathways. Surgical traumatologists, critical care specialists, and rehabilitation professionals should benefit from the information contained in this textbook. It remains one of our primary intentions, however, to provide a resource for spinal surgeons by delineating how to evaluate a specific injury as well as how to treat that injury both nonoperatively and operatively. Specific illustrations are provided to outline the anatomic dissection as well as the technical aspects of operative procedures. This book provides both general knowledge about the spine and spinal cord injury along with specific information about each particular type of spine trauma.

Although this second edition of the text may, at first glance, appear to be more relevant to surgeons who see spine trauma on a daily basis in major trauma centers, the first edition has actually enjoyed wider application, even

Preface (cont.)

among nonsurgeon healthcare providers who evaluate and treat patients with spine trauma in emergency departments, in trauma centers, and in community practice. Because residents, practicing neurosurgeons, and orthopaedic surgeons fairly commonly see patients with both high and low energy trauma injuries to the spine, this text can serve as a specific reference to treating the types of injuries that may be encountered on almost a daily basis.

In selecting the authors of the book, a conscious effort was made to include physicians with extensive experience in the day to day management of these injuries from several different major centers around the country. These physicians all work in multispecialty environments where input from various medical and allied health fields is combined to enhance patient care. This collaboration imparts a breadth of experience that informs and enhances the material in the text, rather than narrowing its scope, as regards decision making and treatment. In addition, we sought to incorporate the work of noted authors in specific areas, and we are clearly indebted to those contributors for their efforts. The final evaluation of a text of this type depends not as much on the concept for the text as on the execution of the plan for each chapter. Thus, the more in-depth the understanding of the injury by the contributor, the more likely the reader will be able to grasp the nuances of evaluation, treatment, and outcome of each injury.

As with the first edition, it is our hope that the text will be of lasting value to all of the professionals treating these injuries and most specifically to those making the decisions and executing the treatment plans.

Alan M. Levine, MD*

Frank J. Eismont, MD

Steven R. Garfin, MD

Jack E. Zigler, MD

Alexander R. Vaccaro, MD, PhD

* Alan M. Levine, MD, died unexpectedly during the process of revising this text to produce the second edition. The work he started was carried on by the remaining original editors and by Dr. Alexander Vaccaro. This preface is based on Dr. Levine's preface from the original text and carries forward the same principles he voiced for the first edition. This second edition is dedicated to Dr. Levine's career as a clinician, educator, and humanitarian.

References

1. Bedbrook GM: *The Care and Management of Spinal Cord Injuries.* New York, Springer-Verlag, 1981, p xiii.

Table of Contents

Section 4: Cervical Injuries

Section 5: Thoracolumbar Injuries

Section 6: Postoperative Care and Rehabilitation

CHAPTER 1
Epidemiology of Spinal Cord Injury

Eli M. Baron, MD Alexander R. Vaccaro, MD, PhD Jack E. Zigler, MD

Spinal cord injury (SCI) with neurologic function loss represents a devastating injury that results in drastic changes in a patient's mobility, independence, and physical and psychological health. Improved health-care delivery systems and advances in the medical management of SCI-associated medical complications have allowed for improvement in the lives of those sustaining a SCI but also have resulted in changes in the epidemiology of SCI.

Incidence

The incidence of SCI varies in different countries. Ackery et al[1] used information from the World Bank and World Health Organization in addition to reviewing 20 published articles from 17 countries to examine SCI epidemiology on a worldwide basis. Nations with similar economic status tended to have similar incidences of injury but diverse classification methods made comparison difficult. They reported that the annual incidence of SCI varies between 11.5 and 57.8 cases per million people in different countries. The reported incidence in Australia was 14.5 per million, while that in North America was 52.5 per million and in Europe 57.8 per million. More recently, the National Spinal Cord Injury Statistical Center in Birmingham, Alabama estimated the annual incidence of SCI in the United States, excluding those who die at the scene of the accident, at approximately 40 cases per million people.[2] This suggests the number often cited, of roughly 30 cases per million, to be a substantial underestimation, especially in the United States. This may be due to persons with spinal column injury but with a mild neurologic deficit or a rapidly improving deficit not being reported. Death due to multiple trauma and head injury may also lead to underreporting of SCI.[3] As of 2007, there was believed to be approximately 262,000 patients in the United States living with a traumatic SCI.[2]

Etiology

Figure 1 reviews etiologies of SCI since 2005 in all age groups combined. Motor vehicle crashes account for 41.3% of reported SCI cases. The next most frequent cause of injury is falls, followed by violence, primarily from firearms, and recreational sporting activities.[2] When stratifying SCI patients

FIGURE 1

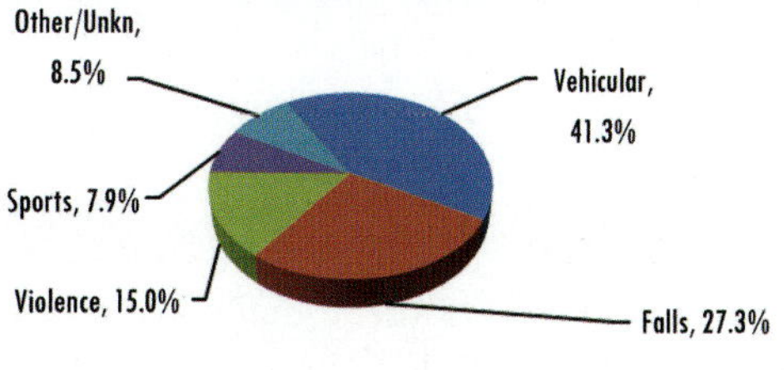

Figure 1 Etiology of SCI. (Reproduced with permission from *Spinal Cord Injury Facts and Figures at a Glance*. Birmingham, AL, National Spinal Cord Injury Statistical Center, 2010.)

Dr. Baron or an immediate family member is a member of a speakers' bureau or has made paid presentations on behalf of Globus Medical and Trans 1; and owns stock or stock options in Savient Pharmaceuticals, Targeted Inc, and NeuroGesX, Inc. Dr. Vaccaro or an immediate family member serves as a board member, owner, officer, or committee member of the North American Spine Society, American Spinal Injury Association, and the Cervical Spine Research Society; has received royalties from Aesculap/B.Braun, DePuy, a Johnson & Johnson company, Globus Medical, Medtronic Sofamor Danek, K2M, Stout Medical, Progressive Spinal Technology, and Applied Spinal Intellectual Properties; serves as a paid consultant to or is an employee of K2M; has received research or institutional support from AO North America, DePuy, a Johnson & Johnson company, Medtronic Sofamor Danek, and Stryker; and owns stock or stock options in Globus Medical, Disk Motion Technology, Progressive Spinal Technologies, Advanced Spinal Intellectual Properties, Computational Biodynamics, Stout Medical, Paradigm Spine, K2M, Replication Medica, Spinology, Spine Medica, Orthovita, Vertiflex, Small Bone Technologies, NeuCore, Crosscurrent, Syndicom, In Vivo, Flagship Surgical, Pearl Driver, Location Based Intelligence, and Gamma Spine. Dr. Zigler or an immediate family member serves as a board member, owner, officer, or committee member of the Cervical Spine Research Society; has received royalties from Zimmer, K2M, and Osprey; serves as a paid consultant to or is an employee of Alphatec Spine and Synthes; owns stock or stock options in Flexuspine; and has received nonincome support (such as equipment or services), commercially derived honoraria, or other non-research-related funding (such as paid travel) from AO and Synthes.

TABLE 1

Etiology of SCI by Age Group

	Age at Injury						
Etiology, n (%)	**< 15 y**	**16-30 y**	**31-45 y**	**46-60 y**	**61-75 y**	**76-98 y**	**Total**
Vehicular accidents	343 (37.4)	6,347 (46.5)	2,809 (44.5)	1,405 (38.5)	535 (30.1)	132 (24.4)	11,571
Violence	214 (23.3)	3,196 (23.4)	1,050 (16.6)	270 (7.4)	47 (2.6)	7 (1.3)	4,784
Sports	219 (23.9)	1,967 (14.4)	435 (6.9)	137 (3.8)	40 (2.2)	3 (0.6)	2,801
Falls	73 (8.0)	1,439 (10.5)	1,438 (22.8)	1,359 (37.3)	880 (49.5)	349 (64.5)	5,538
Other	68 (7.4)	699 (5.1)	568 (9.0)	468 (12.8)	275 (15.5)	47 (8.7)	2,125
Unknown	0 (0.0)	11 (0.1)	10 (0.2)	6 (0.2)	2 (0.1)	3 (0.6)	32
Total	917	13,659	6,310	3,645	1,779	541	26,851

(Reproduced with permission from *2009 Annual Report for the Model Spinal Cord Injury Care Systems*. Birmingham, AL, National Spinal Cord Injury Statistical Center, 2010, p 40.)

by patient age at time of injury, different mechanisms clearly dominate various age brackets; vehicular accidents are the most common in young adults as the cause of SCI, for example, while falls dominate in the elderly (**Table 1**).[4] Over time, the proportion of injuries caused by falls has increased, while acts of violence peaked in the 1990s at 24.8% and declined to 15.0% since 2005.[2]

Demographics

SCI continues to primarily affect young adult males, with 80.8% of those injured being male. Interestingly, in the 1970s, the average age at injury was 28.7 years, with most SCIs occurring between the age of 16 and 30. Since 2005, however, the average age at injury is 40.2, reflecting an increase of approximately 11 years in the median age of the injury population. Possible reasons for the trend toward older age at injury might include changes in referral patterns to the model systems (see appendix at the end of this chapter for an explanation of the spinal cord injury model systems), changes in locations of the model systems, increased survival of the elderly at the scene of the trauma, or age-specific incidence rates.

Race and ethnicity may also play a role in sustaining SCI. In the 1970s, 76.8% of the patients in the National SCI Database were Caucasian, 14.2% were African American, and 9% were listed as other racial or ethnic groups. Since 2005, however, those sustaining new SCIs were listed as 66.2% Caucasian, 27.0% African American, and 6.8% from other racial groups. Hispanic ethnicity has risen from 5.9% in the 1970s to 7.9% since 2005.

The majority of patients sustaining an SCI are single at the time of injury (52%). Those who were married at the time of injury sustained a slightly higher divorce rate than the general population. A total of 57.5% of patients sustaining SCI reported being employed at the time of injury.[2]

SCI continues to occur more commonly with diving than with other sports. Diving contributed to 6.3% of all SCIs in the National SCI Database. This was followed by football, skiing, and horseback riding, each at 0.5% of all injures.[4]

Neurologic Level, Skeletal Level, and Extent of Lesion

Neurologic level is defined as the most caudal segment with normal function on neurologic examination. Quadriplegia or tetraplegia is defined as having a partial or complete loss of any of the cervical segments (cervical level), while paraplegia is defined as a functional loss at the thoracic, lumbar, or sacral levels.[3]

TABLE 2

Trends in Neurologic Category of Injury at Discharge[a]

	Year of Injury, n (%)							
Neurologic Category	**1973-1979**	**1980-1984**	**1985-1989**	**1990-1994**	**1995-1999**	**2000-2004**	**2005-2009**	**Total**
Para, incomplete	805 (17.6)	948 (19.2)	802 (20.9)	642 (19.5)	636 (17.5)	556 (16.1)	592 (18.9)	4,981
Para, complete	1,265 (27.7)	1,231 (24.9)	961 (25.0)	946 (28.7)	973 (26.8)	799 (23.2)	673 (21.5)	6,848
Para, min def	0 (0.0)	19 (0.4)	50 (1.3)	97 (2.9)	56 (1.5)	52 (1.5)	41 (1.3)	315
Tetra, incomplete	1,282 (28.1)	1,599 (32.3)	1,197 (31.2)	821 (24.9)	1,027 (28.3)	1,123 (32.6)	1,070 (34.1)	8,119
Tetra, complete	1,156 (25.3)	1,085 (21.9)	733 (19.1)	626 (19.0)	683 (18.8)	640 (18.6)	497 (15.9)	5,420
Tetra, min def	4 (0.1)	13 (0.3)	62 (1.6)	116 (3.5)	89 (2.5)	63 (1.8)	56 (1.8)	403
Normal, min def	45 (1.0)	38 (0.8)	16 (0.4)	13 (0.4)	19 (0.5)	24 (0.7)	10 (0.3)	165
Unknown	6 (0.1)	17 (0.3)	21 (0.5)	34 (1.0)	141 (3.9)	187 (5.4)	195 (6.2)	601
Total	4,563	4,950	3,842	3,295	3,624	3,444	3,134	26,852

[a]Para = paraplegia; min def = minimal deficit; tetra = tetraplegia. The para and tetra minimal deficit categories were not added until 1987; some records have been updated.

(Reproduced with permission from *2009 Annual Report for the Model Spinal Cord Injury Care Systems*. Birmingham, AL, National Spinal Cord Injury Statistical Center, 2010, p 54.)

In 2009, 53.2% of patients listed in the National SCI Database had cervical level cord injuries at discharge, while 35.6% had thoracic level injuries and 11.1% had lumbosacral lesions. Since 2005, most commonly neurologically incomplete tetraplegia was seen (38.3%), followed by neurologically complete paraplegia (21.5%), neurologically incomplete paraplegia (21.5%), and neurologically complete tetraplegia (16.9%).[2] Neurologically incomplete tetraplegia was most commonly seen regardless of etiology of injury with the exception of violence where complete paraplegia was most commonly seen.[4] In terms of osseous injury, anterior dislocations and fracture-dislocations are more likely to result in complete SCI than compression or burst fractures.[5]

Trends regarding neurologic category of injury at discharge are shown in **Table 2**.[4] The proportion of patients with neurologically incomplete lesions increased from 45.6% in 1973-1979 to 53 since 2005, likely reflecting improved emergency medical services at the injury scene.[4] Also, greater attention to immobilization after injury, the increased use of seatbelts and airbags in motor vehicles, and the attempted avoidance of secondary insults such as systemic hypotension and hypoxia postinjury may be contributory.[5] A decrease in incomplete injuries was seen from 1991-1994, likely reflecting an increase in SCI secondary to gunshot wounds. Since 2005, the percentage of incomplete injuries has risen again, likely due to a decrease in violence.[4] It is difficult to establish whether high-dose methylprednisolone therapy has had any bearing on patterns of injury extent or injury level.

Associated Trauma

Spinal cord trauma may result in isolated SCI, but other substantial organ injuries may occur almost 50% of the time. Common injuries associated with SCI by anatomic region include trunk fractures, long-bone fractures, head and facial trauma, pneumothorax/chest injury, and abdominal injury.

It is important to aggressively treat hypotension and shock as these can potentiate any SCI. An aggressive work-up for associated injuries must ensue without relegating the cause of hypotension to the SCI.

Head injury and SCI occur concurrently between 24% and 59% of the time.[6] Severe traumatic brain injury with cervical spine injury is typically reported as occurring in 4% to 8% of cases but has been reported as high as 20%.[7-9] A concomitant head injury and SCI can mask one another, making an accurate diagnosis difficult. The widespread availability of thin-cut CT with sagittal and coronal reconstruction may reduce the occurrence of missed bony injuries, but a high index of suspicion and a systematic approach to assessment of trauma, as per the Advanced Trauma Life Support Guidelines, is mandatory to reduce the frequency of missed spinal and appendicular injuries.

Abdominal injuries can be a significant source of hypotension. Intra-abdominal injuries have been reported to occur in 2.6% of patients sustaining blunt cervical SCI.[10] Abdominal injuries occur much more frequently in association with lumbar spine injuries. One series looking at flexion-distraction injuries of the lumbar spine noted 67% of these patients also sustained an abdominal injury requiring surgical intervention, primarily for a hollow viscus injury.[11] Similar thoracolumbar spine fractures sustained through a blunt mechanism may be rarely associated with an abdominal aortic dissection and or lacerations. A Canadian review of 11,465 trauma admissions identified 8 patients who sustained a descending aortic injury: 6 of them had also sustained a thoracolumbar spine injuries.[12] In fact, injury to the thoracolumbar spinal column may be associated with an abdominal injury. One series looking at trauma patients sustaining transverse process fractures in the lumbar spine, as identified by helical CT, found that 51% of patients also sustained some degree of intra-abdominal injury.[13] This highlights the importance of a complete trauma evaluation, with a thorough assessment of the abdomen, when working up SCI.

Pelvic and long-bone fractures can also be a source of hypotension associated with SCI. A recent retrospective series of 1,290 patients sustaining SCI found an 11% association between pelvic/extremity fractures and SCI. The most frequently observed skeletal fractures involved the radius (18%), tibia (11%), femur (9%), humerus (8%), fibula (8%), and ulna (7%).[14]

The start of rehabilitation is often delayed in the SCI patient suffering multiple other associated injuries.[3] There has been a trend toward shorter acute hospitalization stays and shorter rehabilitation facility stays. For those patients who entered a model system immediately following injury, the average days hospitalized in the acute care unit declined from 25 days in 1974 to 12 days since 2005. Similarly, rehabilitation stays have decreased from 115 to 38 days. Mean days hospitalized were greater during acute care and rehabilitation for complete injuries.[2]

Medical Problems in SCI

The resulting sensory and motor loss seen with SCI leads to significant changes in multiple organ systems, including the respiratory system, the genitourinary tract, and the integrity of the patient's skin. Changes in the functioning of these systems continue to require major modifications in the SCI patients' lifestyles and considerable efforts on the part of the care providers in terms of complication avoidance.[3]

Respiratory complications continue to be the leading cause of death following SCI, according to data acquired in the Collaborative SCI Survival Study (**Table 3**); 69.7% of these cases were due to pneumonia. The second leading cause was infection and parasitic diseases; 94.3% of these cases were in association with septicemia and usually associated with decubitus ulcers or pulmonary or urinary tract infections.[4] The third leading cause was "other heart disease"; however, these were often listed as unexplained heart attacks, suggesting relatively poor data quality regarding cause of death and poor reporting practice. Years ago, renal failure was the leading cause of death following SCI; improvements in urologic management, however, have resulted in a marked reduction in renal related deaths.[2] There has also been a reduction in deep venous thrombosis and pulmonary embolism, where increased awareness and improved prophylaxis may be resulting in the reduced incidence.[15]

Decubitus ulcers continue to be a significant problem for those sustaining SCI. By far the most common location is the sacrum, where ulcers occur in nearly one-third of patients. Data from the National SCI Database suggested that nearly half the ulcers seen in rehabilitation are grade 1: severe ulcers (grade 3 and 4) were only seen in 9.2% of patients.[16]

TABLE 3

Causes of Death in Patients Sustaining SCI

ICD9CM Codes	Primary Cause of Death	n	%
460-519	Diseases of the respiratory system	1,741	21.2
000-139	Infective and parasitic diseases	912	11.1
420-429	Other heart disease	784	9.5
140-239	Neoplasms	783	9.5
400-414	Hypertensive and ischemic heart disease	769	9.4
E800-E949	Unintentional injuries	517	6.3
520-579	Diseases of the digestive system	390	4.7
430-438	Cerebrovascular disease	315	3.8
415-417	Disease of pulmonary circulation	313	3.8
E950-E959	Suicides	300	3.6
780-799	Symptoms of ill-defined conditions	277	3.4
580-629	Diseases of the genitourinary system	258	3.1
240-279	Endocrine, nutritional, metabolic and immunity disorders (includes AIDS)	252	3.1
320-389	Diseases of the nervous system and sense organs	164	2.0
440-448	Diseases of the arteries, arterioles, and capillaries	106	1.3
E980-E989	Subsequent trauma of uncertain nature (unintentional/suicide/homicide)	96	1.2
E960-E969	Homicides	85	1.0
290-319	Mental disorders	74	0.9
710-739	Diseases of the musculoskeletal system and connective tissue	35	0.4
280-289	Diseases of the blood and blood-forming organs	26	0.3
451-459	Diseases of the veins, lymphatics, and other diseases of the circulatory system	17	0.2
740-759	Congenital anomalies	10	0.1
E970-E979	Legal intervention	1	0.1
	Total known causes of death Total unknown causes of death	8,225 1,549	
	Total deaths	9,774	

(Reproduced with permission from *2009 Annual Report for the Model Spinal Cord Injury Care Systems*. Birmingham, AL, National Spinal Cord Injury Statistical Center, 2010, p 31.)

Depression, Suicide, and Life Satisfaction After SCI

Suicide and depression are very common after SCI. The Collaborative SCI Survival Study reported suicide to be the primary cause of death in 3.6% of the total deaths following SCI.[4] This is increased compared to 1.3% of the total deaths in the United States due to suicide during the year 2001.[17] In another analysis of 9,135 patients treated at model SCI centers between 1973 and 1985, based on age-, sex-, and race-specific rates for the general population, suicide was calculated to occur at 4.9 times the rate of the general population. Suicide was the leading cause of death for persons with complete paraplegia and the second leading cause of death for persons with incomplete paraplegia.[18] Risk factors for suicide after SCI include male sex; having schizoid, depressive, or narcissistic personality traits; alcohol or drug

TABLE 4

Life Expectancy After SCI

Age at Injury	No SCI	Motor Functional Any Level	Paraplegia	Tetraplegia C5-C8	Tetraplegia C1-C4	Ventilator-Dependent Any Level
	Life Expectancy (Years)					
		Not Ventilator-Dependent				
10 years	68.5	61.9	54.0	48.5	43.9	25.2
15 years	63.6	57.0	49.1	43.8	39.2	21.0
20 years	58.8	52.3	44.6	39.4	35.1	18.1
25 years	54.0	47.7	40.3	35.3	31.2	15.9
30 years	49.3	43.0	35.9	31.1	27.2	13.3
35 years	44.5	38.4	31.5	26.9	23.2	10.5
40 years	39.9	33.9	27.2	22.9	19.4	8.0
45 years	35.3	29.5	23.1	19.1	15.9	5.9
50 years	30.9	25.3	19.3	15.7	12.8	4.2
55 years	26.6	21.3	15.8	12.5	10.0	2.9
60 years	22.5	17.5	12.6	9.6	7.5	1.8
65 years	18.7	14.1	9.7	7.2	5.4	1.0
70 years	15.1	11.0	7.2	5.1	3.7	0.3
75 years	11.9	8.3	5.1	3.5	2.3	< 0.1
80 years	9.1	5.9	3.4	2.1	1.3	< 0.1

Life expectancy for SCI patients surviving at least 24 hours postinjury. Values for persons with no SCI are from the 2004 US Life Tables for the general population.

(Reproduced with permission from *2009 Annual Report for the Model Spinal Cord Injury Care Systems*. Birmingham, AL, National Spinal Cord Injury Statistical Center, 2010, p 33.)

abuse; preinjury depression; and family or significant others preferring death as an option after SCI and the development of depression.[19,20]

A recent study of 849 patients 1 year after sustaining SCI found symptoms suggestive of a major depressive disorder in 11.4% of patients. These patients also tended to have poorer subjective health, lower satisfaction with life, and more difficulty in daily role functioning.[21] Depressive symptoms and anxiety are most common in the acute phase following SCI and before being discharged from rehabilitation.[22] Nevertheless, with proper counseling, rehabilitative and psychologic/psychiatric interventions (as needed), good to excellent mental health outcomes can be obtained. Hall et al[23] assessed psychological outcomes in 82 patients with high cervical tetraplegia 14 years after SCI. All patients had undergone acute inpatient SCI rehabilitation. Ninety-five percent of participants reported being "glad to be alive," and the authors concluded that, "quality of life was higher than expected, considering the substantial physical limitations of the group."

Survivability in SCI

The survivability following SCI continues to improve. In the past, longevity was expressed as 5-year survival; at present, it is expressed as percentage of normal life expectancy. Younger patients with paraplegia have nearly a 90% normal life expectancy, while quadriplegia with optimal care has about an 80% life expectancy.[3] Based on data from the National SCI Database, the cumulative 20-year survival rate for patients with SCI was 69.14%. Given the high proportion of losses to follow-up and the underreporting of SCI fatalities occurring soon after injury, this may be an overestimation. The life expectancies for patients with SCI are shown in **Table 4**.

The level and severity of injury both have an effect on long-term survival. Higher injury levels in tetraplegic patients are associated with reduced life expectancies. From the National SCI Database, for patients surviving at least 24 hours after injury, a 25-year-old with tetraplegia at C5-C8 would have a 35.3-year expected survival, while one with an injury at C1-C4 would have a 31.2-year survival. Similarly, an 80-year-old sustaining these injuries would have a 2.1- and 1.3-year expected survival period, respectively.[4] Age at injury is also a major factor predicting life expectancy. As evident from **Table 4**, older patients sustaining SCI have a greater percentage of reduced life expectancies than do younger patients.

Employment After Cord Injury

As mentioned above, only 57.5% of patients with SCI report being employed before injury. This must be taken into account when looking at the employment rate after SCI. A recent study of employment after SCI found an employment rate of 11.9% at 1 year postinjury (N = 5,925), 18.7% at 5 years after injury (N = 2,852), 22% at 10 years postinjury (N = 9,932), and 22.9% at 20 years (N = 162). Significant disparities were seen in employment rates between Caucasians and African Americans after SCI. After SCI, 16.4% of Caucasians were employed, while only 5.9% of African Americans were employed. While significant preinjury disparities were noted in terms of job type of the two groups, at 1 year after SCI, the most common employment seen in both groups was professional subspecialty occupations; no disparities in job types were noted in both groups at 1 year after injury.[24]

Similar results were seen by Krause et al,[25] who noted a 1-year employment rate of 22% to 24.8% depending on the reporting methodology rate used. They also noted men to be more likely employed full time than women after SCI. Young age, increased years of education and injury severity, as well as being Caucasian, correlated with a higher likelihood of employment after SCI as did decreased injury severity.

Programs that encourage employment of disabled individuals, with the additional goal of returning the disabled individual to as normal a life as possible, may provide an environment conducive to employment.[3] The Americans with Disabilities Act (ADA) of 1990 acted to establish a clear and comprehensive prohibition of discrimination on the basis of disability. Title I of the ADA prohibits employment discrimination against those with disabilities. In terms of people sustaining a SCI, these laws serve as a starting point to help them reintegrate socioeconomically into society. Efforts should be made to promote higher education if possible in patients with SCI, especially those injured at a relatively young age. Additionally, the majority of people sustaining SCI were previously employed in fields requiring motor involvement and manual dexterity. These skills are often incompatible with the physical limitations associated with SCI. Unfortunately, despite sustaining an SCI, a large percentage of those affected are unlikely to shift their vocational interests. Finally, interventions geared toward minority populations sustaining SCI may have the largest impact, given the disparities seen in employment after SCI.[25]

Conclusion

Studying the epidemiology of SCI enables the treating physician to anticipate secondary complications in this population. It also enables legislative bodies and policy makers to establish focused programs directed at minimizing the occurrence of SCI and maximizing rehabilitative potential. Clearly there have been changes in the injury patterns seen from the 1970s to the present, where improved life expectancies are seen as well as reduced complications, such as death from renal failure and pulmonary embolism. Nevertheless, improvements need to be made in the rehabilitative efforts for survivors of SCI, especially in terms of employment and societal reintegration. Studying the epidemiology of mental health issues and employment after SCI is most beneficial in understanding ways to better the lives of patients with SCI.

References

1. Ackery A, Tator C, Krassioukov A: A global perspective on spinal cord injury epidemiology. *J Neurotrauma* 2004;21(10):1355-1370.
2. *Spinal Cord Injury Facts and Figures at a Glance*. Birmingham, AL, National Spinal Cord Injury Statistical Center, 2010. Available at https://www.nscisc.uab.edu/public_content/pdf/Facts%20and%20Figures%20at%20a%20Glance%202010.pdf. Accessed August 13, 2010.
3. Zigler JE, Capen DA: Epidemiology of spinal cord injury: A perspective on the problem, in Levine AM, Eismont FJ, Garfin SR, Zigler JE, eds: *Spine Trauma*, ed 1. Philadelphia, PA, WB Saunders Company, 1998, pp 2-8.

4. *2009 Annual Report for the Model Spinal Cord Injury Care Systems*. Birmingham, AL, National Spinal Cord Injury Statistical Center, 2010. Available at https://www.nscisc.uab.edu/public_content/pdf/2009%20NSCISC%20 Annual%20Statistical%20Report%20-%20 Complete%20Public% 20Version.pdf. Accessed August 13, 2010.
5. Sekhon LH, Fehlings MG: Epidemiology, demographics, and pathophysiology of acute spinal cord injury. *Spine (Phila Pa 1976)* 2001;26 (24, Suppl)S2-S12.
6. Sommer JL, Witkiewicz PM: The therapeutic challenges of dual diagnosis: TBI/SCI. *Brain Inj* 2004; 18(12):1297-1308.
7. Davis JW, Parks SN, Detlefs CL, Williams GG, Williams JL, Smith RW: Clearing the cervical spine in obtunded patients: The use of dynamic fluoroscopy. *J Trauma* 1995;39(3):435-438.
8. Holly LT, Kelly DF, Counelis GJ, Blinman T, McArthur DL, Cryer HG: Cervical spine trauma associated with moderate and severe head injury: Incidence, risk factors, and injury characteristics. *J Neurosurg* 2002;96(3 Suppl):285-291.
9. Irwin J, Abbott RJ, Burt AA, Harriman D: Brain stem signs in acute cervical cord trauma. *Paraplegia* 1985;23(2):82-88.
10. Albuquerque F, Wolf A, Dunham CM, Wagner R, Spagnolia T, Rigamonti D: Frequency of intra-abdominal injury in cases of blunt trauma to the cervical spinal cord. *J Spinal Disord* 1992;5(4): 476-480.
11. Rabinovici R, Ovadia P, Mathiak G, Abdullah F: Abdominal injuries associated with lumbar spine fractures in blunt trauma. *Injury* 1999;30(7): 471-474.
12. Inaba K, Kirkpatrick AW, Finkelstein J, et al: Blunt abdominal aortic trauma in association with thoracolumbar spine fractures. *Injury* 2001;32(3): 201-207.
13. Patten RM, Gunberg SR, Brandenburger DK: Frequency and importance of transverse process fractures in the lumbar vertebrae at helical abdominal CT in patients with trauma. *Radiology* 2000; 215(3):831-834.
14. Anderson SD, Anderson DG, Vaccaro AR: Skeletal fracture demographics in spinal cord-injured patients. *Arch Orthop Trauma Surg* 2004;124(3): 193-196.
15. Chen D, Apple DF Jr, Hudson LM, Bode R: Medical complications during acute rehabilitation following spinal cord injury—Current experience of the Model Systems. *Arch Phys Med Rehabil* 1999; 80(11):1397-1401.
16. *The 2004 Statistical Report for the Model Spinal Cord Injury Care Systems*. Birmingham, AL, National Spinal Cord Injury Statistical Center, 2004, p 115.
17. *Suicide Facts and Statistics*. Bethesda, MD, National Institute of Mental Health, 2001.
18. DeVivo MJ, Black KJ, Richards JS, Stover SL: Suicide following spinal cord injury. *Paraplegia* 1991; 29(9):620-627.
19. Charlifue SW, Gerhart KA: Behavioral and demographic predictors of suicide after traumatic spinal cord injury. *Arch Phys Med Rehabil* 1991;72(7): 488-492.
20. Judd FK, Brown DJ: Suicide following acute traumatic spinal cord injury. *Paraplegia* 1992;30(3): 173-177.
21. Bombardier CH, Richards JS, Krause JS, Tulsky D, Tate DG: Symptoms of major depression in people with spinal cord injury: Implications for screening. *Arch Phys Med Rehabil* 2004;85(11): 1749-1756.
22. Kennedy P, Rogers BA: Anxiety and depression after spinal cord injury: A longitudinal analysis. *Arch Phys Med Rehabil* 2000;81(7):932-937.
23. Hall KM, Knudsen ST, Wright J, Charlifue SW, Graves DE, Werner P: Follow-up study of individuals with high tetraplegia (C1-C4) 14 to 24 years postinjury. *Arch Phys Med Rehabil* 1999;80(11): 1507-1513.
24. Meade MA, Lewis A, Jackson MN, Hess DW: Race, employment, and spinal cord injury. *Arch Phys Med Rehabil* 2004;85(11):1782-1792.
25. Krause JS, Kewman D, DeVivo MJ, et al: Employment after spinal cord injury: An analysis of cases from the Model Spinal Cord Injury Systems. *Arch Phys Med Rehabil* 1999;80(11):1492-1500.

Appendix: Spinal Cord Injury Model Systems*

The Model Spinal Cord Injury System program, sponsored by the National Institute on Disability and Rehabilitation Research (NIDRR), Office of Special Education and Rehabilitative Services, US Department of Education, provides assistance to develop innovative projects for the delivery, demonstration, and evaluation of comprehensive medical, vocational, and rehabilitation services to meet the needs of individuals with spinal cord injury. Its centers, which are located across the United States, work together for improved care, maintain a national database, participate in independent and collaborative research, and provide continuing education relating to spinal cord injury.

*Available on the Spinal Cord Injury Information Network, at http://www.spinalcord.uab.edu/show.asp?durki=21392. Accessed August 25, 2010.

CHAPTER 2
Injury Scene Assessment, Extrication, and Transport

S. Babak Kalantar, MD Christopher H. Perkins, MD Charles A. Reitman, MD

Introduction

Trauma is the leading cause of death in patients less than 45 years of age.[1] Injuries to the cervical and thoracolumbar spine represent a significant and important component of blunt trauma. Due to the substantial societal and economic burden, there have been and continue to be significant advances in prevention and management of trauma. The introduction of the Advanced Trauma Life Support (ATLS) program noticeably improved trauma patient outcome in the first hour after admission.[2] The process includes preparation, triage, primary survey, resuscitation, adjuncts to primary survey and resuscitation, secondary survey and adjuncts, continued postresuscitation monitoring, reevaluation, and definitive care.[3] Preparation involves coordination of the emergency medical services (EMS) providers and the receiving hospital before the patient leaves the scene, which allows for mobilization of appropriate resources. Triage refers to the sorting of patients and resources based on need for treatment, as well as sorting of patients to the appropriate medical facility. The American College of Surgeons developed the Field Triage Decision Scheme in 1986 (most recently revised in 2006) that guides EMS providers through four decision steps (physiologic, anatomic, mechanism of injury, and special considerations) to determine field triage to a level I through IV trauma center.[1]

Initial Survey

Care begins with the on-scene initial survey, most often conducted by EMS providers. The initial phase of management is critical to ultimate outcomes, and in general, most of this initial "golden hour" of assessment and resuscitation elapses outside the hospital.[4] Adherence to ATLS protocols is important to optimize the outcomes of trauma patients, but deviations from ATLS protocol are common.[5,6] In one study, the field assessment of the cervical spine by EMS providers and emergency department physicians was found to be in agreement 79% of the time, and cervical immobilization was not initiated when clinically indicated by emergency department physicians 7.7% of the time.[7]

Primary Survey

A review of trauma management cannot be complete without discussion of the ABCs (airway, breathing, and circulation). Although this is basic, it is well worth repeating that it is critical to be thorough and methodical during the evaluation of these patients. Skipping steps leads to missed injuries and worse outcomes. Despite all the new advances, missed injuries are reported in 5% to 10% of patients in a Level I trauma center, and this percentage goes up in patients with high trauma scores.[8,9] It is imperative that providers not only optimally manage the existing problems, but also avoid further iatrogenic injury. The primary survey allows for logical sequential evaluation and treatment of the injured patient based on the mnemonic ABCDE.[3]

Upon initiation of care, all patients should be assumed to have a spine injury until proven otherwise. Assessment of airway and breathing often occurs simultaneously, and is done with cervical spine protection. Intubation should be performed in patients who cannot maintain an adequate airway. Airway patency alone does not ensure ventilation; therefore, chest wall inflation and adequate exchange of gases must be evaluated. Massive chest wall injury, pneumothorax, and hemothorax are the most common reasons for inability to ventilate with an adequate airway. Circulation is then evaluated. In patients with a patent airway, hemorrhage is the leading cause of death.

Dr. Kalantar or an immediate family member has received nonincome support (such as equipment or services), commercially derived honoraria, or other non-research-related funding (such as paid travel) from Persys Medical. Dr. Reitman or an immediate family member serves as a board member, owner, officer, or committee member of North American Spine Society. Neither Dr. Perkins nor any immediate family member has received anything of value from or owns stock in a commercial company or institution related directly or indirectly to the subject of this chapter.

The mnemonic's "D" represents disability, which refers to the neurologic status of the patient. A rapid neurologic examination is performed, along with assessment of level of consciousness by use of the Glasgow Coma Scale (GCS).[10] Patients presenting with a GCS of 3 and fixed and dilated pupils have a low chance for survival while many patients with a GCS of 3 who are not fixed and dilated survive to discharge.[11] The Full Outline of Unresponsiveness (FOUR) score is an alternative to the GCS score that has high interrater reliability and predicts functional outcome similar to the GCS;[12] however, the GCS is much more commonly used and has been incorporated in classification systems in trauma. Decreased level of consciousness can be secondary to many causes, but should be assumed to be from central nervous system trauma until proven otherwise.

The "E" stands for exposure and environmental control. During this phase of the primary survey, the patient should be undressed to facilitate better examination and assessment. Environmental control refers primarily to the maintenance of the patient's body temperature by covering the patient with warm blankets or using an external warming device. In addition, intravenous fluids can be warmed before administration. Control of hemorrhage and resuscitation also contribute to maintenance of body temperature. The primary survey should be repeated if the patient's condition changes or deteriorates. Special populations include pediatric, pregnant, and elderly patients, in which the priorities of the initial survey are the same but differences exist in elements such as medications, response to injury, and medical comorbidities. With regard to patients with cervical spine injuries in particular, early ventilation and differentiation of hemorrhagic from neurogenic shock are key elements of prehospital assessment and resuscitation.[13]

Intubation of Trauma Patients With Cervical Spine Injury

The airway is of critical importance in patients with cervical spine injury, and intubation is often necessary if there is evidence of respiratory compromise. The majority of patients with cervical spinal cord injury (SCI) require intubation.[14] Patients with incomplete cervical SCI require intubation less frequently than patients with complete injuries.[15] Prehospital intubation has been shown to be unsuccessful 31% of the time; however, there was no difference in mortality between successful and failed intubations, suggesting that bag-mask ventilation is acceptable in these circumstances.[16]

Regardless of the injury, traction, flexion, or extension of the neck can all be harmful. Therefore, manual in-line stabilization of the cervical spine has been advocated during intubation of patients with cervical spine injury, recognizing that even then the cervical spine may be vulnerable to further injury.[17,18]

Oral intubation with a Macintosh blade after intravenous induction of anesthesia and muscle relaxation along with in-line stabilization has been advocated as the safest and quickest way to achieve intubation in a patient with suspected cervical spine injury.[19] However, several new technologies for intubation have been developed to improve visualization and reduce cervical spine motion, theoretically resulting in increased safety and accuracy. These devices include the intubating laryngeal mask airway, Combitube (Covidien, Mansfield, MA), lighted intubating stylets, optical laryngoscopes, and fiberoptic laryngoscopes.[18,20-28]

When intubation cannot be obtained by endotracheal means in the prehospital setting, cricothyroidotomy can be performed. Emergency cricothyroidotomy is performed 0.1% of the time by EMS personnel with a success rate of 100%.[29] Cricothyroidotomy results in a small amount of axial distraction and anteroposterior translation across an unstable cervical spine injury that is theoretically less than the threshold for clinical significance.[30] Regardless of the methodology used to secure and maintain the airway, it should be performed in a timely and accurate manner with particular attention to minimizing motion in the cervical spine.

Cardiopulmonary Resuscitation (CPR) in Patients with Spinal Trauma

If the patient is found to be nonresponsive or not breathing, the first maneuver is to open the airway by the head tilt–chin lift or jaw-thrust maneuver and clear the airway by finger sweep. This may be difficult in patients with suspected cervical spine injuries who are immobilized in a collar. The jaw-thrust maneuver may still be possible, but the airway may have to be opened and cleared with an assistant holding in-line cervical stabilization. Rescue breaths are given through a barrier device or bag-mask ventilation is initiated. If the patient is not able to maintain an adequate airway or ventilation is not possible by the above measure, intubation may be necessary.

After the airway has been secured and ventilation is established, attention is drawn to circulation. If signs of circulation and pulses are absent, chest compressions are initiated. Five cycles of 15 chest compressions are performed at a rate of 100 compressions per minute followed by two long rescue breaths.[31] The force required to perform adequate chest compressions in CPR has resulted in thoracic vertebral fractures in older adults with osteoporosis in addition to rib or sternum fractures.[32] This force can also be theoretically transmitted through an unstable thoracic fracture as well, although this has not been formally studied. At the same time circulation is being addressed, an automated external defibrillator (AED) can be connected to the patient to assess for cardiac rhythm abnormalities and defibrillation can be initiated if indicated. Significant force could theoretically be transmitted to the spine with defibrillation. Therefore, it is ideal to have the patient's spine appropriately immobilized before starting CPR and application of a defibrillator in particular.

History and Indications for Spine Immobilization

The early management of the patient with a suspected spine fracture or SCI begins at the scene of the accident and involves early immobilization of the whole spine and the institution of measures to prevent secondary injury from hypoxia, hypoperfusion, or further mechanical disruption. Spinal immobilization was developed due to the concern that neurologic injury may occur or worsen with pathologic motion of injured vertebrae. Some have estimated that between 3% and 29% of those with spinal injuries develop worsening of those injuries due to manipulation early in the course of management.[33-36]

Louis Kossuth has been credited as the first clinician to support the need for extrication standards including cervical spine immobilization in 1965.[37] JD Farrington further explored and helped popularize this concept, outlining the use of the backboard, sandbags, and tape for prehospital extrication and care of patients with spinal injuries.[38] In 1971, the Emergency Medical Services system was initiated and instituted prehospital care and spine immobilization standards. During the 1970s, 55% of patients referred to regional SCI centers arrived with complete neurologic lesions. In the 1980s, 61% of SCI patients arrived with incomplete lesions.[39] This improvement has been attributed to the implementation of these standards.[40,41] Spinal immobilization is now routinely practiced and widely recommended in resuscitation guidelines. This includes formal recommendations by the American College of Surgeons and ATLS.[42-44] Initially, the cervical spine was immobilized with use of a soft collar and rolled up blanket. In 1974, Glen Hare introduced the rigid extrication collar, which has led to development of a plethora of immobilization devices.[45]

Spinal immobilization is one of the most frequent prehospital procedures in the United States. It has been championed by many as integral to reducing mortality and morbidity in trauma patients.[46] However, recent literature has questioned the efficacy and safety of spinal immobilization in all trauma patients. This has led to certain absolute and relative indications to spinal immobilization. Initially, spinal immobilization was implemented based on mechanism of injury. Prospective studies have more recently been performed supporting the use of clinical findings as indicators for prehospital spinal immobilization.[47,48] Although there is little conclusive evidence in the literature that supports prehospital clinical clearance of the spine, the similarities between prehospital immobilization decisions and in-hospital radiography decisions are such that it is likely that clinical clearance will be effective for selected patients. This decision can be made at the scene provided the patient has no evidence of the following: altered level of consciousness or mental status, intoxication, neurologic symptoms or signs of a distracting painful injury (eg, chest injuries, long-bone fracture), or midline spinal pain or tenderness. In general, all intoxicated patients; all unconscious trauma patients; those who report spine pain, paresthesias, weakness, or absent movement; those with language barriers; and those at extremes of age should be immobilized. These criteria were able to predict 95% of spinal injuries independent of mechanism of injury; therefore, mechanism of injury alone is not a useful criterion.[48]

Methods of Immobilization

Initially, the cervical spine was immobilized with use of a soft collar and rolled-up blanket. Hare's introduction of the rigid extrication collar in 1974 led to development of several immobilization devices.[49] However, with regard to the cervical spine, the collar does not provide complete immobilization and should be placed in conjunction with a backboard. There are a few contraindications to placement of a cervical extrication collar. Those patients with a surgical airway (ie, cricothyroidotomy) and those with fixed deformity may preclude its placement. Also, some studies suggest that patients with significant cervical swelling or penetrating trauma to the cervical spine without neurologic deficit may not require spinal immobilization.[50,51] Gunshot wounds to the head are also not considered an indication for routine cervical spine immobilization. In fact, as has been reported, cervical collars may actually raise intracranial pressure.[52]

In discussing methods of spinal immobilization, one must recognize that the best methods of immobilization and the best position in which the injured spine should be held immobile are poorly defined. Several methods have been studied to measure the movement of the cervical spine and determine its ideal position; these include clinical evaluation, radiography, CT, and MRI. Schriger[53] defined the ideal position of placement as the "neutral position," or the anatomic position the head and torso assumes when standing and looking forward. He extrapolated that visual determination to correlate to 12° of cervical extension on a lateral radiograph.[53] De Lorenzo et al[49] used MRI to study 19 patients and found that approximately 2 cm of occiput elevation and neck flexion increased spinal canal diameter at C5 and C6 (a common region of unstable cervical spine injuries). Other investigators have made differing recommendations on occipital padding on backboards that places the head/neck in the ideal position.[53,54] As one can ascertain, there is no formal agreement or recommendation for ideal cervical immobilization position. Therefore, in practice, the goal of immobilization has been to maintain the head in a visually neutral position with 0° of motion in all directions using in-line manual stabilization. This should also be performed in conjunction with immobilization of the entire spine in such a way that circulatory and pulmonary compromises are avoided. This includes application of a cervical collar, supports on either side of the head, and long versus short backboards with straps to attach and immobilize the entire body.

In the prehospital setting, EMS personnel traditionally move the patient onto a backboard using the so-called log-roll maneuver. Log-rolling is not only important for initial assessment and stabilization but also throughout the prehospital care and early work-up once the patient has arrived at the hospital. Using this technique to turn the patient can improve lung function, prevent atelectasis, and prevent skin breakdown, especially in the SCI patient.[55-57] Historically, the log roll is properly performed with at least two medical professionals, but likely requires a minimum of four people to do this with as much safety as is possible. The patient's spine must be properly immobilized, which means those involved need to perform precise and synchronized movements.

Log-rolling, although currently widely practiced in the prehospital setting, is not without risks. Conrad et al[58] performed a cadaver study comparing standard log-rolling technique with that of a RotoRest Delta KTT single-sided turning table (Kinetic Concepts, Inc [KCI], San Antonio, TX). They simulated subaxial cervical instability as well as thoracolumbar instability. They found that for the cervical spine, log-rolling produced three times the angular motion and 50% more lateral bending motion in the cervical spine and five times more axial rotation in the thoracolumbar spine. They also found that log-rolling resulted in rapid and abrupt spinal motions.[58] Similarly McGuire et al[59] evaluated thoracolumbar motion in a volunteer with a stable spine, a cadaver with a simulated thoracolumbar instability, and a patient with a T12-L1 fracture-dislocation. They found that the log-rolling maneuver presented the greatest possibility for movement of the spine in the unstable segment.[59] Alternatives to the log-roll maneuver are the multihand method and the HAINES (High Arm IN Endangered Spine) method. The multihand method involves several rescuers on either side of the patient, each of whom slides their arms underneath the patient and lifts from one position to the extrication board. In the HAINES method, the patient is placed supine, the upper arm away from the kneeling rescuer is abducted to 180°, the near arm is placed across the patient's chest, and both lower limbs are flexed. The rescuers' hands stabilize the head and neck and the patient is rolled away onto the extrication board.[60] As one can imagine, these methods may not be plausible if there are not enough rescuers on the scene and/or if the patient has other distracting or position-limiting injuries.

In summary, the patient has to be moved and transported, but even with the best techniques, this is not without risk. Thus, this should be done in an organized and cautious fashion with as many hands for assistance as possible.

Options for Immobilization

For the cervical spine, an immobilization device should theoretically fix the head, hold the occiput and mandible, and restrict motion at the cervicothoracic junction. This belief and practice has led to the development of cervical extrication collars. Their production has been predicated on the need for easily applicable, affordable, and disposable devices.

Some have proposed strict performance standards for cervical extrication collars but these standards have not been uniformly implemented.[61] There are three types of collars: cervical, head-cervical, and head-cervical-thoracic. Most modern collars are rigid head-cervical-thoracic devices using a five-point support structure: the trapezius muscles posteriorly, the clavicles anteriorly, and the sternum. The Stifneck Collar (Laerdal Medical, Wappinger Falls, NY) is an example of this type of device. Soft collars have no role in spinal immobilization as they provide minimal support and do not significantly reduce cervical motion.[62] In applying the collar, the neck should first be examined for swelling, ecchymosis, deformity, bony tenderness, and penetrating wounds. It should only be applied if the head and neck can be brought to the "neutral" position using in-line manual stabilization. If unable to achieve this position, then a collar should not be placed. If an appropriate-sized collar is not available, then an improvised device can be constructed. Once the patient is secured to a backboard firmly, lateral stabilization should be achieved using foam blocks or sandbags and tape. This should also be supported with occipital padding to prevent excessive cervical extension. Another cervical extrication device is the KED (Kendrick Extrication Device), which consists of nylon mesh impregnated with plywood slats. It has thoracic anterior support panels that can be folded to fit multiple patient sizes and shapes.

Adequate full-body thoracolumbar spine immobilization is best accomplished with a full-length backboard. The key elements of backboard use are proper strapping, which minimizes movement during transport, and backboard tilting, which may be used in the event of emesis. A backboard is made from wood or plastic composite with openings along the edges that can be used for straps. Other full-spine immobilizers are the scoop stretcher, made up of two or four pieces, or full-body splints. The scoop stretcher is more comfortable than the standard backboard and can be applied essentially without moving the patient from the supine position. Its application necessitates a large field space due to its size. Many full-body splints use vacuum technology that consists of a vacuum mattress that conforms to the contours of the patient's body, decreasing sacral pressure and ischemic pain.[63]

With the multitude of extrication devices used in emergency situations, one must consider their efficacy in immobilizing the spine. In 1983, Podolsky et al[64] studied cervical immobilization methods using goniometry. They evaluated flexion, extension, lateral bending, and rotation. They found that sandbags and tape immobilized better than soft collars, rigid collars, and hard collars and that combining sandbags with a rigid collar was the best means to limit cervical motion.[64] More recently, Del Rossi et al[65] used a cadaveric study to test the efficacy of several commercially available collars with simulated cervical instability. They found that although the collars did reduce segmental spine motion, this did not significantly differ from the spinal motion generated without a collar in the control condition. They concluded that while further study is needed, a cervical collar should continue to be used as it can perhaps be most effective in preventing a disproportionate amount of motion that may result in secondary neurologic injury.[65] Perry et al[66] evaluated three cervical spine immobilization devices during simulated motion in adults. Neck motion was assessed by independent observers as to whether motion was clinically significant. They concluded that substantial head motion occurs regardless of device unless the head and trunk were controlled using backboard strapping techniques.[66] These studies underscore that overall immobilization using multiple techniques is the most effective in limiting spine motion after traumatic injury and no one device can be adequately relied upon.

Despite obvious benefits, spine immobilization does have a few drawbacks. Not only can immobilization be uncomfortable, but it can have more serious sequelae as well. In a study of normal volunteers, immobilization using a rigid backboard, rigid collar, and lateral stabilizers was associated with headache, backache, and jaw pain.[67] It can also result in ischemic pain at pressure points and even the development of decubitus ulcers. It has been shown that after 8 hours on a backboard, a patient with an SCI has a 95% chance of a sacral decubitus ulcer and severe ischemic pain, whereas the use of backboard padding significantly decreases that risk and resulting pain.[57,68] Many other studies have shown that rigid collar application and backboard strapping may cause airway difficulties, and increase risk of aspiration, dysphagia, and increased intracranial pressure.[50,52,69-73]

Physiologic Goals During Transport

The trauma patient can exhibit multisystem injuries that will require intensive management. This begins in the prehospital period and includes not only stabilization but physiologic management, most notably involving respiratory and cardiovascular support. This is managed with continuous monitoring with three-lead cardiac and pulse oximetry, which is also of utmost importance in those patients with SCI. These patients are prone to the occurrence of neurogenic shock and risk of ventilatory insufficiency. Continuous pulse oximetry is used to detect hypoxia. Oxygen is given to the patient on arrival to the scene if respiratory effort is in question and before intubation if needed. In the multisystem trauma or SCI patient, intubation should be considered with a GCS of less than 9 or oxygen saturation persistently less than 90%.[55] As previously stated, neurogenic shock is associated with SCI patients. In the trauma patient in general, one must also recognize the presence of hypovolemic shock. In neurogenic shock, there may be hypotension secondary to arteriolar and venous vasodilation, hypotension secondary to loss of the sympathetic outflow, and bradycardia secondary to interruption of the sympathetic innervation of the heart.[74] Although not normally treated in the field, its recognition could be potentially life-saving in the early management of the trauma patient. Episodes of hypotension in SCI patients should be avoided and mean arterial pressure should be maintained at or above 90 mm Hg.[75,76] In neurogenic shock, the patient should also be placed in the Trendelenburg position to prevent blood pooling and be treated with vasopressors. For fluid resuscitation in the prehospital setting, either crystalloids or colloids can be given. Crystalloids are iso-oncotic solutions with varying osmolarities. Colloids have the same osmolarity with differing oncotic pressures. Colloids have been associated with blood coagulation and therefore are not routinely used in the multisystem trauma or SCI patient.[77] Recent literature has examined the use of hypertonic-hyperosmotic solutions in resuscitation of the trauma patient, or "small-volume resuscitation." Vassar et al[78] showed in a randomized double-blinded clinical trial that those multisystem trauma patients with traumatic brain injury receiving hypertonic solution as their initial volume load showed better survival at hospital discharge. While no clinical trial has been performed on SCI patients, use of hypertonic saline in experimental SCIs showed attenuation of leukocyte adhesion, increase in spinal cord perfusion, and improvement in neurologic function.[79,80] Fluid resuscitation in the prehospital setting in the trauma patient should not include glucose. Glucose metabolizes rapidly producing "free" water and resulting edema. Also, due to an increase in anaerobic glycolysis in trauma, glucose infusion can result in hyperglycemia and increased lactate and reduced pH. Although no study has associated blood glucose levels with outcomes in the acute SCI patient, it has been shown to be associated with increased intracranial pressure in the traumatic brain injury patient with a GCS of 8 or below.[81] In the patient without SCI, maintenance of blood pressure and fluid balance is more controversial, and recent trends consider more hypotensive resuscitation and less fluids.[82]

Recent literature has focused on temperature control of the polytrauma and SCI patient. In the polytrauma patient, hypothermia can pose a significant risk, resulting in increased morbidity and mortality. This is likely due to impaired coagulation, peripheral vasoconstriction, elevated oxygen consumption, metabolic acidosis, hemodynamic instability, and cardiac arrhythmias.[83] There has been direct association with hypothermia as an independent contributing factor for multiple organ failure, increased length of stay, and mortality.[84] In addition, fluid resuscitation can result in substantial decreases in core temperature. Initially, treatment should begin with prevention of additional heat loss. In the prehospital setting, this can consist of warming blankets, removal of wet clothes, and removal from cold environment. More invasive measures can include prewarmed fluids given intravenously. This will allow stabilization of core temperature until arrival to higher level of care in the emergency department.

There have been attempts to pursue the potential role of controlled hypothermia in the traumatic SCI or brain injury patient. In theory, hypothermia may prevent the initiation of the cascade of events after injury that can lead to cell death. This may directly be related to the slowing of the metabolic rate, lowering the energy requirements of cells and thus maintaining adenosine triphosphate (ATP) concentrations.[85] Some studies have found that mild hypothermia can be protective in anoxic brain injury following resuscitation from prehospital cardiac arrest.[86] The role of hypothermia in traumatic brain injury is somewhat controversial in the literature, although some authors have found a substantial therapeutic effect;[87] however, a 2002 Cochrane systematic review concluded that there was no evidence that hypothermia is beneficial in head injury.[88] Polderman et al[89] suggest that the successful use of hypothermia in these patients depends on identifying carefully selected patients (those with increased intracranial pressure), strict protocols, and close monitoring to avoid complications such as hypovolemia, hypotension, and hyperglycemia. The literature is less controversial for the use of hypothermia in cardiac arrest. Multiple studies, including a Cochrane review, have concluded that mild hypothermia decreases in-hospital mortality in comatose cardiac arrest patients.[90,91] As for hypothermia use in the SCI patient, due to the lack of randomized clinical data, the American Association of Neurologic Surgeons/Neurologic and Spinal Surgery Joint Sections of the Disorders of the Spine and Joint Section of Trauma have recommended that there is not enough evidence for or against the use of hypothermia.[92,93] There are, however, some experimental data, all in rats, which suggest a potential benefit such as reduced secondary damage to the spinal cord as well as reduced swelling and vasogenic edema.[94-96] Further controlled study will be needed before this can be adopted as a suggested standard of care.

Secondary Survey and Adjuncts to the Primary and Secondary Surveys

The secondary survey does not begin until the primary survey is completed, resuscitation is well underway, and the patient is demonstrating reasonable vital signs.[3] This involves a head-to-toe evaluation with a complete history and physical examination including a more complete neurologic examination. Depending on the condition of the patient, this may or may not occur before arrival at the hospital. The secondary survey and subsequent tertiary surveys additionally reduce the incidence of missed injuries.[97] Other adjuncts to initial evaluation and resuscitation can include the electrocardiogram, urinary catheters, gastric tubes, and pulse oximeters.

Orthopaedic and Spine Examination

The orthopaedic and spine examination begins with exposure of the patient. A superficial examination takes place at the end of the primary survey, but, time permitting, most of this examination occurs with the secondary survey. Systematic inspection and palpation of the entire skeleton is performed and abnormalities noted. In particular, visible trauma above the clavicle may be associated with head trauma and or cervical spine injury. More detailed examination of specific joints can be undertaken during the secondary survey if abnormalities are noted. Moving the patient should be kept to a minimum, but for detailed spine examination and transport, log-rolling is preferred, recognizing that this carries risks as mentioned above. Long-bone fractures can be splinted and open wounds dressed. Peripheral pulses should be palpated and circulation assessed. In a young patient who is awake and alert with no distracting injuries, the absence of pain and tenderness to palpation of the spine suggests the absence of a significant spine injury. As long as the patient's spine is protected and immobilized, evaluation of the spine and exclusion of spine injury may be deferred in the presence of systemic instability.[3]

A more detailed neurologic examination that assesses motor and sensory function in a systematic manner should be undertaken during the secondary survey when possible. A baseline can often be established during this early assessment period, although the complete examination usually does not occur until arrival at the emergency center. When possible, muscle strength in all major spinal levels is tested and graded on a 0 to 5 scale as follows: 0 (no function), 1 (trace contraction), 2 (motion with gravity eliminated), 3 (motion against gravity), 4 (motion against slight resistance), and 5 (motion against full resistance). Evaluation of sensation begins at the neck and proceeds to the feet, assessing for intact sensation in all dermatomal distributions.

Triage and Transport

Once prepared for transport, EMS personnel must determine which hospital is most appropriate for the patient. Most metropolitan ambulance centers have access to Level I, II, and III trauma centers. These designations have been established by the American College of Surgeons based on specific criteria. A Level I trauma center provides the highest level of surgical care to the trauma patient. It must have certain personnel available, including 24-hour in-house general surgery and prompt availability of orthopaedics and neurosurgery. It must also have a program of research and education. Level II centers provide all comprehensive care and availability of all services. They are not required to have a research program or surgical residency. Level III centers are rural or community hospitals that have emergency, surgical, and intensive care resources but do not have the full availability of specialists. General indications for direct transport to a Level I trauma center are: hemodynamic instability in a patient with blunt or penetrating trauma to the torso or head, significant burns, spinal injury with neurologic deficit, significant upper or lower extremity amputation, or injury severity score greater than 14.[98]

Method of transport includes either ground or air transport. The use of air transport of patients dates to World War I but expanded during the Korean and Vietnam wars. The first hospital-based air transport began in Denver at St. Anthony hospital in 1972. The advantages of medical transport by air may include providing a higher level of care at the scene of trauma and improving access and speed of access to high-level trauma centers. They also provide critical care capabilities during interfacility transport.[99] Efficacy of air or helicopter EMS is directly related to the availability and efficiency of ground response. Stringent criteria should be used. The Air Medical Physician Association has established criteria including the following: the closest appropriate facility is too far away; patient's clinical condition requires time spent in transport to be short; patient's condition is time-critical; potential for transport delay associated with ground transport could worsen patient's condition; patient requires critical care life support during transport; patient is located in area inaccessible by ground transport; and local ground units are not available, or use of local ground transport would leave local area without EMS for interfacility transport.[100] The single most important factor in deciding for or against air transport is crew and patient safety. There have been reports of air crashes putting air transport in question. Factors associated with these fatal crashes have been flying at night and during bad weather.[101] There are clear data, however, showing improvements in mortality and morbidity compared to ground transport, especially in the traumatic brain injury patient.[102] An important consideration is the cost-effectiveness of air medical transport. A large Scandinavian study found that the benefits of air transport exceeded the costs by a factor of almost six. This and other studies conclude that air transport is well within the accepted range per quality-adjusted life year saved.[103] As can be seen, the value of air transport is not in question, but rather the determination of whom it would benefit. This fact is the focus of current study and discussion. Clear prognostic identifiers that would help ground personnel triage appropriately are still not uniformly established.

Summary

Protocols to optimize the initial field management of blunt trauma victims have evolved substantially in the past 40 years. In SCI, there are still significant questions regarding efficacy of pharmacologic and hypothermic treatment strategies. Advancements in understanding of spinal instability and immobilization, airway management, fluid and hypotensive resuscitation, better methods of transport, as well as high-level trauma care centers have all contributed to decreased morbidity and mortality for blunt trauma patients in general. Despite these improvements, missed injuries still occur, and iatrogenic harm continues to be a concern.

References

1. Sasser SM, Hunt RC, Sullivent EE, et al: Guidelines for field triage of injured patients: Recommendations of the National Expert Panel on Field Triage. *MMWR Recomm Rep* 2009;58(RR-1):1-35.
2. van Olden GD, Meeuwis JD, Bolhuis HW, Boxma H, Goris RJ: Clinical impact of advanced trauma life support. *Am J Emerg Med* 2004;22(7): 522-525.
3. Committee on Trauma: *Advanced Trauma Life Support Manual*, ed 8. Chicago, IL, American College of Surgeons, 2008.
4. van der Velden MW, Ringburg AN, Bergs EA, Steyerberg EW, Patka P, Schipper IB: Prehospital interventions: Time wasted or time saved? An observational cohort study of management in initial trauma care. *Emerg Med J* 2008;25(7):444-449.
5. Hemmila MR, Nathens AB, Shafi S, et al: The Trauma Quality Improvement Program: Pilot study and initial demonstration of feasibility. *J Trauma* 2010;68(2):253-262.
6. Spanjersberg WR, Bergs EA, Mushkudiani N, Klimek M, Schipper IB: Protocol compliance and time management in blunt trauma resuscitation. *Emerg Med J* 2009;26(1):23-27.
7. Brown LH, Gough JE, Simonds WB: Can EMS providers adequately assess trauma patients for cervical spinal injury? *Prehosp Emerg Care* 1998; 2(1):33-36.
8. Enderson BL, Reath DB, Meadors J, Dallas W, DeBoo JM, Maull KI: The tertiary trauma survey: A prospective study of missed injury. *J Trauma* 1990;30(6):666-670.
9. Brooks A, Holroyd B, Riley B: Missed injury in major trauma patients. *Injury* 2004;35(4): 407-410.
10. Sternbach GL: The Glasgow coma scale. *J Emerg Med* 2000;19(1):67-71.
11. Lieberman JD, Pasquale MD, Garcia R, Cipolle MD, Mark Li P, Wasser TE: Use of admission Glasgow Coma Score, pupil size, and pupil reactivity to determine outcome for trauma patients. *J Trauma* 2003;55(3):437-443.

12. Stead LG, Wijdicks EF, Bhagra A, et al: Validation of a new coma scale, the FOUR score, in the emergency department. *Neurocrit Care* 2009; 10(1):50-54.

13. Inaba K, Teixeira PG, Shulman I, et al: The impact of uncross-matched blood transfusion on the need for massive transfusion and mortality: Analysis of 5,166 uncross-matched units. *J Trauma* 2008;65(6):1222-1226.

14. Velmahos GC, Toutouzas K, Chan L, et al: Intubation after cervical spinal cord injury: To be done selectively or routinely? *Am Surg* 2003;69(10): 891-894.

15. Hassid VJ, Schinco MA, Tepas JJ, et al: Definitive establishment of airway control is critical for optimal outcome in lower cervical spinal cord injury. *J Trauma* 2008;65(6):1328-1332.

16. Cobas MA, De la Peña MA, Manning R, Candiotti K, Varon AJ: Prehospital intubations and mortality: A level 1 trauma center perspective. *Anesth Analg* 2009;109(2):489-493.

17. Gerling MC, Davis DP, Hamilton RS, et al: Effects of cervical spine immobilization technique and laryngoscope blade selection on an unstable cervical spine in a cadaver model of intubation. *Ann Emerg Med* 2000;36(4):293-300.

18. Turner CR, Block J, Shanks A, Morris M, Lodhia KR, Gujar SK: Motion of a cadaver model of cervical injury during endotracheal intubation with a Bullard laryngoscope or a Macintosh blade with and without in-line stabilization. *J Trauma* 2009; 67(1):61-66.

19. Siddiqui AK: Airway management for cervical spine injury. *Saudi Med J* 2009;30(9):1133-1137.

20. Arslan ZI, Yildiz T, Baykara ZN, Solak M, Toker K: Tracheal intubation in patients with rigid collar immobilisation of the cervical spine: A comparison of Airtraq and LMA CTrach devices. *Anaesthesia* 2009;64(12):1332-1336.

21. Turkstra TP, Pelz DM, Jones PM: Cervical spine motion: A fluoroscopic comparison of the AirTraq Laryngoscope versus the Macintosh laryngoscope. *Anesthesiology* 2009;111(1):97-101.

22. Robitaille A, Williams SR, Tremblay MH, Guilbert F, Thériault M, Drolet P: Cervical spine motion during tracheal intubation with manual in-line stabilization: Direct laryngoscopy versus GlideScope videolaryngoscopy. *Anesth Analg* 2008; 106(3):935-941.

23. Gercek E, Wahlen BM, Rommens PM: In vivo ultrasound real-time motion of the cervical spine during intubation under manual in-line stabilization: A comparison of intubation methods. *Eur J Anaesthesiol* 2008;25(1):29-36.

24. Byhahn C, Meininger D, Walcher F, Hofstetter C, Zwissler B: Prehospital emergency endotracheal intubation using the Bonfils intubation fiberscope. *Eur J Emerg Med* 2007;14(1):43-46.

25. Bilgin H, Bozkurt M: Tracheal intubation using the ILMA, C-Trach or McCoy laryngoscope in patients with simulated cervical spine injury. *Anaesthesia* 2006;61(7):685-691.

26. Turkstra TP, Craen RA, Pelz DM, Gelb AW: Cervical spine motion: A fluoroscopic comparison during intubation with lighted stylet, GlideScope, and Macintosh laryngoscope. *Anesth Analg* 2005; 101(3):910-915.

27. Wahlen BM, Gercek E: Three-dimensional cervical spine movement during intubation using the Macintosh and Bullard laryngoscopes, the bonfils fibrescope and the intubating laryngeal mask airway. *Eur J Anaesthesiol* 2004;21(11):907-913.

28. Brimacombe J, Keller C, Künzel KH, Gaber O, Boehler M, Pühringer F: Cervical spine motion during airway management: A cinefluoroscopic study of the posteriorly destabilized third cervical vertebrae in human cadavers. *Anesth Analg* 2000; 91(5):1274-1278.

29. McIntosh SE, Swanson ER, Barton ED: Cricothyrotomy in air medical transport. *J Trauma* 2008; 64(6):1543-1547.

30. Gerling MC, Davis DP, Hamilton RS, et al: Effect of surgical cricothyrotomy on the unstable cervical spine in a cadaver model of intubation. *J Emerg Med* 2001;20(1):1-5.

31. *Advanced Cardiac Life Support Provider Manual.* Dallas, TX, American Heart Association, 2001.

32. Goldberg RM, Rowan L, Anderson RE: Thoracic vertebral fracture as a complication of cardiopulmonary resuscitation. *J Emerg Med* 1988;6(3): 177-178.

33. Bohlman HH: Acute fractures and dislocations of the cervical spine: An analysis of three hundred hospitalized patients and review of the literature. *J Bone Joint Surg Am* 1979;61(8):1119-1142.

34. Davis JW, Phreaner DL, Hoyt DB, Mackersie RC: The etiology of missed cervical spine injuries. *J Trauma* 1993;34(3):342-346.

35. Geisler WO, Wynne-Jones M, Jousse AT: Early management of the patient with trauma to the spinal cord. *Med Serv J Can* 1966;22(7):512-523.

36. Prasad VS, Schwartz A, Bhutani R, Sharkey PW, Schwartz ML: Characteristics of injuries to the cervical spine and spinal cord in polytrauma patient population: Experience from a regional trauma unit. *Spinal Cord* 1999;37(8):560-568.

37. Kossuth LC: The removal of injured personnel from wrecked vehicles. *J Trauma* 1965;5(6): 703-708.

38. Farrington JD: Extrication of victims—surgical principles. *J Trauma* 1968;8(4):493-512.

39. Gunby I: New focus on spinal cord injury. *JAMA* 1981;245(12):1201-1206.

40. Green BA, Eismont FJ, O'Heir JT: Spinal cord injury—a systems approach: prevention, emergency medical services, and emergency room management. *Crit Care Clin* 1987;3(3):471-493.

41. Waters RL, Meyer PR Jr, Adkins RH, Felton D: Emergency, acute, and surgical management of spine trauma. *Arch Phys Med Rehabil* 1999;80(11): 1383-1390.

42. Domeier RM, National Association of EMS Physicians Standards and Clinical Practice Committee: Indications for prehospital spinal immobilization. *Prehosp Emerg Care* 1999;3(3):251-253.

43. Alexander R, Proctor H: *Advanced Trauma Life Support Course for Physicians*. Chicago, IL, American College of Surgeons, 1993, pp 21-22.

44. Spine and spinal cord trauma, in *Advanced Trauma Life Support for Doctors: Student Course Manual*, ed 6. Chicago, IL, American College of Surgeons, 1997, pp 215-242.

45. De Lorenzo RA: A review of spinal immobilization techniques. *J Emerg Med* 1996;14(5):603-613.

46. Garfin SR, Shackford SR, Marshall LF, Drummond JC: Care of the multiply injured patient with cervical spine injury. *Clin Orthop Relat Res* 1989;239:19-29.

47. Domeier RM, Evans RW, Swor RA, Rivera-Rivera EJ, Frederiksen SM: Prospective validation of out-of-hospital spinal clearance criteria: A preliminary report. *Acad Emerg Med* 1997;4(6):643-646.

48. Domeier RM, Evans RW, Swor RA, et al: The reliability of prehospital clinical evaluation for potential spinal injury is not affected by the mechanism of injury. *Prehosp Emerg Care* 1999;3(4):332-337.

49. De Lorenzo RA, Olson JE, Boska M, et al: Optimal positioning for cervical immobilization. *Ann Emerg Med* 1996;28(3):301-308.

50. Haut ER, Kalish BT, Efron DT, et al: Spine immobilization in penetrating trauma: More harm than good? *J Trauma* 2010;68(1):115-121.

51. Connell RA, Graham CA, Munro PT: Is spinal immobilisation necessary for all patients sustaining isolated penetrating trauma? *Injury* 2003; 34(12):912-914.

52. Davies G, Deakin C, Wilson A: The effect of a rigid collar on intracranial pressure. *Injury* 1996; 27(9):647-649.

53. Schriger DL: Immobilizing the cervical spine in trauma: Should we seek an optimal position or an adequate one? *Ann Emerg Med* 1996;28(3):351-353.

54. McSwain NE Jr: Spine management skills, in *Prehospital Trauma Life Support*, ed 2. Akron, OH, Educational Direction, 1990, pp 225-256.

55. Bernhard M, Gries A, Kremer P, Böttiger BW: Spinal cord injury (SCI)—prehospital management. *Resuscitation* 2005;66(2):127-139.

56. Kirschenbaum L, Azzi E, Sfeir T, Tietjen P, Astiz M: Effect of continuous lateral rotational therapy on the prevalence of ventilator-associated pneumonia in patients requiring long-term ventilatory care. *Crit Care Med* 2002;30(9):1983-1986.

57. Krishnagopalan S, Johnson EW, Low LL, Kaufman LJ: Body positioning of intensive care patients: Clinical practice versus standards. *Crit Care Med* 2002;30(11):2588-2592.

58. Conrad BP, Horodyski MB, Wright J, Ruetz P, Rechtine GR II: Log-rolling technique producing unacceptable motion during body position changes in patients with traumatic spinal cord injury. *J Neurosurg Spine* 2007;6(6):540-543.

59. McGuire RA, Neville S, Green BA, Watts C: Spinal instability and the log-rolling maneuver. *J Trauma* 1987;27(5):525-531.

60. Gunn BD, Eizenberg N, Silberstein M, et al: How should an unconscious person with a suspected neck injury be positioned? *Prehosp Disaster Med* 1995;10(4):239-244.

61. Garth G: Proposal for the establishment of minimum performance specifications for cervical extrication collars. *14th Annual Meeting of the Acute Traumatic Stress Management Skeletal Support Committee*, 1988.

62. Karbi OA, Caspari DA, Tator CH: Extrication, immobilization and radiologic investigation of patients with cervical spine injuries. *CMAJ* 1988; 139(7):617-621.

63. Johnson DR, Hauswald M, Stockhoff CY: Comparison of a vacuum splint device to a rigid backboard for spinal immobilization. *Am J Emerg Med* 1996;14(4):369-372.

64. Podolsky S, Baraff LJ, Simon RR, Hoffman JR, Larmon B, Ablon W: Efficacy of cervical spine immobilization methods. *J Trauma* 1983;23(6): 461-465.

65. Del Rossi G, Heffernan TP, Horodyski MB, Rechtine GR: The effectiveness of extrication collars tested during the execution of spine-board transfer techniques. *Spine J* 2004;4(6):619-623.

66. Perry SD, McLellan B, McIlroy WE, Maki BE, Schwartz M, Fernie GR: The efficacy of head immobilization techniques during simulated vehicle motion. *Spine (Phila Pa 1976)* 1999;24(17): 1839-1844.

67. Chan D, Goldberg R, Tascone A, Harmon S, Chan L: The effect of spinal immobilization on healthy volunteers. *Ann Emerg Med* 1994;23(1):48-51.

68. Hauswald M, Hsu M, Stockoff C: Maximizing comfort and minimizing ischemia: A comparison of four methods of spinal immobilization. *Prehosp Emerg Care* 2000;4(3):250-252.

69. Kwan I, Bunn F: Effects of prehospital spinal immobilization: A systematic review of randomized trials on healthy subjects. *Prehosp Disaster Med* 2005;20(1):47-53.

70. Brown JB, Bankey PE, Sangosanya AT, Cheng JD, Stassen NA, Gestring ML: Prehospital spinal immobilization does not appear to be beneficial and may complicate care following gunshot injury to the torso. *J Trauma* 2009;67(4):774-778.

71. Houghton DJ, Curley JW: Dysphagia caused by a hard cervical collar. *Br J Neurosurg* 1996;10(5): 501-502.

72. Butman AM, Schelble DT, Vomacka RW: The relevance of the occult cervical spine controversy and mechanism of injury to prehospital protocols: A review of the issues and literature. *Prehosp Disaster Med* 1996;11(3):228-233.

73. Hewitt S: Skin necrosis caused by a semi-rigid cervical collar in a ventilated patient with multiple injuries. *Injury* 1994;25(5):323-324.

74. Stevens RD, Bhardwaj A, Kirsch JR, Mirski MA: Critical care and perioperative management in traumatic spinal cord injury. *J Neurosurg Anesthesiol* 2003;15(3):215-229.

75. Blood pressure management after acute spinal cord injury. *Neurosurgery* 2002;50(3, Suppl): S58-S62.

76. Vale FL, Burns J, Jackson AB, Hadley MN: Combined medical and surgical treatment after acute spinal cord injury: Results of a prospective pilot study to assess the merits of aggressive medical resuscitation and blood pressure management. *J Neurosurg* 1997;87(2):239-246.

77. Dieterich HJ: Colloids in intensive care. *Anaesthesist* 2001;50(1):54-68.

78. Vassar MJ, Perry CA, Gannaway WL, Holcroft JW: 7.5% sodium chloride/dextran for resuscitation of trauma patients undergoing helicopter transport. *Arch Surg* 1991;126(9):1065-1072.

79. Spera PA, Arfors KE, Vasthare US, Tuma RF, Young WF: Effect of hypertonic saline on leukocyte activity after spinal cord injury. *Spine (Phila Pa 1976)* 1998;23(22):2444-2449.

80. Spera PA, Vasthare US, Tuma RF, Young WF: The effects of hypertonic saline on spinal cord blood flow following compression injury. *Acta Neurochir (Wien)* 2000;142(7):811-817.

81. Rovlias A, Kotsou S: The influence of hyperglycemia on neurological outcome in patients with severe head injury. *Neurosurgery* 2000;46(2): 335-343.

82. Jackson K, Nolan J: The role of hypotensive resuscitation in the management of trauma. *J Intensive Care Soc* 2009;10(2):109-114.

83. Tsuei BJ, Kearney PA: Hypothermia in the trauma patient. *Injury* 2004;35(1):7-15.

84. Eddy VA, Morris JA Jr, Cullinane DC: Hypothermia, coagulopathy, and acidosis. *Surg Clin North Am* 2000;80(3):845-854.

85. Arrica M, Bissonnette B: Therapeutic hypothermia. *Semin Cardiothorac Vasc Anesth* 2007;11(1): 6-15.

86. Bernard SA, Gray TW, Buist MD, et al: Treatment of comatose survivors of out-of-hospital cardiac arrest with induced hypothermia. *N Engl J Med* 2002;346(8):557-563.

87. Marion DW, Penrod LE, Kelsey SF, et al: Treatment of traumatic brain injury with moderate hypothermia. *N Engl J Med* 1997;336(8):540-546.

88. Gadkary CS, Alderson P, Signorini DF: Therapeutic hypothermia for head injury. *Cochrane Database Syst Rev* 2002;1:CD001048.

89. Polderman KH, Tjong Tjin Joe R, Peerdeman SM, Vandertop WP, Girbes AR: Effects of therapeutic hypothermia on intracranial pressure and outcome in patients with severe head injury. *Intensive Care Med* 2002;28(11):1563-1573.

90. Hypothermia after Cardiac Arrest Study Group: Mild therapeutic hypothermia to improve the neurologic outcome after cardiac arrest. *N Engl J Med* 2002;346(8):549-556.

91. Cheung KW, Green RS, Magee KD: Systematic review of randomized controlled trials of therapeutic hypothermia as a neuroprotectant in post cardiac arrest patients. *CJEM* 2006;8(5):329-337.

92. Dietrich WD III: Therapeutic hypothermia for spinal cord injury. *Crit Care Med* 2009;37 (7, Suppl):S238-S242.

93. Kwon BK, Mann C, Sohn HM, et al: Hypothermia for spinal cord injury. *Spine J* 2008;8(6):859-874.

94. Yu CG, Jimenez O, Marcillo AE, et al: Beneficial effects of modest systemic hypothermia on locomotor function and histopathological damage following contusion-induced spinal cord injury in rats. *J Neurosurg* 2000;93(1, Suppl)85-93.

95. Yu WR, Westergren H, Farooque M, Holtz A, Olsson Y: Systemic hypothermia following compression injury of rat spinal cord: Reduction of plasma protein extravasation demonstrated by immunohistochemistry. *Acta Neuropathol* 1999; 98(1):15-21.

96. Shibuya S, Miyamoto O, Janjua NA, Itano T, Mori S, Norimatsu H: Post-traumatic moderate systemic hypothermia reduces TUNEL positive cells following spinal cord injury in rat. *Spinal Cord* 2004;42(1):29-34.

97. Huynh TT, Moran KR, Blackburn AH, Jacobs DG, Thomason MH, Sing RF: Optimal management strategy for incidental findings in trauma patients: An initiative for midlevel providers. *J Trauma* 2008;65(2):331-336.

98. American College of Surgeons: Committee on Trauma: About the Committee on Trauma. Trauma Programs-Consultation/Verification Programs for Hospitals. Chicago, IL, American College of Surgeons. http://www.facs.org/trauma/about.html. Accessed August 16, 2010.

99. Branas CC, MacKenzie EJ, Williams JC, et al: Access to trauma centers in the United States. *JAMA* 2005;293(21):2626-2633.

100. Air Medical Physician Association: Medical condition list and appropriate use of air medical transport: Position statement of the Air Medical Physician Association. *Prehosp Emerg Care* 2002;6(4): 464-470.

101. Baker SP, Grabowski JG, Dodd RS, Shanahan DF, Lamb MW, Li GH: EMS helicopter crashes: What influences fatal outcome? *Ann Emerg Med* 2006; 47(4):351-356.

102. Wang HE, Peitzman AB, Cassidy LD, Adelson PD, Yealy DM: Out-of-hospital endotracheal intubation and outcome after traumatic brain injury. *Ann Emerg Med* 2004;44(5):439-450.

103. Elvik R: Cost-benefit analysis of ambulance and rescue helicopters in Norway: Reflections on assigning a monetary value to saving a human life. *Appl Health Econ Health Policy* 2002;1(2):55-63.

CHAPTER 3
Physical Examination

Robert A. McGuire, MD

Introduction

Every year, spinal injuries occur as a result of motor vehicle accidents, falls, gunshot wounds, and recreational accidents. Many of these injuries are missed in the initial emergency evaluation because of distracting factors such as a head injury, acute intoxication secondary to drugs or alcohol, or multiple trauma. Critical factors such as spinal stability and neurologic compromise become important issues in planning treatment regimens and counseling the patient and family members regarding the prognosis. It is paramount to have an accurate, well-documented physical examination when treating patients with spinal injuries.

The physical examination begins by obtaining a history from the patient, and questioning the investigating officer and paramedical personnel involved in treating the patient. This inquiry should include the circumstances of the accident, the position in which the patient was found, whether or not the patient was wearing a seatbelt or shoulder harness, and the type of treatment provided at the accident scene. It is important to ask for specific information regarding transient motor or sensory loss or the presence of Lhermitte's sign. This information provides insight into the forces involved and the possible mechanisms of injury. A high correlation has been reported between head injury and resulting neck injury.[1-3] These patients must also be thoroughly evaluated for multiple spinal fractures.[4] Children and infants present unique challenges when evaluating for possible spinal injuries; due to the immature skeleton, great vigilance is necessary to avoid missing fractures and soft-tissue injury in this population.[5] In patients with multiple trauma, strict adherence to principles of airway maintenance, breathing, and circulation take precedence over bony injury.

Dr. McGuire or an immediate family member serves as a board member, owner, officer, or committee member of AO Spine; has received royalties from DePuy, a Johnson & Johnson company; and serves as a paid consultant to or is an employee of Synthes.

Inspection

The physical examination begins with inspection of the patient. All clothing should be carefully removed, allowing a systematic visual evaluation to be performed, and all areas of tissue abrasions, contusions, lacerations, and limb asymmetry should be noted. Chest expansion is observed for abnormal motion or paradoxical movement of the thoracic cage, signifying possible pulmonary or cardiac injury.

Palpation

Palpation is then undertaken in a systematic manner. The extremities and joints are evaluated for crepitus, abnormal motion, and malalignment. Careful attention to the peripheral pulses is mandatory because vessel lacerations, transections, and intimal tears often produce either absent or asymmetric pulsations. Low pulse rate with low blood pressure can be indicative of a sympathectomy from a spinal cord injury rather than hypovolemic shock. The abdomen is then evaluated for possible peritoneal signs indicating damaged viscera. Seatbelt injuries causing lumbar fractures have been associated with bowel rupture and major vessel, liver, spleen, and urologic injury.[6] In evaluating the chest, each rib is carefully palpated for continuity or crepitus. Soft-tissue crepitus is indicative of major pulmonary trauma with probable pneumothorax. The pelvis is evaluated for widening of the symphysis pubis or any asymmetry of the iliac wings. The spine is then palpated in a systematic manner.

The cervical collar is carefully removed and the anterior aspect of the neck is evaluated. Evidence of venous congestion such as distended jugular veins should be noted. The carotid pulses are palpated carefully for any evidence of hematoma formation or thrills. The position of the trachea is evaluated for any deviation from the midline, and the anterior aspect of the cervical spine is carefully palpated for malalignment or tenderness. Attention is next directed to the head, occipitocervical junction, and posterior aspect of the cervical spine. If tenderness is encountered, the collar is replaced and the patient carefully rolled to allow palpation of the thoracic and lumbar spine. Great

FIGURE 1

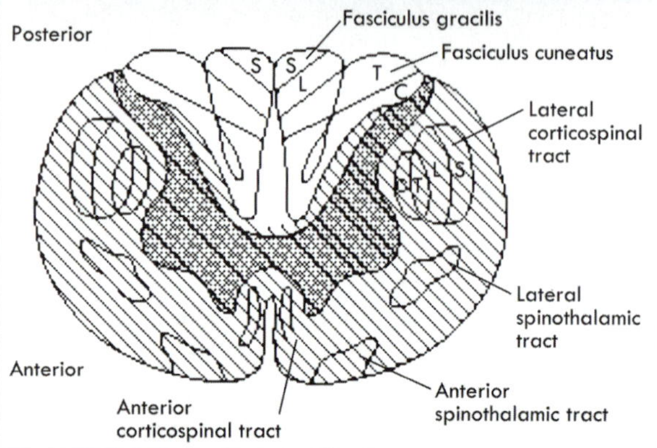

Figure 1 Involvement of the anterior two-thirds of the spinal cord leads to loss of motor and sensory function below the lesion. Only deep sensation is present, with this being mediated through the posterior column. (Reproduced with permission from Keenen TL, Benson DR: Initial evaluation of the spine-injured patient, in Browner BD, Jupiter JB, Levine AM, Trafton PG, eds: *Skeletal Trauma: Fractures, Dislocations, Ligamentous Injuries*. Philadelphia, PA, WB Saunders, 1992, p 588.)

care must be used with the log-roll maneuver because an unstable spine can become displaced and potentially lead to neural compromise.[7] In a comatose patient, the cervical spine must be radiographically evaluated before removal of the collar, because 3% to 5% of these patients will have an associated neck injury. Each spinous process should be palpated, noting tenderness, alignment, asymmetry, or interspinous widening. The sacroiliac joints are evaluated for instability in lateral compression or longitudinal migration. The patient is then carefully rolled back to the supine position and a thorough neurologic examination is performed.

Neurologic Evaluation

The neurologic examination consists of evaluation of the motor, sensory, and reflex portion of the nervous system. Strict attention must be paid to sharp versus dull discrimination, temperature, and the ability to distinguish between light and deep pressure. Evaluation of motor function must include not only the presence or absence of function but also grades of strength.

Muscle grading is important to allow consistency of evaluation between different examiners as well as monitoring improvement or deterioration of function with time. The grading system for muscle strength is as follows: grade 0, no function; grade 1 or trace, palpable contraction without joint motion; grade 2 or poor, complete joint range of motion (ROM) with gravity eliminated; grade 3 or fair, full joint ROM against gravity; grade 4 or good, complete ROM against gravity with slight resistance; and grade 5 or normal, full ROM against gravity and resistance. Using this grading scheme, the motor index score serves as a numeric system to document improvement or deterioration of function (**Appendix 1**).

The Frankel classification also provides a standardized method of evaluation of both motor and sensory function in spinal injury patients.[8] In this scheme, Frankel A represents no motor or sensory function; Frankel B, no motor function, sensory incomplete; Frankel C, motor function useless, sensory incomplete; Frankel D, motor function useful, sensory incomplete; and Frankel E, motor function normal, sensory normal. Bradford and McBride[2] have further divided the Frankel D classification as follows: D1, preserved motor function at lowest functional grade (3+/5+) with or without bowel or bladder paralysis with normal or reduced voluntary motor function; D2, preserved motor function at midfunctional grade (3+ to 4+/5+) and normal voluntary bowel or bladder function; and D3, preserved motor function at high functional grade (4+ to 5+) and normal voluntary bowel or bladder function.

Damage to specific sections of the spinal cord presents as cord syndromes; they are categorized by specific physical findings. These syndromes can also present as a combination of two or more syndromes rather than the "pure" variety described below.

Anterior cord syndrome, which involves the anterior two-thirds of the spinal cord, is manifest as loss of all motor function and sensation below the injured level. Only the posterior columns are spared, which provide crude sensation only. This syndrome has a poor prognosis for recovery (**Figure 1**).

Central cord syndrome is usually seen in older persons who sustain a hyperextension injury to their neck. The spinal cord is injured by a pincer mechanism formed by osteophytes anteriorly and hypertrophied ligamentum flavum posteriorly, which compress the spinal cord in the middle. This injury preferentially involves the central portion of the cord more than the peripheral. Because the anatomic arrangements of the neural tracts providing function to the upper extremity are mostly medial, followed by thoracic, lower extremity, and sacral in a more lateral distribution, these patients will present with more involvement of the hand than of the lower extremity. The ma-

FIGURE 2

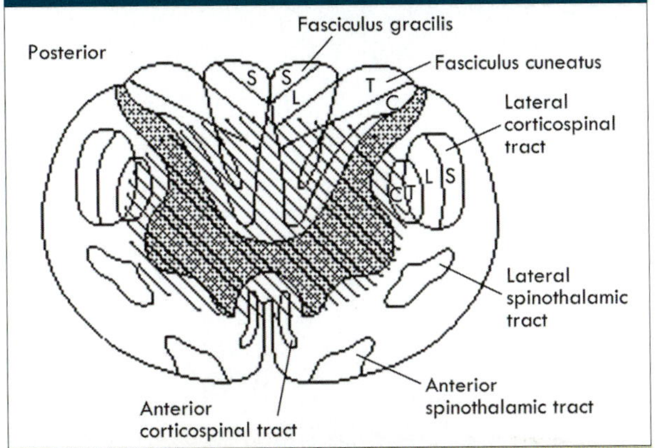

Figure 2 The central portion of the spinal cord is involved, with sacral sparing due to the arrangements of the fibers in the corticospinal and spinothalamic tracts. In the corticospinal and spinothalamic tracts, the fibers innervating the upper extremity are more medial, with the fibers innervating the distal extremity being located more lateral in each tract. (Reproduced with permission from Keenen TL, Benson DR: Initial evaluation of the spine-injured patient, in Browner BD, Jupiter JB, Levine AM, Trafton PG, eds: *Skeletal Trauma: Fractures, Dislocations, Ligamentous Injuries*. Philadelphia, PA, WB Saunders, 1992, p 588.)

FIGURE 3

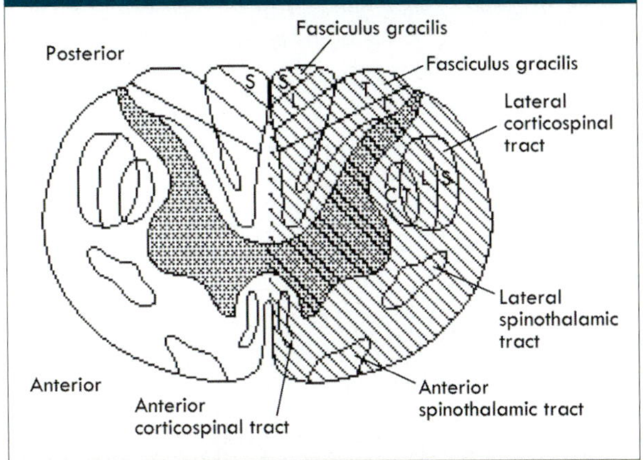

Figure 3 Hemisection of the spinal cord leads to loss of motor function on the same side of the lesion, and loss of pain and the ability to distinguish temperature and light touch on the opposite side. (Reproduced with permission from Keenen TL, Benson DR: Initial evaluation of the spine-injured patient, in Browner BD, Jupiter JB, Levine AM, Trafton PG, eds: *Skeletal Trauma: Fractures, Dislocations, Ligamentous Injuries*. Philadelphia, PA, WB Saunders, 1992, p 588.)

FIGURE 4

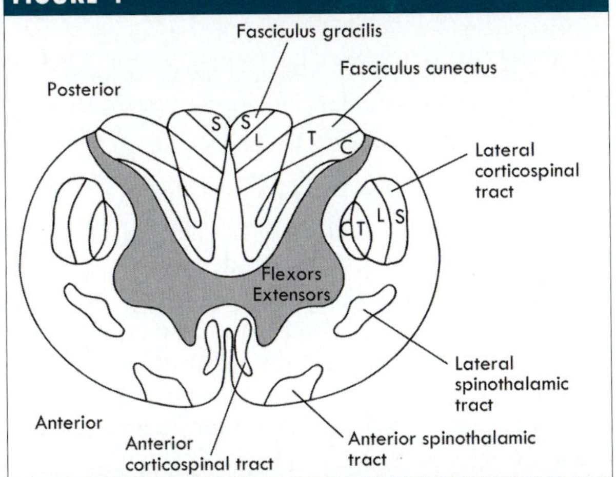

Figure 4 Cross section of the spinal cord noting orientation of the fibers in the spinothalamic and corticospinal tracts. (Reproduced with permission from Keenen TL, Benson DR: Initial evaluation of the spine-injured patient, in Browner BD, Jupiter JB, Levine AM, Trafton PG, eds: *Skeletal Trauma: Fractures, Dislocations, Ligamentous Injuries*. Philadelphia, PA, WB Saunders, 1992, p 588.)

jority will have bowel and bladder control and will be able to ambulate, although often with a spastic gait. Most of these patients do not regain fine motor use of their upper extremities (**Figure 2**).

Brown-Séquard syndrome results from hemisection of the cord. It is manifested by loss of ipsilateral motor function and contralateral pain, inability to distinguish temperature, and loss of light touch sensation. These patients will regain control of their bowel and bladder function and most will be able to ambulate (**Figure 3**).

Posterior cord syndrome is rare and involves loss of posterior column function, which provides proprioception and position sense. These patients maintain the ability to ambulate, but rely on visual input for their spatial orientation.

Root injuries can be isolated in the cervical, lumbar, or sacral spine or may be combined with other cord injury. Nerve root injuries have a more favorable prognosis than cord injuries. In the cervical spine, the complex of a complete cord injury with varying levels of root injury is frequently seen. Those patients with complete high cervical injuries have a 30% chance of recovery of one nerve root level, those with midcervical injuries have a 60% chance, and almost all patients with low cervical injuries will have recovery of one root level and sometimes two.

Sensory Evaluation

Evaluation of the sensory level in each patient should be carefully tested using an alcohol wipe to distinguish temperature and a sterile needle to

FIGURE 5

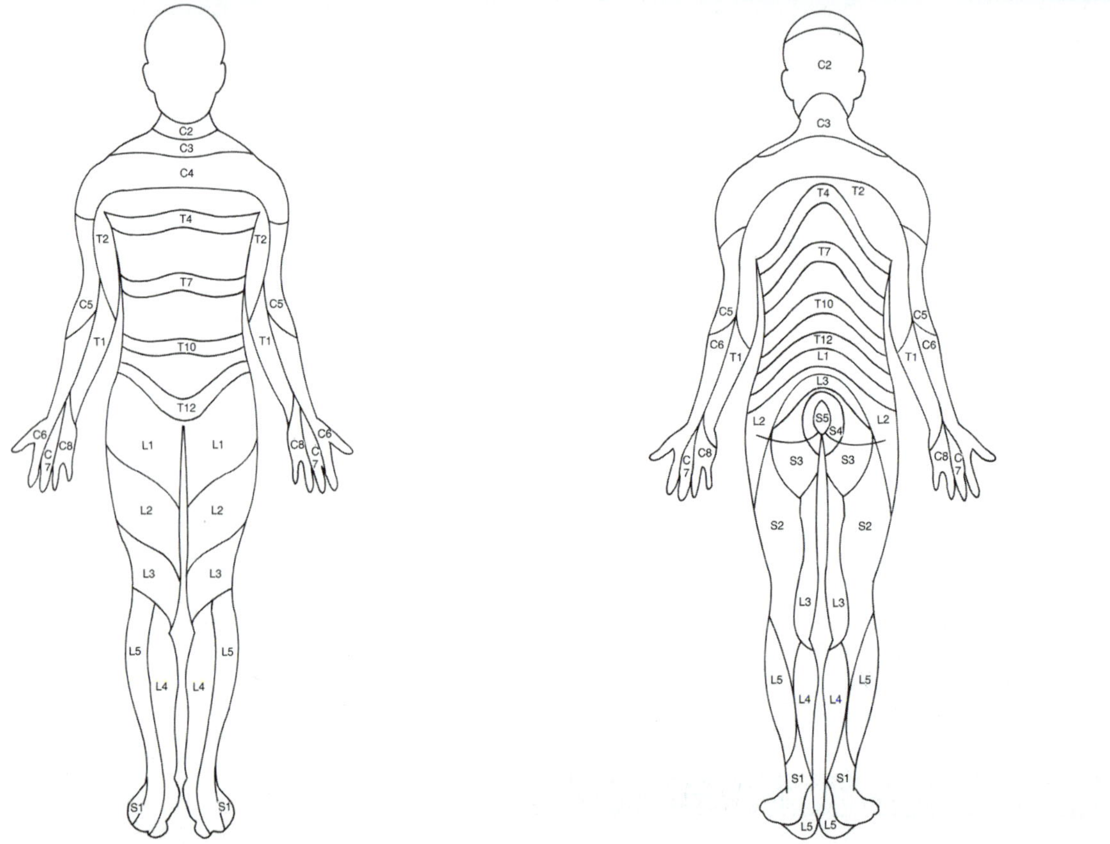

Figure 5 Dermatomes. (Reproduced with permission from Keenen TL, Benson DR: Initial evaluation of the spine-injured patient, in Browner BD, Jupiter JB, Levine AM, Trafton PG, eds: *Skeletal Trauma: Fractures, Dislocations, Ligamentous Injuries.* Philadelphia, PA, WB Saunders, 1992, p 595.)

evaluate pain and light touch. These are functions of the spinothalamic tract, which has fibers in the anterolateral portion of the spinal cord. Posterior column function of the spinal cord can be tested using a tuning fork to detect vibration or the position of the limb in space. The muscles are innervated by the neural tissues in the corticospinal tracts, which are positioned in the anterolateral aspect of the spinal cord (**Figure 4**). The sensory and motor examination must be performed in a sequential and systematic manner.

Evaluation of sensation begins with the cervical region and proceeds distally with evaluation of specific dermatomal regions (**Figure 5**, **Table 1**). Unrestricted access to the patient is mandatory. C1 and C2 roots provide sensation from the occipital region to the nape of the neck. C3 and C4 provide sensation in a cape distribution from the neck and shoulders posteriorly to the anterior chest just inferior to the clavicles. C5 innervates the deltoid region of the shoulder and anterolateral aspect of the upper arm. C6 innervates the radial aspect of the forearm, thumb, and index finger. C7 provides sensation to the long fingers and a small strip of skin on the dorsal aspect of the hand. C8 innervates the ulnar aspect of the hand, including the fourth and fifth digits and the ulnar aspect of the forearm. T1 provides sensation to the medial aspect of the arm, axilla, and pectoral region of the chest.

The thoracic region and abdomen receive sensory innervation from the thoracic nerve roots, with significant sensory overlap in this area due to the dual innervation of the skin. Anatomically, the skin in this area receives input from the fibers of three different spinal nerve levels. Localizing sensory levels in this region are the nipple line, which represents a T5 level, and the umbilicus, representing the T10 level. The inguinal region receives input from the lower thoracic and upper lumbar region.

The lower extremity and perineum are innervated by the roots making up the lumbosacral plexus (**Figure 6**). L1 and L2 innervate the skin

TABLE 1

Major Sensory Levels

Level	Region
C4	Clavicle
C5	Deltoid region
C6	Radial forearm and thumb
C7	Middle finger
C8	Fifth finger
T1	Medial, proximal arm
T5	Nipples
T7	Costal margins
T10	Umbilicus
T12	Inguinal ligament
L3	Anterior thigh
L4	Medial aspect of knee
L5	Lateral calf, dorsum of foot, big toe
S1	Lateral foot, fifth toe
S2	Posterior thighs
S3-S4	Buttocks, perianal region

(Reproduced from McGuire RA Jr: Physical examination in spinal trauma, in Levine AM, Eismont FJ, Garfin SR, Zigler JE, eds: *Spine Trauma*. Philadelphia, PA, WB Saunders, 1998, pp 16-27.)

FIGURE 6

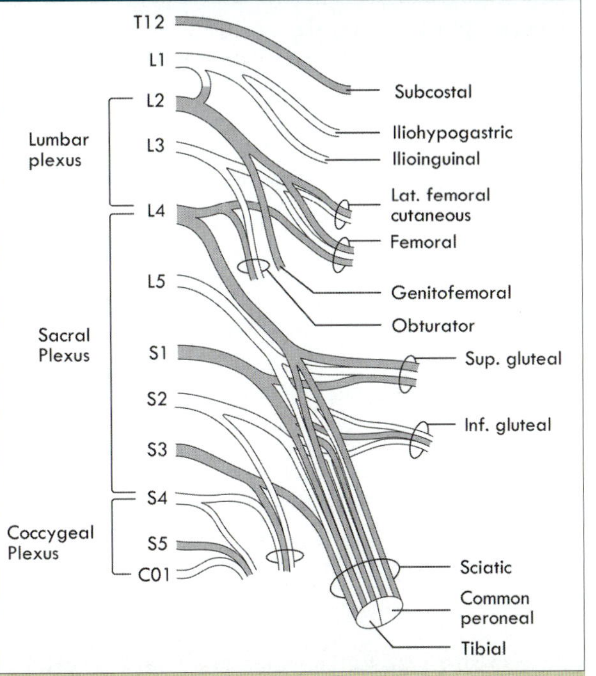

Figure 6 The lumbosacral plexus. (Modified with permission from Gardner E, Gray DJ, O'Rahilly R, eds: *Anatomy*. Philadelphia, PA, WB Saunders, 1975, p 426.)

just below the inguinal ligament and the inner thigh, while L3 and L4 provide sensation to the anterior and anterolateral leg and the knee. L5 provides sensation to the lateral aspect of the calf and the dorsomedial skin of the foot and ankle. S1 innervates the posterior calf and the lateral and plantar aspect of the foot.

The perineum is innervated by sacral nerves S2 through S5, and becomes important as a prognostic indicator of functional recovery in those patients with a spinal cord injury.[9,10]

Motor Evaluation

Following a thorough evaluation of sensory function, muscles are evaluated and carefully documented regarding functional strength (**Table 2**, **Figure 7**). C1 and C2 innervate the musculature of the suboccipital triangle. C3 and C4, in conjunction with the intercostal nerves, provide respiratory function via the diaphragm. Patients with low cervical and thoracic spinal cord injuries often present with paradoxical respiration. The cord injury renders the intercostal and abdominal musculature nonfunctional. With inspiration, the diaphragm contracts, which displaces the abdominal contents inferiorly, resulting in abdominal distention rather than the flattening of the abdomen and expansion of the chest that takes place normally with inspiration in neurologically intact patients. Should the C3 and C4 roots be nonfunctional, the diaphragm will be paralyzed and severe respiratory compromise may result. C5-innervated muscles include the deltoid, the internal and external shoulder rotators, and the biceps. Muscles innervated by C6 include the biceps, brachioradialis, and wrist extensors (extensor carpi radialis longus, extensor carpi radialis brevis). C7 function evaluates the triceps, wrist flexors (flexor carpi radialis, flexor carpi ulnaris), and finger extensors (extensor digitorum communis). Finger flexors (flexor digitorum superficialis, flexor digitorum profundus) and hand intrinsics are innervated by the C8 root, with interossei function being provided by the T1 root.

Thoracic roots innervate the intercostal muscles and the abdominal and paraspinal muscles. Upper abdominal contraction without lower abdominal contraction results in the upward migration of the umbilicus, known as Beevor's sign, which is indicative of paralysis below T10. L1, L2, and L3

TABLE 2

Major Motor Levels

Level	Muscle Group	Action	Deep Tendon Reflex
C5	Deltoid, internal and external shoulder rotators	Abduction of shoulder, external rotation of arm	Biceps jerk (C5-C6)
C6	Biceps, brachialis, wrist extensors	Flexion of elbow	Brachioradialis jerk (C5-C6)
C7	Triceps, wrist flexors	Extension of elbow, wrist	Triceps jerk
C8	Intrinsic hand muscles	Abduction, adduction of fingers	
L2-L3	Iliopsoas	Hip flexion	
L4	Quadriceps	Extension of knee	Knee jerk
L5	Tibialis anterior and posterior, extensor hallucis longus	Dorsiflexion of foot and big toe	
S1	Gastrocnemius	Plantar flexion of foot	Ankle jerk
S4-S5	Anal sphincter	Voluntary contraction of anal sphincter	

(Reproduced from McGuire RA Jr: Physical examination in spinal trauma, in Levine AM, Eismont FJ, Garfin SR, Zigler JE, eds: *Spine Trauma*. Philadelphia, PA, WB Saunders, 1998, pp 16-27.)

FIGURE 7

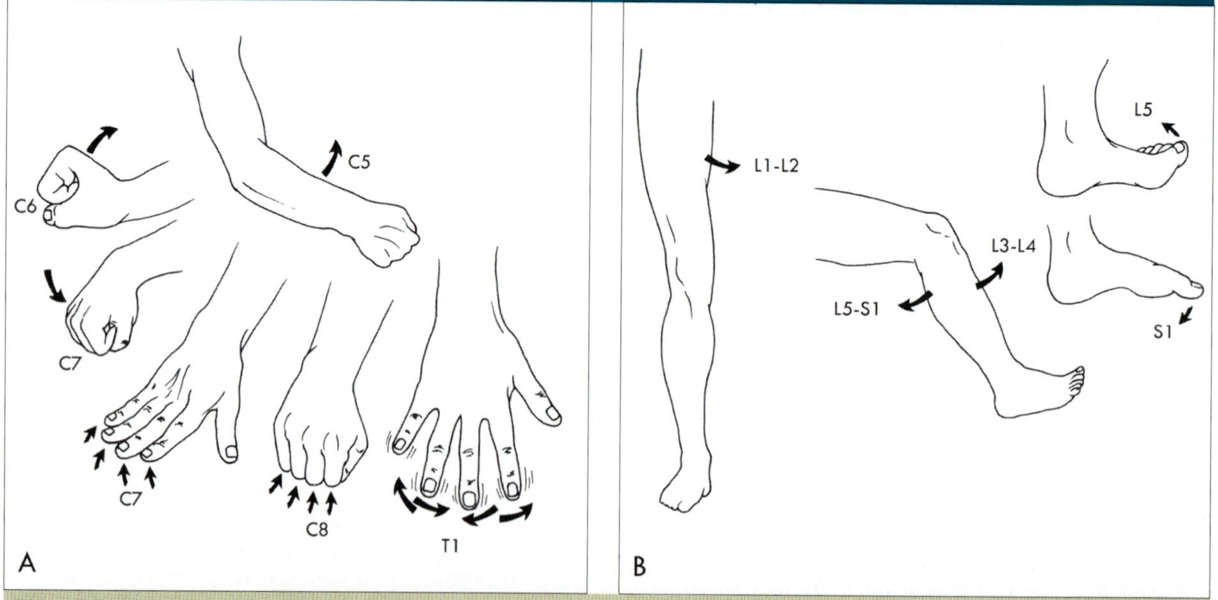

Figure 7 A, An examination of the upper extremities must include, at a minimum, the muscle groups that are designated by their respective nerve root innervation. These are C5, elbow flexion; C6, wrist extension; C7, finger extension; C8, finger flexion; and T1, finger abduction. The strength (0 to 5) should be listed on the time-oriented flow sheet. **B,** An examination of the lower extremities needs to include at least these muscle groups, designated by their respective nerve root innervation: L1-L2, hip abductors; L3-L4, knee extension; L5-S1, knee flexion; L5, great toe extension; and S1, great toe flexion. (Reproduced with permission from Keenen TL, Benson DR: Initial evaluation of the spine-injured patient, in Browner BD, Jupiter JB, Levine AM, Trafton PG, eds: *Skeletal Trauma: Fractures, Dislocations, Ligamentous Injuries*. Philadelphia, PA, WB Saunders, 1992, p 594.)

functions are tested by evaluating the hip flexors and adductors. L4 function includes the quadriceps femoris and anterior tibialis. L5 innervates the hip abductors, the hamstring group, and the extensor hallucis longus. S1 function includes hip extensors, the lateral hamstring group, and the gastrocnemius-soleus complex.

Sacral roots 2 through 5 innervate the sphincter muscles of the perineum.

TABLE 3

Segmental Reflexes

Reflex	Level
Biceps	C6
Triceps	C7
Upper abdominal[a]	T7-T10
Lower abdominal[a]	T10-T12
Cremasteric[a]	L1
Knee jerk	L4
Posterior tibial jerk	L5
Ankle jerk	S1
Bulbocavernosus[b]	S2-S4
Anocutaneous[c]	S4-S5

[a]Cutaneous reflexes: decreased in upper motor neuron lesion.
[b]Contraction of bulbocavernosus muscle after stimulation of the glans penis.
[c]Contraction of anal sphincter after stroking perineal skin.

Reflex Evaluation

Following thorough muscle evaluation, the reflex function is tested (**Table 3**, **Figure 8**). The biceps reflex evaluates C5 function, the brachioradialis evaluates C6 function, and C7 function is evaluated by the triceps reflex.

Important reflex functions in the lower extremity include the L4 quadriceps reflex or knee jerk and the Achilles reflex, which evaluates S1 function (**Table 2**). These deep tendon reflexes are mediated through the anterior horn cells. The cerebral cortex provides an inhibitory function to prevent excessive reaction with stimulation.

The abdominal and cremasteric reflexes are upper motor neuron tests requiring superficial stimulation of the skin, and are mediated through the central nervous system.

The superficial abdominal reflex is elicited by stroking the skin in each quadrant of the abdomen

FIGURE 8

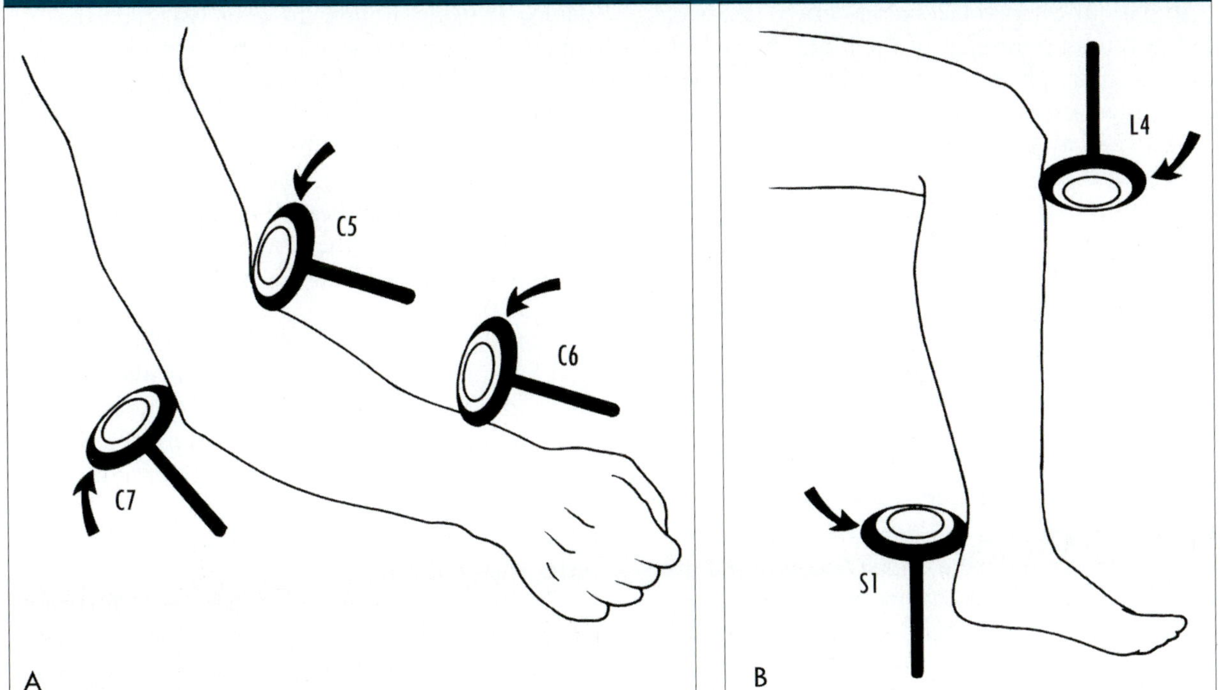

Figure 8 Stretch reflexes and nerve roots of origin. (Reproduced with permission from Keenen TL, Benson DR: Initial evaluation of the spine-injured patient, in Browner BD, Jupiter JB, Levine AM, Trafton PG, eds: *Skeletal Trauma: Fractures, Dislocations, Ligamentous Injuries*. Philadelphia, PA, WB Saunders, 1992, p 596.)

FIGURE 9

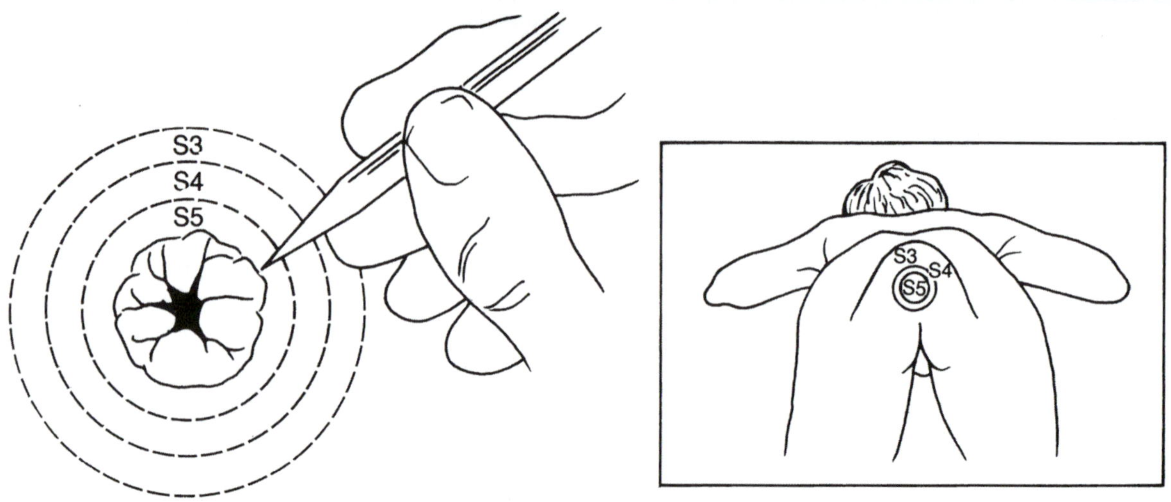

Figure 9 The anal reflex, indicative of S2-S4 function, can be elicited by stimulating the perianal skin. (Reproduced with permission from Keenen TL, Benson DR: Initial evaluation of the spine-injured patient, in Browner BD, Jupiter JB, Levine AM, Trafton PG, eds: *Skeletal Trauma: Fractures, Dislocations, Ligamentous Injuries*. Philadelphia, PA, WB Saunders, 1992, p 591.)

and noting whether the umbilicus is drawn toward the stimulated area. Innervation of the abdominal musculature is segmental, with the upper musculature innervated by T7-T10 and the lower muscles by T10-L1. Asymmetric loss of this reflex may indicate a localized lower motor neuron lesion.

In men, the superficial cremasteric reflex is elicited by stroking the skin of the inner thigh. If the reflex is intact, the scrotum will be drawn upward by the cremasteric muscle. Absence of the reflex is indicative of an upper motor lesion, while unilateral absence suggests a lower motor lesion. Anatomically, this reflex involves T12-L2.

Loss of superficial reflexes combined with an exaggerated response of the deep tendon reflexes due to loss of cerebral inhibition is indicative of an upper motor neuron lesion.

Pathologic reflexes are significant because their presence indicates an upper motor neuron lesion. The Babinski reflex is elicited by stroking the skin on the lateral plantar surface with a sharp object such as a key or the handle of the reflex hammer. A positive response is indicated by extension of the great toe with flexion and splaying of the remaining toes. The Oppenheim reflex is tested in a similar manner. The fingernail or hammer handle is drawn along the tibial crest, with a positive test eliciting the same response as Babinski.

The presence or absence of sacral sparing is extremely important when evaluating spinal trauma patients. It provides an indicator for prognosis of functional recovery in persons sustaining a spinal cord injury.

Sphincter function is tested by inserting a gloved finger into the rectum and noting the resting tone. The patient is then asked to voluntarily contract the sphincter. Sensation to light touch and pin prick are also evaluated at this time. Stimulating the skin around the anus will elicit the superficial anal reflex and contraction of the anal sphincter. This reflex involves S2-S4 function (**Figure 9**).

During the rectal examination in males, the position of the prostate should be noted. An abnormal position is indicative of a possible urethral tear and warrants further evaluation. Special care must be observed during Foley catheter insertion in these patients.

Persons with a neurologic deficit must be evaluated for spinal shock. Spinal shock is often present within 24 hours of injury and is due to edema from the initial trauma to surrounding neural tissues. These patients will exhibit loss of motor, sensory, and reflex function. At this point, determination of whether the neurologic deficit is complete or partial cannot be made.

The bulbocavernosus reflex becomes important in evaluation of the spinal injury patient because its presence signifies resolution of spinal shock and allows the determination of a complete or incomplete neurologic deficit. This reflex is elicited by stimulation of the penis or clitoris by digital pressure or traction on the Foley catheter,

FIGURE 10

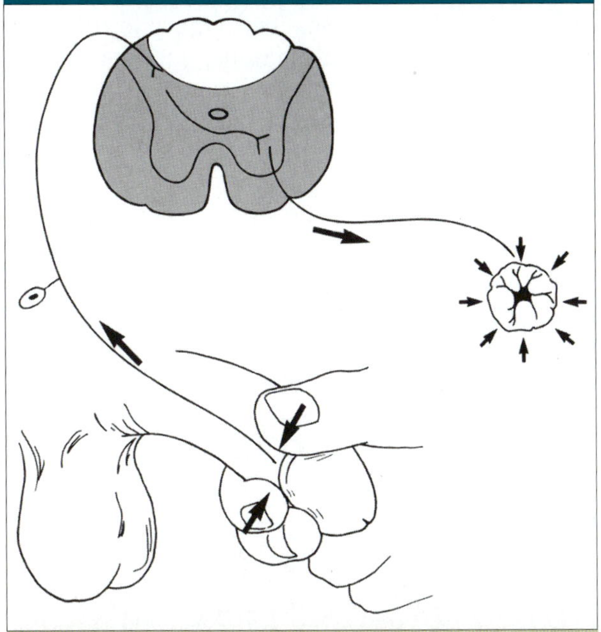

Figure 10 The bulbocavernosus reflex returns following resolution of spinal shock. Once this reflex returns, the determination of whether a neurologic lesion is complete or incomplete can be made. (Reproduced with permission from Keenen TL, Benson DR: Initial evaluation of the spine-injured patient, in Browner BD, Jupiter JB, Levine AM, Trafton PG, eds: *Skeletal Trauma: Fractures, Dislocations, Ligamentous Injuries*. Philadelphia, PA, WB Saunders, 1992, p 588.)

while a gloved finger in the rectum notes a resulting contraction of the anal sphincter. A positive response indicates resolution of spinal shock with return of the reflex arc (**Figure 10**).

Summary

Spinal trauma patients must be visually inspected for external evidence that may indicate severe internal injury. Bony palpation must then be performed, noting associated soft-tissue defects and malalignment. Motor and sensory evaluation requires careful attention to detail and thorough documentation to provide accurate neurologic status.

References

1. Bohlman HH: Acute fractures and dislocations of the cervical spine: An analysis of three hundred hospitalized patients and review of the literature. *J Bone Joint Surg Am* 1979;61(8):1119-1142.
2. Bradford DS, McBride GG: Surgical management of thoracolumbar spine fractures with incomplete neurologic deficits. *Clin Orthop Relat Res* 1987; 218:201-216.
3. Davis D, Bohlman H, Walker AE, Fisher R, Robinson R: The pathological findings in fatal craniospinal injuries. *J Neurosurg* 1971;34(5): 603-613.
4. Vaccaro AR, An HS, Lin S, Sun S, Balderston RA, Cotler JM: Noncontiguous injuries of the spine. *J Spinal Disord* 1992;5(3):320-329.
5. Pieretti-Vanmarcke R, Velmahos GC, Nance ML, et al: Clinical clearance of the cervical spine in blunt trauma patients younger than 3 years: A multi-center study of the American Association for the Surgery of Trauma. *J Trauma* 2009;67(3): 543-550.
6. Gertzbein SD, Court-Brown CM: Flexion-distraction injuries of the lumbar spine: Mechanisms of injury and classification. *Clin Orthop Relat Res* 1988;227:52-60.
7. McGuire RA, Neville S, Green BA, Watts C: Spinal instability and the log-rolling maneuver. *J Trauma* 1987;27(5):525-531.
8. Frankel HL, Hancock DO, Hyslop G, et al: The value of postural reduction in the initial management of closed injuries of the spine with paraplegia and tetraplegia: I. *Paraplegia* 1969;7(3): 179-192.
9. Stauffer ES: Neurologic recovery following injuries to the cervical spinal cord and nerve roots. *Spine (Phila Pa 1976)* 1984;9(5):532-534.
10. Stauffer ES: Spinal cord injury syndromes. *Semin Spine Surg* 1991;3(1):87-90.

Appendix 1 Standard Neurological Classification of Spinal Cord Injury

The American Spinal Injury Association (ASIA) neurologic classification of spinal cord injury form is composed of several sections. The initial portion grades five muscle groups in the upper and five muscle groups in the lower extremities on a score of 1 to 5. A composite motor score is then obtained. The next section grades light touch and pin prick. The final section on the first page specifies the level of injury.

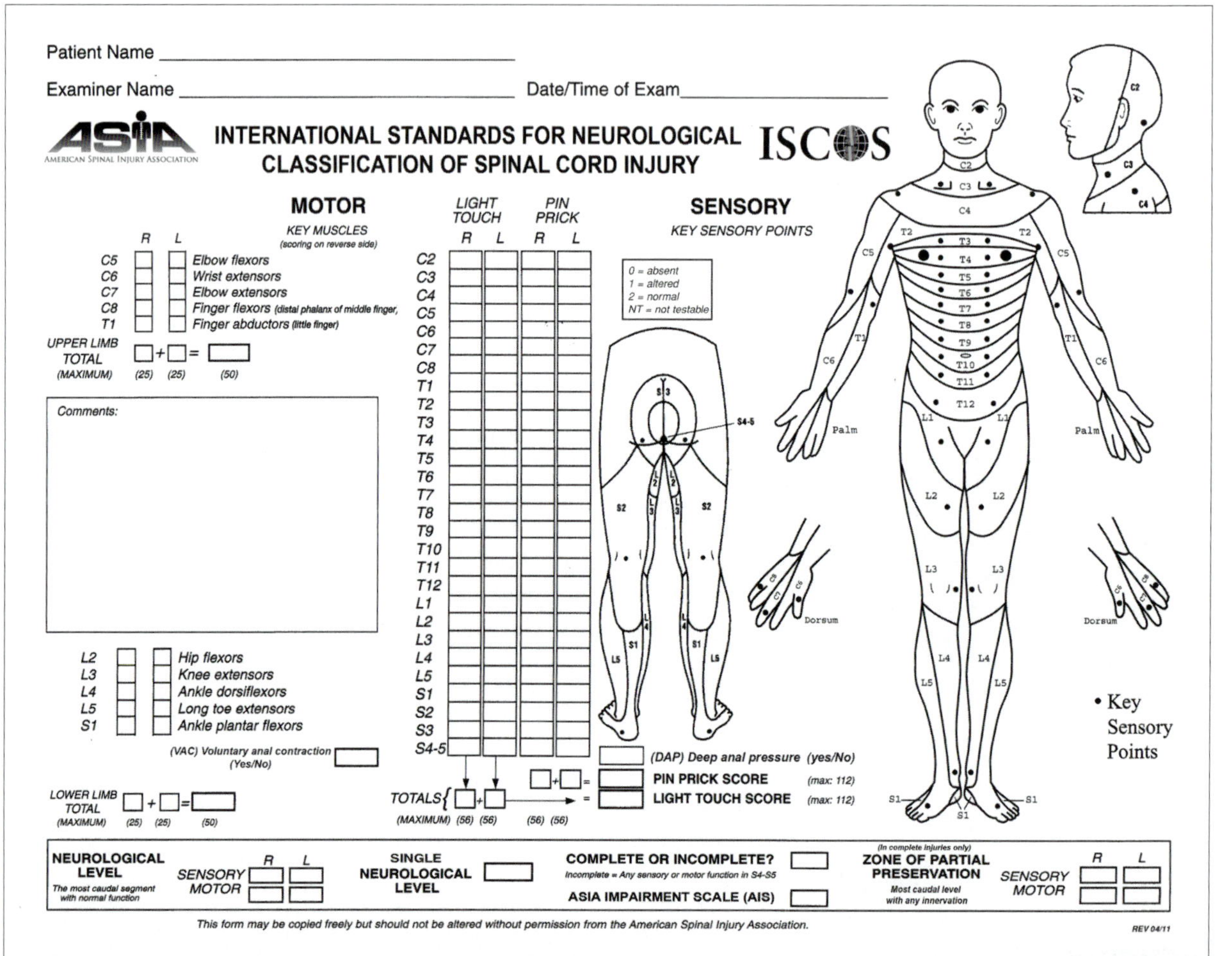

Patient Name ______________________

Examiner Name ______________________ Date/Time of Exam ______________________

ASIA AMERICAN SPINAL INJURY ASSOCIATION

INTERNATIONAL STANDARDS FOR NEUROLOGICAL CLASSIFICATION OF SPINAL CORD INJURY

ISCOS

MOTOR

KEY MUSCLES (scoring on reverse side)

	R	L	
C5			Elbow flexors
C6			Wrist extensors
C7			Elbow extensors
C8			Finger flexors (distal phalanx of middle finger)
T1			Finger abductors (little finger)
UPPER LIMB TOTAL (MAXIMUM)	(25)	(25)	(50)

Comments:

	R	L	
L2			Hip flexors
L3			Knee extensors
L4			Ankle dorsiflexors
L5			Long toe extensors
S1			Ankle plantar flexors
LOWER LIMB TOTAL (MAXIMUM)	(25)	(25)	(50)

(VAC) Voluntary anal contraction (Yes/No)

SENSORY

KEY SENSORY POINTS

	LIGHT TOUCH R	LIGHT TOUCH L	PIN PRICK R	PIN PRICK L
C2				
C3				
C4				
C5				
C6				
C7				
C8				
T1				
T2				
T3				
T4				
T5				
T6				
T7				
T8				
T9				
T10				
T11				
T12				
L1				
L2				
L3				
L4				
L5				
S1				
S2				
S3				
S4-5				
TOTALS (MAXIMUM)	(56)	(56)	(56)	(56)

0 = absent
1 = altered
2 = normal
NT = not testable

(DAP) Deep anal pressure (yes/No)

PIN PRICK SCORE (max: 112)

LIGHT TOUCH SCORE (max: 112)

• Key Sensory Points

NEUROLOGICAL LEVEL (The most caudal segment with normal function)	R	L
SENSORY		
MOTOR		

SINGLE NEUROLOGICAL LEVEL

COMPLETE OR INCOMPLETE? (Incomplete = Any sensory or motor function in S4-S5)

ASIA IMPAIRMENT SCALE (AIS)

ZONE OF PARTIAL PRESERVATION (In complete injuries only) (Most caudal level with any innervation)	R	L
SENSORY		
MOTOR		

This form may be copied freely but should not be altered without permission from the American Spinal Injury Association.

REV 04/11

COPY FREELY – DO NOT CHANGE. American Spinal Injury Association.

Muscle Function Grading

0 = total paralysis

1 = palpable or visible contraction

2 = active movement, full range of motion (ROM) with gravity eliminated

3 = active movement, full ROM against gravity

4 = active movement, full ROM against gravity and moderate resistance in a muscle specific position.

5 = (normal) active movement, full ROM against gravity and full resistance in a muscle specific position expected from an otherwise unimpaired peson.

5* = (normal) active movement, full ROM against gravity and sufficient resistance to be considered normal if identified inhibiting factors (i.e. pain, disuse) were not present.

NT = not testable (i.e. due to immobilization, severe pain such that the patient cannot be graded, amputation of limb, or contracture of >50% of the range of motion).

ASIA Impairment (AIS) Scale

☐ **A = Complete.** No sensory or motor function is preserved in the sacral segments S4-S5.

☐ **B = Sensory Incomplete.** Sensory but not motor function is preserved below the neurological level and includes the sacral segments S4-S5 (light touch, pin prick at S4-S5: or deep anal pressure (DAP)), AND no motor function is preserved more than three levels below the motor level on either side of the body.

☐ **C = Motor Incomplete.** Motor function is preserved below the neurological level**, and more than half of key muscle functions below the single neurological level of injury (NLI) have a muscle grade less than 3 (Grades 0-2).

☐ **D = Motor Incomplete.** Motor function is preserved below the neurological level**, and at least half (half or more) of key muscle functions below the NLI have a muscle grade ≥ 3.

☐ **E = Normal.** If sensation and motor function as tested with the ISNCSCI are graded as normal in all segments, and the patient had prior deficits, then the AIS grade is E. Someone without an initial SCI does not receive an AIS grade.

**For an individual to receive a grade of C or D, i.e. motor incomplete status, they must have either (1) voluntary anal sphincter contraction or (2) sacral sensory sparing with sparing of motor function more than three levels below the motor level for that side of the body. The Standards at this time allows even non-key muscle function more than 3 levels below the motor level to be used in determining motor incomplete status (AIS B versus C).

NOTE: When assessing the extent of motor sparing below the level for distinguishing between AIS B and C, the ***motor level*** on each side is used; whereas to differentiate between AIS C and D (based on proportion of key muscle functions with strength grade 3 or greater) the ***single neurological level*** is used.

Steps in Classification

The following order is recommended in determining the classification of individuals with SCI.

1. Determine sensory levels for right and left sides.
2. Determine motor levels for right and left sides.
   Note: in regions where there is no myotome to test, the motor level is presumed to be the same as the sensory level, if testable motor function above that level is also normal.
3. Determine the single neurological level.
   This is the lowest segment where motor and sensory function is normal on both sides, and is the most cephalad of the sensory and motor levels determined in steps 1 and 2.
4. Determine whether the injury is Complete or Incomplete. (i.e. absence or presence of sacral sparing)
   If voluntary anal contraction = **No** *AND all S4-5 sensory scores =* **0** *AND deep anal pressure =* **No,** *then injury is COMPLETE. Otherwise, injury is incomplete.*
5. Determine ASIA Impairment Scale (AIS) Grade:

Is injury Complete? If **YES,** AIS=A and can record ZPP (lowest dermatome or myotome on each side with some preservation)

NO ↓

Is injury motor Incomplete? If **NO,** AIS=B (Yes=voluntary anal contraction OR motor function more than three levels below the motor level on a given side, if the patient has sensory incomplete classification)

YES ↓

Are at least half of the key muscles below the single neurological level graded 3 or better?

NO ↓ AIS=C

YES ↓ AIS=D

If sensation and motor function is normal in all segments, AIS=E

Note: AIS E is used in follow-up testing when an individual with a documented SCI has recovered normal function. If at initial testing no deficits are found, the individual is neurologically intact; the ASIA Impairment Scale does not apply.

CHAPTER 4
Emergency Management of Spine Injuries in Polytrauma Patients

Sohail K. Mirza, MD, MPH

Introduction

Polytrauma patients require coordinated and comprehensive care. The evaluation and treatment of patients with multiple injuries requires continuous respect for potential interactions among their multisystem injuries, multidisciplinary physicians, and the parallel multiple diagnostic and therapeutic interventions to which these patients are subjected. Survival hinges on expeditious, appropriate treatment within minutes and hours of injury. By necessity, things must move quickly, both at the trauma scene and in the emergency department. Safety concerns are paramount because the risk of iatrogenic harm—from inadequate evaluation or treatment, from unnecessary delay due to overevaluation, or from focused interventions that do not consider other potential injuries—is high. Often, patients and their families are unable to participate in fully informed consent, further increasing the burden of responsibility on the trauma surgeons. Compared to patients with isolated injuries, these concerns greatly increase the challenge of managing polytrauma patients.

This chapter reviews the principles of spine evaluation and treatment in polytrauma patients. All trauma patients need to be fully evaluated for potential spinal injury and protected against neurologic deterioration during the process. In awake trauma patients, even mild reports of pain or posterior midline tenderness should not be dismissed without thorough assessment, including imaging studies. Obtunded patients require imaging of the entire spine. Unclear findings on imaging studies should be assumed to reflect acute injury until further evaluation clarifies their significance. Persistent symptoms despite normal initial imaging studies may require further evaluation with dynamic imaging studies such as upright radiographs or flexion-extension radiographs. Unresolved findings from the patient's history, physical examination, and imaging studies should be clearly and efficiently communicated to all providers involved in the patient's care.

Although initial evaluation and management of patients with a spinal injury is complex, priorities of Advanced Trauma Life Support (ATLS) still apply.[1] Evaluation of the spine follows emergent lifesaving interventions. Critical decisions must be made at each step as more diagnostic information about the patient becomes available. At each stage of evaluation, the patient's further triage is influenced by the injuries identified, both for management of any spinal injury and for management of other injuries. Identification of spinal injuries takes precedence over management of other orthopaedic injuries.

Field Care of Polytrauma Patients

All trauma victims are at risk for spinal injury. Field management of trauma patients requires keeping the possibility of an unstable spine injury in the forefront of active concerns until spinal injury is definitively excluded or treated. Treatment priorities are preserving life, limb, and function. The spine must be protected as treatment priorities are sequentially addressed.

Protection and provisional immobilization of the spine at the accident scene are crucial for minimizing risk of additional neurologic injury.[2] The head and neck should be aligned with the long axis of the trunk and immobilized in this position.[3] Immobilization with cervical collar, sandbags, tape, and spine board is superior to immobilization with a collar alone.[4] Log-rolling still allows motion at the spinal injury site.[5] A scoop-stretcher is a useful adjunct to the spine board.[5] Neutral flexion-extension head and neck alignment is optimal during prehospital transport of cervical spine injury patients.[2] Cervical extension narrows the spinal canal more than flexion and should be avoided.[6] The relatively larger head of pediatric patients should be accommodated by elevating the trunk on padding or using a special pediatric spine board containing a cutout for the occiput.[7]

Neither Dr. Mirza nor any immediate family member has received anything of value from or owns stock in a commercial company or institution related directly or indirectly to the subject of this chapter.

TABLE 1

Steroid Administration Protocol from the National Acute Spinal Cord Injury Studies[12-14]

1. Methylprednisolone bolus 30 mb/kg, then infusion 5.4 mg/kg/h
2. Infusion for 24 h if bolus given within 3 h of injury
3. Infusion for 48 h if bolus given within 3 to 8 h after injury
4. No benefit if methylprednisolone started more than 8 h after injury
5. No benefit with naloxone
6. No benefit with tirilazad

For injured athletes, motorcycle riders, and cyclists, helmet and shoulder gear should be left in position until personnel trained in safe removal techniques are available.[8-11]

Neurologic assessment in the field helps prioritize treatment interventions. The patient's spontaneous physical movements and function should be documented in field records and conveyed to subsequent care providers in the emergency department. These observations are extremely valuable in determining the possibility and sometimes the extent of neurologic injury. Subjective symptoms in alert and communicative patients are an important part of neurologic assessment. Awake patients should be specifically questioned about neck pain, back pain, numbness, and weakness.

If a spinal cord injury (SCI) is suspected, steroids should be started in the field according to the dosage and administration schedule established by three publications from the National Acute Spinal Cord Injury Study (NASCIS) (**Table 1**).[12-14]

Pharmacologic Intervention for Spinal Cord Injury

The secondary events following acute SCI are complex and interdependent.[15] The physiologic responses to spinal injury are both reparative and also contributory to additional injury. Interrupting the cascade of events has the potential to change either aspect of this balance. It is difficult to identify optimal interruption points for preserving neurologic function. Many experimental treatments have investigated agents that block specific pathophysiologic events occurring after the injury, but only a few of these interventions have shown sufficient promise in laboratory studies to prompt clinical trials.[12-14,16-19]

Methylprednisolone has a protective effect against neurologic injury in animal experiments when given in high doses before SCI.[20,21] NASCIS consisted of three large-scale randomized clinical trials investigating methylprednisolone in acute SCI patients.[12-14] The first trial compared low-dose to high-dose methylprednisolone administered within 48 hours of injury.[12] The results showed no difference in outcome and increased infection rate in the high-dose group. The second trial compared methylprednisolone (30 mg/kg loading dose + 5.4 mg/kg/h × 23 h) to naloxone and placebo.[13] Statistically significant improvement in motor and sensory scores in both complete and incomplete injuries occurred in the group given methylprednisolone.[13] The magnitude of effect was small: neurologic change score (improvement in motor score) was 16.0 in the treatment group and 11.2 in the control group, with a P value of 0.03 for the difference.[13] The pin-prick score change was 11.4 in the treatment group and 6.6 in the control group ($P = 0.02$).[13] These differences reached statistical significance but may have little or no clinical significance.

A critical component missing from the acute SCI trials is measurement of function and quality of life. NASCIS showed sufficient neurologic improvement with early administration of high-dose methylprednisolone to establish this intervention as the standard for acute care of SCI patients.[12-14,22-25] Even though statistically significant, the additional improvement of 3 to 7 points in motor score may have limited functional benefit. However, the NASCIS trials demonstrate that large-scale, high-quality randomized clinical trials are methodologically feasible, even when addressing difficult problems such as the emergent management of SCI. This achievement is as significant for future work in this area as the clinical impact of the study findings. Until other such large-scale trials demonstrate otherwise, the intervention established by these studies should be a component of acute care of SCI patients.

Other pharmacologic treatments have not shown sufficient promise in the clinical trial stage to become relevant for clinical usage.[16-18] One category of candidate drugs is lazaroids. Lazaroids are 21-aminosteroid free-radical scavengers.[26] One such agent, 21-aminosteroid U-74006F, inhibits membrane peroxidation. Another category of potential drugs for SCI treatment is gangliosides. Gangliosides are large glycolipid molecules found on the outer surface of most cell membranes.[16] They are highly concentrated in neural tissues and are involved in immunologic processes, binding, transport, and nerve cytogenesis. Gangliosides have a trophic effect on nerve cells. They can stimulate dendritic outgrowth and neuronal recovery. Further research is needed to understand their application to SCI treatment.

Emergency Department Care

Polytrauma patients require serial monitoring to diagnose conditions not readily apparent early in their clinical course. Spinal evaluation takes place concurrently with resuscitative measures. Spine assessment within the first few minutes of arrival in the emergency department includes: (1) determination of potential neurologic function by report from field personnel, direct observation, or initial gross examination during primary survey; (2) identification of severely unstable injuries such as fracture-dislocations or distractive injuries on trauma radiographs that include lateral cervical spine and AP chest radiographs; and (3) evaluation for potential neurogenic shock.

SCI can complicate resuscitation measures.[1] Loss of vasoconstrictive sympathetic control of the peripheral vasculature can accentuate hemodynamic effects of hemorrhage. Nonetheless, recognizing neurogenic shock as distinct from hemorrhagic shock is critical for safe initial resuscitation of a trauma patient.[1,27] Treatment of neurogenic shock is pharmacologic intervention to augment peripheral vascular tone. It may be essential for effective resuscitation. Fluid overload from excessive fluid volume administration, typical in treatment of hemorrhagic shock, can result in pulmonary edema in the setting of neurogenic shock. SCI itself increases the risk for multiple organ system failure in polytrauma patients.[28] Presence of severe hemodynamic parameter abnormalities in the initial phases of resuscitation is associated with a poor prognosis for neurologic recovery.[27] Normal hemodynamics, on the other hand, do not predict neurologic recovery.

Awake and cooperative patients require a complete neurologic examination. The American Spinal Injury Association (ASIA) has identified essential minimal elements of neurologic assessment recommended for all patients with a spinal injury.[29] The essential elements of neurologic function are strength assessment of 5 specific muscles in each limb and pin-prick discrimination assessment at 28 specific sensory locations on each side of the body. On each side of the body, five muscles representing the segments of the cervical cord and five muscles representing segments of the lumbar cord are scored on a 5-point muscle grading scale. The sum of all 20 muscles yields a total motor score for each patient, with a maximum possible score of 100 points for patients with no weakness. For the 28 sensory dermatomes on each side of the body, sensory levels are scored on a scale from 0 to 2 points, yielding a maximum possible pin-prick score of 112 points for a patient with normal sensation. The findings on pin-prick testing of the sacral segments distinguish complete from incomplete SCI. The motor strength and pin-prick testing allow designation of neurologic injury levels for each patient: sensory level, motor level, and neurologic level.

The spine examination includes inspection of the spine and palpation of the spine. The patient must be rolled on his or her side using a log-rolling maneuver. The patient's head and neck are supported by one assistant and the patient's trunk is supported by two to three other assistants. The head and trunk are then rolled by the assistants in unison while the examiner inspects and palpates the spine to check for hemorrhage, abrasion, laceration, malalignment, or palpable gap in the spinous processes. The chest and abdomen are also examined for contusions or abrasions suggestive of a seatbelt or steering wheel–induced injury.

Categorization of a specific patient into a specific division of a classification requires some arbitration and judgment. The variability in these judgments sometimes makes comparisons across different research studies difficult. Older SCI literature contains variable interpretations of many commonly used terms. The ASIA definitions have provided guidance for use of these terms with greater clarity. These specific definitions will hopefully improve categorization of SCI patients in scientific communication and allow more meaningful analyses of collective experience.

According to ASIA definitions, neurologic injury level is the most caudal segment of the spinal cord with normal motor and sensory function on both sides: right and left sensation, and right and left motor function.[29] Complete injury is defined by the absence of sensory and motor function in the lowest sacral segment.[29,30] Sacral sensation refers to sensation at the anal mucocutaneous junction and deep anal sensation. Sacral motor function is voluntary anal sphincter contraction on digital examination. Incomplete injuries have partial preservation of sensory or motor function in the lowest sacral segment. Distal motor function and sacral sparing are important for prognosis.[31] Sacral sensory sparing predicts improvement in neurologic status.[32] Sacral pin-prick sensation carries an improved prognosis of regaining the ability to walk even in patients who are initially motor complete.[33]

Neurologic assessment in unresponsive patients includes a review of observations recorded in the field and during transport by emergency medical system personnel. The neurologic assessment must be systematically reevaluated and updated over time in unresponsive patients until a complete examination is possible. If imaging studies identify a spinal column injury, the treating spine surgeon makes a decision regarding the urgency of assessing the integrity of neurologic structures. In an unresponsive patient, the options for this assessment are serial neurologic examinations, MRI to identify structural neural tissue disruption, and sensory- or motor-evoked potentials to assess function in neural pathways.

Spinal Shock

Spinal shock is a term that accounts for much confusion in the assessment of SCI patients.[34] Spinal shock refers to depressed spinal reflexes caudal to SCI.[34] First, spinal shock should be distinguished from neurogenic shock, which refers to hypotension associated with loss of peripheral vascular resistance in SCI. Second, the etiology and significance of spinal shock are unclear.[34] The confusion surrounding the concept of spinal shock is responsible for some complacency in the management of SCI patients during the initial few hours following injury, the time interval in whcih intervention may have the most beneficial results. Spinal shock may involve immediate depolarization of the axonal membranes from kinetic energy of the injury.[35] Spinal shock disrupts all cord function distal to injury, including reflexes. Early effects of spinal shock typically resolve within 24 hours of injury.[35] During this early period, prognosis for neural recovery is not reliable. Examinations conducted between 72 hours and 1 week after injury more accurately predict functional muscle recovery than examinations conducted within the first 24 hours.[36] For this reason, distinction of SCI as complete or incomplete on the basis of clinical examination is problematic.[30] Suspending treatment interventions until resolution of this depressed reflex state may waste a time-sensitive opportunity to possibly arrest or diminish the secondary injury process in patients with SCI.[37]

Lessons for Spine Evaluation of Polytrauma Patients

Following is a list of principles for spine care in busy trauma centers. Each lesson represents an occurrence avoidable through clinical knowledge, pattern recognition, and attention to detail.

(1) Use all available sources of information to assess neurologic status, including the report from the paramedics on conditions at the scene.
(2) Give steroids if SCI is a possibility.
(3) Review all outside records.
(4) Convey his or her level of concern regarding spine stability and SCI to other providers.
(5) DO NOT base decisions on inadequate radiographs.
(6) Review all radiographs that show the vertebral column, including AP chest and pelvis radiographics. Sometimes these will show a fracture-dislocation.
(7) Perform a neurologic examination at the earliest opportunity.
(8) Record the neurologic examination clearly and record the time of neurologic assessment.
(9) Check sacral sparing.
(10) DO NOT attribute neurologic findings to confounding factors without first excluding spine injury.
(11) Consider incomplete SCI for unusual neurologic deficits.
(12) Investigate discrepancy between neurologic level on examination and radiographic level of injury.
(13) Identify and treat neurogenic shock.
(14) DO NOT delay closed reduction of a dislocated cervical spine in a patient with tetraplegia to obtain nonessential diagnostic tests.
(15) DO NOT apply traction pins in a patient with a skull fracture without consulting a neurosurgeon and reviewing the head CT scan.
(16) Make sure traction tongs, weights, or pins are MRI-compatible.
(17) DO NOT apply traction for distraction injuries.
(18) Recognize associated injury patterns.
(19) Look for additional levels of spinal injury.
(20) Remove the backboard within 2 hours.

Imaging the Spine in Polytrauma Patients

Every trauma patient requires a definitive decision regarding the presence or absence of spine injury. At a minimum, the assessment requires a careful review of history and a thorough examination. Usually, spine evaluation involves serial clinical examinations and review of cervical spine radiographs. Radiographic studies are the primary modalities for identifying a spine injury in unresponsive patients. Spine injury precautions are maintained until a spine injury is identified and treated, or until assessment is complete and injury excluded.

Assessment of the cervical spine is an essential component of the ATLS protocol.[1] The prevalence of cervical spine injury is 1% to 5% in screening radiographs.[38] Standard imaging (three views of the cervical spine and CT as necessary) has a false-negative rate of 0.1%. The radiographic evaluation should be correlated to clinical considerations. The aim of careful decision making is to have a zero missed-injury rate. Ideally, no patient undergoing care for trauma should deteriorate from a missed spine injury. To meet this goal, immediate recognition of a potential cervical spine injury is essential.[38] Patients with missed fractures can develop neurologic deterioration.[38,39]

Plain Radiography

Plain radiographs, if they show complete lateral visualization of the cervical spine and include an open-mouth view, are fairly sensitive in identifying cervical spine fractures. The risk of missing significant fractures is less than 1% of patients.[38] The sensitivity of the lateral radiograph alone is 83% and specificity is 97%.[40] The addition of open-mouth and AP views increases the sensitivity to approximately 100%.[40]

Cervical radiographs in a trauma patient are performed with the patient supine and secure on a backboard. The patient is not moved to position for the various views; rather, the x-ray beam and film position is adjusted to provide the desired image perspective. Opinions for the minimum number of plain radiographs necessary in trauma patients range from 0 to 7 (AP, lateral, open mouth, oblique, flexion-extension).[41]

Accurate interpretation of the lateral cervical spine radiograph is essential, yet this interpretation may frequently be erroneous because of the stressed circumstances in an emergency setting and inexperience of the individuals responsible for initial care. The first step in interpreting radiographs is to make sure they are of adequate quality for the intended purpose. Lower quality films significantly increase error rates.[42] Adequate lateral cervical spine radiographs require clear visualization of the spine from the occiput to the first thoracic vertebra. If the lower cervical spine is not visualized on a lateral radiograph, a swimmer's lateral view or a CT scan can be used to visualize this region.

The AP cervical spine view is less helpful in diagnosing acute injuries. A change in alignment of the uncovertebral joints and spinous processes can indicate an acute injury. The open-mouth view is essential for excluding C1 arch or C2 odontoid process fractures. Tomograms or a CT scan may be necessary to substitute for the open-mouth view in unresponsive patients. Oblique views can identify injuries of the facet joints, pedicles, and lateral masses, particularly at the cervicothoracic junction. For this reason, oblique views in the trauma setting can increase the diagnostic sensitivity of cervical radiographs.

Most spine injuries occur at the junctions—craniocervical, cervicothoracic, and thoracolumbar. They are often the most difficult to see on standard radiographs. Among these injuries, the most serious and most frequently missed is craniocervical dissociation. Harris measurements based on the distance between the dens and the basion are probably the simplest and most reliable measurements for identifying craniocervical dissociation.[43] Suspicion of injury and careful scrutiny of radiographs minimizes errors of missed injury.[44]

In patients with cervical tenderness and normal plain radiographs, flexion-extension views can identify occult cervical ligamentous injury. Flexion-extension views in the acute setting of an emergency department, however, can be nondiagnostic or even dangerous. Patients in acute pain may have limited mobility related to muscle spasm, limiting cervical spine motion on dynamic views. Unsupervised or forceful flexion in a patient with an occult ligamentous injury may precipitate a neurologic injury. When necessary, flexion-extension radiographs should be performed in alert patients, under supervision, and with voluntary unassisted positioning by the patient.

Interpretation of radiographs has limitations. Knowledge of anatomy and clinical experience are important for accurate interpretation of radiographs.[45] Landmarks for measurements can be difficult to identify. A systematic approach to reading cervical radiographs can help reduce the

TABLE 2

Risk Factors for Cervical Spine Fracture

Risk Factor	Odds Ratio
Focal neurologic deficit	34
Unconsciousness	14
Skull fracture	10
Brain/coma contusion	9
Intercranial hematoma	8
Loss of consciousness (transient)	5
Scalp laceration	5
High-speed motor vehicle crash	4
Pedestrian struck by a car	4
Mandible fracture	2
Facial fracture	2
Facial laceration	2
Intoxication	2
Motorcycle crash	1.4
Fall	1
Low-speed motor vehicle crash	0.8
Use of seatbelts	0.4
Struck by a blunt object	0.1

(Reproduced with permission from Blackmore CC, Emerson SS, Mann FA, et al: Cervical spine imaging in patients with trauma: Determination of fracture risk to optimize use. *Radiology* 1999;211:759-765; Blackmore CC, Ramsey SD, Mann FA, et al: Cervical spine screening with CT in trauma patients: A cost-effectiveness analysis. *Radiology* 1999;212:117-125.)

chances of missing an important injury. Alignment of the cervical vertebrae is assessed by examining longitudinal lines along vertebral bodies, lamina, and spinous processes. Examining alignment of the lamina in the upper cervical vertebrae is particularly helpful in excluding injuries of the craniocervical junction in both children and adults.

The prevertebral soft tissues can be useful as an indicator of swelling from acute hemorrhage. Increased thickness and altered contour of the pharyngeal tissue anterior to C2 (ie, convexity instead of concavity caudal to the C1 anterior arch) suggest acute craniocervical injury. The prevertebral soft-tissue shadow thickness, however, becomes unreliable in the presence of oropharyngeal tubes. Also, soft-tissue swelling can occur without bony injury and, conversely, bony injuries can occur without significant soft-tissue swelling.[46] Prevertebral soft-tissue widening resolves to normal after 2 weeks in 50% of patients, and in 3 weeks in 90%.[42]

Computed Tomography

CT and MRI may be useful together in determining the presence and extent of spinal column injury.[47] MRI is superior in demonstrating spinal cord pathology and intervertebral disk herniation. CT is superior to MRI in demonstrating osseous injury. However, injuries purely localized to the transverse plane, such as odontoid fracture, can be missed on axial CT images. For these types of injuries, direct coronal CT can provide superior demonstration of skeletal features in the upper cervical spine.[48]

Magnetic Resonance Imaging

MRI is useful for imaging soft tissues and bone. MRI can show edema and hemorrhage associated with acute SCI. Increased cord signal and parenchymal cord hemorrhage indicate a poor prognosis for neurologic recovery.[49,50] MRI is particularly useful for assessing the craniocervical junction. Edema in the occipitocervical facet capsules and basicervical ligaments or acute cervicomedullary angulation suggests craniocervical injury.[51]

MRI provides noninvasive assessment of the vertebral artery blood flow in cervical trauma, which can be frequently disrupted in cervical spine injuries.[52] Magnetic resonance angiograms are abnormal in 24% of patients.[52] However, MRI diagnosis of patients who have cervical trauma involving the transverse foramen may not be functionally significant.[53]

Clearing the Spine in Polytrauma Patients

A cleared spine in a patient implies that diligent spine evaluation is complete and the patient does not have a spinal injury requiring treatment. All trauma patients are at risk for spinal injury. Two percent to 4.6% of patients with blunt trauma have cervical spine injuries.[54] Systematic evaluation is necessary to achieve the goal of zero missed injuries. Physician judgment, based on mechanism of injury and physical examination, is not accurate in predicting cervical spine fractures.[55] Clinical prediction rules, based on measurement of patient characteristics, injury circumstances, and findings on initial evaluation associated with spinal injuries, however, allow efficient utilization of radiologic imaging studies (**Table 2**).[56]

The necessary elements for a complete spine evaluation are: (1) history to assess for high-risk events and high-risk factors, (2) physical examination to check for physical signs of spinal injury or neurologic deficit, and (3) imaging studies based on an initial evaluation.

Radiographs are not necessary for patients who are alert, are not intoxicated, have an isolated blunt trauma, and have no neck tenderness on physical examination.[57] This estimate of "no false negatives" is based on small numbers of patients with fractures.[57] Each patient with a diagnosed fracture had at least one of the following four characteristics: midline neck tenderness, evidence of intoxication, abnormal level of alertness, or several painful injuries elsewhere.[57] Absence of these clinical findings suggests absence of a spine fracture but does not definitively exclude injury.

Spine injury may be difficult to recognize in a patient with altered mental status.[58,59] Cervical spine injury should be considered in an unconscious patient even in the absence of a definitive history of trauma.[60] The clinical presentation of an unrecognized SCI, such as a neurologic deficit from a cervical injury, may be misinterpreted as a stroke.[61] In obtunded patients found unresponsive at the scene, SCI may present as a medical emergency, such as hydronephrosis, renal failure, or pyelonephritis associated with urinary retention. Focused emergency department evaluation of medical symptoms may overlook the underlying SCI.[62] SCI without an associated cervical fracture or dislocation, advanced age, unusual or changing neurologic deficits, intoxication, and psychiatric problems all contribute to clinical confusion and missed diagnoses of cervical fracture.[63] Neurologic problems in these patients may be attributed to hysteria or intoxication or other disease.

The process of clearing the thoracolumbar spine is similar to that for clearing the cervical spine. Only AP and lateral view radiographs are necessary. Patients with a clear mental status, no back pain, and no other major injuries do not need radiographs of the spine to exclude a spinal fracture.[64] The spine in these patients can be safely cleared by a physical examination alone.

Any physician with adequate training and experience can clear the spine.[65] A specific examination of the patient and careful review of appropriate and adequate quality radiographs is mandatory. Serial examinations and imaging may be necessary to diagnose subtle or occult injuries.

Sequence of Imaging Studies

Clearing the spine frequently requires considerable time, and one study reported a median time of 15 hours.[66] Patients frequently need emergent care and transport before the spine can be cleared. Emergent procedures such as intubation, anesthesia, and abdominal or chest surgery may be safely performed with appropriate precaution in an incompletely evaluated cervical spine.

Plain radiographic studies remain the primary diagnostic spine evaluation. Findings on plain radiographs direct the approach to further diagnostic investigation.[67] Addition of CT adds information in approximately half of all cases.

Obtaining a lateral cervical spine radiograph is part of the initial evaluation of a trauma patient.[1] Obtaining AP chest, AP pelvis, and lateral cervical spine radiographs does not interfere with the urgent management of multiply injured patients during resuscitation and these three images provide crucial information that facilitates resuscitation. They are standard "trauma series" in trauma centers. Additional emergent spinal imaging is only necessary if these initial views demonstrate a spine injury or if the primary survey examination suggests a neurologic deficit. Otherwise, further spinal imaging can follow resuscitation and hemodynamic stabilization.

Complete cervical spine views are obtained once the patient is medically stable. These views are open-mouth, AP, and, in some institutions, right and left oblique radiographs. Alternatively, trauma patients at high risk for cervical spine injury can be screened for a cervical injury with a rapid-sequence helical CT scan.[68] Patients with an incomplete SCI may require emergent MRI to identify the source of cord injury, particularly if radiographs and CT do not show vertebral column injury.[69]

MRI (or CT myelography) should be performed urgently in any patient with an increasing neurologic deficit. One report of six cases with neurologic deterioration during treatment identified an unrecognized disk herniation as a potential contributor to neurologic worsening after reduction of cervical spine facet dislocation.[70] Many surgeons cite this report as justification for obtaining prereduction MRI in patients with SCI associated with cervical facet dislocation. This report, however, acknowledged other treatment-related complications that may have also contributed to deterioration in three of the six reported cases.

Most traumatic disk injuries associated with cervical fractures and dislocations do not adversely influence neurologic function.[71] In patients with

SCI associated with cervical spine fracture-dislocations, the most urgent priority after life-saving measures is mechanical decompression of the spinal cord. This is most expeditiously and efficiently achieved through closed reduction. Rapid closed reduction is successful and safe.[71] Waiting for MRI in this setting should not delay closed reduction. Other interventions or other diagnostic tests for non-life-threatening conditions also should not supersede the priority for closed reduction.

Postreduction MRI, however, is useful to look for disk extrusion if neurologic deterioration occurs or for planning the approach for definitive surgical treatment.[72]

Neurologically intact patients with a cervical spine dislocation do not have the time urgency of SCI. In these patients, MRI may be obtained before reduction without adversely influencing outcome. The disk at the level of dislocation is usually abnormal on these images.[73] These disk abnormalities have been advanced as an argument for decompressing the damaged disk before reduction. However, induction of anesthesia and positioning for surgery are difficult in a patient with a dislocated cervical spine. Furthermore, performing an open reduction through an anterior approach is a difficult task. The improved stability gained from reduction, safer induction of anesthetic, and the option of posterior surgery are arguments for attempted closed reduction even in neurologically intact patients.

Patients with pain and normal initial imaging studies may have an occult fracture. Also, fractures may be difficult to see if patients have severe degenerative disease, osteoporosis, or ankylosis of the spine. In these settings, MRI or a technetium bone scan can facilitate diagnosis of occult fractures.[74,75]

Unresponsive Patients

Spine clearance is a difficult issue in obtunded patients with high-energy injury mechanisms. In these patients, spine clearance is sometimes deferred until the patient is examinable. However, that may be a very long time in some patients. Meanwhile, these patients may develop complications associated with external bracing and mobility restrictions imposed by spine precautions. If good-quality radiographs are completely normal, the spine may be cleared without further imaging or examination. When radiographs are abnormal, from severe degeneration, osteoporosis, diffuse idiopathic skeletal hyperostosis, or ankylosing spondylitis, then additional imaging such as CT, MRI, or bone scan may be needed to rule out injury of the cervical spine. Thoracic and lumbar injuries can be reliably excluded by radiographs alone.

Patient Care Until the Spine is Cleared

Neurologic deterioration after admission occurs in 5% of spine injury patients.[76] An identifiable specific management event is associated with 86% of these deteriorations.[76] Unstable spinal injury should be assumed and the patient protected.[77] Log-rolling does not keep the spine immobile, and unstable injuries should be stabilized immediately when the patient's medical condition permits doing so safely.[5] Extremely combative patients with closed head injury may require intubation and chemical paralysis to protect against neurologic injury from an associated spine fracture. Fiberoptic intubation or a laryngeal mask airway should be considered in the management of patients with cervical spine instability.[78]

Missed Injuries

The rate for missed or delayed diagnosis of cervical spine injury at trauma centers is from < 1% to 4.9%.[38,76,79] Most patients with missed injuries or delayed diagnosis (71%) suffer no adverse consequences.[79] However, patients who deteriorate from a missed injury (29%) may have severe complications.[79] These complications range from death (20%), to quadriplegia (40%) or other new neurologic deficits (40%).[79]

The most frequent reasons for missed injuries are inadequate radiographs (44%) and misinterpretation of adequate-quality radiographs (47%). More frequently than cervical injuries, the diagnosis of thoracolumbar fractures may be delayed in 11% of trauma patients and missed in 5.5%.[64] A thoracolumbar fracture may not be recognized, despite reports of back pain by 66% of these patients during their initial evaluation.[64] Patients with a missed thoracolumbar fracture who do not report back pain have either altered mental status or other major associated injuries.[64] Back pain in trauma patients should be taken seriously and evaluated thoroughly, and the evaluation should include radiographic imaging.

Recommendations for Spine Clearance in Polytrauma Patients

At the regional Level 1 trauma center with which I am affiliated (Dartmouth-Hitchcock Medical Center), we obtain cervical radiographs in all trauma patients brought to the emergency department by ambulance. The cervical spine series consists of five views (lateral, AP, open mouth, right oblique, and left oblique). We obtain a CT scan of the craniocervical junction in intubated patients. We obtain thoracic and lumbar spine radiographs in patients sustaining high-energy injuries. If the patient requires a head CT, we concurrently obtain a screening CT of the cervical spine visualizing the skull to T4. We obtain high-resolution CT of all regions of the spine suspected or recognized to have an injury.

We obtain MRI of the cervical spine in all patients with cervical-level SCI. We also undertake MRI in patients who require surgical stabilization of cervical injuries, even if neurologically intact; it is helpful in deciding between anterior versus posterior surgical approach. We obtain MRI scans after closed reduction in patients with a cervical level neurologic deficit to assess residual neural compression and assess urgency of surgery. MRI of the cervical, thoracic, or lumbar spine is also useful in assessing extent of ligament injury if identification of a clear soft-tissue disruption will alter management. We also obtain MRI of the entire spine in patients with ankylosing spondylitis or other conditions that make radiograph interpretation uncertain.

Dartmouth Spine Clearance Policy

At Dartmouth-Hitchcock Medical Center, the only regional Level 1 trauma center for New Hampshire, we evaluate and treat a substantial number of spine fractures every year. In trying to balance pragmatic management of a high volume of trauma patients against the goal of not missing any unstable spine injuries, Dartmouth has developed the following seven-item spine clearance policy:

(1) Evaluation for spinal injury will be initiated in the emergency department on every trauma patient with clinical evidence or mechanism of injury consistent with spinal trauma.

(2) Spine clearance is established by clinical examination and radiologic studies as indicated by the primary treating service.

(3) Diagnosis or exclusion of spinal injury is determined by the patient's primary service in consultation with radiology. The spine service is consulted for identified injuries or other special considerations.

(4) Spine clearance assessment should be finalized as soon as is clinically feasible (goal is within 24 hours of admission). Spinal evaluation should be expedited to either exclude injury and remove activity restrictions or diagnose injury and institute provisional treatment.

(5) Portable upright cervical spine radiographs may be attempted once in the intensive care unit. If quality is not adequate, subsequent films must be done in the radiology department. If quality is still not adequate, a cervical spine CT may be obtained.

(6) Each time spine precautions are changed, a physician on the primary treating service will revise the spine clearance orders and write a progress note in the patient's medical record reflecting the relevant evaluation and change in activity status.

(7) Once spinal injury has been excluded, it is the responsibility of the patient's primary service to complete the relevant section of the spine clearance order form.

Spine clearance is clarified in a flow diagram (**Figure 1**). This policy was implemented in 2009.

Principles of Treatment of Spine Trauma

The goal of treatment of every spinal injury is restoration of the patient to maximal possible function. In trauma care, this goal implies protecting all patients until a spinal injury is definitively excluded, or identified and treated. Also, caring for a trauma patient requires that associated injuries be expeditiously identified and appropriately treated. For patients sustaining a spinal column injury, the treatment focus is protecting uninjured neural tissues, maximizing recovery of injured neural tissues, and optimizing conditions for the musculoskeletal portions of the spinal column to heal in a satisfactory position.

Treatment Priorities

Errors in the initial care of spinal injury patients can have catastrophic or fatal outcomes.[79] Minimizing these errors requires management of spinal injury patients at highly specialized centers with experienced personnel.[80] SCI patients in particular benefit from early transfer to a trauma center with an SCI unit.[81] Early referral to an SCI center improves patient survival and neurologic recovery.[82]

Management of spinal injuries in multiply injured patients requires concerted activity of a trauma team. Experienced field personnel, emergency department physicians, general surgeons, orthopaedic surgeons, neurosurgeons, radiologists, anesthesiologists, physiatrists, and nursing

FIGURE 1

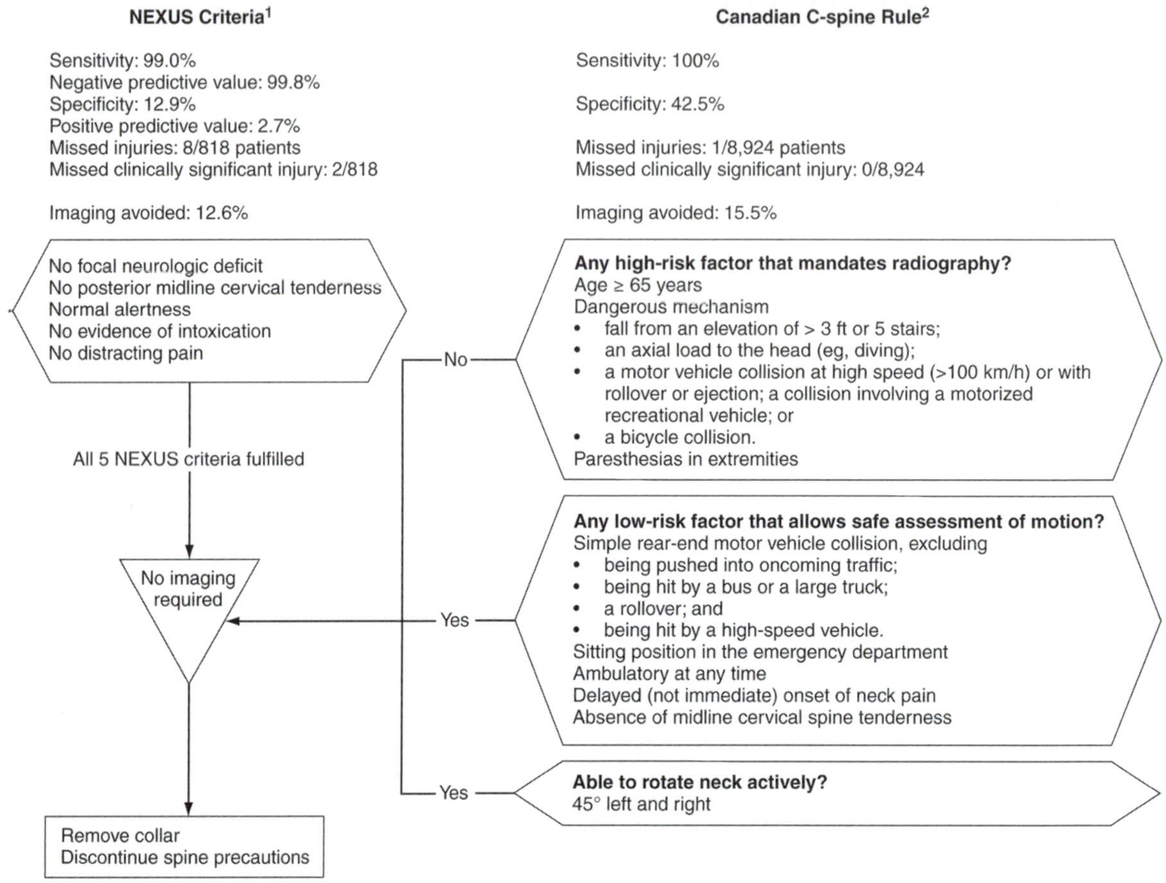

[1] Hoffman JR, Mower WR, Wolfson AB, Todd KH, Zucker MI: Validity of a set of clinical criteria to rule out injury to the cervical spine in patients with blunt trauma: National Emergency X-Radiography Utilization Study Group. *N Engl J Med* 2000;343(2):94-99.

[2] Stiell IG, Wells GA, Vandemheen KL, et al: The Canadian C-spine rule for radiography in alert and stable trauma patients. *JAMA* 2001;286:1841-1848.

A

Figure 1 A, Cervical spine imaging of alert and stable trauma patients.

personnel are integral members of this team. The overriding general principle in effective care of trauma patients is early involvement by appropriate members of this team. Physicians ultimately assuming the long-term management of trauma patients, frequently orthopaedic surgeons and physiatrists, are particularly critical in directing optimal initial care.[83]

Provisional Stabilization

Trauma patients require protection and immobilization of the spine until spinal injury is definitively excluded or treated. This general principle has specific patient-care implications commonly referred to as "spine precautions" (**Table 3**). All trauma patients should be maintained in the supine position at strict bed rest with the bed flat, transfers with a spine board, and frequent logrolling for decubitus ulcer prophylaxis. Alternatively, patients may be placed in a rotating frame for improved pulmonary mechanics and skin care.

Cervical injuries associated with malalignment require skull traction, except for injuries with complete ligamentous disruption, which are usually indicated by distraction between vertebrae on imaging studies. Distraction injuries are the most unstable spine injuries. Skull traction in these patients will lead to catastrophic neurologic deterioration or even fatal vascular injury. Patients with distraction injuries are best immobilized with sandbags and tape or a halo apparatus. Even when immobilized in the halo apparatus, these patients should be maintained in strict bed rest with full spine precautions until definitive surgical stabilization.

FIGURE 1

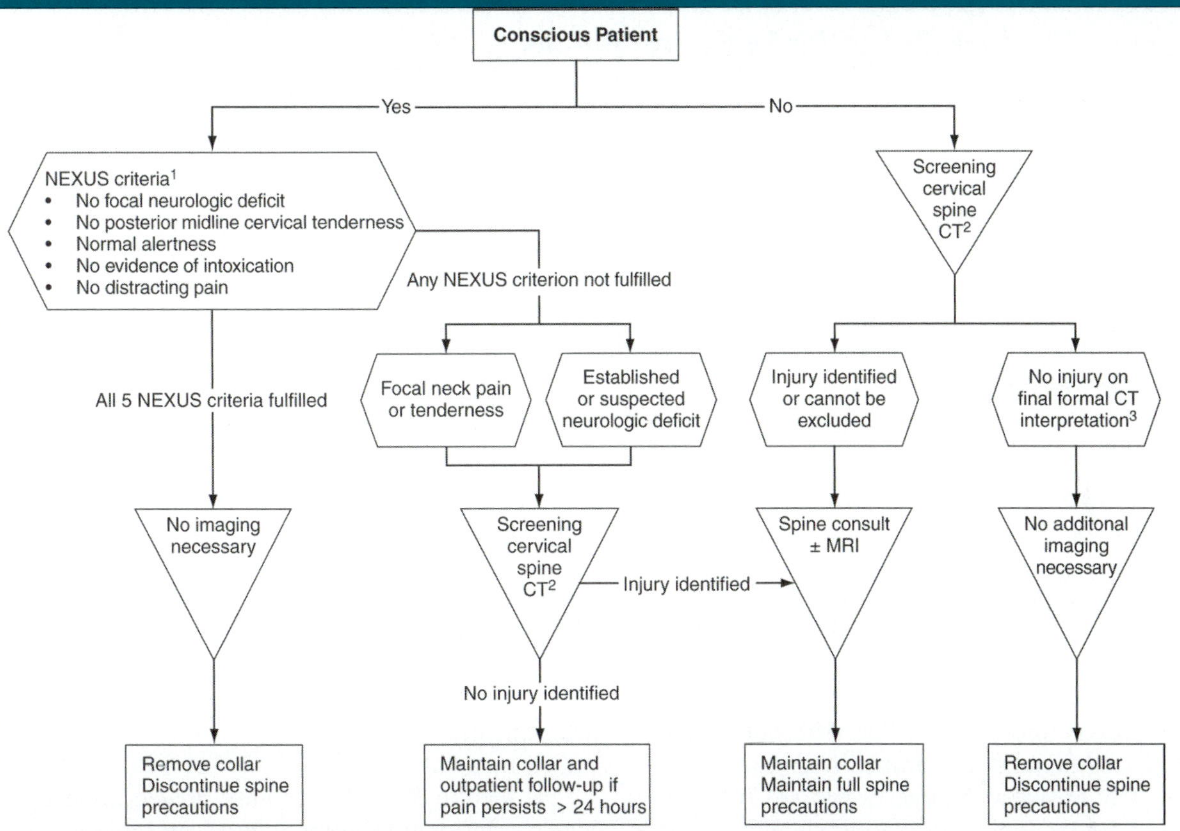

[1] The original NEXUS publication chose not to define the criteria with specific detail to allow broad interpretation and discretionary application by practicing physicians (Hoffman JR, Mower WR, Wolfson AB, Todd KH, Zucker MI: Validity of a set of clinical criteria to rule out injury to the cervical spine in patients with blunt trauma: National Emergency X-Radiography Utilization Study Group. *N Engl J Med* 2000;343(2):94-99.) From a subsequent publication, the following definitions specified the NEXUS criteria (Stiell IG, Clement CM, McKnight RD, et al: The Canadian C-spine rule versus the NEXUS low-risk criteria in patients with trauma. *N Engl J Med* 2003;349:2510-2518.):

- A focal neurologic deficit is any focal neurologic finding on motor or sensory examination.
- Midline posterior bony cervical-spine tenderness is present if the patient reports pain on palpation of the posterior midline neck from the nuchal ridge to the prominence of the first thoracic vertebra, or if the patient evinces pain with direct palpation of any cervical spinous process.
- Patients should be considered intoxicated if they have either of the following: a recent history provided by the patient or an observer of intoxication or intoxicating ingestion, or evidence of intoxication on physical examination such as an odor of alcohol, slurred speech, ataxia, dysmetria, or other cerebellar findings, or any behavior consistent with intoxication. Patients may also be considered intoxicated if tests of bodily secretions are positive for alcohol or drugs that effect the level of alertness.
- An altered level of alertness can include any of the following: a Glasgow Coma Scale score of 14 or less; disorientation to person, place, time, or events; an inability to remember three objects in five minutes; a delayed or inappropriate response to external stimuli; or other findings.
- No precise definition of a painful distracting injury is possible. This category includes any condition thought by the clinician to be producing pain sufficient to distract the patient from a second (neck) injury. Such injuries may include, but are not limited to, any long-bone fracture; a visceral injury requiring surgical consultation, a large laceration, degloving injury, or crush injury, large burns; or any other injury causing acute functional impairment. Physicians may also classify any injury as distracting if it is thought to have the potential to impair the patient's ability to appreciate other injuries.

[2] Screening CT: multichannel, helical CT scan without contrast from occiput to T4 with sagittal and coronal reformatted images.

[3] Formal interpretation may be provided by radiologist, orthopaedic surgeon, or neurosurgeon.

B

Figure 1 B, Dartmouth spine trauma imaging protocol (2009).

Traction pins for skull tongs are placed in line with the external auditory meatus, 1 cm above the pinna. Carbon fiber tongs with titanium pins should be used initially to permit subsequent MRI evaluation if necessary. Carbon-fiber tongs, however, grip the skull less strongly than steel tongs. Pins in carbon-fiber tongs may pull out of the skull with traction weights above 80 lb. Pins in steel tongs can withstand traction up to 140 lb.[84] On occasion, if closed reduction in a cervical injury requires weights greater than 80 lb, carbon fiber-tongs may be exchanged for steel tongs before applying high weights.

Emergent Closed Reduction

Closed reduction in cervical spine injuries is safe and effective.[71,85] Successful reduction may require weights as high as 140 lb.[86] In young patients with no osteoporosis, traction weight up to 70% of body weight is generally safe, provided steel tongs are used and pins are properly placed.[86] Cervical traction at weights greater than 80 lb should not

TABLE 3

Sample Physician Orders for Spine Precautions

Full spine precautions
• Bed rest only.
• Patient requires a hard cervical collar at all times (collar may not be removed to manipulate the neck).
• Log roll every 2 h unless patient is in a rotating bed.
• Log roll with manual cervical stabilization when moving patient.
• DO NOT place patient on any therapeutic air mattress.
• Bed surface must remain flat at all times (reverse Trendelenberg if head requires elevation).
Partial spine precautions
• Bed rest only, patient may not sit or stand except for upright films.
• Bed surface flat (reverse Trendelenberg for head elevation) unless otherwise specified below.
• Patient must wear spine immobilization device indicated below at all times.
• Do not place patient on therapeutic air mattress (risk for patient removal of stabilization device) unless otherwise specified below. Patient requires care when moving, but log-rolling (with cervical stabilization if cervical spine not cleared) not necessary when spine immobilization device in place.

be applied to most carbon-fiber MRI-compatible tongs; traditional steel Gardner-Wells tongs are less likely to slip with larger weights.[84] Traction should not be applied in injuries showing distraction of the spinal column.

Decompression of SCI should proceed as soon as the patient can medically tolerate it.[87] The window of opportunity for maximal neurologic improvement through decompression may be as short as the first few hours following SCI.[87-90] SCI patients may have an excellent capacity for spinal cord recovery regardless of initial presentation.[91] Reduction within the first few hours of injury may lead to dramatic improvement in neurologic status. Reduction within 2 hours of injury has been reported to reverse tetraplegia.[92]

In cervical injuries, closed reduction can achieve decompression. Emergent attempted closed reduction is the treatment of choice for alert, cooperative patients with acute SCI from a cervical spine dislocation.[93] In these patients, MRI is not necessary before reduction and should not delay reduction.[94] Reduction in an unconscious or unexaminable patient should be preceded by an MRI scan. In this situation, the presence of a herniated disk may be treated with surgical decompression before reduction.[69,70]

Patients with highly unstable injuries, such as craniocervical dissociation or a cervical injury that shows distraction at the injured segment, require compression for reduction, not further traction. Compression across the cervical spine can be applied by a halo vest.[95]

Reduction improves stability, preventing neurologic deterioration in the interval preceding definitive treatment.[96] Closed reduction can also improve neurologic recovery.[97] Although case reports have described neurologic deterioration during reduction,[98] larger series of closed reductions have not observed neurologic deterioration.[71,99] In fact, one case in one of these series was of a patient with a large disk herniation seen on a prereduction MRI scan that resolved with closed reduction.[71] Closed reduction also decreases the need for more complicated surgical procedures later.[100]

Timing of Spine Surgery in Polytrauma Patients

Early surgical stabilization of spinal fractures in the multiply injured patient is advocated under the premise that it reduces complications associated with prolonged recumbency. This philosophy is based largely on information available on treatment of long-bone fractures in polytrauma patients. Initial stabilization of long-bone fractures in the multiply injured patient is now the preferred course of action in many trauma centers. Prior to the 1970s, however, the prevailing thought was that early fracture manipulation and stabilization predisposed patients to respiratory deterioration and the accepted treatment was to treat these injuries in balanced skeletal traction during the acute period and delay long-bone stabilization until 10 days to 2 weeks after injury.[101,102] In the late 1960s, the wisdom of this approach began to be questioned and in the early 1970s, the first reports of early long-bone stabilization in multiply injured patients from centers in Europe were published.[103,104] These studies demonstrated that early mobilization decreases complications of recumbency, including respiratory deterioration, thromboembolic disease, skin breakdown, and disuse atrophy. Early surgical stabilization of long-bone fractures, however, continued to be viewed with skepticism by many in the United States.[105]

Treatment in the United States began to change in 1985, when Johnson et al,[106] in a retrospective study of 132 patients, reported a decreased incidence of pulmonary complications in polytrauma patients with femur fractures who underwent surgical stabilization less than 48 hours after injury. Bone et al[107] subsequently conducted a randomized, prospective study of 178 patients with femur fractures treated either within 24 hours (early stabilization) or after 48 hours (late stabilization). Patients who underwent late stabilization were found to have a higher incidence of pulmonary complications (pneumonia and adult respiratory distress syndrome) and had longer intensive care unit stays and hospitalizations. Several other studies confirmed the benefits of early long-bone stabilization, and its role in the care of the multiply injured patient became widely accepted.

Contrary to timing of long-bone stabilization, timing of spinal stabilization in polytrauma patients remains controversial, both with regard to its effect on neurologic outcome as well as prevention of complications of recumbency. Although some studies show an apparent improvement in neurologic status with surgical decompression and stabilization,[108-111] others show no improvement.[112-114] Three studies have examined acute complications of surgically treated spine fractures, but they involved evaluation of a limited number of risk factors, lacked multivariate analysis, and did not examine respiratory failure as a specific outcome.[115-117] With lack of convincing evidence of neurologic improvement or respiratory benefit with surgical treatment, many surgeons advocate delayed surgery, and others argue that aggressive nonsurgical care with rotating beds and deep venous thrombosis prophylaxis yields similar or even lower morbidity than surgical stabilization.[101,102,118]

The utility of surgical stabilization of spinal column injuries is controversial, both with regard to its effect on neurologic outcome as well as prevention of complications of recumbent immobilization. In a Harborview Medical Center (Seattle, WA) review of a large cohort of patients treated surgically for thoracolumbar fractures, surgical stabilization more than 2 days after admission was an independent risk factor by multivariate analysis for the development of respiratory deterioration.[119] This is clinically relevant because the other independent risk factors identified in this study (Glasgow coma score [GCS], injury severity score [ISS], age, and blunt chest trauma) were all determined by the circumstances of the traumatic injury. Although they influence patient management decisions, they are not directly alterable per se. Specifically, GCS ≤ 12 indicates the presence of at least a moderate head injury and ISS > 25 correlates in general terms with more severe trauma. These indices possibly also correlate with the magnitude of the inflammatory process that may mediate acute lung injury and acute respiratory distress syndrome both in multiply injured patients[29,30] and in patients with isolated traumatic brain injury.[31] Other studies have also shown ISS, GCS, age, and blunt chest trauma to be risk factors for respiratory failure in the multiply injured patient.[120-123]

A major limitation of this study was potentially confounding by indication: the same circumstances that delayed surgery may also be associated with respiratory failure. The patients in this study were all treated at a single institution where the prevailing philosophy of spine surgeons is to surgically stabilize severe spine injuries as soon as the patient is cleared by the trauma team to be medically safe for major surgery. The patients who had surgery late were likely to be medically unstable for earlier surgery, possibly due to pulmonary problems. Pearson correlation analysis did demonstrate a modest correlation between surgical delay, abbreviated injury scale (AIS) head, and GCS, and lesser correlations with blunt lung injury, age, ISS, AIS chest and Charlson score. In spite of these correlations, however, surgical delay was found to be an independent risk factor for respiratory failure by multivariate analysis in the cohort matched by propensity analysis.

This study had several other weaknesses. Limitations of the data collected in the trauma registry prevented examination of other risk factors known to influence risk of respiratory failue, such as history of blood transfusion, hypotension on initial presentation, and metabolic acidosis. In addition, clinical interventions such as the use of a rotating bed, could not be evaluated. The authors share concerns many have expressed about data quality in a large administrative database for an outcomes study. Some variables such as age, ISS, trauma diagnoses, and surgical procedures by their nature are mandatory entries into the trauma registry and therefore their documentation is presumably more accurate than entries such as comorbidities and smoking history that are not directly trauma-related. Medical comorbidities and smoking history were, most likely, largely underreported in the database, limiting the authors' analysis of these variables. In particular, the 6.1% incidence of smoking identified in the cohort of patients is far below the current prevalence of smokers in the US population, 22.5%.[124]

Because surgical timing may be in part under the control of the treating physician, Harborview Medical Center developed a clinical prediction rule to determine the relative risk of delaying surgical stabilization in patients with unstable thoracolumbar spine fractures. This algorithm predicts an increase in the relative risk for respiratory failure with surgical delay of greater than 2 days, ranging from a threefold increase for patients less than 35 years of age with minimal head trauma and no blunt chest injury to an over 36-fold increase for patients greater than 35 years of age with significant head trauma and a blunt chest injury.

The question of when to perform stabilization surgery in polytrauma patients with spine fractures would be most clearly answered by a randomized trial. However, given the suspicion that delayed surgery may increase risk of respiratory failure, as observed in this study[119] and also noted in long-bone fracture surgery, a clinical trial that requires intentionally delaying surgery through a random treatment allocation will likely involve difficult ethical choices. As an alternative, more reliable estimates of the risk associated with delayed surgery may be obtained from observational studies that compare patients of surgeons or trauma centers with differing opinions regarding timing of surgery.

Within the limitations of this study, the authors observed a lower rate of respiratory failure in multiply injured patients undergoing surgical stabilization of thoracic and lumbar spine fractures within 2 days of admission.[119] Optimal care of these patients is complex and requires coordinated, multidisciplinary care with many health-care providers, including critical care specialists, general surgeons, anesthesiologists, neurosurgeons, orthopaedic surgeons, nurses, and therapists. Surgical timing in this context must be determined for each patient on an individual basis.

Early surgical stabilization of spine fractures was supported by Schlegel et al[117] in a retrospective analysis of 138 patients who underwent surgical fixation of unstable spinal fractures. For thoracolumbar fractures (98 patients), they found that patients with ISS ≥ 18 had significantly greater collective morbidity if surgery was done after 72 hours. Unfortunately, due to the small number of patients in the study, the significance of surgical timing on individual morbidities such as pulmonary complications, urinary tract infections, and thromboembolic disease could not be determined. Furthermore, the effects of other specific traumatic injuries such as chest and head injuries were not considered.[117]

Croce et al[115] subsequently published additional supportive evidence in an analysis of 291 patients with spinal column injuries who underwent surgical fixation. Several variables were collected including age, ISS, GCS, blood transfusion, chest AIS, neurologic injury, and spinal level of injury. Individuals who underwent surgical fixation within 3 days of injury had a significantly lower incidence of pneumonia and shorter intensive care unit stays. Subgroup analysis of patients with thoracic spine fractures demonstrated that those who underwent surgical fixation in less than 3 days had a lower incidence of pneumonia and fewer ventilator, intensive care unit, and hospital days compared with patients who underwent surgical fixation after 3 days. Statistical analysis consisted of multiple univariate comparisons between patients grouped by injury characteristics. Multivariate analysis was not done.[115]

In 2005, Kerwin et al[116] published a similar analysis of 299 patients with spinal column fractures requiring surgical stabilization. Univariate analysis was done comparing patients who underwent surgical stabilization within 72 hours of injury with those delayed more than 72 hours. Again, multivariate analysis was not done. The early surgery group was found to have a shorter hospital length of stay. No difference in incidence of pneumonia or mortality could be demonstrated between the two groups. Subgroup analysis of the patients with thoracic spine injuries and associated SCI showed this group to have a lower incidence of pneumonia if surgery was performed within 72 hours of injury. The authors concluded that a rigid protocol to determine timing of surgical fixation is not justified and treatment should be individualized to the medical condition of each patient.

The largest study supporting nonsurgical care with rotating beds was a retrospective study of 235 patients by Rechtine et al.[125] A group of 117 patients were treated with surgical stabilization and another 118 underwent nonsurgical care on a kinetic bed for 6 weeks. There were no significant differences in the incidence of decubitus, thromboembolic disease, or mortality between the two groups. The surgical group had an 8% incidence of deep infection. Only three patients in each group developed pneumonia. Forty-eight percent of patients treated surgically and 56% of patients treated nonsurgically were noted to have multiple system injuries, although this was not quantitated by ISS or other means and the severity and extent of their other injuries was not reported.[125]

Conclusions

Optimal management of polytrauma patients requires repeat assessments and continuous communication among the treating physicians. Spinal evaluation is an integral part of the initial care. Early spinal decompression and stabilization is preferred for patients with SCI.

References

1. American College of Surgeons Committee on Trauma: *Advanced Trauma Life Support (ATLS): Advanced Trauma Life Support Student Manual*. Chicago, IL, American College of Surgeons, 1989.
2. Podolsky S, Baraff LJ, Simon RR, Hoffman JR, Larmon B, Ablon W: Efficacy of cervical spine immobilization methods. *J Trauma* 1983;23(6): 461-465.
3. Heckman JD, Rosenthal RE, Worsing RA, McFee AS, eds: *Emergency Care and Transportation of the Sick and Injured*, ed 4. Park Ridge, IL, American Academy of Orthopaedic Surgeons, 1987.
4. Green BA, Eismont FJ, O'Heir JT: Pre-hospital management of spinal cord injuries. *Paraplegia* 1987;25(3):229-238.
5. McGuire RA, Neville S, Green BA, Watts C: Spinal instability and the log-rolling maneuver. *J Trauma* 1987;27(5):525-531.
6. Ching RP, Watson NA, Carter JW, Tencer AF: The effect of post-injury spinal position on canal occlusion in a cervical spine burst fracture model. *Spine (Phila Pa 1976)* 1997;22(15):1710-1715.
7. Apple DF Jr, Anson CA, Hunter JD, Bell RB: Spinal cord injury in youth. *Clin Pediatr (Phila)* 1995; 34(2):90-95.
8. Aprahamian C, Thompson BM, Darin JC: Recommended helmet removal techniques in a cervical spine injured patient. *J Trauma* 1984;24(9): 841-842.
9. Donaldson WF III, Lauerman WC, Heil B, Blanc R, Swenson T: Helmet and shoulder pad removal from a player with suspected cervical spine injury: A cadaveric model. *Spine (Phila Pa 1976)* 1998;23(16):1729-1733.
10. Gastel JA, Palumbo MA, Hulstyn MJ, Fadale PD, Lucas P: Emergency removal of football equipment: A cadaveric cervical spine injury model. *Ann Emerg Med* 1998;32(4):411-417.
11. Metz CM, Kuhn JE, Greenfield ML: Cervical spine alignment in immobilized hockey players: Radiographic analysis with and without helmets and shoulder pads. *Clin J Sport Med* 1998;8(2):92-95.
12. Bracken MB, Collins WF, Freeman DF, et al: Efficacy of methylprednisolone in acute spinal cord injury. *JAMA* 1984;251(1):45-52.
13. Bracken MB, Shepard MJ, Collins WF, et al: A randomized, controlled trial of methylprednisolone or naloxone in the treatment of acute spinal-cord injury: Results of the Second National Acute Spinal Cord Injury Study. *N Engl J Med* 1990; 322(20):1405-1411.
14. Bracken MB, Shepard MJ, Holford TR, et al: Administration of methylprednisolone for 24 or 48 hours or tirilazad mesylate for 48 hours in the treatment of acute spinal cord injury: Results of the Third National Acute Spinal Cord Injury Randomized Controlled Trial. National Acute Spinal Cord Injury Study. *JAMA* 1997;277(20): 1597-1604.
15. Schwab ME, Bartholdi D: Degeneration and regeneration of axons in the lesioned spinal cord. *Physiol Rev* 1996;76(2):319-370.
16. Geisler FH, Dorsey FC, Coleman WP: Recovery of motor function after spinal-cord injury—a randomized, placebo-controlled trial with GM-1 ganglioside. *N Engl J Med* 1991;324(26):1829-1838.
17. Petitjean ME, Pointillart V, Dixmerias F, et al: Medical treatment of spinal cord injury in the acute stage. *Ann Fr Anesth Reanim* 1998;17(2): 114-122.
18. Pitts LH, Ross A, Chase GA, Faden AI: Treatment with thyrotropin-releasing hormone (TRH) in patients with traumatic spinal cord injuries. *J Neurotrauma* 1995;12(3):235-243.
19. Potter PJ, Hayes KC, Segal JL, et al: Randomized double-blind crossover trial of fampridine-SR (sustained release 4-aminopyridine) in patients with incomplete spinal cord injury. *J Neurotrauma* 1998;15(10):837-849.
20. Braughler JM, Hall ED: Pharmacokinetics of methylprednisolone in cat plasma and spinal cord following a single intravenous dose of the sodium succinate ester. *Drug Metab Dispos* 1982;10(5): 551-552.
21. Hall ED, Braughler JM: Effects of intravenous methylprednisolone on spinal cord lipid peroxidation and Na+ + K+)-ATPase activity: Dose-response analysis during 1st hour after contusion injury in the cat. *J Neurosurg* 1982;57(2):247-253.

22. Bracken MB: Pharmacological treatment of acute spinal cord injury: Current status and future prospects. *Paraplegia* 1992;30(2):102-107.
23. Bracken MB, Holford TR: Effects of timing of methylprednisolone or naloxone administration on recovery of segmental and long-tract neurological function in NASCIS 2. *J Neurosurg* 1993; 79(4):500-507.
24. Bracken MB, Shepard MJ, Collins WF Jr, et al: Methylprednisolone or naloxone treatment after acute spinal cord injury: 1-year follow-up data. Results of the second National Acute Spinal Cord Injury Study. *J Neurosurg* 1992;76(1):23-31.
25. Bracken MB, Shepard MJ, Holford TR, et al: Methylprednisolone or tirilazad mesylate administration after acute spinal cord injury: 1-year follow up. Results of the third National Acute Spinal Cord Injury randomized controlled trial. *J Neurosurg* 1998;89(5):699-706.
26. Anderson DK, Braughler JM, Hall ED, Waters TR, McCall JM, Means ED: Effects of treatment with U-74006F on neurological outcome following experimental spinal cord injury. *J Neurosurg* 1988; 69(4):562-567.
27. Levi L, Wolf A, Belzberg H: Hemodynamic parameters in patients with acute cervical cord trauma: Description, intervention, and prediction of outcome. *Neurosurgery* 1993;33(6):1007-1017.
28. Baker SP, O'Neill B, Haddon W Jr, Long WB: The injury severity score: A method for describing patients with multiple injuries and evaluating emergency care. *J Trauma* 1974;14(3):187-196.
29. American Spinal Injury Association (ASIA): *Standards for Neurological Classification of Spinal Injury*. Chicago, IL, American Spinal Injury Association. 1996.
30. Waters RL, Adkins RH, Yakura JS: Definition of complete spinal cord injury. *Paraplegia* 1991; 29(9):573-581.
31. Stauffer ES: Neurologic recovery following injuries to the cervical spinal cord and nerve roots. *Spine (Phila Pa 1976)* 1984;9(5):532-534.
32. Kiwerski J, Weiss M: Neurological improvement in traumatic injuries of cervical spinal cord. *Paraplegia* 1981;19(1):31-37.
33. Crozier KS, Graziani V, Ditunno JF Jr, Herbison GJ: Spinal cord injury: Prognosis for ambulation based on sensory examination in patients who are initially motor complete. *Arch Phys Med Rehabil* 1991;72(2):119-121.
34. Ditunno JF, Little JW, Tessler A, Burns AS: Spinal shock revisited: A four-phase model. *Spinal Cord* 2004;42(7):383-395.
35. Kakulas BA: Pathology of spinal injuries. *Cent Nerv Syst Trauma* 1984;1(2):117-129.
36. Brown PJ, Marino RJ, Herbison GJ, Ditunno JF Jr: The 72-hour examination as a predictor of recovery in motor complete quadriplegia. *Arch Phys Med Rehabil* 1991;72(8):546-548.
37. Mirza SK, Krengel WF III, Chapman JR, et al: Early versus delayed surgery for acute cervical spinal cord injury. *Clin Orthop Relat Res* 1999;359: 104-114.
38. Enderson BL, Reath DB, Meadors J, Dallas W, DeBoo JM, Maull KI: The tertiary trauma survey: A prospective study of missed injury. *J Trauma* 1990;30(6):666-670.
39. Ward WG, Nunley JA: Occult orthopaedic trauma in the multiply injured patient. *J Orthop Trauma* 1991;5(3):308-312.
40. MacDonald RL, Schwartz ML, Mirich D, Sharkey PW, Nelson WR: Diagnosis of cervical spine injury in motor vehicle crash victims: How many X-rays are enough? *J Trauma* 1990;30(4):392-397.
41. Harris JH Jr: What is the minimum number of plain radiographs necessary to evaluate the cervical spine in patients who have had trauma? *AJR Am J Roentgenol* 1994;163(1):217-218.
42. Penning L: Prevertebral hematoma in cervical spine injury: Incidence and etiologic significance. *AJR Am J Roentgenol* 1981;136(3):553-561.
43. Harris JH Jr, Carson GC, Wagner LK, Kerr N: Radiologic diagnosis of traumatic occipitovertebral dissociation: 2. Comparison of three methods of detecting occipitovertebral relationships on lateral radiographs of supine subjects. *AJR Am J Roentgenol* 1994;162(4):887-892.
44. Powers B, Miller MD, Kramer RS, Martinez S, Gehweiler JA Jr: Traumatic anterior atlanto-occipital dislocation. *Neurosurgery* 1979;4(1): 12-17.
45. Neer CS II: Fracture classification systems: Do they work and are they useful? *J Bone Joint Surg Am* 1994;76(5):789-790.
46. Miles KA, Finlay D: Is prevertebral soft tissue swelling a useful sign in injury of the cervical spine? *Injury* 1988;19(3):177-179.
47. Levitt MA, Flanders AE: Diagnostic capabilities of magnetic resonance imaging and computed tomography in acute cervical spinal column injury. *Am J Emerg Med* 1991;9(2):131-135.
48. Peh WC, Cheng P, Chan FL: Direct coronal computed tomography of the upper cervical spine. *Spine (Phila Pa 1976)* 1995;20(8):972-974.
49. Schaefer DM, Flanders A, Northrup BE, Doan HT, Osterholm JL: Magnetic resonance imaging of acute cervical spine trauma: Correlation with severity of neurologic injury. *Spine (Phila Pa 1976)* 1989;14(10):1090-1095.
50. Schaefer DM, Flanders AE, Osterholm JL, Northrup BE: Prognostic significance of magnetic

resonance imaging in the acute phase of cervical spine injury. *J Neurosurg* 1992;76(2):218-223.

51. Bundschuh CV, Alley JB, Ross M, Porter IS, Gudeman SK: Magnetic resonance imaging of suspected atlanto-occipital dislocation: Two case reports. *Spine (Phila Pa 1976)* 1992;17(2):245-248.
52. Friedman D, Flanders A, Thomas C, Millar W: Vertebral artery injury after acute cervical spine trauma: Rate of occurrence as detected by MR angiography and assessment of clinical consequences. *AJR Am J Roentgenol* 1995;164(2): 443-449.
53. Sim E, Schwarz N, Biowski-Fasching I, Biowski P: Color-coded Duplex sonography of vertebral arteries: 11 cases of blunt cervical spine injury. *Acta Orthop Scand* 1993;64(2):133-137.
54. Chan RN, Ainscow D, Sikorski JM: Diagnostic failures in the multiple injured. *J Trauma* 1980; 20(8):684-687.
55. Jacobs LM, Schwartz R: Prospective analysis of acute cervical spine injury: A methodology to predict injury. *Ann Emerg Med* 1986;15(1):44-49.
56. Blackmore CC, Emerson SS, Mann FA, Koepsell TD: Cervical spine imaging in patients with trauma: Determination of fracture risk to optimize use. *Radiology* 1999;211(3):759-765.
57. Hoffman JR, Schriger DL, Mower W, Luo JS, Zucker M: Low-risk criteria for cervical-spine radiography in blunt trauma: A prospective study. *Ann Emerg Med* 1992;21(12):1454-1460.
58. Mace SE: The unstable occult cervical spine fracture: A review. *Am J Emerg Med* 1992;10(2): 136-142.
59. Mace SE: Unstable occult cervical-spine fracture. *Ann Emerg Med* 1991;20(12):1373-1375.
60. Abarbanell NR: Mismanagement of a potential cervical spine injury. *Am J Emerg Med* 1990;8(5): 468-469.
61. Pepin JW, Bourne RB, Hawkins RJ: Odontoid fractures, with special reference to the elderly patient. *Clin Orthop Relat Res* 1985;193:178-183.
62. Barron MM: Cervical spine injury masquerading as a medical emergency. *Am J Emerg Med* 1989; 7(1):54-56.
63. Bicknell JM, Fielder K: Unrecognized incomplete cervical spinal cord injury: Review of nine new and 28 previously reported cases. *Am J Emerg Med* 1992;10(4):336-343.
64. Meldon SW, Moettus LN: Thoracolumbar spine fractures: Clinical presentation and the effect of altered sensorium and major injury. *J Trauma* 1995;39(6):1110-1114.
65. Rizzolo SJ, Vaccaro AR, Cotler JM: Cervical spine trauma. *Spine (Phila Pa 1976)* 1994;19(20): 2288-2298.
66. Cohn SM, Lyle WG, Linden CH, Lancey RA: Exclusion of cervical spine injury: A prospective study. *J Trauma* 1991;31(4):570-574.
67. Clark CR, Igram CM, el-Khoury GY, Ehara S: Radiographic evaluation of cervical spine injuries. *Spine (Phila Pa 1976)* 1988;13(7):742-747.
68. Hanson JA, Blackmore CC, Mann FA, Wilson AJ: Cervical spine injury: A clinical decision rule to identify high-risk patients for helical CT screening. *AJR Am J Roentgenol* 2000;174(3):713-717.
69. Rizzolo SJ, Piazza MR, Cotler JM, Balderston RA, Schaefer D, Flanders A: Intervertebral disc injury complicating cervical spine trauma. *Spine (Phila Pa 1976)* 1991;16(6, Suppl)S187-S189.
70. Eismont FJ, Arena MJ, Green BA: Extrusion of an intervertebral disc associated with traumatic subluxation or dislocation of cervical facets: Case report. *J Bone Joint Surg Am* 1991;73(10): 1555-1560.
71. Grant GA, Mirza SK, Chapman JR, et al: Risk of early closed reduction in cervical spine subluxation injuries. *J Neurosurg* 1999;90(1, Suppl) 13-18.
72. Robertson PA, Ryan MD: Neurological deterioration after reduction of cervical subluxation: Mechanical compression by disc tissue. *J Bone Joint Surg Br* 1992;74(2):224-227.
73. Doran SE, Papadopoulos SM, Ducker TB, Lillehei KO: Magnetic resonance imaging documentation of coexistent traumatic locked facets of the cervical spine and disc herniation. *J Neurosurg* 1993; 79(3):341-345.
74. Finkelstein JA, Chapman JR, Mirza S: Occult vertebral fractures in ankylosing spondylitis. *Spinal Cord* 1999;37(6):444-447.
75. Batillas J, Vasilas A, Pizzi WF, Gokcebay T: Bone scanning in the detection of occult fractures. *J Trauma* 1981;21(7):564-569.
76. Marshall LF, Knowlton S, Garfin SR, et al: Deterioration following spinal cord injury: A multicenter study. *J Neurosurg* 1987;66(3):400-404.
77. Green BA, Eismont FJ, O'Heir JT: Spinal cord injury—a systems approach: Prevention, emergency medical services, and emergency room management. *Crit Care Clin* 1987;3(3):471-493.
78. Brimacombe J, Berry A: Laryngeal mask airway insertion: A comparison of the standard versus neutral position in normal patients with a view to its use in cervical spine instability. *Anaesthesia* 1993;48(8):670-671.
79. Davis JW, Phreaner DL, Hoyt DB, Mackersie RC: The etiology of missed cervical spine injuries. *J Trauma* 1993;34(3):342-346.
80. Rogers NA: Treatment of fractures of vertebral bodies uncomplicated by lesions of the spinal cord. *Arch Surg* 1935;30:284-324.

81. Oakes DD, Wilmot CB, Hall KM, Sherck JP: Benefits of early admission to a comprehensive trauma center for patients with spinal cord injury. *Arch Phys Med Rehabil* 1990;71(9):637-643.
82. Kiwerski J: The results of early conservative and surgical treatment of cervical spinal cord injured patients. *Int J Rehabil Res* 1986;9(2):149-154.
83. Grace TG: The orthopaedist as traumatologist. *J Bone Joint Surg Am* 1991;73(3):319.
84. Krag MH, Byrt W, Pope M: Pull-off strength of gardner-Wells tongs from cadaveric crania. *Spine (Phila Pa 1976)* 1989;14(3):247-250.
85. Kleyn PJ: Dislocations of the cervical spine: Closed reduction under anaesthesia. *Paraplegia* 1984;22(5):271-281.
86. Sabiston CP, Wing PC, Schweigel JF, Van Peteghem PK, Yu W: Closed reduction of dislocations of the lower cervical spine. *J Trauma* 1988; 28(6):832-835.
87. Delamarter RB, Sherman J, Carr JB: Pathophysiology of spinal cord injury: Recovery after immediate and delayed decompression. *J Bone Joint Surg Am* 1995;77(7):1042-1049.
88. Carlson GD, Minato Y, Okada A, et al: Early time-dependent decompression for spinal cord injury: Vascular mechanisms of recovery. *J Neurotrauma* 1997;14(12):951-962.
89. Carlson GD, Warden KE, Barbeau JM, et al: Viscoelastic relaxation and regional blood flow response to spinal cord compression and decompression. *Spine (Phila Pa 1976)* 1997;22(12): 1285-1291.
90. Carlson SL, Parrish ME, Springer JE, Doty K, Dossett L: Acute inflammatory response in spinal cord following impact injury. *Exp Neurol* 1998; 151(1):77-88.
91. Brunette DD, Rockswold GL: Neurologic recovery following rapid spinal realignment for complete cervical spinal cord injury. *J Trauma* 1987;27(4): 445-447.
92. Sussman BJ: Letter: Early management of spinal cord trauma. *J Neurosurg* 1976;44(6):766-767.
93. Star AM, Jones AA, Cotler JM, Balderston RA, Sinha R: Immediate closed reduction of cervical spine dislocations using traction. *Spine (Phila Pa 1976)* 1990;15(10):1068-1072.
94. Lee AS, MacLean JC, Newton DA: Rapid traction for reduction of cervical spine dislocations. *J Bone Joint Surg Br* 1994;76(3):352-356.
95. Montane I, Eismont FJ, Green BA: Traumatic occipitoatlantal dislocation. *Spine (Phila Pa 1976)* 1991;16(2):112-116.
96. Mahale YJ, Silver JR: Progressive paralysis after bilateral facet dislocation of the cervical spine. *J Bone Joint Surg Br* 1992;74(2):219-223.
97. Shrosbree RD: Neurological sequelae of reduction of fracture dislocations of the cervical spine. *Paraplegia* 1979;17(2):212-221.
98. Olerud C, Jónsson H Jr: Compression of the cervical spine cord after reduction of fracture dislocations: Report of 2 cases. *Acta Orthop Scand* 1991;62(6):599-601.
99. Cotler HB, Miller LS, DeLucia FA, Cotler JM, Davne SH: Closed reduction of cervical spine dislocations. *Clin Orthop Relat Res* 1987;214: 185-199.
100. Subin B, Liu JF, Marshall GJ, Huang HY, Ou JH, Xu GZ: Transoral anterior decompression and fusion of chronic irreducible atlantoaxial dislocation with spinal cord compression. *Spine (Phila Pa 1976)* 1995;20(11):1233-1240.
101. Davies WE, Morris JH, Hill V: An analysis of conservative (non-surgical) management of thoracolumbar fractures and fracture-dislocations with neural damage. *J Bone Joint Surg Am* 1980;62(8): 1324-1328.
102. Hartman MB, Chrin AM, Rechtine GR: Nonoperative treatment of thoracolumbar fractures. *Paraplegia* 1995;33(2):73-76.
103. Riska EB, von Bonsdorff H, Hakkinen S, Jaroma H, Kiviluoto O, Paavilainen T: Primary operative fixation of long bone fractures in patients with multiple injuries. *J Trauma* 1977;17(2):111-121.
104. Weller S: Urgency of osteosyntheses in the first aid for combined injuries. *Langenbecks Arch Chir* 1971;329:82-87.
105. Talucci RC, Manning J, Lampard S, Bach A, Carrico CJ: Early intramedullary nailing of femoral shaft fractures: A cause of fat embolism syndrome. *Am J Surg* 1983;146(1):107-111.
106. Johnson KD, Cadambi A, Seibert GB: Incidence of adult respiratory distress syndrome in patients with multiple musculoskeletal injuries: Effect of early operative stabilization of fractures. *J Trauma* 1985;25(5):375-384.
107. Bone LB, Johnson KD, Weigelt J, Scheinberg R: Early versus delayed stabilization of femoral fractures: A prospective randomized study. *J Bone Joint Surg Am* 1989;71(3):336-340.
108. Bohlman HH, Freehafer A, Dejak J: The results of treatment of acute injuries of the upper thoracic spine with paralysis. *J Bone Joint Surg Am* 1985; 67(3):360-369.
109. Bradford DS, Akbarnia BA, Winter RB, et al: Surgical stabilization of fracture and fracture-dislocations of the thoracic spine. *Spine (Phila Pa 1976)* 1977;2:185-196.
110. Krengel WF III, Anderson PA, Henley MB: Early stabilization and decompression for incomplete paraplegia due to a thoracic-level spinal cord in-

jury. *Spine (Phila Pa 1976)* 1993;18(14): 2080-2087.

111. McLain RF, Benson DR: Urgent surgical stabilization of spinal fractures in polytrauma patients. *Spine (Phila Pa 1976)* 1999;24(16):1646-1654.

112. Flesch JR, Leider LL, Erickson DL, Chou SN, Bradford DS: Harrington instrumentation and spine fusion for unstable fractures and fracture-dislocations of the thoracic and lumbar spine. *J Bone Joint Surg Am* 1977;59(2):143-153.

113. McAfee PC, Bohlman HH, Yuan HA: Anterior decompression of traumatic thoracolumbar fractures with incomplete neurological deficit using a retroperitoneal approach. *J Bone Joint Surg Am* 1985; 67(1):89-104.

114. McKinley W, Meade MA, Kirshblum S, Barnard B: Outcomes of early surgical management versus late or no surgical intervention after acute spinal cord injury. *Arch Phys Med Rehabil* 2004;85(11): 1818-1825.

115. Croce MA, Bee TK, Pritchard E, Miller PR, Fabian TC: Does optimal timing for spine fracture fixation exist? *Ann Surg* 2001;233(6):851-858.

116. Kerwin AJ, Frykberg ER, Schinco MA, Griffen MM, Murphy T, Tepas JJ: The effect of early spine fixation on non-neurologic outcome. *J Trauma* 2005;58(1):15-21.

117. Schlegel J, Bayley J, Yuan H, Fredricksen B: Timing of surgical decompression and fixation of acute spinal fractures. *J Orthop Trauma* 1996; 10(5):323-330.

118. Rechtine GR: Nonsurgical treatment of thoracic and lumbar fractures. *Instr Course Lect* 1999;48: 413-416.

119. McHenry TP, Mirza SK, Wang J, et al: Risk factors for respiratory failure following operative stabilization of thoracic and lumbar spine fractures. *J Bone Joint Surg Am* 2006;88(5):997-1005.

120. Bone LB, Anders MJ, Rohrbacher BJ: Treatment of femoral fractures in the multiply injured patient with thoracic injury. *Clin Orthop Relat Res* 1998; 347:57-61.

121. Crowl AC, Young JS, Kahler DM, Claridge JA, Chrzanowski DS, Pomphrey M: Occult hypoperfusion is associated with increased morbidity in patients undergoing early femur fracture fixation. *J Trauma* 2000;48(2):260-267.

122. Miller PR, Croce MA, Kilgo PD, Scott J, Fabian TC: Acute respiratory distress syndrome in blunt trauma: Identification of independent risk factors. *Am Surg* 2002;68(10):845-851.

123. Waydhas C, Nast-Kolb D, Trupka A, et al: Posttraumatic inflammatory response, secondary operations, and late multiple organ failure. *J Trauma* 1996;40(4):624-631.

124. Centers for Disease Control and Prevention (CDC): Cigarette smoking among adults—United States, 2002. *MMWR Morb Mortal Wkly Rep* 2004; 53(20):427-431.

125. Rechtine GR II, Cahill D, Chrin AM: Treatment of thoracolumbar trauma: Comparison of complications of operative versus nonoperative treatment. *J Spinal Disord* 1999;12(5):406-409.

CHAPTER 5
"Clearing" the Cervical Spine in the Trauma Patient

Darren R. Lebl, MD Rajiv K. Sethi, MD Paul A. Anderson, MD
Mitchel B. Harris, MD, FACS

Introduction

The initial evaluation and management of the multiply injured patient requires a multidisciplinary approach. Attention to maintenance of spinal precautions during the complete evaluation of the polytrauma patient is essential to minimize the risk of neurologic injury. This chapter will review the common methods of studying the cervical spine and provide evidence-based recommendations to help guide the clinician through the evaluation of the cervical spine in the trauma patient.

A universally agreed-upon guideline for clearance of the cervical spine has yet to be established. The optimal method of assessment of the cervical spine requires a consistent and methodical approach. Spinal imaging plays an important role in the evaluation of the osseous, ligamentous, and neural structures and ultimately guides treatment. However, controversy persists as to whether a cervical spine can be "cleared" without the patient's active involvement in the physical examination. The intoxicated or obtunded patient in whom a comprehensive physical examination is not reliable provides further challenges for the treating physician.

Dr. Anderson or an immediate family member serves as a board member, owner, officer, or committee member of the American Academy of Orthopaedic Surgeons, the ASTM, the North American Spine Society, the Spine Arthroplasty Society, and the Spine Section of AANS/CNS; has received royalties from Pioneer and Stryker; serves as a paid consultant to or is an employee of Aesculap/B.Braun, Expanding Orthopedics, Medtronic Sofamor Danek, Spertec, and Titan Surgical; and owns stock or stock options in Pioneer Surgical, Spartec, Titan, and Titan Surgical. Dr. Harris or an immediate family member serves as a board member, owner, officer, or committee member of the American Academy of Orthopaedic Surgeons, the North American Spine Society, and the Orthopaedic Trauma Association. None of the following authors or any immediate family member has received anything of value from or owns stock in a commercial company or institution related directly or indirectly to the subject of this chapter: Dr. Lebl and Dr. Sethi.

Advanced Trauma Life Support Guidelines

Advanced Trauma Life Support (ATLS) training provides guidelines for the evaluation of the cervical spine in the adult trauma patient.[1] Although these guidelines reinforce the principle that the trauma patient should initially be considered to have an unstable spinal injury until clinically and/or radiographically proven otherwise, they have not been sufficiently studied with respect to the radiographic evaluation. Spinal precautions should be maintained until the spine is cleared by the treating physician. The current ATLS guidelines include the following:

(1) Patients with quadriplegia or paraplegia are assumed to have spinal instability.

(2) Awake, alert, and sober patients without pain, tenderness, or neurologic deficits may have their cervical collars removed and be tested for pain-induced motion in the presence of the treating physician. If the patient can first laterally rotate his or her neck without pain and then subsequently actively flex and extend without pain, the spine may be cleared without further imaging.

(3) In the obtunded patient, plain radiographs and a CT scan with reformats are the minimum imaging studies required in addition to consultation with a spine specialist. The necessity of plain radiographs in this setting is controversial at this time.

Adverse Consequences of the Screening Process

Extended periods of immobilization are commonly associated with significant morbidity and should be avoided whenever possible. Prolonged immobilization in a cervical collar in the supine position, especially in the intensive care unit (ICU), places the trauma patient at risk for occipital and submental pressure sores. Occipital and submental decubitus formation is directly related to the

FIGURE 1

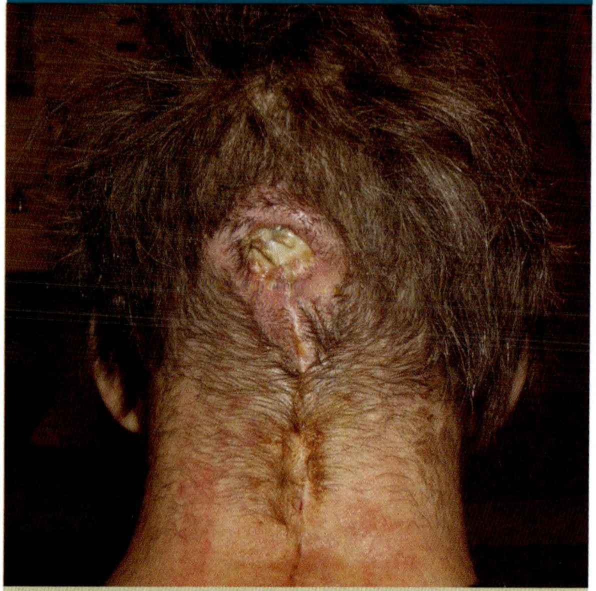

Figure 1 Occipital breakdown after prolonged collar use in a postoperative patient with severe rheumatoid arthritis.

FIGURE 2

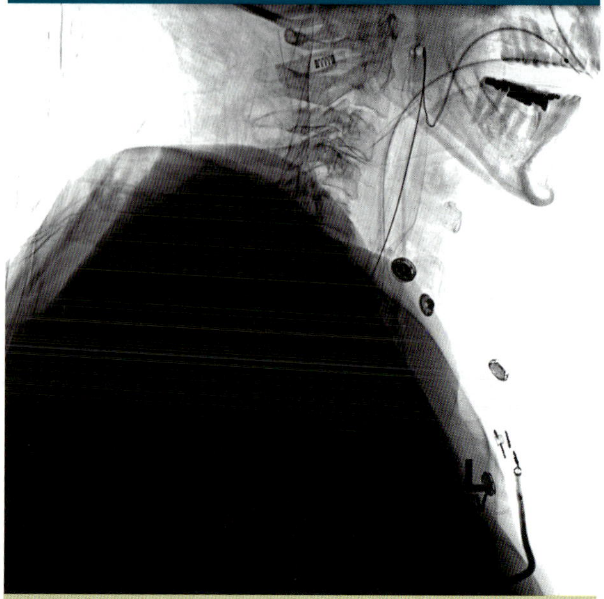

Figure 2 Example of an inadequate lateral cervical spine radiograph, illustrating the necessity for CT scanning with sagittal and coronal reconstructions.

length of time the collar is in place[2] (**Figure 1**). In addition, spinal precautions in the supine position negatively affect pulmonary function, increase the risk of pneumonia,[3] and have been reported to potentially elevate intracranial pressure.[4-8] Daily nursing care, including skin care, pulmonary toilet, and mobilization, is impeded by the presence of a collar and a cervical spine that has not been "cleared."

Timely and accurate diagnosis of cervical spine injuries is therefore an important consideration for the trauma team. Missed or delayed diagnosis of a cervical spine injury can cause a neurologic injury or result in the exacerbation of an incomplete injury.[9,10] Levi et al[11] reported 24 patients treated at Level I trauma centers in whom delayed or missed diagnosis of cervical injuries resulted in neurologic deterioration. The etiology of the delayed or missed diagnosis was attributed to insufficient or poor quality radiographs in 58% of patients (**Figure 2**) and to studies that were misread in 33% of patients. The incidence of delayed diagnosis and neurologic deterioration among all spine-injured patients was 0.21%. The incidence of delayed diagnosis in all blunt trauma patients presenting to the Level I trauma center was 0.025%. The authors noted that older patients, patients with high-energy trauma mechanisms of injury, and patients with inadequate imaging were at risk for this complication. To avoid potentially catastrophic neurologic complications, the authors recommend the following methods be considered carefully by the treating physician.

Methods to Evaluate the Cervical Spine

History

Obtaining a detailed history is a fundamental and important part of the evaluation of the spine in the trauma patient. Important components of the history include the use of intoxicants, a prior history of spinal pathology (eg, prior spinal surgery, ankylosing spondylitis, etc), preinjury functional status, and the presence of transient or persistent neurologic symptoms. The mechanism of injury will provide important information for the clinician. High-energy trauma mechanisms such as high-speed motor vehicle accidents or falls from a substantial height are predictive of an increased risk for spinal injury.

Physical Examination

The patient's spine should be examined for tenderness, palpable step-offs between spinous processes, and/or crepitus. After completion of the examination of the axial skeleton, a comprehensive neurologic examination should be performed. If the patient is asymptomatic, alert, and sober (meets criteria for Group I; see Screening the Cer-

FIGURE 3

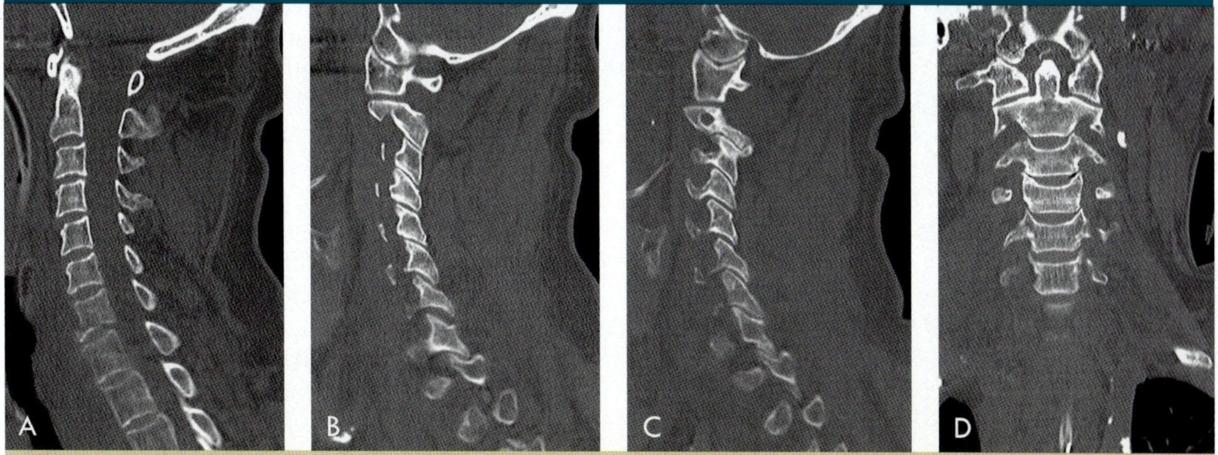

Figure 3 Sagittal (**A**) and parasagittal (**B** and **C**) reformatted CT images have largely replaced traditional lateral radiographs. Coronal reformatted CT scans (**D**) have replaced traditional open-mouth odontoid and AP radiographs.

vical Spine below), the collar may be removed and the patient should be asked to rotate his or her neck 45° laterally to each side. In a patient with midline spinal tenderness, the sensitivity of a complete physical examination to detect the presence of cervical spine fractures is 95%; however, the specificity is low.[12] It should be noted that the sensitivity of a physical examination is decreased in patients who have distracting injuries and/or altered sensorium.

Plain Radiography

Plain radiographs are able to detect only 75% to 95% of clinically significant injuries and therefore have been replaced in most practices by multidetector CT (MDCT) for screening purposes in trauma patients. However, there is still a role for plain radiographs in the acute evaluation of the trauma patient. In the patient found to be in extremis who is too unstable to undergo "pan-scanning," it may be necessary to resort to the previously popular trauma series of AP chest, AP pelvis, and lateral cervical spine plain radiographs. This trauma series will often allow early identification of life-threatening injuries and the potential need to reduce or provide urgent intervention for a significant cervical spine injury. In the subset of patients who will not otherwise require a CT scan, three views of the cervical spine (an AP, a lateral view that is "adequate" [down to T1], and an open-mouth odontoid view) may be obtained for screening purposes. Increasingly, these views are not ordered in the presence of a suspicious history or examination. The sensitivity of plain radiographs increases with the number of views included in the series. Other views such as oblique trauma views have largely been replaced by CT and/or MRI scans in modern practice.

Computed Tomography

In recent years, CT scans with reformatted images have largely replaced the use of plain radiographs in the trauma setting (**Figure 3**). MDCT provides high-quality images in all planes and has become the primary study for the detection of spinal injury in many trauma centers. Brown et al[13] demonstrated that CT identifies 99.3% of all fractures in the cervical, thoracic, and lumbar spine. In their study, fractures that were missed by helical CT required minimal to no treatment. Moreover, helical CT scans have shown to be cost effective in addition to having an increased sensitivity in detecting injuries.[14] The cost effectiveness of helical CT is enhanced when it is used as the only method of radiographic evaluation in patients who are already going into the CT scanner for other indications (eg, traumatic brain injury, or associated chest, abdominal, and/or pelvic injuries). Grogan et al[15] have advocated for CT imaging as the preferred initial screening test for detection of cervical spine fractures among moderate- to high-risk patients seen in urban trauma centers. Similarly, using reformatted spinal images from chest and abdominal CT scans has been shown to increase the sensitivity of identifying thoracolumbar spinal injuries.[16]

Detecting the presence of a ligamentous injury in the trauma patient with altered mental status remains a diagnostic challenge. When used as the primary radiographic instrument, CT is highly

FIGURE 4

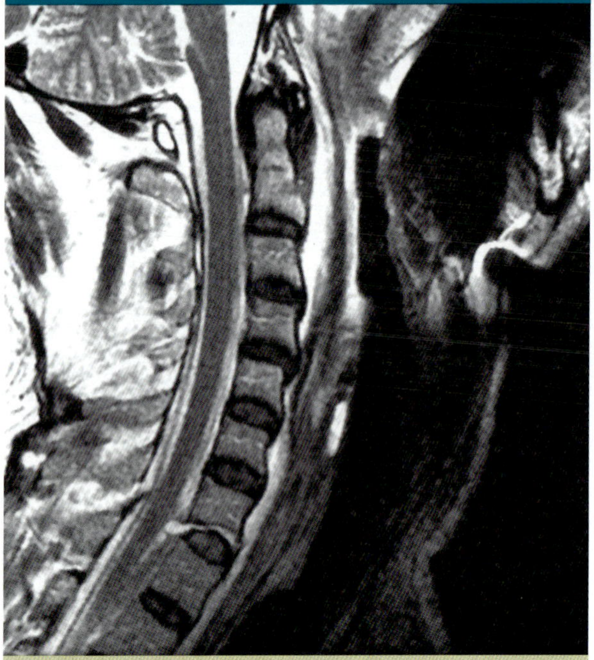

Figure 4 MRI of the cervical spine illustrating posterior ligamentous injury at the cervical thoracic junction.

effective for occult bony injuries but is less sensitive and specific for detecting ligamentous injuries.[17-19] The reasons for this are twofold: (1) the plane of the ligament injury often coincides with the orientation of the acquisition CT cut, and (2) the soft-tissue windows that are commonly used rarely have the sensitivity to identify isolated soft-tissue injuries with any degree of accuracy. Sagittal images reformatted from the acquisition axial cuts can also be misleading due to small amounts of patient movement and disparity between the alignment of the gantry and the alignment of the spine. Further complicating the evaluation of spinal stability by CT is the fact that the study is generally performed with the patient in the supine position, which eliminates any of the deforming forces of gravity that the spine would normally see under a physiologic load.

Magnetic Resonance Imaging

MRI is the most sensitive imaging method to evaluate a suspected soft-tissue injury of the cervical spine. It provides the best imaging of neurologic structures, ligaments, and the intervertebral disk (**Figure 4**). MRI can also demonstrate subtle fractures that are occasionally missed on CT, such as nondisplaced fractures of the dens or fractures through the fused intervertebral disk space in patients with ankylosing spondylitis. However, MRI should not routinely be used in the initial evaluation of the polytrauma patient because of the time required to perform a technically adequate scan and the difficulty of providing adequate patient monitoring in the MRI scanner. Additionally, to incorporate MRI in the screening algorithm of all trauma patients would be prohibitively expensive. MRI is useful in patients whose CT scans do not explain the clinical (neurologic) picture. This is most commonly seen in the neurologically impaired victim with "normal"-appearing plain films. Vaccaro et al[20] reported that 25% of patients with cervicothoracic injuries and a neurologic deficit on presentation had their preliminary treatment plan altered after obtaining an MRI. In the same study cohort, the authors revealed that routine MRI did not alter the treatment plan in the neurologically intact patients.[20]

Muchow et al[21] recently performed a meta-analysis assessing the use of MRI in evaluating symptomatic or obtunded patients. Five studies were identified, which led to a combined analysis of 461 patients.[22-26] MRI was found to have a 100% negative predictive value (meaning a negative examination successfully ruled out a spinal injury 100% of the time). However, the MRI scan is often nonspecific and many false positive findings do occur. False positives are defined by the presence of an abnormal finding on MRI without an accompanying clinical finding or any long-term clinical sequelae. Complicating the picture is the fact that the investigators in these studies treated the patients with "false positive" MRI findings in a collar, making the true value of MRI false positives unknown. In the five studies included in their analysis, MRI identified an abnormality in 20% of cases after a normal CT scan.

MRI can provide valuable information about the status of the ligaments without placing the spinal cord at risk, a common concern with physician-directed flexion-extension evaluations as discussed below.[27] However, there exists no consensus as to which MRI sequence should be used or the specific criteria as to which imaging findings constitute a clinically significant injury. Fat-suppression sequences including T2 fast-spin echo and short-tau inversion recovery (STIR) are believed to be the most sensitive to fluid and hemorrhage. T1 sagittal images will classically demonstrate a black stripe, which represents ligaments such as the anterior and posterior longitudinal ligament, the ligamentum flavum, and the supraspinous ligament. However, in our experience, this is variably present. Findings that indicate ligamentous injury include disruption of the black stripe on T1 and an increased signal that extends through normal ligamentous structures on T2 fat-suppressed images.

Lower strength magnets (< 1.5 T) have a lower signal-to-noise ratio and an increased likelihood of false positive findings. Although 48 to 72 hours postinjury has been cited as the important time interval during which one must obtain MRI to evaluate for ligamentous injury, there are no data to support this hypothesis.[28-30]

Flexion-Extension Radiographs

Physician-directed flexion-extension studies have consistently demonstrated the capacity to identify soft-tissue injuries that are not identified by plain radiographs or CT.[31,32] One group of authors included a stretch test before the flexion-extension motion to further safeguard the patient from injury.[32] Although there are many studies identifying the merits of this technique,[30,32,33] the question arises as to who should be performing this evaluation and in which setting (operating room, ICU, or emergency department).[34-36] The difficulty of fully visualizing the cervicothoracic junction, the inconsistency in the results, and the risk associated with motion of a potentially unstable spine have dulled our enthusiasm for this method of cervical spine evaluation. These controversial issues have basically eliminated this method of study from common use in the acute trauma patient.

Screening the Cervical Spine

Cervical spine clearance is defined as the screening process to rule out any clinically significant (unstable) injuries. Unstable injuries are those with the potential to displace or cause a neurologic deficit if left undiagnosed and unprotected. Occult injuries can often be trivial, stable, and pose little harm to the patient if not immediately diagnosed. Due to the cost, time, and certain facility limitations, it is often considered acceptable to not fully identify a clinically insignificant injury radiographically as long as harm does not come to the patient once the collar is removed. The optimal screening process should have a high sensitivity (identify a significant injury if present) and a high negative predictive value (a negative screen indicates that the patient does not have an injury).

For screening purposes, it is useful to classify patients into four groups based on their presentation. Each group has unique risks and considerations and should be evaluated using different protocols. Group I patients are asymptomatic, awake, alert, and without evidence of intoxication. This subset of patients has a Glasgow Coma Scale (GCS) score of 15 and must be neurologically intact without an injury deemed to be capable of distracting the patient. Distracting injuries commonly include visceral injuries, thoracic injuries, long-bone fractures, and/or dislocations. Group II patients are those individuals with signs or symptoms suggestive of a cervical spine injury (eg, midline spinal tenderness, neurologic deficit). Group III patients are awake and alert patients who have a distracting injury, are intoxicated, or demonstrate a mild head injury that prevents reliable clinical evaluation at the time of presentation but may improve within the next 24 to 48 hours. Group IV patients are obtunded or intubated and cannot be reliably assessed by clinical examination.

Group I: Asymptomatic, Awake, and Alert Patients

Several studies have demonstrated that asymptomatic patients who are alert, oriented, have no midline spinal tenderness, and are without distracting injuries are at low risk for cervical spine injury and do not require radiographic evaluation. The National Emergency X-Radiography Utilization Study (NEXUS) developed a decision-making protocol for asymptomatic patients.[37] The proposed criteria that eliminated the need for radiographs included the following: no neurologic abnormalities, a normal level of alertness, no evidence of intoxication, no cervical spine tenderness, and the absence of clinically apparent pain that might distract the patient from a cervical spine injury. To evaluate this protocol, a multicenter prospective study of 44,450 patients from 21 emergency departments was performed. The emergency departments ranged from Level I to Level III and were both academic and community centers. Patients were followed by phone contact 2 weeks after injury to determine if the screening process correctly identified injuries. Overall, 818 patients (2.4%) sustained a cervical spine injury. Eight patients (< 1 patient in 4,000) were missed by the protocol (ie, the patient did not initially have radiographs and was later found to have a cervical spine injury) for a sensitivity of 99.6% and a negative predictive value of 99.7%. Of those 8 patients with missed injuries by the NEXUS decision instrument, 2 patients had a clinically significant injury.[38]

The Canadian C-spine rule was originally reported by Stiell et al in 2001.[39] This protocol was based on three questions: (1) Is there a "high-risk factor" that mandates radiography (age > 65 years, presumed dangerous mechanism, or paresthesia in the extremity)? (2) Are there any "low-risk factors" that allow safe assessment of range of motion (ie, simple rear-end motor vehicle collision, sitting position in emergency department, ambulatory at any time since injury, delayed onset of neck pain, or absence of midline cervical spine tenderness)? (3) Is the patient able to actively rotate his or her neck 45° to the left and right? Stiell et al reviewed 8,924 patients from ten medical centers in Canada. Overall, the Canadian C-spine rule correctly identified all 151 injuries (1.7%) and had a 100% sensitivity (95% confidence interval, 98% to 100%) and a 100% negative predictive value. The inclusion of a functional test (ie, the range of motion after determining that there is a low likelihood of injury) further improved the negative predictive value and sensitivity.

In a follow-up study, Stiell et al[40] prospectively compared the NEXUS criteria and the Canadian C-spine rule. In 8,283 patients, the ability of both protocols to identify appropriate patients for radiographic evaluation was evaluated. They found that the Canadian C-spine rule had higher specificity and a higher negative predictive value for cervical spine injury than the NEXUS protocol. Multiple studies have addressed the need to radiographically evaluate the cervical spine in asymptomatic trauma patients, all of which had similarly high sensitivity and negative predictive value. Anderson et al[41] performed a comprehensive review of the literature (from 1966 to 2004) and a subsequent meta-analysis. They concluded that an alert and asymptomatic patient without a distracting injury or a neurologic deficit who is able to complete a functional range-of-motion examination may safely be cleared without radiographic evaluation (sensitivity of 98.1% and a negative predictive value of 99.8%).

Trauma patients in general do not require radiographic evaluation if they are asymptomatic, have no midline neck tenderness, do not have a neurologic deficit, and do not have injuries that may distract them from the pain of a cervical spine injury. Group I patients should first and foremost be evaluated by the treating physician. Sound clinical judgment in each individual patient to determine what constitutes a distracting injury and the reliability of a given examination is of paramount importance. Group I patients can generally be cleared of spinal precautions clinically without radiographs and immobilization may be discontinued. The use of a functional test, such as a range-of-motion test, after the initial screening increases the sensitivity and negative predictive value and should be done under physician supervision.

Group II: Symptomatic Patients

Patients having midline neck tenderness or a neurologic deficit require continued hard cervical collar immobilization and further radiographic evaluation. The assessment of these patients is described in chapter 2.

Group III: Patients Who Cannot Be Accurately Evaluated Clinically for 24 to 48 Hours

This subset of trauma patients may potentially be cleared from a cervical collar 24 to 48 hours after presentation once clearance of intoxicants has occurred and/or other distracting injuries have been adequately addressed. If knowledge of spinal stability is essential for the treatment of other injuries, then a full radiographic evaluation as described below for Group IV (obtunded patients) should be performed. Alternatively, if patient care will not be compromised by the lack of an initial comprehensive radiographic evaluation of the spine and continued hard collar immobilization, then the clearance process may be delayed until the physical examination is acceptable. If upright positioning is desired, obtaining an upright lateral cervical radiograph in a collar should be performed to exclude the possibility of significant instability during the time delay until a reliable clinical examination.

Group IV: Obtunded Patients

Despite several well-performed studies in the literature, there is to date no universally agreed-upon cervical spine screening protocol in the obtunded trauma patient. Those patients with altered sensorium (GCS < 15) or who are multiply injured, intubated, or in shock require multidisciplinary collaboration and communication. This subset of patients is at a significantly higher risk for cervical spine injury because of the typically high-energy trauma mechanism and that diagnosis may be challenging due to the lack of a reliable neurologic examination. In some cases, the neurologic function of the spinal cord may be altogether unknown. It is generally accepted that in this patient population, the cervical spine should have some form of radiographic imaging to identify an injury. It should be considered that early removal of a cervical collar and mobilization of the patient and advancement of position from supine to upright has many physiologic advantages.

The Eastern Association for the Surgery of Trauma (EAST)[42] and the American Association of Neurologic Surgeons/Congress of Neurologic Surgeons (AANS/CNS) Committees[43] have established guidelines to evaluate obtunded patients. However, neither of these algorithms has been evaluated or validated in prospective multicenter trials.

The EAST guidelines, revised in 2009, recognize the need for future investigations to further delineate the optimal method of cervical spine evaluation in the obtunded trauma patient and make no definitive recommendations with regard to the role of MRI.

At present, we cannot make a definitive recommendation on the need for cervical spine MRI after a negative cervical spine CT scan in the obtunded patient with blunt trauma. The risk-to-benefit ratio is unclear and the incidence of significant cervical spine injury approaches zero. There are significant, nontrivial risks in bringing a severely injured, mechanically ventilated patient to the MRI suite, which is often far from the ICU. However, prolonged cervical spine immobilization has significant risks as previously noted. These issues must be weighed against the devastating potential of a missed cervical spine injury. Thus, current practice guidelines with regard to this issue are at the discretion of each institution.[44]

The AANS/CNS guidelines for cervical spine evaluation in the obtunded patient indicate that cervical spine immobilization in obtunded patients with normal cervical spine radiographs (including supplemental CT as necessary) may be discontinued (1) after dynamic flexion-extension studies performed under fluoroscopic guidance, (2) after a normal MRI study is obtained within 48 hours of injury, or (3) at the discretion of the treating physician.[43]

The AANS/CNS guidelines recognize that plain radiographs and supplemental CT alone may not be sufficient to clear the cervical spine in the obtunded trauma patient. With regard to these guidelines, two points deserve consideration. First, despite early data that flexion-extension radiographs performed under fluoroscopic visualization appear to be safe and effective for ruling out significant ligamentous injury with a reported negative predictive value of 99%,[45] their routine use remains controversial and uncommonly done in practice. Indeed, case reports using flexion-extension radiographs have documented neurologic deterioration.[46,47] Second, there remains no evidence that MRI must be performed within 48 hours of a trauma to accurately demonstrate ligamentous injury. The notion that MRI must be obtained within 48 hours of injury is based on several studies that arbitrarily chose a 48-hour window as their institutional guideline without the specific purpose of establishing a protocol for MRI usage.[23,24,48,49]

In recent years, progressive improvements in the image resolution of MDCT scans have facilitated the identification of soft-tissue injuries based on subtle intervertebral malalignment or loss of facet joint congruity. The sensitivity of modern MDCT scans for the detection of unstable cervical spine injuries has been reported to be 98% to 100%.[50] This development has led several authors to propose that the use of MDCT alone may be sufficient to clear the cervical spine in the obtunded patient. Stelfox et al[51] conducted a prospective study comparing consecutive patients admitted to the ICU of a Level I trauma center who were evaluated by (1) helical CT with reconstructions and either clinical examination or MRI over a 2-year period (n = 140) and by (2) helical CT with reconstructions alone over a 1-year period (n = 75). They found that cervical spine clearance by helical CT alone resulted in shorter hospital and ICU lengths of stay, shorter periods of mechanical ventilation, and no difference in mortality.

Caution should be used, however, if MDCT is used as the only imaging modality for screening in the obtunded trauma patient. In a retrospective study, Simon et al[52] reviewed 91 obtunded trauma patients with MDCT scans that were officially read as adequate and negative by attending emergency department radiologists. Review of those MDCT studies by two fellowship-trained spine surgeons revealed that only 76 of these 91 studies (84%) were felt to be adequate studies by both spine surgeons. Three of those adequate scans had fractures identified by both spine surgeons, and four had additional fractures identified by one of the two spine surgeons. There were 15 findings suspicious for spinal instability identified by at least one of the spine surgeons. A total of 22 of the 91 MDCT scans read as adequate and normal by the attending emergency department radiologists were felt to be suspicious for an abnormality by the spine surgeons. Of these 22 cases, the MRI reading was positive for a trauma-related abnormality in 17 cases.

There is however, some support in the literature for a CT-alone screening protocol in the obtunded patient. Como et al[53] found that in a prospective evaluation of 115 obtunded blunt trauma patients, the MRI scan did not identify any additional injuries that changed management. They concluded that "MR-CS [MRI of the cervical spine] may be unnecessary in the obtunded trauma patient if the CT-CS [CT of the cervical spine] is negative."[53] At the other end of the spectrum, the meta-analysis by Muchow et al[21] supported the idea that MRI be included for all patients as a conclusive study to confirm a cervical spine as "cleared."

A recent meta-analysis compared CT scan alone to CT and MRI to identify occult injuries to the cervical spine.[54] The authors reported a 6% incidence (96 of 1,550) of occult and clinically significant injuries identified by MRI alone. Clinically significant was defined as an injury that required continued collar immobilization or surgical stabilization. Additionally, the authors identified a 1% incidence (12 of 1,550) of injuries detected only by MRI that required surgical stabilization. In a similar study, Sarani et al[55] reported on 4 of 46 trauma patients who were unexaminable and had clinically significant injuries demonstrated by MRI alone in the setting of a normal CT scan. These data support a continued role for the addition of MRI in evaluating patients who are obtunded or unexaminable despite a negative CT scan.

Despite enormous advancements in medical technology, imaging modalities alone still cannot demonstrate the complex anatomy and dynamic nature of the cervical spine to the extent necessary to precisely determine stability. Quite recently, Brandenstein et al[56] reported on a series of four cases in which an unstable subaxial cervical spine injury was identified despite initial acquisition of both "normal" MDCT and MRI. They demonstrated a cumulative incidence of 0.04% to 0.2% of undetected cervical injuries requiring surgical stabilization in their Level I trauma center despite normal plain radiographs, CT scans, and MRI scans.[56]

As such, there is agreement that radiographic examination is needed for the obtunded blunt trauma patient; however, there has not yet been consensus on an evidence-based protocol to clear the cervical spine in the Group IV patient population. Increasing the number of radiographic examinations increases the likelihood of identifying an injury, but at the cost of increased expenditure and increased radiation exposure.[57]

Clearance of the cervical spine in the obtunded patient should be done through a multidisciplinary approach in consultation with the spine surgery team. The time and cost of MRI must be weighed and considered by the treating physician with the risk of missing a clinically significant injury and the resultant potential for catastrophic neurologic injury. These considerations are the basis for the following screening protocols that we recommend.

Authors' Recommendations

Until clinical evaluation is complete, all trauma patients should be initially treated as if they have a cervical spine injury. This includes supine positioning, the maintenance of cervical collar immobilization, and in-line spinal precautions. If the patient is on a backboard, this should be removed by a log-roll technique as soon as possible.

For screening purposes, patients can be stratified into the following four groups: asymptomatic, alert, sober patients without a distracting injury; symptomatic patients with neck pain, tenderness, or a neurologic deficit; asymptomatic patients who have a temporary change in sensorium, intoxication, or a distracting injury; and obtunded, intubated, or unexaminable patients.

The awake, alert, and asymptomatic patient without a distracting injury may be cleared of cervical spine precautions without radiographs. A simple functional test—having the patient rotate the head 45° to each side in the presence of the examiner—to assess for pain increases the sensitivity of this screening process.

The patient who is symptomatic with neck pain, tenderness, or neurologic symptoms requires maintenance of cervical collar immobilization and radiographic evaluation. This scenario is discussed in chapter 2.

Patients who are asymptomatic and cannot be clinically evaluated at the present time but may have cleared sensorium, sobriety, or treatment of painful distracting injuries within 24 to 48 hours should have continued immobilization in a cervical collar until such time as a reliable clinical evaluation is possible. If the patient remains asymptomatic once the examination is reliable, and a satisfactory range of motion 45° to each side can be performed, then the spine may be cleared. Alternatively, if the patient does not become alert and stabilized from other distracting injuries, they will require diagnostic imaging as described below for the obtunded patient.

The obtunded, intubated, or unexaminable patient presents the greatest diagnostic dilemma for potential cervical spine injury. These patients should be screened radiographically. A cervical MDCT scan with reconstruction views should be performed and plain radiographs can be avoided. If the MDCT and/or plain radiographs are negative for injury, several alternatives are available. The patient can simply be cleared at this point and immobilization and restrictions removed. However, as previously discussed, there are risks of missed injuries with this method. As such, at this stage of the protocol we recommend MRI and/or consultation with a spine surgeon before removal of the cervical collar. A general rule of thumb for the successful and safe clearance of the cervical spine in the obtunded or cognitively compromised patient is to successfully complete the "2/3 rule" as proposed by Simon et al.[52] This rule requires the presence of a negative MDCT and either a normal clinical examination or a negative MRI scan to safely remove the collar.

References

1. Spine and spinal cord trauma, in American College of Surgeons Committee on Trauma: *Advanced Trauma Life Support Program for Doctors: Student Course Manual*, ed 7. Chicago, IL, First Impression Publishing, 2004, pp 177-203.
2. Chendrasekhar A, Moorman DW, Timberlake GA: An evaluation of the effects of semirigid cervical collars in patients with severe closed head injury. *Am Surg* 1998;64(7):604-606.
3. Dodd FM, Simon E, McKeown D, Patrick MR: The effect of a cervical collar on the tidal volume of anaesthetised adult patients. *Anaesthesia* 1995; 50(11):961-963.
4. Davis JW, Phreaner DL, Hoyt DB, Mackersie RC: The etiology of missed cervical spine injuries. *J Trauma* 1993;34(3):342-346.
5. Fazl M, LaFebvre J, Willinsky RA, Gertzbein S: Posttraumatic ligamentous disruption of the cervical spine, an easily overlooked diagnosis: Presentation of three cases. *Neurosurgery* 1990;26(4): 674-678.
6. Gerrelts BD, Petersen EU, Mabry J, Petersen SR: Delayed diagnosis of cervical spine injuries. *J Trauma* 1991;31(12):1622-1626.
7. Webb JK, Broughton RB, McSweeney T, Park WM: Hidden flexion injury of the cervical spine. *J Bone Joint Surg Br* 1976;58(3):322-327.
8. Raphael JH, Chotai R: Effects of the cervical collar on cerebrospinal fluid pressure. *Anaesthesia* 1994; 49(5):437-439.
9. Reid DC, Henderson R, Saboe L, Miller JD: Etiology and clinical course of missed spine fractures. *J Trauma* 1987;27(9):980-986.
10. Stiell IG, Wells GA, Vandemheen K, et al: Variation in emergency department use of cervical spine radiography for alert, stable trauma patients. *CMAJ* 1997;156(11):1537-1544.
11. Levi AD, Hurlbert RJ, Anderson P, et al: Neurologic deterioration secondary to unrecognized spinal instability following trauma—a multicenter study. *Spine (Phila Pa 1976)* 2006;31(4):451-458.
12. Gonzalez RP, Fried PO, Bukhalo M, Holevar MR, Falimirski ME: Role of clinical examination in screening for blunt cervical spine injury. *J Am Coll Surg* 1999;189(2):152-157.
13. Brown CV, Antevil JL, Sise MJ, Sack DI: Spiral computed tomography for the diagnosis of cervical, thoracic, and lumbar spine fractures: Its time has come. *J Trauma* 2005;58(5):890-896.
14. McCulloch PT, France J, Jones DL, et al: Helical computed tomography alone compared with plain radiographs with adjunct computed tomography to evaluate the cervical spine after high-energy trauma. *J Bone Joint Surg Am* 2005;87(11): 2388-2394.
15. Grogan EL, Morris JA Jr, Dittus RS, et al: Cervical spine evaluation in urban trauma centers: Lowering institutional costs and complications through helical CT scan. *J Am Coll Surg* 2005;200(2):160-165.
16. Berry GE, Adams S, Harris MB, et al: Are plain radiographs of the spine necessary during evaluation after blunt trauma? Accuracy of screening torso computed tomography in thoracic/lumbar spine fracture diagnosis. *J Trauma* 2005;59(6): 1410-1413.
17. Blacksin MF, Lee HJ: Frequency and significance of fractures of the upper cervical spine detected by CT in patients with severe neck trauma. *AJR Am J Roentgenol* 1995;165(5):1201-1204.
18. Schleehauf K, Ross SE, Civil ID, Schwab CW: Computed tomography in the initial evaluation of the cervical spine. *Ann Emerg Med* 1989;18(8): 815-817.
19. Tehranzadeh J, Bonk RT, Ansari A, Mesgarzadeh M: Efficacy of limited CT for nonvisualized lower cervical spine in patients with blunt trauma. *Skeletal Radiol* 1994;23(5):349-352.
20. Vaccaro AR, Kreidl KO, Pan W, Cotler JM, Schweitzer ME: Usefulness of MRI in isolated upper cervical spine fractures in adults. *J Spinal Disord* 1998;11(4):289-294.
21. Muchow RD, Resnick DK, Abdel MP, Munoz A, Anderson PA: Magnetic resonance imaging (MRI) in the clearance of the cervical spine in blunt trauma: A meta-analysis. *J Trauma* 2008;64(1): 179-189.
22. Albrecht RM, Kingsley D, Schermer CR, Demarest GB, Benzel EC, Hart BL: Evaluation of cervical spine in intensive care patients following blunt trauma. *World J Surg* 2001;25(8):1089-1096.
23. Benzel EC, Hart BL, Ball PA, Baldwin NG, Orrison WW, Espinosa MC: Magnetic resonance imaging for the evaluation of patients with occult cervical spine injury. *J Neurosurg* 1996;85(5): 824-829.

24. D'Alise MD, Benzel EC, Hart BL: Magnetic resonance imaging evaluation of the cervical spine in the comatose or obtunded trauma patient. *J Neurosurg* 1999;91(1, Suppl)54-59.

25. Keiper MD, Zimmerman RA, Bilaniuk LT: MRI in the assessment of the supportive soft tissues of the cervical spine in acute trauma in children. *Neuroradiology* 1998;40(6):359-363.

26. Schuster R, Waxman K, Sanchez B, et al: Magnetic resonance imaging is not needed to clear cervical spines in blunt trauma patients with normal computed tomographic results and no motor deficits. *Arch Surg* 2005;140(8):762-766.

27. Harris MB, Shilt J: The potentially unstable cervical spine: Evaluation and techniques. *Tech Orthop* 2002;17(3):278-286.

28. Green RA, Saifuddin A: Whole spine MRI in the assessment of acute vertebral body trauma. *Skeletal Radiol* 2004;33(3):129-135.

29. Hogan GJ, Mirvis SE, Shanmuganathan K, Scalea TM: Exclusion of unstable cervical spine injury in obtunded patients with blunt trauma: Is MR imaging needed when multi-detector row CT findings are normal? *Radiology* 2005;237(1):106-113.

30. Morris CG, McCoy E: Clearing the cervical spine in unconscious polytrauma victims, balancing risks and effective screening. *Anaesthesia* 2004;59(5):464-482.

31. Geusens E, Van Breuseghem I, Pans S, Brys R: Some tips and tricks in reading cervical spine radiographs in trauma patients. *JBR-BTR* 2005;88(2):87-92.

32. Harris MB, Kronlage SC, Carboni PA, et al: Evaluation of the cervical spine in the polytrauma patient. *Spine (Phila Pa 1976)* 2000;25(22):2884-2892.

33. Sees DW, Rodriguez Cruz LR, Flaherty SF, Ciceri DP: The use of bedside fluoroscopy to evaluate the cervical spine in obtunded trauma patients. *J Trauma* 1998;45(4):768-771.

34. Anglen J, Metzler M, Bunn P, Griffiths H: Flexion and extension views are not cost-effective in a cervical spine clearance protocol for obtunded trauma patients. *J Trauma* 2002;52(1):54-59.

35. Bolinger B, Shartz M, Marion D: Bedside fluoroscopic flexion and extension cervical spine radiographs for clearance of the cervical spine in comatose trauma patients. *J Trauma* 2004;56(1):132-136.

36. Sliker CW, Mirvis SE, Shanmuganathan K: Assessing cervical spine stability in obtunded blunt trauma patients: Review of medical literature. *Radiology* 2005;234(3):733-739.

37. Hoffman JR, Wolfson AB, Todd K, Mower WR: Selective cervical spine radiography in blunt trauma: Methodology of the National Emergency X-Radiography Utilization Study (NEXUS). *Ann Emerg Med* 1998;32(4):461-469.

38. Hoffman JR, Mower WR, Wolfson AB, Todd KH, Zucker MI, National Emergency X-Radiography Utilization Study Group: Validity of a set of clinical criteria to rule out injury to the cervical spine in patients with blunt trauma. *N Engl J Med* 2000;343(2):94-99.

39. Stiell IG, Wells GA, Vandemheen KL, et al: The Canadian C-spine rule for radiography in alert and stable trauma patients. *JAMA* 2001;286(15):1841-1848.

40. Stiell IG, Clement CM, McKnight RD, et al: The Canadian C-spine rule versus the NEXUS low-risk criteria in patients with trauma. *N Engl J Med* 2003;349(26):2510-2518.

41. Anderson PA, Muchow RD, Munoz A, Tontz WL, Resnick DK: Clearance of the asymptomatic cervical spine: A meta-analysis. *J Orthop Trauma* 2010;24(2):100-106.

42. Pasquale M, Fabian TC: Practice management guidelines for trauma from the Eastern Association for the Surgery of Trauma. *J Trauma* 1998;44(6):941-957.

43. Hadley MN, Walters BC, Grabb PA, et al: Guidelines for the management of acute cervical spine and spinal cord injuries. *Clin Neurosurg* 2002;49:407-498.

44. Como JJ, Diaz JJ, Dunham CM, et al: Practice management guidelines for identification of cervical spine injuries following trauma: Update from the eastern association for the surgery of trauma practice management guidelines committee. *J Trauma* 2009;67(3):651-659.

45. Davis JW, Parks SN, Detlefs CL, Williams GG, Williams JL, Smith RW: Clearing the cervical spine in obtunded patients: The use of dynamic fluoroscopy. *J Trauma* 1995;39(3):435-438.

46. Budorick TE, Anderson PA, Rivara FP, Cohen W: Flexion-distraction fracture of the cervical spine: A case report. *J Bone Joint Surg Am* 1991;73(7):1097-1100.

47. Ralston ME, Chung K, Barnes PD, Emans JB, Schutzman SA: Role of flexion-extension radiographs in blunt pediatric cervical spine injury. *Acad Emerg Med* 2001;8(3):237-245.

48. Emery SE, Pathria MN, Wilber RG, Masaryk T, Bohlman HH: Magnetic resonance imaging of posttraumatic spinal ligament injury. *J Spinal Disord* 1989;2(4):229-233.

49. Katzberg RW, Benedetti PF, Drake CM, et al: Acute cervical spine injuries: Prospective MR imaging assessment at a level 1 trauma center. *Radiology* 1999;213(1):203-212.

50. Crim JR, Tripp D: Multidetector CT of the spine. *Semin Ultrasound CT MR* 2004;25(1):55-66.

51. Stelfox HT, Velmahos GC, Gettings E, Bigatello LM, Schmidt U: Computed tomography for early and safe discontinuation of cervical spine immobilization in obtunded multiply injured patients. *J Trauma* 2007;63(3):630-636.

52. Simon JB, Schoenfeld AJ, Katz JN, et al: Are "normal" multidetector computed tomographic scans sufficient to allow collar removal in the trauma patient? *J Trauma* 2010;68(1):103-108.

53. Como JJ, Thompson MA, Anderson JS, et al: Is magnetic resonance imaging essential in clearing the cervical spine in obtunded patients with blunt trauma? *J Trauma* 2007;63(3):544-549.

54. Schoenfeld AJ, Bono CM, McGuire KJ, Warholic N, Harris MB: Computed tomography alone versus computed tomography and magnetic resonance imaging in the identification of occult injuries to the cervical spine: A meta-analysis. *J Trauma* 2010;68(1):109-114.

55. Sarani B, Waring S, Sonnad S, Schwab CW: Magnetic resonance imaging is a useful adjunct in the evaluation of the cervical spine of injured patients. *J Trauma* 2007;63(3):637-640.

56. Brandenstein D, Molinari RW, Rubery PT, Rechtine GR II: Unstable subaxial cervical spine injury with normal computed tomography and magnetic resonance initial imaging studies: A report of four cases and review of the literature. *Spine (Phila Pa 1976)* 2009;34(20):E743-E750.

57. Smith-Bindman R, Lipson J, Marcus R, et al: Radiation dose associated with common computed tomography examinations and the associated lifetime attributable risk of cancer. *Arch Intern Med* 2009;169(22):2078-2086.

CHAPTER 6
Pharmacologic Treatments for Spinal Cord Injury

Michelle T.L. Ng, BSc   Brian K. Kwon, MD, PhD, FRCSC

Introduction

Spinal cord injury (SCI) is one of the most physically and psychologically devastating injuries one can suffer. Despite decades of intense research effort, robust therapeutic treatments of this catastrophic condition remain elusive. Many promising experimental therapeutic treatments that have shown encouraging results in animal models of SCI have failed to produce significant neurologic improvements for patients when evaluated in human clinical trials.[1,2] The appreciation for the complexity of SCI pathophysiology that has emerged over the past few decades of study has led to the belief that a multifaceted, interdisciplinary combination of strategies will be necessary to treat the paralysis resulting from SCIs. Such strategies will be aimed at minimizing secondary damage, stimulating axonal regeneration, and promoting plasticity of residual neural tissue.

This chapter will focus on pharmacologic treatments of SCI. First, it will review treatments that have previously been studied in clinical trials. Second, it will discuss emerging drug therapies that have either begun clinical testing, or may soon initiate human trials.

Previously Evaluated Pharmacologic Therapies

Methylprednisolone Sodium Succinate

Methylprednisolone sodium succinate (MPSS) remains the most extensively studied pharmacologic treatment of SCI. Steroids have long been used in neurologic disorders, and the neuroprotective properties of MPSS are thought to include inhibition of lipid peroxidation, modulation of the inflammatory response, reduction of spinal cord edema with improved perfusion, and prevention of calcium influx.[3,4] Three landmark, multicenter human clinical trials of MPSS for acute SCI were conducted in the 1980s and 1990s.[5-10] The first National Acute Spinal Cord Injury Study (NASCIS 1) randomized 330 patients to either 100 mg or 1,000 mg of MPSS.[5] No control group was included, as the assumed benefits of steroids made it seem unethical to randomize patients to receive a placebo.[6] The failure to demonstrate a significant neurologic improvement was attributed to the dose of MPSS, which was deemed in subsequent laboratory studies to be too low to reach therapeutic levels.[11] Thus, NASCIS 2 was initiated to test the efficacy of high doses of MPSS.[7] NASCIS 2 randomized 487 patients to MPSS (30-mg/kg bolus followed by 5.4 mg/kg/h for 23 hours), naloxone (an opioid antagonist), or placebo, within 24 hours of injury. In the primary analysis of all randomized patients, MPSS did not confer any neurologic benefit. However, in a small subset of patients who received treatment within 8 hours of injury (MPSS n = 65, placebo n = 62), there was a significant improvement with MPSS.[7] This study was the first ever to suggest that a pharmacologic treatment might change the neurologic outcome of SCI. The subsequent NASCIS 3 study evaluated whether extending the MPSS infusion to 48 hours might be beneficial.[9] A total of 499 patients within 8 hours of injury were randomized to either a 23- or 47-hour MPSS infusion of 5.4 mg/kg/h (after the initial 30-mg/kg bolus), or to tirilazad mesylate, a 21-aminosteroid.[9] Again, the primary outcome analysis of all randomized patients revealed no significant differences, and only the post hoc analyses revealed a small functional benefit in those who received the 48-hour infusion between 3 and 8 hours of injury.[9,10] The extended infusion of MPSS was also associated with increases in wound infection, gastrointestinal hemorrhage, sepsis, pulmonary embolism, and death.[12]

The NASCIS trials (NASCIS 2 in particular) made MPSS the "standard of care" for patients with acute SCI. Intense criticism has subsequently been leveled at the NASCIS trials, pointing out flaws in both the methodology and the

Dr. Kwon or an immediate family member serves as a paid consultant to or is an employee of Medtronic Sofamor Danek. Neither Ms. Ng nor any immediate family member has received anything of value from or owns stock in a commercial company or institution related directly or indirectly to the subject of this chapter.

interpretation of these studies, the small (if any) therapeutic effect, and the rate of adverse events.[12-14] Extensive reviews of the MPSS literature have concluded that it should not be considered a "standard of care," but rather a "treatment option" only.[15] Many Canadian surgeons have since abandoned it,[16] while many American physicians continue to administer it out of fear of litigation.[17] Of interest, a recent systematic review of the preclinical literature on MPSS in animal models of SCI has revealed that the majority of published studies (58%) reported no beneficial effects with MPSS.[18]

Tirilazad Mesylate

Tirilazad mesylate (TM) is noteworthy from a historical perspective because it was tested alongside MPSS in the NASCIS 3 clinical trial. TM is a synthetic 21-aminosteroid that has antioxidant effects similar to MPSS but without glucocorticoid activity and immunologic and metabolic effects.[19-21] TM has antioxidant properties and protects the integrity of cell membranes by scavenging free radicals and limiting lipid peroxidation.[22,23] The TM-treated group (n = 166) in NASCIS 3 was shown to be comparably effective as the 24-hour regimen of MPSS.[9] However, the interpretation of these data is made difficult by the absence of a placebo arm in NASCIS 3, and conclusions regarding the efficacy of TM are reliant on the contentious assumption that MPSS treatment was indeed superior to placebo in NASCIS 2. However, lower complication rates in the TM-treated versus MPSS-treated groups suggest that TM's lack of glucocorticoid effect indeed has some therapeutic value. To our knowledge, no further development of this drug has occurred since the NASCIS 3 study.

Naloxone

Like tirilazad mesylate, naloxone holds some historical significance, as it was evaluated alongside MPSS in the NASCIS 2 study. Naloxone is a nonspecific opioid receptor antagonist, which has been shown in various animal studies to improve spinal cord blood flow,[24] reduce edema,[25,26] and inhibit production of reactive oxygen species,[27] with associated functional and electrophysiologic outcomes.[26,28] After SCI, a marked increase in the endogenous opiate, dynorphin A, and opioid receptor activation has been implicated in the propagation of secondary injury,[29] thus rationalizing the application of opioid antagonists such as naloxone. In the NASCIS 2 study, initial analysis suggested no therapeutic benefits of naloxone over placebo,[7] but a post hoc analysis indicated some benefit when applied within 8 hours of injury.[30] To our knowledge, no further development of naloxone as a therapeutic agent for SCI has occurred since the NASCIS 2 study.

GM-1 Ganglioside

Gangliosides are complex sialic acid–containing glycosphingolipids abundant in the outer cell membrane of central nervous system tissue. GM-1 ganglioside has been reported to decrease edema,[31] increase neurite outgrowth,[32] and inhibit excitotoxicity[33] and apoptosis after brain injury or SCI.[34,35] A small, prospective randomized placebo-controlled study of 37 patients conducted in Maryland reported beneficial effects of GM-1 ganglioside even when treatment did not commence until 48 hours after SCI.[34] These promising results prompted the initiation of the largest prospective randomized clinical trial in SCI to date.[34-36] The Sygen multicenter acute SCI study (Fidia Pharmaceutical Corporation, Abano Terme, Italy) investigated the effects of GM-1 in patients treated with the NASCIS 2 MPSS regimen followed by either placebo, low-dose GM-1, or high-dose GM-1 (n = 797, 300-mg bolus and 100 mg/d or 600-mg bolus and 200 mg/d for 56 days).[36] Like the previous NASCIS studies, the primary outcome measure of GM-1 was negative. However, promising trends were observed in recovery rate, motor and sensory scores, and bowel and bladder function in incomplete SCI patients compared to placebo.[36] Despite these improvements in important secondary outcome measures, US Food and Drug Administration (FDA) approval was not granted because of the failure to achieve a significant improvement on the primary outcome, which was based on two-level improvements on a modified American Spinal Injury Association (ASIA) impairment scale at 26 weeks after injury. No further development of Sygen as a neuroprotective agent has since occurred. Importantly, however, the data on spontaneous neurologic recovery from the Sygen trial have been extensively used to provide guidelines for further study design of clinical trials.[37]

Nimodipine

Excessive intracellular calcium is known to be a mediator of excitotoxic damage, and holds a crucial role in the activation of calpains resulting in apoptotic cell death.[38] Inhibiting such intracellular calcium influx therefore has great rationale as a neuroprotective strategy. Nimodipine is an L-type calcium channel antagonist that has been shown in *in vivo* studies to enhance spinal cord blood flow and reverse spinal cord hypoperfusion.[39] Subsequent animal models have reported no significant improvement in neurologic recovery when nimodipine was administered after SCI.[40] Nonetheless, a human clinical trial was initiated in France (n = 106, 0.15 mg/kg/h for 2 hours, then 0.03 mg/kg/h for 7 days), which tested the efficacy of nimodipine with or without MPSS (NASCIS 2 regimen) versus placebo. This study failed to show significant neurologic benefits, although it was likely underpowered to do so.[41,42] Furthermore, one of the challenges for calcium channel blockade as a therapeutic strategy is the assumption that calcium influx starts very soon after injury, making for a very limited window of opportunity for neuroprotective intervention.[43] This consideration of the narrow time window for intervention is likely to be applicable to most neuroprotective strategies.

Gacyclidine

Gacyclidine or GK-11 (Beaufour-Ipsen Pharma, Paris, France) is a noncompetitive N-methyl-D-aspartic acid (NMDA) receptor antagonist. Overactivation of NMDA receptors due to excess glutamate released after SCI can also result in massive calcium influx and "excitotoxicity" leading to cell death. Gacyclidine has been reported to be neuroprotective in several animal studies, with reduced lesion size and improved functional outcome in a dose-dependent manner.[44-46] These promising animal data encouraged researchers in France to initiate a randomized placebo-controlled trial of gacyclidine in acute SCI patients (n = 280). Although preliminary data were optimistic,[47] this trial unfortunately failed to show any neurologic benefit with gacyclidine at the 1-year end point.[48] In retrospect, the multiple treatment arms in this trial limited the number of patients for analysis and sufficient statistical power to demonstrate a benefit was not reached. Gacyclidine was last reported in a prospective, randomized placebo-controlled study aimed at improving neurologic and functional recovery after acute traumatic brain injury.[49]

Fampridine

Fampridine is included here in this chapter as a "pharmacologic intervention for SCI," but differs importantly from the other agents because it has been developed not as an acute neuroprotective intervention, but rather as a treatment to enhance function in chronic SCI. Fampridine (4-aminopyridine) is a voltage-gated potassium channel antagonist that enhances electrophysiologic conduction across demyelinated axon nodes, and improves neuroneural and neuromuscular transmission.[50,51] Promising animal data led to human clinical trials for the use of fampridine in the treatment of chronic SCI. Because of the proposed mechanism of action, the use of fampridine appeared to be most justified for patients with incomplete SCI, where there would presumably be more axons in continuity across the injury site, but with inefficient conduction due to demyelination.[52,53] Although no significant improvements in motor and sensory scores were found across all patients,[52,53] significant increases in important qualitative clinical observations such as patient satisfaction and quality-of-life scores were reported.[52] Further studies have been conducted on the safety and efficacy of sustained release (SR) fampridine in chronic SCI patients.[54-57] Although significant functional improvements have been reported in motor function, sensation, and independence, mild (nausea, dry mouth) to moderate (posterior tibial artery vasospasm) adverse side effects were also reported in the same study.[55]

SR fampridine has recently completed a phase III clinical trial for multiple sclerosis, showing improved walking ability of some patients,[58] and is expected to be released in March 2010 by Acorda Therapeutics, New York, New York as AMPRYA.

Thyrotropin-Releasing Hormone

Aside from its obvious hormonal effects, thyrotropin-releasing hormone (TRH) has also been reported to antagonize various secondary injury mediators after SCI, such as excitotoxic amino acids, peptidoleukotrienes, endogenous opioids, and platelet-activating factor, all contributing to the prevention of lipid peroxidation after SCI.[59,60] It also has potent systemic metabolic effects to help maintain blood pressure, blood flow, and body temperature.[61] *In vivo* studies in the use of TRH after SCI have reported significant neurologic benefits, even when treatment was initiated 7 days after injury.[62,63] In light of the beneficial therapeutic effects shown in animal studies, a small clinical trial of 20 patients was conducted to test the efficacy of TRH in complete and incomplete SCI patients who received a 0.2-mg/kg intravenous bolus followed by 0.2 mg/kg/h for 6 hours.[64] Although the 4-month follow-up revealed promising results with improvements in motor, sensory, and the Sunnybrook score for incomplete SCI patients, further investigation was discontinued due to high patient default rates in the 1-year follow-up.[64]

TABLE 1

Previously Evaluated Pharmacologic Therapies for the Treatment of SCI

Therapy	Logic/Mechanism of Action	Results
Methylprednisolone	Corticosteroid/anti-inflammatory, antioxidant, inhibit lipid peroxidation, reduce edema, improve blood flow, prevent calcium influx	NASCIS 1-3, no significant neurologic recovery in primary analysis[5-10]
Tirilazad mesylate	Aminosteroid/antioxidant, membrane protection by scavenging free radicals	NASCIS 3, as effective as MPSS with lower complication rates[9,10]
Naloxone	Opioid receptor antagonist/reduce edema, improve blood flow, inhibit reactive oxygen species production	NASCIS 2, no significant therapeutic benefits versus placebo[7,8]
GM-1 ganglioside (Sygen)	Glycosphingolipid/decrease edema, increase neurite growth, inhibit excitotoxicity, antiapoptosis	GM-1 Maryland, beneficial effects Sygen multicenter acute SCI trial, negative primary outcome measure (ASIA grade) but with promising trends[34,36]
Nimodipine	L-type calcium channel antagonist/inhibit calcium influx, enhance blood flow, reverse hypoperfusion	Nimodipine with or without MPSS versus placebo, no significant neurologic benefit[41,42]
Gacyclidine	NMDA receptor antagonist/limit glutamate excitotoxicity, inhibit calcium influx, antiapoptosis	GK-11 versus placebo, no significant neurologic benefit at 1-year outcome[47,48]
Fampridine	Voltage-gated potassium channel antagonist/stimulate axonal electrophysiological signals across demyelinated axon nodes, enhance synaptic transmission	Sustained release fampridine versus placebo in chronic SCI[52-57,64]
Thyrotropin-releasing hormone	Pituitary hormone/antagonize excitotoxic amino acids, peptidoleukotrienes, endogenous opioids, and platelet-activating factor to prevent lipid peroxidation	TRH versus placebo in complete and incomplete SCI, promising data at 4 months, discontinued due to patient default[64]

Summary of Previously Evaluated Pharmacologic Agents (Table 1)

The past clinical trials in SCI that have evaluated methylprednisolone, GM-1 ganglioside, naloxone, tirilazad mesylate, TRH, nimodipine, gacyclidine, and fampridine have unfortunately failed to establish and validate a convincingly efficacious pharmacologic treatment of SCI. Important lessons have been learned, however. We understand now that it is unlikely that any specific neuroprotective drug will be a "magic bullet," and that "significant improvements" will likely be measured in terms of relatively small gains in motor/sensory function in a modest number of patients. Additionally, we understand much better now (from large trials such as the Sygen multicenter study) the vexing extent of variability in spontaneous neurologic recovery—particularly in patients assessed very early after injury. These two issues—the anticipation of a relatively small effect size and the recognition of high variability in spontaneous neurologic recovery—mandate that fairly large numbers of patients be enrolled in clinical trials. The converse is true as well, which is why small clinical trials will be highly unlikely to demonstrate significant improvements with the therapy in question, as exemplified by the clinical trials of TRH, nimodipine, and even gacyclidine. An analysis of the GM-1 ganglioside trial has provided the field with important statistical guidance regarding the numbers of patients required to recruit, given different anticipated effect sizes.[37] Such guidance is invaluable in planning subsequent clinical trials. Additionally, the fact that some agents have shown promise in animal models and not in human studies speaks to the disquieting possibility that important biologic differences exist between these two conditions.

TABLE 2

Pharmacologic Therapies Currently Under Investigation for the Treatment of SCI

Therapy	Logic/Mechanism of Action	Current Use/Status of Ongoing Clinical Trials
Minocycline	Tetracycline antibiotic/antioxidant, antiapoptosis, inhibit excitotoxicity and inflammatory mediators	Treatment of acne and chronic peritonitis. Phase I/II pilot study for SCI in Calgary, Alberta, Canada now complete.
Riluzole	Voltage-gated sodium channel antagonist/decrease intracellular sodium and calcium, inhibit glutamate release	Treatment of ALS. Phase IIa clinical trial for acute SCI sponsored by the North American Clinical Trials Network is currently recruiting participants.
Erythropoietin	Hematopoietic growth factor/anti-inflammatory, antioxidant, antiapoptosis, limits lipid peroxidation	Treatment of anemia. Phase III clinical trial for traumatic SCI in Milan, Italy.
Magnesium	NMDA receptor blockade	Treatment of pre-eclampsia and cardiac arrest. Phase I safety study complete, phase II clinical trial has received FDA approval but has not yet started.

Pharmacologic Therapies Currently Under Investigation for Treatment of SCI (Table 2)

Minocycline

Another prominent strategy against secondary damage after SCI is to limit the neuroinflammatory response that occurs after injury. Minocycline is a broad-spectrum tetracycline antibiotic that can inhibit bacterial protein synthesis and is used for the treatment of acne and chronic periodontitis.[65] More recently, it has been shown to promote neuroprotection in Parkinson disease,[66,67] multiple sclerosis,[66] amyotrophic lateral sclerosis (ALS),[68] and cerebral ischemia.[69] It has been postulated that minocycline exerts its effects by a combination of increasing interleukin-10 while decreasing tumor necrosis factor–α expression, to prevent the exacerbation of secondary injury.[70,71] Minocycline inhibits excitotoxicity, oxidative stress, both caspase-dependent and caspase-independent apoptotic pathways, and inflammatory mediators released by activated microglia.[71] Furthermore, it has been shown to reduce microglial activation and decrease tissue damage, lesion size, and apoptosis at the injury site, resulting in improved functional outcome.[70,72]

These promising results from animal studies prompted investigators in Calgary, Alberta, Canada, to initiate a prospective randomized controlled pilot study of intravenous minocycline in acute SCI patients. The study has now been completed, with 52 patients (both cervical and thoracic complete and incomplete SCI) enrolled. At the time of this writing, the results of this trial have not been published, although the suggestion of trends toward neurologic benefit in minocycline-treated patients has prompted the investigators to propose a definitive, multicenter study.

Erythropoietin

Erythropoietin (EPO) is a glycoprotein hormone involved in survival, differentiation, and proliferation of erythroid progenitor cells.[73] It is a hematopoietic growth factor that has been reported to also have anti-inflammatory, antioxidant, and antiapoptotic properties.[74] EPO initiates tissue protective strategies in response to hypoxia by upregulating the production of red blood cells.[74] EPO is used as a treatment of anemia due to chemotherapy, chronic renal failure, and autologous blood donations,[75] and has also been studied extensively in animal models of multiple sclerosis, Parkinson disease, myocardial infarction, stroke, and SCI.[65,76] Of interest, one study reported both neurologic and histologic improvements in experimental stroke in rats following an injection of recombinant human EPO (rhEPO),[77] prompting a small phase I/IIa clinical study evaluating EPO administration after acute stroke.[78] This pilot study reported the safety and efficacy of rhEPO in reducing infarct size and improving clinical outcome when compared with placebo,[78] while a subsequent phase II/III clinical trial suggested no significant beneficial effects of rhEPO but raised safety concerns for the use of systemic thrombolytic agents, an established treatment of acute stroke.[78,79]

Several investigators have reported that intravenous and subcutaneous administration of EPO in animal models of SCI promotes tissue protection and improves locomotor performance when compared with controls.[80-84] Furthermore, EPO has shown superior anti-lipid peroxidation properties when compared with MPSS treatment using the NASCIS 2 regimen *in vivo*.[85] Interestingly, one study reported that rats receiving lower doses of EPO achieved a greater improvement in functional outcome than those receiving higher doses.[82] This is possibly due to the fact that EPO-induced increases in hematocrit may exacerbate secondary injury after SCI as well as other detrimental effects caused by prolonged elevation of the hematocrit.[86] This has prompted the development of synthetic EPO derivatives devoid of erythrogenic properties to avoid this problem. Such derivatives have shown neuroprotective promise in animal models of stroke, peripheral neuropathy, and SCI.[47,87,88]

Some of the original preclinical work on EPO in SCI was performed in Italy,[80,81,84,89] and this has prompted the initiation of an Italian phase III multicenter prospective randomized clinical trial of MPSS versus EPO in patients with ASIA A or B SCI. At the time of this writing, a total of 14 patients have been enrolled in this trial.

Riluzole

Riluzole (or Rilutek, Sanofi-Aventis, Laval, Quebec, Canada) is a benzothiazole anticonvulsant currently FDA-approved for the treatment of ALS.[90] It is a potent antagonist of voltage-sensitive sodium channels, and thus is postulated to attenuate secondary damage by decreasing intracellular sodium,[91] and inhibiting presynaptic calcium-dependent glutamate release.[92] The approach of using riluzole or other sodium channel blockers has been shown to be neuroprotective in animal models of SCI, increasing both spared white and gray matter,[91] and improving locomotor function.[93] It has been reported to be neuroprotective of motor neurons in a model of anterior root avulsion.[94]

The North American Clinical Trials Network has planned a small phase IIa multicenter study to evaluate the safety and pharmacokinetics of orally administered riluzole in traumatic SCI. At the time of this writing, this study is actively recruiting participants.

Magnesium

Magnesium is a physiologic antagonist of NMDA receptors. It is currently used as a treatment of many conditions, such as preeclampsia, cardiac arrest, severe asthma, and migraine.[95] The administration of magnesium as a neuroprotective agent has been reported to attenuate excitotoxicity by limiting free radical production and glutamate release, and reducing apoptosis.[96] Magnesium depletion after brain injury has been postulated to exacerbate secondary damage.[97] It has been found that magnesium (in the form of magnesium sulfate or magnesium chloride) pretreatment or administration after experimental traumatic brain injury has led to improved functional outcome and an improved cellular bioenergetic state in a dose-dependent manner.[97,98] Its potential neuroprotective effects have recently been evaluated in clinical studies in acute stroke, with no significant effect in reducing the occurrence of death or disability after magnesium treatment.[99] A randomized clinical trial of magnesium sulfate in traumatic brain injury reported no benefit, and rather a higher mortality rate in magnesium-treated patients—indicating that despite a long track record of clinical safety, deviating from this to administer extremely high doses of magnesium is dangerous (and ineffective).[100]

Studies on the efficacy of magnesium after SCI in animal models have found that a high-dose magnesium administration after SCI resulted in a significant improvement in functional recovery as well as a significant reduction in apoptosis and lipid peroxidation.[101] To translate this to human SCI, a combination of magnesium with polyethylene glycol has been developed. This has been shown to promote neuroprotection in an acute SCI model,[102] and has allowed for much lower doses of magnesium to be administered.[103] This combination has been also found to be effective in an animal model of cervical SCI.[104] A phase I safety study of healthy human volunteers has been concluded on this magnesium–polyethylene glycol formulation (NeuroShield; Medtronic, Minneapolis, MN), and a phase II study in cervical SCI patients has received FDA approval to proceed. At the time of this writing, this clinical trial in SCI patients had not been initiated.

Pharmacologic Therapies With High Translational Potential for Treatment of SCI (Table 3)

In addition to the drugs that have entered into clinical trials, there are others that are being ac-

TABLE 3

Pharmacologic Therapies With High Translational Potential for the Treatment of SCI

Therapy	Logic/Mechanism of Action	Current Use
NSAIDs	Anti-inflammatory, inhibit cyclo-oxygenase	Analgesic agent
Statins	Anti-inflammatory, modulate immune response	Treatment of hypercholesterolemia

tively explored because of their long-standing track record for safety in human patients. The fact that clinically used compounds may also have potential neuroprotective properties introduces the possibility for such therapies to enter clinical trials with fewer safety concerns. Minocycline, riluzole, erythropoietin, and magnesium are all good examples of this, although the magnesium–polyethylene glycol combination had never been used in humans before (and hence, the phase I study in healthy human volunteers). Other drugs of a similar nature include ibuprofen and the statins.

Nonsteroidal Anti-Inflammatory Drugs

Cyclo-oxygenases COX-1 and COX-2 have been reported to be significantly upregulated after SCI to mediate inflammatory prostaglandins.[105,106] Many commercial nonsteroidal anti-inflammatory drugs (NSAIDs) such as ibuprofen, naproxen, and celecoxib exert their effects via the inhibition of cyclo-oxygenases to relieve pain and inflammation. The use of NSAIDs in animal models of SCI has been suggested to be beneficial in reducing prostaglandin-mediated inflammation and maintaining normal spinal cord blood flow after trauma.[107] Recently, the implication of ibuprofen as a proregeneration agent via the inhibition of the RhoA pathway and its effectiveness in chronic SCI models *in vivo* has renewed the interest in the development of NSAIDs as a pharmacologic treatment of chronic SCI.[108,109] Furthermore, ibuprofen has been reported to have significant histologic and neurologic benefits in animal models of SCI even when administered 3[110] or 7[108] days after injury, making it a more relevant potential therapy for clinical situations.

Statins

Statins are a group of drugs that have long been used in lowering cholesterol. They inhibit HMG-CoA reductase activity, which is required for the synthesis of cholesterol.[111] More recently, statins have also been recognized to have anti-inflammatory and immunomodulatory properties by increasing eNOS expression while suppressing expression of several inflammatory cytokines.[112,113] Recent studies investigating the role of atorvastatin in rats after SCI have reported significant reduction in inflammatory cytokines, Rho activity, glial fibrillary acidic protein (GFAP) expression (representing reactive astrogliosis), caspase-3 activation, and neuronal and oligodendrocyte apoptosis.[114,115] Increased tissue-sparing and locomotor recovery over control animals was also reported, although these findings could not be repeated in a subsequent study comparing the efficacy of atorvastatin and simvastatin.[112] Nevertheless, because many statins are already commercially available, the development of a statin as a pharmacologic treatment of SCI appears to be an attractive option if their neuroprotective properties can be more conclusively confirmed.

Summary of Current Ongoing Clinical Trials and Pharmacologic Agents With High Translational Potential

The few highlighted ongoing clinical trials investigating minocycline, riluzole, erythropoietin, and magnesium hold promise that at least one of these treatments will successfully make the translation from bench to bedside for the treatment of SCI. Furthermore, many more pharmacologic agents such as NSAIDs and the statins are currently undergoing preclinical evaluation. The reality that biologic differences exist between the pathophysiology of animal and human SCI will be one hurdle for researchers to overcome. Nonetheless, it is now widely accepted that any neuroprotective strategy to alleviate secondary injury mechanisms or any small gains of axonal conduction from regeneration strategies may yield functionally relevant neurologic recovery that will improve the lives of SCI patients tremendously. A model using a larger animal with greater anatomic and biophysiologic similarities to humans or a more objective prediction model using biomarkers could help to stratify preclinical results and facilitate a successful translation from bench to bedside.

References

1. Tator CH: Review of treatment trials in human spinal cord injury: Issues, difficulties, and recommendations. *Neurosurgery* 2006;59(5):957-987.
2. Hawryluk GW, Rowland J, Kwon BK, Fehlings MG: Protection and repair of the injured spinal cord: A review of completed, ongoing, and planned clinical trials for acute spinal cord injury. *Neurosurg Focus* 2008;25(5):E14.
3. Hall ED, Braughler JM: Glucocorticoid mechanisms in acute spinal cord injury: A review and therapeutic rationale. *Surg Neurol* 1982;18(5): 320-327.
4. Ducker TB, Zeidman SM: Spinal cord injury: Role of steroid therapy. *Spine (Phila Pa 1976)* 1994; 19(20):2281-2287.
5. Bracken MB, Collins WF, Freeman DF, et al: Efficacy of methylprednisolone in acute spinal cord injury. *JAMA* 1984;251(1):45-52.
6. Bracken MB, Shepard MJ, Hellenbrand KG, et al: Methylprednisolone and neurological function 1 year after spinal cord injury: Results of the National Acute Spinal Cord Injury Study. *J Neurosurg* 1985;63(5):704-713.
7. Bracken MB, Shepard MJ, Collins WF, et al: A randomized, controlled trial of methylprednisolone or naloxone in the treatment of acute spinal-cord injury: Results of the Second National Acute Spinal Cord Injury Study. *N Engl J Med* 1990; 322(20):1405-1411.
8. Bracken MB, Shepard MJ, Collins WF Jr, et al: Methylprednisolone or naloxone treatment after acute spinal cord injury: 1-year follow-up data. Results of the second National Acute Spinal Cord Injury Study. *J Neurosurg* 1992;76(1):23-31.
9. Bracken MB, Shepard MJ, Holford TR, et al: Administration of methylprednisolone for 24 or 48 hours or tirilazad mesylate for 48 hours in the treatment of acute spinal cord injury: Results of the Third National Acute Spinal Cord Injury Randomized Controlled Trial. National Acute Spinal Cord Injury Study. *JAMA* 1997;277(20): 1597-1604.
10. Bracken MB, Shepard MJ, Holford TR, et al: Methylprednisolone or tirilazad mesylate administration after acute spinal cord injury: 1-year follow up. Results of the third National Acute Spinal Cord Injury randomized controlled trial. *J Neurosurg* 1998;89(5):699-706.
11. Braughler JM, Hall ED: Correlation of methylprednisolone levels in cat spinal cord with its effects on (Na+ + K+)-ATPase, lipid peroxidation, and alpha motor neuron function. *J Neurosurg* 1982;56(6):838-844.
12. Hurlbert RJ: Methylprednisolone for acute spinal cord injury: An inappropriate standard of care. *J Neurosurg* 2000;93(1, Suppl)1-7.
13. Coleman WP, Benzel D, Cahill DW, et al: A critical appraisal of the reporting of the National Acute Spinal Cord Injury Studies (II and III) of methylprednisolone in acute spinal cord injury. *J Spinal Disord* 2000;13(3):185-199.
14. Short DJ, El Masry WS, Jones PW: High dose methylprednisolone in the management of acute spinal cord injury - a systematic review from a clinical perspective. *Spinal Cord* 2000;38(5): 273-286.
15. Pharmacological therapy after acute cervical spinal cord injury. *Neurosurgery* 2002;50(3, Suppl) S63-S72.
16. Hurlbert RJ, Hamilton MG: Methylprednisolone for acute spinal cord injury: 5-year practice reversal. *Can J Neurol Sci* 2008;35(1):41-45.
17. Eck JC, Nachtigall D, Humphreys SC, Hodges SD: Questionnaire survey of spine surgeons on the use of methylprednisolone for acute spinal cord injury. *Spine (Phila Pa 1976)* 2006;31(9): E250-E253.
18. Akhtar AZ, Pippin JJ, Sandusky CB: Animal studies in spinal cord injury: A systematic review of methylprednisolone. *Altern Lab Anim* 2009;37(1): 43-62.
19. Braughler JM: Lipid peroxidation-induced inhibition of gamma-aminobutyric acid uptake in rat brain synaptosomes: Protection by glucocorticoids. *J Neurochem* 1985;44(4):1282-1288.
20. Hall ED: Effects of the 21-aminosteroid U74006F on posttraumatic spinal cord ischemia in cats. *J Neurosurg* 1988;68(3):462-465.
21. Hall ED: Neuroprotective actions of glucocorticoid and nonglucocorticoid steroids in acute neuronal injury. *Cell Mol Neurobiol* 1993;13(4): 415-432.
22. Anderson DK, Braughler JM, Hall ED, Waters TR, McCall JM, Means ED: Effects of treatment with U-74006F on neurological outcome following experimental spinal cord injury. *J Neurosurg* 1988; 69(4):562-567.
23. Liu D, Liu J, Sun D, Alcock NW, Wen J: Spinal cord injury increases iron levels: Catalytic production of hydroxyl radicals. *Free Radic Biol Med* 2003;34(1):64-71.
24. Faden AI, Jacobs TP, Mougey E, Holaday JW: Endorphins in experimental spinal injury: Therapeutic effect of naloxone. *Ann Neurol* 1981;10(4): 326-332.

25. Winkler T, Sharma HS, Stålberg E, Olsson Y, Nyberg F: Naloxone reduces alterations in evoked potentials and edema in trauma to the rat spinal cord. *Acta Neurochir Suppl (Wien)* 1994;60: 511-515.

26. Winkler T, Sharma HS, Stålberg E, Olsson Y, Nyberg F: Opioid receptors influence spinal cord electrical activity and edema formation following spinal cord injury: Experimental observations using naloxone in the rat. *Neurosci Res* 1994;21(1): 91-101.

27. Chang RC, Rota C, Glover RE, Mason RP, Hong JS: A novel effect of an opioid receptor antagonist, naloxone, on the production of reactive oxygen species by microglia: A study by electron paramagnetic resonance spectroscopy. *Brain Res* 2000; 854(1-2):224-229.

28. Young W, Flamm ES, Demopoulos HB, Tomasula JJ, DeCrescito V: Effect of naloxone on posttraumatic ischemia in experimental spinal contusion. *J Neurosurg* 1981;55(2):209-219.

29. Long JB, Martinez-Arizala A, Petras JM, Holaday JW: Endogenous opioids in spinal cord injury: A critical evaluation. *Cent Nerv Syst Trauma* 1986; 3(4):295-315.

30. Bracken MB, Holford TR: Effects of timing of methylprednisolone or naloxone administration on recovery of segmental and long-tract neurological function in NASCIS 2. *J Neurosurg* 1993; 79(4):500-507.

31. Karpiak SE, Mahadik SP: Reduction of cerebral edema with GM1 ganglioside. *J Neurosci Res* 1984; 12(2-3):485-492.

32. Ferrari G, Fabris M, Gorio A: Gangliosides enhance neurite outgrowth in PC12 cells. *Brain Res* 1983;284(2-3):215-221.

33. Skaper SD, Leon A, Facci L: Ganglioside GM1 prevents death induced by excessive excitatory neurotransmission in cultured hippocampal pyramidal neurons. *Neurosci Lett* 1991;126(1):98-101.

34. Geisler FH, Dorsey FC, Coleman WP: Recovery of motor function after spinal-cord injury—a randomized, placebo-controlled trial with GM-1 ganglioside. *N Engl J Med* 1991;324(26):1829-1838.

35. Geisler FH: GM-1 ganglioside and motor recovery following human spinal cord injury. *J Emerg Med* 1993;11(Suppl 1):49-55.

36. Geisler FH, Coleman WP, Grieco G, Poonian D, Sygen Study Group: The Sygen multicenter acute spinal cord injury study. *Spine (Phila Pa 1976)* 2001;26(24, Suppl)S87-S98.

37. Fawcett JW, Curt A, Steeves JD, et al: Guidelines for the conduct of clinical trials for spinal cord injury as developed by the ICCP panel: Spontaneous recovery after spinal cord injury and statistical power needed for therapeutic clinical trials. *Spinal Cord* 2007;45(3):190-205.

38. Schanne FA, Kane AB, Young EE, Farber JL: Calcium dependence of toxic cell death: A final common pathway. *Science* 1979;206(4419):700-702.

39. Fehlings MG, Tator CH, Linden RD: The effect of nimodipine and dextran on axonal function and blood flow following experimental spinal cord injury. *J Neurosurg* 1989;71(3):403-416.

40. Ford RW, Malm DN: Failure of nimodipine to reverse acute experimental spinal cord injury. *Cent Nerv Syst Trauma* 1985;2(1):9-17.

41. Petitjean ME, Pointillart V, Dixmerias F, et al: Medical treatment of spinal cord injury in the acute stage. *Ann Fr Anesth Reanim* 1998;17(2): 114-122.

42. Pointillart V, Petitjean ME, Wiart L, et al: Pharmacological therapy of spinal cord injury during the acute phase. *Spinal Cord* 2000;38(2):71-76.

43. Stokes BT, Fox P, Hollinden G: Extracellular calcium activity in the injured spinal cord. *Exp Neurol* 1983;80(3):561-572.

44. Gaviria M, Privat A, d'Arbigny P, Kamenka JM, Haton H, Ohanna F: Neuroprotective effects of gacyclidine after experimental photochemical spinal cord lesion in adult rats: Dose-window and time-window effects. *J Neurotrauma* 2000;17(1): 19-30.

45. Gaviria M, Privat A, d'Arbigny P, Kamenka J, Haton H, Ohanna F: Neuroprotective effects of a novel NMDA antagonist, Gacyclidine, after experimental contusive spinal cord injury in adult rats. *Brain Res* 2000;874(2):200-209.

46. Hirbec H, Gaviria M, Vignon J: Gacyclidine: A new neuroprotective agent acting at the N-methyl-D-aspartate receptor. *CNS Drug Rev* 2001;7(2):172-198.

47. Tadie M, d'Arbigny P, Mathe JF, et al: Acute spinal cord injury: Early care and treatment in a multicenter study with gacyclidine. *Proceedings of the 29th Annual Meeting of the Society for Neuroscience*. Miami Beach, FL, October 23-38, 1999.

48. Mitha AP, Maynard KI: Gacyclidine (Beaufour-Ipsen). *Curr Opin Investig Drugs* 2001;2(6): 814-819.

49. Lepeintre JF, D'Arbigny P, Mathé JF, et al: Neuroprotective effect of gacyclidine: A multicenter double-blind pilot trial in patients with acute traumatic brain injury. *Neurochirurgie* 2004; 50(2-3 Pt 1):83-95.

50. Blight AR: Effect of 4-aminopyridine on axonal conduction-block in chronic spinal cord injury. *Brain Res Bull* 1989;22(1):47-52.

51. Shi R, Blight AR: Differential effects of low and high concentrations of 4-aminopyridine on axonal conduction in normal and injured spinal cord. *Neuroscience* 1997;77(2):553-562.

52. Potter PJ, Hayes KC, Segal JL, et al: Randomized double-blind crossover trial of fampridine-SR (sustained release 4-aminopyridine) in patients with incomplete spinal cord injury. *J Neurotrauma* 1998;15(10):837-849.
53. Hayes KC, Katz MA, Devane JG, et al: Pharmacokinetics of an immediate-release oral formulation of Fampridine (4-aminopyridine) in normal subjects and patients with spinal cord injury. *J Clin Pharmacol* 2003;43(4):379-385.
54. Cardenas DD, Ditunno J, Graziani V, et al: Phase 2 trial of sustained-release fampridine in chronic spinal cord injury. *Spinal Cord* 2007;45(2):158-168.
55. Grijalva I, Guízar-Sahagún G, Castañeda-Hernández G, et al: Efficacy and safety of 4-aminopyridine in patients with long-term spinal cord injury: A randomized, double-blind, placebo-controlled trial. *Pharmacotherapy* 2003;23(7):823-834.
56. Hayes KC, Potter PJ, Hansebout RR, et al: Pharmacokinetic studies of single and multiple oral doses of fampridine-SR (sustained-release 4-aminopyridine) in patients with chronic spinal cord injury. *Clin Neuropharmacol* 2003;26(4):185-192.
57. DeForge D, Nymark J, Lemaire E, et al: Effect of 4-aminopyridine on gait in ambulatory spinal cord injuries: A double-blind, placebo-controlled, crossover trial. *Spinal Cord* 2004;42(12):674-685.
58. Goodman AD, Brown TR, Krupp LB, et al: Sustained-release oral fampridine in multiple sclerosis: A randomised, double-blind, controlled trial. *Lancet* 2009;373(9665):732-738.
59. Faden AI, Jacobs TP, Smith MT: Thyrotropin-releasing hormone in experimental spinal injury: Dose response and late treatment. *Neurology* 1984;34(10):1280-1284.
60. Faden AI, Jacobs TP: Effect of TRH analogs on neurologic recovery after experimental spinal trauma. *Neurology* 1985;35(9):1331-1334.
61. Sirén AL, Lake CR, Feuerstein G: Hemodynamic and neural mechanisms of action of thyrotropin-releasing hormone in the rat. *Circ Res* 1988;62(1):139-154.
62. Hashimoto T, Fukuda N: Effect of thyrotropin-releasing hormone on the neurologic impairment in rats with spinal cord injury: Treatment starting 24 h and 7 days after injury. *Eur J Pharmacol* 1991;203(1):25-32.
63. Hashimoto T, Fukuda N: Effect of thyrotropin-releasing hormone on the time course of neurologic recovery after spinal cord injury in the rat. *Jpn J Pharmacol* 1990;53(4):479-486.
64. Pitts LH, Ross A, Chase GA, Faden AI: Treatment with thyrotropin-releasing hormone (TRH) in patients with traumatic spinal cord injuries. *J Neurotrauma* 1995;12(3):235-243.
65. Kwon BK, Fisher CG, Dvorak MF, Tetzlaff W: Strategies to promote neural repair and regeneration after spinal cord injury. *Spine (Phila Pa 1976)* 2005;30(17, Suppl):S3-S13.
66. Zhang Y, Metz LM, Yong VW, et al: Pilot study of minocycline in relapsing-remitting multiple sclerosis. *Can J Neurol Sci* 2008;35(2):185-191.
67. NINDS NET-PD Investigators: A randomized, double-blind, futility clinical trial of creatine and minocycline in early Parkinson disease. *Neurology* 2006;66(5):664-671.
68. Gordon PH, Moore DH, Miller RG, et al: Efficacy of minocycline in patients with amyotrophic lateral sclerosis: A phase III randomised trial. *Lancet Neurol* 2007;6(12):1045-1053.
69. Yrjänheikki J, Tikka T, Keinänen R, Goldsteins G, Chan PH, Koistinaho J: A tetracycline derivative, minocycline, reduces inflammation and protects against focal cerebral ischemia with a wide therapeutic window. *Proc Natl Acad Sci U S A* 1999;96(23):13496-13500.
70. Stirling DP, Khodarahmi K, Liu J, et al: Minocycline treatment reduces delayed oligodendrocyte death, attenuates axonal dieback, and improves functional outcome after spinal cord injury. *J Neurosci* 2004;24(9):2182-2190.
71. Stirling DP, Koochesfahani KM, Steeves JD, Tetzlaff W: Minocycline as a neuroprotective agent. *Neuroscientist* 2005;11(4):308-322.
72. Wells JE, Hurlbert RJ, Fehlings MG, Yong VW: Neuroprotection by minocycline facilitates significant recovery from spinal cord injury in mice. *Brain* 2003;126(Pt 7):1628-1637.
73. Jelkmann W, Metzen E: Erythropoietin in the control of red cell production. *Ann Anat* 1996;178(5):391-403.
74. Brines M, Cerami A: Emerging biological roles for erythropoietin in the nervous system. *Nat Rev Neurosci* 2005;6(6):484-494.
75. Coleman T, Brines M: Science review: Recombinant human erythropoietin in critical illness. A role beyond anemia? *Crit Care* 2004;8(5):337-341.
76. Kwon BK, Okon E, Hillyer J, et al: A systematic review of non-invasive pharmacologic neuroprotective treatments for acute spinal cord injury. *J Neurotrauma* 2010 Apr 14 [Epub ahead of print].
77. Wang L, Zhang Z, Wang Y, Zhang R, Chopp M: Treatment of stroke with erythropoietin enhances neurogenesis and angiogenesis and improves neurological function in rats. *Stroke* 2004;35(7):1732-1737.
78. Ehrenreich H, Hasselblatt M, Dembowski C, et al: Erythropoietin therapy for acute stroke is both safe and beneficial. *Mol Med* 2002;8(8):495-505.

79. Ehrenreich H, Weissenborn K, Prange H, et al: Recombinant human erythropoietin in the treatment of acute ischemic stroke. *Stroke* 2009; 40(12):e647-e656.

80. Gorio A, Gokmen N, Erbayraktar S, et al: Recombinant human erythropoietin counteracts secondary injury and markedly enhances neurological recovery from experimental spinal cord trauma. *Proc Natl Acad Sci U S A* 2002;99(14):9450-9455.

81. Gorio A, Madaschi L, Di Stefano B, et al: Methylprednisolone neutralizes the beneficial effects of erythropoietin in experimental spinal cord injury. *Proc Natl Acad Sci U S A* 2005;102(45): 16379-16384.

82. Kontogeorgakos VA, Voulgaris S, Korompilias AV, et al: The efficacy of erythropoietin on acute spinal cord injury: An experimental study on a rat model. *Arch Orthop Trauma Surg* 2009;129(2): 189-194.

83. Matis GK, Birbilis TA: Erythropoietin in spinal cord injury. *Eur Spine J* 2009;18(3):314-323.

84. Vitellaro-Zuccarello L, Mazzetti S, Madaschi L, Bosisio P, Gorio A, De Biasi S: Erythropoietin-mediated preservation of the white matter in rat spinal cord injury. *Neuroscience* 2007;144(3): 865-877.

85. Kaptanoglu E, Solaroglu I, Okutan O, Surucu HS, Akbiyik F, Beskonakli E: Erythropoietin exerts neuroprotection after acute spinal cord injury in rats: Effect on lipid peroxidation and early ultrastructural findings. *Neurosurg Rev* 2004;27(2): 113-120.

86. Wiessner C, Allegrini PR, Ekatodramis D, Jewell UR, Stallmach T, Gassmann M: Increased cerebral infarct volumes in polyglobulic mice overexpressing erythropoietin. *J Cereb Blood Flow Metab* 2001; 21(7):857-864.

87. Sirén AL, Fasshauer T, Bartels C, Ehrenreich H: Therapeutic potential of erythropoietin and its structural or functional variants in the nervous system. *Neurotherapeutics* 2009;6(1):108-127.

88. Leist M, Ghezzi P, Grasso G, et al: Derivatives of erythropoietin that are tissue protective but not erythropoietic. *Science* 2004;305(5681):239-242.

89. Vitellaro-Zuccarello L, Mazzetti S, Madaschi L, et al: Chronic erythropoietin-mediated effects on the expression of astrocyte markers in a rat model of contusive spinal cord injury. *Neuroscience* 2008; 151(2):452-466.

90. Bensimon G, Doble A: The tolerability of riluzole in the treatment of patients with amyotrophic lateral sclerosis. *Expert Opin Drug Saf* 2004;3(6): 525-534.

91. Schwartz G, Fehlings MG: Evaluation of the neuroprotective effects of sodium channel blockers after spinal cord injury: Improved behavioral and neuroanatomical recovery with riluzole. *J Neurosurg* 2001;94(2, Suppl):245-256.

92. Wang SJ, Wang KY, Wang WC: Mechanisms underlying the riluzole inhibition of glutamate release from rat cerebral cortex nerve terminals (synaptosomes). *Neuroscience* 2004;125(1): 191-201.

93. Stutzmann JM, Pratt J, Boraud T, Gross C: The effect of riluzole on post-traumatic spinal cord injury in the rat. *Neuroreport* 1996;7(2):387-392.

94. Nógrádi A, Szabó A, Pintér S, Vrbová G: Delayed riluzole treatment is able to rescue injured rat spinal motoneurons. *Neuroscience* 2007;144(2): 431-438.

95. Guerrera MP, Volpe SL, Mao JJ: Therapeutic uses of magnesium. *Am Fam Physician* 2009;80(2): 157-162.

96. Lee JS, Han YM, Yoo DS, et al: A molecular basis for the efficacy of magnesium treatment following traumatic brain injury in rats. *J Neurotrauma* 2004;21(5):549-561.

97. McIntosh TK, Faden AI, Yamakami I, Vink R: Magnesium deficiency exacerbates and pretreatment improves outcome following traumatic brain injury in rats: 31P magnetic resonance spectroscopy and behavioral studies. *J Neurotrauma* 1988; 5(1):17-31.

98. McIntosh TK, Vink R, Yamakami I, Faden AI: Magnesium protects against neurological deficit after brain injury. *Brain Res* 1989;482(2):252-260.

99. Muir KW, Lees KR, Ford I, Davis S, Intravenous Magnesium Efficacy in Stroke (IMAGES) Study Investigators: Magnesium for acute stroke (Intravenous Magnesium Efficacy in Stroke trial): Randomised controlled trial. *Lancet* 2004;363(9407): 439-445.

100. Temkin NR, Anderson GD, Winn HR, et al: Magnesium sulfate for neuroprotection after traumatic brain injury: A randomised controlled trial. *Lancet Neurol* 2007;6(1):29-38.

101. Süzer T, Coskun E, Islekel H, Tahta K: Neuroprotective effect of magnesium on lipid peroxidation and axonal function after experimental spinal cord injury. *Spinal Cord* 1999;37(7):480-484.

102. Ditor DS, John SM, Roy J, Marx JC, Kittmer C, Weaver LC: Effects of polyethylene glycol and magnesium sulfate administration on clinically relevant neurological outcomes after spinal cord injury in the rat. *J Neurosci Res* 2007;85(7): 1458-1467.

103. Kwon BK, Roy J, Lee JH, et al: Magnesium chloride in a polyethylene glycol formulation as a neuroprotective therapy for acute spinal cord injury: Preclinical refinement and optimization. *J Neurotrauma* 2009;26(8):1379-1393.

104. Lee JH, Roy J, Sohn HM, et al: Magnesium in a polyethylene glycol formulation provides neuroprotection after unilateral cervical spinal cord injury. *Spine (Phila Pa 1976)* 2010;35(23): 2041-2048.

105. Resnick DK, Nguyen P, Cechvala CF: Selective cyclooxygenase 2 inhibition lowers spinal cord prostaglandin concentrations after injury. *Spine J* 2001;1(6):437-441.

106. Resnick DK, Graham SH, Dixon CE, Marion DW: Role of cyclooxygenase 2 in acute spinal cord injury. *J Neurotrauma* 1998;15(12):1005-1013.

107. Hall ED, Wolf DL: A pharmacological analysis of the pathophysiological mechanisms of posttraumatic spinal cord ischemia. *J Neurosurg* 1986; 64(6):951-961.

108. Fu Q, Hue J, Li S: Nonsteroidal anti-inflammatory drugs promote axon regeneration via RhoA inhibition. *J Neurosci* 2007;27(15):4154-4164.

109. Zhou Y, Su Y, Li B, et al: Nonsteroidal anti-inflammatory drugs can lower amyloidogenic Abeta42 by inhibiting Rho. *Science* 2003; 302(5648):1215-1217.

110. Wang X, Budel S, Baughman K, Gould G, Song KH, Strittmatter SM: Ibuprofen enhances recovery from spinal cord injury by limiting tissue loss and stimulating axonal growth. *J Neurotrauma* 2009; 26(1):81-95.

111. Schachter M: Chemical, pharmacokinetic and pharmacodynamic properties of statins: An update. *Fundam Clin Pharmacol* 2005;19(1):117-125.

112. Mann CM, Lee JH, Hillyer J, Stammers AM, Tetzlaff W, Kwon BK: Lack of robust neurologic benefits with simvastatin or atorvastatin treatment after acute thoracic spinal cord contusion injury. *Exp Neurol* 2010;221(2):285-295.

113. Stüve O, Youssef S, Steinman L, Zamvil SS: Statins as potential therapeutic agents in neuroinflammatory disorders. *Curr Opin Neurol* 2003;16(3): 393-401.

114. Déry MA, Rousseau G, Benderdour M, Beaumont E: Atorvastatin prevents early apoptosis after thoracic spinal cord contusion injury and promotes locomotion recovery. *Neurosci Lett* 2009;453(1): 73-76.

115. Pannu R, Barbosa E, Singh AK, Singh I: Attenuation of acute inflammatory response by atorvastatin after spinal cord injury in rats. *J Neurosci Res* 2005;79(3):340-350.

CHAPTER 7

Considerations of Timing and Sequencing of Treatment

Jamie Purzner, MD   Teresa Purzner, MD   Michael G. Fehlings, MD, PhD, FRCSC, FACS

Introduction

An appreciation of the timing and frequency of posttraumatic changes following spinal cord injury (SCI) allows clinicians to anticipate foreseeable problems and provide timely and appropriate intervention. Early optimization of medical management, including well-sustained blood pressure, assurance of adequate oxygenation, and avoidance of medical complications, has been shown to benefit the overall outcome of the patient. The timing of definitive surgical management, however, remains controversial. Although there is a large body of literature reporting changes in outcome in relation to the timing of surgery, the results are often conflicting. While the ultimate decision of whether and when to intervene relies on the experience of the surgeon and the characteristics of each case, understanding the existing literature will provide an evidence-based guide that aids in decision making. In this chapter, we will review the literature surrounding the timing of medical and surgical intervention in spine trauma to help provide a rationale behind the timing of management of SCI.

Medical Optimization of SCI

Patients with SCI require close medical attention in the acute period. In order to ensure optimal outcomes, potential sources of complications must be recognized. **Figure 1** shows a general timeline of the common complications following SCI. The following sections describe the timing of medical management and strategies for complication avoidance in spine trauma.

Dr. Fehlings or an immediate family member has received royalties from DePuy, a Johnson & Johnson company; serves as a paid consultant to or is an employee of Covidien; and has received research or institutional support from DePuy, a Johnson & Johnson company. Neither of the following authors or any immediate family member has received anything of value from or owns stock in a commercial company or institution related directly or indirectly to the subject of this chapter: Dr. Jamie Purzner and Dr. Teresa Purzner.

Blood Pressure Optimization

Following SCI, the local microvasculature of the spine is disrupted, producing an area of surrounding ischemia. In animal studies, it has been shown that the extent of ischemia is significantly affected by systemic blood pressure, in part due to loss of local vascular autoregulation. Maintenance of normotension is required to maintain adequate spinal cord blood flow and to minimize the ischemic insult.[1] Unfortunately, SCI patients can often become hypotensive as a result of hypovolemia from associated injuries or from neurogenic shock. Neurogenic shock develops in patients with cervical or upper thoracic spine injuries and is thought to result from disruption of preganglionic sympathetic neurons, resulting in an absence of supraspinal control of the heart, vessels, and kidneys.[2]

Hypotension is typically deemed significant when a patient's systolic blood pressure drops below 85 to 90 mm Hg. The incidence of hypotension upon arrival at the emergency department is approximately 25.8% in patients with cervical SCI and 11.8% in patients with thoracic SCI.[3] The rate of neurogenic shock reaches a maximum at day 4[4,5] and can extend up to 5 weeks following the injury.[6] Hypotension as a result of neurogenic shock is often refractory to volume replacement, particularly in complete cord injuries, where it was found to be 5.5 times greater than in incomplete cord injuries.[7]

Several studies have suggested a trend toward increased neurologic improvement when early hemodynamic monitoring and correction are used. These studies describe using arterial and central venous pressure monitoring as well as maintaining normotension. In a study published in 1976, 117 patients were monitored in the intensive care unit (ICU) and treated with volume expansion and pharmacologic blood pressure control.[8] These patients were stratified by the time of their admission to hospital. Patients admitted < 12 hours showed a 67% improvement in neurologic examination as opposed to a 59% improvement for those admitted between 12 and 48 hours and a

FIGURE 1

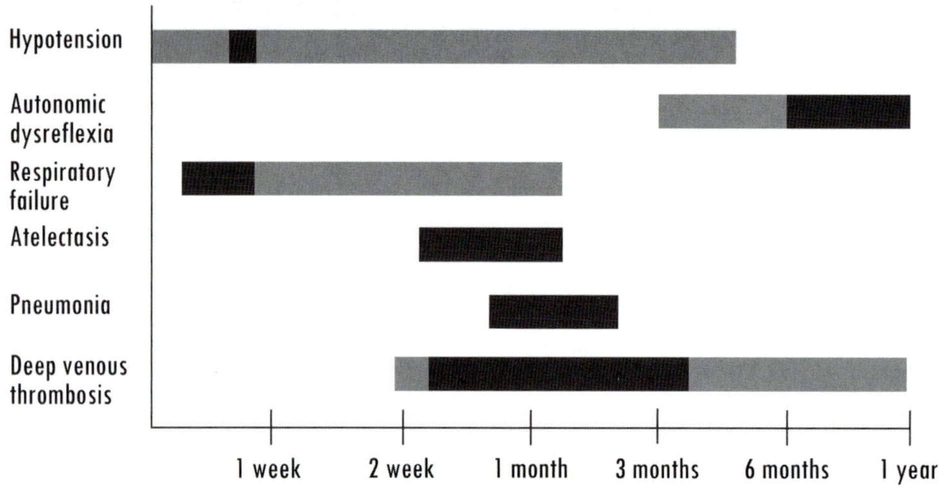

Figure 1 Time line of complications secondary to blunt spine trauma.

50% improvement in patients admitted after 48 hours.[8] Further studies have demonstrated similar improvement with no associated increase in mortality or major morbidity from use of fluids, vasopressors, or insertion of vascular catheters.[7,9] Ploumis et al[10] and Casha and Christie[11] provide two detailed reviews of the evidence pertaining to the use of vasopressors in SCI. They found that overall there was some limited evidence in support of early and invasive monitoring and treatment of hypotension in a special care unit.

Hypotension and bradycardia occur early and can persist for weeks in the SCI patient. Although the evidence that blood pressure control enhances an SCI patient's outcome is not strong, given the reasonable safety and sound physiologic basis for maintaining normotension, early and aggressive blood pressure management is advised. This should be assessed upon admission and should drive early transfer to hospitals capable of invasive monitoring. This is reflected in the guidelines on SCI from the Section on Disorders of the Spine and Peripheral Nerves of the American Association of Neurological Surgeons and the Congress of Neurological Surgeons, which recommend maintaining a mean arterial blood pressure at 85 mm Hg to 95 mm Hg for the first 7 days posttrauma.[12]

Respiratory Management

Respiratory complications are the most common cause of mortality in patients following SCI.[13] They include atelectasis (29% to 36%), pneumonia (31% to 36%), pulmonary edema, and aspiration.[14,15] Jackson and Groomes[14] subdivided the timing of the individual complications and found that atelectasis occurred with a mean onset of 17.7 days and duration of 12.8 days. Pneumonia began later, with an onset of 24.5 days and duration of 15.5 days. Vigilance during at-risk periods may help prevent respiratory decline. Following 1 year posttrauma, respiratory complications occur in 3.2% to 5.6% of patients and remain stable for the remaining time period. Significantly more late respiratory complications occur in older patients.[16]

Generally patients who develop respiratory failure following spine trauma or SCI fall into two groups: patients with respiratory decline as a result of cervical SCI and patients with concomitant thoracic injuries. Respiratory failure was documented in 23% to 49% of patients with cervical SCI. These patients have significant alteration in lung volume secondary to weakness and paralysis in muscles controlling respiration as well as changes to the pattern of breathing. The time course of pulmonary function in this group has a characteristic early decline over the first 2 to 5 days and then recovers after approximately 5 weeks. The incidence of respiratory failure varies with the level and degree of SCI.[14,17] Patients with thoracolumbar injuries also have a 21.6% chance of developing pulmonary complications and subsequent respiratory failure. Cotton et al[18] further subdivided the population into high thoracic and low thoracic fractures showing respiratory failure of 42.4% and 30.7%, respectively. These high rates of respiratory failure are likely related to the considerable associated chest injuries such as rib fractures, pulmonary contusions, and hemo/pneumothorax, which are demonstrated by the high injury severity score (ISS) found in this study.[18] The complications in thoracic trauma occur on average earlier than in cervical injuries.[14]

Early tracheotomy should be considered in patients who will require prolonged intubation. A tracheotomy is required in 9% to 11% of all SCI patients.[19,20] Early tracheotomy (usually considered before 7 days) is associated with shorter ICU stays, a reduction in tracheal stenosis, and a reduced length of mechanical ventilation from an average of 48.75 days to 26.07 days.[21] There was not a significant difference in the number of patients who developed pneumonia.

Venous Thromboembolism

Patients with SCI and spinal fractures are highly prone to developing deep venous thrombosis (DVT) and pulmonary embolism (PE). Posttraumatic SCIs fulfill all of Virchow's triad of stasis, hypercoagulability, and endothelial damage, making them highly prone to thrombosis. In patients without prophylaxis, 12% to 64% developed clinically identifiable DVT or PE.[22] With routine screening of all SCI patients, the rates of DVT are up to 81%.[23] With pharmacologic prophylaxis, the rate varies from 5.3% to 38.6% depending upon the type of prophylaxis and the specific trial.[22]

Despite the extensive literature on venous thromboembolism in SCI, few studies have stratified results over time. In a retrospective review of 101 patients with SCI, Thumbikat et al describe two peak times for DVT formation.[24] The first peak was noted at 20 to 50 days after injury and the second at 90 to 110 days after injury. A second study examining the trend of complications following SCI showed that DVT and PE began to occur at approximately 2 weeks from injury and continued to increase until the study concluded at 2 months.[25] In a study that examined the long-term risk of venous thromboembolism, 287 patients were followed for an average of 13.7 years.[26] In the first 6 months, 83% of events were noted. The rate drops to 0.17% per year in the subsequent period. This suggests that after 6 months, patients have a normal risk profile. McKinley et al[16] examined late complications in SCI in the rehabilitation setting and showed that 2.1% of patients had a symptomatic DVT at 1 year and 1% of patients at 2 years. Similarly, the PE rate at 1 year posttrauma was 0.5% and dropped to 0.2% by year 2.[16] Overall, these data suggest that the risk of thromboembolism remains elevated for 6 months following injury and returns to near-normal by year 1.

The guidelines for the management of SCI recommend DVT prophylactic therapy for a period of 3 months.[12] This is echoed by the 2008 American College of Chest Physicians' guidelines on prevention of venous thromboembolism, which support a 3-month duration of therapy by use of low molecular-weight heparin (LMWH) as the primary thromboprophylaxis.[27] These guidelines also propose using a combination of LMWH with a sequential compression device. For details regarding the evidence supporting the specific regimen, a detailed meta-analysis and review articles are available.[10,28] The 3-month duration suggested in the guidelines arises primarily because it is the duration of follow-up for the majority of trials.

Aito et al[29] examined the effect of initiating DVT prophylaxis early (before 72 hours posttrauma) compared to late (averaging 12 days posttrauma) in 275 patients with SCI. Prophylaxis included LMWH, gradient elastic stockings, external sequential pneumatic compression, and early ambulation. Patients underwent routine Doppler ultrasound screening. The early group had a DVT rate of 2% as opposed to the late group, which had a rate of 26%. This supports beginning thromboprophylaxis as early as possible in patients with no contraindications to anticoagulation (uncontrolled bleeding, unstable intracranial hematoma, spinal epidural hematoma, or previous heparin-induced thrombocytopenia).

Medical Therapy for SCI

Steroids

The use of steroids following SCI remains controversial.[30-32] The National Acute Spinal Cord Injury Study (NASCIS) I trial used a 100 mg or a 1,000 mg of methylprednisolone for 10 days and showed no change in neurologic performance.[33] NASCIS II and III both used a 30 mg/kg bolus followed by a 5.4 mg/kg/h infusion. NASCIS II continued the infusion for 23 hours while NASCIS III had one arm with methylprednisolone for 24 hours and another for 48 hours.[34,35] The only positive effect on neurologic outcome noted in these trials was when administration occurred less than 8 hours following injury. The clinical applicability of these trials is a source of great debate. A common criticism is that the findings were based solely on post hoc analysis and the degree of neurologic improvement is of questionable clinical significance. These trials noted a significant increase in rates of pneumonia, sepsis, and death in patients receiving a 48-hour methylprednisolone infusion as opposed to a 24-hour infusion.[36]

Therefore, if methylprednisolone is to be given, it should be administered within 8 hours of the injury and continued for up to 24 hours.

Timing of Surgical Management for Blunt Trauma

There are several classically accepted indications for urgent surgical correction of a spine fracture. The most universally agreed-upon indication is a progressive neurologic deficit with compression of the spine. Others include unreduced spinal dislocation with neurologic deficit and severe deformity or kyphosis compromising the overlying skin or ability to position the patient. Several comprehensive reviews and meta-analyses of the basic science and clinical research regarding early decompression have been published.[37-40] In general, patients are divided into an early decompression group and a delayed decompression group. Early decompression in the literature has ranged from less than 6 hours to greater than 72 hours. For the purpose of this chapter, late surgery refers to surgery greater than 72 hours; intermediate surgery, before 72 hours; early surgery, less than 24 hours; and emergency surgery, less than 8 hours. The sheer amount of data and the variability in outcomes make synthesizing reasonable conclusions that could be used in clinical decision-making difficult. The majority of these studies were retrospective case series. In addition, the literature spans a large time period and thus represents very different surgical techniques and access to technology. A large number of studies are reviewed in this chapter to reflect the variability in literature results.

Impact on Mortality

Patients who have undergone significant trauma are often medically unstable. Even following initial resuscitation, these patients can be poor surgical candidates. Several studies have examined the impact of early versus late surgery on mortality, with conflicting results. A study by Kerwin et al[41] showed a significantly higher mortality at 7.6% in the < 48-hours-to-surgery group compared with 2.5% in the delayed-surgery group. The majority of these deaths are associated with acute respiratory distress syndrome that occurred postoperatively and there was no documented case of a patient dying during the surgical procedure. There have been several studies demonstrating no difference in mortality between early and later surgery.[42-45] One study assessed 142 patients who underwent surgery in < 72 hours and 149 patients who underwent late surgery.[46] The mortality was not statistically significantly different between earlier and later groups, although the late group had significantly higher abbreviate injury scale (AIS) chest scores, which may have presented a bias. In a subgroup analysis, patients with ISS > 25 demonstrated a higher mortality in the < 72 hours group (12% compared to 2%), while other subgroups such as age > 50 years and Glasgow Coma Scale (GCS) ≤ 10 showed no difference in mortality.[46] McLain and Benson[45] followed spine-injured patients with polytrauma and compared early surgery (< 24 hours) with intermediate surgery (< 72 hours). No significant difference was noted between these groups in terms of mortality. In patients where an anterior or combined approach was required, the average blood loss was 6.8 L in the urgent group as opposed to 4 L in the early group. When a posterior approach was used, the estimated blood loss was 1.4 L in the urgent group and 1.6 L in the early group.[45] Regardless of the significant blood loss, no patient in the urgent group who underwent an anterior approach died.

In contrast, the results from the German Trauma Registry showed the late surgery group to have a higher mortality than early surgery at 17% and 6.3%, respectively.[47] Overall, there is limited evidence to suggest that earlier surgery has a higher risk, if patients have significant associated injuries. Careful evaluation of hemodynamic state and preoperative stabilization should be performed before attempting an urgent anterior or combined approach.

Neurologic Outcome

The effect of early decompression on neurologic improvement is contentious. Several trials have directly compared neurologic recovery in patients who underwent surgical decompression with timing stratified into late (> 72 hours), intermediate (< 72 hours) and early (< 24 hours). These trials have been summarized in **Table 1**. The majority of studies show no significant difference in neurologic outcome.[9,48,46,49-53] However, a notable minority showed significantly greater improvement in patients who underwent early surgery. Most of these showed improvement in the range of 0.29 to 1.8 Frankel grades.[54-57] This is a considerable increase; however, no study has shown a difference in an SCI functional outcome scale, which may better reflect the impact on quality of life for the patient. The greatest improvement occurred in patients with incomplete SCI, but several patients did have improvement following a complete injury. Unfortunately, a convincing subgroup has not

TABLE 1

Studies Investigating the Timing of Surgery on Neurologic Improvement[a]

Superior Neurologic Improvement	Amount of Neurologic Improvement	No Difference in Improvement
Intermediate Surgery (< 72 h)		
Clohisy et al (1992)[54]	N = 20 Δ Frankel = 0.83 Δ ASIA-M = 21.1	Croce et al (2001)[46]
Mirza et al (1999)[56]	N = 15 Δ Frankel = 1.8 Δ ASIA-M = 37.9	Vaccaro et al (1997)[53]
Papadopoulos et al (2002)[57]	N = 91 Δ Frankel = 0.69	Chipman et al (2004)[49]
Rath et al (2005)[55b]	N = 7 Δ Frankel = 0.29	McKinley et al (2004)[50]
		Kerwin et al (2005)[48]
		Sapkas and Papadakis (2007)[51]
		Vale et al (1997)[9]
		Schlegel et al (1996)[52]
Early Surgery (< 24 h)		
McLain and Benson (1999)[45]	N_{urgent} = 14 Δ Frankel = 1.12 N_{early} = 13 Δ Frankel = 0.65	Levi et al (1991)[59]
Rath et al (2005)[55]	N = 11 Δ Frankel = 1.64	Duh et al (1994)[58]
		Vale et al (1997)[9]
		Pollard and Apple (2003)[60]
Emergency Surgery (< 8 h)		
Cengiz et al (2008)[43]	N = 12 Δ ASIA = 1.67	Pointillart et al (2000)[61]

[a]N = number of patients. Δ Frankel indicates the change in Frankel score between early and late surgery. Δ ASIA-M indicates the change in the American Spinal Injury Association (ASIA) motor score between early and late surgery.

[b]Rath et al is subgrouped into < 24 h, 24-48 h and > 48 h; the intermediate group in this table is composed of the 24-48 h subgroup.

been found across studies that can be targeted to reliably show neurologic improvement. No study to date has shown a significant neurologic deterioration secondary to early surgical deterioration.

The effect of surgical decompression sooner than 72 hours is also debatable. One study examined early surgery (< 24 hours; average, 9.7 hours) compared to intermediate surgery (24 to 72 hours; average, 35 hours). The early surgery group showed a higher percentage of patients with neurologic improvement than the intermediate surgery group at 88% and 50%, respectively.[45] The mean change in Frankel grades was 1.12 in the early group and 0.65 in the intermediate group. These findings were validated by a second study that showed significantly greater improvement in patients operated on in < 24 hours.[55] The mean change in Frankel grades was 1.64 when < 24 hours, 0.29 when between 24 and 48 hours, and 0.71 when > 48 hours. Both of these studies focused on patients with exclusively thoracolumbar spine pathology.

In contrast, four studies showed no additional neurologic improvement from surgery in < 24 hours.[9,58-60] Levi et al[59] compared urgent anterior decompression and stabilization of subaxial cervical spine fractures and found no difference in neurologic change. Another study followed patients with cervical and thoracic injuries in a protocol with strict blood pressure monitoring and correction. No significant impact on the timing of surgery was observed.[9] This may be related to the small number of patients who were decompressed before 24 hours.

Few studies have assessed the benefit of emergency surgery, where patients are operated on within 8 hours of injury. One trial examined 27 patients with thoracic and lumbar injuries who were randomized to laminectomy with instrumented fusion before 8 hours postinjury or a delayed group in which the surgery would occur 3 days later.[43] The emergency surgery group showed a significant improvement in the American Spinal Injury Association (ASIA) scale by 1.67, whereas the delayed surgery showed no significant difference. Within this trial, 83% of patients with emergency surgery had neurologic improvement, compared to 26.6% in the late group.[43] Patients with other injuries or biomechanical abnormalities were excluded from the trial. Another study focused on the effect of methylprednisolone and nimodipine on neurologic improvement evaluated the effect of emergency surgery as a secondary outcome.[61] This showed no significant difference in emergency versus late surgery.[61] A possible explanation for the discrepancy may be that the delayed group in this study was from 8 hours to 24 hours, as opposed to 3 days in the study by Cengiz et al.[43]

Given these data, there is some evidence that rapid decompression has a chance to improve neurologic improvement. Determining the optimal time based on the current literature is difficult. Some studies comparing decompression within 24 hours or even 8 hours appeared to be superior to surgery within 72 hours. It is important to understand the specific population that is being studied. For example, the results of Cengiz et al may support surgery within 8 hours for well patients, but this may not translate to a severely ill polytrauma patient.

Nonneurologic Advantages of Early Surgery

A consistent finding in the literature is that early surgery allows the patient to spend less time in hospital. The majority of studies showed a significant reduction in hospital length of stay favoring patients operated on before 72 hours.[41,46,47,49,50,56,57] A summary of the results and studies is found in **Table 2**. The reduction in times spent in hospital ranged from 0 to 52 days. The duration of ICU stay was also decreased by up to 14 days, although less reliably than hospital stay. Decreased duration of mechanical ventilation was less reliable, but positive studies showed a decrease of up to 9 days.

In subgroup analyses, Frangen et al[44] found that patients with complete paraplegia had the greatest benefit from early surgery. The average decrease in hospital length of stay was 31 days. Similarly, patients with preoperative respiratory issues experienced a substantial benefit, with a reduction of length of stay of 45 days.[44] Patients with thoracic injuries or severe injuries also demonstrated an additional benefit.[44,46,52,57]

Several studies have assessed the impact of early surgery on complication rates. A summary of these results can be found in **Table 3**. The most consistent trend was a decrease in respiratory complications, with a benefit of 10.8% to 43.5%.[46,47,50,52] This includes atelectasis, pneumonia, and other causes of respiratory failure. The benefit was greatest in patients with thoracic injuries, where a decrease in respiratory complications has been shown in 34% of patients. Two of three studies showed a decrease in thromboembolic complications of 6% to 16%.[46,52] Early surgery has also shown a benefit in decreased rate of urinary tract infections (33.2%), pressure sores (22.3%), and wound infections (8%).[52]

Overall, there is good evidence that early surgery accelerates the patient's movement through the acute care system. There appears to be a reduction to pulmonary complications that is greatest in patients with severe injuries or thoracic injuries. Increased respiratory performance may be explained by early mobilization and participation in physiotherapy.

Polytrauma

Multisystem trauma is common in thoracolumbar fractures. Injuries commonly associated with SCI include head trauma (17.2%), chest injury (2.9%), abdominal trauma (1.5%), pelvic injury or fracture (2.5%), upper limb fracture (4.4%), and lower limb fracture (5.9%).[62] The severity of injuries and number of systems involved is often expressed in the ISS. Scores for each region range from 1 (minor) to 5 (critical) and 6 (unsurvivable). The three most injured regions are then squared and summed. ISS scores greater than 26 are considered polytrauma. Definitive surgical management of damage to the spine is complex in patients with multiple injuries. Often these patients are hemodynamically unstable and other injuries often provide practical barriers to surgery. Prioritization of

TABLE 2

Effect of Intermediate (< 72 h), Early (< 24 h), and Emergency Surgery (< 8 h) on the Duration of Care[a]

Study	N	Hospital Stay	ICU Stay	Mechanical Ventilation
Intermediate Surgery (< 72 h)				
Croce et al (2001)[46]	291	↓ 8.7 d	↓ 6 d	NS
→ ISS > 25	156	NS	NS	NS
→ Thoracic	79	↓ 17.3 d	↓ 8.1 d	↓ 6.4 d
Mirza et al (1999)[56]	30	↓ 14.9 d	NS	NS
Papadopoulos et al (2002)[57]	91	↓ 28.5 d	↓ 13.9 d	
Chipman et al (2004)[49]				
→ ISS < 15	58	↓ 7.4 d	NS	
→ ISS ≥ 15	88	↓ 9.2 d	↓ 6.4 d	NS
McKinley et al (2004)[50]	779	↓ 5.2 d		
Kerwin et al (2007)[41]	361	↓ 3.2 d	NS	NS
Schinkel et al (2006)[47]	205	↓ 3.8	↓ 7.4 d	↓ 5.9 d
→ ISS < 26	84	NS	NS	NS
→ ISS 26 to 38	80	NS	↓ 7.8 d	NS
→ ISS > 38	40	NS	↓ 0.5 d	↓ 6 d
Schlegel et al (1996)[52]				
→ ISS < 18	57	NS	NS	NS
→ ISS ≥ 18	60	↓ 15.5 d	↓ 11.3 d	↓ 8.9 d
Frangen et al (2009)[44]	160	NS	NS	NS
→ ISS ≤ 25	109	NS	NS	NS
→ ISS 26 to 37	28	NS	NS	↓ 3 d
→ ISS ≥ 38	23	↓ 52 d	↓ 6 d	NS
→ Paraplegia	38	↓ 31 d	↓ 7 d	↓ 7 d
→ Preop lung failure	30	↓ 45 d	↓ 9 d	↓ 5 d
Early Surgery (< 24 h)				
Campagnolo et al (1997)[42]	64	↓ 17.2 d		
Emergency Surgery (< 8 h)				
Cengiz et al (2008)[43]	27	↓ 13.5 d	NS	

[a]NS = no significant change; ISS = injury severity score.

care requires close coordination with other specialties.

A study analyzing patient data from the German National Trauma Database have addressed the effect of injury severity on early and intermediate (< 72 hours) versus late (> 72 hours) spine decompression and stabilization. Groups were stratified based upon ISS scores of < 25, 26 to 37 and > 38.[44] No significant difference in mortality was noted. In the severely injured group (ISS > 38) there was a significant decrease in ICU stay (20 to 14 days) and hospital admission (56 to 108 days) when comparing earlier and delayed surgery.[44] Shorter ICU stays[47,49,52] and equal mortality[45] were consistent findings throughout the literature. The advantage of early surgery appears to be greater in the most severely injured patients. This likely reflects the fact that in patients with multiple

TABLE 3

Effect of Intermediate (< 72 h), Early (< 24 h), and Emergency Surgery (< 8 h) on Complication and Mortality Rates[a]

Study	N	Complications	Respiratory	Infection
Intermediate Surgery (< 72 h)				
Croce et al (2001)[46]	291		↓ 12%	
→ ISS > 25	156		NS	
→ Thoracic	79		↓ 34%	
Mirza et al (1999)[56]	30	NS		
Chipman et al (2004)[49]				
→ ISS < 15	58	NS	NS	NS
→ ISS ≥ 15	88	↓ 26.2	NS	NS
McKinley et al (2004)[50]	779		↓10.8%	
Kerwin et al (2007)[41b]	361		NS	
Schinkel et al (2006)[47]	205		↓ 12%	
Schlegel et al (1996)[52]				
→ ISS < 18	57		NS	
→ ISS ≥ 18	60		↓ 43.5%	↓ 8%
Frangen et al (2009)[44]	160		NS	
→ ISS ≤ 25	109		NS	
→ ISS 26 to 37	28		NS	
→ ISS ≥ 38	23		NS	
→ Paraplegia	38		NS	
→ Preop lung failure	30		NS	
Early Surgery (< 24 h)				
Campagnolo et al (1997)[42]	64		NS	NS
McLain and Benson (1999)[45]	27			
Emergency Surgery (< 8 h)				
Cengiz et al (2008)[43]	27		NS	

[a]NS = no significant change; GU, genitourinary.

[b]Kerwin et al divided group into surgery in < 48 h and surgery in > 48 h.

injuries, mobility restrictions from unstable spine injuries can delay patient progress and increase their susceptibility to complications.

Certain associated injuries make definitive surgical repair difficult to accomplish. For instance, it is very difficult to perform a posterior decompression and stabilization on a patient with extensive rib and sternum fractures. This is reflected by the finding that patients who underwent earlier surgical decompression had significantly lower chest AIS scores and fewer rib fractures.[46] Other injuries that prevent appropriate positioning include abdominal injuries precluding primary closure or pelvic and other fractures with external fixators. Excessive bleeding or hemodynamic instability may also delay surgical treatment.

In polytrauma patients, there is always a balance between early mobilization and surgical risk. These patients are frequently hemodynamically unstable and have compromised ventilation. The decision to delay surgery should be made on a case-to-case basis. However, the literature suggests that early surgery is safe in patients with severe and numerous injuries and that the benefit of

TABLE 3 *(CONTINUED)*

Ulcers	GU	DVT	Mortality
Intermediate Surgery (< 72 h)			
		↓ 6%	NS
			↑ 10%
			NS
NS		NS	
			↑ 5.1%
			↓ 10.7%
NS	NS	NS	
↓ 22.3%	↓ 33.2	↓ 16%	
			NS
			NS
			NS
			NS
			NS
			NS
Early Surgery (< 24 h)			
NS	NS	NS	NS
			NS
Emergency Surgery (< 8 h)			
			NS

early intervention is in fact greatest in the polytrauma patient.

Feasibility of Early Surgery

In a large multicenter study, Tator et al[63] examined the timing of surgery in patients with SCI. Surgical management was attained in less than 24 hours in 23.5% and between 25 to 48 hours in 15.8%. Another study of 255 patients with traumatic SCI showed that 51.4% could be accomplished in less than 24 hours.[64] Several causes of surgical delay exist: patients must be hemodynamically stabilized, some will require transfer to an appropriate surgical center, or associated injuries may take precedence over spinal stabilization. Tuli et al[65] showed that hypotension following SCI significantly delayed definitive surgical management. In patients who presented with an ASIA-A SCI and hypotension, surgical management occurred at 80.9 hours as opposed to 58 hours in patients without hypotension.[65]

The barriers to early surgery are becoming fewer. Transfers to major surgical centers are more rapid and access to neuroimaging is becoming widespread and easily available. Dedicated trauma teams provide rapid treatment to multiple injuries, thus making a patient medically stable for spine surgery more rapidly. We recommend early surgery (< 24 hours) whenever medically feasible.

Applying the Concepts of Early Surgery to Clinical Care

A great deal of data exist regarding the timing of medical and surgical care in patients with spine trauma. Because of the variability in practice, it is difficult to establish a concrete algorithm for the care of these patients. **Figure 2** presents an overview of the care plan in patients who have sustained a blunt injury to the spine. To demonstrate the clinical approach of early surgery, we summarize a case under the care of one of us. A 20-year-old male who was involved in a motor vehicle rollover was transferred to a tertiary care neurosurgical center. At the to hospital, he had an incomplete SCI with an ASIA score of 47 of 100 with significant motor deficits below C7. Imaging showed a C6-C7 flexion distraction injury with significant cord compression (**Figure 3**). Closed reduction was achieved shortly after initial imaging was completed. Following closed reduction, an anterior decompression with C7 corpectomy was performed. An autologous tricortical bone graft and plate system was used for reconstruction. The time from injury to decompression was approximately 12 hours. A comparison of the preoperative and postoperative MRI shows the extent of decompression of the spinal cord (**Figure 4**). The patient showed some improvement on postoperative day 8 with an ASIA score of 53 of 100. He had excellent neurologic improvement throughout follow-up, and at 1 year, his ASIA score was 96. Facilitating early management of spinal trauma requires rapid transfer to specialized centers, immediate access to appropriate neuroimaging, and prioritization of definitive surgical management.

FIGURE 2

Injury — ATLS protocol

Indications for surgical intervention

- Progressive neurologic deterioration
- Significant dislocation with neurologic deficit
- Spinal cord injury without polytrauma

8 hours

24 hours — Consider early surgery for patients with spinal trauma in the setting of polytrauma and isolated injuries

72 hours — Hemodynamically unstable during early Injuries preclude surgical positioning

Anterior or combined approach required in a patient with significant medical comorbidity

Medical optimization

Spinal cord injury
- Maintain MAP 85-95 mm Hg for 7 days
- Follow respiratory failure

DVT prophylaxis for 3 months using low molecular-weight heparin

Follow for late complications

Consider early tracheostomy

Figure 2 Algorithm of treatment options for blunt spine trauma. ATLS = Advanced Trauma Life Support; MAP = mean arterial pressure.

FIGURE 3

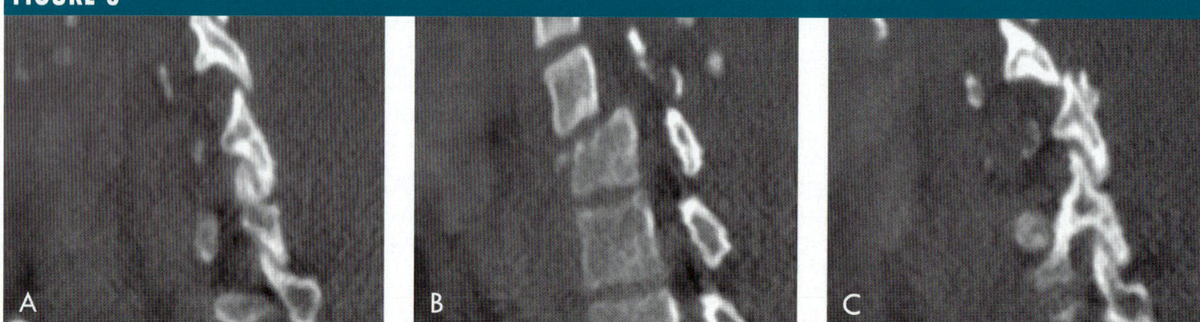

Figure 3 Case example of early reduction and decompression following spinal trauma. This CT scan of the cervical spine with sagittal reconstructions shows a C6-C-7 flexion-distraction injury.

FIGURE 4

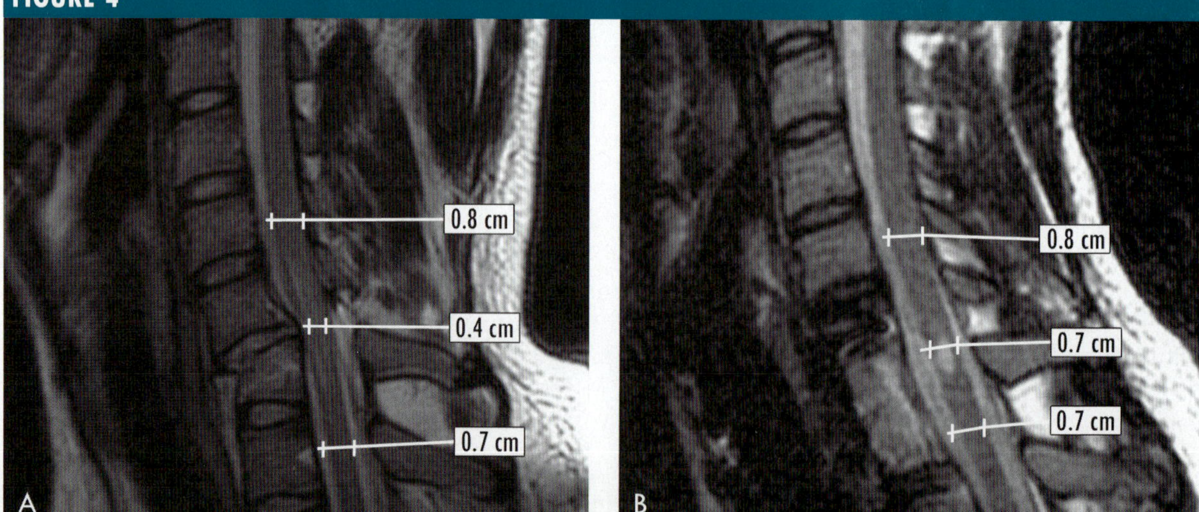

Figure 4 **A,** Preoperative MRI scan showing significant compromise of the spinal canal. **B,** Postoperative image showing good decompression of the spinal canal.

Penetrating Trauma to the Spine

Although the majority of spine trauma results from blunt injury, 13% to 17% of injuries result from penetrating trauma,[66] typically a result of gunshot wounds or other projectile weapons. As with all trauma, prioritization is placed on treatment of immediately life-threatening injuries. These injuries often require surgery to repair or explore other systems. In SCI, the management of gunshot wounds varies depending upon the missile trajectory, associated injuries, and degree of spinal instability.

Unlike with blunt trauma, few studies have focused on timing of surgery in penetrating trauma. The timing and type of surgery depends upon several factors. Immediate decompression is indicated, with rapid neurologic decline associated with compression of the spinal cord by displaced bone, foreign body, or epidural hematoma. Outside of those indications, several studies have shown no significant neurologic improvement as a result of routine spinal exploration when compared with conservative management in low-velocity gunshot injuries.[67-69] Of these, the study by Aarabi et al[67] was the only one that recorded surgical timing and showed an average time to surgery of 6.3 days. Early surgery does not appear to be beneficial in the context of penetrating trauma.[70] Cybulski et al[71] showed no significant difference in percentage of neurologic improvement between decompression before 72 hours (47.5%) and after 72 hours (48.1%). In addition, an increased rate of complications was noted in the earlier surgery group (eg, abscess formation).[71]

When clear spinal instability is noted, surgical stabilization is warranted. Detailed imaging of the spine should always be performed to assess bony and ligamentous stability. Side-to-side injuries often produce damage to the facet and pedicles bilaterally, resulting in an unstable spine. Duz et al[66] showed that significant improvement in the Frankel grade was observed when the goals of surgery were both to decompress the spinal cord and stabilize the spine. Increased neurologic function was seen in 87.5% for decompression, in 70% for stabilization, and 88.9% when the indication was both decompression and stabilization.[66]

A subgroup that did show potential benefit from decompression and removal of bullets was patients with injuries at the level of the conus or below. Patients with complete injuries of the cauda equina showed improvement in neurologic function following surgical exploration in 28.6% of patients as compared with 16.6% patients managed conservatively. The improvement was also greater than in patients with injuries to the spinal cord.[67]

High-velocity gunshot wounds produce larger areas of necrosis and cavitation, thereby increasing the likelihood of developing trauma-related spinal complications. Splavski et al[72] describe early laminectomy and dural repair producing a complication rate of 14.5%. In comparison, with conservative management, the complication rate has been found to be 34.6%, including meningitis, osteomyelitis, and wound infections. Therefore, early surgical exploration is warranted in patients with injuries to the spine secondary to high-velocity projectile.

Complications following gunshot wounds involving the spine are common and typically present in a delayed fashion. Infectious complications depend upon associated injuries. Patients with transperitoneal incursion will invariably require immediate surgical exploration to determine and control injuries. Further management depends upon whether or not enteric contamination of the wound has occurred. When hollow viscus perforation occurs in association with spinal injuries, a high rate of spinal infection occurs. For low-velocity injuries, several studies have shown that a prolonged 7- to 14-day course of intravenous broad-spectrum antibiotics reduces the risk of late infection[73-75] such that surgical débridement of the spine is not necessary. **Figure 5** outlines the basic management of patients with penetrating injuries to the spine. Shorter courses of antibiotics (48 hours) do not appear to be effective and were associated with an 87.5% rate of osteomyelitis.[76]

Dural damage can be caused by any trajectory. Cerebral spinal fluid (CSF) fistula develops in 9.4% of patients following gunshot wounds to the spine and meningitis arises in 20% of patients with CSF leaks.[77] CSF fistula is a delayed complication and should be repaired when identified. If enteric contamination has occurred the repair should be delayed until a prolonged course of antibiotics is completed.

Summary

- From first patient contact, maintain mean arterial pressure > 90 mm Hg for at least 7 days.
- Follow pulmonary performance closely in patients with cervical SCI and patients with thoracic spine fractures; correct any hypoxemia.
- Consider early tracheostomy for prolonged intubation.

FIGURE 5

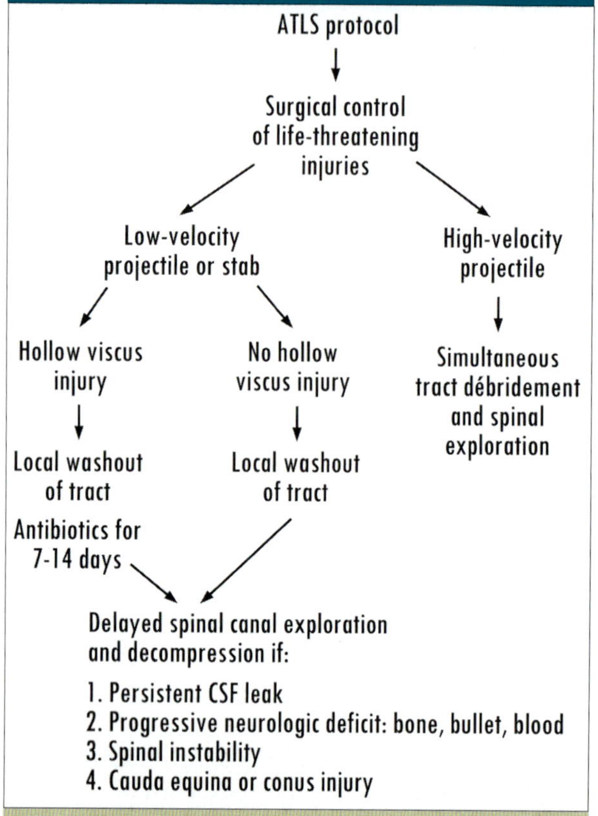

Figure 5 Algorithm of treatment options for penetrating spine trauma. ATLS = Advanced Trauma Life Support; CSF = cerebrospinal fluid.

- Initiate pharmacologic DVT prophylaxis as soon as possible and continue for 3 months.
- If using steroids, begin as soon as possible and not after 8 hours. Duration should not exceed 24 hours.
- Following blunt trauma, if a patient is hemodynamically stable and there are no other medical contraindications, we recommend early surgery (< 24 hours) for decompression and stabilization.
- Benefits from early surgery in blunt trauma include shortened hospital stay, decreased complications, and the possibility of neurologic improvement.
- Patients with more severe injuries and thoracic injuries receive the most benefit from early surgery.
- Following penetrating trauma, high-velocity injuries should undergo urgent tract exploration and débridement.
- Following low-velocity penetrating trauma, patients should undergo delayed surgery for stabilization or CSF fistula repair.
- Any patient with enteric contamination should undergo a prolonged 7- to 14-day course of antibiotics.

References

1. Tator CH, Fehlings MG: Review of the secondary injury theory of acute spinal cord trauma with emphasis on vascular mechanisms. *J Neurosurg* 1991;75(1):15-26.
2. Furlan JC, Fehlings MG: Cardiovascular complications after acute spinal cord injury: Pathophysiology, diagnosis, and management. *Neurosurg Focus* 2008;25(5):E13.
3. Guly HR, Bouamra O, Lecky FE, Trauma Audit and Research Network: The incidence of neurogenic shock in patients with isolated spinal cord injury in the emergency department. *Resuscitation* 2008;76(1):57-62.
4. Lehmann KG, Lane JG, Piepmeier JM, Batsford WP: Cardiovascular abnormalities accompanying acute spinal cord injury in humans: Incidence, time course and severity. *J Am Coll Cardiol* 1987;10(1):46-52.
5. Piepmeier JM, Lehmann KB, Lane JG: Cardiovascular instability following acute cervical spinal cord trauma. *Cent Nerv Syst Trauma* 1985;2(3):153-160.
6. Furlan JC, Fehlings MG, Shannon P, Norenberg MD, Krassioukov AV: Descending vasomotor pathways in humans: Correlation between axonal preservation and cardiovascular dysfunction after spinal cord injury. *J Neurotrauma* 2003;20(12):1351-1363.
7. Levi L, Wolf A, Belzberg H: Hemodynamic parameters in patients with acute cervical cord trauma: Description, intervention, and prediction of outcome. *Neurosurgery* 1993;33(6):1007-1017.
8. Zäch GA, Seiler W, Dollfus P: Treatment results of spinal cord injuries in the Swiss Paraplegic Centre of Basle. *Paraplegia* 1976;14(1):58-65.
9. Vale FL, Burns J, Jackson AB, Hadley MN: Combined medical and surgical treatment after acute spinal cord injury: Results of a prospective pilot study to assess the merits of aggressive medical resuscitation and blood pressure management. *J Neurosurg* 1997;87(2):239-246.
10. Ploumis A, Yadlapalli N, Fehlings MG, Kwon BK, Vaccaro AR: A systematic review of the evidence supporting a role for vasopressor support in acute SCI. *Spinal Cord* 2010;48(5):356-362.
11. Casha S, Christie S: A systematic review of intensive cardiopulmonary management after spinal cord injury. *J Neurotrauma* 2010 Apr 8. [Epub ahead of print].

12. Hadley MN, Walters BC, Grabb PA, et al: Guidelines for the management of acute cervical spine and spinal cord injuries. *Clin Neurosurg* 2002;49: 407-498.
13. Frankel HL, Coll JR, Charlifue SW, et al: Long-term survival in spinal cord injury: A fifty year investigation. *Spinal Cord* 1998;36(4):266-274.
14. Jackson AB, Groomes TE: Incidence of respiratory complications following spinal cord injury. *Arch Phys Med Rehabil* 1994;75(3):270-275.
15. Lemons VR, Wagner FC Jr: Respiratory complications after cervical spinal cord injury. *Spine (Phila Pa 1976)* 1994;19(20):2315-2320.
16. McKinley WO, Jackson AB, Cardenas DD, DeVivo MJ: Long-term medical complications after traumatic spinal cord injury: A regional model systems analysis. *Arch Phys Med Rehabil* 1999;80(11): 1402-1410.
17. Ledsome JR, Sharp JM: Pulmonary function in acute cervical cord injury. *Am Rev Respir Dis* 1981;124(1):41-44.
18. Cotton BA, Pryor JP, Chinwalla I, Wiebe DJ, Reilly PM, Schwab CW: Respiratory complications and mortality risk associated with thoracic spine injury. *J Trauma* 2005;59(6):1400-1409.
19. Biering-Sørensen F, Charlifue S, DeVivo M, et al: International Spinal Cord Injury Data Sets. *Spinal Cord* 2006;44(9):530-534.
20. Reines HD, Harris RC: Pulmonary complications of acute spinal cord injuries. *Neurosurgery* 1987; 21(2):193-196.
21. Griffiths J, Barber VS, Morgan L, Young JD: Systematic review and meta-analysis of studies of the timing of tracheostomy in adult patients undergoing artificial ventilation. *BMJ* 2005;330(7502): 1243.
22. Furlan JC, Fehlings MG: Role of screening tests for deep venous thrombosis in asymptomatic adults with acute spinal cord injury: An evidence-based analysis. *Spine (Phila Pa 1976)* 2007;32(17): 1908-1916.
23. Geerts WH, Code KI, Jay RM, Chen E, Szalai JP: A prospective study of venous thromboembolism after major trauma. *N Engl J Med* 1994;331(24): 1601-1606.
24. Thumbikat P, Poonnoose PM, Balasubrahmaniam P, Ravichandran G, McClelland MR: A comparison of heparin/warfarin and enoxaparin thromboprophylaxis in spinal cord injury: The Sheffield experience. *Spinal Cord* 2002;40(8):416-420.
25. Aito S, Gruppo Italiano Studio Epidemiologico Mielolesioni GISEM Group: Complications during the acute phase of traumatic spinal cord lesions. *Spinal Cord* 2003;41(11):629-635.
26. Lamb GC, Tomski MA, Kaufman J, Maiman DJ: Is chronic spinal cord injury associated with increased risk of venous thromboembolism? *J Am Paraplegia Soc* 1993;16(3):153-156.
27. Geerts WH, Bergqvist D, Pineo GF, et al: Prevention of venous thromboembolism: American College of Chest Physicians Evidence-Based Clinical Practice Guidelines (8th Edition). *Chest* 2008; 133(6, Suppl)381S-453S.
28. Teasell RW, Hsieh JT, Aubut JA, et al: Venous thromboembolism after spinal cord injury. *Arch Phys Med Rehabil* 2009;90(2):232-245.
29. Aito S, Pieri A, D'Andrea M, Marcelli F, Cominelli E: Primary prevention of deep venous thrombosis and pulmonary embolism in acute spinal cord injured patients. *Spinal Cord* 2002;40(6):300-303.
30. Bracken MB: Steroids for acute spinal cord injury. *Cochrane Database Syst Rev* 2002;3:CD001046.
31. Hurlbert RJ: The role of steroids in acute spinal cord injury: An evidence-based analysis. *Spine (Phila Pa 1976)* 2001;26(24, Suppl)S39-S46.
32. Hurlbert RJ: Strategies of medical intervention in the management of acute spinal cord injury. *Spine (Phila Pa 1976)* 2006;31(11, Suppl)S16-S21, discussion S36.
33. Bracken MB, Collins WF, Freeman DF, et al: Efficacy of methylprednisolone in acute spinal cord injury. *JAMA* 1984;251(1):45-52.
34. Bracken MB, Shepard MJ, Collins WF, et al: A randomized, controlled trial of methylprednisolone or naloxone in the treatment of acute spinal-cord injury: Results of the Second National Acute Spinal Cord Injury Study. *N Engl J Med* 1990; 322(20):1405-1411.
35. Bracken MB, Shepard MJ, Holford TR, et al: Methylprednisolone or tirilazad mesylate administration after acute spinal cord injury: 1-year follow up. Results of the third National Acute Spinal Cord Injury randomized controlled trial. *J Neurosurg* 1998;89(5):699-706.
36. Bracken MB, Shepard MJ, Holford TR, et al: Administration of methylprednisolone for 24 or 48 hours or tirilazad mesylate for 48 hours in the treatment of acute spinal cord injury: Results of the Third National Acute Spinal Cord Injury Randomized Controlled Trial. National Acute Spinal Cord Injury Study. *JAMA* 1997;277(20): 1597-1604.
37. Fehlings MG, Perrin RG: The role and timing of early decompression for cervical spinal cord injury: Update with a review of recent clinical evidence. *Injury* 2005;36(Suppl 2):B13-B26.
38. Furlan JC, Noonan V, Cadotte DW, Fehlings MG: Timing of decompressive surgery of spinal cord after traumatic spinal cord injury: An evidence-based examination of pre-clinical and clinical studies. *J Neurotrauma* 2010 Mar 4. [Epub ahead of print].

39. Rutges JP, Oner FC, Leenen LP: Timing of thoracic and lumbar fracture fixation in spinal injuries: A systematic review of neurological and clinical outcome. *Eur Spine J* 2007;16(5):579-587.
40. Schinkel C, Anastasiadis AP: The timing of spinal stabilization in polytrauma and in patients with spinal cord injury. *Curr Opin Crit Care* 2008; 14(6):685-689.
41. Kerwin AJ, Frykberg ER, Schinco MA, et al: The effect of early surgical treatment of traumatic spine injuries on patient mortality. *J Trauma* 2007; 63(6):1308-1313.
42. Campagnolo DI, Esquieres RE, Kopacz KJ: Effect of timing of stabilization on length of stay and medical complications following spinal cord injury. *J Spinal Cord Med* 1997;20(3):331-334.
43. Cengiz SL, Kalkan E, Bayir A, Ilik K, Basefer A: Timing of thoracolomber spine stabilization in trauma patients; impact on neurological outcome and clinical course: A real prospective (RCT) randomized controlled study. *Arch Orthop Trauma Surg* 2008;128(9):959-966.
44. Frangen TM, Ruppert S, Muhr G, Schinkel C: The beneficial effects of early stabilization of thoracic spine fractures depend on trauma severity. *J Trauma* 2010;68(5):1208-1212.
45. McLain RF, Benson DR: Urgent surgical stabilization of spinal fractures in polytrauma patients. *Spine (Phila Pa 1976)* 1999;24(16):1646-1654.
46. Croce MA, Bee TK, Pritchard E, Miller PR, Fabian TC: Does optimal timing for spine fracture fixation exist? *Ann Surg* 2001;233(6):851-858.
47. Schinkel C, Frangen TM, Kmetic A, Andress HJ, Muhr G, German Trauma Registry: Timing of thoracic spine stabilization in trauma patients: Impact on clinical course and outcome. *J Trauma* 2006;61(1):156-160.
48. Kerwin AJ, Frykberg ER, Schinco MA, Griffen MM, Murphy T, Tepas JJ: The effect of early spine fixation on non-neurologic outcome. *J Trauma* 2005;58(1):15-21.
49. Chipman JG, Deuser WE, Beilman GJ: Early surgery for thoracolumbar spine injuries decreases complications. *J Trauma* 2004;56(1):52-57.
50. McKinley W, Meade MA, Kirshblum S, Barnard B: Outcomes of early surgical management versus late or no surgical intervention after acute spinal cord injury. *Arch Phys Med Rehabil* 2004;85(11): 1818-1825.
51. Sapkas GS, Papadakis SA: Neurological outcome following early versus delayed lower cervical spine surgery. *J Orthop Surg (Hong Kong)* 2007; 15(2):183-186.
52. Schlegel J, Bayley J, Yuan H, Fredricksen B: Timing of surgical decompression and fixation of acute spinal fractures. *J Orthop Trauma* 1996; 10(5):323-330.
53. Vaccaro AR, Daugherty RJ, Sheehan TP, et al: Neurologic outcome of early versus late surgery for cervical spinal cord injury. *Spine (Phila Pa 1976)* 1997;22(22):2609-2613.
54. Clohisy JC, Akbarnia BA, Bucholz RD, Burkus JK, Backer RJ: Neurologic recovery associated with anterior decompression of spine fractures at the thoracolumbar junction (T12-L1). *Spine (Phila Pa 1976)* 1992;17(8, Suppl):S325-S330.
55. Rath SA, Kahamba JF, Kretschmer T, Neff U, Richter HP, Antoniadis G: Neurological recovery and its influencing factors in thoracic and lumbar spine fractures after surgical decompression and stabilization. *Neurosurg Rev* 2005;28(1):44-52.
56. Mirza SK, Krengel WF III, Chapman JR, et al: Early versus delayed surgery for acute cervical spinal cord injury. *Clin Orthop Relat Res* 1999;359: 104-114.
57. Papadopoulos SM, Selden NR, Quint DJ, Patel N, Gillespie B, Grube S: Immediate spinal cord decompression for cervical spinal cord injury: Feasibility and outcome. *J Trauma* 2002;52(2): 323-332.
58. Duh MS, Shepard MJ, Wilberger JE, Bracken MB: The effectiveness of surgery on the treatment of acute spinal cord injury and its relation to pharmacological treatment. *Neurosurgery* 1994;35(2): 240-249.
59. Levi L, Wolf A, Rigamonti D, Ragheb J, Mirvis S, Robinson WL: Anterior decompression in cervical spine trauma: Does the timing of surgery affect the outcome? *Neurosurgery* 1991;29(2):216-222.
60. Pollard ME, Apple DF: Factors associated with improved neurologic outcomes in patients with incomplete tetraplegia. *Spine (Phila Pa 1976)* 2003;28(1):33-39.
61. Pointillart V, Petitjean ME, Wiart L, et al: Pharmacological therapy of spinal cord injury during the acute phase. *Spinal Cord* 2000;38(2):71-76.
62. Chu D, Lee YH, Lin CH, Chou P, Yang NP: Prevalence of associated injuries of spinal trauma and their effect on medical utilization among hospitalized adult subjects—A nationwide data-based study. *BMC Health Serv Res* 2009;9:137.
63. Tator CH, Fehlings MG, Thorpe K, Taylor W: Current use and timing of spinal surgery for management of acute spinal surgery for management of acute spinal cord injury in North America: Results of a retrospective multicenter study. *J Neurosurg* 1999;91(1, Suppl)12-18.
64. Bötel U, Gläser E, Niedeggen A: The surgical treatment of acute spinal paralysed patients. *Spinal Cord* 1997;35(7):420-428.

65. Tuli S, Tuli J, Coleman WP, Geisler FH, Krassioukov A: Hemodynamic parameters and timing of surgical decompression in acute cervical spinal cord injury. *J Spinal Cord Med* 2007;30(5): 482-490.

66. Duz B, Cansever T, Secer HI, Kahraman S, Daneyemez MK, Gonul E: Evaluation of spinal missile injuries with respect to bullet trajectory, surgical indications and timing of surgical intervention: A new guideline. *Spine (Phila Pa 1976)* 2008;33(20):E746-E753.

67. Aarabi B, Alibaii E, Taghipur M, Kamgarpur A: Comparative study of functional recovery for surgically explored and conservatively managed spinal cord missile injuries. *Neurosurgery* 1996;39(6): 1133-1140.

68. Simpson RK Jr, Venger BH, Narayan RK: Treatment of acute penetrating injuries of the spine: A retrospective analysis. *J Trauma* 1989;29(1):42-46.

69. Venger BH, Simpson RK, Narayan RK: Neurosurgical intervention in penetrating spinal trauma with associated visceral injury. *J Neurosurg* 1989; 70(4):514-518.

70. Robertson DP, Simpson RK: Penetrating injuries restricted to the cauda equina: A retrospective review. *Neurosurgery* 1992;31(2):265-270.

71. Cybulski GR, Stone JL, Kant R: Outcome of laminectomy for civilian gunshot injuries of the terminal spinal cord and cauda equina: Review of 88 cases. *Neurosurgery* 1989;24(3):392-397.

72. Splavski B, Vranković D, Sarić G, Blagus G, Mursić B, Rukovanjski M: Early management of war missile spine and spinal cord injuries: Experience with 21 cases. *Injury* 1996;27(10):699-702.

73. Lin SS, Vaccaro AR, Reisch S, Devine M, Cotler JM, Reich SM: Low-velocity gunshot wounds to the spine with an associated transperitoneal injury. *J Spinal Disord* 1995;8(2):136-144.

74. Quigley KJ, Place HM: The role of debridement and antibiotics in gunshot wounds to the spine. *J Trauma* 2006;60(4):814-820.

75. Roffi RP, Waters RL, Adkins RH: Gunshot wounds to the spine associated with a perforated viscus. *Spine (Phila Pa 1976)* 1989;14(8):808-811.

76. Romanick PC, Smith TK, Kopaniky DR, Oldfield D: Infection about the spine associated with low-velocity-missile injury to the abdomen. *J Bone Joint Surg Am* 1985;67(8):1195-1201.

77. Kahraman S, Gonul E, Kayali H, et al: Retrospective analysis of spinal missile injuries. *Neurosurg Rev* 2004;27(1):42-45.

CHAPTER 8
Pediatric Spinal Cord Injury

Patrick J. Cahill, MD Terrence Cahill, MD Steven Hwang, MD Amer Samdani, MD
Martin J. Herman, MD

Introduction

Management of children with a spinal cord injury (SCI) presents unique acute and long-term medical, surgical, and rehabilitative challenges. Advancements in medicine, technology, and public policy related to disabilities have combined to increase the life expectancy of these children.[1,2] A clear understanding of the anatomic, biomechanical, and physiologic differences between the pediatric and adult spine is essential to the provision of care to the pediatric spine patient. While management principles and the complications encountered are similar to those seen in adults after an SCI, some aspects of care are distinctly different for children and adolescents compared with adults. This chapter presents established principles regarding the acute and chronic surgical management of pediatric SCI and highlights the problems of the skeletally immature patient with an SCI.

Incidence

Spinal injury in the pediatric age group is rare. Because there are no standardized reporting guidelines or a comprehensive database for reporting pediatric SCI in the United States, determination of the true incidence of this injury is difficult.[3,4] The reported incidence of pediatric SCI ranges from 0.65% to 10% of all reported spinal injuries,[5-13] with two notable age peaks: patients younger than 5 years of age and those older than 10 years of age.[5,6] Several states have reported statewide population data, and these ranges also vary widely, from 1.0 to 16.7 per million.[14-18] A more recent US population-based study reports an incidence of 19 per million.[19] The Scandinavian countries of Finland and Sweden report an incidence of 1.9 to 2.4 per million.[3,4] Such a relatively low rate of SCI in these countries suggests that most of the SCIs in the United States may be secondary to societal differences in the way motor vehicles are operated and the violence rates.

Rate of SCI also varies with gender and ethnicity. In the United States, boys have an injury rate of 27.9 per million and girls a rate of 11.5 per million.[20] In children younger than 6 years of age, the incidence is equal for boys and girls. In older children and teenagers, boys are two to three times more likely to sustain an SCI compared with girls. African Americans are about two times as likely as Hispanics and four times as likely as Asians to sustain an SCI.[3,20]

There is also significant variation in the spinal level and type of injury with age. Two-thirds of injuries that occur in children younger than 6 years of age occur in the thoracic, lumbar, or sacral spine and result in paraplegia.[20,21] In older children and teenagers, more than half of the SCIs occur in the cervical spine and result in tetraplegia. Mixed SCIs, such as anterior cord syndrome, are exceedingly rare in the pediatric population.

The incidence of SCI without radiographic evidence of abnormality (SCIWORA) is greatest in children compared to all other age groups and accounts for up to 67% of SCIs in children.[9,11,13,22-30] SCIWORA occurs most commonly in those younger than 5 years of age[29,31,32] and results in complete cord injury in over 40% of patients.[33] SCIWORA is diagnosed by MRI, which demonstrates cord edema, hemorrhage, or disruption, as well as ligamentous, vertebral end-plate, or disk injuries. Flexion-extension lateral cervical radiography, cineradiography, and flexion-

Dr. Patrick J. Cahill or an immediate family member serves as a paid consultant to or is an employee of DePuy, a Johnson & Johnson company, Osteotech, and Synthes; and has received research or institutional support from DePuy, a Johnson & Johnson company. Dr. Hwang or an immediate family member has received research or institutional support from DePuy, a Johnson & Johnson company. Dr. Samdani or an immediate family member is a member of a speakers' bureau or has made paid presentations on behalf of DePuy, a Johnson & Johnson company, Synthes, and Spinevision; serves as a paid consultant to or is an employee of DePuy, a Johnson & Johnson company, Synthes, and Spinevision; and has received research or institutional support from DePuy, a Johnson & Johnson company. Dr. Herman or an immediate family member serves as a board member, owner, officer, or committee member of the American Academy of Orthopaedic Surgeons and the Pediatric Orthopaedic Society of North America. Neither Dr. Terrence Cahill nor any immediate family member has received anything of value from or owns stock in a commercial company or institution related directly or indirectly to the subject of this chapter.

TABLE 1

Patients at Highest Risk for Pediatric SCI

1. Unrestrained children of all ages involved in motor vehicle crashes
2. Adolescent males who participate in sports such as diving and collision sports, and who ride motorized recreational vehicles
3. African-American adolescent and young adult males who are victims of street violence
4. Infants and toddlers who are victims of child abuse

extension MRI are useful to assess the degree of instability in children who sustain SCIWORA, but instability is not seen in all cases.[4,20,21,29,34,35]

Mechanisms of SCI

Motor vehicle collision is the most common cause of SCI in all children older than 1 year (**Table 1**).[4,19,20] Two-thirds of these children are not wearing seat belts.[4] Driver impairment by alcohol or drugs is believed to be a factor in one-third of these collisions. In all age groups, paraplegia from the SCI is most common after a motor vehicle collision injury, although with increasing age, the rate of tetraplegia from these collision injuries increases.[20]

Among teenagers, sports-related injuries are the second most common cause of SCI.[3,20] Diving accidents are the most common cause of sports-related SCIs. American football, snow skiing, ice hockey, and horseback riding are other sports that result in SCI in this age group. Since the 1970s, the incidence of SCI from sports-related injuries has declined as a result of safer techniques, improved equipment, and a generally increased awareness of the risk of these catastrophic injuries.[36]

Motor vehicle sports, such as riding all-terrain vehicles and motorcycles, are increasingly recognized as causes of severe injuries in children and adolescents, including SCIs. Children younger than 16 years of age are particularly at risk because they may not have sufficient strength or motor coordination to control the vehicle and lack experience or proper judgment to operate it safely.[37] The American Academy of Pediatrics and the American Academy of Orthopaedic Surgeons have established specific recommendations regarding the operation of these vehicles and have them available on their respective Web sites (aap.org and aaos.org).

Violence from firearms, stabbing, and assault are common causes of SCI, particularly for minority groups. The most common mechanism of SCI in African-American and Hispanic teenagers is violence.[20] African Americans of all ages are more likely than any other ethnicity to sustain an SCI from violence. Nearly two-thirds of all SCIs that occur in African Americans who are in their late teens and early 20s result from violence against the victim.

Birth trauma and child abuse (**Figure 1**) are the most common causes of SCI in children younger than 1 year.[20] SCI secondary to birth trauma has been reported as the result of difficult cephalic or breech delivery with distraction and hyperextension of the head and neck resulting in injury to the spine.[7,11,25,26,38-42] Spinal injury may be an unrecognized cause of death in the newborn.[10,43] Autopsy studies of stillborn infants have documented evidence of cord damage, including extradural and intradural hemorrhage, nerve root avulsion, cord transection,[38,44-47] and SCIWORA.[9,18,48,49] Spinal fracture-dislocation with paraplegia resulting from intentional trauma has been reported.[50] The infant and young child who presents with an SCI or any traumatic injury to the spinal column not consistent with the mechanism of injury and history provided by the caregiver should be carefully evaluated to rule out child abuse.[6,11] Other stigmata of child abuse include retinal hemorrhages, skull fractures, posterior rib fractures, long-bone corner fractures, and multiple fractures or skin lesions in various stages of healing. No vertebral radiographic findings are specific for abuse.[6,10,11]

Evaluation of the Child With a Potential SCI

Emergency Department Management

When a child presents with multiple organ system trauma, a high index of suspicion should be exercised with regard to potential injury of the spinal column. After careful assessment of the patient's cardiopulmonary status, strict immobilization of the spinal column must be initiated at the scene of the injury. In children younger than 8 years of age, adult spine boards must be avoided.[11] Because of the relatively large size of the child's head in relation to body size, the standard spine board places the neck in relative flexion, potentially causing further injury to the spinal cord. Elevation

FIGURE 1

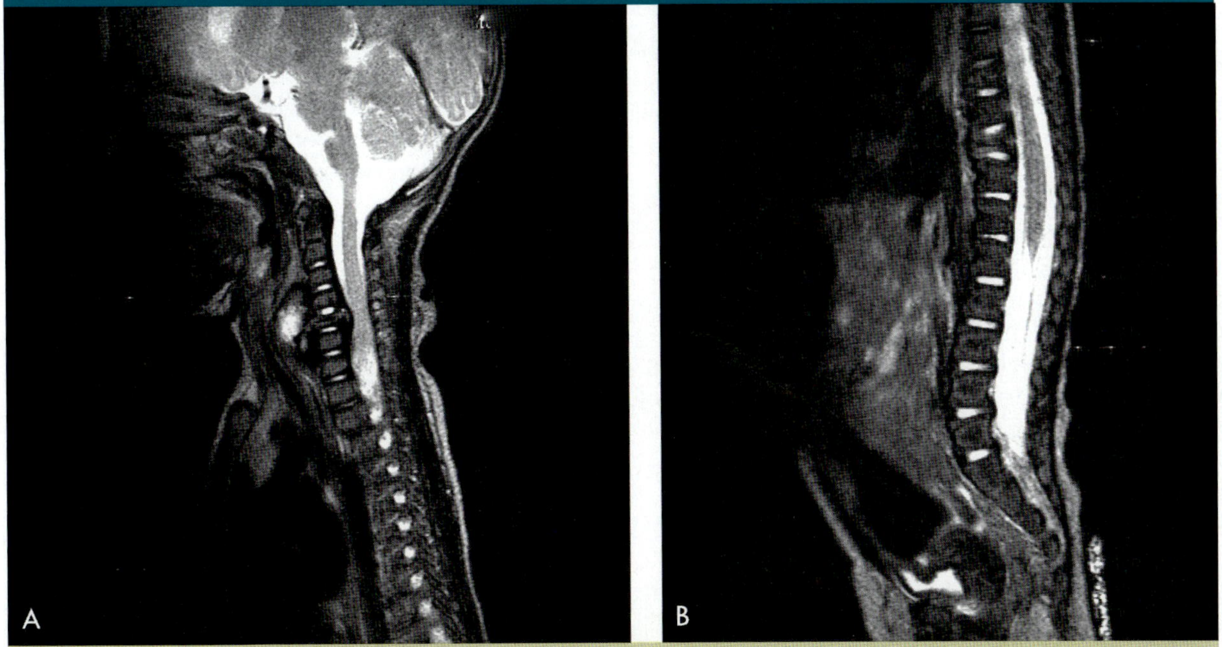

Figure 1 Sagittal cervical (**A**) and thoracic (**B**) MRI scans of a 2-year-old girl who was the victim of child abuse. There is a compression fracture of the C5 vertebral body with a surrounding paravertebral soft-tissue mass and anterior cord impingement with mild cord edema. There are also compression fractures of the T9 and T11 vertebral bodies without associated paraspinal mass or associated cord signal abnormality. Clinically, she had signs of an anterior cord syndrome but was difficult to fully assess because of her young age.

FIGURE 2

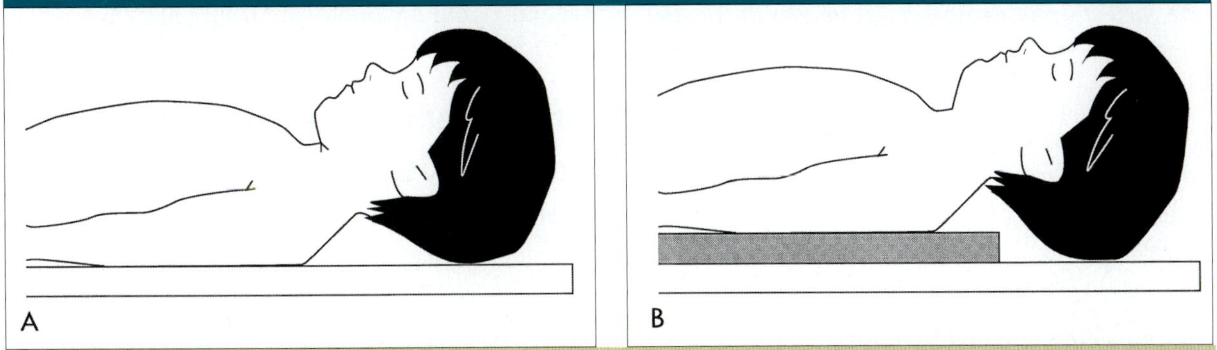

Figure 2 A, Because of the disproportionately large head-to-chest ratio in children younger than 8 years of age, standard spine boards result in flexion of the cervical spine. **B,** Simple modifications to accommodate the large head size allow neutral positioning of the cervical spine. (Reproduced from Vaccaro AR, Pizzutillo PD: Management of pediatric spinal cord injury patients, in Levine AM, Eismont FJ, Garfin SF, Zigler JE, eds: *Spine Trauma*. Philadelphia, PA, WB Saunders, 1998, pp 544-559.)

of the shoulders and thorax with bolsters or use of a spinal board that is recessed in the area of the head is necessary to prevent flexion of the cervical spine (**Figure 2**). The use of tape and sandbags provides superior immobilization of the cervical spine compared with a hard collar. In patients wearing a helmet, removal ideally occurs not on the field but in the emergency department while the head is manually stabilized. For the patient with compromised pulmonary function that requires airway support, orotracheal or nasotracheal intubation may safely be performed in a controlled manner.[51] The role of intravenous steroid infusion in the emergency department for a pediatric patient with an SCI remains unclear. Although Bracken et al[52] reported that methylprednisolone improved spinal cord recovery up to 5 motor points if administered within 8 hours of injury, only 15% of patients in the study were between 13 years and 19 years of age.

Diagnosing SCI is particularly challenging in the child with a concomitant closed head injury who is unresponsive. Head injury occurs with SCI in 25% to 50% of patients.[53,54] Important clinical signs of SCI in the emergency setting include a step-off that is palpable along the spine, torticollis, generalized flaccidity, diaphragmatic breathing without the use of accessory muscles of inspiration, dermatomal pattern sensory loss, the absence of sacral reflexes, bradycardia with hypotension, autonomic hyperreflexia, poikilothermia, priapism, unexplained urinary retention, and the presence of clonus in an unconscious patient without decerebrate rigidity.[55] Patients presenting with severe hypotension not explained by an obvious site of blood loss,[33] hypoxic encephalopathy,[55] or cardiac arrest should also be evaluated carefully to differentiate injury to the high cervical cord, a potential etiology for these findings, from other injuries.

Neurologic Examination

Following a complete physical examination, a thorough and well-documented neurologic examination should be performed on all patients with a suspected SCI. This examination should be repeated at short and regular intervals to ensure early detection of neurologic deterioration or the presence of transient neurologic findings. The International Standards for Neurological Classification of Spinal Cord Injury (ISCSCI) provide a method for the examination of myotomes and dermatomes and classification of the neurologic consequence of SCI.[56] This system is routinely used for assessing pediatric patients with SCI and is considered the gold-standard assessment for both prognosis and outcomes despite little study of its appropriateness for children. Mulcahey et al[57-60] showed strong test and retest reliability of the ISCSCI in a sample of 74 children and youth with chronic SCI. No reliable method for complete assessment of infants and toddlers with SCI has been established. The type and level of injury must be approximated in this age group. Serial neurologic examinations in the months and years after injury allow for more accurate determination of function with maturity.

Imaging

AP and lateral radiographs of the entire spine are required when spinal injury is suspected.[28] CT is used in conjunction with plain radiographs to define the extent of spinal column injuries. CT evaluation is also used to rule out head, thoracoabdominal, and pelvic injuries,[8] which are frequently seen in association with an SCI. The role of MRI in the acute setting is limited but may be an important tool to assess the child with a suspected SCIWORA or who cannot cooperate with a neurologic examination because of a head injury or developmental deficits. Flexion-extension MRI is useful to assess for occult instability. Diffusion tensor imaging is a relatively new noninvasive MRI technique that quantifies the diffusion of water molecules in neural tissue in directions parallel and transverse to the axis of axons and may be useful in determining the precise level and type of SCI when the clinical examination is unreliable.[61,62]

Team Evaluation

After acute cardiopulmonary stabilization, identification of associated injuries, and careful evaluation of the extent of the spinal column and neurologic injury, management of the child with SCI is a multidisciplinary effort initiated upon admission. Complete care of the child is best provided by a team that includes the general trauma surgeon, the orthopaedic surgeon, and the neurosurgeon, working in conjunction with a rehabilitation specialist and others, including an otolaryngologist, a pulmonologist, a urologist, a gastroenterologist, a nutritionist, and a wound care team with experience in the care of the child with an SCI.[63]

Orthopaedic Considerations for the Pediatric SCI Patient

Basic Management Principles

The goals of treatment of spinal injuries in the pediatric patient do not differ from those for the adult with SCI. Restoration of spinal column alignment and stability, prevention of progressive neurologic deterioration, and improvement of existing neurologic function when possible are the basic tenets of acute SCI management. Young patients are a unique challenge because the pathoanatomy of specific types of injury differs from adults, primarily because of the osteochondral nature of the vertebral column and increased soft-tissue mobility. SCIWORA is a particularly unique problem for children because of anatomic considerations (**Table 2**).[64-66] The difficulty in accurately determining the presence of instability in the immature spine after SCI makes management decisions difficult.[67] Because of increased capacity for healing, external immobilization and supportive care is more commonly used for injuries without severe spinal malalignment.[6,7,68] When spinal instrumentation is necessary, the wide variation in vertebral sizes makes selection of spinal instrumentation sometimes challenging. While the available options for instrumentation of the entire spinal column have increased in the last decade, children younger than 3 years of age who require stabilization pose a particularly difficult problem.

Halo fixation, one of the most fundamental forms of immobilization of the cervical spine, is a good example of the problem of managing young children with a cervical injury and SCI. As with adults, proper halo-ring application in children is critical in preventing complications including pin loosening and infection.[69] Anterior pins should be placed superior to and at the level of the middle or lateral one-third of the orbit to avoid the supraorbital and supratrochlear nerves. The ring should lie below the greatest circumference of the cranium.[70] For the patient older than 12 years of age, pins should be torqued to 8 in-lb, a value that has been shown to reduce pin loosening and infection as compared to 5 in-lb to 6 in-lb of pin torque.[71] When pin drainage is noted, the site should be prepped sterilely and swabbed for culture before initiation of antibiotics. The torque on the potentially infected pin should then be rechecked. If the pin cannot be tightened to the appropriate number of inch-pounds after three turns, the pin should be removed or replaced.

Children younger than 12 years of age present a unique problem with halo fixation. A custom-sized halo ring secured with multiple pins torqued to 2 in-lb can be safely used in infants; as many as ten pins can be placed compared with the standard of four used for adults.[72] For children 2 to 12 years of age, the torque may range from 4 in-lb to 6 in-lb. For children under 6 years of age, CT of the skull is useful before pin placement so that variations in skull thickness at the potential sites of the pins may be identified.[73] When halo removal is necessary because of loosening and/or infection, a custom-molded Minerva-type cervicothoracolumbosacral orthosis (CTLSO) is an effective alternative to provide continued cervical immobilization. Frequent skin inspection beneath the halo vest or orthosis by experienced caregivers is essential to prevent pressure ulcers and other skin complications commonly seen in insensate patients.

Spine Deformity After SCI

The paralyzed, skeletally immature patient is at a high risk for developing spine deformity. These deformities are the result of several factors, including asymmetric truncal weakness, injury to growth plates leading to asymmetric growth, postlaminectomy deformity, and chronic instability at the site of the injury (**Figure 3**). Osteoporotic bone, spasticity, and posttraumatic changes in the spinal cord such as development of syringomyelia are other contributory etiologies. A child injured more than a year before skeletal maturity has a 98% chance of developing scoliosis and a 67% chance of requiring surgery to manage the deformity.[74-76] By contrast, those injured within a year of skeletal maturity have only a 20% chance of developing scoliosis, and only 5% of these patients will require surgery.

TABLE 2

Characteristics of the Pediatric Spine That Predispose to SCIWORA

1. High head-to-torso ratio
2. Underdeveloped cervical musculature
3. High water content of the intervertebral disks and anulus
4. Shallow and horizontally oriented facet joints and underdeveloped uncinate processes
5. Generalized laxity of spinal ligaments and facet capsules
6. Incompletely ossified and wedge-shaped vertebral bodies

Prophylactic bracing, in the form of a lightweight thoracolumbosacral orthosis (TLSO), may be effective in delaying or preventing surgery. In one important retrospective study, Mehta et al[77] evaluated the effect of bracing on development of scoliosis in 123 skeletally immature children with SCI. Of 42 patients with less than 10° of scoliosis, 29 were braced. Only 13 (45%) of the braced patients required surgery while 10 patients (77%) in the nonbraced group required a spinal fusion. A similar trend was observed for patients with curves measuring 10° to 20°. In addition, the braced group demonstrated a longer time period to surgical fusion, thus allowing for maximal truncal growth before the procedure.

Based on these findings and our experience, prophylactic bracing of all skeletally immature patients with SCI should be considered. For those younger than 10 years of age, a TLSO is prescribed for curves as large as 80° if the curve is flexible enough to permit adequate curve correction without discomfort, pulmonary restrictions, or skin complications. For children older than

FIGURE 3

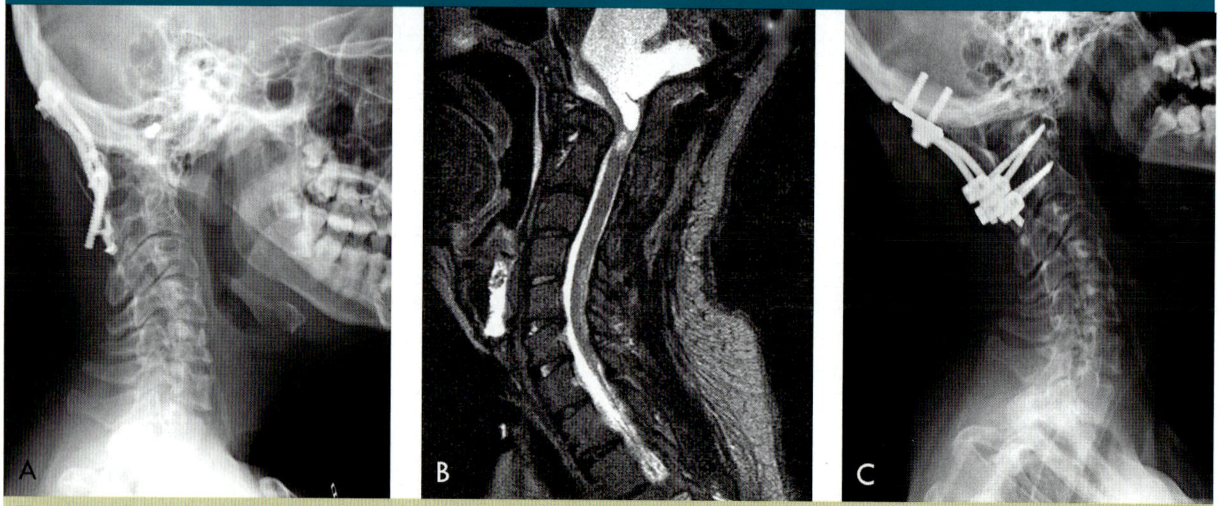

Figure 3 **A,** Lateral radiograph of a 15-year-old tetraplegic girl who had sustained a traumatic occipital cervical dislocation and SCI 8 years earlier. She had begun to develop torticollis with cervical kyphosis and diminished ability to shrug her shoulders. **B,** MRI revealed expansion of her fourth ventricle and an upper cervical syrinx. **C,** She underwent revision cervical fusion and within 3 months, her shoulder shrug returned.

10 years of age, surgery is recommended for deformity measuring greater than 40°. Curves larger than 40° in the pediatric SCI patient are generally progressive, despite careful brace interventions, and require surgical intervention.[28,78,79]

Although fusionless options such as vertebral wedge osteotomies have been used for this patient population,[80] spinal fusion is the preferred method of spinal deformity management. Surgical correction and fusion in this population carry a high complication rate.[75] The incidence of pseudarthrosis requiring revision surgery is reported to be as high as 29%.[81] Infection rates are also higher in children and adolescents with SCI compared with other causes of scoliosis. In one recent study, Cahill et al[82] reported a 16% infection rate after fusion surgery for patients with SCI. Lack of protective sensation, fecal contamination because of genitourinary colonization and frequent catheterization, incontinence, immobility, and nutritional deficits contribute to the development of wound infections after spinal surgery.

Paralytic Hip Dysplasia

Children younger than 5 years of age with spastic paralysis after SCI are at risk for hip instability and subluxation. McCarthy et al[83] reported that at least one hip developed dysplasia and subluxation in almost half of children who sustained SCI. Age at injury correlated with the risk of hip subluxation, as 93% of patients 10 years of age or younger had at least one subluxated hip compared to only 9% of those older than 10 years of age. Hip instability may cause pelvic obliquity that creates challenges in proper seating and positioning in the wheelchair (**Figure 4**), limb-length discrepancy that inhibits ease of walking in long leg braces, compensatory spine deformity, and, for many patients, increasing spasticity in the affected extremity.

Strategies for prevention of spastic hip dysplasia include maintaining the hips in abduction through the use of wheelchair inserts, abduction pillows, and other devices; prone sleep positioning to diminish flexion contractures of the hip, which may worsen instability; and range-of-motion exercises. Botox injections and antispasticity medications are sometimes helpful to slow progression of this deformity. Surgical reconstruction of paralytic hip dysplasia includes soft-tissue releases and capsulorrhaphy of the hip in combination with femoral and pelvic osteotomies, such as Chiari or posterior augmentation of the acetabulum with allograft.[84]

Heterotopic Ossification

Heterotopic ossification (HO) is the formation of bone at ectopic sites and is the most common orthopaedic complication after SCI. HO occurs in 3% to 18% of pediatric patients with SCI, compared with as many as 50% of adult patients.[85-87] The most common site of HO is the hip but it also occurs about the knee, elbow, and shoulder. Generally, the onset of HO is approximately 1 year from injury in pediatric patients, a time frame lon-

FIGURE 4

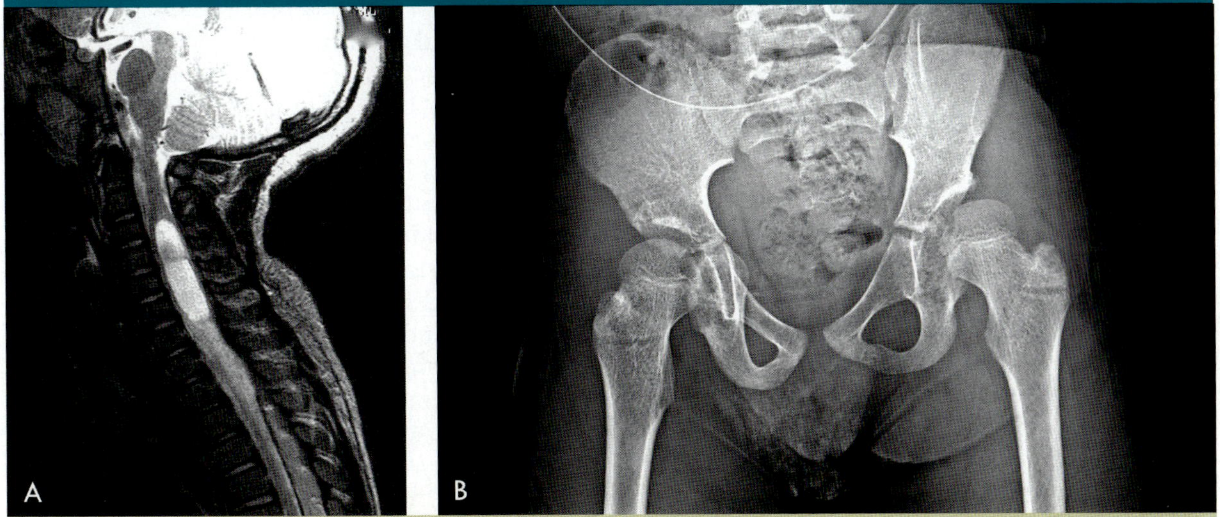

Figure 4 A, Midline sagittal cervical spine MRI scan of a 6-year-old girl with SCI from a birth injury with a stable syrinx. She has incomplete tetraplegia and increasing difficulty with seating. **B,** AP pelvis radiograph reveals left hip subluxation and acetabular dysplasia.

ger than the 1 to 4 months in which HO typically develops in adults. The etiology of HO after SCI is not known. Fever is the earliest symptom. Joint pain, swelling, and stiffness are also seen as the HO begins to develop. Separating impending HO from other diagnoses can sometimes be difficult because, in addition to the nonspecific clinical findings, increased levels of inflammatory markers, such as erythrocyte sedimentation rate, C-reactive protein, and serum alkaline phosphatase can be found in the early stages of HO. Differential diagnosis for HO includes deep vein thrombosis, cellulitis, fracture, impending ulcer, and septic arthritis. Urinary levels of prostaglandin E2 have been shown to increase concomitantly with the progression of HO[88] and may serve as a marker for the disease. Prophylaxis against the development of HO in pediatric patients with SCI is not routinely prescribed due to the relatively lower risk for HO and the potential for complications from editronate disodium, the most commonly used medication for prophylaxis.[89] Surgical resection of HO may be considered when HO severely limits joint motion. This is best done after bone maturation, when alkaline phosphatase levels have normalized and a bone scan of the affected area shows little isotope uptake, typically at least 1 year after development of HO.

Osteopenia

Osteopenia occurs in all patients with SCI. There is rapid loss of trabecular bone in the lower extremity and pelvis. Calcium homeostasis is reached by approximately 16 months after injury. For the typical pediatric patient, bone mass after SCI is only 50% to 70% of the normal preinjury mass and the degree of osteopenia puts most patients at risk for fractures.[90,91]

Pathologic fractures of the long bones occur commonly in patients with SCI.[92-95] Fracture diagnosis in patients with SCI is sometimes subtle, particularly because of the absence of pain. A child with an SCI who sustains a pathologic fracture typically presents with a swollen limb, malaise, and a low-grade fever. Radiographs should be taken for any child with this constellation of symptoms to confirm the fracture. Fracture management most commonly consists of nonsurgical care by immobilization with well-padded splinting or casting. Immobilization time varies based on the type and location of the fracture. Rapid mobilization of the child out of bed, early weight bearing when safe, and careful range of motion of the affected joint after bone healing are critical to minimize complications of these injuries.

Medical Complications in the Pediatric SCI Patient

Pulmonary

Vocal cord dysfunction, direct tracheal injury, and diaphragm weakness or paralysis are common with upper cervical SCI and predispose the patient to recurrent hypoxemia and respiratory failure.[96,97]

Decreased inspiratory ventilation is the result of loss of intercostal muscle function. Decreased expiratory pressure occurs because the diaphragm cannot be passively pushed upward by the contracting abdominal muscles. Patients are at risk for aspiration pneumonia and pulmonary sepsis. Postural maneuvers and breathing exercises are essential to train accessory muscles to assist in breathing and to help clear secretions. Prevention of respiratory infections, including pneumococcus, by caregivers' attention to hand washing and use of masks when indicated; aggressive and well-coordinated regular pulmonary care; and yearly influenza vaccinations are some of the steps necessary to avoid respiratory complications.

For injuries at or above C6, early tracheostomy can be life-saving and shorten inpatient stays. All children with cervical injuries should be evaluated completely for airway injury and dysfunction and for diaphragmatic paresis or paralysis, which may be unilateral. Theophylline, a phosphodiesterase inhibitor that increases intracellular cyclic AMP (adenosine monophosphate), has been shown experimentally to improve diaphragm function in animals with hemitransection of the cervical cord, suggesting both direct and indirect beneficial effects on the diaphragm and the respiratory system as a whole.[98,99] There is insufficient evidence to support the routine use of theophylline in patients with SCI and diaphragm dysfunction, although in refractory cases it may be beneficial.[100]

Cardiovascular

In the days immediately following an SCI, a sympathetic stress response occurs that may result in a disturbance of cardiovascular homeostasis, potentially causing secondary insults to the injured cord and other organ systems.[101,102] Spinal or neurogenic shock following traumatic SCI is a well-recognized but poorly understood phenomenon.[103,104] Neurogenic shock is defined as a state of inadequate tissue oxygen delivery with resultant end-organ failure in the presence of a complete SCI above the sixth thoracic vertebra, a response to the loss of sympathetic outflow and cardiac accelerators that originate from the T1-T5 spinal levels. The most common manifestation is hypotension. Tachycardia predominates in the immediate postinjury period, followed by bradycardia in the weeks to months after the SCI. Bradycardia results from the loss of sympathetic input and the eventual development of unopposed vagal tone.[105,106] The cardiovascular changes are usually managed successfully with administration of intravenous fluids and vasopressors such as dopamine and other medications.

One of the most dangerous late complications of SCI is autonomic dysreflexia. This complication is characterized by a sudden exaggerated reflex increase in blood pressure, sometimes accompanied by bradycardia, in response to a noxious stimulus originating below the level of injury.[107-109] Although this is seen in as many as 85% of all SCI patients with injury at T6 and above, the true incidence in children is unknown.[108,109] A strong painful stimulus ascends through the spinothalamic tract and posterior columns below the level of the lesion and incites sympathetic discharge from the preganglionic sympathetic neurons in the intermediolateral cell column resulting in the release of large quantities of norepinephrine, dopamine-β-hydroxylase, and dopamine. The patient may experience hypertension, pounding headache, sweating, and flushing. The most common cause of autonomic dysreflexia is bladder irritation as a result of overdistension, bladder/renal calculi, or urinary tract infections. Other common causes include bowel distension, pressure ulcers, tight clothing, deep vein thrombosis, menses, pregnancy, labor, trauma, HO, surgery/invasive procedures, hyperthermia, or painful stimuli. Clinical manifestations of autonomic dysreflexia in children may be more subtle or vague. All caregivers should be educated on the detection and management of autonomic dysreflexia. The mainstay of treatment is elimination of the irritation, such as bladder emptying or bowel evacuation. Failing that, medication may be needed.

Genitourinary

Immediately after SCI, the bladder becomes atonic. Careful management of a neurogenic bladder reduces the risk of renal injury by reducing bladder reflux and hydronephrosis. Initial management is Foley catheter placement to prevent bladder overdistension, followed shortly by a program of frequent intermittent catheterizations. Intermittent catheterization can be initiated as early as 3 years of age and self-catheterization may be taught to patients who are developmentally 5 to 7 years old.[110,111] Timed voidings and careful administration of intravenous fluids are other useful management strategies for a neurogenic bladder. Prophylactic antibiotics should be given to patients with recurrent and severe urinary tract infections, obstructive uropathy, or compromised renal function, including vesicoureteral reflux hydronephrosis. Patients with asymptomatic bacteriuria are generally not treated unless they have compromised renal function.

Gastrointestinal

Gastrointestinal motility may cease for several days after an SCI, increasing the risk of gastric reflux, a potential cause of stress ulcers and gastrointestinal bleeding. Patients with SCI should prophylactically receive a proton pump inhibitor or other types of medications designed to reduce the risk of developing these complications. Most patients develop an ileus for several days after the injury as well. Enteral feeding can be started orally or via an orogastric or nasogastric tube after the ileus has resolved, based on the return of normal bowel sounds and lack of abdominal distension. A regular bowel program should be instituted as soon as the patient receives enteral nutrition to diminish the risk of constipation and impaction that may result from the lack of reflex neural control of the bowel secondary to the SCI. The goals of a standard bowel regime are regular bowel movements, continence, and prevention of impaction.[112]

Neuromuscular

Between 65% and 78% of patients with a chronic SCI (≥ 1 year postinjury) develop muscle spasticity.[113-115] This complication may result in pain, joint contractures, pressure ulcers from difficulty with seating, and problems with perineal care, and may inhibit rehabilitation efforts. Many options for treatment of spasticity are available and applied on a case-by-case basis. The effect of physical therapy on diminishing spasticity has not been well documented. This modality is most frequently used in combination with other modalities that control spasticity and is used to preserve joint range of motion and ensure proper patient positioning and maintenance of seating systems and other equipment. For patients with spasticity that impairs functioning and is refractory to physical therapy alone, antispasticity medications are the first line of management. Oral baclofen and botulinum toxin for patients with localized spasticity[114,116] are the most commonly used medications. For diffuse spasticity that is unresponsive to oral baclofen or other oral medications, intrathecal baclofen is an option. Baclofen is delivered directly into the cerebrospinal fluid through a catheter that connects the drug reservoir to the intrathecal space.[117] Intrathecal baclofen more effectively diminishes diffuse muscle spasticity compared with oral baclofen but has more side effects. Although some patients are functionally better with use of these agents, reduction of spasticity does not correlate with improved function in every patient.

Dermatologic

Pressure ulcers are one of the most common complications in patients who sustain an SCI. Children and adolescents with pressure ulcers may require extensive care for management of this problem including periods of immobilization, hospitalization for acute wound care issues, and surgical management. Serious complications such as systemic sepsis, osteomyelitis, and malnutrition may also result from skin breakdown.[118,119] Preventative measures are paramount to prevent dermatologic complications. Some strategies include frequent weight shifting, proper seating equipment with adequate cushioning, and proper brace fitting, all with the important goal of reducing pressure, friction, and shear forces that cause pressure ulcers. Thermal injuries may also occur to insensate areas. Prevention includes avoiding hot car heaters, radiators, hair dryers, curling irons, and hot plates or cups placed in the lap.

Other Medical Considerations

Hypercalcemia is a frequent cause of nonspecific gastrointestinal complaints in adolescents with SCI. This complication typically presents in males within 3 months after injury and affects 10% to 23% of patients.[120,121] Clinical symptoms and signs are nausea, vomiting, abdominal pain, poor appetite, polydipsia and mental status change. The increase in bone turnover characteristic of growing children, combined with increased bone resorption from immobility and other factors after an SCI, are believed to be the causes of this effect. Intravenous hydration and furosemides, both of which enhance the renal excretion of calcium, are the recommended treatment. Symptoms generally resolve within 3 to 4 days of initiation of treatment.

Venous thromboembolism and pulmonary embolism occur less frequently in children and adolescents compared with adults with SCI. Only 1% of patients younger than 14 years of age with SCI develop clinically significant deep vein thrombi or pulmonary embolism. However, the incidence in the adolescent is almost 5%, a percentage approaching that which is seen in adults.[122] Anticoagulation is the mainstay of prevention and therapy for thromboembolism after SCI. Subcutaneous low molecular-weight heparin is the drug most commonly prescribed for prophylaxis and treatment of these complications because its pharmacokinetics are more predictable than unfractionated heparin or oral anticoagulants.[123] Most cases of deep vein thrombosis occur during the first

3 months after injury. Increased risk is seen after surgery that requires bed rest postoperatively, such as plastic surgery for decubiti, and after spinal surgery.

Conclusion

Understanding the normal variations in the growth and development of the immature spinal column serves as a foundation for appropriate diagnosis and management of the acute pediatric SCI patient. The goal of medical treatment of any SCI patient is to protect the central nervous system from further injury by appropriate support and stabilization while facilitating, through aggressive rehabilitation, the reintroduction of the patient into society as a productive, functioning member. Through appreciation of the various anatomic, biomechanical, and physiologic differences between adult and pediatric spinal injury patients, the surgeon can anticipate potential problems unique to the growing patient and minimize or prevent the complications of this catastrophic injury and its long-term sequelae.

References

1. Shavelle RM, DeVivo MJ, Paculdo DR, Vogel LC, Strauss DJ: Long-term survival after childhood spinal cord injury. *J Spinal Cord Med* 2007; 30(Suppl 1):S48-S54.
2. Shavelle RM, DeVivo MJ, Strauss DJ, Paculdo DR, Lammertse DP, Day SM: Long-term survival of persons ventilator dependent after spinal cord injury. *J Spinal Cord Med* 2006;29(5):511-519.
3. Augutis M, Levi R: Pediatric spinal cord injury in Sweden: Incidence, etiology and outcome. *Spinal Cord* 2003;41(6):328-336.
4. Puisto V, Kääriäinen S, Impinen A, et al: Incidence of spinal and spinal cord injuries and their surgical treatment in children and adolescents: A population-based study. *Spine (Phila Pa 1976)* 2010;35(1):104-107.
5. Asher MA, Jacobs RR: Pediatric thoracolumbar spine trauma, in Bradford DS, Hensinger RN, eds: *The Pediatric Spine*. New York, NY, Thieme, 1985, pp 105-117.
6. Crawford AH: Operative treatment of spine fractures in children. *Orthop Clin North Am* 1990; 21(2):325-339.
7. Henrys P, Lyne ED, Lifton C, Salciccioli G: Clinical review of cervical spine injuries in children. *Clin Orthop Relat Res* 1977;129:172-176.
8. Hill SA, Miller CA, Kosnik EJ, Hunt WE: Pediatric neck injuries: A clinical study. *J Neurosurg* 1984;60(4):700-706.
9. Kewalramani LS, Tori JA: Spinal cord trauma in children: Neurologic patterns, radiologic features, and pathomechanics of injury. *Spine (Phila Pa 1976)* 1980;5(1):11-18.
10. Mann DC: Spine fractures in children and adolescents. *Spine State Art Rev* 1990;4(1):25-47.
11. Price AE: Unique aspects of pediatric spine injuries, in Ervico TJ, Bauer RO, Waugh T, eds: *Spinal Trauma*. Philadelphia, PA, JB Lippincott, 1991, pp 581-625.
12. Ransohoff J: Lesions of the cauda equina. *Clin Neurosurg* 1970;17:331-344.
13. Ruge JR, Sinson GP, McLone DG, Cerullo LJ: Pediatric spinal injury: The very young. *J Neurosurg* 1988;68(1):25-30.
14. Surkin J, Gilbert BJ, Harkey HL III, Sniezek J, Currier M: Spinal cord injury in Mississippi: Findings and evaluation, 1992-1994. *Spine (Phila Pa 1976)* 2000;25(6):716-721.
15. Buechner JS, Speare MC, Fontes J: Hospitalizations for spinal cord injuries, 1994-1998. *Med Health R I* 2000;83(3):92-93.
16. Warren S, Moore M, Johnson MS: Traumatic head and spinal cord injuries in Alaska (1991-1993). *Alaska Med* 1995;37(1):11-19.
17. Price C, Makintubee S, Herndon W, Istre GR: Epidemiology of traumatic spinal cord injury and acute hospitalization and rehabilitation charges for spinal cord injuries in Oklahoma, 1988-1990. *Am J Epidemiol* 1994;139(1):37-47.
18. Woodruff BA, Baron RC: A description of nonfatal spinal cord injury using a hospital-based registry. *Am J Prev Med* 1994;10(1):10-14.
19. Vitale MG, Goss JM, Matsumoto H, Roye DP Jr: Epidemiology of pediatric spinal cord injury in the United States: Years 1997 and 2000. *J Pediatr Orthop* 2006;26(6):745-749.
20. DeVivo MJ, Vogel LC: Epidemiology of spinal cord injury in children and adolescents. *J Spinal Cord Med* 2004;27(Suppl 1):S4-S10.
21. Lee JH, Sung IY, Kang JY, Park SR: Characteristics of pediatric-onset spinal cord injury. *Pediatr Int* 2009;51(2):254-257.
22. Anderson JM, Schutt AH: Spinal injury in children: A review of 156 cases seen from 1950 through 1978. *Mayo Clin Proc* 1980;55(8): 499-504.
23. Andrews LG, Jung SK: Spinal cord injuries in children in British Columbia. *Paraplegia* 1979; 17(4):442-451.
24. Choi JU, Hoffman HJ, Hendrick EB, Humphreys RP, Keith WS: Traumatic infarction of the spinal cord in children. *J Neurosurg* 1986;65(5): 608-610.
25. Hachen HJ: Spinal cord injury in children and adolescents: Diagnostic pitfalls and therapeutic

considerations in the acute stage [proceedings]. *Paraplegia* 1977;15(1):55-64.

26. Jones L: Birth trauma and the cervical spine. *Arch Dis Child* 1970;45(239):147.
27. Melzak J: Paraplegia among children. *Lancet* 1969;2(7610):45-48.
28. Ogden JA: Spine, in Wickland E, ed: *Skeletal Injury in the Child*, ed 2. Philadelphia, PA, WB Saunders, 1990, pp 571-625.
29. Pang D, Wilberger JE Jr: Spinal cord injury without radiographic abnormalities in children. *J Neurosurg* 1982;57(1):114-129.
30. Yngve DA, Harris WP, Herndon WA, Sullivan JA, Gross RH: Spinal cord injury without osseous spine fracture. *J Pediatr Orthop* 1988;8(2): 153-159.
31. Hadley MN, Zabramski JM, Browner CM, Rekate H, Sonntag VK: Pediatric spinal trauma: Review of 122 cases of spinal cord and vertebral column injuries. *J Neurosurg* 1988;68(1):18-24.
32. Walsh JW, Stevens DB, Young AB: Traumatic paraplegia in children without contiguous spinal fracture or dislocation. *Neurosurgery* 1983;12(4): 439-445.
33. Bohn D, Armstrong D, Becker L, Humphreys R: Cervical spine injuries in children. *J Trauma* 1990; 30(4):463-469.
34. Platzer P, Jaindl M, Thalhammer G, et al: Cervical spine injuries in pediatric patients. *J Trauma* 2007;62(2):389-396.
35. Jagannathan J, Dumont AS, Prevedello DM, Shaffrey CI, Jane JA Jr: Cervical spine injuries in pediatric athletes: Mechanisms and management. *Neurosurg Focus* 2006;21(4):E6.
36. Torg JS, Guille JT, Jaffe S: Injuries to the cervical spine in American football. *J Bone Joint Surg Am* 2002;84-A(1):112-122.
37. Kellum E, Creek A, Dawkins R, Bernard M, Sawyer JR: Age-related patterns of injury in children involved in all-terrain vehicle accidents. *J Pediatr Orthop* 2008;28(8):854-858.
38. Allen JP: Birth injury to the spinal cord. *Northwest Med* 1970;69(5):323-326.
39. Bresnan MJ, Abroms IF: Neonatal spinal cord transection secondary to intrauterine hyperextension of the neck in breech presentation. *J Pediatr* 1974;84(5):734-737.
40. De Souza SW, Davis JA: Spinal cord damage in a newborn infant. *Arch Dis Child* 1974;49(1):70-71.
41. Shulman ST, Madden JD, Esterly JR, Shanklin DR: Transection of spinal cord: A rare obstetrical complication of cephalic delivery. *Arch Dis Child* 1971;46(247):291-294.
42. Towbin A: Latent spinal cord and brain stem injury in newborn infants. *Dev Med Child Neurol* 1969;11(1):54-68.
43. Allen JP, Meyers GG, Condon VR: Laceration of the spinal cord related to breech delivery. *JAMA* 1969;208(6):1019-1022.
44. Allen B, Ferguson RL: Cervical spinal trauma in children, in Bradford DS, Hensinger RN, eds: *The Pediatric Spine*. New York, NY, Thieme, 1985, pp 89-104.
45. Burke DC: Spinal cord trauma in children. *Paraplegia* 1971;9(1):1-14.
46. Caffey J: The whiplash shaken infant syndrome: Manual shaking by the extremities with whiplash-induced intracranial and intraocular bleedings, linked with residual permanent brain damage and mental retardation. *Pediatrics* 1974;54(4):396-403.
47. Stern WE, Rand RW: Birth injuries to the spinal cord: A report of 2 cases and review of the literature. *Am J Obstet Gynecol* 1959;78:498-512.
48. Ahmann PA, Smith SA, Schwartz JF, Clark DB: Spinal cord infarction due to minor trauma in children. *Neurology* 1975;25(4):301-307.
49. LeBlanc HJ, Nadell J: Spinal cord injuries in children. *Surg Neurol* 1974;2(6):411-414.
50. Gabos PG, Tuten HR, Leet A, Stanton RP: Fracture-dislocation of the lumbar spine in an abused child. *Pediatrics* 1998;101(3 Pt 1): 473-477.
51. Holley J, Jorden R: Airway management in patients with unstable cervical spine fractures. *Ann Emerg Med* 1989;18(11):1237-1239.
52. Bracken MB, Shepard MJ, Collins WF, et al: A randomized, controlled trial of methylprednisolone or naloxone in the treatment of acute spinal-cord injury: Results of the Second National Acute Spinal Cord Injury Study. *N Engl J Med* 1990; 322(20):1405-1411.
53. Cirak B, Ziegfeld S, Knight VM, Chang D, Avellino AM, Paidas CN: Spinal injuries in children. *J Pediatr Surg* 2004;39(4):607-612.
54. Betz RR, Mulcahey MJ, D'Andrea LP, Clements DH: Acute evaluation and management of pediatric spinal cord injury. *J Spinal Cord Med* 2004; 27(Suppl 1):S11-S15.
55. Sneed RC, Stover SL: Undiagnosed spinal cord injuries in brain-injured children. *Am J Dis Child* 1988;142(9):965-967.
56. Maynard FM Jr, Bracken MB, Creasey G, et al: International standards for neurological and functional classification of spinal cord injury. *Spinal Cord* 1997;35(5):266-274.
57. Mulcahey MJ, Gaughan J, Betz RR, Johansen KJ: The International Standards for Neurological Classification of Spinal Cord Injury: Reliability of data when applied to children and youths. *Spinal Cord* 2007;45(6):452-459.

58. Chafetz RS, Vogel LC, Betz RR, Gaughan JP, Mulcahey MJ: International Standards for Neurological Classification of Spinal Cord Injury: Training effect on accurate classification. *J Spinal Cord Med* 2008;31(5):538-542.

59. Chafetz RS, Gaughan JP, Vogel LC, Betz R, Mulcahey MJ: The International Standards for Neurological Classification of Spinal Cord Injury: Intra-rater agreement of total motor and sensory scores in the pediatric population. *J Spinal Cord Med* 2009;32(2):157-161.

60. Mulcahey MJ, Gaughan J, Betz RR: Agreement of repeated motor and sensory scores at individual myotomes and dermatomes in young persons with complete spinal cord injury. *Spinal Cord* 2009;47(1):56-61.

61. Bhadelia RA, Price LL, Tedesco KL, et al: Diffusion tensor imaging, white matter lesions, the corpus callosum, and gait in the elderly. *Stroke* 2009;40(12):3816-3820.

62. Kim JH, Loy DN, Wang Q, et al: Diffusion tensor imaging at 3 hours after traumatic spinal cord injury predicts long-term locomotor recovery. *J Neurotrauma* 2010;37(3):587-598.

63. Denis F, Krach L: Spinal injuries in the growing person, in Lovell WW, Winter RB, eds: *Pediatric Orthopaedics*. Philadelphia, PA, JB Lippincott, 1986, pp 499-529.

64. Bailey DK: The normal cervical spine in infants and children. *Radiology* 1952;59(5):712-719.

65. Sullivan CR, Bruwer AJ, Harris LE: Hypermobility of the cervical spine in children; a pitfall in the diagnosis of cervical dislocation. *Am J Surg* 1958; 95(4):636-640.

66. Fesmire FM, Luten RC: The pediatric cervical spine: Developmental anatomy and clinical aspects. *J Emerg Med* 1989;7(2):133-142.

67. McPhee IB: Spinal fractures and dislocations in children and adolescents. *Spine (Phila Pa 1976)* 1981;6(6):533-537.

68. Fielding JW, Hawkins RJ, Ratzan SA: Spine fusion for atlanto-axial instability. *J Bone Joint Surg Am* 1976;58(3):400-407.

69. Dormans JP, Criscitiello AA, Drummond DS, Davidson RS: Complications in children managed with immobilization in a halo vest. *J Bone Joint Surg Am* 1995;77(9):1370-1373.

70. Garfin SR, Botte MJ, Waters RL, Nickel VL: Complications in the use of the halo fixation device. *J Bone Joint Surg Am* 1986;68(3):320-325.

71. Botte MJ, Byrne TP, Garfin SR: Application of the halo device for immobilization of the cervical spine utilizing an increased torque pressure. *J Bone Joint Surg Am* 1987;69(5):750-752.

72. Mubarak SJ, Camp JF, Vuletich W, Wenger DR, Garfin SR: Halo application in the infant. *J Pediatr Orthop* 1989;9(5):612-614.

73. Letts M, Kaylor D, Gouw G: A biomechanical analysis of halo fixation in children. *J Bone Joint Surg Br* 1988;70(2):277-279.

74. Lancourt JE, Dickson JH, Carter RE: Paralytic spinal deformity following traumatic spinal-cord injury in children and adolescents. *J Bone Joint Surg Am* 1981;63(1):47-53.

75. Mayfield JK, Erkkila JC, Winter RB: Spine deformity subsequent to acquired childhood spinal cord injury. *J Bone Joint Surg Am* 1981;63(9): 1401-1411.

76. Dearolf WW III, Betz RR, Vogel LC, Levin J, Clancy M, Steel HH: Scoliosis in pediatric spinal cord-injured patients. *J Pediatr Orthop* 1990;10(2): 214-218.

77. Mehta S, Betz RR, Mulcahey MJ, McDonald C, Vogel LC, Anderson C: Effect of bracing on paralytic scoliosis secondary to spinal cord injury. *J Spinal Cord Med* 2004;27(Suppl 1):S88-S92.

78. Audic B, Maury M: Secondary vertebral deformities in childhood and adolescence. *Paraplegia* 1969;7(1):11-16.

79. Bedbrook GM: Correction of scoliosis due to paraplegia sustained in paediatric age-group [proceedings]. *Paraplegia* 1977;15(1):90-96.

80. McCarthy KP, Chafetz RS, Mulcahey MJ, Frisch RF, D'Andrea LP, Betz RR: Clinical efficacy of the vertebral wedge osteotomy for the fusionless treatment of paralytic scoliosis. *Spine (Phila Pa 1976)* 2010;35(4):403-410.

81. Tsirikos AI, Markham P, McMaster MJ: Surgical correction of spinal deformities following spinal cord injury occurring in childhood. *J Surg Orthop Adv* 2007;16(4):174-186.

82. Cahill PJ, Warnick DE, Lee MJ, et al: Infection after spinal fusion for pediatric spinal deformity: Thirty years of experience at a single institution. *Spine (Phila Pa 1976)* 2010;35(12):1211-1217.

83. McCarthy JJ, Chafetz RS, Betz RR, Gaughan J: Incidence and degree of hip subluxation/dislocation in children with spinal cord injury. *J Spinal Cord Med* 2004;27(Suppl 1):S80-S83.

84. Betz RR, Mulcahey MJ, Smith BT, Triolo RJ, McCarthy JJ: Implications of hip subluxation for FES-assisted mobility in patients with spinal cord injury. *Orthopedics* 2001;24(2):181-184.

85. Garland DE, Shimoyama ST, Lugo C, Barras D, Gilgoff I: Spinal cord insults and heterotopic ossification in the pediatric population. *Clin Orthop Relat Res* 1989;245:303-310.

86. Garland DE: A clinical perspective on common forms of acquired heterotopic ossification. *Clin Orthop Relat Res* 1991;263:13-29.

87. Betz RR: Unique management needs of pediatric spinal cord injury patients: Orthopedic problems in the child with spinal cord injury. *J Spinal Cord Med* 1997;20(1):14-16.

88. Schurch B, Capaul M, Vallotton MB, Rossier AB: Prostaglandin E2 measurements: Their value in the early diagnosis of heterotopic ossification in spinal cord injury patients. *Arch Phys Med Rehabil* 1997;78(7):687-691.

89. Silverman SL, Hurvitz EA, Nelson VS, Chiodo A: Rachitic syndrome after disodium etidronate therapy in an adolescent. *Arch Phys Med Rehabil* 1994; 75(1):118-120.

90. Garland DE, Stewart CA, Adkins RH, et al: Osteoporosis after spinal cord injury. *J Orthop Res* 1992; 10(3):371-378.

91. Moynahan M, Betz RR, Triolo RJ, Maurer AH: Characterization of the bone mineral density of children with spinal cord injury. *J Spinal Cord Med* 1996;19(4):249-254.

92. Jiang SD, Dai LY, Jiang LS: Osteoporosis after spinal cord injury. *Osteoporos Int* 2006;17(2): 180-192.

93. McMaster WC, Stauffer ES: The management of long bone fracture in the spinal cord injured patient. *Clin Orthop Relat Res* 1975;112:44-52.

94. Nottage WM: A review of long-bone fractures in patients with spinal cord injuries. *Clin Orthop Relat Res* 1981;155:65-70.

95. Garland DE, Jones RC, Kunkle RW: Upper extremity fractures in the acute spinal cord injured patient. *Clin Orthop Relat Res* 1988;233:110-115.

96. Padman R, Alexander M, Thorogood C, Porth S: Respiratory management of pediatric patients with spinal cord injuries: Retrospective review of the duPont experience. *Neurorehabil Neural Repair* 2003;17(1):32-36.

97. Winslow C, Rozovsky J: Effect of spinal cord injury on the respiratory system. *Am J Phys Med Rehabil* 2003;82(10):803-814.

98. Nantwi KD, Basura GJ, Goshgarian HG: Effects of long-term theophylline exposure on recovery of respiratory function and expression of adenosine A1 mRNA in cervical spinal cord hemisected adult rats. *Exp Neurol* 2003;182(1):232-239.

99. Nantwi KD: Recovery of respiratory activity after C2 hemisection (C2HS): Involvement of adenosinergic mechanisms. *Respir Physiol Neurobiol* 2009; 169(2):102-114.

100. Bascom AT, Lattin CD, Aboussouan LS, Goshgarian HG: Effect of acute aminophylline administration on diaphragm function in high cervical tetraplegia: A case report. *Chest* 2005; 127(2):658-661.

101. Guha A, Tator CH: Acute cardiovascular effects of experimental spinal cord injury. *J Trauma* 1988; 28(4):481-490.

102. Krassioukov A, Claydon VE: The clinical problems in cardiovascular control following spinal cord injury: An overview. *Prog Brain Res* 2006; 152:223-229.

103. Ko HY, Ditunno JF Jr, Graziani V, Little JW: The pattern of reflex recovery during spinal shock. *Spinal Cord* 1999;37(6):402-409.

104. Ditunno JF, Little JW, Tessler A, Burns AS: Spinal shock revisited: A four-phase model. *Spinal Cord* 2004;42(7):383-395.

105. Teasell RW, Arnold JM, Krassioukov A, Delaney GA: Cardiovascular consequences of loss of supraspinal control of the sympathetic nervous system after spinal cord injury. *Arch Phys Med Rehabil* 2000;81(4):506-516.

106. Bravo G, Guízar-Sahagún G, Ibarra A, Centurión D, Villalón CM: Cardiovascular alterations after spinal cord injury: An overview. *Curr Med Chem Cardiovasc Hematol Agents* 2004;2(2):133-148.

107. Vogel LC, Krajci KA, Anderson CJ: Adults with pediatric-onset spinal cord injury: Part 1. Prevalence of medical complications. *J Spinal Cord Med* 2002;25(2):106-116.

108. Hickey KJ, Vogel LC, Willis KM, Anderson CJ: Prevalence and etiology of autonomic dysreflexia in children with spinal cord injuries. *J Spinal Cord Med* 2004;27(Suppl 1):S54-S60.

109. McGinnis KB, Vogel LC, McDonald CM, et al: Recognition and management of autonomic dysreflexia in pediatric spinal cord injury. *J Spinal Cord Med* 2004;27(Suppl 1):S61-S74.

110. McLaughlin JF, Murray M, Van Zandt K, Carr M: Clean intermittent catheterization. *Dev Med Child Neurol* 1996;38(5):446-454.

111. Silveri M, Salsano L, Pierro MM, Mosiello G, Capitanucci ML, De Gennaro M: Pediatric spinal cord injury: Approach for urological rehabilitation and treatment. *J Pediatr Urol* 2006;2(1):10-15.

112. Lynch AC, Frizelle FA: Colorectal motility and defecation after spinal cord injury in humans. *Prog Brain Res* 2006;152:335-343.

113. Maynard FM, Karunas RS, Waring WP III: Epidemiology of spasticity following traumatic spinal cord injury. *Arch Phys Med Rehabil* 1990;71(8): 566-569.

114. Adams MM, Hicks AL: Spasticity after spinal cord injury. *Spinal Cord* 2005;43(10):577-586.

115. Fleuren JF, Voerman GE, Snoek GJ, Nene AV, Rietman JS, Hermens HJ: Perception of lower limb spasticity in patients with spinal cord injury. *Spinal Cord* 2009;47(5):396-400.

116. Kirshblum S: Treatment alternatives for spinal cord injury related spasticity. *J Spinal Cord Med* 1999;22(3):199-217.

117. Plassat R, Perrouin Verbe B, Menei P, Menegalli D, Mathé JF, Richard I: Treatment of spasticity with intrathecal Baclofen administration: Long-term follow-up, review of 40 patients. *Spinal Cord* 2004;42(12):686-693.

118. McKinley WO, Gittler MS, Kirshblum SC, Stiens SA, Groah SL: Spinal cord injury medicine: 2. Medical complications after spinal cord injury: Identification and management. *Arch Phys Med Rehabil* 2002;83(3, Suppl 1)S58-S64, S90-S98.

119. Wu SS, Ahn C, Emmons KR, Salcido RS: Pressure ulcers in pediatric patients with spinal cord injury: A review of assessment, prevention, and topical management. *Adv Skin Wound Care* 2009; 22(6):273-286.

120. Maynard FM: Immobilization hypercalcemia following spinal cord injury. *Arch Phys Med Rehabil* 1986;67(1):41-44.

121. Massagli TL, Cardenas DD: Immobilization hypercalcemia treatment with pamidronate disodium after spinal cord injury. *Arch Phys Med Rehabil* 1999;80(9):998-1000.

122. Jones T, Ugalde V, Franks P, Zhou H, White RH: Venous thromboembolism after spinal cord injury: Incidence, time course, and associated risk factors in 16,240 adults and children. *Arch Phys Med Rehabil* 2005;86(12):2240-2247.

123. Deep K, Jigajinni MV, McLean AN, Fraser MH: Prophylaxis of thromboembolism in spinal injuries—results of enoxaparin used in 276 patients. *Spinal Cord* 2001;39(2):88-91.

CHAPTER 9
Vascular Anatomy of the Spine

Christopher Bono, MD Wesley W. Parke, PhD Steven R. Garfin, MD Mark Valente, DO

Arterial Blood Supply of the Bone and Joints

Notwithstanding regional variations, the basic vascularity of the spinal column can be first understood by considering the repetitive, homologous features that are common to each vertebral level. A segmental artery or its equivalent (eg, segmental branches from the vertebral arteries in the cervical spine) gives rise to several branches that provide the main arterial blood supply. These include the anterior central, posterior central, prelaminar, and postlaminar branches. The anterior central and postlaminar branches supply the bone through its external (outer) surface and provide the minority of the blood supply to the vertebral body and posterior arch. The posterior central and prelaminar vessels are branches within the spinal canal. They provide the majority of the arterial blood supply to the vertebral body and posterior arch as well as arterial inflow to the neural, meningeal, and epidural tissues. In the cervical spine, however, the outer vessels (ie, the anterior central and postlaminar branches) can be the predominant supplier to the bone.

Vertebral vascularity is most uniform between the second thoracic and fourth lumbar vertebrae. At each level, paired segmental arteries arise directly from the aorta along its posterior surface (**Figure 1**). These left and right branches then course posteriorly within the middle aspect of the vertebral body. Near the transverse processes, they

FIGURE 1

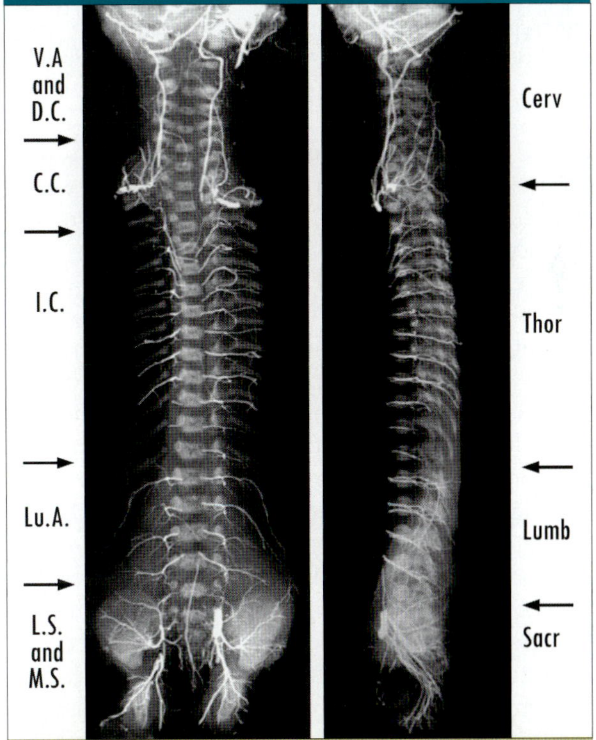

Figure 1 AP and lateral radiographs of the spine of an 8-month fetus injected with finely divided barium sulfate. The traditional regional subdivisions of the spine are indicated on the left, and the regional arteries that provide the segmental branches to the individual vertebrae are shown on the right. The upper cervical region is supplied by vertebral and deep cervical arteries (V.A. and D.C.). The lower cervical and upper two thoracic segments are supplied by the costocervical trunk (C.C.), while the remaining thoracic vertebrae receive intercostal vessels (I.C.). The lumbar arteries (Lu.A.) supply their regional vertebrae, and the sacral segments are provided with branches from the lateral sacral (L.S.) and middle sacral (M.S.) arteries.

Dr. Bono or an immediate family member serves as a board member, owner, officer, or committee member of American Academy of Orthopaedic Surgeons and the North American Spine Society; and has received nonincome support (such as equipment or services), commercially derived honoraria, or other non-research-related funding (such as paid travel) from Barricaid. Dr. Garfin or an immediate family member serves as a board member, owner, officer, or committee member of the Spine Arthroplasty Society; has received royalties from DePuy, a Johnson & Johnson company and Lippincott; is a member of a speakers' bureau or has made paid presentations on behalf of DePuy, a Johnson & Johnson company; serves as a paid consultant to or is an employee of Applied Spine, Benvenue Medical, Cytonics Corp, DePuy, a Johnson & Johnson company, Disc Dynamics, EBI, Globus Medical, Magnifi Group, Nuvasive, SI Bone, Spinal Kinetics, SpineMark, SpineMedica, and Vertiflex; has received research or institutional support from AO North America, DePuy, a Johnson & Johnson company, EBI, Medtronic, and Synthes; and owns stock or stock options in Cytonics Corp, Orthovita, SI Bone, SpineMark, and SpineMedica. Dr. Valente or an immediate family member serves as a paid consultant to or is an employee of Salient Surgical Technologies. Dr. Parke is deceased. At the time this chapter was written, disclosure information was unavailable for Dr. Parke.

FIGURE 2

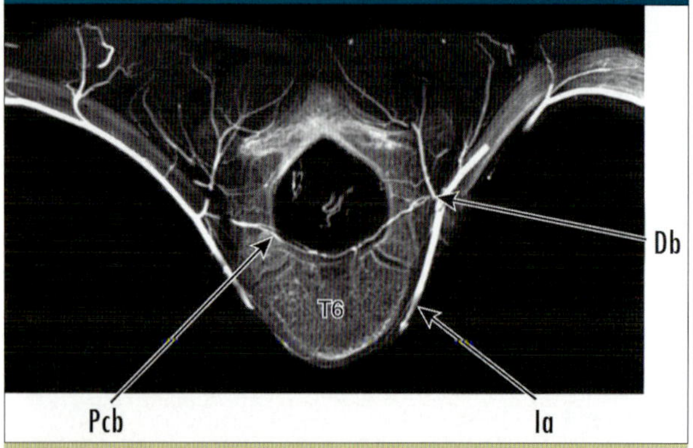

Figure 2 Ventral radiograph of a section through T6 of a specimen from a 6-year-old child injected with barium sulfate. The intercostal arteries (Ia) give rise to dorsal branches (Db) that provide spinal branches to the vertebral canal and posterior branches to the arch and dorsal musculature. The posterior central branches (Pcb) are well shown as they send vessels into the vertebral body. Fine anterior central and anterior laminar and posterior laminar vessels can be seen. Note the neurocentral synchondrosis.

FIGURE 3

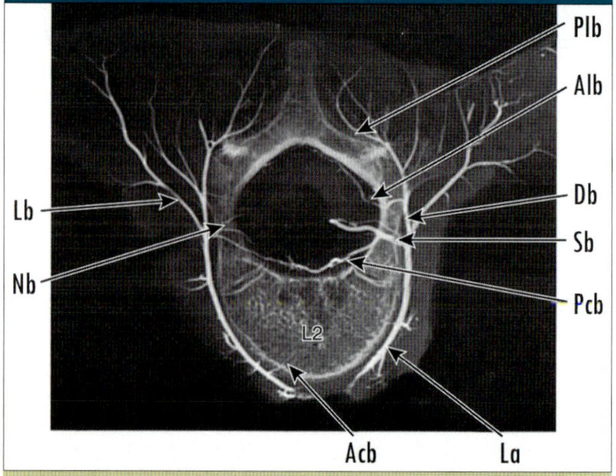

Figure 3 Vertical radiograph of a section through the lumbar vertebra of a 6-year-old child. The vascularity of the lumbar vertebra may be regarded as the archetypal pattern from which other regions evolved variations. The segmental lumbar artery (La) gives rise to several anterior central branches (Acb) that penetrate the cortical bone of the body. The spinal branch (sb) sends prominent posterior central branches (Pcb) to the dorsum of the body, while the dorsal branch (Db) supplies both the anterior (Alb) and posterior (Plb) laminar branches. Neural branches (Nb) follow the nerve roots to the cord. In this section, the arteria radicularis magna is seen as a neural branch on the right side. Lb = lumbar branches.

divide into lateral (intercostal or lumbar) and dorsal branches. The dorsal branch continues posterior, lying lateral to the intervertebral foramen and the facet joint, to supply the posterior spinal muscles.

The first branches of the segmental arteries are the anterior central branches, which, as described above, provide some supply to the vertebral body spongiosa (**Figures 2** and **3**). Smaller branches from the segmental arteries also supply the anterior longitudinal ligament (**Figure 4**).

Originating from the dorsal branch of the segmental artery are the posterior central and prelaminar arteries. These enter the spinal canal through the intervertebral foramina. The posterior central branch courses along the posterolateral aspect of the intervertebral disk. It then proceeds to divide into superior and inferior branches that lie along the posterior aspect of the adjacent cranial and caudal vertebral bodies. This is the major source of blood supply to this structure. Smaller branches supply the posterior longitudinal ligament (PLL) and the overlying dura mater before entering into a large nutrient foramen within the central aspect of the vertebral body. Considering this arrangement, the posterior vertebral body is therefore supplied by four arteries derived from two intervertebral levels (**Figure 5**), providing a rich collateral arterial anastomosis. The prelaminar branch courses within the spinal canal along the anterior aspect of the vertebral arch. It provides several fine penetrating nutrient branches that supply the laminae, ligamenta flava, and regional epidural and dural tissues.

Posterior to the intervertebral foramen, the dorsal branch passes between the transverse processes. The dorsal branch yields a fine array of branches to the facet joint capsule. Next, it further divides into dorsal and medial branches. The larger dorsal branch pierces and supplies the bulk of the paraspinal musculature. The medial branch passes along the posterior cortical surface of the laminae and spinous process and is known as the postlaminar artery. In addition to supplying the adjacent bone, it also feeds the smaller intersegmental musculature overlying the laminae and spinous processes. The largest of these branches penetrate the lamina through a nutrient foramen located along the posteromedial aspect of the facet joint.

Regional Arterial Variations

The aorta is not present at the cervical, upper thoracic, and sacral regions. Thus, developmental analogs of segmental vessels provide the blood supply. In the cervical region, segmental analogs

FIGURE 4

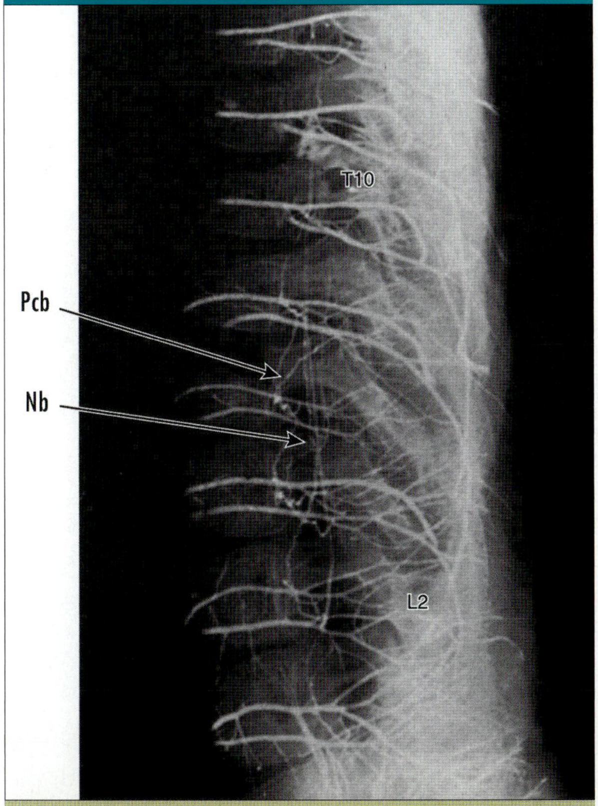

Figure 4 Lateral view of the section in Figure 3. The longitudinal anastomoses of the posterior central branches (Pcb) can be appreciated, and the disposition of neural branches (Nb) is clarified. The lumbar arteries also supply small longitudinal branches to the anterior longitudinal ligament.

FIGURE 5

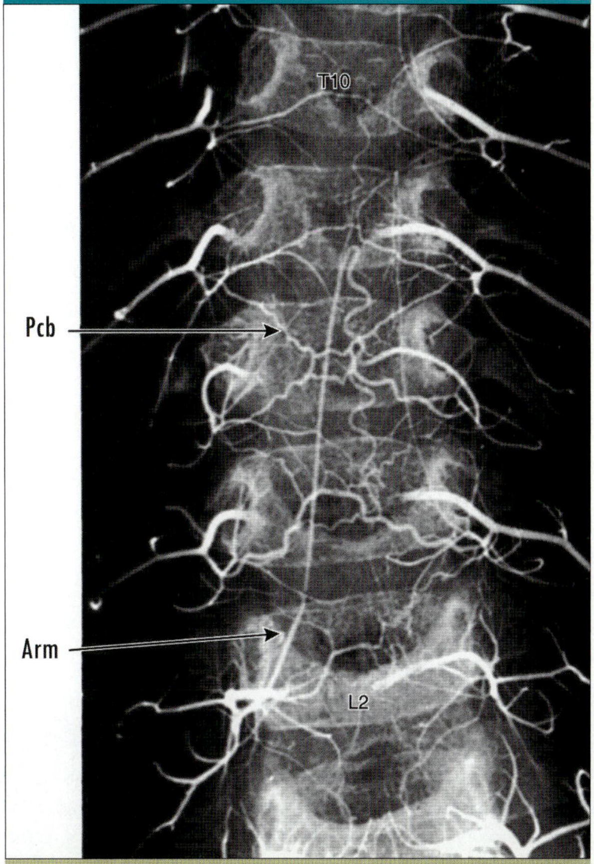

Figure 5 AP arteriogram of the lower thoracic and upper lumbar vertebrae in a 6-year-old child. The interlocking anastomotic pattern formed by the posterior central branches (Pcb), and the manner in which four branches converge over the center of the dorsum of the body of each vertebra, are well shown. The arteria radicularis magna (Arm), which forms a major contribution to the anterior spinal artery of the cord, can be seen arising at L2.

arise from the vertebral arteries. At the cervicothoracic junction, costocervical branches of the subclavian artery are present. In the sacral area, lateral sacral branches of the internal iliac artery and branches of the middle sacral artery provide segmental arterial supply.

Cervical Region

Subaxial Cervical Spine

Developmentally, the longitudinally coursing vertebral arteries actually represent fusion of embryologic segmental vessels. An anterior central artery and a medially directed posterior central vessel arise from the vertebral arteries at each subaxial cervical level. The anterior spinal plexus represents an anastomosis of the transverse anterior central arteries, from which smaller branches supply the anterior longitudinal ligament, prevertebral musculature, anterior vertebral body and anulus. In the lower cervical spine, the thyrocervical and costocervical trunks provide contributions. The upper plexus receives branches from the ascending pharyngeal arteries as well.

Upper Cervical Spine

Paralleling its unique bony and developmental anatomy, the upper cervical spine demonstrates various regional differences compared to its subaxial counterparts.

The odontoid process, a component of C2, developmentally represents the centrum of C1. Therefore, its segmental blood supply is derived from vessels originating at the level of the atlas. The body of C2, though the structural pedestal of the odontoid process, is supplied by C2 segmental branches. This leads to a "watershed" region

FIGURE 6

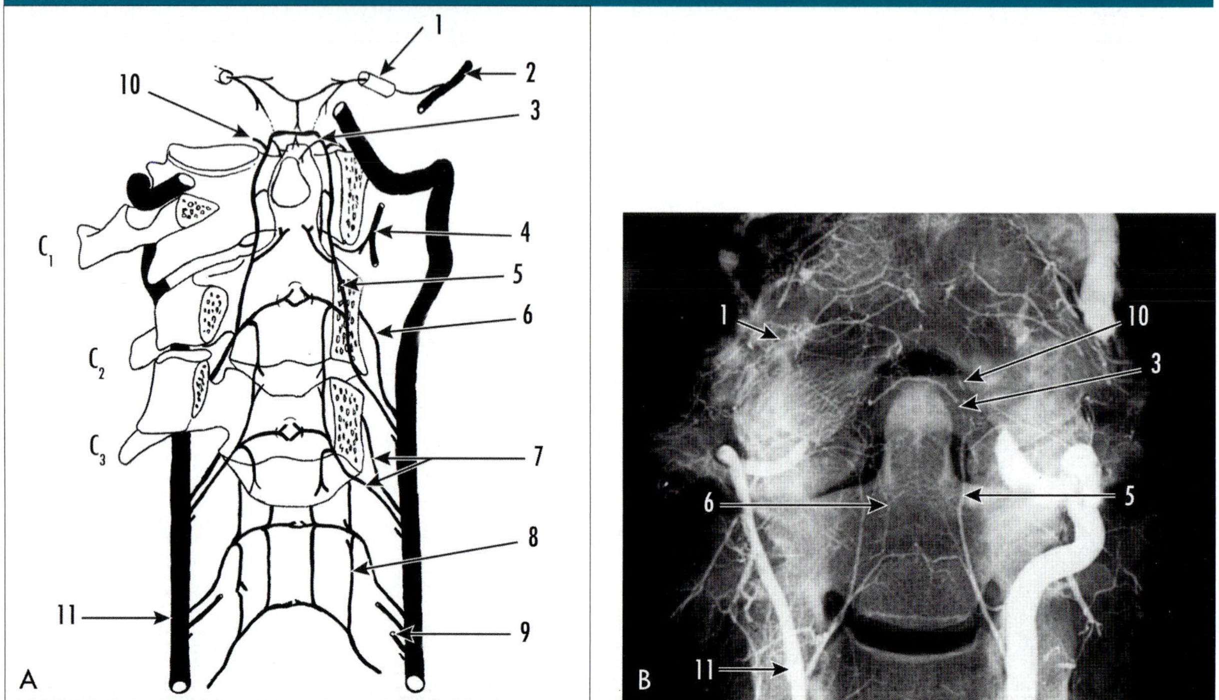

Figure 6 **A,** Illustration of the arterial supply to the bodies of the upper cervical vertebrae and the odontoid process. **B,** Latex-barium arterially injected radiograph of the upper cervical vertebrae. 1 = hypoglossal canal passing meningeal artery; 2 = occipital artery; 3 = apical arcade of odontoid process; 4 = ascending pharyngeal artery with collateral branch beneath anterior arch of atlas; 5 = posterior ascending artery; 6 = anterior ascending artery; 7 = precentral and postcentral arteries to typical cervical vertebral body; 8 = anterior spinal plexus; 9 = medullary branch of vertebral artery (Radicular, prelaminar, and meningeal branches are also found at each level.) 10 = collateral to ascending pharyngeal artery passing rostral to anterior arch of atlas; 11 = left vertebral artery. (Adapted with permission from Parke WW: The vascular relations of the upper cervical vertebrae. *Orthop Clin North Am* 1978;9:879-889.)

located at the junction of the dens and body of C2, in which few, if any, crossing arterial anastomoses are present. This is further aggravated by the presence of a transient cartilaginous plate that represents an incipient intervertebral disk between the atlas and axis. It does not calcify until the latter half of the first decade and effectively prevents the development of any significant vascular communication between the odontoid process and the C2 body. The penultimate example of persistence of this cartilaginous plate is the presence of an os odontoideum.

In the adult spine, the odontoid process is supplied primarily by pairs of anterior and posterior central branches that course upward from the surfaces of the C2 body.[1] They are branches of the vertebral artery that enter the spinal canal through the C2-C3 neural foramina. The larger posterior ascending arteries arise independently from the posteromedial sides of their respective vertebral arteries. Within the canal, the posterior ascending arteries trifurcate along the posterior aspect of the C2 vertebral body. Branching perforators penetrate deep to the tectorial membrane (the PLL analog in the upper cervical spine) as well as the bone itself. A small descending branch connects distally with vessels of the next adjacent caudal segment.

The posterior ascending artery crosses the posterior surface of the transverse ligament about 1.5 mm lateral to the odontoid process (**Figure 6**). Its injury can contribute to the inevitable epidural hematoma present after sagittal atlantoaxial dislocation (transverse ligament disruption). The posterior ascending artery sends an anterior anastomotic branch over the superior aspect of the alar ligament to collateralize with branches of the anterior ascending artery. It then courses medially to meet its contralateral counterpart, and forms an apical arcade that arches over the tip of the odontoid process.

The anterior ascending arteries are smaller than the posterior ascending arteries. They arise from the anteromedial aspect of the vertebral arteries. Passing along the anterior aspect of the C2 body, they provide fine medial branches that perforate into the bone. They eventually converge into a median anastomosis. The anterior ascending arteries continue cranially along the anterior arch of C1. Perforating branches from this vessel supply the C1 ring as well as the odontoid neck.

Terminal branches supply blood to the midline atlanto-dens articulation. Small branches from the anterior and posterior ascending arteries also supply the craniovertebral (occipitoatlantal) articulations. The main blood supply to the lateral occipitoatlantal joints is provided by a complex of vessels derived from the vertebral and occipital arteries.

Collateral vessels pass both above and below the anterior C1 arch to anastomose with the apical arcade and ascending arteries, respectively.[1] These vessels are branches of the ascending pharyngeal artery, which arises from the external carotid artery. The ascending pharyngeal artery sends a branch along the inner aspect of the carotid sheath that, on reaching the base of the skull, becomes recurrent and descends deep to the prevertebral fascia to supply the upper prevertebral cervical muscles and anastomose with the anterior spinal plexus. The tectorial membrane and alar and apical ligaments are also supplied by several small vessels that branch from the occipital artery (above the foramen magnum) that go on to anastomose with the apical arcade (below the foramen magnum) in this region.

Sacroiliolumbar Region

The aorta ends at approximately the level of the L4 vertebral body. It then bifurcates into a left and right common iliac (or hypogastric) artery. Each then subsequently divides into an internal and external iliac vessel. In lieu of direct aortic branches, analogs of segmental vessels stem from a "sacroiliolumbar system" that consists of contributions from the fourth lumbar artery, the iliolumbar artery, and the middle and lateral sacral arteries.

Within the confines of the vertebral column, the sacroiliolumbar system supplies the lower lumbosacral elements of the spine and the inferior half of the lumbosacral spinal nerve roots (cauda equina), as well as the paraspinal musculature below L4. This system is also a major contributor to various extraspinal structures, such as the lumbosacral plexus, to which it supplies blood via the vasa nervorum. Significant medullary branches to the spinal cord are seldom found below L4. However, if they are present, ligation of both internal iliac arteries can result in spinal cord ischemia.[2]

Fourth Lumbar Arteries

The fourth lumbar artery can have nearly twice the diameter of more cranial segmental vessels because of a greater muscular and intersegmental distribution and demand. The lateral muscular branch, which is analogous to the thoracic intercostals, can be very large. It passes anterior, instead of posterior, to the quadratus lumborum. It then courses along the superior aspect of the iliac crest to supply the lower posterolateral abdominal wall.

The dorsal branch and its ramifications supply the external aspects of the facet joints, neural arch components, and adjacent paraspinal musculature. The vertebromedullary (spinal) branches of the fourth lumbar artery are also similar to other levels (**Figure 7**). They are sorted into three divisions: (1) ventral periosteal and osseous branches that supply the PLL and the vertebral body; (2) a radiculomedullary division that comprises the individual radicular branches to the nerve roots (or, rarely, a significant spinal cord medullary feeder); and (3) a dorsal division that supplies the deep aspects of the facet joints, the intracanal surfaces of the laminae, and associated ligaments. The first two divisions usually originate from a common branch of the segmental artery that enters the intervertebral foramen anterior to the nerve root. This is in contrast to the dorsal division, which arises from the musculocutaneous branch of the segmental artery and enters the foramen posterior to the nerve root. As in other regions, the dura mater is supplied by fine branches from adjacent vessels.

In addition to the usual segmental branches (as described above), the fourth lumbar artery has some unique ramifications. Its major peculiarity is that it has a relatively large, caudally directed intersegmental branch that arises near the level of the intervertebral foramen. This anastomoses with the lumbar branch of the iliolumbar artery (**Figures 7** and **8**).

Iliolumbar and Lateral Sacral Arteries

The internal iliac artery divides into an anterior (supplying mostly visceral structures) and posterior division. The posterior division gives rise to the iliolumbar and lateral sacral branches.

The iliolumbar artery is usually the first branch. It is directed in a posterosuperior direction, passing over the anterolateral surface of S1 and then coursing cranially superiorly behind the obturator nerve and in front of the lumbosacral trunk. Just lateral to the lower part of the L5-S1 disk, it

FIGURE 7

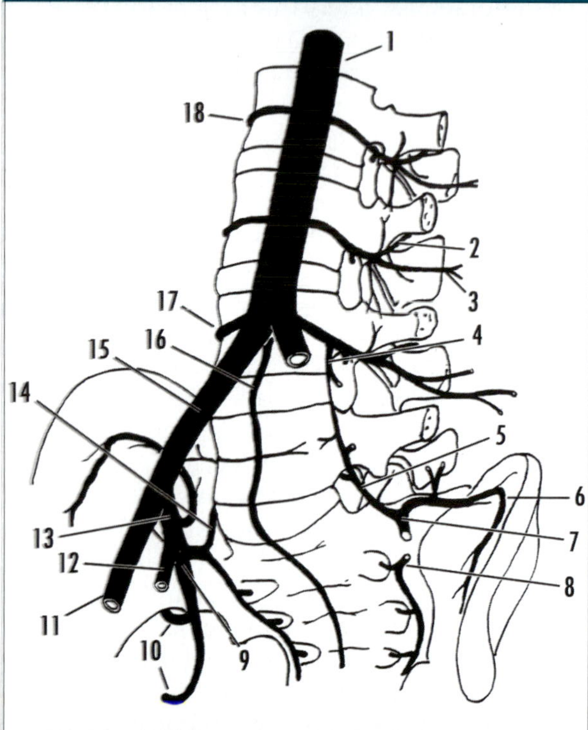

Figure 7 Illustration of the distribution and major variations of the sacroiliolumbar system of arteries that supply the vertebrae and their associated structures inferior to the fourth lumbar vertebra. These patterns of the vessels were derived from radiographs of perinatal specimens and dissections of adults, and then drawn against a tracing of the lumbosacral region taken from a left anterior oblique radiograph of a male adult. Note that the aorta lies to the left of center as it approaches the bifurcation ventral to the fourth lumbar vertebra. This schema shows the more frequent arrangement of the sacroiliolumbar system on the right side of the illustration, where the iliolumbar vessel (7) has a single origin from the dorsum of the posterior division of the (removed) internal iliac artery. The left side shows the common variation where the iliac artery and the lumbar artery (14) are derived separately. The middle sacral artery (16) is in its typical position, and the anastomotic contribution from the fourth lumbar artery (4) shows its most frequent form. 1 = aorta; 2 = musculocutaneous branch of the third lumbar artery; 3 = muscular branch to posterior abdominal wall; 4 = anastomotic contribution of fourth lumbar artery to sacroiliolumbar system; 5 = lumbar branch of iliolumbar artery; 6 = iliac branch of iliolumbar artery; 7 = iliolumbar artery; 8 = left lateral sacral artery; 9 = posterior division of internal iliac artery; 10 = superior and inferior gluteal arteries; 11 = external iliac artery; 12 = anterior (visceral) division of internal iliac artery; 13 = internal iliac artery; 14 = variant origin of lumbar branch of iliolumbar artery from lateral sacral artery; 15 = common iliac artery; 16 = middle sacral artery; 17 = left fourth lumbar segmental artery; 18 = left second lumbar segmental artery.

FIGURE 8

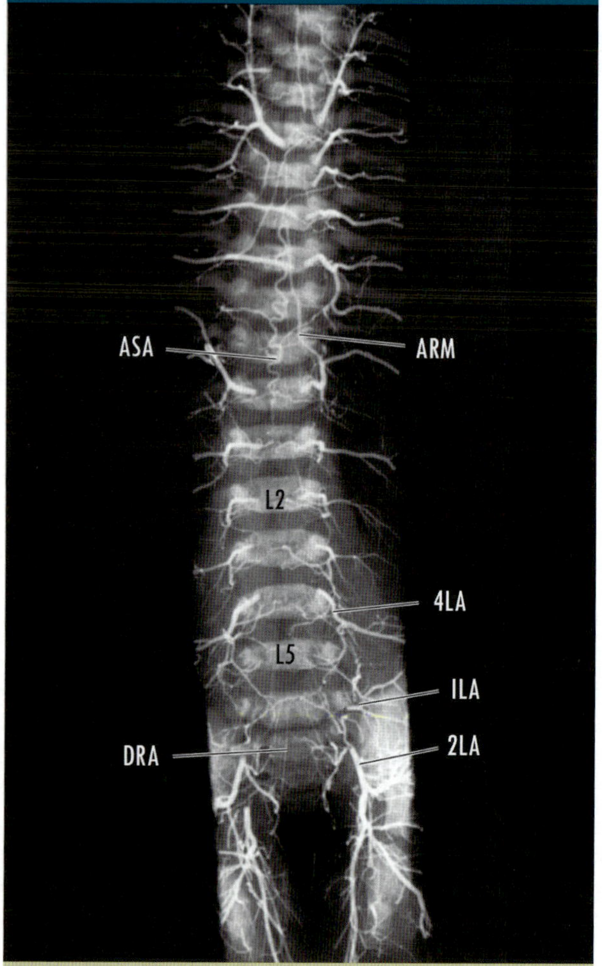

Figure 8 AP radiograph of a spine from a perinatal cadaver injected with barium sulfate. The aorta and common iliac vessels have been removed before radiography. This specimen was chosen because it showed considerable variation between the two sides of the sacroiliolumbar system. Note that on the right side of the illustration, both a small lumbar branch and a descending branch from the fourth lumbar artery (4LA) enter the L5-S1 intervertebral foramen. On the left side, there is no lumbar branch, and a descending branch of the L4 artery supplies all of the vessels to the L5-S1 intervertebral foramen. Also, the middle sacral artery is absent and other branches of the system supply its domain. The radicular branches of the vertebromedullary vessels supply the distal radicular arteries (DRA) and reveal the positions of the lower ends of the lumbosacral nerve roots. ASA = anterior spinal artery; ARM = arteria radicularis magna; ILA = first lumbar artery; 2LA = second lumbar artery.

FIGURE 9

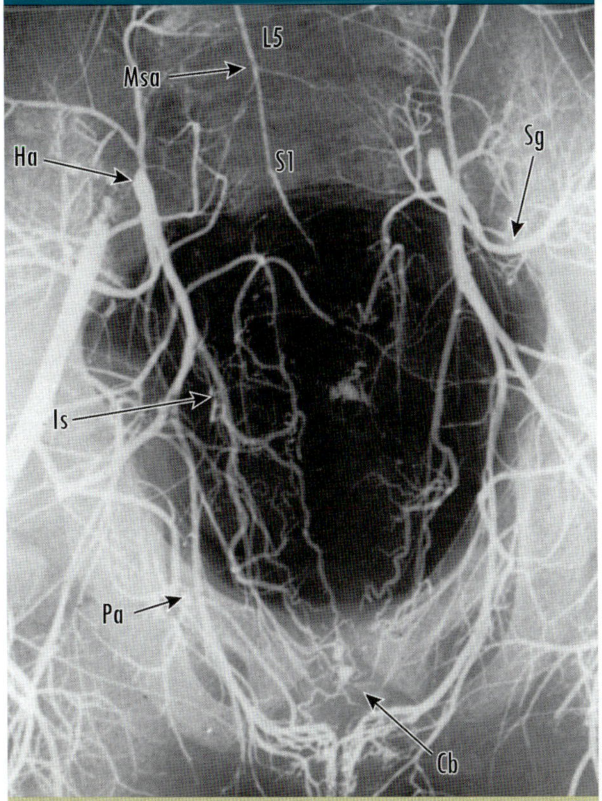

Figure 9 AP arteriogram of the sacral region in a 7-year-old child. The lateral sacral arteries (Is) can be seen coming from the hypogastric vessels (Ha). The middle sacral artery (Msa) is atypical in this specimen because it stops at S1. Just anterior to the coccyx, the coccygeal bodies (Cb) are indicated as small knots of arteriovenous anastomoses. Pudendal arteries (Pa) are well injected. Sg = superior gluteal.

FIGURE 10

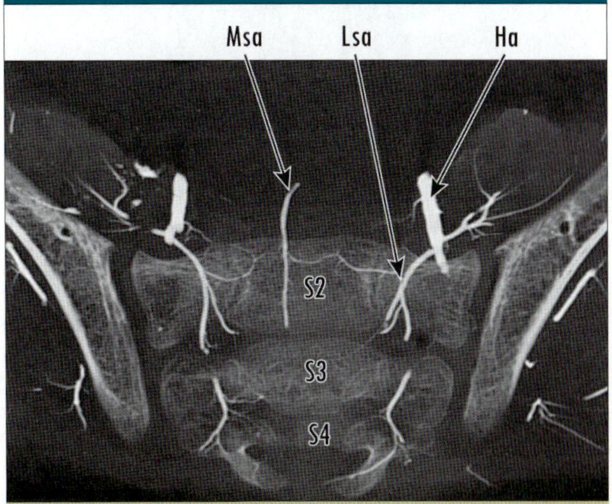

Figure 10 Radiograph of a horizontal section through the sacroiliac joint. The natural curvature of the sacrum provided oblique sections through segments 2, 3, and 4. The hypogastric artery (Ha) gives off the lateral sacral artery (Lsa) that sends anastomotic branches to join the middle sacral artery (Msa); from these, the sacral segments receive the penetrating anterior central branches. The dorsal branches pass into the anterior sacral foramina to provide posterior, central, neural, and prelaminar branches. The dorsal branches then leave through the posterior sacral foramina to supply the muscles and posterior laminar branches.

divides into a laterally directed iliac branch and an ascending lumbar branch. The iliac branch passes over the sacroiliac joint to enter the pelvis and courses along the internal aspect of the iliac crest. It provides muscular branches to the iliac muscle as well as articular branches that descend to the acetabulum. The latter eventually anastomoses with the deep circumflex branch of the femoral artery.

The lumbar branch passes along the posterolateral aspect of the L5-S1 disk between the obturator nerve and the lumbosacral trunk. It provides vertebromedullary branches to the L5-S1 intervertebral foramen (**Figures 7** through **9**). Usually, the lumbar branch has a superior branch that joins the descending branch of the fourth lumbar artery. This vessel provides regional blood supply to the psoas and quadratus lumborum muscles.

The second branch of the posterior division of the internal iliac artery is the lateral sacral artery. It courses along the pars lateralis of the sacrum on each side. The lateral sacral artery yields medial branches that enter the spinal canal through their respective foramina. The artery continues posteriorly, exiting the posterior sacral foramen, to provide dorsal muscular branches that supply the sacral origins of the (paraspinal) erector spinae muscles.

Middle Sacral Artery

The middle sacral artery is the last branch of the aorta. This median unpaired vessel stems from the posterior surface of the aorta just above its bifurcation (**Figures 7** and **10**). It descends along the anterior longitudinal ligament over the L4 and L5 vertebral bodies and anterior sacrum to terminate at the sacrococcygeal junction in a vascular glomus (sacrococcygeal body). The middle sacral artery can be a significant component of the sacroiliolumbar system; its first lateral branch along the L5 vertebral body can provide segmental blood supply in the absence of a well-developed iliolumbar or fourth lumbar vessel. In the absence of neuroforaminal branches from the lateral sacral

FIGURE 11

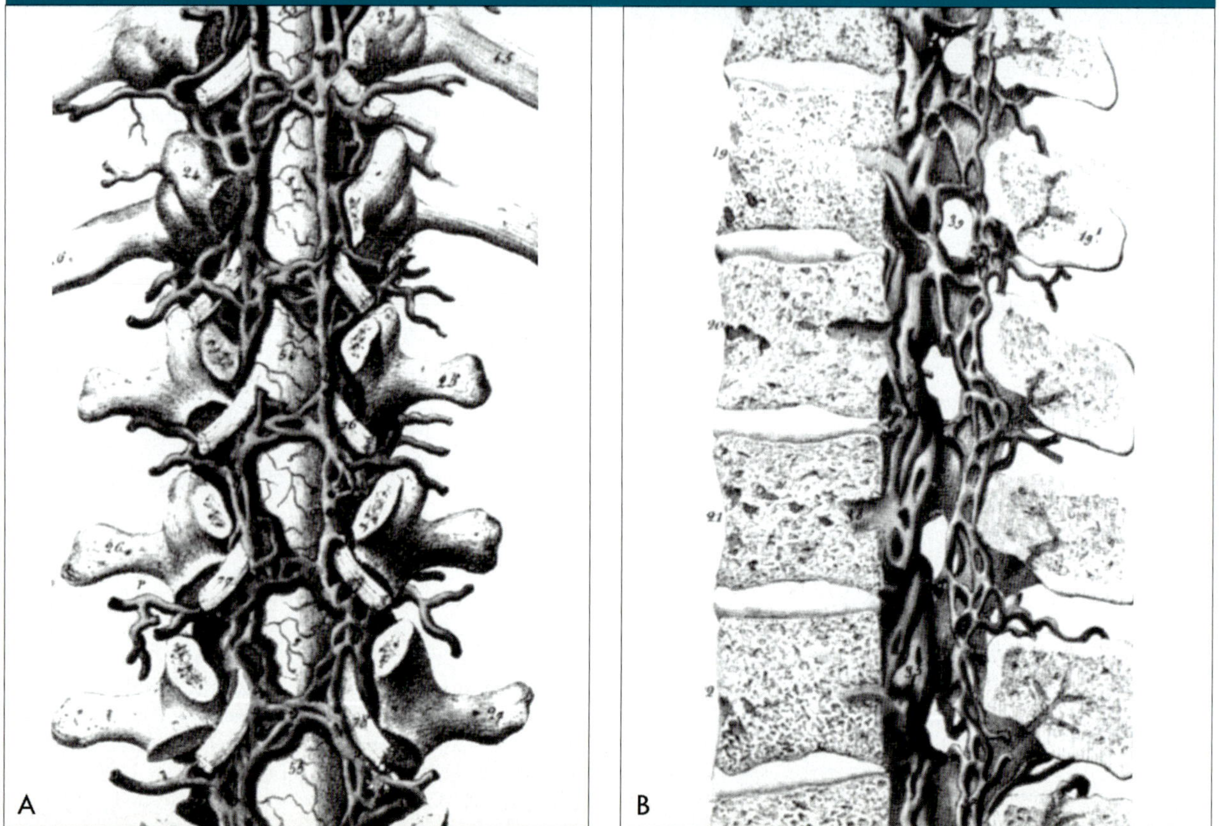

Figure 11 Posterior (**A**) and lateral (**B**) illustrations of the spinal epidural venous plexus taken from hand-colored copies of Gilbert Breschet's original work. (ca 1835; Courtesy of Scott Memorial Library, Jefferson Medical College, Philadelphia, PA.)

arteries, it may also contribute vertebromedullary branches to each anterior sacral foramen.

Venous Anatomy

An external and an internal plexus of veins roughly follow the paths served by the external and internal vertebral arteries. Like the arterial system, the external venous plexus has anterior and posterior divisions. The smaller anterior plexus follows the anterior central arteries and receives tributaries that perforate the anterior and lateral sides of the vertebral body.

The posterior plexus is more extensive. It drains the regions supplied by the posterior branches of the segmental artery. The paired posterior external veins lie in two vertebrocostal grooves, but have anastomotic branches between the spinous processes. The posterior plexus is a valveless venous system that receives the draining segmental tributaries of the internal veins through the intervertebral foramina, and communicates ultimately with the lumbar and intercostal tributaries of the caval and azygos system. The plexus is most extensive in the posterior nuchal region, where it receives the tributaries from the vertebral veins and drains into the deep cervical and jugular veins.

The internal venous plexus is essentially a series of irregular, valveless epidural sinuses that extend from the coccyx to the foramen magnum. They are embedded within the epidural fat and supported by a network of collagenous fibers. Their walls, however, are so thin that their extent cannot be discerned by gross dissection (**Figure 11**). The plexus is arranged in a series of cross-connected expansions that produce anterior and posterior ladder-like configurations up the vertebral canal. The anterior epidural plexus consists of two continuous channels that course along the posterior surface of the vertebral bodies just medial to the pedicles. These channels cross-anastomose over the central dorsal area of each vertebral body and are thinnest over the intervertebral disks. Chaynes et al[3] found that anterior veins were located in a "dehiscence" within the periosteum along the lateral aspect of the spinal canal, and that veins of each side communicated with each other through a retrocorporeal vein. In the cervical spine, the retrocorporeal vein is deep to the PLL. In the thoracic and lumbar regions, it is superficial to the PLL. Large, unpaired basivertebral sinuses that arise within a dorsal central concavity of the vertebral body drain the intraosseous labyrinth of sinusoids.

The epidural plexus communicates with external vessels through veins that pass through the intervertebral foramen, which eventually empty into segmental intercostal or lumbar veins (**Figure 12**). Since they are valveless, however, the direction of flow can vary with shifting intra-abdominal and intrathoracic pressures. Importantly, the plexus is capable of passing large quantities of blood without developing varices, possibly because of an intricate network of collagenous fibers that supports the thin walls of the sinuses.[4] Passive congestion of the spinal cord is prevented by minute valves in the radicular branches draining the spinal cord.[4] As a point of interest, valves exist nowhere else in the venous channels of the central nervous system.

Along with the epidural fat, an additional function of the epidural venous plexus might be to act as a hydraulic shock-absorbing buffer for the neural elements during movements of the vertebral column. The vertebral sinuses are largest in the suboccipital and upper cervical region, where they also receive numerous nerve endings from the sinuvertebral nerves, suggesting a possible baroceptive function.[5]

The pharyngovertebral veins drain the superior posterolateral regions of the nasopharynx and coalesce into two or more veins that penetrate the anterior occipitoatlantal membrane. These drain into the venous complex surrounding the median and lateral atlantoaxial joints.[6] As posterior pharyngeal infections have been linked with atlantoaxial rotatory subluxations (ie, Grisel's syndrome[7]), it is believed that the pharyngovertebral veins are instrumental in transporting infectious processes that may produce a hyperemic relaxation of the atlantoaxial ligaments.

Blood Supply to the Spinal Cord

Three distinct longitudinal vessels, receiving blood from the medullary branches of the segmental arteries, supply the substance of the spinal cord. These are a single median anterior spinal artery (ASA) and two smaller dorsolateral spinal arteries (DSAs) (**Figure 13**). However, not all medullary branches were created equal, as the major contributions to the cord are found at irregular intervals.

FIGURE 12

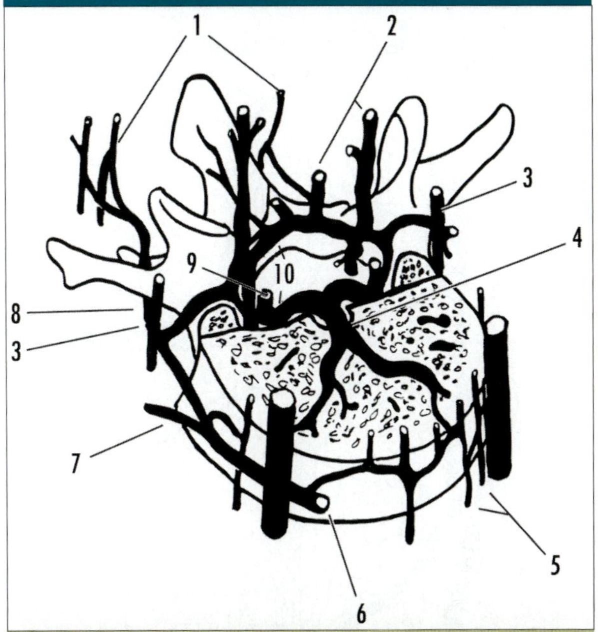

Figure 12 Illustration showing the venous relations of a lumbar vertebra. Engorgement and a relative venous hypertension in the epidural vessels exacerbate neuroischemic conditions in the lumbosacral roots. 1 = dorsal external vertebral plexus; 2 = dorsal epidural plexus; 3 = ascending lumbar veins; 4 = basivertebral vein; 5 = ventral external vertebral plexus; 6 = lumbar segmental vein; 7 = muscular vein from posterior abdominal wall; 8 = circumferential channels (sinuses) of epidural plexus; 9 = anterior internal venous plexus; 10 = posterior internal venous plexus.

Several larger radicular arteries are discernible in the cervical and upper thoracic regions. The largest, the arteria radicularis magna (ARM, also known as the artery of Adamkiewicz[8]), is an asymmetric branch from one of the upper lumbar or lower thoracic segmental arteries. It courses obliquely upward with a ventral spinal root to join the anterior spinal artery in the region of the conus medullaris. One must not take this branch for granted, as ligation of a single segmental vessel, in some cases, can lead to catastrophic iatrogenic spinal cord ischemia.

The DSAs arise from the posterior inferior cerebellar vessels. They are of smaller caliber and less physiologic significance than the ASA. They are often present in a plexiform distribution over the dorsum of the cord and are less likely to be longitudinally continuous. The larger intradural spinal arteries have no significant vasa vasorum. They likely derive their nutritional supply from metabolic exchange with the cerebrospinal fluid across their thin walls.

FIGURE 13

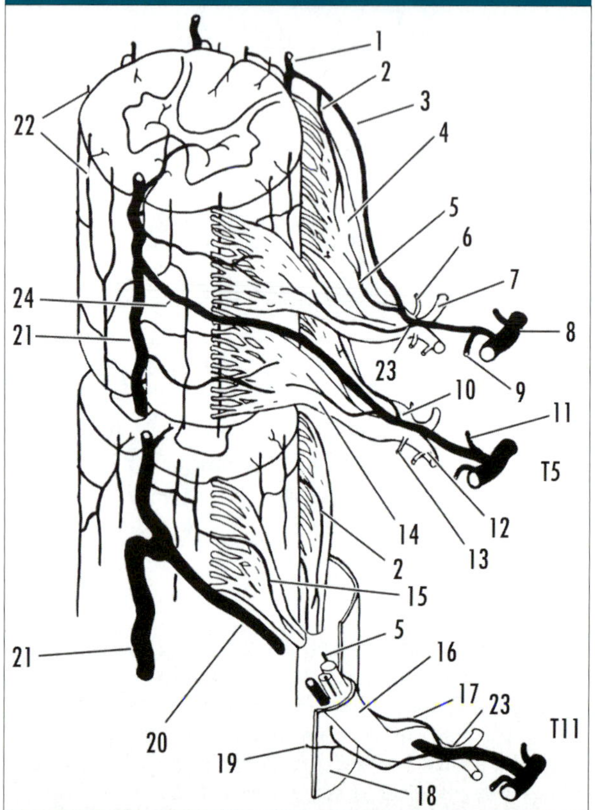

Figure 13 Composite schema of the blood supply to the spinal cord and nerve roots showing two regions of the cord. Note the distinction between medullary arteries and true radicular arteries and that the medullary arteries usually run a course that is independent of the roots. 1 = dorsolateral longitudinal artery; 2 = proximal radicular artery (of dorsal root); 3 = dorsal medullary artery; 4 = dorsal root of thoracic spinal nerve; 5 = distal radicular artery (of dorsal root); 6 = sinuvertebral nerve; 7 = dorsal ramus of spinal nerve; 8 = segmental artery; 9 = dorsal central artery; 10 = dorsal root ganglion; 11= anterior laminar artery; 12 = ventral ramus of spinal nerve; 13 = rami communicantes; 14 = ventral root of spinal nerve; 15 = proximal radicular artery of ventral root; 16 = periradicular theca of dura; 17 = dorsal meningeal branch of vertebromedullary artery; 18 = dura; 19 = ventral meningeal plexus; 20 = great ventral radicular artery (great "radicular" artery of Adamkiewicz); 21 = anterior (ventral) spinal artery; 22 = vasa corona of spinal cord; 23 = spinal nerve; 24 = ventral medullary artery of thoracic cord.

FIGURE 14

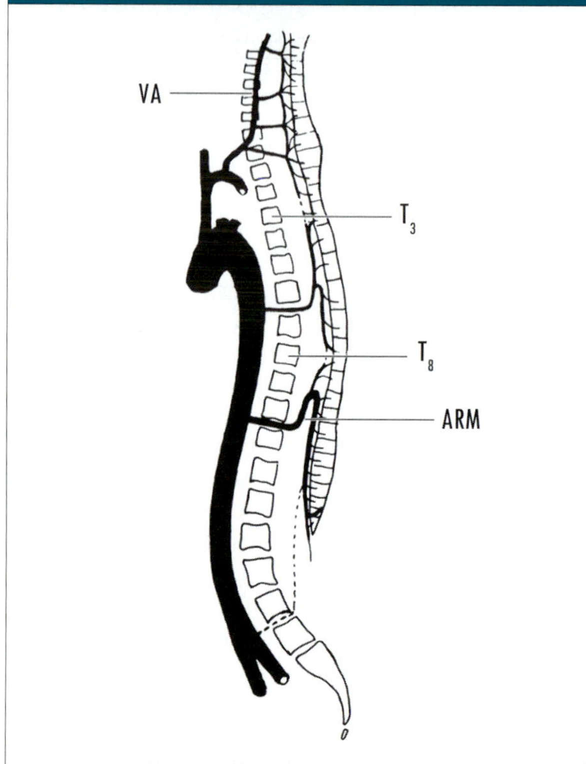

Figure 14 Diagram illustrating the sources and relationships of the medullary feeder arteries to the spine and the spinal cord. The anterior spinal artery (ASA) is shown to be formed by an anastomotic chain of ascending and descending branches of medullary feeders. The cervicothoracic, midthoracic, and thoracolumbar (includes sacral cord) regions are indicated, and their usual boundaries at vertebral levels T3 and T8 are shown. Medullary feeders may be as few as 6 or as many as 14, but the respective domains persist. VA = vertebral artery; ARM = arteria radicularis magna (artery of Adamkiewicz). The dotted line indicates the frequent position of a smaller accessory medullary feeder to the thoracolumbar area. (Reproduced with permission from Parke WW, Whalen JL, Bunger PC, Settles HE: Intimal musculature of the lower anterior spinal artery. *Spine (Phila Pa 1976)* 1995;20(19):2073-2079.)

Anterior Spinal Artery

The ASA is derived from the fusion of bilateral pairs of ascending and descending anastomotic branches of the segmental arteries of the developing spinal cord.[9] This median vessel accounts for approximately 80% of the intrinsic spinal cord blood supply. While it is often depicted in texts as a single continuous artery of nearly uniform caliber extending from the medulla oblongata to the conus, it is actually a longitudinal series of functionally independent vessels with varying luminal diameters and discontinuities.[9-11]

The spinal cord has three major arterial domains along its vertical axis: (1) the cervicothoracic region (C1-T3), (2) the midthoracic region (T3-T8), and (3) the thoracolumbar region (including the sacral portion of the cord) (T8-conus). Particularly significant after traumatic injury, these areas have little anastomotic exchange between them (**Figure 14**).

Interruptions or narrowings of the ASA in the midthoracic region influence the potential collateral blood flow along the longitudinal axis of the cord.[10,11] However, lumen size is not the only important factor. The spinal cord has been demonstrated to exhibit precise autoregulatory control of its intrinsic blood flow.[12,13] A layer of predominantly longitudinal intimal musculature is thought to be a crucial controller of this dynamic function.[14] Located between the internal elastic lamina and the endothelium, this layer ranges in thickness from one-fifth to one-half that of the tunica media (**Figure 15**). At the mouth of the central (sulcal) arteries, which are the largest ASA derivatives, the intimal musculature stops abruptly, often forming a lip-like projection over the opening of the branch vessel. Although no intimal muscle fibers extend into the central arteries, a sphincter-like thickening of the central artery tunica media, seen at the ostium of the vessels, indicates that this conventional muscle layer has a greater contractile influence at this point (**Figure 15**). The intimal musculature, in addition to enhancing the luminal control of the ASA, also is involved in controlling the blood flow into the central arteries. Where the intimal layer shows the lip-like projections, the longitudinally disposed intimal muscle fibers form an ellipsoidal buttonhole-shaped orifice whose long axis is parallel to that of the fiber orientation. The physiologic importance of this arrangement is that it allows exquisite muscular control of the blood flow from the ASA to its central artery branches.

At the arch-shaped junction of the ARM and the descending ASA branches, the intimal layer, in most cases, is organized into prominent intimal cushions. These muscular thickenings are erratically distributed along the lumen and could exert considerable influence over the quantity of blood flow between the thoracolumbar and midthoracic vascular domains. This intimal control system, when coupled with the intramedullary arteriovenous anastomoses (described below), provides an anatomic basis for the dramatic range of blood flow regulation of the spinal cord. Furthermore, it helps explain the not-infrequent failure of the ARM to provide adequate blood supply to the midthoracic spinal cord (above the ARM-ASA junction) with proximal aortic cross-clamping.

Regional Arterial Variation to the Cervical Spinal Cord

The spinal cord from C1 to C4 is supplied by a unique set of lateral spinal arteries. Developmentally, they represent the most rostral expressions of the DSAs; however, they have a much greater role than the DSAs at more caudal levels. The lateral spinal arteries can arise from the intradural parts of the vertebral arteries near the origins of the posterior inferior cerebellar arteries or from the proximal regions of the posterior inferior cerebellar arteries themselves. They typically course anterior to the posterior C1 to C4 nerve roots but dorsal to the denticulate ligaments. Their general distribution is to the posterolateral and anterolateral spinal cord below the olives.

FIGURE 15

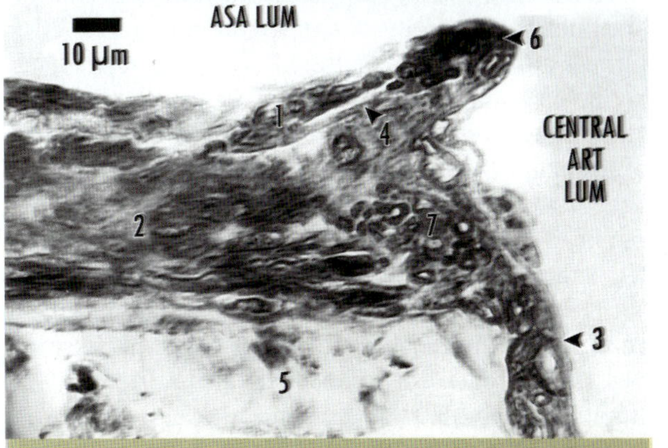

Figure 15 High-power cross section of thoracolumbar ASA wall at the junction with one side of a central artery (CENTRAL ART). Note the intimal musculature (1) may extend as a lip-like projection (6) over the central artery orifice. This muscle layer stops at this point and does not extend into branch vessels. A sphincter-like enlargement of the conventional circular muscle of the central artery (7) is indicated. 2 = tunica media; 3 = endothelium; 4 = internal elastic lamina; 5 = adventitia-pia; LUM = lumbar. (Reproduced with permission from Parke WW, Whalen JL, Bunger PC, Settles HE: Intimal musculature of the lower anterior spinal artery. *Spine (Phila Pa 1976)* 1995;20(19):2073-2079.)

Intrinsic Vascularity of the Spinal Cord

Arterial Vascularity

There are two intrasubstance vascular systems within the tissues of the spinal cord. One is a centripetal arrangement of arteries that supplies the superficial tracts of the ventral and lateral funiculi, the entire dorsal funiculus, and the extremities of the dorsal horns. These arteries are radially penetrating branches of the vasa corona and the dorsolateral spinal arteries. They serve just over one-fourth of the spinal cord.

The second is a centifugal system of vessels derived from the sulcal (or central) arteries that supplies the majority of the spinal cord (and almost all of its gray matter).[15] This is a repetitive series of branches from the dorsal aspect of the ASA. These vessels penetrate the depths of the anterior median fissure. In the midsagittal plane, they form a close palisade of vessels that are densest in the lumbar region. The average diameters of the sulcal arteries are greater in the cervical (0.21 mm) and lumbosacral (0.23 mm) regions than in the thoracic cord (0.14 mm).[16] As these vessels approach the anterior commissure, they turn to either the right or left and supply only that side of the cord,[17-19] which reflects their embryologic origins. However, bilateral distributions are present in 9%, 7%, and 14% of the cervical, thoracic, and lumbar vessels, respectively.[16,20]

The sulcal arteries enter the substance of the cord, just ventral to the anterior white commissure. After they divide into their individual right and left arteries, they then subdivide into dorsal and ventral branches. The ventral branches supply the ventral horns but also provide vessels to Clarke's column and the deeper fibers of the anterior and lateral funiculi. The smaller dorsal branches supply the gray commissure and the ventral one-half to two-thirds of the dorsal horns. All of these vessels then provide finer arterioles that eventually form the spinal cord capillary beds.

Capillary density is four to five times greater within spinal gray matter than white matter, a reflection of greater metabolic demands.[21] However, capillary distribution is not homogeneous and varies with the regional concentrations of the nuclei. While the nuclei of the dorsal horn are fairly uniformly distributed, those of the ventral horn demonstrate segmental nuclear clusters that in turn display distinct nerve cell groups.

Unlike most other bodily tissues, the capillary densities of the white and gray matter of the central nervous system are established at a minimally requisite level for metabolic needs.[22] Thus, they have no capillary "reserve." Despite this, autoregulation of blood flow can make dramatic shifts to suffice metabolic requirements throughout a wide range of systemic blood pressure alterations.[12,13,23] As transection of the upper cervical cord has no effect on this autoregulative capacity, it may be assumed that this reflex is local and independent of autonomic nerve control.

Numerous sulcal artery branches communicate directly with veins through convoluted anastomoses located at the junction of the ventral two-thirds and dorsal one-third of the dorsal horn and in the more central regions of the ventral horn. They do not have contractile elements, but instead have an "epithelioid" type of media that is capable of swelling and diminishing its thickness. Since this action could rapidly control the caliber of the anastomotic lumina in immediate response to local metabolic changes, these anastomotic convolutions may be the site of the reflex adjustment in the flow resistance of the spinal cord vasculature.[24]

Perhaps most importantly, one should recognize individual variability of the vascular supply of the spinal cord. Surgical cases in which the ARM has been inadvertently ligated without producing a disastrous spinal cord ischemia demonstrate that the presence of an adequate collateral arterial blood supply protects the viability of the spinal cord in most individuals. However, in procedures involving the interruption of blood flow of numerous consecutive segmental branches of the aorta, such as that produced with aortic cross-clamping, the maintenance of adequate spinal cord blood flow appears to be more dependent on the regional competence of the ASA than the number of collateral sources to the spinal cord. Spinal cord injury after aortic cross-clamping without adjunctive vascular support has been reported in 15% to 25% of cases.[25,26] Proximal-to-distal aortic shunting may alleviate these problems.

Intrinsic Venous Drainage

In contrast to other organ systems, the veins of the central nervous system are generally less numerous than the arteries. To compensate, they are larger than their corresponding arteries. However, the larger branches may not show a pattern paralleling greater arterial distribution. They are also not accompanied by lymphatics.

A centrifugal arrangement of intrinsic venous vessels drains the dorsal half of the spinal cord. They empty, via venous vasa coronae, to a large median dorsal longitudinal spinal vein. The ventral half of the cord sends tributaries to sulcal veins that empty into a large median ventral longitudinal vein, which runs parallel to the ASA. The ventral and dorsal longitudinal veins are circumferentially connected by a prominent venous vasa corona. These vessels empty into the epidural venous plexus by medullary (radicular) veins.[27] It should be noted that the proximal region of the spinal nerve roots drain centripetally into the vasa corona and longitudinal veins of the spinal cord, subsequently emptying into the epidural system via the medullary veins.

FIGURE 16

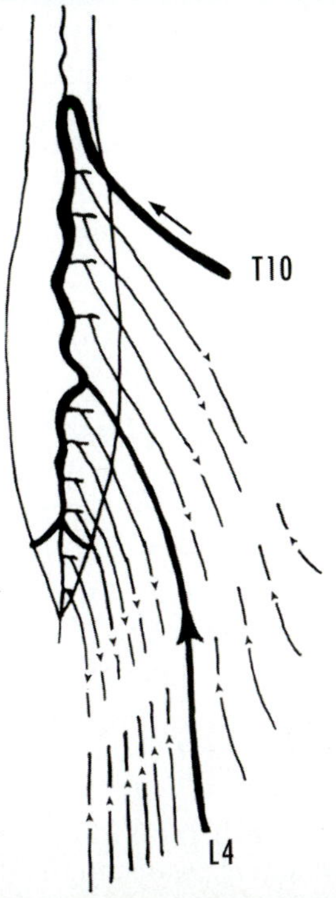

Figure 16 Diagram indicating the directions of normal blood flow in the cauda equina. Note that the ASA of the lumbosacral part of the cord is supplied by medullary arteries and, in turn, supplies 75% at the cord substance and the upper parts of the cauda equina via the proximal radicular arteries. This accounts for the enlargement of the ASA in the lumbosacral region.

FIGURE 17

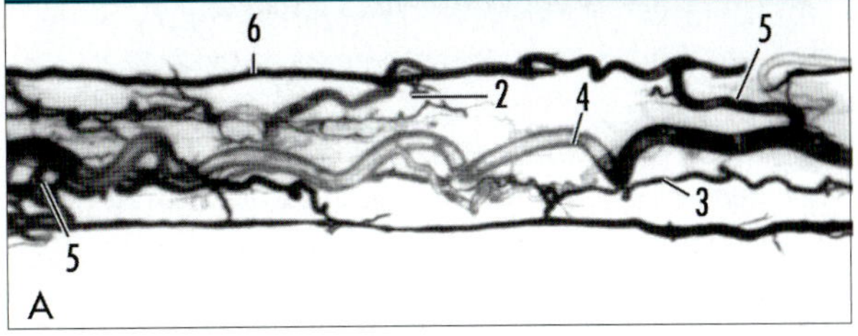

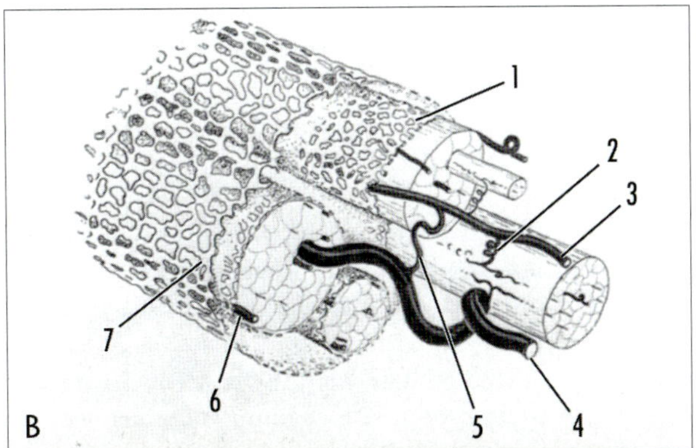

Figure 17 **A,** Low-power (×20) transillumination photomicrograph of a midsection from part of an L4 nerve root that had been treated with hydrogen peroxide after vascular injection with latex–India ink but before clearing in a solution of tributyl-tricresyl phosphates. The peroxidases within the residual blood elements inflated the radicular veins (4) to provide a temporary contrast medium. Note the frequency of the large arteriovenous anastomoses (5) that permitted the latex–India ink to enter the veins. **B,** Graphic compilation showing the structure of a typical lumbosacral nerve root derived from data obtained by injection studies and scanning electron microscopy. The gauze-like pia-arachnoid membranes permit the cerebrospinal fluid to percolate into nerve tissues and assist metabolic support. 1 = fascicular pia; 2 = inter- and intrafascicular arteries showing compensating coils to allow interfascicular movement; 3 = longitudinal radicular artery; 4 = large radicular vein (does not course with arteries); 5 = arteriovenous anastomosis; 6 = collateral radicular artery; 7 = gauze-like pia-arachnoid that permits percolation of cerebrospinal fluid to assist in metabolic support. (Reproduced with permission from Parke WW, Watanabe R: Lumbosacral nerve roots. *Spine (Phila Pa 1976)* 1985;10: 508-515.

Blood Supply to Spinal Nerve Roots

Spinal nerve roots receive arterial blood supply from both their cranial and caudal ends (**Figures 13** and **16**).[28-30] Multiple coils along the branches of the radicular arteries provide for redundancy so that stresses and stretching of the nerve roots with intervertebral movements do not normally interrupt blood flow. Large arteriovenous anastomoses exist throughout the length of the root (**Figure 17**). These vascular cross connections might allow maintenance of blood flow in areas above and below a point of compression. However, the exact role of these anastomoses in autoregulation of the intrinsic radicular vasculature remains unknown.

References

1. Schiff DC, Parke WW: The arterial supply of the odontoid process (dens). *Anat Rec* 1972;172: 399-400.
2. Kaisary AV, Smith P: Spinal cord ischemia after ligation of both internal iliac arteries during radical cystoprostatectomy. *Urology* 1985;25(4): 395-397.
3. Chaynes P, Verdié JC, Moscovici J, Zadeh J, Vaysse P, Becue J: Microsurgical anatomy of the internal vertebral venous plexuses. *Surg Radiol Anat* 1998;20(1):47-51.
4. Clemens HJ: *Die Venesysteme der menschlichen Wirbelsaule*. Berlin, Germany, Walter de Gruyter, 1961.
5. Parke WW, Valsamis MP: The ampulloglomerular organ: An unusual neurovascular complex in the suboccipital region. *Anat Rec* 1967;159(2): 193-198.
6. Parke WW, Rothman RH, Brown MD: The pharyngovertebral veins: An anatomic rationale for Grisel's syndrome. *J Bone Joint Surg Am* 1984; 66(4):568-574.
7. Wetzel FT, La Rocca H: Grisel's syndrome. *Clin Orthop Relat Res* 1989;(240):141-152.
8. Milen MT, Bloom DA, Culligan J, Murasko K: Albert Adamkiewicz (1850-1921)—his artery and its significance for the retroperitoneal surgeon. *World J Urol* 1999;17(3):168-170.
9. Corbib JL: *Anatomie et Pathologie Arterielles de la Moelleed*. Paris, France, Masson et Cie, 1961.
10. Brewer LA III, Fosburg RG, Mulder GA, Verska JJ: Spinal cord complications following surgery for coarctation of the aorta: A study of 66 cases. *J Thorac Cardiovasc Surg* 1972;64(3):368-381.
11. Lazorthes G, Gouaze A, Zadeh JO, et al: Arterial vascularization of the spinal cord: Recent studies of the anastomotic substitution pathways. *J Neurosurg* 1971;35:253-262.
12. Kobrine AI, Doyle TF, Rizzoli HV: Spinal cord blood flow as affected by changes in systemic arterial blood pressure. *J Neurosurg* 1976;44(1): 12-15.
13. Marcus ML, Heistad DD, Ehrhardt JC, Abboud FM: Regulation of total and regional spinal cord blood flow. *Circ Res* 1977;41(1):128-134.
14. Parke WW, Whalen JL, Bunger PC, Settles HE: Intimal musculature of the lower anterior spinal artery. *Spine (Phila Pa 1976)* 1995;20(19): 2073-2079.
15. Gillilan LA: The arterial blood supply of the human spinal cord. *J Comp Neurol* 1958;110(1): 75-103.
16. Hassler O: Blood supply to human spinal cord: A microangiographic study. *Arch Neurol* 1966;15(3): 302-307.
17. Ferguson WR: Some observations on the circulation in foetal and infant spines. *J Bone Joint Surg Am* 1950;32(3):640-648.
18. Herren RY, Alexander L: Sulcal and intrinsic blood vessels of human spinal cord. *Arch Neurol Psychiat* 1939;41:678-683.
19. Kadyi H: *Über die Blutgefäasse des menschlichen Ruckenmarkes*. Lemberg, Poland, Grubryonowisz & Schmidt, 1889.
20. Turnbull IM, Brieg A, Hassler O: Blood supply of cervical spinal cord in man: A microangiographic cadaver study. *J Neurosurg* 1966;24(6):951-965.
21. Ireland WP, Fletcher TF, Bingham C: Quantification of microvasculature in the canine spinal cord. *Anat Rec* 1981;200(1):102-113.
22. Feeney JF, Watterson RL: The development of the vascular pattern within the walls of the central nervous system of the chick embryo. *J Morphol* 1946;78:231-303.
23. Lobosky JM, Hitchon PW, Torner JC, Yamada T: Spinal cord autoregulation in the sheep. *Curr Surg* 1984;41(4):264-267.
24. Parke WW: Arteriovenous anastomoses in the spinal cord: Probable role in blood flow autoregulation. *Anat Rec* 1989;223:87.
25. Molina JE, Cogordon J, Einzig S, et al: Adequacy of ascending aorta-descending aorta shunt during cross-clamping of the thoracic aorta for prevention of spinal cord injury. *J Thorac Cardiovasc Surg* 1985;90(1):126-136.
26. Wadouh F, Arndt CF, Oppermann E, Borst HG, Wadouh R: The mechanism of spinal cord injury after simple and double aortic cross-clamping. *J Thorac Cardiovasc Surg* 1986;92(1):121-127.
27. Gillilan LA: Veins of the spinal cord: Anatomic details; suggested clinical applications. *Neurology* 1970;20(9):860-868.
28. Parke WW, Gammell K, Rothman RH: Arterial vascularization of the cauda equina. *J Bone Joint Surg Am* 1981;63(1):53-62.
29. Parke WW, Watanabe R: The intrinsic vasculature of the lumbosacral spinal nerve roots. *Spine (Phila Pa 1976)* 1985;10(6):508-515.
30. Yamamoto H: Quantitative measurements of blood flow in cauda equina in spinal cords of monkeys by using radioactive microspheres. *J Jap College Angiol* 1982;22:35-42.

CHAPTER 10
The Anatomy and Physiology of the Spinal Cord in Injury and Repair

Douglas G. Chang, MD, PhD   Kevin D. Gerhart, MD, PhD

Key Points

- The spinal cord connects the brain neurologically with the body. The cord is enveloped within cerebrospinal fluid and the pia, arachnoid, and dural membranes, and anchored by denticulate ligaments, filum terminale, exiting spinal nerve roots, and surrounding epidural fat.
- Spinal gray matter contains posterior, intermediate, and anterior horns that contain the motor neuron cell bodies but also contain some sensory pathways.
- Spinal white matter has ascending tracts (with posterior, lateral, and anterior sensory pathways), descending tracts (with posterior, lateral, and anterior motor pathways), and intersegmental tracts.
- Intersegmental fibers help connect and coordinate the different spinal cord levels.
- Motor "engrams," or central pattern generators, are complex collections of sensorimotor reflexes and adaptable, plastic networks.
- Experimental spinal cord injury mechanics research demonstrates inhomogeneous, viscoelastic material properties. Posttraumatic imaging may significantly underestimate the actual amount of spinal deformation which occurs during an injury process.
- The spinal cord response to trauma has early, intermediate, late, and chronic phases, with primary necrotic and secondary reperfusion and apoptotic injury mechanisms.
- Spinal cord protection and repair strategies involve pharmacologic interventions, molecular biologic intra- and extracellular approaches, graft technologies, and rehabilitation protocols.

Dr. Chang or an immediate family member has received research or institutional support from Kimberly Clark; and owns stock or stock options in Merck. Neither Dr. Gerhart nor any immediate family member has received anything of value from or owns stock in a commercial company or institution related directly or indirectly to the subject of this chapter.

Introduction

Although spinal cord injuries (SCIs) have been recognized since ancient times, the revolutionary advances in the field have occurred over the past 50 years in particular.[1] During this time, there have been developments in many areas—epidemiology, injury biomechanics, neurologic classification (the most often quoted is the American Spinal Cord Injury Association [ASIA] scheme), acute treatment protocols, medications, radiological imaging, surgical techniques, and outcome measures. This growing knowledge base has improved clinical outcomes overall. During World War II, the life expectancy of SCI patients was about 3 months. In 1966, the life expectancy was 20 years, with renal failure (the sequela of inadequately treated neurogenic bladder, recurrent urinary tract infections, and stones) contributing to the majority of deaths.[1,2] Currently, SCI patients have a life expectancy of 25 to 30 years beyond the initial injury, with the primary causes of death now being pulmonary and cardiac in nature.[2,3] Recently, new energy is pouring into the tantalizing field of spinal cord repair. How much this research will help patients remains to be seen.

In the acutely injured SCI patient, the neurologic status is not permanently established until approximately 3 to 30 days after injury, with some recovery possible for about 1 year.[4,5] In the meantime, the treatment goals for patients with acute spinal cord trauma involve the prevention of medical and neurologic deterioration, with supportive medical care and appropriate surgical intervention to improve spinal column stability, and the use of strategies to possibly improve neurologic function. Subacutely, the treatment focus is on therapies to maximize the functional independence of patients within the context of their existing neurologic state. For the patient, this involves many physical, emotional, and environmental changes. Chronically, the treatment goals continue to focus on maximal functional independence. Some patients may benefit from technological advances in prosthetic technology. However, for most, the emphasis of treatment is the prevention, recognition, and treatment of the unique, but predictable, medical complications of SCI. All of these goals depend fundamentally upon an understanding of the anatomy and physiology of the spinal cord.

A Brief History of Spinal Cord Medicine

Knowledge of spinal cord anatomy and function can be dated back to the Smith papyrus (1600 BC), in which Imhotep and at least two other Egyptian priests described six cervical spine trauma cases and correlated the loss of motor and bladder function. Hippocrates (460-377 BC) described spinal cord vascular anatomy and categorized spinal injuries, diseases, and treatments.[6] Herophilus of Alexandria (325-255 BC) distinguished cranial from spinal nerves.[8] Galen, in the second century AD, transected animal spinal cords to experimentally produce paralysis. Syringomyelia, the presence of abnormal fluid collection within the spinal cord, was first described by Charles Estienne in 1546. Marcello Malpighi (1628-1694) used a microscope to describe the bundles of nerve fibers connected to the brain by the spinal cord. Bell distinguished spastic from flaccid paralysis in 1824. Anatomic localization of spinal cord function was described by Brown-Séquard in the mid-19th century. A spinal tumor was removed by means of a laminectomy in 1887 by Sir Victor Horsley. In 1928, Nobel laureate Santiago Ramon y Cajal suggested that central nervous system (CNS) neurons could regenerate within an environment of nutritive and orienting substances. These are just some of the pioneers who laid the groundwork for our current understanding of the spinal cord.[6-10]

Spinal Cord Anatomy

The spinal cord begins as a continuation of the brainstem, at the base of the skull, and usually terminates near the L1 vertebral body. The human adult spinal cord measures approximately 44 cm in length, 1 cm in diameter, and weighs about 35 g.[11] The nerves that lie within the spinal cord are termed upper motor neurons, while spinal nerves that branch out from the cord to innervate the body are called lower motor neurons. The spinal nerves exit and enter at specific vertebral levels. The cord contains 31 such levels, each with a pair of nerve roots (8 cervical, 12 thoracic, 5 lumbar, 5 sacral, and 1 coccygeal). On each side, the nerve roots have an anterior motor and posterior sensory branch, which join laterally into a spinal nerve. Nerves from each of the 31 segments connect to specific regions of the body. For example, the cervical segments, referred to as C1 through C8, provide innervation to the neck and upper extremities. The thoracic segments, T1 through T12, control signaling in the torso and some parts of the arms and hands. Lumbar segments, L1 through L5, provide innervation to the lower extremities. Finally, the sacral segments, S1 through S5, control signals in the feet, posterior thigh, and perineal region. The deleterious effects of SCI to these different segments reflect this organization.

The spinal cord itself is enclosed within membranes. The innermost layers, the leptomeninges or "pia-arachnoid mater," are delicate structures that contain blood vessels and the cerebrospinal fluid. The pia mater lies on the surface of the spinal cord and has two specialized attachments, the denticulate ligament and filum terminale. The denticulate ligaments are radial projections that attach to the outer dura. The filum terminale are inferior extensions of the membrane that extend beyond the spinal cord to the coccyx. The blood vessels supplying the spinal cord are lined with endothelial cells linked together by tight junctions, continuing the blood-brain barrier, which limits the transport of metabolically active substances into and out of the CNS. The pachymeninx, or "dura mater," is made of strong connective tissue and forms a tough, gray outer layer of the spinal cord and nerve roots.

Between the dura–cerebral spinal fluid (CSF)–cord complex and the spinal canal is the epidural space, which contains loose areolar connective tissue, fat, lymphatics, arteries, venous plexuses, and the spinal nerve roots as they exit the dural sac and pass through the intervertebral foramina.[12] The lumbar epidural space in adults is segmented and discontinuous, separated by areas of contact between the dura and the vertebral lamina and pedicles. In adult males, the anterior-posterior dimension in the posterior space is about 5 mm to 6 mm in diameter. At the thoracic and cervical levels, the epidural contents are diminished in size but are less septated. Solutions injected into the space typically flow as rivulets through numerous small channels in a nonuniform fashion.[13] Substantial barriers do not appear to partition the posterior and lateral epidural space. However, the lateral spaces may not communicate with each other directly, and remain separated at the posterior, midline aspect of the spinal canal.[14] The lateral epidural space does communicate freely with the intervertebral foramina and paravertebral space. Therefore, solution injected into the epi-

FIGURE 1

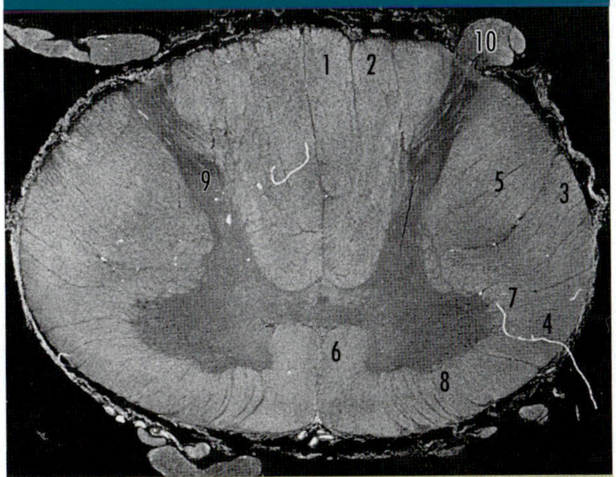

Figure 1 A transverse section through the cervicothoracic junction of the normal adult spinal cord. The posterior funiculus shows the anatomic appearance of the fasciculus gracilis (**1**) and fasciculus cuneatus (**2**). The lateral funiculus shows the posterior (**3**) and anterior spinocerebellar tracts (**4**), and the lateral (**5**) and anterior (**6**) corticospinal tracts. Also shown are the lateral spinothalamic tract (**7**) and the anterior lateral sulcus (**8**), which contains the exiting anterior horn motor cell fibers. The substantia gelatinosa (**9**), the nuclei where primary afferents of the spinothalamic tract become second-order neurons, is well visualized in the dorsal horn of the gray matter. Well visualized in this specimen is the dorsal root entering the dorsal horn (**10**). (Reproduced from Vaccaro AR, Ahmad SS, Rauschning W, Garfin SR: Anatomy and pathophysiology of spinal cord injury, in Levine AM, Eismont FJ, Garfin SR, Zigler JE, eds: *Spine Trauma*. Philadelphia, PA, WB Saunders, 1998, pp 75-86.)

FIGURE 2

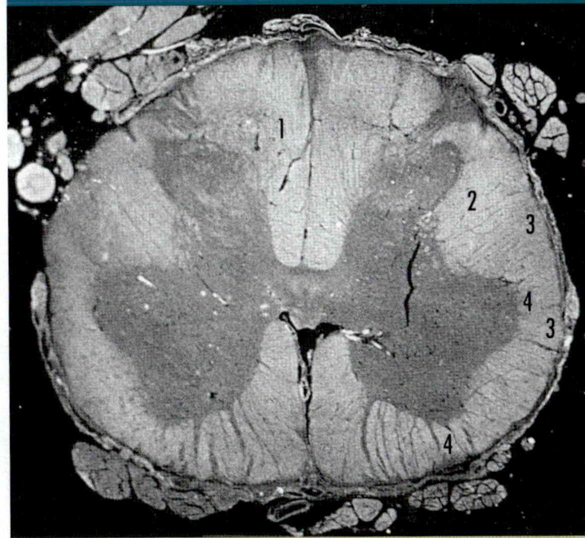

Figure 2 This photograph depicts a transverse section through the lumbar spinal cord. Note the increased proportion of gray matter in the caudal lumbar cord compared with more rostral sections of the spinal cord. The posterior funiculus of the lumbar cord is solely composed of the fasciculus gracilis (**1**), for the fasciculus cuneatus commences rostral to T6. The lateral corticospinal (**2**) tract makes up a large proportion of the lateral funiculus. However, contributions from the spinocerebellar (**3**) and spinothalamic (**4**) tracts can be seen along the periphery of the white matter. The dorsal and ventral nerve roots enter and exit the gray matter via the dorsal and ventral horns. (Reproduced from Vaccaro AR, Ahmad SS, Rauschning W, Garfin SR: Anatomy and pathophysiology of spinal cord injury, in Levine AM, Eismont FJ, Garfin SR, Zigler JE, eds: *Spine Trauma*. Philadelphia, PA, WB Saunders, 1998, pp 75-86.)

dural space extends circumferentially about the spinal canal and tends to course preferentially outwards, along the nerve root sheaths and the dorsal root ganglia. At some levels, the anterior epidural space is almost entirely filled by a rich venous plexus. In the T10-L2 region, the basivertebral vein communicates between the vertebral bodies and the plexus.

Macroscopically, the spinal cord has two predominant enlargements in the cervical and lumbosacral regions, which correspond to areas of greatest spinal nerve function. The enlargements provide innervation in the upper and lower extremities, respectively. A transverse section (**Figures 1** and **2**) through the spinal cord reveals a deep anterior median fissure and a posterior median sulcus. On the anterior surface, just lateral to the anterior median fissure on either side, lies the anterior lateral sulcus, through which the anterior horn motor cell fibers exit to the ventral nerve root (**Figure 1,** *number 8*). On the posterior surface of the spinal cord, just lateral to the posterior median sulcus on either side, lies a posterior lateral sulcus through which nerve fibers enter from the dorsal root (**Figure 1,** *number 10*).

The adult spinal cord tapers caudally, referred to as the conus medullaris; this section terminates at about the L1-2 disk space. From there, it is replaced by a remnant, called the conus terminalis, which anchors the spinal cord to the coccyx. Because the spinal cord ends at about the L1-2 disk space, it is some 25 cm shorter than the vertebral column. Thus, the lower segments of the spinal cord do not align next to their correspondingly named vertebral bodies. Instead, the lumbar and sacral nerve roots are very long and extend from the spinal cord segments inferiorly, within the spinal canal, to the lumbar and sacral intervertebral foramina. The nerve roots descend in a bundle

2: General Principles

FIGURE 3

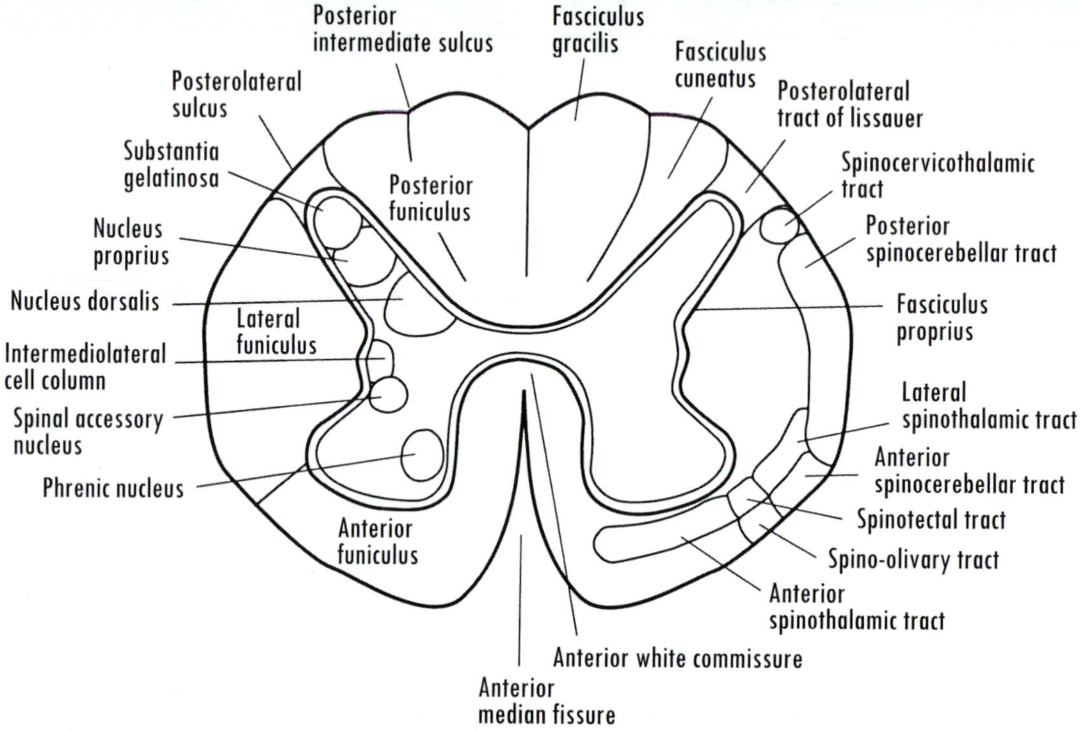

Figure 3 Transverse section of the spinal cord showing the various ascending tracts of the three funiculi (anterior, lateral, and posterior) of the spinal white matter. The various subdivisions of the anterior, intermediate, and posterior horns of the spinal gray matter are also shown. (Reproduced from Vaccaro AR, Ahmad SS, Rauschning W, Garfin SR: Anatomy and pathophysiology of spinal cord injury, in Levine AM, Eismont FJ, Garfin SR, Zigler JE, eds: *Spine Trauma*. Philadelphia, PA, WB Saunders, 1998, pp 75-86.)

from the conus terminalis, resembling the tail of a horse and referred to as the cauda equina.

The internal structure of the spinal cord is comprised of gray matter and white matter. Horizontal sections of the spinal cord reveal an H- or butterfly-shaped area of central gray matter, surrounded by peripheral white matter (**Figure 3**). The central gray matter is composed of unmyelinated cell bodies, interneurons, short nerve cell processes (axons and dendrites), connective tissues, and vascular components. The gray matter is divided into symmetric columns, containing the anterior and dorsal horns. In general, the anterior horns contain efferent motor nerve fibers, and the dorsal horns contain afferent sensory nerve fibers. Left-right communication between the horns is made across the center of the cord through a thin commissure. The peripheral white matter contains myelinated neurons and houses the principal fiber tracts of the ascending and descending neural pathways of the spinal cord (**Figures 1** through **5**). Disruption of these structures in a spinal cord lesion leads to well-recognized patterns of clinical loss, which are explainable by the location and type of fibers involved (see chapter 13, Classification of Spinal Injury).

The spinal cord is perfused by an intraneural microvascular system. At most, 7 or 8 of the 62 radicular artery branches participate in the vascularization of the cord. The cervical area is richly vascularized by the anterior artery of the intracranial vertebral artery, two or three arteries from the vertebral artery, and an artery from the costocervical trunk. A rich, superficial network of peripheral arteries descend from the radicular artery branches to supply the pia mater and spinal cord white matter. The central gray matter is supplied by numerous large central arteries that descend from the spinal artery branches. Substitution pathways are available to vascularize the cord. However, these networks are incomplete and appear mainly to supply the peripheral cord.[15] The nerve roots, ganglia, and spinal nerves are supplied from spinal branches of the segmental arteries and medullary vessels. Arteries enter the dorsal root ganglia by penetrating the dural sheath. Veins drain into a periganglionic plexus. Within the ganglion, there are arterioles, capillaries, and venules. Almost every nerve cell in the ganglion appears surrounded by a capillary loop. An intrinsic control mechanism for autoregulation of spinal cord blood flow in response to blood pressure and carbon dioxide levels has been suggested.[16]

Spinal Gray Matter

The spinal gray matter is composed of nerve cell bodies, connective tissue, and vascular components. The quantity of gray matter, and the shape on transverse section, varies dramatically at the different levels of the spinal cord. In the thoracic region, the quantity is small. In the cervical and lumbar enlargements, it is greatly increased. Nevertheless, all along the spinal cord, there are three distinct regions, or horns, which are identified within the gray matter: the posterior, intermediate, and anterior. A less clinically useful classification scheme divides the gray matter into 10 groups of nuclei (**Figure 5**).[17] Viewed longitudinally, the nuclei are seen to be cell columns, or laminae. According to Rexed's classification, lamina I is the posterior margin of the posterior gray matter, lamina IX involves the motor neurons of the anterior gray matter, and lamina X corresponds to the intermediate gray matter around the central canal.

FIGURE 4

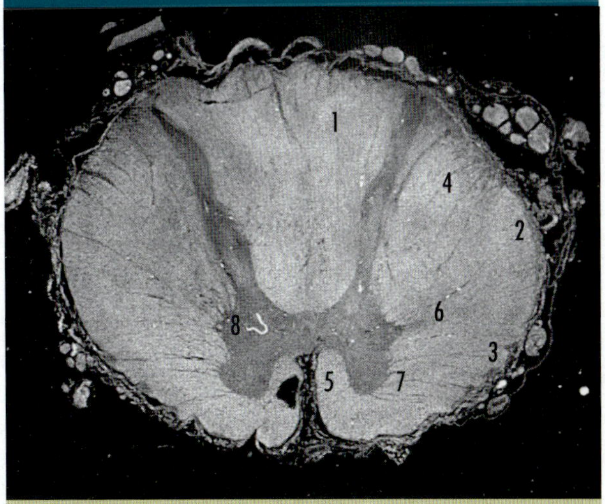

Figure 4 A transverse section through the thoracic spinal cord. Because the fasciculus cuneatus commences rostral to T6, the posterior funiculus is solely composed of the fasciculus gracilis (**1**). The lateral funiculus consists of the posterior (**2**) and anterior (**3**) spinocerebellar tracts, the lateral (**4**) and anterior (**5**) corticospinal tracts, and the lateral (**6**) and anterior (**7**) spinothalamic tracts. The intermediolateral cell column (**8**), composed of preganglionic sympathetic nerve cell bodies, is easily seen in sections through the thoracic cord. (Reproduced from Vaccaro AR, Ahmad SS, Rauschning W, Garfin SR: Anatomy and pathophysiology of spinal cord injury, in Levine AM, Eismont FJ, Garfin SR, Zigler JE, eds: *Spine Trauma*. Philadelphia, PA, WB Saunders, 1998, pp 75-86.)

Posterior Gray Matter

The posterior horn of gray matter in the spinal cord is long and slender, directed backward and laterally. The horn contains cells whose axons form the various tracts of the sensory columns, the most important of which are the substantia gelatinosa, nucleus proprius, body of the posterior column, and nucleus dorsalis/fasciculus cuneatus.

The most dorsal aspect of the posterior horn contains a crescent mass of translucent, gelatinous neuroglia, termed the substantia gelatinosa of Rolando (**Figures 1** and **3**). This area contains fine, myelinated and unmyelinated sensory fibers that ascend and descend to relay information on pain, temperature, and touch. Ventral to the substantia gelatinosa is the nucleus proprius, which relays information on proprioception, two-point discrimination, and body movement. Both of these areas traverse the entire length of the spinal cord. The body of the posterior column (or nucleus proprius) is composed of cells concerned with somatic and visceral sensory functions, and is located from the spinal segments T1 to L3. Lastly, the nucleus dorsalis cell group and tracts (or Clarke's nucleus) are located approximately at spinal levels C8 to L3, and relay proprioceptive information from the lower extremities to the thalamus and cerebellum. Proprioceptive information from the upper extremities enters the spinal cord above the C8 spinal segment in a region of the posterior gray matter called the fasciculus cuneatus.

Intermediate Gray Matter

This region lies intermediate to the anterior and posterior horns, and lies in two regions of the spinal cord to control autonomic function. From T1 through L2 or L3, there are preganglionic sympathetic neurons. In the segments S2 to S4, there are preganglionic parasympathetic fibers. Surrounding neural tissue in this region is composed of tracts and sensory neurons that communicate with cells of the anterior gray matter ventral roots.

Anterior Gray Matter

The anterior horns contain the motor neuron cell bodies. The primary motor neurons are multipolar-shaped alpha motor neurons. There are

2: General Principles

FIGURE 5

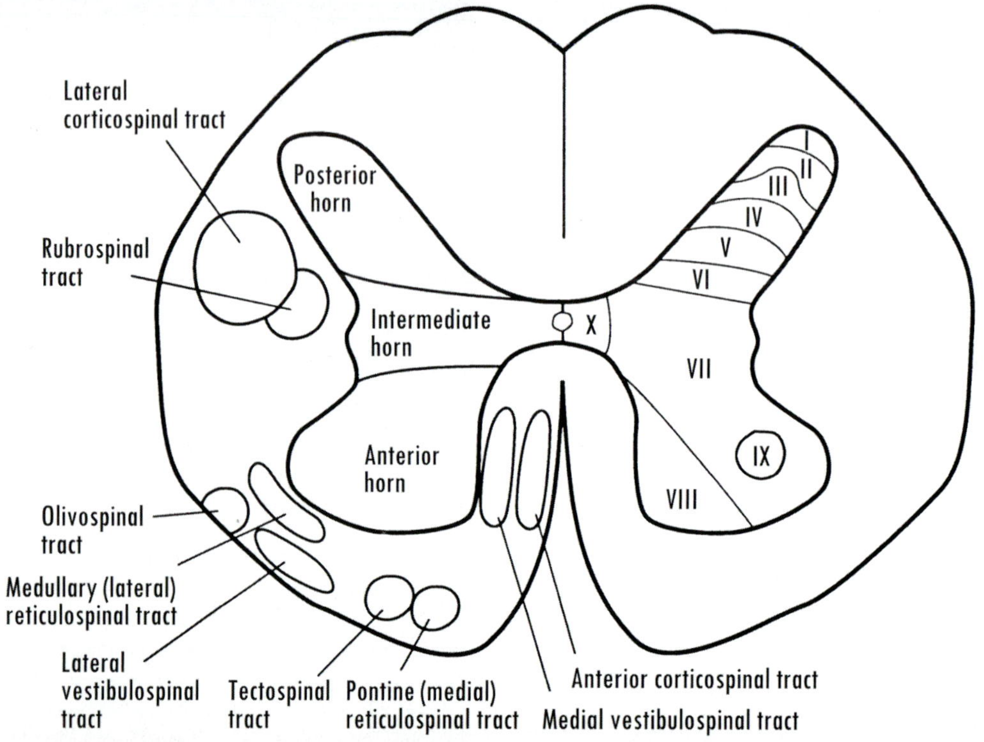

Figure 5 The transverse section of the spinal cord, illustrating the various descending tracts of the spinal white matter. The laminae of Rexed are illustrated contralateral to the three horns (posterior, intermediate, and anterior) of the spinal gray matter. (Reproduced from Vaccaro AR, Ahmad SS, Rauschning W, Garfin SR: Anatomy and pathophysiology of spinal cord injury, in Levine AM, Eismont FJ, Garfin SR, Zigler JE, eds: *Spine Trauma*. Philadelphia, PA, WB Saunders, 1998, pp 75-86.)

secondary gamma efferent neurons, which are smaller, and innervate the intrafusal muscle fibers of neuromuscular spindles.[11] These are the cells affected in "anterior horn diseases," such as polio, amyotrophic lateral sclerosis, spinal muscular atrophy, and Charcot-Marie-Tooth disease.

The cell bodies lie in three main groups, the medial, central, and lateral cell columns.[18]

The medial column consists of cells that innervate the axial, spinal, abdominal, and intercostal muscles. The central column is present in certain locations of the spinal cord, mainly in the medullary brainstem to cervical C5 or C6 region, and the lumbosacral region. The cervical portion (**Figure 3**) contains both the phrenic nucleus (C3 to C5), innervating the diaphragm, and the spinal accessory nucleus (lower medulla to C6), innervating the trapezius and sternocleidomastoid muscles. The lateral column of the anterior horn, present in the cervical and lumbosacral regions, is composed of motor neurons that innervate the appendicular skeletal muscles of the extremities.

Spinal White Matter

The spinal cord white matter in the periphery of the cord is composed of the nerve tracts of the motor and sensory nerves, vascular tissue, and connective tissue. On axial cross-section, three groups of spinal white matter are seen, and these are separated by portions of the spinal gray matter (**Figure 3**). The three groups are the posterior, lateral, and anterior funiculi.[18] However, it is easier to discuss the tracts in terms of those with ascending, descending, and intersegmental connections.

Ascending Tracts

The majority of the ascending white matter tracts of the human spinal cord have been identified, although newer tracts are continually discovered and their function clarified with continued research. They provide the brain with information about the body and the environment. These data are perceived consciously by the cortex, as well as unconsciously.

Posterior Column

The posterior white column is regarded as the high-speed "data link" to the brain. Large myelinated fiber tracts relay information regarding pain, temperature, proprioception, kinesthesia (sense of body movement), tactile discrimination, pressure, and vibration from the extremities to the brainstem, thalamus, and cerebellum. Tactile discrimination involves a wide array of fine-touch sensory information, including two-point discrimination and stereognosis, the appreciation of shape, patterns, and textures by touch. Muscle and joint information is relayed by nerve fibers from the Golgi tendon organs (1b fibers) and muscle spindles (1a fibers).

Two important columns are the fasciculus gracilis and cuneatus. The gracilis transmits information from the sacral, lumbar and lower thoracic segments (**Figures 2** and **4**). The cuneatus appears cephalad to the level of T6, and contains sensory information from the cervical and upper-middle thoracic segments. The fasciculus gracilis and cuneatus convey their information to the medulla oblongata, where the axons terminate respectively in the nucleus gracilis and the nucleus cuneatus. There is a somatotopic arrangement of the ascending fibers, with the more cephalad fibers adding on laterally to the posterior column.

In summary, the posterior white column supplies the brain with important data regarding position in space, muscular action, and the environment. Damage to the posterior columns results in impairment to complex tactile sensibilities and to the sense of kinesthesia, which results in a distinctive broad-based, ataxic gait pattern.

Lateral Column

There are several ascending tracts of the lateral column[11] (**Figure 3**). These are the spinocerebellar, spinothalamic, spinoreticular, spinotectal, spino-olivary, and spinocervicothalamic tracts, and the posterolateral tract of Lissauer. The tracts help coordinate the transmission of pain, temperature, and tactile information from the extremities and somatic system.

The anterior and posterior spinocerebellar tracts relay painful stimuli and unconscious proprioception, touch, and pressure information. The anterior spinocerebellar tract is mostly concerned with information from the lower limbs and with the control of posture. These fibers ascend from the lower cord and are divided into a few ipsilateral (uncrossed) and mostly contralateral (crossed) fibers. The rostral spinocerebellar tract is the analog equivalent for the upper extremities, arising from the nucleus centralis basis of the spinal cord and projecting to the cerebellum.[19] The posterior spinocerebellar tract, below L3, ascends first to the upper lumbar segments where they end in Clarke's nuclei. Impulses from the upper part of the body are mostly transmitted through the posterior spinocerebellar tract.

The spinothalamic system transmits sensory information to the brain, but the transmission is slower and less precise than in the dorsal column system. The lateral spinothalamic tract is found next to the anterior spinocerebellar tract, and carries somatic sensations of pain and temperature, as well as simple touch and itching. The tract is somatotopically arranged, such that cephalad nerve fibers are added anteromedially by axons that cross in the anterior commissure. Pain sensation is always found anterior to those fibers carrying temperature. This tract belongs to the anterolateral system of the somatosensory afferents, which includes the anterior (see section on Anterior Column below) and lateral spinothalamic tracts, as well as the spinoreticular tract. The spinoreticular tract terminates before reaching the thalamus and, therefore, is not technically a spinothalamic tract. However, the spinoreticular fibers are mixed within the fibers of the spinothalamic tract. These fibers carry sensory information to the reticular formation from the muscles, joints, and skin. They appear to respond to noxious stimuli.

The spinotectal tract is positioned between the anterior and lateral spinothalamic tracts. Functionally, it is similar to the spinothalamic tract because both transmit pain, temperature, and tactile information. The spinotectal tract does not terminate in the thalamus. Instead, it synapses in the midbrain and helps integrate the information into the spinovisual reflexes. For example, the spinotectal tract is involved in reflex head gaze to a location of noxious sensory input on the body surface. The spino-olivary tract is positioned next to the spinotectal and anterior spinocerebellar tracts. It relays the cutaneous and proprioceptive information typical of the spinothalamic system directly to the cerebellum instead of the thalamus.

The spinocervicothalamic tract lies in the posterior horn between the posterolateral tract of Lissauer and the posterior spinocerebellar tract. It relays information on touch and pain sensation from the skin and hair, as well as vibratory and position senses. Lastly, the posterolateral tract of Lissauer caps the substantia gelatinosa in the posterior horn. The tract is composed of short ascending and descending nerve branches and relays information from noxious stimuli via A-delta and

C peripheral nerve fibers to the underlying dorsal column in the spinal cord.

Anterior Column

The anterior spinothalamic tract fibers ascend in the anterior white column of the spinal cord. These fibers carry sensation from tactile, pain, and pressure receptors, and are somatotopically arranged with the more cephalad fibers entering the spinal cord more medially.

Descending Tracts

Pathways from the brain to the spinal cord involve motor pathways originating from neurons in the motor cortex and several other areas of the cerebrum. The descending fibers pass down through the brainstem, with most fibers crossing in the medulla to the contralateral side, to enter the spinal cord. About 90% of the descending fibers cross at this so-called pyramidal tract decussation, and descend through the spinal cord as the lateral corticospinal tract. The 10% of fibers that do not decussate in the medulla descend in the anterior corticospinal tract.

Posterior Column

The descending tracts of the posterior column are not well identified, but there is evidence that small descending fiber tracts exist.

Lateral Column

The lateral column contains several descending pathways (**Figure 5**). The largest is the lateral corticospinal or pyramidal tract. This tract is composed of small myelinated, relatively slow-conducting, crossed nerve fibers concerned mainly with the control and delivery of voluntary motor function. More than 80% of its axons are said to exert an inhibitory influence on the interneurons and motor neurons of the spinal cord.[20] The tract is involved in the skilled movements of the distal muscles of the limbs, and facilitation of the alpha and gamma motor neurons that innervate the distal flexor musculature.[19] The tract is organized with the more cephalad fibers positioned medially, and more caudad fibers located laterally. In the so-called "central cord syndrome," an injury to the central spinal cord preferentially affects these medial fibers and clinically, the patients exhibit more weakness in the upper extremities than in the lower extremities. In the spinal cord, the lateral corticospinal tract lies in the posterior portion of the lateral column, near the descending posterior spinocerebellar tract.

There are several bulbospinal pathways which originate in the brainstem and terminate in the spinal cord, including the olivospinal, lateral medullary reticulospinal, and rubrospinal tracts. These are small pathways, thought to be more important in the fetus and neonate than at any other time, after which their function is supplanted by the large corticospinal tract.[20] The olivospinal tract is located only in the upper cervical cord at the periphery of the lateral column close to the anterior column. The tract modulates motor neurons in the anterior gray column. The medullary reticulospinal tract originates in the reticular formation and is also thought to be located at the juncture of the lateral and anterior white columns. This tract is mostly uncrossed and carries information to the preganglionic sympathetic and parasympathetic autonomic nervous systems. It also modulates the alpha, beta, and gamma motor neurons of the anterior gray column. The red nucleus gives rise to the crossed fibers of the rubrospinal tract, which is found between the reticulospinal tract and lateral corticospinal tract. The rubrospinal tract generally facilitates flexor and inhibits extensor motor neurons, particularly those for the distal arm.

Anterior Column

There are several descending pathways in the anterior column (**Figure 5**), including the anterior corticospinal tract and a group of pathways collectively known as the medial longitudinal fasciculus. The anterior corticospinal tract contains uncrossed fibers and is located in the cervical and upper thoracic spinal cord next to the anterior median fissure. At their respective level of termination, the anterior corticospinal tract fibers cross through the anterior white commissure before synapsing with interneurons and motor neurons. The medial longitudinal fasciculus is used to describe a bundle of several tracts that descend in the anterior funiculus of the spinal cord. These tracts include the tectospinal, medial pontine reticulospinal, vestibulospinal, and the interstitiospinal tracts. The function of the medial longitudinal fasciculus centers on head and neck reflex movements in response to visual and vestibular stimuli.

The tectospinal tract arises from the superior colliculus, crosses to the contralateral side near the oculomotor nucleus, and passes caudally to the upper thoracic spinal cord. The fibers are involved in coordinated eye muscle movements and help coordinate the pupillary light reflex response via the sympathetic neurons. The uncrossed fibers of the medial pontine reticulospinal tract are located next to the tectospinal tract. These fibers facilitate extensor alpha motor neurons to the axial trunk and proximal limb musculature.[19] The lateral vestibulospinal tract descends the entire length of the spinal cord, while the medial vestibulospinal tract descends only to upper thoracic levels. These fibers relay information from the inner ear and cerebellum to the muscles of the body, controlling postural tone and adjustments to accompany head movements. The lateral tract involves excitatory facilitation of the extensor motor neurons of the neck, back, and extremity muscles, and reciprocal inhibition of the flexor motor neurons. The medial tract involves inhibition and excitation of the neck and back muscles only. The interstitiospinal tract originates from the nucleus of Cajal, an accessory oculomotor nucleus. It has a brief course, supplying only the upper cervical cord.

Intersegmental Fibers

The intersegmental nerve fibers are grouped posteriorly, laterally, and anteriorly around the gray matter. They are referred to as the propriospinal tracts, or fasciculus proprius, and are responsible for connecting the different spinal cord levels to coordinate complex movements. Long propriospinal neurons descend in the anterior fasciculus proprius at all levels of the spinal cord, influencing medial musculature. Intermediate propriospinal neurons reside in the lateral aspect of the fasciculus proprius and influence proximal limb muscles. Short propriospinal neurons are located in the cervical and lumbosacral enlargements in the lateral funiculus proprius and modulate distal limb muscles.[21]

Spinal Plasticity

In the past two decades, clinical experience with motor learning during rehabilitation has been supplemented with new research from the neurosciences on neural development, cell networks, activity-dependent synaptic remodeling, and motor control systems.[22] The existence of central pattern generators, or motor engrams, in the spinal cord and the rest of the CNS has been observed in various animal and human models. These pattern generators direct subconscious repetitive motion such as respiration and gut motility. In the mammalian spinal cord, central pattern generators can direct crude locomotion without cortical involvement.[23] Such pattern generators involve the coordinated activity of neuronal populations that have not been identified anatomically as discrete tracts or nuclei within the CNS. Instead, they appear as complex collections of sensorimotor reflexes and plastic networks that are adaptable.[24] Their activity is influenced by direct electrical stimulation of the spinal cord horn cells, skeletal muscle firing patterns, noradrenergic and glycinergic neurotransmitters, and various neuropeptides such as serotonin, glutamate, and gamma-aminobutyric acid (GABA).[25] A major challenge will be to unravel the secrets of these intriguing circuits using new molecular biology, functional imaging, and rehabilitation protocols.[26]

Pathophysiology of SCI

The severity of neurologic injury incurred during spinal trauma is contingent on several variables. These variables contribute to the pathophysiologic response of the spinal cord to injury, and include the mechanism of injury, the time course, the energy of trauma, the premorbid health and functioning of the patient, the type of environmental safety precautions in effect around the patient, the level of the SCI, any evidence of cord disruption, continued posttraumatic cord compression, or medical comorbidities. As with an acute stroke, the SCI is a dynamic process; the full extent of injury may not be apparent initially. Incomplete cord lesions can evolve into complete lesions. Injuries that initially appear to be complete often improve to an incomplete status over time. More commonly, the injury level initially raises one or two spinal levels in the hours to days after the initial trauma. Such clinical deterioration is related to altered blood flow, edema, inflammation, and mechanical instability of the spine.[27]

Physicians treating SCI must recognize these variables and optimize patient health, halt or reverse neurologic deterioration, decompress the spinal cord from any impinging structures, and prevent complications in the peritrauma period. These goals have been facilitated by newer and more rapid imaging modalities, and newer surgical procedures and fixation technology. However, meticulous attention must still be paid to the critical parameters of normal oxygenation, perfusion, and acid-base balance to prevent worsening of an acute SCI.[27]

Experimental Spinal Canal and Cord Biomechanics

Some information is available regarding the geometry of the cervical spinal canal during trauma,[28] physiologic range of motion,[29] and acceleration/deceleration.[30] In these studies, no significant spinal distraction is seen. Additionally, cervical spinal canal size does not change appreciably during range of motion in physiologic or whiplash simulations. However, the postinjury spinal canal appearance that might be seen with clinical imaging after a serious injury can significantly underestimate the extent of transient canal diameter changes and occlusion that occurred during the actual injury event.[28]

Less is known about the mechanics of the spinal cord itself. MRI studies have shown that the human cervical spinal cord elongates 5% to 15% in physiologic flexion, with significantly greater stretch of the posterior cord compared to the anterior cord.[31] In degenerated cervical spines, the spinal cord tends to exhibit more compression from encroaching intervertebral disk and ligamentum flavum with the neck in extension. Conversely, there can be spinal cord decompression with the neck in flexion.[32]

With 33% spinal canal occlusion, the thoracolumbar spinal cord has been shown to compress with 6 kPa of pressure and demonstrate a 15% viscoelastic stress relaxation within 10 seconds. Strain is distributed inhomogeneously along the cord, and the cord is stiffer when stretched in distraction.[33,34] Viscoelastic stress-strain behavior was described in tensile testing of the spinal cord at low (< 5%) strains. Lastly, the modulus of elasticity for spinal cord gray and white matter was estimated to be about 3 kPa in finite-element analysis and micropipette experiments. However, the effects of fluid pressurization or stiffening have not been studied.[35-38]

Overview of the Biochemical and Histologic Changes in Injury

The tissue changes occurring during traumatic injury to the spinal cord have been studied in decades of patient autopsies[39,40] and various animal models. Most of the animal studies involve an impact blow,[41-43] compression,[44-46] or ischemia.[47,48] Other studies have used pulsed ultrasound[49] and axial cord distraction.[50,51] In all such studies, a threshold trauma initiates a process of tissue destruction which was monitored and described.

Briefly, basic biologic research and clinical experience demonstrate several points. The gray matter and white matter of the spinal cord respond differently to trauma. The central gray matter appears to have an early susceptibility to injury, owing to increased metabolic requirements, regional perfusion differences, and the loss of intrinsic biologic repair mechanisms at the site of injury.[52] In contrast, there is a delayed and milder response from the surrounding white matter. For example, irreversible damage can occur to the gray matter within an hour after trauma, but the potential for salvage of white matter neural function is possible up to 3 days postinjury.[53] Furthermore, research has demonstrated that the spread of damage is related to the magnitude and duration of the trauma, and time after injury. Mild injuries may be reversible. Histopathologic changes in the spinal cord can take place even in the presence of clinical improvement. Lastly, damage seems to be mediated by direct mechanical injury to neuronal tissues, inflammation, vascular ischemia, and reperfusion. Recently, there has been more attention to the molecular biology of SCI,[54] which will be discussed in more detail below.

SCI Response in Closed Trauma

In clinical SCI, the spinal cord typically suffers a contusion or compression injury. The cord can also be lacerated or transected (knife or gunshot wounds).[2,3] Closed spinal trauma with compression of the spinal cord initiates a sequence of events that can be divided into acute, intermediate, and chronic/late histological phases (**Table 1**). These phases involve several cellular players (**Table 2**).

Early or Acute Phase

The acute phase of SCI lasts from the initial injury event to about 3 days postinjury. Changes in the tissue matrix, vasculature, and cells become evident within minutes.[41]

Five minutes after injury, increased water content is seen in the spinal cord, and this remains persistently elevated for weeks. Edema is seen first in the central gray matter, and may progress into the surrounding white matter.[42,55,56] Intracellular swelling is also seen, primarily in the astrocytes, and this may persist for 3 days postinjury.[4,40] At first, the tissue edema is characterized as nonproteinaceous, but with time, a primary vasogenic edema with protein extravasation becomes evident. This is due to the breakdown of the vascular endothelial spinal cord barrier, tissue electrolyte disturbances, and cell membrane dysfunction. Macroscopically, engorged edematous tissue extension may be seen caudally and cephalad, over several spinal segments, within 18 hours.[10]

Central gray matter areas of punctate hemorrhage appear from disrupted endothelial junctions in the thin capillaries and thin-walled muscular venules within 15 minutes of injury. The hemorrhage is progressive over 8 hours after injury,

TABLE 1

Major Features of SCI Response in Closed Trauma

Acute/Early (Seconds to ~ 3 Days)	Intermediate (Days to Weeks)	Chronic/Late (Months to Years)
• Edema, intracellular swelling • Hemorrhage • Vasospasm • Regional cord perfusion shifts • Inflammatory response with free-radical production, lipid peroxidation, and cytokine release • Membrane instability with shifts in electrolytes and accumulation of neurotransmitters • Demyelination • Cell necrosis • Apoptosis	• Caudal and cephalad extension of edema, necrosis, and apoptosis • Continued inflammatory response • Vascular angiopathy • Peak levels of astrocyte and macrophage activity • Scar formation • Neural plastic changes, spasticity	• Formation of fluid-filled cavity • Wallerian degeneration • Astroglial and collagenous scar formation • Demyelination • Schwann cell proliferation • Syringomyelia • Tethered cord • Schwannosis and neurite sprouting • Altered neurocircuits, chronic pain syndromes • Degenerative disease of the spine

spreading in a central-to-peripheral fashion that can involve the surrounding white matter, depending on the magnitude of the trauma. Within the gray matter, hemorrhagic lesions and neuronal damage is especially marked at 4 hours postinjury. In contrast, the white matter retains a normal structure at this time.[57-59] In the minutes following trauma, there are marked differences in the regional perfusion of the spinal cord.[52,60-62] Immediately, gray matter perfusion drops by 80%. In contrast, white matter flow increases slightly and remains elevated for several hours. Within the first 24 hours, a milieu of ischemia and edema is seen with vascular dilation, leakage, thrombosis, and disruption. The spread of hemorrhagic necrosis and edema may obscure the gray and white matter boundaries within 24 hours, with extension to the leptomeninges and obliteration of the subarachnoid and subdural spaces.[10]

Several hours after the initial traumatic event, there is an influx of polymorphonuclear cells, followed by the appearance of mononuclear lymphocytes, plasma B cells, and then macrophages at about 24 hours after injury. At this time, a rim of leukocytes may be seen along the remaining periphery of intact white matter surrounding areas of hemorrhagic necrosis. Histologically, the first 2 to 4 hours are characterized by neural injury, with axonal, myelin, and periaxonal swelling. This is followed by myelin breakdown and fragmentation, with axonal process disruption and neuronal cell central chromatolysis.[39] The remaining axonal processes are swollen and contain multiple organelles because of transport stasis. During this time, necrosis and apoptosis lead to neuronal and glial cell death. This process involves immediate early gene expression, and the induction of heat shock proteins.[54]

Spinal-evoked response and evoked potential conduction properties seem to depend directly on the severity of mechanical trauma to these neural processes and not directly on vascular changes.[45,63] The initial core of cell death, with a perimeter of cells at risk for death, may involve a larger region over time.[3] Depending on the injury severity, the ventral horn cells may show neuronal cell chromatolysis and ischemic changes about 1 hour after injury.[58] Dorsal column demyelination can be seen as early as 21 hours after injury (**Figures 6** and **7**). By day 3, macrophages take on a characteristic fat-laden appearance, due to the ingestion of degenerated myelin fragments.[4,10] With continued disturbances of the microcirculation and tissue necrosis over the next 3 to 4 days, a central cord cystic structure filled with cellular debris, blood, or clear fluid may develop.

In conjunction with the immediate mechanical and ischemic damage to neural and vascular tissues, there are significant biochemical shifts. Injured nerve cells respond initially with injury-induced barrages of action potentials. This process involves membrane instability to sodium, potassium, and toxic levels of intracellular calcium that eventually contribute to neural failure and spinal shock.[3] Within 15 minutes of injury, there are toxic extracellular concentrations of glutamate and

TABLE 2

A Few Important Cell Types Involved in SCI

Cell Type	Function and Description
Neuron	• Relays information between the brain and the rest of the body by conducting electrochemical signals • Several neuron types: motor, sensory, autonomic, and interneuron
Glial	• Nonneuronal cells that provide support, nutrition, immune protection, and structure • Microglia are the smallest kind of glial cell in the CNS. They are involved in phagocytosis, removing microbes, and tissue debris • Macroglia include astrocytes, oligodendrocytes, Schwann cells.
Astrocyte	• A star-shaped glial cell type found in the CNS • Provides physical structure in the brain • Provides neurons with nutrients • Forms part of the blood-brain barrier • Regulates ion concentration in the extracellular space • Reacts to injury with hypertrophy and proliferation, and formation of a glial scar • May also secrete molecules, such as chondroitin sulfate proteglycans, which inhibit CNS regenerative activity
Oligodendrocyte	• A glial cell type found in the CNS • Forms the myelin sheath around axons in the central nervous system • One oligodendrocyte myelinates multiple axons
Schwann cell	• A glial cell type found in the peripheral nervous system • Forms the myelin sheath around axons in the peripheral nervous system • One Schwann cell myelinates only one axon • Migrates into the spinal cord after injury, where it is involved in remyelination and laminin production
Endothelial	• Forms the interior lining of blood vessels • Involved in inflammation and edema, releasing cytokines • Controls the passage of materials in and out of the blood stream, maintaining the blood-brain/spinal cord barrier • May also secrete molecules, such as chondroitin sulfate proteglycans, which inhibit CNS regenerative activity
Neutrophil	• A highly motile type of granular white blood cell • During acute inflammation, neutrophils leave the vasculature and migrate by chemotaxis. • Involved in phagocytosis, removing microbes and tissue debris • Secretes serine proteases, permeability-increasing proteins, and defensins • Their activity and death forms pus.
Lymphocyte	• A white blood cell with two broad categories: large and small • Large granular natural killer cells • Small lymphocytes (T helper and B cells) • Secretes cytokines, growth factors, and antibodies
Macrophage	• Another type of agranular white blood cell • Derived from circulating monocytes, which have migrated from the bloodstream and entered tissue • Involved in phagocytosis, removing microbes and tissue debris • Secretes enzymes, complement proteins, and interleukins • Stimulates lymphocytes and other immune responders

(Adapted with permission from Liverman C, Altevogt B, Joy J, Johnson R, eds: *Spinal Cord Injury: Progress, Promise and Priorities*. Washington, DC, The National Academies Press, 2005.)

FIGURE 6

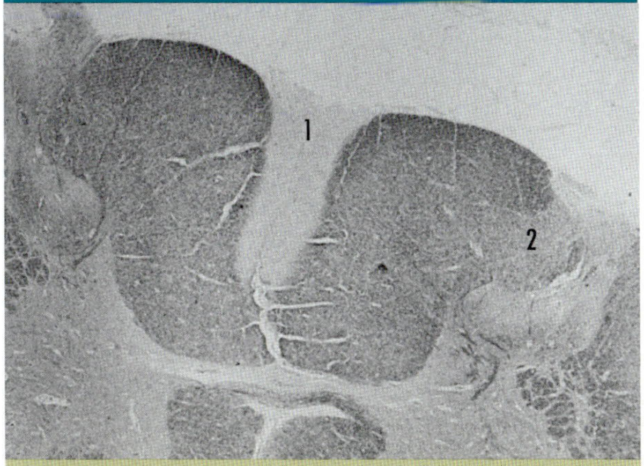

Figure 6 A high-powered view of the spinal cord cephalad to the original injury. This cervical section reveals a sharply demarcated area of demyelination evidenced by decreased staining in the major ascending tract, the fasciculus gracilis (**1**), with relative sparing of the adjacent tracts. Focal, less complete demyelination is also noted in the fasciculus cuneatus (**2**). (Reproduced from Vaccaro AR, Ahmad SS, Rauschning W, Garfin SR: Anatomy and pathophysiology of spinal cord injury, in Levine AM, Eismont FJ, Garfin SR, Zigler JE, eds: *Spine Trauma.* Philadelphia, PA, WB Saunders, 1998, pp 75-86.)

FIGURE 7

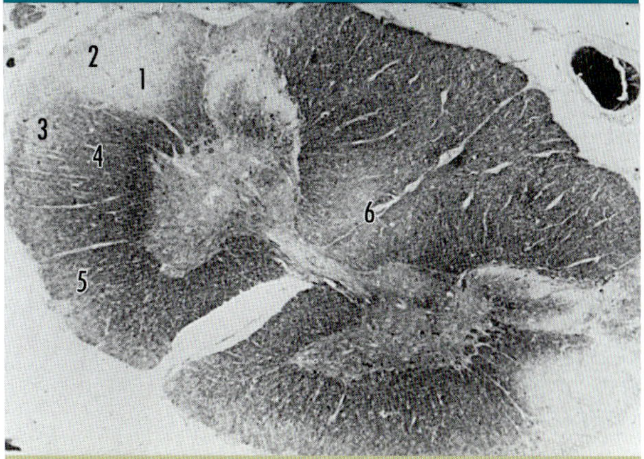

Figure 7 A histologic section obtained from the spinal cord caudal to the site of injury. This thoracic section demonstrates demyelination of both ascending and descending tracts. More specifically, nearly complete obliteration of the corticospinal (**1**) and posterior spinocerebellar (**2**) tracts is evidenced as sharply circumscribed areas of nonstaining, with less but significant involvement of the anterior spinocerebellar tract (**3**). Patchy demyelination of the lateral (**4**) and anterior (**5**) spinothalamic tracts is also evident. Note the presence of retrograde demyelination apparent in the most ventral portion of the fasciculus gracilis (**6**). (Reproduced from Vaccaro AR, Ahmad SS, Rauschning W, Garfin SR: Anatomy and pathophysiology of spinal cord injury, in Levine AM, Eismont FJ, Garfin SR, Zigler JE, eds: *Spine Trauma.* Philadelphia, PA, WB Saunders, 1998, pp 75-86.)

other excitatory amino acids[43] as a result of cell lysis and synaptic and nonsynaptic transport. Additionally, glutamate receptor-activated and mediated pathways initiate an excitotoxic cascade with lipid peroxidation and free-radical production. The influx of cells to the injury site brings other chemical mediators; neutrophils secrete myeloperoxidase, and lymphocytes secrete cytokines and growth factors.

In summary, acute SCI changes originate from a cascade of edema, hemorrhage, ischemia, inflammation, and cell injury that involves mediators such as nitric oxide, free radicals, intracellular calcium, and bioactive peptides.[54] Traditionally, the research focus has been on the necrotic death pathways following tissue damage and inflammation. Recently, the occurrence of programmed cell death also is increasingly recognized as an actively mediated cellular process following acute SCI.[4] All of this research implies that there may be a treatment window, between the time of injury and onset of pathology, for physiologic interventions. However, the best circumstances bring an SCI patient to the hospital at about 3 hours after injury. Therefore, clinically useful therapeutic interventions in the acute phase must be adapted for use with emergency medical services.[3]

Intermediate Phase

The intermediate phase starts a few days after injury, and continues for several weeks. The transverse spread of hemorrhagic necrosis and edema is complete by about 48 hours, but superior and inferior extension may continue for 6 days after injury. Apoptotic cell death continues in both orthograde and retrograde directions. Above and below the level of injury, there will also be demyelination and disintegration of injured axonal segments. A variety of tissue receptors and cellular ion channels are altered in expression levels and activation states.[3] Much of this occurs at the synaptic level with changes in excitatory, or inhibitory, signals and release of neurotransmitters and neuroendocrine substances. These neural plastic changes continue over time. About 4 weeks postinjury, signs of vascular angiopathy occur, which is the obliteration of a vessel's lumen because of intimal proliferation as an aftereffect of endothelial thrombosis and necrosis. Over time, degeneration of long fiber tracts and swelling of the axonal processes near the injury zone occurs. This is seen up to 2 years after injury.[10]

FIGURE 8

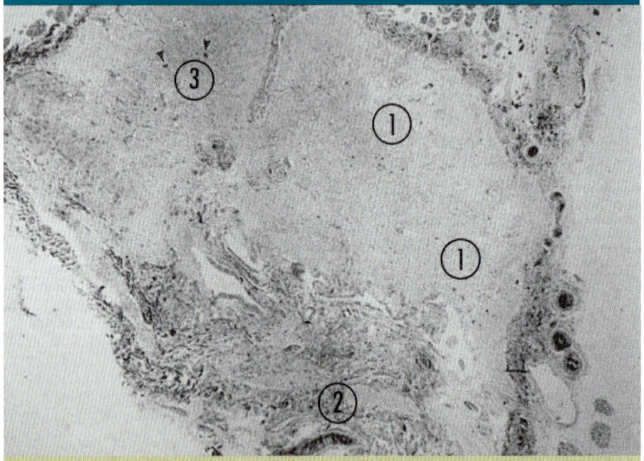

Figure 8 A histologic transverse section obtained through the level of cord injury (cervicothoracic) demonstrating an architecture distorted by compression with subsequent atrophic loss of cord matter. Demyelination and cystic degeneration are evidenced by lack of staining and the spongiform appearance of most of the section (**1**). Additionally, focal areas of reactive gliosis are revealed as darker areas, secondary to an increased number of activated astrocytes, particularly in the peripheral portions of the cord (**2**). Foci of old hemorrhage are punctate, demarcated by small clusters of macrophages laden with phagocytosed hemosiderin (**3**). (Reproduced from Vaccaro AR, Ahmad SS, Rauschning W, Garfin SR: Anatomy and pathophysiology of spinal cord injury, in Levine AM, Eismont FJ, Garfin SR, Zigler JE, eds: *Spine Trauma*. Philadelphia, PA, WB Saunders, 1998, pp 75-86.)

During the intermediate phase, there are peak levels of astrocyte and macrophage activity. They participate in the gradual decrease in soft-tissue edema with removal of necrotic debris and blood products over the weeks. By the second or third week, many astrocytes around the lesion have proliferated and hypertrophied. The astrocytes elongate and form a glial scar that walls off areas of necrotic tissue.[40] If the tissue damage is severe, the astrocyte response is not present. Instead, there is a proliferation of fibroblastic activity that forms collagenous scar in proportion to the amount of hemorrhage.[4] This collagenous scar is thought to impede axonal regeneration.

Clinically, one significant development is the evolution of spasticity. The syndrome accompanies the muscle weakness or paresis seen as a result of the initial injury. Spasticity is the increase in skeletal muscle tone and hyperreflexia seen in the weeks after a CNS injury. The muscle tone is velocity-dependent, meaning there is increased tone with increased speed through a range of motion. Other signs include clonus, clasp-knife phenomenon, positive release signs (Hoffman, Babinski), flexor reflexes, and flexor spasms. Clearly, there is hyperexcitability of the stretch reflexes. However, the pathophysiology is incompletely understood. Muscle tone changes likely arise from imbalances in the reticulospinal and other descending motor and interneuron circuitry of the spinal cord, which would otherwise provide inhibitory signals. In addition, there appear to be important intrinsic muscle changes that may involve the protein titin. A more complete discussion of spasticity may be found in other references.[64,65]

Chronic and Late Phases

In the chronic phase, further histologic changes are seen in the spinal cord tissue. The resorption of hemorrhagic regions leaves behind phagocytes laden with hemosiderin. Further macrophage activity leads to cavity formation, with cystic regions surrounded by vascularized granulation tissue. These cavities may support vascular-glial bundles and regenerated nerve roots, but they impede axon regeneration. Above and below the lesion site, there is Wallerian degeneration, seen for up to a year postinjury. Astroglial and collagenous scars are formed. The astroglial scarring is not extensive or impenetrable when growth-promoting molecules such as laminin are present, but the reactive astrocytes may also secrete molecules such as chondroitin sulfate proteglycans that inhibit regenerative activity.[4,66] The extent of scar formation involves the surrounding leptomeningeal tissues as well as the scarred fibrotic spinal cord.[10] On a macroscopic level, there is atrophy and sclerosis, with complete obliteration of the subarachnoid space. Collagenous or glial islands are seen embedded within the scarred spinal cord parenchyma, and hemosiderin deposits are seen in a thickened dura (**Figures 8** and **9**).

Late clinical effects in SCI include (1) syringomyelia and arachnoiditis, (2) tethered cord, (3) schwannosis, (4) chronic pain syndromes, and (5) degenerative disease of the spine.

Syringomyelia is a tubular cavity within the spinal cord and is seen as a late sequela of spinal cord trauma and/or meningeal scarring (arachnoiditis). Adhesive spinal arachnoiditis is a chronic inflammatory process in the pia-arachnoid space of the spinal cord. Among other causes, spinal surgery is one known factor. Arachnoiditis may occur in absence of a syrinx, but often they are observed together.

Several mechanisms have been proposed for syrinx formation. They include vascular compromise of spinal cord vessels with cord ischemia and necrosis, and meningeal scarring with CSF block.

FIGURE 9

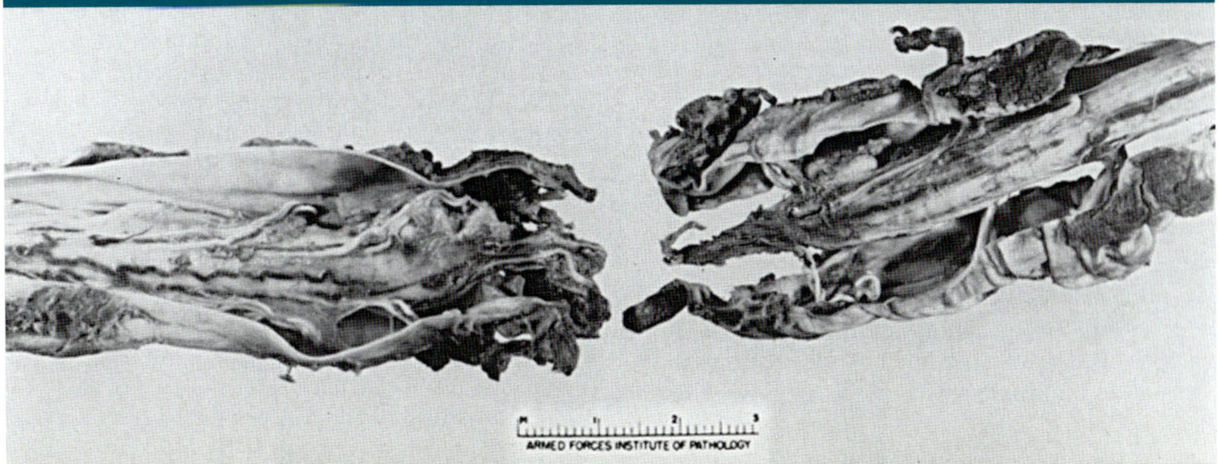

Figure 9 A pathologic specimen of a transected spinal cord with its dural sheath opened and reflected, revealing the late appearance or final phase of SCI. Normal remnants of spinal cord tissue may be seen above and below the level of cord transection. (Reproduced from Vaccaro AR, Ahmad SS, Rauschning W, Garfin SR: Anatomy and pathophysiology of spinal cord injury, in Levine AM, Eismont FJ, Garfin SR, Zigler JE, eds: *Spine Trauma*. Philadelphia, PA, WB Saunders, 1998, pp 75-86.)

Other factors include the edema and cystic formation, which occur in the acute and intermediate phases of SCI. A syrinx tends to occur in watershed regions within the cord, suggesting an ischemic infarction etiology. Syrinx enlargement results from an imbalance between CSF inflow and outflow. Such fluid flow may be influenced by respiratory or arterial pulse–induced CSF pressure waves, changes in subarachnoid space compliance, spinal stenosis, cord compression, and arachnoid adhesions.[9,67] Posttraumatic syringomyelia presents between 3 months and 35 years after injury. The risk factors for symptomatic syrinx include increased age, cervical and thoracic injury (compared with lumbar), displaced fractures, and surgery using spinal instrumentation without decompression.[68]

In 80% of the cases, the syrinx originates at the injury level and extends rostrally. About a quarter of SCI patients have a syrinx present, but only about 5% of the spinal-injured population is symptomatic.[9] The clinical progression is usually gradual, with segmental pain and dissociative sensory loss. The pain reflects injury to the spinothalamic tracts and is described as dull, aching, or burning. Valsalva maneuvers may exacerbate the pain. Later, there is a gradual loss of motor function above the level of previous injury. In the cervicothoracic level, syringomyelia with arachnoiditis is characterized by progressive myelopathic weakness. In the lumbosacral region, the main symptom is radicular pain due to cauda equina involvement.[69] The MRI findings in syringomyelia cases due to adhesive spinal arachnoiditis have been shown to include cord deformity at the site of arachnoiditis, a blurred syrinx wall, a flow void within the syrinx cavity, and a lack of abnormal contrast enhancement.[70] The cornerstone of treatment is interventional in nature, but overall the problem remains difficult to treat.[9]

Noncystic, posttraumatic, spinal cord tethering with subarachnoid adhesions has been described as another cause of late neurologic deterioration in SCI patients.[3,71-74] Tethering of the spinal cord by scar to surrounding dura, in the area near an injury site, has been suggested to occur in all SCIs. It causes pathologic symptoms when there is abnormal traction on the spinal cord and nerve roots, and obstruction to normal CSF pulsatile flow.[73]

Other late spinal cord effects include a process called schwannosis, a proliferation of Schwann cells and axons that replace portions of the damaged spinal cord. The Schwann cells enter the cord from the spinal nerve roots and seem to be involved in remyelination and production of the extracellular matrix protein laminin. Laminin is known to promote neurite sprouting.[66] Sprouting of dorsal root ganglia central processes is seen extending into spinal cord tissue. Cut and nearby uncut axons demonstrate sprouting responses,[3] but travel no farther than 1 mm. This distance may be sufficient, as there is some clinical improvement in many SCI patients during the first year after injury. For example, about one-half of incomplete SCI patients (ASIA classes B, C, and

D) ultimately are able to ambulate.[5] This figure improves to 87% if ASIA B patients are not considered.

Chronic pain syndromes are seen in a majority (ie, 70%) of SCI patients,[75] and they involve both nociceptive and neuropathic pain types. Nociceptive pain after an SCI most commonly involves the musculoskeletal system. Examples include chronic use injuries to the shoulders, elbow, and hand. Back pain has been identified in about 60% of chronic SCI patients, and may be caused by muscle weakness and prolonged sitting. Age-related changes of the spine continue to affect SCI patients at an increased prevalence compared with the able-bodied population. Disk degeneration, osteoporosis, atherosclerotic changes of spinal blood vessels, facet joint arthropathy, so-called "adjacent-level disease," and ligamentum flavum hypertrophy may all lead to worsening spinal stenosis, possibly with further deterioration of neurologic status.[4,76,77] Visceral pain from urinary tract infections, bowel impaction, and renal calculi can be another source of nociceptive pain.

Neuropathic pain is present in about 40% of chronic SCI patients. It is often refractory to standard treatment.[78] The pain is thought to arise from permanent hyperexcitability in the neural cells and circuits of the pain pathways.[3,79,80] Sodium channels are thought to play an important role in such neuropathic and central pain syndromes after SCI.[81] Additionally, damage to nerve root segments may induce sprouting and lead to activity in primary afferent fibers.

Neuropathic pain usually evolves about 12 to 18 months after an SCI. Pain below the neurologic level of injury is usually bilateral. It is characterized as burning, aching, and throbbing, and may be provoked by normal tactile stimuli (allodynia). Pain at the level of the neurologic injury may be unilateral or bilateral, with characteristics of both allodynia and hyperalgesia (increased response to normally painful stimuli). Pain at the injury level is not generally associated with activity or position.

Regeneration in SCI

For about 50 years, it has been known that CNS neurons possess some capacity to regenerate.[3] Over 30 years ago, it was shown that adult mammalian CNS neurons could regenerate across long distances if a favorable environment of peripheral nerves was provided.[82,83] These landmark studies demonstrated that physical substances in the CNS environment specifically inhibited, or promoted, the regenerative process. Later, a specific inhibitory matrix protein in the white matter, NOGO-A, was identified.[84,85] However, SCI models using a knockout mouse (without the presence of NOGO-A) show only promising, but not dramatic, examples of axonal regrowth. Contradictory results have also been observed.[86] In addition to NOGO-A, there seem to be other inhibitory components that prohibit regeneration, including the physical presence of scar tissue, through which a tissue bridge or scaffold may be required to guide regenerating axons. Stimulatory neurotrophic factors are involved as well. These factors seem to involve extracellular matrix molecules, but many seem to work intracellularly. To this end, there is intense interest in the study of intracellular molecular switches to promote cell survival. Specifically, the apoptotic pathways involving the caspase proteases and the Bcl-2 protein family seem particularly intriguing.[87] Separately, neuromuscular electrical activity, in itself, has been shown to enhance neuronal survival in vitro, possibly by membrane depolarization and cyclic adenosine monophosphate elevation. This research may provide the biologic basis for so-called neurorehabilitative protocols that encourage gait training after SCI.[88]

Neuroprotection

The acute support of neuron survival, or "neuroprotection," is an obvious research focus in the field of SCI. These efforts involve the pharmacologic control of edema and the inflammatory response, as well as molecular biologic studies of apoptosis and neural tissue rescue.

The only approved pharmacologic intervention in acute SCI is methylprednisolone (MP). The cellular mechanism of action is not entirely clear. The anti-inflammatory effects seem to arise from free-radical scavenging, and the inhibition of various processes such as lipid membrane peroxidation, calcium influx, ischemia, wallerian degeneration, and apoptosis.[3,4,89] The National Acute Spinal Cord Injury Studies (NASCIS I, II, and III) were clinical trials, with results supporting the use of MP in reducing the extent of a patient's disabilities and providing a chance of better recovery.[90,91] The recommendations are for acute, nonpenetrating, closed SCIs only. The dosing involves an intravenous bolus (30 mg/kg) given over 15 minutes with a 45-minute gap, followed by a 5.4 mg/kg drip given over 23 hours. If the MP is given within the first 3 hours after injury, no further treatment is necessary. For patients presenting between 3 and 8 hours after the initial injury, another 24 hours of the 5.4 mg/kg drip is advised.

The results of these trials have been challenged by some for several reasons.[92,93] There are concerns about deficiencies in the statistical analysis, poorly defined clinical end points, and only relatively modest attributable gains within the context of increased risk of sepsis, pneumonia, wound infection, and pulmonary embolus. However, acute treatment of closed, nonpenetrating SCI with MP is commonly used.

Besides glucocorticoids, there are several other neuroprotective pharmacologic interventions worth mentioning. These agents remain largely experimental, and have no formal guidelines or indications for use. The ganglioside, monosialotetrahexosylganglioside GM1 sodium salt, has shown benefits in experimental models of injury. The salt is thought to be involved in several CNS cellular processes. However, in a large multicenter trial, acute SCI patients given GM1 did not show improved outcome compared to MP.[53,94] Opiate antagonists, such as thyrotropin-releasing hormone (TRH) and naloxone, block the release of spinal cord opioids. Such opioids are thought to contribute to injury-induced systemic hypotension and decreased cord perfusion. However, there was no clinical benefit seen using naloxone in the National Acute Spinal Cord Injury Study.[90] The potassium channel blocker, 4-aminopyridine, can be given orally or intrathecally, and has been shown to improve pulmonary muscle strength and function in humans.[95] It seems to be active primarily at synapses and at the neuromuscular junction. The sodium channel blocker, phenytoin, has been shown in rat models of SCI to minimize the cord tissue destruction seen histologically, preserve axonal conduction through injury sites, and improve overall functional motor recovery.[96] The physiologic basis appears to be an alteration of intracellular sodium levels, which is an important early event in the SCI cascade leading to cytotoxic edema and cell death. Lastly, glutamate receptor antagonists, nitric oxide inhibitors, erythropoietin, minocycline, and anti-inflammatory agents such as the selective cyclo-oxygenase (COX)-2 inhibitors are other pharmacologic agents researched to control the SCI response.[3,86]

To increase neuronal survival, there are several molecular biologic attempts to inhibit programmed cell death (ie, apoptosis). This secondary injury cascade appears to be important in SCI. Apoptotic cell death in vertebrates occurs mostly through intrinsic mitochondrial pathways. During this process, the execution phase of apoptosis seems mediated largely by the caspase proteases. The apoptotic process has been stopped in motor neuron cell cultures derived from chick embryos by using specific peptide inhibitors of caspase-1 and caspase-3, known as YVAD and DEVD-CHO, respectively.[97] Additionally, before caspase activation, the family of intracellular peptides related to the proto-oncogene, Bcl-2, also helps regulate the apoptotic pathways. Bcl-2 is localized to mitochondria, endoplasmic reticulum, and nuclear membranes. Certain proteins of the Bcl-2 family, like Bcl-2 itself or Bcl-Xl, are antiapoptotic and have a strong cytoprotective effect. They inhibit the release of cytochrome C (which participates in caspase activation) and mitochondrial calcium, suppress lipid peroxidation, and also may inhibit oxidant and hypoxia-induced necrosis.[4,98-101] Caspase activation can also be triggered by the direct activation of transmembrane death receptors on cell surfaces. For instance, the Fas ligand from killer lymphocytes will bind to the death receptor Fas (also known as CD95/APO-1) on a target cell surface, with caspase-mediated apoptosis being the result. Such pathways have been observed in motor neuron cell death after nerve transaction and ischemia.[102] Furthermore, the neutralization of the Fas ligand by several methods seems to promote neuronal survival, axonal regeneration, and functional recovery in rodent models of SCI.[103,104] Lastly, the calcium-activated calpains represent another family of proteases that play a role in cellular necrosis and apoptosis. In SCI, calpain activity modulates the degradation of cytoskeletal and membrane proteins of damaged cells. It appears to activate proapoptotic Bax levels, which make the mitochondrial membranes more permeable to cytochrome C. Neuroprotective effects have been seen with the administration of the calpain inhibitor, E-64-d, in a rat model of SCI.[105]

Efforts to inhibit caspase, calpain, and Fas receptors, and increase Bcl-2, are the current focus of tremendous molecular biologic efforts to protect cells, preserve axon-myelin structure, and restore neuromotor function in SCI patients. However, blocking apoptosis may not be entirely desirable; cells otherwise doomed in the initial trauma that are rescued may not be able to perform normally.[104]

Promoting Regeneration in the Injured Spinal Cord

The creation of a favorable environment for spinal cord nerve fiber tract regeneration is another research focus. In neural development, there are a variety of neurite-promoting and guidance molecules present within the extracellular matrix. In the adult, these molecules are downregulated. Furthermore, the adult CNS produces specific inhibitory factors that block neurite outgrowth.[106,107] These mechanisms may provide stability of the neural circuitry. Despite this regulation, injured CNS nerve fibers in the adult do respond with short-lived regenerative attempts with sprouting, but this is ultimately abortive.[108]

Many molecules inhibitory to axonal growth have been identified. The NOGO-A protein was already discussed. Additionally, there are other matrix molecules such as the netrins, semaphorins, ephrins, tenascins, and integrins.[3] Inhibitory chondroitin sulfate proteoglycans (eg, phosphacan, brevican, neurocan, and NG2) are upregulated in responsive astrocytes and endothelial cells in the intermediate phase after SCI.[109-111] These proteoglycans act mainly to reduce axonal growth after injury. Their inhibition seems to promote regeneration. For instance, rats treated with intrathecal chondroitinase ABC, which degrades these proteoglycans, show improved functional recovery after an SCI.[112] Axonal growth may also be stimulated by certain neurotrophic factors, which are small proteins secreted by cells that enhance nerve fiber growth during embryonic development.[108] More than 30 neurotrophic factors are known, but only a few seem promising as treatments of injured spinal cords. These include neurotrophic factor-3 (NT-3) and brain-derived neurotrophic factor (BDNF). These have been delivered to a lesion site by injections or pump systems. Genetically altered cell transplants have also been considered for neurotrophic delivery systems.[4] The main limitation is that the neurotrophic factors are exquisitely specific for certain embryonic nerve cell populations, but these specificities are simply not known in the adult CNS at this time.[108] Also, there are challenging pharmacokinetic considerations when considering the timing, dosing, and delivery of such specific factors. Ultimately, it appears that axonal growth across a region of SCI depends upon a highly localized balance of cues, both inhibitory and stimulatory, which determine the fate of the regenerative process.[109] Such complexities require additional study in animal models.

The dense glial scar tissue at an injury site is filled with disorganized matrix, growth-inhibiting factors, and physical gaps that may respond to several strategies for nerve fiber growth.[110,111,113] Many types of cells, tissues, and artificial materials have been used to bridge spinal cord scars and cysts.[114] Some of these cell replacement strategies have looked into embryonic stem cells, fetal CNS tissue, activated macrophages, and genetically altered fibroblasts.[3,113] The success of these approaches has been muted, in general, because the bridges are walled off as "foreign objects" by the astrocytes, and functional regrowth of nerve fibers into the spinal cord is inhibited. However, implants of glial cells have shown unique and promising characteristics. Glial cells are the only CNS neuronal cells that spontaneously regenerate axons after being sectioned. They also produce several trophic factors, including BDNF, and cell adhesion molecules.[4] Purified populations can be prepped in suitable numbers for use in graft constructs.[113] In an SCI rat model, olfactory nerve glial cells seem to align themselves within spinal cord lesion sites, migrate long distances, and guide regenerating axons through the lesion. In addition, some functional motor recovery has been observed.[115] The use of peripheral nerve glial cells, which produce myelin sheaths (aka Schwann cells), and peripheral nerve grafts have also been studied.[83,113,116] In rats, these implants are invaded by regenerating axons and may bridge even anatomically complete lesions.[4,117] However, human applications of glial cell technology may be limited. These glial cells are intrinsically foreign to the spinal cord, and there are theoretical immunologic concerns about glial cell–mediated damage to native spinal cord tissue.[108]

Apart from the research on specific cells to transplant, there is also attention on the delivery or carrier mechanisms, with mechanically engineered scaffolds. A nonbiodegradable hydrogel, poly (2-hydroxyethyl methacrylate), or PHEMA, has a water content and compressive modulus similar to spinal cord tissue. In rats, it elicits a transient, modest cellular inflammatory response with minimal scar tissue formation, and considerable angiogenesis with axonal penetration into the gel.[118] Biodegradable synthetic polymer (various poly alphahydroxyl, lactic, and glycolic acids), natural polymer (eg, collagen, alginate, polyhydroxyalkanoate, and chitins), and carbon filament implants have also been researched. Such implants can be seeded with permissive cell types or therapeutic agents during rather complex fabrication processes.[113,119]

Enhancing Plasticity: Recovery of Function Through Physical Therapy

It is possible to grow axons in the spinal cord, and they appear to make functionally meaningful connections. Is there a way to encourage and promote such functional growth? It is well known that many people with incomplete SCIs continue to show significant functional recovery in the years after the injury. Much of this recovery does not appear to be related to significant spinal cord regeneration, as might be seen histologically. Instead, it is becoming apparent that neural function is promoted when associated with physical therapy regimens that "retrain" the neural circuitry.[120] This recovery process seems to depend on the central pattern generators, and the reorganization of neural circuits in a process of synaptic plasticity. Plasticity is commonly seen in noninjury situations, such as the acquisition and perfection of new motor skills. It is seen dramatically in the fetus and newborn infant. This redistributive process is much less prominent in the adult CNS, but significant reorganization does occur after SCI, head injury, and other CNS pathologies.[110] The process is thought to involve both an activation of neuronal connections, which are usually kept inhibited, and a regrowth of fibers which affect the afferent input paths, interneuronal pathways, and the efferent motor neurons. Additionally, there seem to be intrinsic changes in the properties of both the synapses and the neurons themselves. There is anatomic[121] and functional[122] evidence that such plasticity is potentiated by the flow of electrical impulses, and the active practice of specific skills.[110] Such is the basis for research in the field of functional electrical stimulation and the development of neural prosthetic devices to facilitate mobility or self-care activities such as micturition.[26,121] Treadmill training with a partial weight-bearing apparatus has been used with incomplete SCI patients.[123] The protocols have combined functional electrical stimulation and/or medications, resulting in improved coordination, speed, endurance, and reliance on assistive devices. It remains to be determined what the exact molecular mechanisms are that relate functionally meaningful nerve regeneration with activity and, ultimately, what is the optimal training regimen for treating SCI patients.

Summary

There are many intriguing approaches to spinal cord regeneration and repair. These include pharmacologic interventions, tissue-environment manipulation, growth-inhibitory molecules, neurotrophic factors, intracellular signaling pathways, and the use of so-called permissive substrates of cells, grafts, and bridges.[124] Physical rehabilitation approaches are also important.[1] However, the leap into human applications remains large. For example, molecular biology and gene therapy techniques to manipulate cell behavior have some genotoxic concerns in general. There is the possibility of collateral damage from unrestricted intracellular enzymatic activity, and the potential for dangerous mutations from the semirandom insertion of transgenes into heterogenous cell populations. Indeed, the clonal dominance of otherwise benign stem cells and malignant transformation resulting in overt leukemia are adverse events that have been reported in some experimental models.[125] Clearly, we need to know more about these complex cellular mechanisms before the efficacy and safety of so-called "tissue engineering" interventions in the spinal cord can be determined clinically. This restraint is especially difficult when many of our patients are desperate to participate in any human experiment that holds the promise for increased mobility. Overall, the basic and clinical research so far has been exciting, giving hope that one day we will be able to mitigate, and even reverse, the devastating consequences of SCIs.

References

1. Lin V, ed: *Spinal Cord Medicine*, ed 2. New York, NY, Demos Medical Publishing, 2010.
2. DeVivo M, Stover S: Long-term survival and causes of death, in Stover S, DeLisa J, Whiteneck G, eds: *Spinal Cord Injury Clinical Outcomes from the Model Systems*. Gaithersburg, MD, Aspen Publishers, 1995, p 355.
3. Hulsebosch CE: Recent advances in pathophysiology and treatment of spinal cord injury. *Adv Physiol Educ* 2002;26(1-4):238-255.
4. Frisch RF, Antonacci MD: Spinal cord injury repair strategies. *Top Spinal Cord Inj Rehabil* 2005; 10(4):1-31.
5. Gittler MS, McKinley WO, Stiens SA, Groah SL, Kirshblum SC: Spinal cord injury medicine: 3. Rehabilitation outcomes. *Arch Phys Med Rehabil* 2002;83(3, Suppl 1):S65-S71.
6. Marketos SG, Skiadas P: Hippocrates: The father of spine surgery. *Spine (Phila Pa 1976)* 1999; 24(13):1381-1387.
7. Knoeller SM, Seifried C: Historical perspective: History of spinal surgery. *Spine (Phila Pa 1976)* 2000;25(21):2838-2843.
8. Wiltse LL, Pait TG: Herophilus of Alexandria (325-255 B.C.): The father of anatomy. *Spine (Phila Pa 1976)* 1998;23(17):1904-1914.
9. Brodbelt AR, Stoodley MA: Post-traumatic syringomyelia: A review. *J Clin Neurosci* 2003;10(4): 401-408.

10. Vaccaro AR, Ahmad SS, Rauschning W, Garfin SR: Anatomy and pathophysiology of spinal cord injury, in Levine AM, Eismont FJ, Garfin SR, Zigler JE, eds: *Spine Trauma*. Philadelphia, PA, WB Saunders, 1998, pp 75-86.
11. Nolte J: Spinal cord, in Nolte J, ed: *The Human Brain: An Introduction to its Functional Anatomy*, ed 5. St. Louis, MO, Mosby, 2001, pp 223-261.
12. Hogan QH: Epidural anatomy examined by cryomicrotome section: Influence of age, vertebral level, and disease. *Reg Anesth* 1996;21(5): 395-406.
13. Hogan Q: Distribution of solution in the epidural space: Examination by cryomicrotome section. *Reg Anesth Pain Med* 2002;27(2):150-156.
14. Harrison GR: Topographical anatomy of the lumbar epidural region: An in vivo study using computerized axial tomography. *Br J Anaesth* 1999; 83(2):229-234.
15. Lazorthes G, Gouaze A, Zadeh JO, Santini JJ, Lazorthes Y, Burdin P: Arterial vascularization of the spinal cord: Recent studies of the anastomotic substitution pathways. *J Neurosurg* 1971;35: 253-262.
16. Kindt GW: Autoregulation of spinal cord blood flow. *Eur Neurol* 1971-1972;6(1):19-23.
17. Rexed B: The cytoarchitectonic organization of the spinal cord in the cat. *J Comp Neurol* 1952;96(3): 415-495.
18. Snell R: *Clinical Neuroanatomy for Medical Students*, ed 5. Philadelphia, PA, Lippincott Williams & Wilkins, 2001.
19. Gilman S, Newman S: *Manter and Gatz's Essentials of Clinical Neuroanatomy and Neurophysiology*, ed 9. Philadelphia, PA, FA Davis, 1996.
20. Sarnat H: Functions of the corticospinal and corticobulbar tracts in the human newborn. *J Pediatr Neurol* 2003;1(1):3-8.
21. de Assis Aquino Gondim F, Thomas F: Spinal cord, topographical and functional anatomy. emedicine from WebMD. http://www.emedicine.com/neuro/topic657.htm. Accessed April 16, 2006.
22. Dobkin BH: Neurobiology of rehabilitation. *Ann N Y Acad Sci* 2004;1038:148-170.
23. Dietz V: Spinal cord pattern generators for locomotion. *Clin Neurophysiol* 2003;114(8): 1379-1389.
24. Rossignol S, Dubuc R, Gossard JP: Dynamic sensorimotor interactions in locomotion. *Physiol Rev* 2006;86(1):89-154.
25. Alford S, Schwartz E, Viana di Prisco G: The pharmacology of vertebrate spinal central pattern generators. *Neuroscientist* 2003;9(3):217-228.
26. Grillner S, Markram H, De Schutter E, Silberberg G, LeBeau FE: Microcircuits in action—from CPGs to neocortex. *Trends Neurosci* 2005;28(10): 525-533.
27. Schreiber D: Spinal cord injuries. emedicine from WebMD. http://www.emedicine.com/EMERG/topic553.htm. Accessed April 18, 2005.
28. Chang DG, Tencer AF, Ching RP, Treece B, Senft D, Anderson PA: Geometric changes in the cervical spinal canal during impact. *Spine (Phila Pa 1976)* 1994;19(8):973-980.
29. Nuckley DJ, Konodi MA, Raynak GC, Ching RP, Mirza SK: Neural space integrity of the lower cervical spine: Effect of normal range of motion. *Spine (Phila Pa 1976)* 2002;27(6):587-595.
30. Ito S, Panjabi MM, Ivancic PC, Pearson AM: Spinal canal narrowing during simulated whiplash. *Spine (Phila Pa 1976)* 2004;29(12):1330-1339.
31. Yuan Q, Dougherty L, Margulies SS: In vivo human cervical spinal cord deformation and displacement in flexion. *Spine (Phila Pa 1976)* 1998; 23(15):1677-1683.
32. Chen CJ, Hsu HL, Niu CC, et al: Cervical degenerative disease at flexion-extension MR imaging: Prediction criteria. *Radiology* 2003;227(1): 136-142.
33. Tencer AF, Allen BL Jr, Ferguson RL: A biomechanical study of thoracolumbar spinal fractures with bone in the canal: Part I. The effect of laminectomy. *Spine (Phila Pa 1976)* 1985;10(6): 580-585.
34. Tencer AF, Ferguson RL, Allen BL Jr: A biomechanical study of thoracolumbar spinal fractures with bone in the canal: Part II. The effect of flexion angulation, distraction, and shortening of the motion segment. *Spine (Phila Pa 1976)* 1985; 10(6):586-589.
35. Bilston LE, Thibault LE: The mechanical properties of the human cervical spinal cord in vitro. *Ann Biomed Eng* 1996;24(1):67-74.
36. Fiford RJ, Bilston LE: The mechanical properties of rat spinal cord in vitro. *J Biomech* 2005;38(7): 1509-1515.
37. Ozawa H, Matsumoto T, Ohashi T, Sato M, Kokubun S: Comparison of spinal cord gray matter and white matter softness: Measurement by pipette aspiration method. *J Neurosurg* 2001;95 (2, Suppl):221-224.
38. Chang GL, Hung TK, Feng WW: An in-vivo measurement and analysis of viscoelastic properties of the spinal cord of cats. *J Biomech Eng* 1988; 110(2):115-122.
39. Bailey FW: Histological changes in the spinal cord of man in cases of fatal injury: II. Alterations in the neurocytons. *Bull Los Angel Neuro Soc* 1959; 24:204-213.
40. Bailey FW: Histological changes in the spinal cord of man in cases of fatal injury: IV. Alteration in

the classical neuroglia. *Bull Los Angel Neuro Soc* 1961;26.32-40.

41. Dohrmann GJ, Wagner FC Jr, Bucy PC: Transitory traumatic paraplegia: Electron microscopy of early alterations in myelinated nerve fibers. *J Neurosurg* 1972;36(4):407-415.
42. Yashon D, Bingham WG Jr, Faddoul EM, Hunt WE: Edema of the spinal cord following experimental impact trauma. *J Neurosurg* 1973;38(6): 693-697.
43. Hedeman LS, Shellenberger MK, Gordon JH: Studies in experimental spinal cord trauma: 1. Alterations in catecholamine levels. *J Neurosurg* 1974;40(1):37-43.
44. Griffiths IR, Trench JG, Crawford RA: Spinal cord blood flow and conduction during experimental cord compression in normotensive and hypotensive dogs. *J Neurosurg* 1979;50(3):353-360.
45. Kobrine AI, Evans DE, Rizzoli HV: Experimental acute balloon compression of the spinal cord: Factors affecting disappearance and return of the spinal evoked response. *J Neurosurg* 1979;51(6): 841-845.
46. Eidelberg E, Staten E, Watkins JC, McGraw D, McFadden C: A model of spinal cord injury. *Surg Neurol* 1976;6(1):35-38.
47. Akizuki T, Harii K: A histopathologic study of spinal cord ischemia using an isohistogenic rat upper-half-body transplantation model. *Spine (Phila Pa 1976)* 1990;15(11):1104-1109.
48. Fried LC, Aparicio O: Experimental ischemia of the spinal cord: Histologic studies after anterior spinal artery occlusion. *Neurology* 1973;23(3): 289-293.
49. Taylor KJ: Ultrasonic damage to spinal cord and the synergistic effect of hypoxia. *J Pathol* 1970; 102(1):41-47.
50. Dolan EJ, Transfeldt EE, Tator CH, Simmons EH, Hughes KF: The effect of spinal distraction on regional spinal cord blood flow in cats. *J Neurosurg* 1980;53(6):756-764.
51. Cusick JF, Myklebust J, Zyvoloski M, Sances A Jr, Houterman C, Larson SJ: Effects of vertebral column distraction in the monkey. *J Neurosurg* 1982; 57(5):651-659.
52. Bingham WG Jr, Goldman H, Friedman SJ, Murphy S, Yashon D, Hunt WE: Blood flow in normal and injured monkey spinal cord. *J Neurosurg* 1975;43(2):162-171.
53. Geisler FH: GM-1 ganglioside and motor recovery following human spinal cord injury. *J Emerg Med* 1993;11(Suppl 1):49-55.
54. Sharma HS: Pathophysiology of blood-spinal cord barrier in traumatic injury and repair. *Curr Pharm Des* 2005;11(11):1353-1389.
55. Goodman JH, Bingham WG Jr, Hunt WE: Edema formation and central hemorrhagic necrosis following impact injury to primate spinal cord. *Surg Forum* 1974;25(0):440-442.
56. Green BA, Wagner FC Jr: Evolution of edema in the acutely injured spinal cord: A fluorescence microscopic study. *Surg Neurol* 1973;1(2):98-101.
57. Osterholm JL, Mathews GJ: Altered norepinephrine metabolism following experimental spinal cord injury: 1. Relationship to hemorrhagic necrosis and post-wounding neurological deficits. *J Neurosurg* 1972;36(4):386-394.
58. Wagner F Jr, Dohrmann G, Bucy P: Histopathology of transitory traumatic paraplegia in the monkey. *J Neurosurg* 1971;35(3):272-276.
59. Ducker TB, Kindt GW, Kempf LG: Pathological findings in acute experimental spinal cord trauma. *J Neurosurg* 1971;35(6):700-708.
60. Dohrmann GJ, Wick KM, Bucy PC: Spinal cord blood flow patterns in experimental traumatic paraplegia. *J Neurosurg* 1973;38(1):52-58.
61. Kobrine AI, Doyle TF, Martins AN: Local spinal cord blood flow in experimental traumatic myelopathy. *J Neurosurg* 1975;42(2):144-149.
62. Griffiths IR: Spinal cord blood flow after acute experimental cord injury in dogs. *J Neurol Sci* 1976;27(2):247-259.
63. Larson SJ, Walsh PR, Sances A Jr, Cusick JF, Hemmy DC, Mahler H: Evoked potentials in experimental myelopathy. *Spine (Phila Pa 1976)* 1980;5(4):299-302.
64. Adams MM, Hicks AL: Spasticity after spinal cord injury. *Spinal Cord* 2005;43(10):577-586.
65. Foran JR, Steinman S, Barash I, Chambers HG, Lieber RL: Structural and mechanical alterations in spastic skeletal muscle. *Dev Med Child Neurol* 2005;47(10):713-717.
66. Hagg T, Oudega M: Degenerative and spontaneous regenerative processes after spinal cord injury. *J Neurotrauma* 2006;23(3-4):264-280.
67. Levy LM: MR imaging of cerebrospinal fluid flow and spinal cord motion in neurologic disorders of the spine. *Magn Reson Imaging Clin N Am* 1999; 7(3):573-587.
68. Vannemreddy SS, Rowed DW, Bharatwal N: Posttraumatic syringomyelia: Predisposing factors. *Br J Neurosurg* 2002;16(3):276-283.
69. Koyanagi I, Iwasaki Y, Hida K, Houkin K: Clinical features and pathomechanisms of syringomyelia associated with spinal arachnoiditis. *Surg Neurol* 2005;63(4):350-356.
70. Inoue Y, Nemoto Y, Ohata K, et al: Syringomyelia associated with adhesive spinal arachnoiditis: MRI. *Neuroradiology* 2001;43(4):325-330.
71. Ragnarsson TS, Durward QJ, Nordgren RE: Spinal cord tethering after traumatic paraplegia with late

neurological deterioration. *J Neurosurg* 1986; 64(3):397-401.

72. Osborne DR, Vavoulis G, Nashold BS Jr, Dubois PJ, Drayer BP, Heinz ER: Late sequelae of spinal cord trauma: Myelographic and surgical correlation. *J Neurosurg* 1982;57(1):18-23.
73. Falci SP, Lammertse DP, Best L, et al: Surgical treatment of posttraumatic cystic and tethered spinal cords. *J Spinal Cord Med* 1999;22(3): 173-181.
74. Lee TT, Alameda GJ, Gromelski EB, Green BA: Outcome after surgical treatment of progressive posttraumatic cystic myelopathy. *J Neurosurg* 2000;92(2 Suppl):149-154.
75. Cardenas DD, Felix ER: Pain after spinal cord injury: A review of classification, treatment approaches, and treatment assessment. *PM R* 2009; 1(12):1077-1090.
76. Groah SL, Stiens SA, Gittler MS, Kirshblum SC, McKinley WO: Spinal cord injury medicine: 5. Preserving wellness and independence of the aging patient with spinal cord injury: A primary care approach for the rehabilitation medicine specialist. *Arch Phys Med Rehabil* 2002;83 (3, Suppl 1):S82-S89.
77. Maynard F, Karunas R, Adkins R, Richards J, Waring W III: Management of the neuromusculoskeletal systems, in Stover S, DeLisa J, Whiteneck G, eds: *Spinal Cord Injury Clinical Outcomes from the Model Systems*. Gaithersburg, MD, Aspen Publishers, 1995.
78. Siddall P, Wrigley P: Pain following spinal cord injury, in Fishman S, Ballantyne J, Rathmell J, eds: *Bonica's Management of Pain*, ed 4. Philadelphia, PA, Wolters Kluwer/Lippincott Williams & Wilkins, 2010, p 1661.
79. Christensen MD, Hulsebosch CE: Chronic central pain after spinal cord injury. *J Neurotrauma* 1997; 14(8):517-537.
80. McKinley WO, Gittler MS, Kirshblum SC, Stiens SA, Groah SL: Spinal cord injury medicine: 2. Medical complications after spinal cord injury: Identification and management. *Arch Phys Med Rehabil* 2002;83(3, Suppl 1):S58-S64.
81. Waxman SG, Hains BC: Fire and phantoms after spinal cord injury: Na+ channels and central pain. *Trends Neurosci* 2006;29(4):207-215.
82. David S, Aguayo AJ: Axonal elongation into peripheral nervous system "bridges" after central nervous system injury in adult rats. *Science* 1981; 214(4523):931-933.
83. Richardson PM, McGuinness UM, Aguayo AJ: Axons from CNS neurons regenerate into PNS grafts. *Nature* 1980;284(5753):264-265.
84. Caroni P, Schwab ME: Antibody against myelin-associated inhibitor of neurite growth neutralizes nonpermissive substrate properties of CNS white matter. *Neuron* 1988;1(1):85-96.
85. Chen MS, Huber AB, van der Haar ME, et al: Nogo-A is a myelin-associated neurite outgrowth inhibitor and an antigen for monoclonal antibody IN-1. *Nature* 2000;403(6768):434-439.
86. Kwon BK, Fisher CG, Dvorak MF, Tetzlaff W: Strategies to promote neural repair and regeneration after spinal cord injury. *Spine (Phila Pa 1976)* 2005;30(17 Suppl):S3-S13.
87. Goldberg JL, Barres BA: The relationship between neuronal survival and regeneration. *Annu Rev Neurosci* 2000;23:579-612.
88. Pinter MM, Dimitrijevic MR: Gait after spinal cord injury and the central pattern generator for locomotion. *Spinal Cord* 1999;37(8):531-537.
89. Vaquero J, Zurita M, Oya S, Aguayo C, Bonilla C: Early administration of methylprednisolone decreases apoptotic cell death after spinal cord injury. *Histol Histopathol* 2006;21(10):1091-1102.
90. Bracken MB, Shepard MJ, Collins WF, et al: A randomized, controlled trial of methylprednisolone or naloxone in the treatment of acute spinal-cord injury: Results of the Second National Acute Spinal Cord Injury Study. *N Engl J Med* 1990; 322(20):1405-1411.
91. Bracken MB, Shepard MJ, Holford TR, et al: Administration of methylprednisolone for 24 or 48 hours or tirilazad mesylate for 48 hours in the treatment of acute spinal cord injury: Results of the Third National Acute Spinal Cord Injury Randomized Controlled Trial. National Acute Spinal Cord Injury Study. *JAMA* 1997;277(20): 1597-1604.
92. Hurlbert RJ: Methylprednisolone for acute spinal cord injury: An inappropriate standard of care. *J Neurosurg* 2000;93(1, Suppl):1-7.
93. Nesathurai S: Steroids and spinal cord injury: Revisiting the NASCIS 2 and NASCIS 3 trials. *J Trauma* 1998;45(6):1088-1093.
94. Geisler FH, Coleman WP, Grieco G, Poonian D, Sygen Study Group: The Sygen multicenter acute spinal cord injury study. *Spine (Phila Pa 1976)* 2001;26(24, Suppl)S87-S98.
95. Segal JL, Pathak MS, Hernandez JP, Himber PL, Brunnemann SR, Charter RS: Safety and efficacy of 4-aminopyridine in humans with spinal cord injury: A long-term, controlled trial. *Pharmacotherapy* 1999;19(6):713-723.
96. Hains BC, Saab CY, Lo AC, Waxman SG: Sodium channel blockade with phenytoin protects spinal cord axons, enhances axonal conduction, and improves functional motor recovery after contusion SCI. *Exp Neurol* 2004;188(2):365-377.
97. Li L, Prevette D, Oppenheim RW, Milligan CE: Involvement of specific caspases in motoneuron

cell death in vivo and in vitro following trophic factor deprivation. *Mol Cell Neurosci* 1998;12(3): 157-167.

98. Seki T, Hida K, Tada M, Koyanagi I, Iwasaki Y: Role of the bcl-2 gene after contusive spinal cord injury in mice. *Neurosurgery* 2003;53(1):192-198.
99. Wingrave JM, Schaecher KE, Sribnick EA, et al: Early induction of secondary injury factors causing activation of calpain and mitochondria-mediated neuronal apoptosis following spinal cord injury in rats. *J Neurosci Res* 2003;73(1): 95-104.
100. Green DR, Kroemer G: Pharmacological manipulation of cell death: Clinical applications in sight? *J Clin Invest* 2005;115(10):2610-2617.
101. Green DR, Reed JC: Mitochondria and apoptosis. *Science* 1998;281(5381):1309-1312.
102. Ugolini G, Raoul C, Ferri A, et al: Fas/tumor necrosis factor receptor death signaling is required for axotomy-induced death of motoneurons in vivo. *J Neurosci* 2003;23(24):8526-8531.
103. Ackery A, Robins S, Fehlings MG: Inhibition of Fas-mediated apoptosis through administration of soluble Fas receptor improves functional outcome and reduces posttraumatic axonal degeneration after acute spinal cord injury. *J Neurotrauma* 2006; 23(5):604-616.
104. Demjen D, Klussmann S, Kleber S, et al: Neutralization of CD95 ligand promotes regeneration and functional recovery after spinal cord injury. *Nat Med* 2004;10(4):389-395.
105. Ray SK, Hogan EL, Banik NL: Calpain in the pathophysiology of spinal cord injury: Neuroprotection with calpain inhibitors. *Brain Res Brain Res Rev* 2003;42(2):169-185.
106. Filbin MT: Myelin-associated inhibitors of axonal regeneration in the adult mammalian CNS. *Nat Rev Neurosci* 2003;4(9):703-713.
107. Schwab ME: Nogo and axon regeneration. *Curr Opin Neurobiol* 2004;14(1):118-124.
108. Schwab ME: Repairing the injured spinal cord. *Science* 2002;295(5557):1029-1031.
109. Jones LL, Sajed D, Tuszynski MH: Axonal regeneration through regions of chondroitin sulfate proteoglycan deposition after spinal cord injury: A balance of permissiveness and inhibition. *J Neurosci* 2003;23(28):9276-9288.
110. Verma P, Fawcett J: Spinal cord regeneration. *Adv Biochem Eng Biotechnol* 2005;94:43-66.
111. Silver J, Miller JH: Regeneration beyond the glial scar. *Nat Rev Neurosci* 2004;5(2):146-156.
112. Bradbury EJ, Moon LD, Popat RJ, et al: Chondroitinase ABC promotes functional recovery after spinal cord injury. *Nature* 2002;416(6881): 636-640.
113. Bunge MB: Bridging areas of injury in the spinal cord. *Neuroscientist* 2001;7(4):325-339.
114. Schmidt CE, Leach JB: Neural tissue engineering: strategies for repair and regeneration. *Annu Rev Biomed Eng* 2003;5:293-347.
115. Ramón-Cueto A, Cordero MI, Santos-Benito FF, Avila J: Functional recovery of paraplegic rats and motor axon regeneration in their spinal cords by olfactory ensheathing glia. *Neuron* 2000;25(2): 425-435.
116. Xu XM, Zhang SX, Li H, Aebischer P, Bunge MB: Regrowth of axons into the distal spinal cord through a Schwann-cell-seeded mini-channel implanted into hemisected adult rat spinal cord. *Eur J Neurosci* 1999;11(5):1723-1740.
117. Fouad K, Schnell L, Bunge MB, Schwab ME, Liebscher T, Pearse DD: Combining Schwann cell bridges and olfactory-ensheathing glia grafts with chondroitinase promotes locomotor recovery after complete transection of the spinal cord. *J Neurosci* 2005;25(5):1169-1178.
118. Bakshi A, Fisher O, Dagci T, Himes BT, Fischer I, Lowman A: Mechanically engineered hydrogel scaffolds for axonal growth and angiogenesis after transplantation in spinal cord injury. *J Neurosurg Spine* 2004;1(3):322-329.
119. Friedman JA, Windebank AJ, Moore MJ, Spinner RJ, Currier BL, Yaszemski MJ: Biodegradable polymer grafts for surgical repair of the injured spinal cord. *Neurosurgery* 2002;51(3):742-752.
120. Fouad K, Pearson K: Restoring walking after spinal cord injury. *Prog Neurobiol* 2004;73(2): 107-126.
121. Wolpaw JR, Tennissen AM: Activity-dependent spinal cord plasticity in health and disease. *Annu Rev Neurosci* 2001;24:807-843.
122. Borgens RB, Toombs JP, Breur G, et al: An imposed oscillating electrical field improves the recovery of function in neurologically complete paraplegic dogs. *J Neurotrauma* 1999;16(7): 639-657.
123. Carhart MR, He J, Herman R, D'Luzansky S, Willis WT: Epidural spinal-cord stimulation facilitates recovery of functional walking following incomplete spinal-cord injury. *IEEE Trans Neural Syst Rehabil Eng* 2004;12(1):32-42.
124. Horner PJ, Gage FH: Regenerating the damaged central nervous system. *Nature* 2000;407(6807): 963-970.
125. Baum C, Kustikova O, Modlich U, Li Z, Fehse B: Mutagenesis and oncogenesis by chromosomal insertion of gene transfer vectors. *Hum Gene Ther* 2006;17(3):253-263.

CHAPTER 11
Experimental Spinal Cord Injury

Ted Brindle, MD Alberto Martinez-Arizala, MD Allan Levi, MD, PhD, FRCSC, FACS
Barth A. Green, MD, FACS

Key Points

- Several spinal cord injury models have been developed in animals to investigate the histopathology and biochemical changes that occur after injury. Weight-drop devices and clip-compression techniques are the most commonly used. Although the biomechanics of these models may differ from human spinal cord injury, they are reliable methods and produce consistent injuries.
- The pathophysiology of spinal cord injury can be divided into primary and secondary components. The primary injury occurs at the time of trauma. Mediators of secondary spinal cord injury include edema, calcium, cellular inflammation, and excitatory amino acids. Experimental therapies targeting these mediators have been successful in animal models.
- High-dose steroids in the form of methylprednisolone have been routinely administered following acute spinal cord injury in humans over the last 15 years. Currently, it is recommended as a treatment option in patients with acute spinal cord injuries but should only be undertaken with the knowledge that the evidence suggesting harmful side effects is more consistent than any suggestion of clinical benefit.
- Clinical trials assessing the safety and feasibility of pharmacologic agents, modest hypothermia, and cellular transplantation strategies after human spinal cord injury are still actively being evaluated. No single treatment has become a standard of care at this time.

Introduction

Although advancements in the surgical techniques for spinal stabilization and the clinical care of the patient in specialized spinal cord injury (SCI) units have effectively reduced the morbidity and mortality associated with spinal injuries, our capability to prevent the loss, or to promote the restoration, of neural function following spinal trauma remains limited. Since the early 1970s, skillfully planned laboratory research has provided knowledge that has dramatically improved our understanding of the pathophysiology of SCI. These experimental studies have provided the groundwork for some of the clinical trials to be described in this chapter. Specifically, the National Acute Spinal Cord Injury Study[1] was the first documented multicenter prospective trial in the pharmacologic treatment of human SCI. Although initial reports of successful outcomes from this trial have been questioned, it was an important step in translational research. The Sygen multicenter randomized trial investigating the use of GM-1 ganglioside in SCI was another landmark study with good interrater reliability.[2] In addition to these large multicenter clinical trials using pharmacotherapeutic strategies for SCI, there have now been several smaller clinical trials using cellular transplantation paradigms.

Spinal Cord Injury Models

Our understanding of SCI will continue to rely on the use of experimental animal models to get a better handle on the cellular consequences of the injury cascade. Animal models of SCI attempt to mimic human SCI as closely as possible. This in itself is quite complex because human injuries are multifactorial. The following are examples of the variables involved in human SCI: (1) age, (2) sex (most human injuries occur in males), (3) level of injury, (4) open versus closed injuries, (5) completeness of injury, (6) force of impact and type of force (eg, flexion, extension, compression, distraction, rotation),[3,4] (7) rate of compression of the spinal cord tissue, (8) presence of associated bony and ligamentous damage producing vertebral column disruption and instability, (9) duration of compression, (10) occurrence of other associated injuries, and (11) presence of preexisting conditions (eg, vascular disease, hypertension, spinal stenosis). In addition, animal models of SCI

Dr. Martinez-Arizala or an immediate family member serves as a paid consultant to or is an employee of Xenoport; and owns stock or stock options in Pfizer. None of the following authors or any immediate family member has received anything of value from or owns stock in a commercial company or institution related directly or indirectly to the subject of this chapter: Dr. Brindle, Dr. Levi, and Dr. Green.

FIGURE 1

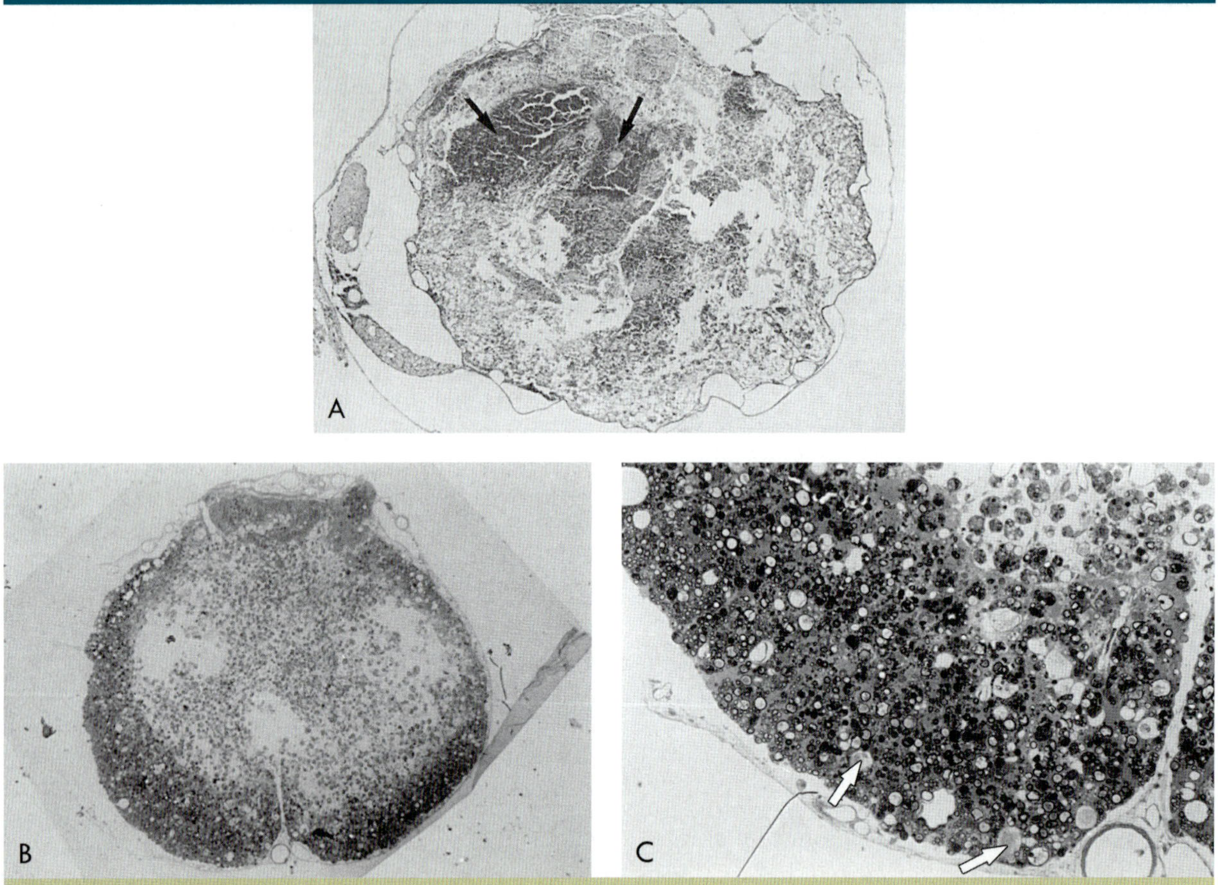

Figure 1 Morphologic changes following weight-drop contusions to the rat thoracic spinal cord (T8). **A,** Thoracic spinal cord 3 days after a moderately severe contusive lesion. The spinal cord tissue has undergone extensive necrosis at the epicenter. Edema and scattered hemorrhages are evident (arrows) (paraffin section stained with hematoxylin-eosin). **B,** Thoracic spinal cord 1 month after a moderate contusive lesion. A typical posttraumatic cystic cavity is identified in the injured segment, and its central portion contains numerous macrophages. Although there is a fair amount of tissue preservation in the ventral and lateral aspects of the spinal cord, the white matter in these areas contains numerous abnormalities (see **C**) (semithin plastic section stained with toluidine blue). **C,** High-powered view of the ventral white matter in **B.** The white matter shows microcystic changes and scattered degenerating fibers (arrows). (Reproduced from Martinez-Arizala A, Green BA: Experimental spinal cord injury, in Levine AM, Eismont FJ, Garfin SR, Zigler JE, eds: *Spine Trauma.* Philadelphia, PA, WB Saunders, 1998, pp 87-101.)

usually require certain conditions that produce deviation from the human condition (eg, using a posterior approach via laminectomy to create the injury and use of anesthesia).

The majority of human SCIs are closed. They rarely involve direct severance of cord tissue; they more commonly derive from contusive forces that do not interrupt the continuity of the cord but lead to internal tissue loss.[5] Contusive types of injuries, in which hemorrhage and tissue necrosis evolve into a fluid-filled cyst, are mimicked by several animal models. **Figure 1** shows such a lesion produced by the Allen, or weight-drop, technique.

Although early models of experimental SCI provided information about the neurologic and histopathologic changes associated with experimental spinal cord lesions, the first model that allowed quantification of the severity of SCI was introduced by A.R. Allen in 1911.[6] Allen produced SCI in dogs by dropping a known weight through a tube that was placed on the exposed thoracic cord. This model thus become known as the Allen or "weight-drop" model of SCI. In this model, the severity of the spinal injury can be graded by varying either the weight or the height of the drop, and the magnitude of the injuries are expressed as the gram-centimeters product. This method allows investigators to produce fairly reproducible graded injuries and has been modified to successfully produce contusive spinal cord lesions in various species.[7-13] The New York University (NYU) weight-drop device consists of a 10-g impactor that can be raised 6.25 mm, 12.5 mm, 25 mm, 50 mm, or 75 mm above the surface of the cord, producing a range of chronic injuries from very mild to complete paraplegia.[14] This model incorporates optical potentiometers that can measure impact parameters and tissue response to injury. Despite its wide acceptance, the weight-drop technique has some disadvantages: (1) compression of the cord occurs from the posterior aspect, which differs from the more common anterior or circumferential compression seen in human injuries; and (2) the weight-drop technique has been noted by some investigators to produce variable results.[15,16] Despite this, the weight-drop mimics some of the biomechanics of the human SCI and has been effectively used by investigators who have carefully controlled experimental variables.[13,17-21]

Besides the weight drop, a variety of other models have also been developed to produce SCI in animals. A highly sophisticated device, consisting of a feedback-controlled electromechanical impactor, has been reported to produce highly reproducible and graded lesions in the rat.[22,23] An electromagnetic injury device developed in Ohio has been modified to produce spinal cord contusions in mice.[24,25] This model creates injuries by the rapid, calibrated vertical displacement of a lucite-tipped impounder positioned to exert a fixed starting force on the surface of the exposed dura. Controlled displacement of this impounder is produced using an electromagnetic vibration generator with increased displacement amplitude corresponding to increased injury severity. More recently, a contusion device developed in Kentucky produces injury to the exposed spinal cord by rapidly applying a force-defined impact with a stainless steel-tipped impounder.[26] The major difference between this device and other models such as the NYU impactor is that force is used as the variable to measure the severity of injury as opposed to the degree of spinal cord displacement.

Balloon or cuff compression techniques were first described in detail by Tarlov et al,[27] who inserted an inflatable balloon in the spinal extradural space of dogs to produce paralysis. The technique was modified by Tator[28] in 1973 for the monkey, and by Khan et al[29] in 1985 for the rat. This technique also has disadvantages: (1) it is difficult to verify proper balloon position in some animals, and the techniques are difficult to perform in small animals; (2) the pressure on the cord itself cannot be measured; and (3) the technique does not closely mimic the biomechanics of the human injury.

Models of static-load compression, in which large weights are placed for varying periods on the exposed cord, have also been described in cats,[30] ferrets,[31] and rats.[32] Another fairly common model in which SCI is created in the rat via compression of the cord with a modified Kerr-Lougheed aneurysm clip was introduced by Rivlin and Tator.[33,34] In this model, the precise delivery of a known force and graded injuries were produced by varying either the force or the duration of the compression;[33,35] and unlike the weight-drop technique, it produced a circumferential compression of the cord. Modified aneurysm clips have also been used in creating extradural cord compression injuries in the mouse.[36] Three clips with different springs were made to produce differing magnitudes of closing force (3 g, 8 g, and 24 g). This method has the following disadvantages: (1) the cord is more extensively manipulated because the clip must be placed under its ventral aspect; (2) the biomechanics of the initial component of the injury do not mimic the human condition; (3) the histopathologic and functional correlates of this injury have not been defined as extensively as in the weight-drop method; and (4) this method has been reported to produce greater hemorrhagic changes than the weight-drop technique.[29]

These observations pertain to acute traumatic spinal injury and should not be generalized to models of other types of spinal injury, such as slow-graded cord compressions that are used to mimic tumor masses, or to models of spinal ischemia.[37] In addition, certain aspects of cord function and plasticity are often better addressed in transection or in vitro models.

Pathophysiology of Acute Experimental Spinal Cord Injury

Experimental SCI can be divided into primary and secondary components. The primary injury is clinically manifested by acute paralysis and is accompanied by shifts in electrolytes, a decrease in the membrane-bound sodium-potassium adenosine triphosphatase (Na^+-K^+ ATPase), loss of energy stores, and morphologic alterations.[38-41] Secondary injury SCI consists of a series of autodestructive

TABLE 1

Secondary Mediators of Spinal Cord Injury

Secondary Mediators of Spinal Cord Injury
Edema
Ischemia
Calcium
Free radical–lipid peroxidation
Endogenous opiates
Excitatory amino acids
Eicosanoids
Inflammatory cells

(Reproduced from Martinez-Arizala A, Green BA: Experimental spinal cord injury, in Levine AM, Eismont FJ, Garfin SR, Zigler JE, eds: *Spine Trauma*. Philadelphia, PA, WB Saunders, 1998, pp 87-101.)

processes that are activated following trauma and promote neural dysfunction and tissue damage for hours or days (**Table 1**).[38,41]

Primary Mediators of Spinal Cord Injury

Electrolytes

Significant injuries of the spinal cord are accompanied by a loss of neurophysiologic conduction across the lesion site,[30,42-45] which has been hypothesized to be associated with the intracellular leakage of sodium.[46] Eidelberg et al,[43] however, reported large increases in the potassium concentration in superfusants obtained from spinal cords subjected to prolonged compression. Because extracellular potassium levels greater than 10 mmol/L can block axonal conduction,[47] their findings suggested that the axonal conduction block was caused by the rise in extracellular potassium. These findings were corroborated by Young et al,[48] who, using ion-sensitive microelectrodes, recorded acute rises in the extracellular potassium from a preinjury level of less than 4 mmol/L to a postinjury mean level of 54 mmol/L in the white matter of the lateral columns. Furthermore, they found that evoked potentials, which disappeared immediately after injury, would return as the extracellular potassium levels fell below 15 mmol/L. Similar findings were also reported by Stokes et al.[49]

Failure of calcium homeostasis has also been associated with SCI. Intracellular calcium concentrations are normally a thousandfold less than extracellular concentrations (< 1 μmol/L compared to > 1 mmol/L), and maintenance of this gradient is necessary to maintain normal neuronal function.[50] Following acute SCI, the extracellular calcium concentration falls within a few minutes from levels of 1.2 mmol/L to levels of about 0.01 mmol/L, which implies a brisk and significant movement of calcium into the intracellular compartment.[49,51,52] The accumulation of intracellular calcium has been implicated in the mediation of secondary injury.

Metabolites

-A variety of metabolic alterations have been noted following experimental spinal trauma. A rapid decline in tissue partial pressure of oxygen (pO_2) occurs in both the gray and white matter of the spinal cord as early as 15 minutes following trauma.[49,53] This is not unexpected in view of the reduction in spinal cord blood flow (SCBF) that is associated with spinal trauma. The decrease in tissue oxygen tension has been reported to last for several hours following injury, implicating tissue hypoxia as a major factor in SCI.[54-56] Studies of energy metabolism in SCI have also shown that a rapid and marked depletion of high-energy phosphates (adenosine triphosphate [ATP] and phosphocreatine) occurs following injury.[57-60] The energy depletion is accompanied by lactic acidosis in spinal cord tissue and oxidative shifts of NAD/NADH (nicotinamide adenine dinucleotide[NAD]/NAD carrying two electrons and bonded with a hydrogen [H] ion) ratios.[57-63] In addition, marked reductions in the specific activity of the critical membrane-bound enzyme Na^+-K^+ ATPase have been reported to occur within 5 minutes after injury.[64]

Rawe et al[65] described increases in both gray and white matter glucose utilization for up to 1 hour after moderate traumatic spinal injuries in dogs. Following this initial increase, glucose utilization in the gray matter progressively decreased and remained low from 3 to 8 hours, and returned toward baseline in the white matter. Severe traumatic injuries produced progressive decreases in gray matter glucose utilization and transient increases in white matter glucose utilization, followed by a progressive deterioration to levels below baseline from 4 to 8 hours after injury. The transient increase in glucose utilization was hypothesized to be secondary to the continued delivery of substrate in the presence of ischemia and an enhancement in anaerobic glycolysis.

Morphology

Morphologic changes become evident within minutes after spinal injury and consist of petechial hemorrhages in the gray matter, small ruptures in the walls of the muscular venules, increases in the size of the extracellular spaces in the gray and white matter, attenuation of the myelin sheaths, enlargement of periaxonal spaces, the appearance of tubulovesicular invaginations into the axoplasm, and disruption of the axoplasm.[10,66-70] By 1 hour after SCI, changes characteristic of central chromatolysis and ischemia begin to appear in the anterior ventral horn cells.[71] By 4 hours postinjury, hemorrhagic changes progress centrifugally and coalesce to form an area of hemorrhagic necrosis that extends along the longitudinal axis of the cord in a spindle-shaped form.[10,39,67,72] The acute damage is located more centrally and, depending on the severity of the injury, it may progress to involve the adjacent white matter.[10,40] Although minor white matter changes have been identified at the ultrastructural level as early as 15 minutes after injury,[70] progressive edema is eventually manifested at the level of light microscopy as spongiform changes. These are secondary to axonal fragmentation and axonal and periaxonal swelling.[68] The axonal enlargements contain multiple organelles (mitochondria, neurofilaments, lysosomes, and smooth endoplasmic reticulum), which Balentine and Hilton[73] and Bresnahan et al[9,74] attributed to the occurrence of axoplasmic stasis. White matter changes begin in the areas closer to gray matter and spread out in a centrifugal fashion.[9,74] The acute cellular infiltration by polymorphonuclear leukocytes is replaced by an invasion of macrophages within days from the injury,[75,76] and by the end of first week after injury, cystic degeneration of the necrotic areas begins to be evident.[10] At 4 weeks, a cystic cavity is better defined, and the surviving white matter displays demyelination and microcysts.[12,19] At 4 months, astrocytic gliosis surrounds the cyst and the region of injury shows thickening of the dura mater.[12]

Secondary Mediators of Spinal Cord Injury

The progressive nature of the morphologic changes that follow acute SCI suggests that damage to the spinal cord is progressive over time,[10,40,67] and several observations support the existence of secondary injury processes: (1) the onset of significant decreases in white matter blood flow are delayed until 1 to 4 hours following severe SCI;[55,77-80] (2) evoked potentials, which transiently recover after acute SCI in some animals, disappear again hours or days later;[80-82] and (3) treatment of the acute phase of SCI directed against these secondary processes can be effective, which suggests that the deleterious effects of these processes can be ameliorated.[80,82-92] The existence of secondary processes in human SCI has been speculative because the progressive deterioration of neurologic deficits following SCI in humans is uncommon.[93,94] Until recently, the application of these findings to the human condition remained a significant question. However, the beneficial effects of steroids in certain types of human SCIs demonstrate that these treatments are also effective in humans.[1,95]

Edema

Following trauma to the spinal cord, a disruption of the blood-brain barrier (or, in the case of the spinal cord, the blood-spinal cord barrier) occurs, thereby impairing the selective permeability of the normal endothelium of the central nervous system (CNS). The endothelial damage promotes the formation of vasogenic edema, which is the accumulation of protein-rich plasma-like fluid in the extravascular space.[96] The presence of edema following SCI was identified histologically as early as 1914 by Allen.[66] Edema is confined to the central portions of the cord immediately after injury, and over hours it progressively spreads into the white matter in a centrifugal fashion.[2,40,97] The severity of the spinal injury has correlated with the longitudinal extension of the edema.[98] The temporal association of the onset of white matter edema with white matter hypoperfusion has implicated edema in the promotion of secondary tissue injury. Studies of acute spinal injury have shown that edema maximizes at 6 to 8 hours postinjury, but increases in spinal cord tissue water occurring at 3 to 5 days postinjury have also been reported.[99] In support of this finding, Němecek et al[97] described the existence of a secondary type of edema in SCI that had the characteristics of a plasma ultrafiltrate, appeared more gradually, and outlasted vasogenic edema. The pathogenesis of posttraumatic edema includes capillary leakage secondary to loosening of the endothelial cell tight junctions[100] and increases in vesicular transport across the endothelium.[101,102]

Ischemia

Alterations in spinal cord vasculature that have been observed in the histopathology of SCI suggest a role for ischemia in SCI, and numerous investigations have documented this.[67,103-105] Several findings support the role of ischemia in SCI: (1) significant elevations in the lactate levels occur following SCI;[61] (2) ischemic models of SCI produce pathologic changes comparable to those produced by spinal trauma;[37,106] (3) the degree of

TABLE 2

Techniques for Measuring Spinal Cord Blood Flow

Radiolabeled microspheres[a]
Hydrogen clearance[b]
^{14}C-iodoantipyrine[c]
Laser Doppler flowmetry[d]

[a]Data from Heymann et al[119] and Smith et al.[113]

[b]Data from Aukland et al,[120] Hayashi et al,[55] and Kobrine et al.[121]

[c]Data from Bingham et al[331] and Reivich et al.[123]

[d]Data from Lindsberg et al[124] and Stern.[125]

(Modified from Martinez-Arizala A, Green BA: Experimental spinal cord injury, in Levine AM, Eismont FJ, Garfin SR, Zigler JE, eds: *Spine Trauma*. Philadelphia, PA, WB Saunders, 1998, pp 87-101.)

posttraumatic ischemia correlates with the changes in spinal cord neurophysiologic function, specifically with changes in evoked potentials;[107] and (4) tissue oxygen content decreases significantly after trauma.[54-56,108]

Unfortunately, the reported alterations in studies of SCBF following SCI have been variable. Their differences are probably secondary to the interactions of various experimental conditions that can affect SCBF, such as the animal species and the injury model used, the severity of injury studied, the technique chosen to measure SCBF, the particular anesthetic used, and changes in the systemic blood pressure. Normally, the spinal cord autoregulates blood flow within the same arterial pressure range (approximately 50 mm Hg to 130 mm Hg) as that of the brain.[109-111] When SCI impairs SCBF autoregulation, the systemic blood pressure becomes an important variable in the perfusion of the injured cord segments.[112-114]

Early techniques of SCBF assessments were limited because they relied on direct visualization to measure the changes in the vessels of the cord[115] or on outlining spinal blood vessels via fluorescent tracers or microangiographic techniques.[116-118] The first quantitative techniques consisted of measuring the clearance of inert gases such as xenon or argon;[54,81] however, these methods are invasive and offer poor resolution between the white and gray matter. Current methods offer a better degree of resolution and accuracy (**Table 2**).[55,113,119-125]

The relative merit of each technique depends on the specific questions each particular study is attempting to answer, and the specific injury model employed. Although the ^{14}C-iodoantipyrine technique offers the best resolution, it allows only one measurement from each animal and it requires that the animal be killed. The hydrogen clearance technique allows multiple measurements over time and offers a reasonable degree of resolution in the spinal cords of large animals (eg, monkeys, cats), but it is more invasive and offers a lesser degree of resolution in small animals (rats). Laser Doppler flowmetry provides continuous online measurement of SCBF, but it is limited to reporting relative changes in SCBF instead of absolute values.

Not all studies of posttraumatic SCBF agree in their results (**Table 3**), but the occurrence of posttraumatic hypoperfusion of the gray matter has been a consistent finding.[34,48,54,77-79,105,121,122,126] Many investigations have focused on white matter SCBF changes following SCI for the following reasons: (1) this area contains the critical fibers for controlling function below the level of the lesion; (2) it is the last area to undergo histologic change; and (3) evoked potentials have been noted to transiently recover, but are subsequently lost concomitant with the onset of white matter ischemia in some models of spinal cord contusion.[77-80] It must be noted that the reported posttraumatic white matter blood flow changes are not all in agreement because the occurrence of both hyperemia and ischemia have been noted (**Table 3**). Furthermore, the significance of posttraumatic white matter hypoperfusion is unclear, because ischemic levels for the spinal cord white matter have not been defined. In fact, several experiments suggest that the spinal cord white matter is fairly resistant to the effects of ischemia or hypoxia.[127-129]

The etiology of the delayed white matter hypoperfusion in SCI is unclear, but it has been attributed to the actions of other vasoactive substances. It was initially ascribed by Osterholm and Mathews[130,131] in 1972 to an alteration in catecholamines (norepinephrine in particular), but their findings could not be substantiated by other investigators.[132-139] Changes in the levels of other transmitters, such as dopamine and serotonin, have also been inconsistent.[130,133,135,137,139-142] The bulk of the data support posttraumatic spinal ischemia as more than just an epiphenomenon; however, its precise contribution to the neurologic deficits and the resultant pathologic changes remains to be defined.

Calcium

It is evident that calcium plays an important role in the mediation of cell injury and cell death.[143-145] Calcium overload was first suggested as a mechanism of cellular injury in liver cells by McLean et al[146] in 1965, and the phenomenon of the "calcium paradox" as a mechanism of cell death in the heart was described by Zimmerman et al.[147,148] They demonstrated that perfusion of isolated rat hearts with a calcium-free medium produced electromechanical dissociation without significant morphologic changes. However, the introduction of calcium into the medium produced substantial intracellular calcium influx, cellular contracture, and cell death.

The initial observation of the potential involvement of calcium in SCI was made by Balentine and Spector in 1977; they described the occurrence of selective intra-axonal calcification in SCI in rats.[149] Calcium accumulation was noted to occur as early as 30 minutes after trauma and became more profuse in the late necrotic phases of the injury.[68,149] Similar findings were also reported in injured spinal cords of monkeys, cats, and humans.[150] Additional observations support the detrimental role of calcium in spinal cord injury: (1) a rapid decrease in the extracellular calcium concentration occurs in the injured cord,[49,51,52] (2) the total calcium concentration in the injured spinal cord segment is significantly elevated after injury,[151] and (3) dripping calcium chloride onto the exposed spinal cord produces morphologic alterations and behavioral deficits similar to those seen following spinal cord trauma.[73,152] In addition, posttraumatic spinal cord ischemia is likely to potentiate the role of calcium in SCI because calcium has also been implicated as a mediator of cellular death in CNS hypoxic-ischemic injury.[153,154] Although the mechanisms for calcium accumulation in the injured spinal cord are not well defined, the following hypotheses have been advanced: (1) leakage through either the voltage-dependent calcium channels or the excitatory amino acid, N-methyl-D-aspartate (NMDA) receptor channel; (2) failure of Ca^{2+}-ATPase–mediated calcium extrusion; and (3) release of calcium from intracellular organelles (ie, endoplasmic reticulum and mitochondria), which normally bind cytosolic calcium.[143]

Excess intracellular calcium produces deleterious effects on cellular function because increases in free cytosolic calcium disrupt the normal regulation of the function of calcium-dependent proteases and nucleases and adversely affect mitochondrial energy production.[155] Activation of calcium-dependent proteases can lead to the degradation of neurofilament and myelin proteins.[156,157] In addition, activation of the calcium-dependent phospholipase enzymes, phospholipase C and A_2, results in the breakdown of cellular membranes and the production of arachidonate by phospholipase A_2.[158] The metabolism of arachidonate yields thromboxanes, leukotrienes, and free radicals, which promote tissue injury via their effects on the vasculature and the inflammatory response.

Endogenous Opiates

While studying spinal shock in 1980, Holaday and Faden[159] observed that the opioid antagonist naloxone reversed the hypotension produced by cervical spinal cord transection. Based on this observation, it was hypothesized that if naloxone would raise arterial pressure following SCI, SCBF would improve and the extent of the injury would be reduced. Indeed, several investigations found naloxone to be beneficial in the treatment of experimental SCI,[80,84] and although it improved posttraumatic SCBF, this effect was independent of its effect on systemic blood pressure.[80] These findings suggested the possibility of the involvement of endogenous opiates in SCI. In support of this, large elevations in plasma of the endogenous opiate β-endorphin have been found to occur following SCI.[85]

The exact nature of opiate involvement in SCI is unclear, because when naloxone is given in the high doses used to treat SCI, it is active at the three principal types of opiate receptors, the mu, delta, and kappa receptors.[160,161] In lower doses, naloxone is typically more selective for the opiate mu receptor. The results from studies from Faden and others have implicated the endogenous opioid dynorphin A (1–17), the ligand for the kappa opioid receptor, as the opioid most likely to be involved in SCI for the following reasons: (1) dynorphin immunoreactivity selectively increased following SCI and the increase correlated with the severity of injury,[162] (2) significant time-dependent increases in kappa opioid receptor occur with spinal trauma,[163] (3) opiate antagonists more selective for the kappa receptor have been increasingly effective in the treatment of experimental SCI and ischemia,[164-166] and (4) dynorphin is the only endogenous opioid that produces hindlimb paralysis in the rat following its intrathecal injection into lumbar subarachnoid space.[167-169] It is clear, however, that dynorphin-induced hindlimb paralysis is in part a nonopiate effect, as it is not reversible by either naloxone or other more specific kappa antagonists.[170-172] Furthermore, unlike the paralysis produced by spinal trauma, dynorphin-induced paralysis is not affected by pretreatment with thyrotropin-releasing hormone (TRH).[172] The intrathecal injection of dynorphin in paralytic doses

TABLE 3

Spinal Cord Blood Flow Changes Following Spinal Cord Injury[a]

Study	Year	Animal	Model
Bingham et al[122]	1975	Monkey	Weight drop
Kobrine et al[121b]	1975	Monkey	Weight drop
Sandler and Tator[105]	1976	Monkey	Cuff compression
Ducker et al[54c]	1978	Dog	Weight drop
Rivlin and Tator[34]	1978	Rat	Clip compression
Senter and Venes[79d]	1978	Cat	Weight drop
Lohse et al[78]	1980	Cat	Weight drop
Cawthon et al[126e]	1980	Cat	Weight drop
Young et al[48]	1982	Cat	Weight drop
Hall and Wolf[77]	1987	Cat	Weight drop

[a]— = no significant change from baseline; ↓ = mild decrease; ↓↓ = moderate decrease; ↓↓↓ = marked decrease; ↑ = mild increase; ↑↑ = moderate increase; ↑↑↑ = marked increase.

[b]The reported gray matter blood flows were low, which suggests they also reflect white matter flow.

[c]Flow was measured at the center of the cord, but the low values suggest it also reflects white matter flow.

[d]Some animals had hyperemic values at < 1 h.

[e]Some animals had hyperemic values at 1 h.

(Modified with permission from Martinez-Avizala A, Green BA, Bunge RP: Experimental spinal cord injury: Pathophysiology and treatment, in Rothman RH, Simeone FA, eds: *The Spine*, ed 3. Philadelphia, PA, WB Saunders, 1992, p 1247.)

in the rat is associated with marked decrease in SCBF, and this may in part explain its paralytic actions.[173]

Free Radicals

Free radicals are molecules that possess an unusual reactivity due to the presence of unpaired electrons in their outer orbits. A peculiar aspect of this reactivity is their ability to propagate via chain reactions.[174] Phospholipid and cholesterol components of biologic membranes are very susceptible to damage by free radical reactions,[175] and the involvement of fatty acids in oxygen free radical chain reactions is known as lipid peroxidation. Normal cellular metabolic pathways for oxygen reduction generate the following oxygen free radi-

TABLE 3 (CONTINUED)

Technique	Severity	Time	SCBF Gray Matter	SCBF White Matter
^{14}C-iodoantipyrine	Moderate	5 min	↓	—
		15 min	—	↑↑
		1 h	↓↓	—
		2–4 h	↓↓	↑
^{2}H washout (clearance)	Severe	1 h	↓	↑↑
		4 h	↓↓	↑
		8–24 h		—
^{14}C-iodoantipyrine	Moderate	15 min	↓↓	↓↓
	Severe	1–6 h	↓	↓
		24 h	↓	↑
		2 h	↓↓↓	↓↓↓
		24 h	↓↓↓	↓↓↓
Xe washout (clearance)	Severe	1 h	↓	
		1–3 h	↓↓	
^{14}C-iodoantipyrine	Severe	15 min	↓↓↓	↓↓
		2 h	↓↓↓	↓↓
		24 h	↓↓↓	↓↓
^{2}H washout (clearance)	Severe	1 h		—
		1–6 h		↓
^{2}H washout (clearance)	Mild	1–6 h		—
	Moderate	1–6 h		↑
^{14}C-iodoantipyrine	Severe	1 h		—
^{2}H washout (clearance)		2–6 h		↓
^{2}H washout (clearance)	Severe	30 min–1 h		—
		2–3 h		↓
^{2}H washout (clearance)	Moderate	< 30 min		↑
	Severe	30 min–4 h		—
		30 min		↓
		2–4 h		↓↓

cals: superoxide anion (O_2^-), hydroxyl radical OH–, and hydrogen peroxide (H_2O_2). Normally, cells control the harmful effects of free radical production with several naturally occurring antioxidant compounds such as superoxide dismutases, catalases, glutathione peroxidase, ascorbic acid, α-tocopherol, steroids, cysteine, and selenium. Superoxide dismutases scavenge the superoxide anion by catalyzing its conversion into hydrogen peroxide and oxygen, whereas catalases reduce hydrogen peroxide to water.

Lipid peroxidation can result in the fragmentation of cellular membranes in pathologic states such as CNS ischemia, in which excess free radicals are generated.[175-177] In addition, these processes have also been implicated in brain and spinal cord trauma.[175,178] Several observations support the role of free radical lipid peroxidation in SCI because of the observation of the following after spinal trauma: (1) increase in peroxidized polyunsaturated fatty acid breakdown products;[179,180] (2) decrease in cholesterol accompanied by the appearance of cholesterol oxidation products;[181] (3) activation of guanylate cyclase and increase in cyclic guanosine monophosphate (cGMP);[179,182] (4) decrease in levels of tissue antioxidants, such as α-tocopherol, and ascorbic acid;[183,184] and (5) inhibition of the phospholipid-dependent membrane-bound Na^+-K^+ATPase.[64] In addition, antioxidants have been shown to be effective in the treatment of experimental SCI.[91,181,185]

Among the possible potential sources of oxygen radicals in SCI is the depletion of ATP and production of adenosine monophosphate (AMP), which is degraded to hypoxanthine.[186] During ischemia, xanthine dehydrogenase converts to its oxidase form, and in the presence of hypoxanthine catalyzes the formation of O_2.[187] Two other potential sources of oxygen free radicals are coenzyme Q (a component of the electron transport chain), and the metabolism of arachidonate in the cyclooxygenase pathway, which generates superoxide radicals. This effect is probably enhanced by the calcium-mediated activation of phospholipase A_2 that occurs following injury. In addition, the respiratory burst of invading neutrophils, the autooxidation of catecholamines, and the release of hemoglobin from the hemorrhage that accompanies SCI are also potential sources of oxygen free radicals.[188,189] Hemoglobin can also stimulate lipid peroxidation and provide a source of iron to catalyze oxygen radical and lipid peroxidation reactions.[190-192] Besides injury to cellular membranes, free radicals can contribute to tissue injury by disrupting lysosomal membranes,[193] promoting tissue edema,[194,195] and inhibiting mitochondrial function.[175]

Excitatory Amino Acids

The concept of excitatory amino acid–mediated cell death, or excitotoxicity, was introduced in 1969 when Olney[196] described the neurotoxic effects of systemically administered glutamate on the endocrine hypothalamus. This concept now embraces the deleterious actions of the excitatory amino acid transmitters, glutamate and aspartate, at their receptors. Specific evidence now implicates excitotoxicity in the pathophysiology of CNS hypoxic-ischemic injury[197] as well as in brain and spinal trauma.[88,198-202]

Of the three well-characterized excitatory amino acid receptors, the majority of data suggest that the NMDA receptor complex is predominantly involved in excitotoxicity in spinal trauma.[154,203,204] However, it must be emphasized that glutamate also acts as an agonist at the kainate and the quisqualate receptors, and recent evidence suggests that non-NMDA receptors are also involved in SCI.[201,202] The following observations support the role of excitatory amino acid toxicity in SCI: (1) excitatory amino acid concentrations increase following spinal trauma;[205] (2) spinal ischemia is associated with SCI, and excitotoxicity has been shown to occur in models of CNS ischemia; and (3) administration of excitatory amino acid receptor antagonists as a form of treatment in experimental SCI and ischemia is effective in improving neurologic outcome.[206-208]

Other

Animal studies have shown that systemic hyperthermia after SCI can have detrimental effects on locomotor recovery. Elevation of systemic temperature from fever or infection may add to the severity of secondary injury following traumatic SCI and significantly affect neurologic outcome. Hyperthermia may exacerbate secondary mediators of SCI by increasing free radical production, excitotoxic neurotransmitters, calcium influx into cells, and ischemic cellular damage. Animal models have shown that moderate systemic hypothermia (32° to 33°C) reduces the area of spinal cord tissue damage at both 7 and 44 days after injury.[209,210]

Studies in the histologic evolution of SCI have shown that an infiltration by polymorphonuclear leukocytes occurs early.[76] In fact, polymorphonuclear leukocytes are deleterious because they can actively engage in neuronophagia acutely after spinal injury,[76] and their respiratory burst serves as a source of free radicals.[188] The macrophage, which heavily infiltrates the lesions after the acute period, may also play a role in the demyelination that occurs in SCI. The eicosanoids thromboxane and leukotrienes may also play a role in SCI. Levels of thromboxane, which stimulates platelet aggregation and vasoconstriction, are elevated in SCI.[211,212] Leukotrienes are potent mediators of inflammation and have been reported to either increase or remain unchanged after SCI.[211,213]

Therapy of Acute Experimental Spinal Cord Injury

Unfortunately, studies in the therapy of experimental SCI have occasionally yielded conflicting results, and this raises difficulties when trying to transfer specific therapies from the laboratory to the clinical arena. In large part, these conflicts are due to the different injury models, animal species, anesthetics, and methods used to measure neurologic outcome by the various investigators. The anatomic and physiologic bases for the recovery function following SCI are unclear because most studies do not include detailed morphologic analysis. Our understanding of the anatomic requirements for the preservation of locomotive capacity in animals suggests that as little as 10% of the white matter permits locomotion.[7,214,215] Following SCI in cats, a preferential loss of the axons, which are large and are located toward the center of the lesion, occurs.[7] Moreover, conduction across the lesion for the surviving axons is absent or abnormal,[8] which suggests that demyelination plays an important role in SCI.

The first measures employed in the treatment of experimental SCI were surgical, not pharmacologic. Allen described the beneficial effects of myelotomies as early as 1911.[6,66] The application of hypothermia was based on the observation that it decreased cerebral metabolic demand and reduced brain volume,[216,217] and it became popular in the treatment of experimental SCI in the 1960s.[83,218-220] The technique of hypothermia fell out of favor because it is technically difficult to implement in humans.[83,219,220] Recently, modest systemic hypothermia has been safely implemented with the use of various cooling blankets and intravascular catheters. Temperature control using these techniques has been investigated in patients with traumatic brain injury,[221] stroke,[222] and cardiac arrest.[223] A phase I clinical trial is in progress to determine the safety and efficacy of moderate intravascular hypothermia in patients with American Spinal Injury Association (ASIA) grade A acute SCI.

Cellular Transplantation

The use of cell transplants and bridges have been studied as an effective therapy in experimental models of SCI. When implanted into the area of the injured spinal cord, these cellular grafts can provide a framework for axonal regeneration and facilitate remyelination.[224] A variety of cell types have been used for these studies including: Schwann cells,[225] olfactory ensheathing cells,[226,227] bone marrow stromal cells,[228] and embryonic stem cells.[229] In order for these grafts to be effective, they must possess certain characteristics. Careful methods of isolating these cells should be in place to consistently yield a population of cells with the highest possible purity. After transplantation, the cells should not have the capability of harming the host by either becoming neoplastic or mounting a significant immune response. Finally, implanted cells should be confined to the injury environment without migrating to surrounding tissues and possibly causing harm.

Successful therapies in experimental SCI may include a combination approach, using cellular implants in conjunction with neurotrophic factors shown to promote neurite regrowth. Various neurotrophins including nerve growth factor (NGF), neurotrophin-3 (NT-3), and brain-derived neurotrophic factor (BDNF) have been used.[230] Therapeutic gene delivery has also been used as a method of transducing the implanted cells with the genes needed to secrete one or a combination of neurotrophic factors. A multineurotrophin molecule called D15A contains both BDNF and NT-3 activities and has been used in combination with cellular transplantation. Glial-restricted precursor cells infected by retroviruses expressing D15A were shown to improve functional recovery in animals with SCI after transplantation.[224,231]

Despite the successful use of cellular transplants in improving histologic and functional outcomes in animal models, few published clinical trials have assessed the safety and efficacy of cellular transplants in humans with SCI. A small phase I clinical trial involving three patients with complete thoracic level SCIs who received transplantation of olfactory ensheathing cells was performed in Australia.[226] The autologous olfactory ensheathing cells were isolated from cultures of a nasal biopsy and then transplanted into the injury site and adjacent areas of the patient's spinal cord. After 1 year of follow-up, no complications such as neuropathic pain, neurologic deterioration, or evidence of spinal cord damage on MRI were noted. A 3-year follow-up of these patients is pending.

A pilot study assessing the safety and feasibility of transplanting fetal spinal cord tissue has been described in two patients with posttraumatic syringomyelia.[232] Both of these patients underwent syrinx decompression followed by injection of donor tissue directly into the cyst cavity. Follow-up was reported up to 18 months and included neurologic function outcome measures, MRI scans, and neurophysiologic testing. Following the transplantation procedure, no negative changes were observed in any of the neurophysiologic measures in either patient.[233] The study concluded that the clinical outcomes for both patients appeared to be no worse than after their previous operations. Although MRI scans showed solid tissue at the graft sites with no evidence of donor-tissue overgrowth, the survival of the transplanted cells could not be confirmed.

The inflammatory response following injury to most parts of the body, including the nervous system, plays an important role in initiating the healing process. Although uncontrolled inflammation following SCI can exacerbate neuronal loss, a controlled inflammatory response may be beneficial. Specifically, the activation of macrophages when coincubated in skin has been shown to secrete elevated levels of the beneficial trophic factors interleukin-1β (IL-1β) and BDNF, and reduces the secretion of neurotoxic tumor necrosis factor–α (TNF-α) in rats.[234] Implantation of autologous macrophages, after prestimulation by exposure to a regenerative (sciatic) nerve, into completely transected spinal cords of adult rats resulted in partial motor recovery.[235]

These results led to a phase I nonrandomized study assessing the safety and tolerability of incubated autologous macrophages administered to patients with acute complete SCI.[236] The procedure involved isolating monocytes from patient blood and incubating them ex vivo with autologous dermis. The resulting incubated autologous macrophages were injected into the patient's spinal cord immediately caudal to the lesion within 14 days of injury. All patients had complete SCIs (ASIA grade A) before treatment. Of the eight patients in the study, three recovered clinically significant neurologic motor and sensory function (ASIA grade C). A phase II multicenter trial is currently underway in the United States.

Surgical Decompression

The beneficial role of early surgical decompression for acute SCI has yet to be firmly established in the literature. The vast majority of studies addressing this issue are retrospective. A meta-analysis of the literature from 1966 through 2000 was conducted to determine whether neurologic outcome is improved in traumatic spinal cord–injured patients who had surgery within 24 hours as compared with those who had late surgery or conservative treatment.[237] Although early decompression resulted in significantly better outcome compared with both conservative ($P < 0.001$) and late management ($P < 0.001$), the evidence was not conclusive and early surgery could be considered only as a practice option rather than a standard of care.[237,238] A prospective, randomized study in Philadelphia assessing the outcome of early (< 72 hours) and late (> 5 days) surgical decompression after cervical SCI was reported in 1997.[239] Comparison of the two groups showed no significant difference in length of acute postoperative intensive care stay, length of inpatient rehabilitation, or improvement in ASIA grade or motor score between early versus late surgery.[239] Currently a large, prospective, longitudinal, multicenter study is underway that is looking at the outcomes of patients undergoing early surgery (< 24 hours) or late surgery (> 24 hours) for SCI.

Steroids

Steroids were one of the earlier pharmacologic agents used in the treatment of both experimental and human SCI based on their anti-inflammatory actions and their effectiveness in treating cerebral edema.[240,241] Reviews of studies that assessed some form of functional outcome, such as the neurologic status of the animal, have shown the beneficial effects of steroids in the treatment of experimental SCI.[31,80,83,89,92,242-247] Some studies have reported negative or no effects.[31,248-250] Conflicting results are secondary to the following factors: (1) the use of different injury models, (2) the use of different measures of outcome, and (3) the use of different treatment protocols. For example, investigators used different steroids (methylprednisolone versus dexamethasone), doses, routes of administration (intravenous versus intrathecal), and/or combinations with surgical therapeutic modalities (myelotomy or dural decompression).[245,250]

The particular actions of the different steroids have become important because it has been shown that methylprednisolone is a stronger inhibitor of lipid peroxidation.[242] The fact that a specific dose is required to obtain the desired effect was also shown in studies in which high doses of methylprednisolone (30 mg/kg) improved neurologic recovery following SCI. This led to its incorporation into the second human SCI cooperative study.[1,52,251]

The beneficial actions of steroids in SCI include the following: (1) prevention of the loss of potassium from the injured cord tissue and facilitation of the recovery of the extracellular level of calcium ions;[52,252] (2) amelioration of posttraumatic spinal cord ischemia;[52,253,254] (3) enhancement of the postinjury activity of neuronal Na^+-K^+–ATPase;[251]; (4) enhancement of the excitability of the CNS, including the motor neuron;[251,255,256] and (5) inhibition of lipid peroxidation,[90,251] which is perhaps the most significant beneficial action of steroids in SCI.

A class of steroid compounds, the 21-aminosteroids, which are potent inhibitors of lipid peroxidation and are devoid of glucocorticoid activity, has been developed.[257,258] These compounds have already shown efficacy in the treatment of experimental brain ischemia and brain and spinal trauma.[15,259] In fact the prototype of these compounds, tirilazad mesylate, was incorporated into the National Acute Spinal Cord Injury Study (NASCIS) III clinical trial.[260] This study compared the efficacy of methylprednisolone administered for 24 hours with methylprednisolone administered for 48 hours or tirilazad mesylate administered for 48 hours in patients with acute SCI. Patients treated with tirilazad had motor recovery rates equivalent to patients who received methylprednisolone for 24 hours. Although this study did not provide a rationale for the clinical use of tirilazad to treat SCI, it showed that patients who received the 48-hour methylprednisolone protocol between 3 and 8 hours after injury had slightly better motor scores than the 24-hour methylprednisolone group.

In recent years, there has been debate in the literature on whether the use of steroids is indeed beneficial in treating SCI. The first NASCIS trial showed a significantly higher incidence of wound infection in the high-dose methylprednisolone group. Although not statistically significant, there was also a higher incidence of sepsis, pulmonary emboli, and death in this group.[261] A randomized double-blind clinical trial in Japan studied the medical complications of high-dose methylprednisolone administration for SCI.[262] The methylprednisolone-treated group had a higher incidence of complications compared to the placebo group (56.5% versus 34.8%). Pulmonary and respiratory complications were the most significant between the two treatment populations.[262]

In a survey of 60 Canadian spine surgeons about their reasons for methylprednisolone administration in SCI, 70% reported doing so because of the perception that everyone else does or out of fear of litigation, while only 17% prescribe steroids because they believe them to be efficacious.[263] Currently, the use of steroids for the treatment of acute SCI is recommended as an option that should only be undertaken with the knowledge that the evidence suggesting harmful side effects is more consistent than the suggestion of clinical benefit.[264]

The full dataset from NASCIS II was never available for peer review until more recently, when several centers across North America and around the world intensively reviewed the data. These authors were in agreement that most of the conclusions of the study were not based on solid statistical data. Therefore, in the United States, as well as around the world, most SCI centers no longer administer high-dose methylprednisolone to acute SCI patients.

Opiate Antagonists

Based on the initial observations of the effect of naloxone on spinal shock, Faden et al[166] showed it was beneficial in the treatment of experimental SCI (see section above on secondary mediators). Various investigators also confirmed the positive effects of naloxone in SCI;[80,82,84,85,87] however, as in the case of steroids, conflicting results have been obtained.[32,265,266] The differences in methodologies, therapeutic regimens, and SCI models must be taken into consideration when interpreting these conflicting results.

The actions of naloxone are not necessarily at opiate receptors, because naloxone has also been demonstrated to have the following effects: (1) reversal of posttraumatic calcium and ascorbic acid derangements,[49,267] (2) inhibition of neutrophil superoxide release and iron-catalyzed lyposomal lipid peroxidation,[268,269] and (3) inhibition of proteolysis and stabilization of lysosomal membranes.[270] Because recent evidence has implicated the endogenous opioid dynorphin A in SCI, more selective kappa opiate receptor (the receptor for dynorphin A) antagonists have been developed and proved to be efficacious in the treatment of experimental SCI.[164,166,206] Results from the NASCIS II study did not show naloxone to be beneficial in human injury;[1] however, antagonists more selective for the kappa receptor may be efficacious.

Like naloxone, TRH was beneficial in models of circulatory shock and spinal injury,[86,271] and various studies have shown TRH to be effective in the treatment of experimental SCI.[272] Because TRH has a short half-life, more stable analogs have been developed and successfully used in the treatment of experimental SCI.[164,273-275] As in other drug studies, there have been negative results in the treatment of SCI with TRH.[16,276] Although it was initially hypothesized that TRH acted as a physiologic opiate antagonist,[271] the actual mechanisms by which TRH improves neurologic function in SCI are unknown. It has been documented to potentiate spinal reflexes and to have trophic effects on cholinergic spinal neurons.[277,278] Subcutaneous treatment with TRH once daily for 7 consecutive days starting 24 hours or 7 days after injury has been shown to improve the neurologic function in rats with cord injury in a dose-related manner.[279] A small clinical study was performed in 20 patients who received either placebo or TRH infusions after SCI.[280] A variety of physiologic variables were followed during this treatment in these patients who had both complete and incomplete injuries. Treatment with TRH was associated with significantly higher motor and sensory scores than placebo treatment, although follow-up was less than 1 year in this study.

Excitatory Amino Acid Antagonists

Excitotoxicity, specifically the actions of glutamate and aspartate at the NMDA receptor complex, have been implicated in the pathophysiology of SCI. Two types of NMDA receptor antagonists have been used in the therapy of experimental SCI: competitive antagonists that act at the glutamate's binding site, and noncompetitive antagonists that act at a site located in the NMDA receptor ion channel.[281] Theoretically, noncompetitive antagonists offer the advantage of functioning in an agonist-dependent fashion (ie, the receptor must be activated for the antagonist to bind). This is favorable for the treatment of pathologic conditions such as CNS trauma and ischemia, in which excessive receptor activation is thought to occur.[282] A variety of competitive and noncompetitive NMDA receptor antagonists have been tested and shown to be protective in models of spinal cord trauma and ischemia.[88,202,207,208] In addition, one study has reported beneficial effects in SCI treated with non-NMDA receptor antagonists.[202] Gacyclidine is a noncompetitive NMDA receptor antagonist that has been shown to improve motor function and somatosensory-evoked potential amplitudes after being administered to rats following spinal cord contusion.[283]

Calcium Channel Antagonists

As discussed in previous sections, the intracellular accumulation of calcium plays an important role in the mediation of neural injury, and calcium channel blockers have been successfully used in certain models of brain ischemia.[284,285] The actions of calcium channel–blocking drugs cannot be ascribed to the prevention of calcium movement into the neuron because calcium may enter cells via other receptor channels (such as the NMDA receptor) or by nonspecific leakage through the damaged cell membrane. Moreover, calcium that is normally bound to intracellular organelles may be released into the cytosol after injury. The actions of calcium channel blockers on the vascular smooth muscle can also produce a vasodilatory improvement in perfusion and thereby improve neurologic outcome.[286] These effects, however, raise concerns over their application in the treatment of SCI, because mean arterial pressure could be lowered to the point of being detrimental to the perfusion of the injured cord (which cannot autoregulate). The significance of this issue is greater in cervical and high thoracic cord lesions, in which neurogenic hypotension is likely to occur. Although nimodipine has been reported to increase blood flow and restore neurophysiologic function in the traumatized spinal cord,[107,287] it has not improved neurologic function in models of spinal cord trauma or ischemia.[16,276,288,289] A clinical trial of 100 patients following acute SCI in France investigated the efficacy of nimodipine on neurologic outcome.[290] The authors found no neurologic benefit with this treatment after 1-year follow-up over the placebo group.

GM_1-Ganglioside

GM_1-ganglioside, a major component of the neuronal membranes in the CNS, was found to be beneficial in models of CNS ischemia,[291-293] in clinical stroke trials, and, on a more limited basis, in models of SCI.[294,295] Based on these observations, it was used in a human SCI study that contained a small number of subjects with positive results.[95] An interesting aspect was that it appeared to be of benefit when administered up to 72 hours after injury. This study had several limitations and its results have been questioned. In addition, a clinical trial of GM_1-ganglioside in stroke in a limited number of patients did not find it to be of value.[296] The randomized double-blind Sygen multicenter acute SCI study[297] evaluated patients divided into placebo, low-dose GM_1, or high-dose GM_1 groups. Although the primary outcome of marked recovery for this trial was negative, patients receiving either low- or high-dose GM_1 showed a more accelerated recovery over the first 3 months postinjury.

The actions of GM_1-ganglioside in SCI are not known, and the following theories have been proposed: (1) it increases neurite outgrowth in vitro,[298,299] (2) it can reduce retrograde and anterograde fiber degeneration,[300,301] (3) it can induce regeneration and sprouting in neurons,[300] and (4) it reduces amino acid–induced neurotoxicity.[302] At present, GM_1-ganglioside, when initiated after the administration of methylprednisolone given within 8 hours of injury (NASCIS II protocol), is recommended as an option in the treatment of adult patients with acute SCI without demonstrated clinical benefit.[264]

Sodium Channel Blockers

Activation of voltage-sensitive Na^+ channels has been associated with cellular toxicity and may contribute to the secondary pathophysiology of neural tissue following traumatic SCI. Accumulation of intracellular calcium contributes to secondary injury by activating damaging enzymes and triggering processes leading to the formation of free radicals. One mechanism of calcium influx involves the initial leakage of sodium into the cell through voltage-gated channels, which drives the sodium-calcium exchanger to import damaging levels of calcium.[303,304] Therefore, various treatments targeting the influx of sodium after acute injury have been investigated.[305]

Phenytoin is a sodium channel blocker that has a protective effect on axons within white matter after anoxia. Studies using phenytoin-treated animals have demonstrated reductions in the degree of destruction of gray and white matter surrounding the lesion epicenter and that phenytoin provides significant protection during prolonged spinal cord ischemia.[306,307] Tetrodotoxin is a potent neurotoxin that blocks action potentials by binding to pores of voltage-gated sodium channels in cell membranes. This toxin has been shown to significantly reduce the loss of large-diameter axons when administered after thoracic spinal cord contusions in rats.[308] Riluzole is a drug that has been used as a treatment of amyotrophic lateral sclerosis and acts as an inhibitor of presynaptic calcium-dependent glutamate release.[309,310] It is also a sodium channel blocker that has neuroprotective properties and promotes functional neurologic recovery following SCI in rodents.[311,312]

Minocycline

Minocycline is a lipophilic semisynthetic broad-spectrum antibiotic derived from tetracycline that is capable of crossing the blood-brain barrier. This drug has been studied for the treatment of neurodegenerative diseases including Parkinson disease and Huntington disease, due to evidence that it protects brain and nerve cells from damage.[313] Laboratory studies have shown that the neuroprotective effects of minocycline can be partially explained by its inhibition of mitochondrial cytochrome C release and reactive microgliosis.[314] Other possible mechanisms for its beneficicial actions include decreased TNF-α concentration and decreased caspase-3 mRNA expression, which is a mediator of the apoptosis cascade.[315] Administration of minocycline has been associated with statistically significant tissue-sparing, reduced microgliosis, and less activated caspase-3 and substrate cleavage following contusion SCI. A current single-center trial in Calgary is underway.

Rho Inhibitors

Ras homology protein (Rho) GTPases (guanosine triphosphatases) are a group of related proteins present in all cells acting as important signaling switches. After SCI, Rho is part of a biochemical pathway mediating growth inhibitors embedded in CNS myelin and glial scar tissue.[316] Studies have shown that Rho inhibition promotes axonal regeneration and increases functional recovery after experimental SCI.[261,317-319] A phase I multicenter clinical trial (37 patients) has been completed in North America examining the safety of a Rho inhibitor after SCI. In this study, the drug is administered as a one-time application onto the dura mater of the injured spinal cord. Preliminary analysis has shown this drug to be safe and suggests efficacy. A large phase II study is planned.

Nogo Antibody

Researchers in the early 1990s described the existence of molecules found within CNS myelin that inhibit the growth of neural fibers. Specifically, a myelin protein called Nogo (NI-250) has been targeted with monoclonal antibodies to neutralize its axonal growth inhibitory properties.[320] Nogo has been identified as a member of the reticulon family of proteins (4-A), and is expressed by oligodendrocytes but not by Schwann cells.[321] The Nogo gene encodes at least three major protein products (Nogo-A, -B, and -C).[322]

Rats with SCI had regeneration and anatomic plasticity of corticospinal axons after treatment with the monoclonal antibody IN-1 directed against Nogo.[323] In a study using unilateral thoracic spinal lesions in Marmoset monkeys, the intrathecal application of IN-1 antibody against Nogo-A resulted in increased regenerative sprouting and growth of spinal cord axons.[324] An ongoing clinical trial in Europe is looking at the safety and efficacy of intrathecal administration of the Nogo antibody after human SCI.

Other Therapies

Based on the monoamine theory of SCI,[130,131] catecholamine blockade has been tried in SCI with compounds such as α-methyltyrosine, phenoxybenzamine, or clonidine. Results from these experiments have been inconsistent.[131,220,249,325] Several other pharmacologic therapies have been used in the treatment of acute experimental SCI, and they have provided either limited data or conflicting results: urea,[326] levothyroxine,[327,328] dimethyl sulfoxide,[244,329] enzymes,[330] erythropoietin,[331] polyethylene glycol,[332] cyclosporine-A,[333] leupeptin,[334] and electrical fields.[335] Other potential therapies include the use of monoclonal antibodies directed against mediators of the secondary inflammatory response following SCI.[311]

Conclusion

Several promising compounds aimed at specific deleterious processes in SCI are presently on the horizon. Carefully conducted clinical trials of these various treatments are indicated after their efficacy is demonstrated from sound laboratory research. Annually, thousands of patients from the United States and around the world subject themselves to experimental treatments that are not only without good basic science justification, but also often result in doing more harm than good to the volunteer patients. We feel strongly that it is the moral and ethical obligation of the scientific and medical community to put their heads together and come up with more rigid guidelines regarding human experimentation that will not only potentially lead to better design and more effective studies, but, most important, safer opportunities for well-meaning patients and volunteers.

References

1. Bracken MB, Shepard MJ, Collins WF, et al: A randomized, controlled trial of methylprednisolone or naloxone in the treatment of acute spinal-cord injury: Results of the Second National Acute Spinal Cord Injury Study. *N Engl J Med* 1990; 322(20):1405-1411.
2. Griffiths IR, Miller R: Vascular permeability to protein and vasogenic oedema in experimental concussive injuries to the canine spinal cord. *J Neurol Sci* 1974;22(3):291-304.
3. Cook PL: Radiology of spine and spinal cord injury, in Illis LS, ed: *Spinal Cord Dysfunction: Assessment*. New York, NY, Oxford University Press, 1988, pp 41-103.
4. Tator CH: Spine-spinal cord relationships in spinal cord trauma. *Clin Neurosurg* 1983;30:479-494.
5. Jellinger K: Neuropathology of spinal cord injuries, in Vinken PJ, Bruyn GW, eds: *The Handbook of Clinical Neurology*. New York, NY, Elsevier, 1976, vol 25, pp 43-121.
6. Allen AR: Surgery of experimental lesion of spinal cord equivalent to crush injury of fracture dislocation of spinal column. *JAMA* 1911;57:878-880.
7. Blight AR: Cellular morphology of chronic spinal cord injury in the cat: Analysis of myelinated axons by line-sampling. *Neuroscience* 1983;10(2): 521-543.
8. Blight AR: Axonal physiology of chronic spinal cord injury in the cat: Intracellular recording in vitro. *Neuroscience* 1983;10(4):1471-1486.
9. Bresnahan JC, King JS, Martin GF, Yashon D: A neuroanatomical analysis of spinal cord injury in the rhesus monkey (Macaca mulatta). *J Neurol Sci* 1976;28(4):521-542.
10. Ducker TB, Kindt GW, Kempf LG: Pathological findings in acute experimental spinal cord trauma. *J Neurosurg* 1971;35(6):700-708.
11. Ford RW: A reproducible spinal cord injury model in the cat. *J Neurosurg* 1983;59(2): 268-275.
12. Wagner FC Jr, VanGilder JC, Dohrmann GJ: Pathological changes from acute to chronic in experimental spinal cord trauma. *J Neurosurg* 1978; 48(1):92-98.
13. Wrathall JR, Pettegrew RK, Harvey F: Spinal cord contusion in the rat: Production of graded, reproducible, injury groups. *Exp Neurol* 1985;88(1): 108-122.
14. Gruner JA: A monitored contusion model of spinal cord injury in the rat. *J Neurotrauma* 1992; 9(2):123-128.
15. Hall ED, Yonkers PA, McCall JM, Braughler JM: Effects of the 21-aminosteroid U74006F on experimental head injury in mice. *J Neurosurg* 1988; 68(3):456-461.
16. Holtz A, Nyström B, Gerdin B: Blocking weight-induced spinal cord injury in rats: Effects of TRH or naloxone on motor function recovery and spinal cord blood flow. *Acta Neurol Scand* 1989; 80(3):215-220.
17. Finkelstein SD, Gillespie JA, Markowitz RS, Johnson DD, Black P: Experimental spinal cord injury: Qualitative and quantitative histopathologic evaluation. *J Neurotrauma* 1990;7(1):29-40.
18. Gale K, Kerasidis H, Wrathall JR: Spinal cord contusion in the rat: Behavioral analysis of functional neurologic impairment. *Exp Neurol* 1985;88(1): 123-134.
19. Noble LJ, Wrathall JR: Spinal cord contusion in the rat: Morphometric analyses of alterations in the spinal cord. *Exp Neurol* 1985;88(1):135-149.
20. Noble LJ, Wrathall JR: Correlative analyses of lesion development and functional status after graded spinal cord contusive injuries in the rat. *Exp Neurol* 1989;103(1):34-40.
21. Panjabi MM, Wrathall JR: Biomechanical analysis of experimental spinal cord injury and functional loss. *Spine (Phila Pa 1976)* 1988;13(12): 1365-1370.
22. Bresnahan JC, Beattie MS, Todd FD III, Noyes DH: A behavioral and anatomical analysis of spinal cord injury produced by a feedback-controlled impaction device. *Exp Neurol* 1987; 95(3):548-570.
23. Noyes DH: Electromechanical impactor for producing experimental spinal cord injury in animals. *Med Biol Eng Comput* 1987;25(3):335-340.
24. Jakeman LB, Guan Z, Wei P, et al: Traumatic spinal cord injury produced by controlled contusion in mouse. *J Neurotrauma* 2000;17(4):299-319.
25. Stokes BT: Experimental spinal cord injury: A dynamic and verifiable injury device. *J Neurotrauma* 1992;9(2):129-134.
26. Scheff SW, Rabchevsky AG, Fugaccia I, Main JA, Lumpp JE Jr: Experimental modeling of spinal cord injury: Characterization of a force-defined injury device. *J Neurotrauma* 2003;20(2):179-193.

27. Tarlov IM, Klinger H, Vitale S: Spinal cord compression studies: I. Experimental techniques to produce acute and gradual compression in dogs. *AMA Arch Neurol Psychiatry* 1953;70(6):813-819.

28. Tator CH: Acute spinal cord injury in primates produced by an inflatable extradural cuff. *Can J Surg* 1973;16(3):222-231.

29. Khan M, Griebel R, Rozdilsky B, Politis M: Hemorrhagic changes in experimental spinal cord injury models. *Can J Neurol Sci* 1985;12(3): 259-262.

30. Croft TJ, Brodkey JS, Nulsen FE: Reversible spinal cord trauma: A model for electrical monitoring of spinal cord function. *J Neurosurg* 1972;36(4): 402-406.

31. Eidelberg E, Staten E, Watkins CJ, Smith JS: Treatment of experimental spinal cord injury in ferrets. *Surg Neurol* 1976;6(4):243-246.

32. Black P, Markowitz RS, Cooper V, et al: Models of spinal cord injury: Part 1. Static load technique. *Neurosurgery* 1986;19(5):752-762.

33. Rivlin AS, Tator CH: Effect of duration of acute spinal cord compression in a new acute cord injury model in the rat. *Surg Neurol* 1978;10(1): 39-43.

34. Rivlin AS, Tator CH: Regional spinal cord blood flow in rats after severe cord trauma. *J Neurosurg* 1978;49(6):844-853.

35. Dolan EJ, Tator CH: A new method for testing the force of clips for aneurysms or experimental spinal cord compression. *J Neurosurg* 1979;51(2): 229-233.

36. Joshi M, Fehlings MG: Development and characterization of a novel, graded model of clip compressive spinal cord injury in the mouse: Part 1. Clip design, behavioral outcomes, and histopathology. *J Neurotrauma* 2002;19(2):175-190.

37. Zivin JA, DeGirolami U: Spinal cord infarction: A highly reproducible stroke model. *Stroke* 1980; 11(2):200-202.

38. Balentine JD: Hypotheses in spinal cord trauma research, in Becker DP, Povlishock JT, eds: *Central Nervous System Trauma Status Report*. Bethesda, MD, National Institute of Neurological and Communicative Disorders and Stroke, 1985, pp 455-461.

39. Ducker TB: Experimental injury of the spinal cord, in Vinken PJ, Bruyn GW, eds: *Handbook of Clinical Neurology*. New York, NY, Elsevier, 1976, pp 9-26.

40. Green BA, Wagner FC Jr: Evolution of edema in the acutely injured spinal cord: A fluorescence microscopic study. *Surg Neurol* 1973;1(2):98-101.

41. Young W: Blood flow, metabolic and neurophysiological mechanisms in spinal cord injury, in Becker PB, Povlishock JT, eds: *Central Nervous System Trauma Status Report*. National Institute of Neurological and Communicative Disorders and Stroke, Bethesda, MD, 1985, pp 463-473.

42. D'Angelo CM, Van Gilder JC, Taub A: Evoked cortical potentials in experimental spinal cord trauma. *J Neurosurg* 1973;38(3):332-336.

43. Eidelberg E, Sullivan J, Brigham A: Immediate consequences of spinal cord injury: Possible role of potassium in axonal conduction block. *Surg Neurol* 1975;3(6):317-321.

44. Martin SH, Bloedel JR: Evaluation of experimental spinal cord injury using cortical evoked potentials. *J Neurosurg* 1973;39(1):75-81.

45. Singer JM, Russell GV, Coe JE: Changes in evoked potentials after experimental cervical spinal cord injury in the monkey. *Exp Neurol* 1970; 29(3):449-461.

46. Kobrine AI: The neuronal theory of experimental spinal cord dysfunction. *Surg Neurol* 1975;3(5): 261-264.

47. Vyklický L, Sykova E: The effects of increased extracellular potassium in the isolated spinal cord on the flexor reflex of the frog. *Neurosci Lett* 1980;19(2):203-207.

48. Young W, Koreh I, Yen V, Lindsay A: Effect of sympathectomy on extracellular potassium ionic activity and blood flow in experimental spinal cord contusion. *Brain Res* 1982;253(1-2):115-124.

49. Stokes BT, Fox P, Hollinden G: Extracellular metabolites: Their measurement and role in the acute phase of spinal cord injury, in Dacey RG Jr, Winn HR, Rimmel RW, et al, eds: *Trauma of the Central Nervous System*. New York, NY, Raven Press, 1985, pp 309-323.

50. Baker PF: The regulation of intracellular calcium. *Symp Soc Exp Biol* 1976;30:67-88.

51. Young W, Yen V, Blight AR: Extracellular calcium ionic activity in experimental spinal cord contusion. *Brain Res* 1982;253(1-2):105-113.

52. Young W, Flamm ES: Effect of high-dose corticosteroid therapy on blood flow, evoked potentials, and extracellular calcium in experimental spinal injury. *J Neurosurg* 1982;57(5):667-673.

53. Stokes BT, Garwood M: Traumatically induced alterations in the oxygen fields in the canine spinal cord. *Exp Neurol* 1982;75(3):665-677.

54. Ducker TB, Salcman M, Perot PL Jr, Ballantine D: Experimental spinal cord trauma, I: Correlation of blood flow, tissue oxygen and neurologic status in the dog. *Surg Neurol* 1978;10(1):60-63.

55. Hayashi N, de la Torre JC, Green BA: Regional spinal cord blood flow and tissue oxygen content after spinal cord trauma. *Surg Forum* 1980;31: 461-463.

56. Kelly DL Jr, Lassiter KR, Calogero JA, Alexander E Jr: Effects of local hypothermia and tissue oxygen

studies in experimental paraplegia. *J Neurosurg* 1970;33(5):554-563.

57. Anderson DK, Means ED, Waters TR, Spears CJ: Spinal cord energy metabolism following compression trauma to the feline spinal cord. *J Neurosurg* 1980;53(3):375-380.
58. Kahn T, Green B, Raimondi AJ: Energy metabolism of acutely injured spinal cord of cat. *J Neuropathol Exp Neurol* 1975;34:84-85.
59. Walker JG, Yates RR, O'Neill JJ, Yashon D: Canine spinal cord energy state after experimental trauma. *J Neurochem* 1977;29(5):929-932.
60. Walker JG, Yates RR, Yashon D: Regional canine spinal cord energy state after experimental trauma. *J Neurochem* 1979;33(1):397-401.
61. Locke GE, Yashon D, Feldman RA, Hunt WE: Ischemia in primate spinal cord injury. *J Neurosurg* 1971;34(5):614-617.
62. Rosenthal M, LaManna J, Yamada S, Younts W, Somjen G: Oxidative metabolism, extracellular potassium and sustained potential shifts in cat spinal cord in situ. *Brain Res* 1979;162(1):113-127.
63. Yamada S, Sanders DC, Maeda G: Oxidative metabolism during and following ischemia of cat spinal cord. *Neurol Res* 1981;3(1):1-16.
64. Clendenon NR, Allen N, Gordon WA, Bingham WG Jr: Inhibition of Na+-K+-activated ATPase activity following experimental spinal cord trauma. *J Neurosurg* 1978;49(4):563-568.
65. Rawe SE, Lee WA, Perot PL: Spinal cord glucose utilization after experimental spinal cord injury. *Neurosurgery* 1981;9(1):40-47.
66. Allen AR: Remarks on the histopathological changes in the spinal cord due to impact: An experimental study. *J Nerv Ment Dis* 1914;41:141-147.
67. Balentine JD: Pathology of experimental spinal cord trauma: I. The necrotic lesion as a function of vascular injury. *Lab Invest* 1978;39(3):236-253.
68. Balentine JD: Pathology of experimental spinal cord trauma: II. Ultrastructure of axons and myelin. *Lab Invest* 1978;39(3):254-266.
69. Dohrmann GJ, Wagner FC Jr, Bucy PC: The microvasculature in transitory traumatic paraplegia: An electron microscopic study in the monkey. *J Neurosurg* 1971;35:263-271.
70. Dohrmann GJ, Wagner FC Jr, Bucy PC: Transitory traumatic paraplegia: Electron microscopy of early alterations in myelinated nerve fibers. *J Neurosurg* 1972;36(4):407-415.
71. Wagner FC, Dohrmann GJ, Bucy PC: Histopathology of transitory traumatic paraplegia in the monkey. *J Neurosurg* 1971;35:272-276.
72. McVeigh JF: Experimental cord crushes with special references to the mechanical factors involved and subsequent changes in the areas affected. *Arch Surg* 1923;7:573-600.
73. Balentine JD, Hilton CW: Ultrastructural pathology of axons and myelin in calcium-induced myelopathy. *J Neuropathol Exp Neurol* 1980;39:339-345.
74. Bresnahan JC: An electron-microscopic analysis of axonal alterations following blunt contusion of the spinal cord of the rhesus monkey (Macaca mulatta). *J Neurol Sci* 1978;37(1-2):59-82.
75. Blight AR: Delayed demyelination and macrophage invasion: A candidate for secondary cell damage in spinal cord injury. *Cent Nerv Syst Trauma* 1985;2(4):299-315.
76. Means ED, Anderson DK: Neuronophagia by leukocytes in experimental spinal cord injury. *J Neuropathol Exp Neurol* 1983;42(6):707-719.
77. Hall ED, Wolf DL: Post-traumatic spinal cord ischemia: Relationship to injury severity and physiological parameters. *Cent Nerv Syst Trauma* 1987;4(1):15-25.
78. Lohse DC, Senter HJ, Kauer JS, Wohns R: Spinal cord blood flow in experimental transient traumatic paraplegia. *J Neurosurg* 1980;52(3):335-345.
79. Senter HJ, Venes JL: Altered blood flow and secondary injury in experimental spinal cord trauma. *J Neurosurg* 1978;49(4):569-578.
80. Young W, Flamm ES, Demopoulos HB, Tomasula JJ, DeCrescito V: Effect of naloxone on posttraumatic ischemia in experimental spinal contusion. *J Neurosurg* 1981;55(2):209-219.
81. Ducker TB, Salcman M, Lucas JT, Garrison WB, Perot PL Jr: Experimental spinal cord trauma, II: Blood flow, tissue oxygen, evoked potentials in both paretic and plegic monkeys. *Surg Neurol* 1978;10(1):64-70.
82. Flamm ES, Young W, Demopoulos HB, DeCrescito V, Tomasula JJ: Experimental spinal cord injury: Treatment with naloxone. *Neurosurgery* 1982;10(2):227-231.
83. Black P, Markowitz RS: Experimental spinal cord injury in monkeys: Comparison of steroids and local hypothermia. *Surg Forum* 1971;22:409-411.
84. Faden AI, Jacobs TP, Holaday JW: Opiate antagonist improves neurologic recovery after spinal injury. *Science* 1981;211(4481):493-494.
85. Faden AI, Jacobs TP, Mougey E, Holaday JW: Endorphins in experimental spinal injury: Therapeutic effect of naloxone. *Ann Neurol* 1981;10(4):326-332.
86. Faden AI, Jacobs TP, Holaday JW: Thyrotropin-releasing hormone improves neurologic recovery after spinal trauma in cats. *N Engl J Med* 1981;305(18):1063-1067.

87. Faden AI, Jacobs TP, Holaday JW: Comparison of early and late naloxone treatment in experimental spinal injury. *Neurology* 1982;32(6):677-681.

88. Faden AI, Simon RP: A potential role for excitotoxins in the pathophysiology of spinal cord injury. *Ann Neurol* 1988;23(6):623-626.

89. Green BA, Kahn T, Klose KJ: A comparative study of steroid therapy in acute experimental spinal cord injury. *Surg Neurol* 1980;13(2):91-97.

90. Hall ED, Braughler JM: Acute effects of intravenous glucocorticoid pretreatment on the in vitro peroxidation of cat spinal cord tissue. *Exp Neurol* 1981;73(1):321-324.

91. Hall ED, Braughler JM: Glucocorticoid mechanisms in acute spinal cord injury: A review and therapeutic rationale. *Surg Neurol* 1982;18(5): 320-327.

92. Means ED, Anderson DK, Waters TR, Kalaf L: Effect of methylprednisolone in compression trauma to the feline spinal cord. *J Neurosurg* 1981;55(2):200-208.

93. Marshall LF, Knowlton S, Garfin SR, et al: Deterioration following spinal cord injury: A multicenter study. *J Neurosurg* 1987;66(3):400-404.

94. Philippi R, Kuhn W, Zäch GA, Jacob-Chia D, Dollfus P, Molé JP: Survey of the neurological evolution of 300 spinal cord injuries seen within 24 hours after injury. *Paraplegia* 1980;18(5): 337-346.

95. Geisler FH, Dorsey FC, Coleman WP: Recovery of motor function after spinal-cord injury—a randomized, placebo-controlled trial with GM-1 ganglioside. *N Engl J Med* 1991;324(26):1829-1838.

96. Klatzo I: Presidental address: Neuropathological aspects of brain edema. *J Neuropathol Exp Neurol* 1967;26(1):1-14.

97. Němecek S, Petr R, Suba P, Rozsival V, Mělka O: Longitudinal extension of oedema in experimental spinal cord injury—evidence for two types of post-traumatic oedema. *Acta Neurochir (Wien)* 1977;37(1-2):7-16.

98. Wagner FC Jr, Stewart WB: Effect of trauma dose on spinal cord edema. *J Neurosurg* 1981;54(6): 802-806.

99. Yashon D, Bingham WG Jr, Faddoul EM, Hunt WE: Edema of the spinal cord following experimental impact trauma. *J Neurosurg* 1973;38(6): 693-697.

100. Studer RK, Welch DM, Siegel BA: Transient alteration of the blood-brain barrier: Effect of hypertonic solutions administered via carotid artery injection. *Exp Neurol* 1974;44(2):266-273.

101. Beggs JL, Waggener JD: Transendothelial vesicular transport of protein following compression injury to the spinal cord. *Lab Invest* 1976;34(4):428-439.

102. Hirano A, Becker NH, Zimmerman HM: Pathological alterations in the cerebral endothelial cell barrier to peroxidase. *Arch Neurol* 1969;20(3): 300-308.

103. Assenmacher DR, Ducker TB: Experimental traumatic paraplegia: The vascular and pathological changes seen in reversible and irreversible spinal-cord lesions. *J Bone Joint Surg Am* 1971;53(4): 671-680.

104. Dohrmann GJ, Wick KM, Bucy PC: Spinal cord blood flow patterns in experimental traumatic paraplegia. *J Neurosurg* 1973;38(1):52-58.

105. Sandler AN, Tator CH: Review of the effect of spinal cord trama on the vessels and blood flow in the spinal cord. *J Neurosurg* 1976;45(6): 638-646.

106. Fried LC, Aparicio O: Experimental ischemia of the spinal cord: Histologic studies after anterior spinal artery occlusion. *Neurology* 1973;23(3): 289-293.

107. Fehlings MG, Tator CH, Linden RD: The relationship among the severity of spinal cord injury, motor and somatosensory evoked potentials and spinal cord blood flow. *Eletroencephalogr Clin Neurophysiol* 1989;74(4):241-259.

108. Kelly DL Jr, Lassiter KR, Vongsvivut A, Smith JM: Effects of hyperbaric oxygenation and tissue oxygen studies in experimental paraplegia. *J Neurosurg* 1972;36(4):425-429.

109. Hickey R, Albin MS, Bunegin L, Gelineau J: Autoregulation of spinal cord blood flow: Is the cord a microcosm of the brain? *Stroke* 1986;17(6): 1183-1189.

110. Kobrine AI, Doyle TF, Martins AN: Autoregulation of spinal cord blood flow. *Clin Neurosurg* 1975;22:573-581.

111. Marcus ML, Heistad DD, Ehrhardt JC, Abboud FM: Regulation of total and regional spinal cord blood flow. *Circ Res* 1977;41(1):128-134.

112. Senter HJ, Venes JL: Loss of autoregulation and posttraumatic ischemia following experimental spinal cord trauma. *J Neurosurg* 1979;50(2): 198-206.

113. Smith DR, Smith HJ, Rajjoub RK: Measurement of spinal cord blood flow by the microsphere technique. *Neurosurgery* 1978;2(1):27-30.

114. Smith AJ, McCreery DB, Bloedel JR, Chou SN: Hyperemia, CO2 responsiveness, and autoregulation in the white matter following experimental spinal cord injury. *J Neurosurg* 1978;48(2): 239-251.

115. Ducker TB, Assenmacher DR: Microvascular response to experimental spinal cord trauma. *Surg Forum* 1969;20:428-430.

116. Dohrmann GJ, Wick KM: Intramedullary blood flow patterns in transitory traumatic paraplegia. *Surg Neurol* 1973;1(4):209-215.

117. Fairholm DJ, Turnbull IM: Microangiographic study of experimental spinal cord injuries. *J Neurosurg* 1971;35:277-286.

118. Fried LC, Goodkin R: Microangiographic observations of the experimentally traumatized spinal cord. *J Neurosurg* 1971;35(6):709-714.

119. Heymann MA, Payne BD, Hoffman JI, Rudolph AM: Blood flow measurements with radionuclide-labeled particles. *Prog Cardiovasc Dis* 1977;20(1): 55-79.

120. Aukland K, Bower BF, Berliner RW: Measurement of local blood flow with hydrogen gas. *Circ Res* 1964;14:164-187.

121. Kobrine AI, Doyle TF, Martins AN: Local spinal cord blood flow in experimental traumatic myelopathy. *J Neurosurg* 1975;42(2):144-149.

122. Bingham WG, Goldman H, Friedman SJ, Murphy S, Yashon D, Hunt WE: Blood flow in normal and injured monkey spinal cord. *J Neurosurg* 1975; 43(2):162-171.

123. Reivich M, Jehle J, Sokoloff L, Kety SS: Measurement of regional cerebral blood flow with antipyrine-14C in awake cats. *J Appl Physiol* 1969; 27(2):296-300.

124. Lindsberg PJ, O'Neill JT, Paakkari IA, Hallenbeck JM, Feuerstein G: Validation of laser-Doppler flowmetry in measurement of spinal cord blood flow. *Am J Physiol* 1989;257(2 Pt 2):H674-H680.

125. Stern MD: In vivo evaluation of microcirculation by coherent light scattering. *Nature* 1975; 254(5495):56-58.

126. Cawthon DF, Senter HJ, Stewart WB: Comparison of hydrogen clearance and 14C-antipyrine autoradiography in the measurement of spinal cord blood flow after severe impact injury. *J Neurosurg* 1980;52(6):801-807.

127. Gelfan S, Tarlov IM: Differential vulnerability of spinal cord structures to anoxia. *J Neurophysiol* 1955;18(2):170-188.

128. Kobrine AI, Evans DE, Rizzoli HV: The effects of ischemia on long-tract neural conduction in the spinal cord. *J Neurosurg* 1979;50(5):639-644.

129. Kobrine AI, Evans DE, Rizzoli HV: Effects of progressive hypoxia on long tract neural conduction in the spinal cord. *Neurosurgery* 1980;7(4): 369-375.

130. Osterholm JL, Mathews GJ: Altered norepinephrine metabolism following experimental spinal cord injury: 1. Relationship to hemorrhagic necrosis and post-wounding neurological deficits. *J Neurosurg* 1972;36(4):386-394.

131. Osterholm JL, Mathews GJ: Altered norepinephrine metabolism, following experimental spinal cord injury: 2. Protection against traumatic spinal cord hemorrhagic necrosis by norepinephrine synthesis blockade with alpha methyl tyrosine. *J Neurosurg* 1972;36(4):395-401.

132. Albin MS, Bunegin L: Catecholamine synthesis rates in traumatized spinal cord. *Anat Rec* 1974; 178:296-297.

133. Bingham WG, Ruffolo R, Friedman SJ: Catecholamine levels in the injured spinal cord of monkeys. *J Neurosurg* 1975;42(2):174-178.

134. Bunegin L, Albin MS, Jannetta PJ: Catecholamine responses to experimental spinal cord impact injury: I. Intrinsic spinal cord synthesis rates. *Exp Neurol* 1976;53(1):274-280.

135. de la Torre JC, Johnson CM, Harris LH, Kajihara K, Mullan S: Monoamine changes in experimental head and spinal cord trauma: Failure to confirm previous observations. *Surg Neurol* 1974;2(1): 5-11.

136. Felten DL, Hall PV, Campbell RL, Kalsbeck JE: A histochemical investigation of catecholamines in spinal cord injury. *J Neural Transm* 1976;39(3): 209-221.

137. Hedeman LS, Shellenberger MK, Gordon JH: Studies in experimental spinal cord trauma: 1. Alterations in catecholamine levels. *J Neurosurg* 1974;40(1):37-43.

138. Rawe SE, Roth RH, Boadle-Biber M, Collins WF: Norepinephrine levels in experimental spinal cord trauma: Part 1. Biochemical study of hemorrhagic necrosis. *J Neurosurg* 1977;46(3):342-349.

139. Rawe SE, Roth RH, Collins WF: Norepinephrine levels in experimental spinal cord trauma: Part 2. Histopathological study of hemorrhagic necrosis. *J Neurosurg* 1977;46(3):350-357.

140. Brodner RA, Dohrmann GJ, Roth RH: Intramedullary serotonin patters following experimental spinal cord trauma. *Mt Sinai J Med* 1977;44(2): 213-217.

141. Naftchi NE, Demeny M, DeCrescito V, Tomasula JJ, Flamm ES, Campbell JB: Biogenic amine concentrations in traumatized spinal cords of cats: Effect of drug therapy. *J Neurosurg* 1974;40(1): 52-57.

142. Zivin JA, Doppman JL, Reid JL, et al: Biochemical and histochemical studies of biogenic amines in spinal cord trauma. *Neurology* 1976;26(2):99-107.

143. Cheung JY, Bonventre JV, Malis CD, Leaf A: Calcium and ischemic injury. *N Engl J Med* 1986; 314(26):1670-1676.

144. Farber JL: Biology of disease: Membrane injury and calcium homeostasis in the pathogenesis of coagulative necrosis. *Lab Invest* 1982;47(2): 114-123.

145. Schanne FA, Kane AB, Young EE, Farber JL: Calcium dependence of toxic cell death: A final common pathway. *Science* 1979;206(4419):700-702.

146. McLean AE, McLean E, Judah JD: Cellular necrosis in the liver induced and modified by drugs. *Int Rev Exp Pathol* 1965;4:127-157.

147. Zimmerman AN, Hülsmann WC: Paradoxical influence of calcium ions on the permeability of the cell membranes of the isolated rat heart. *Nature* 1966;211(5049):646-647.

148. Zimmerman AN, Daems W, Hülsmann WC, et al: Morphological changes of heart muscle caused by successive perfusion with calcium-free and calcium-containing solutions (calcium paradox). *Cardiovasc Res* 1967;1:201-209.

149. Balentine JD, Spector M: Calcification of axons in experimental spinal cord trauma. *Ann Neurol* 1977;2(6):520-523.

150. Balentine JD: Axonal calcification in spinal cord injury of humans, monkeys and cats. *Lab Invest* 1980;42:99.

151. Happel RD, Smith KP, Banik NL, Powers JM, Hogan EL, Balentine JD: Ca2+-accumulation in experimental spinal cord trauma. *Brain Res* 1981; 211(2):476-479.

152. Balentine JD, Dean DL Jr: Calcium-induced spongiform and necrotizing myelopathy. *Lab Invest* 1982;47(3):286-295.

153. Dienel GA: Regional accumulation of calcium in postischemic rat brain. *J Neurochem* 1984;43(4): 913-925.

154. Simon RP, Griffiths T, Evans MC, Swan JH, Meldrum BS: Calcium overload in selectively vulnerable neurons of the hippocampus during and after ischemia: An electron microscopy study in the rat. *J Cereb Blood Flow Metab* 1984;4(3): 350-361.

155. Lehninger AL: Mitochondria and calcium ion transport. *Biochem J* 1970;119(2):129-138.

156. Banik NL, Hogan EL, Powers JM, Whetstine LJ: Degradation of cytoskeletal proteins in experimental spinal cord injury. *Neurochem Res* 1982; 7(12):1465-1475.

157. Banik NL, Hogan EL, Whetstine LJ, Balentine JD: Changes in myelin and axonal proteins in CaCl2-induced myelopathy in rat spinal cord. *Cent Nerv Syst Trauma* 1984;1(2):131-137.

158. Rasmussen H: The calcium messenger system (1). *N Engl J Med* 1986;314(17):1094-1101.

159. Holaday JW, Faden AI: Naloxone acts at central opiate receptors to reverse hypotension, hypothermia and hypoventilation in spinal shock. *Brain Res* 1980;189(1):295-300.

160. Long JB, Martinez-Arizala A, Petras JM, Holaday JW: Endogenous opioids in spinal cord injury: A critical evaluation. *Cent Nerv Syst Trauma* 1986; 3(4):295 315.

161. Paterson SJ, Robson LE, Kosterlitz HW: Classification of opioid receptors. *Br Med Bull* 1983;39(1): 31-36.

162. Faden AI, Molineaux CJ, Rosenberger JG, Jacobs TP, Cox BM: Endogenous opioid immunoreactivity in rat spinal cord following traumatic injury. *Ann Neurol* 1985;17(4):386-390.

163. Krumins SA, Faden AI: Traumatic injury alters opiate receptor binding in rat spinal cord. *Ann Neurol* 1986;19(5):498-501.

164. Behrmann DL, Bresnahan JC, Beattie MS: A comparison of YM-14673, U-50488H, and nalmefene after spinal cord injury in the rat. *Exp Neurol* 1993;119(2):258-267.

165. Faden AI, Jacobs TP: Opiate antagonist WIN44,441-3 stereospecifically improves neurologic recovery after ischemic spinal injury. *Neurology* 1985;35(9):1311-1315.

166. Faden AI, Takemori AE, Portoghese PS: Kappa-selective opiate antagonist nor-binaltorphimine improves outcome after traumatic spinal cord injury in rats. *Cent Nerve Syst Trauma* 1987;4(4): 227-237.

167. Faden AI, Jacobs TP: Dynorphin-related peptides cause motor dysfunction in the rat through a non-opiate action. *Br J Pharmacol* 1984;81(2): 271-276.

168. Long JB, Petras JM, Mobley WC, Holaday JW: Neurological dysfunction after intrathecal injection of dynorphin A (1-13) in the rat: II. Nonopioid mechanisms mediate loss of motor, sensory and autonomic function. *J Pharmacol Exp Ther* 1988;246(3):1167-1174.

169. Przewłocki R, Shearman GT, Herz A: Mixed opioid/nonopioid effects of dynorphin and dynorphin related peptides after their intrathecal injection in rats. *Neuropeptides* 1983;3(3):233-240.

170. Long JB, Rigamonti DD, de Costa B, Rice KC, Martinez-Arizala A: Dynorphin A-induced rat hindlimb paralysis and spinal cord injury are not altered by the kappa opioid antagonist nor-binaltorphimine. *Brain Res* 1989;497(1):155-162.

171. Stevens CW, Yaksh TL: Dynorphin A and related peptides administered intrathecally in the rat: A search for putative kappa opiate receptor activity. *J Pharmacol Exp Ther* 1986;238(3):833-838.

172. Martinez-Arizala A, Long JB, Holaday JW: TRH fails to antagonize the acute paralytic effects of intrathecal dynorphin A and substance P antagonists in the rat. *Brain Res* 1988;473(2):385-388.

173. Long JB, Kinney RC, Malcolm DS, Graeber GM, Holaday JW: Intrathecal dynorphin A1-13 and

dynorphin A3-13 reduce rat spinal cord blood flow by non-opioid mechanisms. *Brain Res* 1987; 436(2):374-379.

174. Del Maestro RF: An approach to free radicals in medicine and biology. *Acta Physiol Scand Suppl* 1980;492:153-168.

175. Demopoulos HB, Flamm ES, Pietronegro DD, Seligman ML: The free radical pathology and the microcirculation in the major central nervous system disorders. *Acta Physiol Scand Suppl* 1980;492: 91-119.

176. Watson BD, Busto R, Goldberg WJ, Santiso M, Yoshida S, Ginsberg MD: Lipid peroxidation in vivo induced by reversible global ischemia in rat brain. *J Neurochem* 1984;42(1):268-274.

177. Yoshida S, Abe K, Busto R, Watson BD, Kogure K, Ginsberg MD: Influence of transient ischemia on lipid-soluble antioxidants, free fatty acids and energy metabolites in rat brain. *Brain Res* 1982; 245(2):307-316.

178. Kontos HA, Povlishock JT: Oxygen radicals in brain injury. *Cent Nerv Syst Trauma* 1986;3(4): 257-263.

179. Kurihara M: Role of monoamines in experimental spinal cord injury in rats: Relationship between Na+-K+-ATPase and lipid peroxidation. *J Neurosurg* 1985;62(5):743-749.

180. Milvy P, Kakari S, Campbell JB, Demopoulos HB: Paramagnetic species and radical products in cat spinal cord. *Ann N Y Acad Sci* 1973;222: 1102-1111.

181. Anderson DK, Saunders RD, Demediuk P, et al: Lipid hydrolysis and peroxidation in injured spinal cord: Partial protection with methylprednisolone or vitamin E and selenium. *Cent Nerv Syst Trauma* 1985;2(4):257-267.

182. Hall ED, Braughler JM: Effects of intravenous methylprednisolone on spinal cord lipid peroxidation and Na+ + K+)-ATPase activity: Dose-response analysis during 1st hour after contusion injury in the cat. *J Neurosurg* 1982;57(2):247-253.

183. Pietronigro DD, Hovsepian M, Demopoulos HB, Flamm ES: Loss of ascorbic acid from injured feline spinal cord. *J Neurochem* 1983;41(4): 1072-1076.

184. Saunders RD, Dugan LL, Demediuk P, Means ED, Horrocks LA, Anderson DK: Effects of methylprednisolone and the combination of alpha-tocopherol and selenium on arachidonic acid metabolism and lipid peroxidation in traumatized spinal cord tissue. *J Neurochem* 1987;49(1):24-31.

185. Anderson DK, Hall ED, Braughler JM, McCall JM, Means ED: Effect of delayed administration of U74006F (tirilazad mesylate) on recovery of locomotor function after experimental spinal cord injury. *J Neurotrauma* 1991;8(3):187-192.

186. Kleihues P, Kobayashi K, Hossmann KA: Purine nucleotide metabolism in the cat brain after one hour of complete ischemia. *J Neurochem* 1974; 23(2):417-425.

187. McCord JM, Fridovich I: The reduction of cytochrome c by milk xanthine oxidase. *J Biol Chem* 1968;243(21):5753-5760.

188. McCord JM: Oxygen-derived radicals: A link between reperfusion injury and inflammation. *Fed Proc* 1987;46(7):2402-2406.

189. Misra HP, Fridovich I: The role of superoxide anion in the autoxidation of epinephrine and a simple assay for superoxide dismutase. *J Biol Chem* 1972;247(10):3170-3175.

190. Anderson DK, Means ED: Lipid peroxidation in the spinal cord: FeCl2 induction and protection with antioxidants. *Neurochem Pathol* 1983;1: 249-264.

191. Aust SD, Morehouse LA, Thomas CE: Role of metals in oxygen radical reactions. *J Free Radic Biol Med* 1985;1(1):3-25.

192. Sadrzadeh SM, Graf E, Panter SS, Hallaway PE, Eaton JW: Hemoglobin: A biologic fenton reagent. *J Biol Chem* 1984;259(23):14354-14356.

193. Fong KL, McCay PB, Poyer JL, Keele BB, Misra H: Evidence that peroxidation of lysosomal membranes is initiated by hydroxyl free radicals produced during flavin enzyme activity. *J Biol Chem* 1973;248(22):7792-7797.

194. Chan PH, Fishman RA: Brain edema: Induction in cortical slices by polyunsaturated fatty acids. *Science* 1978;201(4353):358-360.

195. Chan PH, Fishman RA: Transient formation of superoxide radicals in polyunsaturated fatty acid-induced brain swelling. *J Neurochem* 1980;35(4): 1004-1007.

196. Olney JW: Brain lesions, obesity, and other disturbances in mice treated with monosodium glutamate. *Science* 1969;164(880):719-721.

197. Rothman SM, Olney JW: Glutamate and the pathophysiology of hypoxic-ischemic brain damage. *Ann Neurol* 1986;19(2):105-111.

198. Faden AI, Demediuk P, Panter SS, Vink R: The role of excitatory amino acids and NMDA receptors in traumatic brain injury. *Science* 1989; 244(4906):798-800.

199. Hao JX, Watson BD, Xu XJ, Wiesenfeld-Hallin Z, Seiger A, Sundström E: Protective effect of the NMDA antagonist MK-801 on photochemically induced spinal lesions in the rat. *Exp Neurol* 1992;118(2):143-152.

200. Pencalet P, Ohanna F, Poulat P, Kamenka JM, Privat A: Thienylphencyclidine protection for the spinal cord of adult rats against extension of lesions secondary to a photochemical injury. *J Neurosurg* 1993;78(4):603-609.

201. Wrathall JR, Teng YD, Choiniere D, Mundt DJ: Evidence that local non-NMDA receptors contribute to functional deficits in contusive spinal cord injury. *Brain Res* 1992;586(1):140-143.

202. Wrathall JR, Bouzoukis J, Choiniere D: Effect of kynurenate on functional deficits resulting from traumatic spinal cord injury. *Eur J Pharmacol* 1992;218(2-3):273-281.

203. Rothman SM, Olney JW: Excitotoxicity and the NMDA receptor. *Trends Neurosci* 1987;10: 299-302.

204. Simon RP, Swan JH, Griffiths T, Meldrum BS: Blockade of N-methyl-D-aspartate receptors may protect against ischemic damage in the brain. *Science* 1984;226(4676):850-852.

205. Panter SS, Yum SW, Faden AI: Alteration in extracellular amino acids after traumatic spinal cord injury. *Ann Neurol* 1990;27(1):96-99.

206. Faden AI, Sacksen I, Noble LJ: Opiate-receptor antagonist nalmefene improves neurological recovery after traumatic spinal cord injury in rats through a central mechanism. *J Pharmacol Exp Ther* 1988;245(2):742-748.

207. Kochhar A, Zivin JA, Lyden PD, Mazzarella V: Glutamate antagonist therapy reduces neurologic deficits produced by focal central nervous system ischemia. *Arch Neurol* 1988;45(2):148-153.

208. Martinez-Arizala A, Rigamonti DD, Long JB, Kraimer JM, Holaday JW: Effects of NMDA receptor antagonists following spinal ischemia in the rabbit. *Exp Neurol* 1990;108(3):232-240.

209. Yu CG, Jagid J, Ruenes G, Dietrich WD, Marcillo AE, Yezierski RP: Detrimental effects of systemic hyperthermia on locomotor function and histopathological outcome after traumatic spinal cord injury in the rat. *Neurosurgery* 2001;49(1): 152-159.

210. Yu CG, Jimenez O, Marcillo AE, et al: Beneficial effects of modest systemic hypothermia on locomotor function and histopathological damage following contusion-induced spinal cord injury in rats. *J Neurosurg* 2001;93(1, Suppl):85-93.

211. Demediuk P, Faden AI: Traumatic spinal cord injury in rats causes increases in tissue thromboxane but not peptidoleukotrienes. *J Neurosci Res* 1988;20(1):115-121.

212. Hsu CY, Halushka PV, Hogan EL, Banik NL, Lee WA, Perot PL Jr: Alteration of thromboxane and prostacyclin levels in experimental spinal cord injury. *Neurology* 1985;35(7):1003-1009.

213. Moreland DB, Soloniuk DS, Feldman MJ: Leukotrienes in experimental spinal cord injury. *Surg Neurol* 1989;31(4):277-280.

214. Eidelberg E, Straehley D, Ersparmer R, Watkins CJ: Relationship between residual hindlimb-assisted locomotion and surviving axons after incomplete spinal cord injuries. *Exp Neurol* 1977; 56(2):312-322.

215. Windle WF, Smart JO, Beers JJ: Residual function after subtotal spinal cord transection in adult cats. *Neurology* 1958;8(7):518-521.

216. Meyer JS, Hunter J: Effects of hypothermia on local blood flow and metabolism during cerebral ischemia and hypoxia. *J Neurosurg* 1957;14(2): 210-227.

217. Rosomoff HL, Gilbert R: Brain volume and cerebrospinal fluid pressure during hypothermia. *Am J Physiol* 1955;183(1):19-22.

218. Albin MS, White RJ, Acosta-Rua G, Yashon D: Study of functional recovery produced by delayed localized cooling after spinal cord injury in primates. *J Neurosurg* 1968;29(2):113-120.

219. Green BA, Khan T, Raimondi AJ: Local hypothermia as treatment of experimentally induced spinal cord contusion: Quantitative analysis of beneficient effect. *Surg Forum* 1973;24:436-438.

220. Howitt WM, Turnbull IM: Effects of hypothermia and methysergide on recovery from experimental paraplegia. *Can J Surg* 1972;15(3):179-186.

221. Clifton GL, Miller ER, Choi SC, et al: Lack of effect of induction of hypothermia after acute brain injury. *N Engl J Med* 2001;344(8):556-563.

222. Polin RA, Randis TM, Sahni R: Systemic hypothermia to decrease morbidity of hypoxic-ischemic brain injury. *J Perinatol* 2007;27 (Suppl 1):S47-S58.

223. Friberg H, Rubertsson S: Therapeutic hypothermia after cardiac arrest seems to protect the brain: Treatment should be according to protocol, and treatment data registered. *Lakartidningen* 2007; 104(8):570-571.

224. Pearse DD, Barakat DJ: Cellular repair strategies for spinal cord injury. *Expert Opin Biol Ther* 2006; 6(7):639-652.

225. Bunge MB: Bridging the transected or contused adult rat spinal cord with Schwann cell and olfactory ensheathing glia transplants. *Prog Brain Res* 2002;137:275-282.

226. Féron F, Perry C, Cochrane J, et al: Autologous olfactory ensheathing cell transplantation in human spinal cord injury. *Brain* 2005;128(Pt 12): 2951-2960.

227. Lu J, Féron F, Mackay-Sim A, Waite PM: Olfactory ensheathing cells promote locomotor recovery after delayed transplantation into transected spinal cord. *Brain* 2002;125(Pt 1):14-21.

228. Syková E, Homola A, Mazanec R, et al: Autologous bone marrow transplantation in patients with subacute and chronic spinal cord injury. *Cell Transplant* 2006;15(8-9):675-687.

229. Reier PJ, Stokes BT, Thompson FJ, Anderson DK: Fetal cell grafts into resection and contusion/

compression injuries of the rat and cat spinal cord. *Exp Neurol* 1992;115(1):177-188.

230. Ruitenberg MJ, Plant GW, Hamers FP, et al: Ex vivo adenoviral vector-mediated neurotrophin gene transfer to olfactory ensheathing glia: Effects on rubrospinal tract regeneration, lesion size, and functional recovery after implantation in the injured rat spinal cord. *J Neurosci* 2003;23(18): 7045-7058.
231. Cao Q, Xu XM, Devries WH, et al: Functional recovery in traumatic spinal cord injury after transplantation of multineurotrophin-expressing glial-restricted precursor cells. *J Neurosci* 2005; 25(30):6947-6957.
232. Wirth ED III, Reier PJ, Fessler RG, et al: Feasibility and safety of neural tissue transplantation in patients with syringomyelia. *J Neurotrauma* 2001; 18(9):911-929.
233. Thompson FJ, Reier PJ, Uthman B, et al: Neurophysiological assessment of the feasibility and safety of neural tissue transplantation in patients with syringomyelia. *J Neurotrauma* 2001;18(9): 931-945.
234. Bomstein Y, Marder JB, Vitner K, et al: Features of skin-coincubated macrophages that promote recovery from spinal cord injury. *J Neuroimmunol* 2003;142(1-2):10-16.
235. Rapalino O, Lazarov-Spiegler O, Agranov E, et al: Implantation of stimulated homologous macrophages results in partial recovery of paraplegic rats. *Nat Med* 1998;4(7):814-821.
236. Knoller N, Auerbach G, Fulga V, et al: Clinical experience using incubated autologous macrophages as a treatment for complete spinal cord injury: Phase I study results. *J Neurosurg Spine* 2005;3(3):173-181.
237. La Rosa G, Conti A, Cardali S, Cacciola F, Tomasello F: Does early decompression improve neurological outcome of spinal cord injured patients? Appraisal of the literature using a meta-analytical approach. *Spinal Cord* 2004;42(9):503-512.
238. Tator CH: Review of treatment trials in human spinal cord injury: Issues, difficulties, and recommendations. *Neurosurgery* 2006;59(5):957-987.
239. Vaccaro AR, Daugherty RJ, Sheehan TP, et al: Neurologic outcome of early versus late surgery for cervical spinal cord injury. *Spine (Phila Pa 1976)* 1997;22(22):2609-2613.
240. Fishman RA: *Cerebrospinal Fluid in Diseases of the Nervous System*. Philadelphia, PA, WB Saunders, 1980, pp 107-128.
241. Haynes RC, Murad F: Adrenocortical steroids and their synthetic analogs: Inhibitors of adrenocortical steroid biosynthesis, in Goodman AG, Goodman LS, Rall TW, et al, eds: *The Pharmacological Basis of Therapeutics*. New York, NY, Macmillan, 1985, pp 1459-1489.
242. Braughler JM: Lipid peroxidation-induced inhibition of gamma-aminobutyric acid uptake in rat brain synaptosomes: Protection by glucocorticoids. *J Neurochem* 1985;44(4):1282-1288.
243. Campbell JB, DeCrescito V, Tomasula JJ, Demopoulos HB, Flamm ES, Ransohoff J: Experimental treatment of spinal cord contusion in the cat. *Surg Neurol* 1973;1(2):102-106.
244. De La Torre JC, Johnson CM, Goode DJ, Mullan S: Pharmacologic treatment and evaluation of permanent experimental spinal cord trauma. *Neurology* 1975;25(6):508-514.
245. Ducker TB, Hamit HF: Experimental treatments of acute spinal cord injury. *J Neurosurg* 1969; 30(6):693-697.
246. Hansebout RR, Kuchner EF, Romero-Sierra C: Effects of local hypothermia and of steroids upon recovery from experimental spinal cord compression injury. *Surg Neurol* 1975;4(6):531-536.
247. Xu J, Qu ZX, Hogan EL, Perot PL Jr: Protective effect of methylprednisolone on vascular injury in rat spinal cord injury. *J Neurotrauma* 1992;9(3): 245-253.
248. Faden AI, Jacobs TP, Patrick DH, Smith MT: Megadose corticosteroid therapy following experimental traumatic spinal injury. *J Neurosurg* 1984; 60(4):712-717.
249. Hedeman LS, Sil R: Studies in experimental spinal cord trauma: 2. Comparison of treatment with steroids, low molecular weight dextran, and catecholamine blockade. *J Neurosurg* 1974;40(1): 44-51.
250. Rucker NC, Lumb WV, Scott RJ: Combined pharmacologic and surgical treatments for acute spinal cord trauma. *Am J Vet Res* 1981;42(7):1138-1142.
251. Braughler JM, Hall ED: Correlation of methylprednisolone levels in cat spinal cord with its effects on (Na+ + K+)-ATPase, lipid peroxidation, and alpha motor neuron function. *J Neurosurg* 1982;56(6):838-844.
252. Lewin MG, Hansebout RR, Pappius HM: Chemical characteristics of traumatic spinal cord edema in cats: Effects of steroids on potassium depletion. *J Neurosurg* 1974;40(1):65-75.
253. Anderson DK, Means ED, Waters TR, Green ES: Microvascular perfusion and metabolism in injured spinal cord after methylprednisolone treatment. *J Neurosurg* 1982;56(1):106-113.
254. Hall ED, Wolf DL, Braughler JM: Effects of a single large dose of methylprednisolone sodium succinate on experimental posttraumatic spinal cord ischemia: Dose-response and time-action analysis. *J Neurosurg* 1984;61(1):124-130.
255. Hall ED: Glucocorticoid effects on the electrical properties of spinal motor neurons. *Brain Res* 1982;240(1):109-116.

256. Woodbury DM, Vernadakis A: Effects of steroids on the central nervous system. *Methods Horm Res* 1966;5:1-57.

257. Braughler JM, Chase RL, Neff GL, et al: A new 21-aminosteroid antioxidant lacking glucocorticoid activity stimulates adrenocorticotropin secretion and blocks arachidonic acid release from mouse pituitary tumor (AtT-20) cells. *J Pharmacol Exp Ther* 1988;244(2):423-427.

258. Jacobsen EJ, McCall JM, Ayer DE, et al: Novel 21-aminosteroids that inhibit iron-dependent lipid peroxidation and protect against central nervous system trauma. *J Med Chem* 1990;33(4):1145-1151.

259. Anderson DK, Braughler JM, Hall ED, Waters TR, McCall JM, Means ED: Effects of treatment with U-74006F on neurological outcome following experimental spinal cord injury. *J Neurosurg* 1988;69(4):562-567.

260. Bracken MB, Shepard MJ, Holford TR, et al: Administration of methylprednisolone for 24 or 48 hours or tirilazad mesylate for 48 hours in the treatment of acute spinal cord injury: Results of the Third National Acute Spinal Cord Injury Randomized Controlled Trial. National Acute Spinal Cord Injury Study. *JAMA* 1997;277(20):1597-1604.

261. Hurlbert RJ: Strategies of medical intervention in the management of acute spinal cord injury. *Spine (Phila Pa 1976)* 2006;31(11, Suppl)S16-S36.

262. Matsumoto T, Tamaki T, Kawakami M, Yoshida M, Ando M, Yamada H: Early complications of high-dose methylprednisolone sodium succinate treatment in the follow-up of acute cervical spinal cord injury. *Spine (Phila Pa 1976)* 2001;26(4):426-430.

263. Hurlbert RJ, Moulton R: Why do you prescribe methylprednisolone for acute spinal cord injury? A Canadian perspective and a position statement. *Can J Neurol Sci* 2002;29(3):236-239.

264. Hadley MN, Walters BC, Grabb PA, et al: Guidelines for the management of acute cervical spine and spinal cord injuries: Pharmacological therapy after acute cervical spinal cord injury. *Neurosurgery* 2002;50(3, Suppl):S63-S72.

265. Haghighi SS, Chehrazi BB, Higgins RS, Remington WJ, Wagner FC: Effect of lidocaine treatment on acute spinal cord injury. *Neurosurgery* 1987;20(4):536-541.

266. Wallace MC, Tator CH: Failure of blood transfusion or naloxone to improve clinical recovery after experimental spinal cord injury. *Neurosurgery* 1986;19(4):489-494.

267. Pietronigro DD, DeCrescito V, Tomasula JJ, Demopoulos HB, Flamm ES: Ascorbic acid: A putative biochemical marker of irreversible neurologic functional loss following spinal cord injury. *Cent Nerv Syst Trauma* 1985;2(2):85-90.

268. Koreh K, Seligman ML, Flamm ES, Demopoulos HB: Lipid antioxidant properties of naloxone in vitro. *Biochem Biophys Res Commun* 1981;102(4):1317-1322.

269. Simpkins CO, Alailima ST, Tate EA: Inhibition by naloxone of neutrophil superoxide release: A potentially useful antiinflammatory effect. *Circ Shock* 1986;20(3):181-191.

270. Curtis MT, Lefer AM: Protective actions of naloxone in hemorrhagic shock. *Am J Physiol* 1980;239(3):H416-H421.

271. Holaday JW, D'Amato RJ, Faden AI: Thyrotropin-releasing hormone improves cardiovascular function in experimental endotoxic and hemorrhagic shock. *Science* 1981;213(4504):216-218.

272. Faden AI, Jacobs TP, Smith MT, Holaday JW: Comparison of thyrotropin-releasing hormone (TRH), naloxone, and dexamethasone treatments in experimental spinal injury. *Neurology* 1983;33(6):673-678.

273. Faden AI, Jacobs TP: Effect of TRH analogs on neurologic recovery after experimental spinal trauma. *Neurology* 1985;35(9):1331-1334.

274. Faden AI: TRH analog YM-14673 improves outcome following traumatic brain and spinal cord injury in rats: Dose-response studies. *Brain Res* 1989;486(2):228-235.

275. Puniak MA, Freeman GM, Agresta CA, Van Newkirk L, Barone CA, Salzman SK: Comparison of a serotonin antagonist, opioid antagonist, and TRH analog for the acute treatment of experimental spinal trauma. *J Neurotrauma* 1991;8(3):193-203.

276. Holtz A, Nyström B, Gerdin B: Spinal cord injury in rats: Inability of nimodipine or anti-neutrophil serum to improve spinal cord blood flow or neurologic status. *Acta Neurol Scand* 1989;79(6):460-467.

277. Ono H, Fukuda H: Ventral root depolarization and spinal reflex augmentation by a TRH analog in rat spinal cord. *Neuropharmacology* 1982;21(8):739-744.

278. Schmidt-Achert KM, Askanas V, Engel WK: Thyrotropin-releasing hormone enhances choline acetyltransferase and creatine kinase in cultured spinal ventral horn neurons. *J Neurochem* 1984;43(2):586-589.

279. Hashimoto T, Fukuda N: Effect of thyrotropin-releasing hormone on the neurologic impairment in rats with spinal cord injury: Treatment starting 24 h and 7 days after injury. *Eur J Pharmacol* 1991;203(1):25-32.

280. Pitts LH, Ross A, Chase GA, Faden AI: Treatment with thyrotropin-releasing hormone (TRH) in pa-

tients with traumatic spinal cord injuries. *J Neurotrauma* 1995;12(3):235-243.

281. Kemp JA, Foster AC, Wong EH: Non-competitive antagonists of excitatory amino acid receptors. *Trends Neurosci* 1987;10:294-298.
282. Wong EH, Knight AR, Woodruff GN: [3H]MK-801 labels a site on the N-methyl-D-aspartate receptor channel complex in rat brain membranes. *J Neurochem* 1988;50(1):274-281.
283. Gaviria M, Privat A, d'Arbigny P, Kamenka J, Haton H, Ohanna F: Neuroprotective effects of a novel NMDA antagonist, Gacyclidine, after experimental contusive spinal cord injury in adult rats. *Brain Res* 2000;874(2):200-209.
284. Steen PA, Newberg LA, Milde JH, Michenfelder JD: Nimodipine improves cerebral blood flow and neurologic recovery after complete global ischemia in the dog. *J Cereb Blood Flow Metab* 1983; 3(1):38-43.
285. Steen PA, Gisvold SE, Milde JH, et al: Nimodipine improves outcome when given after complete cerebral ischemia in primates. *Anesthesiology* 1985;62(4):406-414.
286. Van Neuten JM, Wauquier A, De Clerk F, et al: Vascular reactivity of selective calcium-entry blockers, in Lenzi S, Descovich GC, eds: *Atherosclerosis and Cardiovascular Disease*. Boston, MA, MTP Press, 1984, pp 93-105.
287. Ross IB, Tator CH: Further studies of nimodipine in experimental spinal cord injury in the rat. *J Neurotrauma* 1991;8(4):229-238.
288. Faden AI, Jacobs TP, Smith MT: Evaluation of the calcium channel antagonist nimodipine in experimental spinal cord ischemia. *J Neurosurg* 1984; 60(4):796-799.
289. Ford RW, Malm DN: Failure of nimodipine to reverse acute experimental spinal cord injury. *Cent Nerv Syst Trauma* 1985;2(1):9-17.
290. Petitjean ME, Pointillart V, Dixmerias F, et al: Medical treatment of spinal cord injury in the acute stage. *Ann Fr Anesth Reanim* 1998;17(2): 114-122.
291. Argentino C, Sacchetti ML, Toni D, et al: GM1 ganglioside therapy in acute ischemic stroke: Italian Acute Stroke Study—Hemodilution + Drug. *Stroke* 1989;20(9):1143-1149.
292. Karpiak SE, Li YS, Mahadik SP: Gangliosides (GM1 and AGF2) reduce mortality due to ischemia: Protection of membrane function. *Stroke* 1987;18(1):184-187.
293. Tanaka K, Dora E, Urbanics R, Greenberg JH, Toffano G, Reivich M: Effect of the ganglioside GM1, on cerebral metabolism, microcirculation, recovery kinetics of ECoG and histology, during the recovery period following focal ischemia in cats. *Stroke* 1986;17(6):1170-1178.
294. Bose B, Osterholm JL, Kalia M: Ganglioside-induced regeneration and reestablishment of axonal continuity in spinal cord-transected rats. *Neurosci Lett* 1986;63(2):165-169.
295. Gorio A, Guillo AM, Young W, et al: GM1 effects on chemical, traumatic and peripheral nerve induced lesions to the spinal cord, in Goldberger ME, Gorio A, Murray M, eds: *Development and Plasticity of the Mammalian Spinal Cord*. Padua, Italy, Liviana Press, 1986, pp 227-242.
296. Hoffbrand BI, Bingley PJ, Oppenheimer SM, Sheldon CD: Trial of ganglioside GM1 in acute stroke. *J Neurol Neurosurg Psychiatry* 1988;51(9): 1213-1214.
297. Geisler FH, Coleman WP, Grieco G, Poonian D, Sygen Study Group: The Sygen multicenter acute spinal cord injury study. *Spine (Phila Pa 1976)* 2001;26(24, Suppl)S87-S98.
298. Di Gregorio F, Ferrari G, Marini P, Siliprandi R, Gorio A: The influence of gangliosides on neurite growth and regeneration. *Neuropediatrics* 1984; 15 Suppl:93-96.
299. Jonsson G, Gorio A, Hallman H, et al: GM1 ganglioside treatment enhances regrowth of central and peripheral noradrenaline neurons after selective 6-hydroxydopamine-induced lesions, in Gilad GM, Gorio A, Kreutzberg GW, eds: *Processes of Recovery from Neural Trauma*. Berlin, Germany, Springer-Verlag, 1986, pp 275-293.
300. Sabel BA, DelMastro R, Dunbar GL, Stein DG: Reduction of anterograde degeneration in brain damaged rats by GM1-gangliosides. *Neurosci Lett* 1987;77(3):360-366.
301. Sofroniew MV, Pearson RC, Cuello AC, Tagari PC, Stephens PH: Parenterally administered GM1 ganglioside prevents retrograde degeneration of cholinergic cells of the rat basal forebrain. *Brain Res* 1986;398(2):393-396.
302. Nicoletti F, Cavallaro S, Bruno V, et al: Gangliosides attenuate NMDA receptor-mediated excitatory amino acid release in cultured cerebellar neurons. *Neuropharmacology* 1989;28(11): 1283-1286.
303. Stys PK, Waxman SG, Ransom BR: Ionic mechanisms of anoxic injury in mammalian CNS white matter: Role of Na+ channels and Na(+)-Ca2+ exchanger. *J Neurosci* 1992;12(2):430-439.
304. Stys PK: White matter injury mechanisms. *Curr Mol Med* 2004;4(2):113-130.
305. Gangemi JJ, Kern JA, Ross SD, Shockey KS, Kron IL, Tribble CG: Retrograde perfusion with a sodium channel antagonist provides ischemic spinal cord protection. *Ann Thorac Surg* 2000;69(6): 1744-1749.
306. Fern R, Ransom BR, Stys PK, Waxman SG: Pharmacological protection of CNS white matter during anoxia: Actions of phenytoin, carbamazepine

and diazepam. *J Pharmacol Exp Ther* 1993;266(3): 1549-1555.

307. Hains BC, Saab CY, Lo AC, Waxman SG: Sodium channel blockade with phenytoin protects spinal cord axons, enhances axonal conduction, and improves functional motor recovery after contusion SCI. *Exp Neurol* 2004;188(2):365-377.

308. Rosenberg LJ, Teng YD, Wrathall JR: Effects of the sodium channel blocker tetrodotoxin on acute white matter pathology after experimental contusive spinal cord injury. *J Neurosci* 1999;19(14): 6122-6133.

309. Bensimon G, Lacomblez L, Meininger V, ALS/ Riluzole Study Group: A controlled trial of riluzole in amyotrophic lateral sclerosis. *N Engl J Med* 1994;330(9):585-591.

310. Wang SJ, Wang KY, Wang WC: Mechanisms underlying the riluzole inhibition of glutamate release from rat cerebral cortex nerve terminals (synaptosomes). *Neuroscience* 2004;125(1): 191-201.

311. Baptiste DC, Fehlings MG: Pharmacological approaches to repair the injured spinal cord. *J Neurotrauma* 2006;23(3-4):318-334.

312. Schwartz G, Fehlings MG: Evaluation of the neuroprotective effects of sodium channel blockers after spinal cord injury: Improved behavioral and neuroanatomical recovery with riluzole. *J Neurosurg* 2001;94(2, Suppl)245-256.

313. Thomas M, Le WD, Jankovic J: Minocycline and other tetracycline derivatives: A neuroprotective strategy in Parkinson's disease and Huntington's disease. *Clin Neuropharmacol* 2003;26(1):18-23.

314. Teng YD, Choi H, Onario RC, et al: Minocycline inhibits contusion-triggered mitochondrial cytochrome c release and mitigates functional deficits after spinal cord injury. *Proc Natl Acad Sci U S A* 2004;101(9):3071-3076.

315. Festoff BW, Ameenuddin S, Arnold PM, Wong A, Santacruz KS, Citron BA: Minocycline neuroprotects, reduces microgliosis, and inhibits caspase protease expression early after spinal cord injury. *J Neurochem* 2006;97(5):1314-1326.

316. McKerracher L, Higuchi H: Targeting Rho to stimulate repair after spinal cord injury. *J Neurotrauma* 2006;23(3-4):309-317.

317. Dergham P, Ellezam B, Essagian C, Avedissian H, Lubell WD, McKerracher L: Rho signaling pathway targeted to promote spinal cord repair. *J Neurosci* 2002;22(15):6570-6577.

318. Fournier AE, Takizawa BT, Strittmatter SM: Rho kinase inhibition enhances axonal regeneration in the injured CNS. *J Neurosci* 2003;23(4): 1416-1423.

319. Hata K, Fujitani M, Yasuda Y, et al: RGMa inhibition promotes axonal growth and recovery after spinal cord injury. *J Cell Biol* 2006;173(1):47-58.

320. Schnell L, Schwab ME: Axonal regeneration in the rat spinal cord produced by an antibody against myelin-associated neurite growth inhibitors. *Nature* 1990;343(6255):269-272.

321. GrandPré T, Nakamura F, Vartanian T, Strittmatter SM: Identification of the Nogo inhibitor of axon regeneration as a Reticulon protein. *Nature* 2000;403(6768):439-444.

322. Chen MS, Huber AB, van der Haar ME, et al: Nogo-A is a myelin-associated neurite outgrowth inhibitor and an antigen for monoclonal antibody IN-1. *Nature* 2000;403(6768):434-439.

323. Bregman BS, Kunkel-Bagden E, Schnell L, Dai HN, Gao D, Schwab ME: Recovery from spinal cord injury mediated by antibodies to neurite growth inhibitors. *Nature* 1995;378(6556): 498-501.

324. Fouad K, Klusman I, Schwab ME: Regenerating corticospinal fibers in the Marmoset (Callitrix jacchus) after spinal cord lesion and treatment with the anti-Nogo-A antibody IN-1. *Eur J Neurosci* 2004;20(9):2479-2482.

325. Naftchi NE: Functional restoration of the traumatically injured spinal cord in cats by clonidine. *Science* 1982;217(4564):1042-1044.

326. Joyner JJ, Freeman LW: Urea and spinal cord trauma. *Neurology* 1963;13:69-72.

327. Harvey JE, Srebnik HH: Locomotor activity and axon regeneration following spinal cord compression in rats treated with L-thyroxine. *J Neuropathol Exp Neurol* 1967;26(4):661-668.

328. Tator CH, van der Jagt RH: The effect of exogenous thyroid hormones on functional recovery of the rat after acute spinal cord compression injury. *J Neurosurg* 1980;53(3):381-384.

329. Kajihara K, Kawanaga H, De la Torre JC, Mullan S: Dimethyl sulfoxide in the treatment of experimental acute spinal cord injury. *Surg Neurol* 1973; 1(1):16-22.

330. Guth L, Albuquerque EX, Deshpande SS, Barrett CP, Donati EJ, Warnick JE: Ineffectiveness of enzyme therapy on regeneration in the transected spinal cord of the rat. *J Neurosurg* 1980;52(1): 73-86.

331. Grasso G, Sfacteria A, Cerami A, Brines M: Erythropoietin as a tissue-protective cytokine in brain injury: What do we know and where do we go? *Neuroscientist* 2004;10(2):93-98.

332. Borgens RB, Bohnert D, Duerstock B, Spomar D, Lee RC: Subcutaneous tri-block copolymer produces recovery from spinal cord injury. *J Neurosci Res* 2004;76(1):141-154.

333. Ibarra A, Correa D, Willms K, et al: Effects of cyclosporin-A on immune response, tissue protection and motor function of rats subjected to spinal cord injury. *Brain Res* 2003;979(1-2):165-178.

334. Iwasaki Y, Iizuka H, Yamamoto T, Konno H, Kadoya S: Alleviation of axonal damage in acute spinal cord injury by a protease inhibitor: Automated morphometric analysis of drug-effects. *Brain Res* 1985;347(1):124-126.

335. Politis MJ, Zanakis MF: The short-term effects of delayed application of electric fields in the damaged rodent spinal cord. *Neurosurgery* 1989;25(1):71-75.

CHAPTER 12
Biomechanics of Spinal Instrumentation: Applications for Trauma

Ahmad Faizan, PhD Nathaniel R. Ordway, MS, PE Vijay K. Goel, PhD
Amir H. Fayyazi, MD Hansen A. Yuan, MD

Introduction

The other chapters of this text examine the epidemiology, management, physical examination, types of fractures, surgical approaches, and complications of spinal trauma. When the integrity of the spinal column is threatened by complete or partial loss of stability, surgical intervention may be the best, or possibly the only, option to treat spinal trauma. Understanding the biomechanics of spinal constructs and associated instrumentation becomes very important from the clinical perspective in terms of achieving stability. Although there is a wealth of information on the biomechanics of injury mechanisms, the purpose of this chapter is to describe the biomechanics of spinal instrumentation used to restore stability, correct deformities, and preserve mobility, when possible, to the spinal column following trauma.

Dr. Faizan or an immediate family member serves as a paid consultant to or is an employee of Custom Spine, Inc. Dr. Ordway or an immediate family member has received research or institutional support from Synthes; and owns stock or stock options in Pioneer Surgical Technology. Dr. Goel or an immediate family member has received royalties from X-Spine, Inc.; and has received research or institutional support from DePuy, a Johnson & Johnson company. Dr. Fayyazi or an immediate family member serves as a paid consultant to or is an employee of Synthes, Baxter, Kuros, and Amedica; serves as an unpaid consultant to LifeSpine; owns stock or stock options in Exactech, Inc. and Alphatec Spine; and has received nonincome support (such as equipment or services), commercially derived honoraria, or other non-research-related funding (such as paid travel) from Synthes. Dr. Yuan or an immediate family member has received royalties from DePuy, a Johnson & Johnson company, Stryker, Zimmer, and Pioneer Surgical; is a member of a speakers' bureau or has made paid presentations on behalf of Nuvasive and Pioneer Surgical; serves as a paid consultant to or is an employee of Nuvasive and Pioneer Surgical; serves as an unpaid consultant to Theracell and Anglefix; and owns stock or stock options in Nuvasive and Pioneer Surgical.

The *New Oxford American Dictionary* defines biomechanics as the study of the mechanical laws relating to the movement or structure of living organisms. The focus of this chapter is not to delve deeply into the principles of the mechanical laws, but rather to apply these principles in clinically relevant terms. In the case of movement and structure, the mechanical laws of statics, dynamics, materials science, and mechanics of materials will determine the stability and mobility as measured by range of motion, neutral zone, stiffness, and failure mechanisms of constructs following spinal instrumentation. The latter terms are important factors for evaluating and understanding spinal instrumentation and the associated constructs that can be formed during surgery.

Cervical Trauma and Instrumentation

Occipitocervical

Traditionally, occipitocervical fixation has involved the use of wiring techniques. However, with the evolution of newer, more rigid, screw–rod/plate devices, wire fixation into the occiput can no longer be recommended for a variety of clinical reasons. Biomechanically, experimental cadaveric studies have shown that both rod/plate and wire fixation increase the stability following fracture; however, rod/plate fixation (**Figure 1**) increases stiffness and decreases range of motion in flexion-extension and torsion compared to wire fixation.[1-3] These differences become more pronounced following fatigue testing.[2] As far as attachment to the occiput, the failure strength is highest at the occipital protruberance. Bicortical screws have been shown to have the highest strength in comparison to either wires or unicortical screws.[4] However, unicortical screws have enough strength in the majority of cases and are clinically safer.

Puttlitz[5] used a finite element model of the occipito-atlanto-axial (C0-C1-C2) complex to investigate the biomechanics of a novel hardware system. Finite element models representing combinations of cervical anchor type (C1-C2 transarticular screws versus C2 pedicle screws) and unilateral versus bilateral instrumentation were evaluated. All models were subjected to compression plus pure moments in flexion, extension, or lateral bending. Bilateral instrumentation provided greater motion reductions than the unilateral hardware. When used bilaterally, C2 pedicle screws approximate the kinematic reductions and hardware stresses (except in lateral bending) that are seen with C1-C2 transarticular screws. The finite element model predicted that the maximum stress was always located in the region where the plate transformed into the rod. Thus, the author felt that C2 pedicle screws should be considered as an alternative to C1-C2 transarticular screw usage when bilateral instrumentation is applied.

FIGURE 1

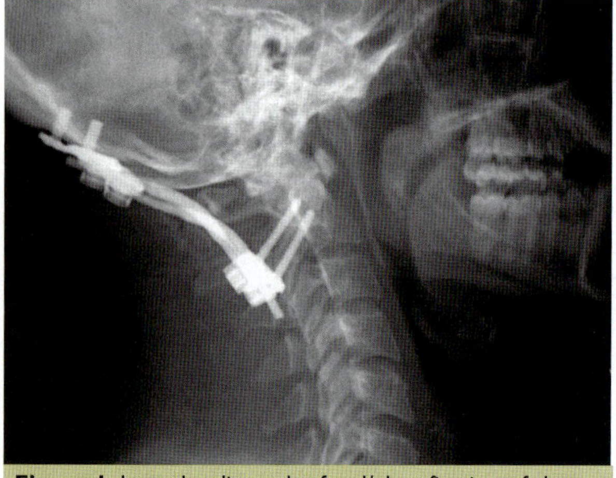

Figure 1 Lateral radiograph of rod/plate fixation of the occipitocervical junction.

Atlantoaxial

Fractures of the odontoid process of the second cervical vertebra comprise 9% to 15% of all cervical spine fractures.[6] Most published reports involving odontoid fracture use the classification system detailed by Anderson and D'Alonzo.[7] Type I is an oblique fracture near the superior tip of the odontoid process and is thought to involve an avulsion defect associated with the alar/apical complex. Fracture of the odontoid process at the juncture of the process and vertebral body in the region of the accessory ligaments is classified as type II. Type III fractures involve the junction of the odontoid process and the anterior portion of the vertebral body (**Figure 2**). However, a more detailed classification of injury types is provided by Maak and Grauer,[6] who further subdivided type II fractures into three categories: type IIA is a minimally or nondisplaced type II fracture with no comminution; type IIB is a displaced fracture extending from anterior-superior to posterior-inferior or a transverse fracture; and type IIC has a fracture line extending from anterior-inferior to posterior-superior or a fracture with significant comminution.

Type I and type III fractures are treated with collar immobilization in most cases. Halo vests are

FIGURE 2

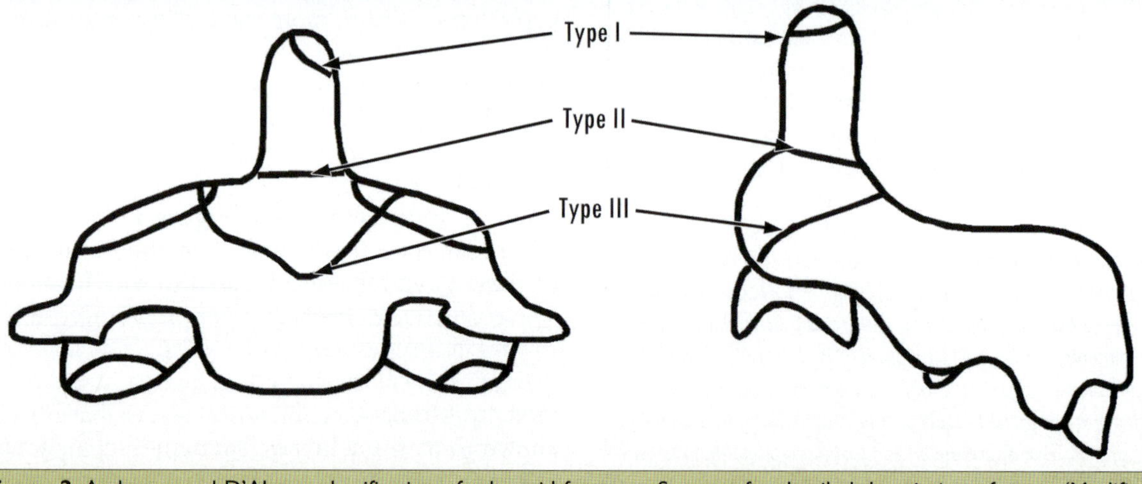

Figure 2 Anderson and D'Alonzo classification of odontoid fractures. See text for detailed description of types. (Modified with permission from Grauer JN, Shafi B, Hilibrand AS, et al: Proposal of a modified, treatment-oriented classification of odontoid fractures. *Spine J* 2005;5(2):123-129.)

FIGURE 3

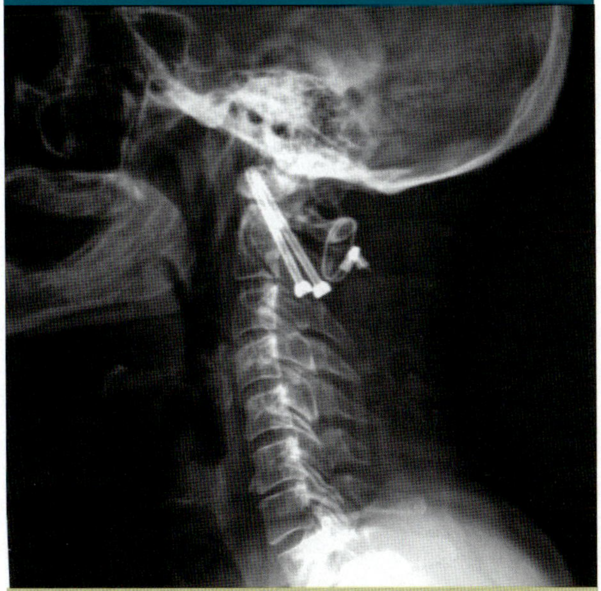

Figure 3 Lateral radiograph of transarticular screw fixation of the upper cervical spine.

FIGURE 4

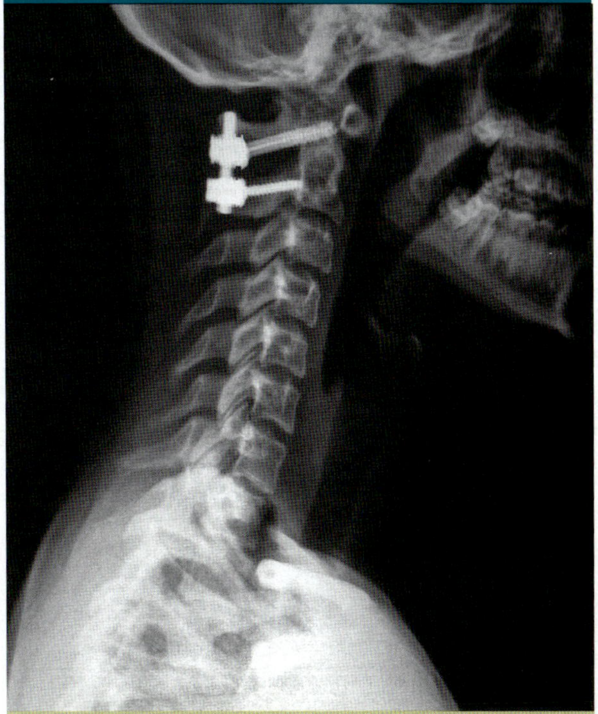

Figure 4 Lateral radiograph of C1 lateral mass–C2 pedicle screw fixation of the upper cervical spine.

also often used to treat type III fractures.[6] However, if these injuries are accompanied with anterior/posterior dislocations or displacement of the joint, then internal fixation or fusion methods are used for treatment. Type II fractures lead to greater instability; therefore, external immobilization techniques may not always be sufficient. Frequent nonunion has been reported in the literature when nonsurgical techniques were used to treat type II fractures.[8] Surgical fixation methods are used when external fixation is not effective.

Posterior fixation systems include wiring and screw-based techniques, and are popular among surgeons. The aim is to achieve fusion of C1-C2 vertebrae to provide stability. Posterior wiring techniques were initially described by Gallie[9] at the C1-C2 level. The technique used a single central wire that provided support and also held a large block autograft in position. Later, Brooks and Jenkins[10] described bilateral sublaminar wires with two autografts to provide greater stability. In an in vitro biomechanical study, this technique has been shown to be more stable than Gallie's technique under physiologic loading.[11]

Transarticular screw fixation (TSF), on the other hand, affords a stiffer atlantoaxial arthrodesis (**Figure 3**). Screws are placed into the C1 lateral mass along the isthmus of C2. Biomechanical testing suggests that TSF has about ten times the torsional stiffness and similar bending stiffness to that of posterior wiring techniques. TSF does have some drawbacks, however, including injury of the vertebral artery, malposition, and screw breakage.[12] Furthermore, body habitus (obesity or thoracic hyperkyphosis) may prohibit achieving the low angle needed for screw placement across C1 and C2. The addition of posterior wiring to the transarticular screw construct increases the stiffness of the construct in flexion/extension, and it holds the graft in place. Recently, a new technique of screw and rod fixation (SRF) that minimizes the risk of injury to the vertebral artery and allows intraoperative reduction has been reported.[13,14] The configuration of this technique, which achieves rigid fixation of the atlantoaxial complex, consists of lateral mass screws at C1 and pedicle screws at C2 linked via longitudinal rods with constrained coupling devices (**Figure 4**).

Kuroki et al[15] studied the biomechanical stability imparted to the atlantoaxial complex by comparing the TSF to the SRF techniques. They assessed how well these methods withstood fatigue in a cadaver model.[15] The results of this study suggested that in unilateral fixation, the SRF group was statistically stiffer than the TSF group in flexion loading, but there were no evident differences in other directions. In bilateral fixation, SRF was more stable than TSF except in flexion and

FIGURE 5

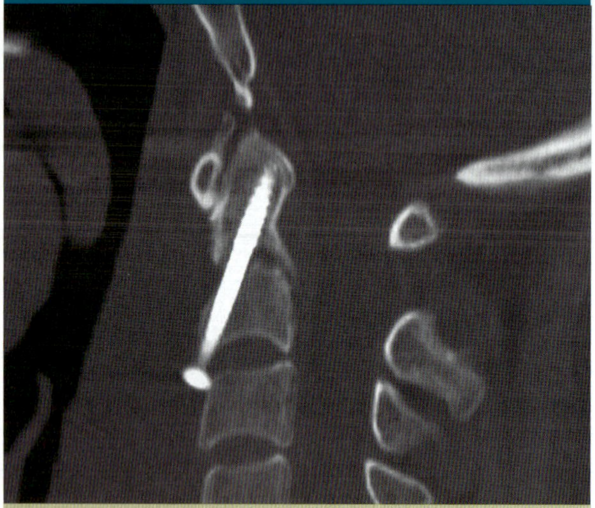

Figure 5 Sagittal image from a CT scan of anterior odontoid screw fixation.

FIGURE 6

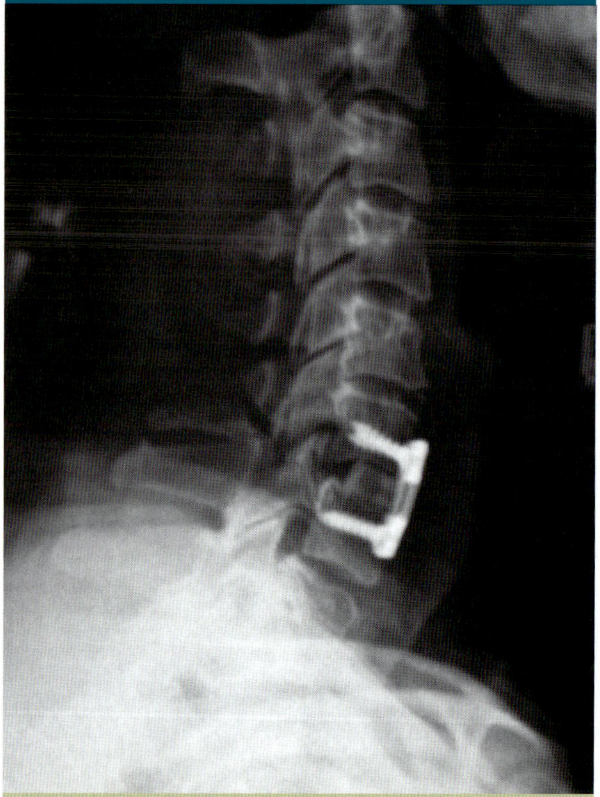

Figure 6 Lateral radiograph of anterior cervical fixation for treatment of subaxial cervical injury.

extension. These results were similar to those reported by Melcher et al[16] and Richter et al,[17] yet different from Lynch et al.[18] The instrumentation (screw length and type of constrained coupling device), the destabilization technique, and the condition of the specimens might have an influence on the results. In the Kuroki study, when stabilizing the atlantoaxial segments, all screws were placed bicortically in both TSF and SRF techniques similar to that reported by Melcher et al.[16] Previous work has demonstrated that bicortical cervical vertical screws are superior to unicortical screws in terms of pullout strength and decreased wobble.[19,20] Most surgeons, however, prefer unicortical screws at C1 and C2 levels to reduce the risk of injury to the internal carotid artery.

In certain odontoid fractures, an anterior screw can be used to stabilize the fracture (**Figure 5**). The advantages of using either one or two screws over conventional posterior C1-C2 fusion are immediate rigid fixation, preservation of the axial rotation at the C1-2 facet articulation, minimal postoperative bracing, and the avoidance of the complications associated with bone grafting. This surgical approach has gradually gained acceptance in the United States as the preferred technique in the management of some types of odontoid fractures.[21] Biomechanical studies have shown that fixation with one or two screws provides 50% of the stability of the unfractured state.[22,23] The two-screw technique increased stiffness in extension compared to the single-screw technique, but there was no significant difference in failure load based on the number of screws used.[23] In addition, the failure load has been shown to be 31% of the unfractured state following fixation with an odontoid screw.[24] McBride et al[25] showed that using a single Herbert screw instead of two cannulated screws resulted in significantly higher torsional stiffness and no significant difference in shear. Clinically, Jenkins et al[26] have shown no significant difference in fusion rate when comparing the one- and two-screw techniques. Rao and Apfelbaum[27] reported an 88% fusion rate if the anterior screw surgery was performed within the first 6 months of injury as compared to a 25% fusion rate if surgery occurred 18 months after injury. In general, the stability of this fixation will be dependent upon the compression achieved during screw insertion and the bone fragment interface quality.

Subaxial (C3-C7)

Anterior Approach

The anterior approach to achieve arthrodesis of the lower cervical spine has become widely used for correcting and stabilizing cervical injuries (**Figure 6**). However, many of these techniques rely on insertion of a bone graft only anteriorly and the use of an external immobilization device, such as a halo vest, or posterior fixation to allow for sufficient fixation. Problems encountered with these methods include dislodging of the bone graft (potentially causing neural compromise), loss of angular correction, and failure to maintain spinal reduction.[28,29] The use of anterior plates has become popular in part because they address some of the complications listed above. In traumatic injuries that involve predominantly the anterior vertebral body or the disk and require surgical stabilization, a stand-alone anterior graft and plate may be sufficient and can potentially decrease the complication rate associated with posterior instrumentation. The use of anterior surgery in the treatment of posterior instability is not an established indication. It can, however, be used in selected patients with good bone quality, or as a part of circumferential fusions. Do Koh et al[30] demonstrated that biomechanically, anterior plating may be effective in treatment of cervical burst fracture; however, these devices are not as stable as posterior plating for treatment of flexion-distraction injuries. The efficacy of anterior plates alone is still debated by some authors, particularly in multilevel reconstruction techniques, due to rates of failure up to 50% in some cases.[31-34]

Clausen et al[35] reported the results of biomechanical testing comparing the Cervical Spine Locking Plate (CSLP) system (Synthes, West Chester, PA) with unicortical locking screws and the Caspar plate system (Aesculap, San Francisco, CA) with unlocked bicortical screws. Fifteen cadaveric human spines were tested intact in flexion, extension, lateral bending, and axial rotation loading modes to determine stiffness characteristics. Next, C5-C6 instability was introduced, consisting of a C5-C6 diskectomy with posterior longitudinal ligament (PLL) removal. An iliac crest bone graft was then introduced into the C5-6 disk space and the spine was instrumented with either the CSLP or Caspar system. Once instrumented, each of the spines was further destabilized through surgical disruption of the interspinous and supraspinous ligaments, the ligamentum flavum, facet capsules, and lateral anulus. After initial postinstrumentation testing was done, biomechanical stability of the specimens was reassessed following cyclic fatigue for 5,000 cycles of flexion/extension. Finally, failure testing of each specimen was performed in flexion. The Caspar system stabilized significantly in flexion before, but not after, fatigue, and it stabilized significantly in extension before and after fatigue. The CSLP system stabilized significantly in flexion before, but not after, fatigue, and it did not stabilize in extension before or after fatigue. The failure moment did not differ between the two systems. Biomechanical stability discrepancy between the two devices was attributed to differences in bone-screw fixation.

Traynelis et al[36] performed biomechanical testing to compare anterior plating versus posterior wiring in a cadaver instability model involving a simulated C5 teardrop fracture with posterior disruption and fixation across C4-C6. Study results showed that bicortical anterior plating provided significantly more stability than posterior wiring in extension and lateral bending, and was slightly more stable than posterior wiring in flexion. Both provided equivalent stability in axial rotation.

Rao et al[37] performed biomechanical evaluation of posterior wiring as a supplement to anterior cervical plate fixation. Six human cadaver cervical spines (C3-T1) were loaded in flexion, extension, lateral bending, and torsion under a maximum moment of 2.5 Nm. The spines were tested in four stages. The first stage involved biomechanical testing of an intact spine, while in the second stage, testing was done after complete diskectomy and interbody strut grafting of the C5-C6 motion segment. Interbody grafting with the Orion anterior cervical plate (Medtronic Sofamor Danek, Memphis, TN) was done and tested in a third stage. Finally, in the fourth stage, spines were tested after interbody grafting with an anterior plate and posterior interspinous process wiring. The results showed that after anterior diskectomy, strut grafting, and anterior plating of the C5-6 interspace, the range of motion was significantly reduced in flexion (60%), extension (52%), and left and right bending (30% and 40%). Further motion reduction was observed after anterior plating and posterior wiring when compared to plating alone. Percentage reductions were 49% in flexion, 48% in extension, and 33% and 39% in left and right bending. The difference in lateral bending was not statistically significant. Therefore, the authors concluded that combined fixation reduces motion significantly at the involved level but does not significantly alter the motion and intradiskal pressure at adjacent levels.

Brodke et al[38] documented the effect of the plate design on the load-sharing ability following a single-level corpectomy and placement of full-length strut graft, and the effects following 10% subsidence of the graft. The three types of plates tested were static plates with fixed-angle screws, rotationally dynamic plates that allowed the screws to toggle in the plate, and translationally dynamic plates that allowed screws to both toggle and translate vertically. A total of 21 cadaveric cervical spines (C2-T1) were randomized into 3 treatment groups and were tested for initial range of motion. A C5 corpectomy was performed, reconstruction was done with a full-length interbody spacer containing a load-cell, and an anterior cervical plate was applied. Load-sharing data was recorded with incremental axial loads. The range of motion was measured with ± 2.5 Nm of torque in flexion-extension, lateral bending, and axial rotation. Then, the total length of the interbody spacer was reduced by 10% to simulate subsidence, and load sharing and range of motion were retested. The authors found that with the full-length interbody spacer, there were no significant differences in the ability of the constructs to share load or limit motion. Following shortening of the interbody spacer, the static plate construct lost nearly 70% of its load-sharing capability, while neither of the dynamic plate constructs lost load-sharing capabilities. Also, the static plate construct allowed significantly more motion in flexion-extension following simulated subsidence than did either of the dynamic plate constructs. They concluded that the static plate system lost its ability to share load and limit motion following simulated subsidence of the spacer. However, both dynamic plate systems maintained load sharing and stiffness despite simulated subsidence.

Clinically, anterior plating is very successful in short fusion, but the success rate decreases (approximate range, 50% to 80%) as the length of the plate system increases. Panjabi et al[39] performed a biomechanical study to evaluate the screw-vertebra interface in single- and three-level corpectomy models of the cervical spine. They found there was excessive motion at the lower-end vertebra-screw junction in the three-level model during fatigue testing. It was observed that in the long plates, fatigue loading makes the vertebra-screw junction weaker. They concluded that the mechanism of clinically observed failure of long anterior plates may be a progressive loosening of the vertebra-screw junction at the lower end of the plate caused by repetitive in situ loading after surgery. The authors suggested that attention should be directed to developing enhanced screw-vertebra fixation, especially at the lower end of long plates, by the use of longer and larger diameter screws and/or supplemental posterior fixation. They believe that this may decrease screw-vertebra loosening.

Scifert[40] developed an experimentally validated C4-C6 cervical spine finite element model to examine stress levels and load-sharing characteristics in an anterior plate and graft. Model predictions demonstrated good agreement with the in vitro data. The rotations across the stabilized segment significantly decreased in the presence of a plate as compared with the graft alone. Much like the in vitro studies, the model also predicted that the compressive load in the graft increased in extension in the presence of a plate as compared with the graft alone. Depending on the load type, stresses in the graft were concentrated in the anterior or posterior region and became more uniformly distributed in the presence of a plate. The predicted load-displacement data and load-sharing results reveal that a plate is very effective in maintaining alignment. Increase in the load borne by the graft in the presence of a plate in the extension mode suggests that pistoning of the graft would be a possible outcome. However, the stress data showed that pistoning of the graft was not likely to happen due to stresses being low. This observation agrees with the clinical outcome data. For optimal healing, the stress results suggest that the tricortical bone graft should be placed with its cortical region toward the canal when used with a plate. For the graft alone, this parameter does not seem to be that critical. A more uniform stress distribution in the graft in the presence of a plate would tend to promote bone fusion in a more uniform fashion, as compared to the graft alone. In the latter case, fusion may initiate in a selective region.

Posterior Approach

Subaxial posterior cervical instrumentation can be achieved by wiring techniques or screw–rod/plate fixation. Presence of, or prevention of, postoperative instability is the main indication for instrumentation of the posterior subaxial cervical spine. The goal of internal fixation is to allow for reduction and maintenance of alignment, rigid stabilization, and early mobilization. Most cervical fusions can be achieved with simple wiring techniques. Wire techniques for fusion of the lower cervical spine have been the time-tested method in both biomechanical and clinical studies since the concept was initially described by Rogers in 1942.[41] They are safe, relatively easy to perform, and do not require sophisticated instrumentation for application. Bohlman's triple-wire technique, which is a modification of Rogers' initial method, and the Robinson-Southwick technique have become the main forms of cervical stabilization using wire techniques.[42]

In cases of postlaminectomy instability or incompetent posterior elements from fracture, simple wiring techniques cannot be used. Lateral mass plate fixation of the cervical spine was initially popularized by Roy-Camille and later modified by Magerl using the hook plate.[43,44] Since its initial description, multiple instrumentation systems have been developed. Initial devices used a plate-screw interface; these devices are very difficult to use given the variability of the anatomy, the constraint associated with the available screw position, and the inability to apply coronal contouring. Newer devices use a rod-screw interface that allows three-dimensional contouring and are much easier to apply.

Biomechanical in vitro studies have examined the efficacy of wiring and posterior plates for posterior subaxial cervical spine stabilization. In general, both techniques have been shown to be effective in terms of stabilizing the spine.[45,46] Others have specifically compared wiring and plating techniques. Roy-Camille et al[47] used a cadaveric model to compare posterior lateral mass plating to spinous process wiring. They found that posterior plates increased stability by 92% in flexion and 60% in extension, while spinous process wiring enhanced flexion stability by only 33% and did not stabilize in extension. Scifert et al[48] found that posterior plates were superior to posterior facet wiring in the majority of loading modes for both short cycle and cyclic fatigue testing, excluding extension. Raftopoulos[49] found that both posterior wiring and posterior plating resulted in significant stability following severe spinal destabilization, although posterior plating provided superior stability compared to that of interfacet wiring. Similar to the results of anterior plates, Gill et al[50] found that bicortical lateral posterior plate screw fixation provided greater stability than unicortical fixation. However, Grubb et al[51] found that unicortical fixation of a destabilized spine using a cervical rod device provided stability in torsion and lateral bending equivalent to bicortical fixation using an AO lateral mass plate (**Figure 7**).

As stated previously, both anterior and posterior plating procedures contain inherent difficulties and drawbacks. Some authors have examined the use of both techniques concomitantly to ensure adequate stabilization. Do Koh et al[30] examined anterior only, posterior only, and combined techniques in vitro to determine the efficacy of these techniques in stabilizing either a C4-C5 flexion-distraction injury or an injury simulating a C5 burst fracture involving a C5 corpectomy. The AXIS and Orion plates (Medtronic Sofamor Danek) were used for posterior and anterior stabilization, respectively. In the C4-C5 flexion-distraction injury, both posterior and combined fixation reduced motion significantly from the intact case in flexion. Only the combined procedure was able to reduce motion effectively in extension. In lateral bending and axial rotation, posterior fixation alone and combined fixation were able to significantly reduce motion as compared with the intact case. In the C5 corpectomy model, all constructs exhibited significantly less motion compared with the intact case in flexion, although the combined fixation was the most rigid. In extension, all constructs, except the posterior fixation with bone graft, were able to reduce motion significantly compared with the intact case. In lateral bending, only the posterior-only fixation and combined fixation were able to provide enhanced stability compared with the intact case. In axial rotation, only the combined fixation was able to significantly reduce motion compared to the intact case. Thus, the authors concluded that combined fixation provided the most rigid stability for both surgical cases tested. In a clinical study of multilevel anterior cervical reconstruction surgical techniques, Doh and Heller[32] found a 0% pseudar-

FIGURE 7

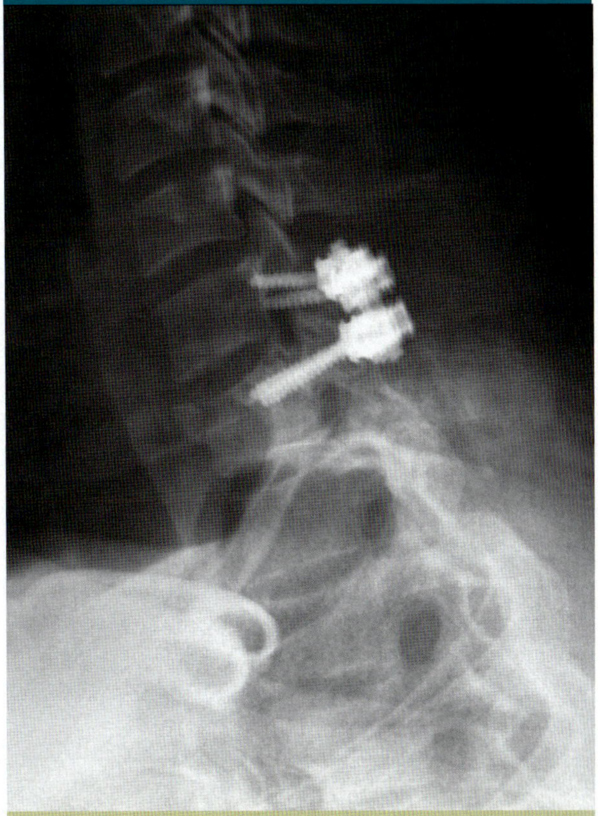

Figure 7 Lateral radiograph of posterior cervical fixation for treatment of subaxial cervical injury.

throsis rate for the combined fixation system only.

Although combined fixation almost certainly allows for the most rigid fixation in most unstable cervical spine injuries, there are other factors to consider, such as the necessity for an additional surgery, possibility of severely reduced range of motion, and neck pain. Jónsson et al[32] found a propensity for patients (22 of 26) with combined fixation to have pain related to the posterior surgery. Additionally, patients with the combined fixation were found to have considerably restricted motion compared with normal. These and other factors must be weighed against the additional advantages of almost assured stability with the combined fixation technique.

Thoracolumbar Trauma and Instrumentation

Thoracolumbar trauma is often associated with motor vehicle collisions, falls, and other blunt injuries. The majority of spine injuries do not require surgical intervention. Despite this, the economic burden is significant. There is usually a wide age distribution seen in patients with these injuries. Elderly patients with osteoporosis are more likely to suffer these injuries. Many of these injuries can be described as major, leading to surgical stabilization. The thoracolumbar junction is the most commonly involved area due to its position between the stiff thoracic spine and the hypermobile lumbar spine. These conditions are often accompanied with spinal cord injuries resulting in neurologic deficit.

Surgical treatment of thoracolumbar spine fractures is usually indicated for pain control, prevention of neurologic injury, and/or spinal instability. White and Panjabi defined instability as the "loss of the ability of the spine under physiologic loads to maintain its pattern of displacement so that there is no initial or additional neurologic deficit, no major deformity, and no incapacitating pain."[53] Additionally, an injury that results in incapacitating deformity or pain can be assumed to be unstable and may require stabilization. Unfortunately, in the clinical setting, spinal stability is not easily defined and multiple classification systems have been developed to address this issue.

The first attempt to define spinal stability can be credited to Holdsworth.[54] In this classification system, five fracture patterns were described: pure flexion, flexion and rotation, extension, vertical compression fracture, and shear fracture. Internal fixation was recommended only for lumbar rotational fracture-dislocation with paraplegia. Holdsworth divided the spinal column into two parts: anterior, which consisted of the disk and anterior body and the PLL; and posterior, which consisted of all spinal structures posterior to the PLL. In this classification system, instability was defined as injury to the posterior column.

The three-column classification system was proposed in 1983 by Denis.[55] In this classification, the spine was divided into three columns. The anterior column was defined as the anterior vertebral body, anterior anulus, and anterior longitudinal ligament. The middle column consisted of the posterior vertebral body and the PLL, and the posterior column was defined as the structures posterior to the PLL. In this classification system, injury to two of the three columns was defined as instability. Denis classified thoracolumbar fractures into four categories: compression fractures, burst fractures, flexion distraction injuries, and fracture-dislocation injuries.

Unfortunately, neither the two-column model of Holdsworth nor the three-column model of Denis reliably predicts an unstable injury. Other attempts to classify thoracolumbar fractures include the mechanistic classification described by Ferguson and Allen[56] and the comprehensive fracture classification described by the AO group.[57] In the AO classification, thoracolumbar fractures are divided into vertebral body compression fractures (type A), anterior and posterior injuries (type B), and anterior and posterior injuries with rotation (type C). Each of these fractures are later subdivided into three types (1 through 3) and further divided into three subtypes. Great care has been taken to describe every possible fracture in the AO classification system.

Panjabi et al[58] performed in vitro biomechanical tests to validate the three-column theory of fractures in the thoracolumbar spine using cadaveric specimens with simulated burst fractures. The specimens were subjected to trauma by dropping increasingly heavier weight on them at a speed of 5.1 m/s until the burst fracture occurred. Physiologic motions were measured by multidirectional flexibility tests before and after trauma. Injury to each of the three columns was visualized by CT scans, and linear correlations were obtained between the flexibility parameters and the injury data. Based on the correlation coefficients, this study supported the three-column theory of thoracolumbar fractures, thus proving the importance of the middle column in providing stability to the spinal column.

The treatment of spinal fractures continues to be controversial. The treatment should result in a spine that maintains sagittal and coronal alignment, protects the neural elements, and is painless. This can be accomplished with either bracing or internal fixation, and the treatment of choice depends mostly on the fracture pattern and the clinical findings. It has been recommended that no more than 30° of segmental kyphosis can be corrected with bracing and fractures that result in further sagittal imbalance should be treated surgically.[59] Multiple techniques are available and can be used for treatment of thoracolumbar instability. These include anterior, posterior, or combined instrumentation, and short versus long posterior instrumentation. Each construct offers certain advantages that will be described further in the following sections.

Anterior Instrumentation

Because of the magnitude of loading in the anterior column and the length of time necessary for maintaining stability, hardware failure of anterior instrumentation has been, and continues to be, a major concern. Dick et al[60] undertook the task of evaluating fatigue strength and stiffness of four anterior thoracolumbar fixation devices using a corpectomy model, without a load-sharing graft, to test the devices under a worst-case scenario. Four types of implants were tested: the Synthes Anterior Thoracolumbar Locking Plate (ATLP), the Kaneda device (Acromed, DePuy Spine, Raynham, MA), a Texas Scottish Rite Hospital anterior construct, and the Z-Plate (Sofamor Danek). The anterior thoracolumbar locking plate was the stiffest in compression, flexion, and torsion, and the Texas Scottish Rite Hospital anterior construct was least stiff in flexion and extension. No significant differences in the stiffness of the thoracolumbar locking plate, Kaneda device, and Z-Plate were reported. In addition, the fatigue life was greatest for the TL locking plate, followed by the Z-Plate, and then the other two systems. These data confirmed the lower failure rate of the TL locking plate and Z-plate observed clinically.

Similar studies performed by Gurr et al[61] found that the Kaneda device used in augmentation with a strut graft restored the spine to a strength comparable to those provided by Cotrel-Dubousset and Steffee posterior pedicle screw–based systems. Several other studies have also shown that different anterior devices restore the spinal column to near normal strength. A study by Harris et al[62] evaluated the effect of anterior thoracolumbar plate application on the compressive loading of a strut graft. Strains were recorded at various locations of the graft, and strain patterns were compared before and after the application of plates. Bovine spines were used to test the two plate types (Amset ALPS Anterior Locking Plate System [AMS, Hayward, California] and Synthes ATLP system) under 500 N of compressive loading. The authors found that with application of the ALPS plate, the compressive strain through the graft adjacent to the plate averaged 77% of the graft-alone construct. With application of the Synthes plate, the compressive strain through the graft adjacent to the plate averaged 34% of the graft-alone construct. Therefore, when either of the plates was applied and a known amount of compression was introduced to the construct, the graft experienced a significantly lower load than did the isolated bone graft. This would support the theory of device-related osteoporosis because plates shield the graft from experiencing the load. However, the investigators only examined the strains in the graft and assumed that the loading would be in the same proportion as the strain.

A more detailed investigation into stiffness and load sharing characteristics of anterior plate and rod systems was performed by Brodke et al.[63] They compared three rod types (Synthes Ventrofix, Acromed Kaneda Device, and Acromed ALC static) and three plate-type anterior instrumentation systems (Synthes ATLP, Sofamor Danek Z-Plate, and DePuy Profile [DePuy Spine, Raynham, MA]) for stabilizing the thoracolumbar spine. Testing was performed on a spine simulator under flexion, extension, lateral bending, and axial rotation loads. Axial load sharing was measured through a range of applied axial loads from 50 N to 500 N with rotational moments maintained at 0 Nm. The bending stiffness of each construct was calculated in response to ± 5 Nm moments about each axis of rotation and a 50-N compressive axial load with a full-length corpectomy graft in place (simulating reconstruction of the anterior column) and with no graft in place (simulating a catastrophic graft failure). Load-sharing results ranged from 63% to 89%. There was an inverse relationship between load sharing and stiffness, and no correlation was found between load sharing and implant style (rod versus plate). However, with the graft in place, stiffness results varied by instrumentation system rather than by plate/rod style. Without the graft, the stiffness of the construct decreased dramatically, underlying the importance of the graft. This study showed that for load sharing and stiffness, the design of the instrumentation system has more influence than implant style (rod versus plate).

Anterior Instrumentation: Interbody Cages

Use of interbody implants to achieve fusion has been popular in the thoracolumbar spine as well. Dvorak at al[64] studied the effectiveness of titanium cylindrical cages in anterior column reconstruction after thoracic and lumbar vertebral body resection. The study was a retrospective review of patients who underwent anterior column reconstruction with a titanium mesh cylindrical cage after single-level or multilevel thoracic or lumbar vertebrectomy. In general, surgeons use structural allograft or autograft bone with anterior, posterior, or a combination of both types of instrumentation for reconstruction. The titanium mesh cages were implanted in vertical orientation between end plates following resection of the vertebral body, and adjacent disks and plate/rods were used to provide initial stability to the column. The mesh cages provide great flexibility to the surgeon because of their variable size and diameter. Based on their study, the authors concluded that titanium mesh cages, supplemented with nonstructural autogenous bone graft, provided an effective method for reconstruction of the anterior column. Radiographs showed that there was a loss of < 5% of sagittal alignment in association with some cage subsidence into the end plates. A high proportion (93%) of reconstructions resulted in solid osseous union, suggesting that after a period of settling, the cage achieves sufficient stability to facilitate bone healing.

There are a variety of cage designs available for lumbar interbody fusion surgery, including circular, tapered, and rectangular with or without curvature. Vadapalli et al[65] performed cadaveric testing to study the effect of lumbar interbody cage geometry on construct stability. Lumbar specimens were subjected to pure moments in sagittal bending, coronal bending, and axial rotation, and the motions were measured sequentially for intact, bilateral spacer placement across L4-L5, supplemented with pedicle screw–rod system fixation, and after cyclic loading. The authors found no statistically significant difference in stability between the intact state and after bilateral spacer placement. Following the addition of posterior fixation using a pedicle screw–rod system, the stability significantly increased in all directions. Cyclic loading did not have any significant effect on the stability. They concluded that stand-alone cages restore motion to near-intact levels at best, and supplemental instrumentation is essential for significantly increasing the stability of the decompressed segment. The effects of cage geometry and Young's modulus of cage material do not seem to influence the stability as compared to the other cage designs, especially after supplemental fixation with a posterior system.

Posterior Instrumentation

Long Versus Short Constructs

Compression or burst fractures generally lead to severe instability of the spinal column. Initially, long fixation systems such as Harrington rods and Drummond wires were used.[66] The Harrington rod, which uses high distraction forces to provide stability, has successfully been used especially to stabilize the thoracic spine. However, high distraction forces sometimes destabilize the spine or cause rod failures. In the lumbar spine, Harrington instrumentation results in overdistraction, loss of lordosis, and flat-back syndrome, and is no longer used. The addition of posterior wiring to Harrington rods to bolster the stability of the construct has been studied. However, this is no longer used given the development of pedicle screw instrumentation systems.[67,68]

Unlike long constructs, the function of short constructs is based on cantilever bending forces.[66] Also, the stability depends on the integrity of the anterior column. Without anterior column support, the biomechanical deficiencies of short-segment constructs have been shown.[69] Short-segment constructs use pedicle screw–based systems most of the time and are now being widely used for thoracolumbar fractures. The short-segment pedicle screw–based instrumentation system provides more stability than do the Harrington rods, wire, or hook systems. In addition, because the system is shorter, the procedure is surgically easier and more efficient. An et al[70] performed a biomechanical study of L2 burst fractures to compare the stability of pedicle screws to hooks and found that pedicle screws provided better stability than hooks in all planes. It is important to note that load sharing by the disk and facets is critical in determining the life span of a pedicle screw construct.

Even with the advantages of short-segment fixation, clinically, there has been evidence of failure based on loss of sagittal balance or breakage of the screws.[71] Many alternatives have been proposed to avoid such failure, such as use of longer constructs, anterior strut graft reconstruction, and use of offset sublaminar hooks at the end of a standard short-segment pedicle instrumentation construct. Chiba et al[72] performed a cadaver-based biomechanical study to determine the relative benefit of adding offset sublaminar hooks to standard pedicle screw constructs to reduce screw bending moments and prevent fixation failure and sagittal collapse. The results of this study showed a significant increase in stiffness after offset laminar hooks were added. For example, with the addition of offset laminar hooks, supralaminar at T11 and infralaminar at L2, to standard short-segment pedicle instrumentation, the construct increased stiffness in flexion by 268%, in extension by 223%, in lateral bending by 161%, and in torsion by 155%. All of the above differences were significant except for the torsion case. Sublaminar hooks also reduced pedicle screw bending moments to roughly 50% of standard in both flexion and extension. Therefore, the authors concluded that supplemental offset hooks significantly increase the construct stiffness without sacrificing principles of short-segment pedicle instrumentation. In addition, the hooks absorb a portion of the construct strain, thereby reducing the pedicle screw bending moments and the likelihood of clinical failure.

Another potential short-segment technique, which does not provide anterior column support, has been examined, adding an additional set of pedicle screws at the fractured level.[73] Biomechanically, this would provide support for an intact posterior column and indirect support for healing at the fractured level. In this combined biomechanical and clinical study, the authors showed improvement in biomechanical stability and feasibility. Clinically, however, these short-segment techniques will have to be examined because other studies have shown better sagittal correction over time with long constructs or anterior constructs when compared with short constructs.[74,75]

Murakami et al[76] biomechanically assessed infralaminar hooks as an alternative to supralaminar hooks in thoracolumbar fixation. Their study consisted of nine vertebrae (T9-L2) on which pedicle screw loosening and stiffness tests were performed. The loosening test showed that a pedicle screw combined with an infralaminar hook offered significantly greater fixation strength as compared to a pedicle screw alone. Also, fixation by pedicle screw combined with infralaminar hooks, placed on the vertebra fixed by pedicle screws at both the cranial and caudal ends, offered a stiffer construct compared with fixation by pedicle screw alone.

Some authors have performed biomechanical studies to evaluate the effectiveness of systems other than traditional pedicle screw systems. Ferrara et al[77] compared the biomechanics of transfacet pedicle screw fixation and pedicle screw fixation. The lumbar constructs were loaded with 6 Nm of flexion bending and tested for 180,000 cycles. Under these testing conditions, stability provided by both transfacet pedicle screw fixation and traditional pedicle screw fixation was not compromised. Hence, the transfacet pedicle screw fixation system appears equivalent biomechanically to traditional pedicle screw fixation. Another such study was one in which the authors evaluated thoracic extrapedicular fixation systems.[78] Pedicles in the thoracic spine are smaller, and thus pose greater challenges for pedicle screw insertion. However, extrapedicular fixation is safer because the screw insertion points are away from the neural canal. The authors found that extrapedicular screw fixation systems were as rigid as the conventional pedicle screw systems.

Vertebral Augmentation

Compression fractures cause severe injury to the vertebral body and intervertebral disk. However, the disk in comparison to the end plates is better equipped to take the compression loads, and therefore fractures of end plates are seen first in most of the cases.[79] Percutaneous vertebroplasty and kyphoplasty procedures in the appropriately selected patient have shown short-term favorable clinical outcomes. These results are due in part to the enhanced biomechanical alterations following the procedure. Injection of the cement into the vertebra can result in initial stability and the exothermic reaction can reduce pain.

Use of polymethylmethacrylate (PMMA) vertebroplasty has been suggested with short-segment pedicle screw fixation for treatment of burst fractures. Cho et al[80] clinically evaluated the performance of such reinforced pedicle screw fixation systems. Two groups of patients with thoracolumbar burst fractures were treated with pedicle screw fixation. Fractures in group A (n = 20) were reinforced with PMMA vertebroplasty while fractures in group B (n = 50) were not reinforced with vertebroplasty. The factors they compared between the two groups were kyphotic deformity, anterior vertebral height, instrument failure rates, and neurologic function. Kyphosis correction was achieved in both groups postoperatively, but at the end of the follow-up period, group A maintained the correction while group B lost the correction. Greater anterior vertebral height was achieved in group A than in group B, but again, at the end of follow-up, only group A maintained the height. In terms of pain control, group A showed better results than group B based on the Denis pain scale grades. Out of the 50 patients in group B, 11 had some kind of instrument failure including screw

FIGURE 8

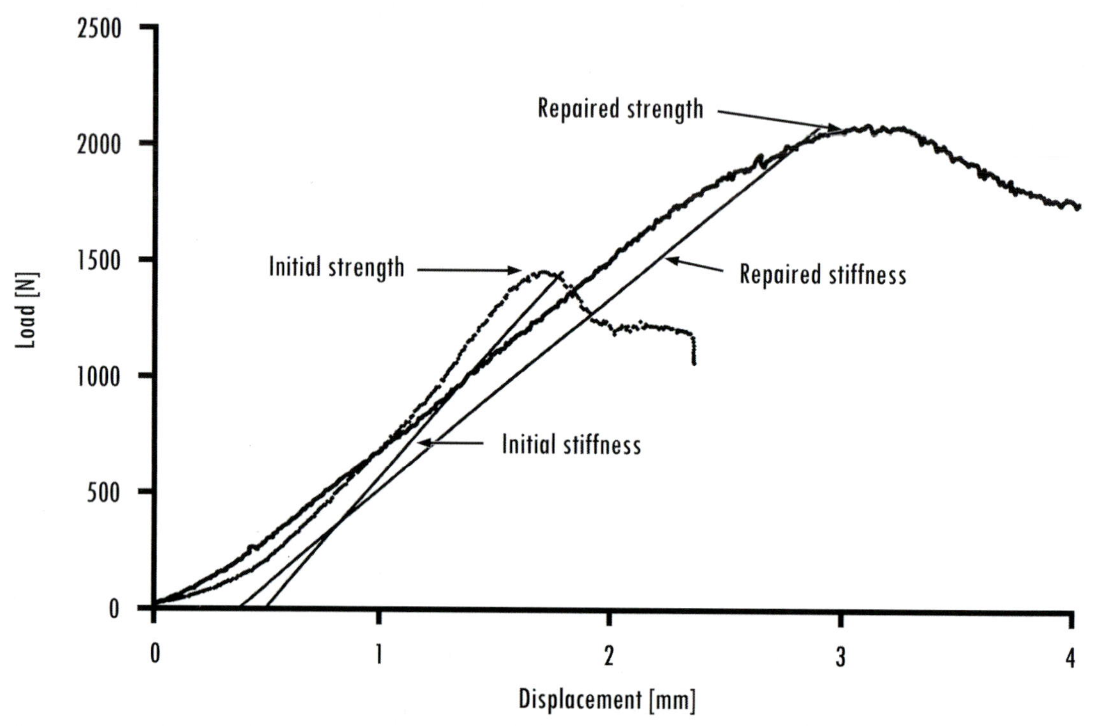

Figure 8 Typical force versus deformation response curves for T9 vertebral body compressed initially and after repair by using 6 mL of hydroxyapatite cement. (Reproduced with permission Belkoff SM, Mathis JM, Jasper LE: Ex vivo biomechanical comparison of hydroxyapatite and polymethylmethacrylate cements for use with vertebroplasty. *AJNR Am J Neuroradiol* 2002;23(10):1647-1651.)

pullout, breakage, disconnection, or dislodgment. There was no implant failure observed in group A. Later, three patients from group B required implant removal. Based on these findings, the authors concluded that reinforcement of short-segment pedicle fixation with PMMA vertebroplasty for the treatment of patients with thoracolumbar burst fracture may achieve and maintain kyphosis correction and may also increase and maintain anterior vertebral height.

In vitro biomechanical studies have been performed on osteoporotic vertebral segments to examine the differences in vertebroplasty and kyphoplasty procedures, the effect of different formulations of cement, the effect of different approaches (unipedicular compared to bipedicular), and the effect of multilevel augmentation. Both procedures result in stabilization of the fractured body and have shown increased compressive strength of the augmented vertebra in comparison to the unaltered vertebra using osteoporotic specimens.[81-83] However, the stiffness following injection of cement under compressive load has been shown to be less than intact controls.[81,83] Thus, for a given compressive load, the axial displacement of an augmented vertebra would be increased in comparison to the intact vertebra (**Figure 8**).[84]

When comparing the differences between vertebroplasty and kyphoplasty, kyphoplasty has resulted in vertebral height restoration whereas vertebroplasty has not.[81,83] The type of cement used for either procedure does not seem to have an effect.[82,83] In addition, increasing the amount of injected cement through either a unipedicular or bipedicular approach does not necessarily result in improved mechanical characteristics, but it can result in increased risk for cement extravasation.[85,86] Multilevel augmentations are advocated in cases where adjacent-level vertebral fracture risk is determined to be high. Kayanja et al[87] have shown that the multilevel segment biomechanics are dependent on the bone mineral density and not the pattern of augmentation (examining 1, 2, or 3 levels), and therefore augmentation of the fractured vertebra can be extended to adjacent levels to assist in preventing further fractures.

Motion-Preservation Systems

Motion-preservation devices have gained popularity in recent years because of their obvious advantage over rigid systems. Vishnubhotla has done finite element–based studies on various dynamic stabilization systems.[88] A validated three-dimensional nonlinear finite element model of the intact L3-S1 lumbar spine was used to biomechanically compare various dynamic stabilization systems to the rigid screw–rod system that is used in a conventional fusion. The intact model was modified at L4-L5 to simulate stabilization with the rigid screw–rod system, rigid screw–flexible rod system, Dynesys system (Zimmer Spine, Minneapolis, MN), Cosmic system (Ulrich Medical, Ulm, Germany), and Wallis system (Zimmer Spine International, Bordeaux, France). These devices were also simulated in decompression surgery to evaluate their stability. Load control and hybrid protocols were used to evaluate these devices. Various biomechanically relevant parameters, including range of motion, facet loading, disk stresses, implant stresses, instantaneous axis of rotation, and load sharing were evaluated. Results show that the flexible rod systems do not vary much in terms of stiffness and load sharing capabilities from the rigid screw-rod system. Dynesys, Cosmic, and Wallis systems are more flexible than the rigid systems, but not flexible enough to clearly demonstrate that they preserve motion. However, they have the ability to allow for loading through the intervertebral disk. All the flexible stabilization systems were capable of stabilizing the decompression surgery in flexion, extension, and lateral bending, but were not as effective in axial rotation. Future biomechanical studies will have to be performed before advocating the use of motion preservation instruments in the setting of trauma.

Minimally Invasive Techniques

Rampersaud et al[89] published a review of management of thoracolumbar trauma using minimally invasive surgical techniques. They discussed the current knowledge in orthopaedics to treat trauma patients and indicated that there is a significant failure rate due to infection, and hence advocated the minimal invasive approach in trauma. Current surgeries involve open procedures where instrumentation is used with bone graft, as well as cages, for fusion. Verlaan et al[90] performed a literature review of the procedures and found that posterior, anterior, or a combination of both procedures, led to an average blood loss of about 1,000 mL. They also reported an average infection rate of 0.7% for anterior and 3.1% for posterior procedures. The traditional approach can also cause other types of problems. For instance, perioperative pain or shoulder girdle dysfunction may occur during anterior transthoracic or transdiaphragmatic approaches. Muscle morbidity has also been reported after these procedures.

To avoid the above mentioned problems caused by traditional open exposure approaches, minimally invasive surgery (MIS) in spinal trauma is slowly gaining some momentum. The initial results have been promising in terms of time to return to work and pain relief. However, the success of MIS depends heavily on anatomic knowledge, radiographic techniques used to visualize the area of interest, and the experience of the surgeon.

There are a few MIS techniques that are promising and are being used by some surgeons to treat thoracolumbar trauma. Anterior endoscopic decompression and stabilization is one of them and is used for decompression or reconstruction of the anterior column. Posterior percutaneous screw fixation is another MIS technique and is used to restore posterior bands or in cases where it is not possible to use anterior fixation. There are techniques to restore the vertebral height as well by using percutaneous balloon-assisted augmentation. Also, there are temporary stabilization techniques that help mobilize the spine along with preventing further injuries when direct fixation is difficult to achieve. These are done by posterior percutaneous fixation. The above MIS techniques seem to have great potential, but associated technical problems are presently keeping surgeons from using them widely. Technical problems may be overcome with time, expertise, and experience to bring down the cost of these procedures in the future.

References

1. Dvorak MF, Sekeramayi F, Zhu Q, et al: Anterior occiput to axis screw fixation: Part II. A biomechanical comparison with posterior fixation techniques. *Spine (Phila Pa 1976)* 2003;28(3):239-245.
2. Hurlbert RJ, Crawford NR, Choi WG, Dickman CA: A biomechanical evaluation of occipitocervical instrumentation: Screw compared with wire fixation. *J Neurosurg* 1999;90(1, Suppl)84-90.
3. Sutterlin CE III, Bianchi JR, Kunz DN, Zdeblick TA, Johnson WM, Rapoff AJ: Biomechanical evaluation of occipitocervical fixation devices. *J Spinal Disord* 2001;14(3):185-192.
4. Haher TR, Yeung AW, Caruso SA, et al: Occipital screw pullout strength: A biomechanical investigation of occipital morphology. *Spine (Phila*

Pa 1976) 1999;24(1):5-9.

5. Puttlitz CM: *A Biomechanical Investigation of the Craniovertebral Junction*. Iowa City, IA, University of Iowa, 1999. Thesis.
6. Maak TG, Grauer JN: The contemporary treatment of odontoid injuries. *Spine (Phila Pa 1976)* 2006;31(11, Suppl):S53-S61.
7. Anderson LD, D'Alonzo RT: Fractures of the odontoid process of the axis. *J Bone Joint Surg Am* 1974;56(8):1663-1674.
8. Chiba K, Fujimura Y, Toyama Y, Fujii E, Nakanishi T, Hirabayashi K: Treatment protocol for fractures of the odontoid process. *J Spinal Disord* 1996;9(4):267-276.
9. Gallie WE: Fractures and dislocations of the cervical spine. *Am J Surg* 1939;46:495-499.
10. Brooks AL, Jenkins EB: Atlanto-axial arthrodesis by the wedge compression method. *J Bone Joint Surg Am* 1978;60(3):279-284.
11. Grob D, Crisco J, Panjabi M, et al: Comparative in vitro evaluation of the multidirectional stability of three dorsal atlanto-axial fusions. *Proceedings of the 17th Annual Meeting of the Cervical Spine Research Society*. New Orleans, LA, 1989.
12. Jun BY: Anatomic study for ideal and safe posterior C1-C2 transarticular screw fixation. *Spine (Phila Pa 1976)* 1998;23(15):1703-1707.
13. Goel A, Desai KI, Muzumdar DP: Atlantoaxial fixation using plate and screw method: A report of 160 treated patients. *Neurosurgery* 2002;51(6): 1351-1357.
14. Goel A, Laheri V: Plate and screw fixation for atlanto-axial subluxation. *Acta Neurochir (Wien)* 1994;129(1-2):47-53.
15. Kuroki H, Rengachary SS, Goel VK, Holekamp SA, Pitkänen V, Ebraheim NA: Biomechanical comparison of two stabilization techniques of the atlantoaxial joints: Transarticular screw fixation versus screw and rod fixation. *Neurosurgery* 2005; 56(1, Suppl):151-159.
16. Melcher RP, Puttlitz CM, Kleinstueck FS, Lotz JC, Harms J, Bradford DS: Biomechanical testing of posterior atlantoaxial fixation techniques. *Spine (Phila Pa 1976)* 2002;27(22):2435-2440.
17. Richter M, Schmidt R, Claes L, Puhl W, Wilke HJ: Posterior atlantoaxial fixation: Biomechanical in vitro comparison of six different techniques. *Spine (Phila Pa 1976)* 2002;27(16):1724-1732.
18. Lynch JJ, Crawford NR, Chamberlain RH, et al: Biomechanics of lateral mass/pedicle screw fixation at C1-2. *Proceedings of the 70th Annual Meeting of the Neurosurgical Society of America*. 2002.
19. Naderi S, Crawford NR, Song GS, Sonntag VK, Dickman CA: Biomechanical comparison of C1-C2 posterior fixations: Cable, graft, and screw combinations. *Spine (Phila Pa 1976)* 1998;23(18): 1946-1956.
20. Paramore CG, Dickman CA, Sonntag VK: The anatomical suitability of the C1-2 complex for transarticular screw fixation. *J Neurosurg* 1996; 85(2):221-224.
21. Aebi M, Etter C, Coscia M: Fractures of the odontoid process: Treatment with anterior screw fixation. *Spine (Phila Pa 1976)* 1989;14(10): 1065-1070.
22. Doherty BJ, Heggeness MH, Esses SI: A biomechanical study of odontoid fractures and fracture fixation. *Spine (Phila Pa 1976)* 1993;18(2): 178-184.
23. Sasso R, Doherty BJ, Crawford MJ, Heggeness MH: Biomechanics of odontoid fracture fixation: Comparison of the one- and two-screw technique. *Spine (Phila Pa 1976)* 1993;18(14):1950-1953.
24. Ames CP, Crawford NR, Chamberlain RH, Deshmukh V, Sadikovic B, Sonntag VK: Biomechanical evaluation of a bioresorbable odontoid screw. *J Neurosurg Spine* 2005;2(2):182-187.
25. McBride AD, Mukherjee DP, Kruse RN, Albright JA: Anterior screw fixation of type II odontoid fractures: A biomechanical study. *Spine (Phila Pa 1976)* 1995;20(17):1855-1860.
26. Jenkins JD, Coric D, Branch CL Jr: A clinical comparison of one- and two-screw odontoid fixation. *J Neurosurg* 1998;89(3):366-370.
27. Rao G, Apfelbaum RI: Odontoid screw fixation for fresh and remote fractures. *Neurol India* 2005; 53(4):416-423.
28. Bell GD, Bailey SI: Section II: General orthopaedics. Anterior cervical fusion for trauma. *Clin Orthop Relat Res* 1977;128:155-158.
29. Stauffer ES, Kelly EG: Fracture-dislocations of the cervical spine: Instability and recurrent deformity following treatment by anterior interbody fusion. *J Bone Joint Surg Am* 1977;59(1):45-48.
30. Do Koh Y, Lim TH, Won You J, Eck J, An HS: A biomechanical comparison of modern anterior and posterior plate fixation of the cervical spine. *Spine (Phila Pa 1976)* 2001;26(1):15-21.
31. Bolesta M, Rechtine G: Three and four level anterior cervical diskectomy and fusion with plate fixation: A prospective study. *Proceedings of the 26th Annual Meeting of the Cervical Spine Research Society*. Atlanta, GA, 1998.
32. Doh E, Heller J: Multi-level anterior cervical reconstruction: Comparison of surgical techniques and results. *Proceedings of the 26th Annual Meeting of the Cervical Spine Research Society*. Atlanta, GA, 1998.
33. Panjabi M, Isomi T, Wang J: Loosening at screw-bone junction in multi-level anterior cervical plate construct. *Proceedings of the 26th Annual Meeting of the Cervical Spine Research Society*. Atlanta, GA,

1998.
34. Swank ML, Lowery GL, Bhat AL, McDonough RF: Anterior cervical allograft arthrodesis and instrumentation: Multilevel interbody grafting or strut graft reconstruction. *Eur Spine J* 1997;6(2): 138-143.
35. Clausen JD, Ryken TC, Traynelis VC, Sawin PD, Dexter F, Goel VK: Biomechanical evaluation of Caspar and Cervical Spine Locking Plate systems in a cadaveric model. *J Neurosurg* 1996;84(6): 1039-1045.
36. Traynelis VC, Donaher PA, Roach RM, Kojimoto H, Goel VK: Biomechanical comparison of anterior Caspar plate and three-level posterior fixation techniques in a human cadaveric model. *J Neurosurg* 1993;79(1):96-103.
37. Rao RD, Wang M, Singrakhia MD, McGrady LM: Mechanical evaluation of posterior wiring as a supplement to anterior cervical plate fixation. *Spine (Phila Pa 1976)* 2004;29(20):2256-2259.
38. Brodke DS, Klimo P Jr, Bachus KN, Braun JT, Dailey AT: Anterior cervical fixation: Analysis of load-sharing and stability with use of static and dynamic plates. *J Bone Joint Surg Am* 2006;88(7): 1566-1573.
39. Panjabi MM, Isomi T, Wang JL: Loosening at the screw-vertebra junction in multilevel anterior cervical plate constructs. *Spine (Phila Pa 1976)* 1999; 24(22):2383-2388.
40. Scifert JL: *Biomechanics of the Cervical Spine*. Iowa City, IA, University of Iowa, 2000. Thesis.
41. Rogers W: Treatment of fractures and dislocations of the cervical spine. *J Bone Joint Surg Am* 1942; 24A:245-258.
42. Abdu WA, Bohlman HH: Techniques of subaxial posterior cervical spine fusions: An overview. *Orthopedics* 1992;15(3):287-295.
43. Roy-Camille R: Methods of osteosynthesis with posterior screw plates, in Laurin CA, Riley LH, Roy-Camille R: *Atlas of Orthopaedic Surgery*. Chicago, IL, Year-Book Medical Publishers, 1989, vol 1, pp 373-376.
44. Ulrich C, Wörsdörfer O, Claes L, Magerl F: Comparative study of the stability of anterior and posterior cervical spine fixation procedures. *Arch Orthop Trauma Surg* 1987;106(4):226-231.
45. Mihara H, Cheng BC, David SM, Ohnari K, Zdeblick TA: Biomechanical comparison of posterior cervical fixation. *Spine (Phila Pa 1976)* 2001; 26(15):1662-1667.
46. Smith ME, Cibischino M, Langrana NA, Lee CK, Parsons JR: A biomechanical study of a cervical spine stabilization device: Roy-Camille plates. *Spine (Phila Pa 1976)* 1997;22(1):38-43.
47. Roy-Camille R, Saillant G, Mazel C: Internal fixation of the unstable cervical spine by posterior osteosynthesis with plates and screws, in Cervical Spine Reseach Society Editorial Committee, ed: *The Cervical Spine*. Philadelphia, PA, Lippincott, 1989, pp 390-404.
48. Scifert JL, Goel V, Smith D, et al: In vitro biomechanical comparison of a posterior plate versus facet wiring in quasi-static and cylic modes. *Trans Orthop Res Soc* 1998;23:255.
49. Raftopoulos D: Comparative stability of posterior cervical plates and interfacet fusion. *Trans Orthop Res Soc* 1991;16:630.
50. Gill K, Paschal S, Corin J, Ashman R, Bucholz RW: Posterior plating of the cervical spine: A biomechanical comparison of different posterior fusion techniques. *Spine (Phila Pa 1976)* 1988;13(7): 813-816.
51. Grubb MR, Currier BL, Shih JS, Bonin V, Grabowski JJ, Chao EY: Biomechanical evaluation of anterior cervical spine stabilization. *Spine (Phila Pa 1976)* 1998;23(8):886-892.
52. Jónsson H Jr, Cesarini K, Petrén-Mallmin M, Rauschning W: Locking screw-plate fixation of cervical spine fractures with and without ancillary posterior plating. *Arch Orthop Trauma Surg* 1991; 111(1):1-12.
53. White AA III, Panjabi MM, eds: *Clinical Biomechanics of the Spine*, ed 2. Philadelphia, PA, JB Lippincott Co, 1990.
54. Holdsworth F: Fractures, dislocations, and fracture-dislocations of the spine. *J Bone Joint Surg Am* 1970;52(8):1534-1551.
55. Denis F: The three column spine and its significance in the classification of acute thoracolumbar spinal injuries. *Spine (Phila Pa 1976)* 1983;8(8): 817-831.
56. Ferguson RL, Allen BL Jr: A mechanistic classification of thoracolumbar spine fractures. *Clin Orthop Relat Res* 1984;189:77-88.
57. Magerl F, Aebi M, Gertzbein SD, Harms J, Nazarian S: A comprehensive classification of thoracic and lumbar injuries. *Eur Spine J* 1994;3(4): 184-201.
58. Panjabi MM, Oxland TR, Kifune M, Arand M, Wen L, Chen A: Validity of the three-column theory of thoracolumbar fractures: A biomechanic investigation. *Spine (Phila Pa 1976)* 1995;20(10): 1122-1127.
59. Tezer M, Ozturk C, Aydogan M, Mirzanli C, Talu U, Hamzaoglu A: Surgical outcome of thoracolumbar burst fractures with flexion-distraction injury of the posterior elements. *Int Orthop* 2005; 29(6):347-350.
60. Dick JC, Brodke DS, Zdeblick TA, Bartel BD, Kunz DN, Rapoff AJ: Anterior instrumentation of the thoracolumbar spine: A biomechanical comparison. *Spine (Phila Pa 1976)* 1997;22(7):

744-750.

61. Gurr KR, McAfee PC, Shih CM: Biomechanical analysis of posterior instrumentation systems after decompressive laminectomy: An unstable calf-spine model. *J Bone Joint Surg Am* 1988;70(5): 680-691.

62. Harris MB, Thomas KA, Igram CM, Bearden CM: The effect of anterior thoracolumbar plate application on the compressive loading of the strut graft. *Spine (Phila Pa 1976)* 1996;21(13): 1487-1493.

63. Brodke DS, Gollogly S, Bachus KN, Alexander Mohr R, Nguyen BK: Anterior thoracolumbar instrumentation: Stiffness and load sharing characteristics of plate and rod systems. *Spine (Phila Pa 1976)* 2003;28(16):1794-1801.

64. Dvorak MF, Kwon BK, Fisher CG, Eiserloh HL III, Boyd M, Wing PC: Effectiveness of titanium mesh cylindrical cages in anterior column reconstruction after thoracic and lumbar vertebral body resection. *Spine (Phila Pa 1976)* 2003;28(9): 902-908.

65. Vadapalli S, Robon M, Biyani A, Sairyo K, Khandha A, Goel VK: Effect of lumbar interbody cage geometry on construct stability: A cadaveric study. *Spine (Phila Pa 1976)* 2006;31(19): 2189-2194.

66. McLain RF: The biomechanics of long versus short fixation for thoracolumbar spine fractures. *Spine (Phila Pa 1976)* 2006;31(11, Suppl)S70-S79.

67. Bryant CE, Sullivan JA: Management of thoracic and lumbar spine fractures with Harrington distraction rods supplemented with segmental wiring. *Spine (Phila Pa 1976)* 1983;8(5):532-537.

68. Sullivan JA: Sublaminar wiring of Harrington distraction rods for unstable thoracolumbar spine fractures. *Clin Orthop Relat Res* 1984;189:178-185.

69. Gurwitz GS, Dawson JM, McNamara MJ, Federspiel CF, Spengler DM: Biomechanical analysis of three surgical approaches for lumbar burst fractures using short-segment instrumentation. *Spine (Phila Pa 1976)* 1993;18(8):977-982.

70. An HS, Singh K, Vaccaro AR, et al: Biomechanical evaluation of contemporary posterior spinal internal fixation configurations in an unstable burst-fracture calf spine model: Special references of hook configurations and pedicle screws. *Spine (Phila Pa 1976)* 2004;29(3):257-262.

71. Alanay A, Acaroglu E, Yazici M, Oznur A, Surat A: Short-segment pedicle instrumentation of thoracolumbar burst fractures: Does transpedicular intracorporeal grafting prevent early failure? *Spine (Phila Pa 1976)* 2001;26(2):213-217.

72. Chiba M, McLain RF, Yerby SA, Moseley TA, Smith TS, Benson DR: Short-segment pedicle instrumentation: Biomechanical analysis of supplemental hook fixation. *Spine (Phila Pa 1976)* 1996; 21(3):288-294.

73. Mahar A, Kim C, Wedemeyer M, et al: Short-segment fixation of lumbar burst fractures using pedicle fixation at the level of the fracture. *Spine (Phila Pa 1976)* 2007;32(14):1503-1507.

74. Sasso RC, Renkens K, Hanson D, Reilly T, McGuire RA Jr, Best NM: Unstable thoracolumbar burst fractures: Anterior-only versus short-segment posterior fixation. *J Spinal Disord Tech* 2006;19(4):242-248.

75. Tezeren G, Kuru I: Posterior fixation of thoracolumbar burst fracture: Short-segment pedicle fixation versus long-segment instrumentation. *J Spinal Disord Tech* 2005;18(6):485-488.

76. Murakami H, Tsai KJ, Attallah-Wasif ES, Yamazaki K, Shimamura T, Hutton WC: A biomechanical assessment of infra-laminar hooks as an alternative to supra-laminar hooks in thoracolumbar fixation. *Spine (Phila Pa 1976)* 2006;31(9): 967-971.

77. Ferrara LA, Secor JL, Jin BH, Wakefield A, Inceoglu S, Benzel EC: A biomechanical comparison of facet screw fixation and pedicle screw fixation: Effects of short-term and long-term repetitive cycling. *Spine (Phila Pa 1976)* 2003;28(12): 1226-1234.

78. Morgenstern W, Ferguson SJ, Berey S, Orr TE, Nolte LP: Posterior thoracic extrapedicular fixation: A biomechanical study. *Spine (Phila Pa 1976)* 2003;28(16):1829-1835.

79. Oner FC, Verlaan JJ, Verbout AJ, Dhert WJ: Cement augmentation techniques in traumatic thoracolumbar spine fractures. *Spine (Phila Pa 1976)* 2006;31(11, Suppl)S89-S95.

80. Cho DY, Lee WY, Sheu PC: Treatment of thoracolumbar burst fractures with polymethyl methacrylate vertebroplasty and short-segment pedicle screw fixation. *Neurosurgery* 2003;53(6): 1354-1361.

81. Belkoff SM, Mathis JM, Fenton DC, Scribner RM, Reiley ME, Talmadge K: An ex vivo biomechanical evaluation of an inflatable bone tamp used in the treatment of compression fracture. *Spine (Phila Pa 1976)* 2001;26(2):151-156.

82. Tomita S, Kin A, Yazu M, Abe M: Biomechanical evaluation of kyphoplasty and vertebroplasty with calcium phosphate cement in a simulated osteoporotic compression fracture. *J Orthop Sci* 2003; 8(2):192-197.

83. Tomita S, Molloy S, Jasper LE, Abe M, Belkoff SM: Biomechanical comparison of kyphoplasty with different bone cements. *Spine (Phila Pa 1976)* 2004;29(11):1203-1207.

84. Belkoff SM, Mathis JM, Jasper LE: Ex vivo biomechanical comparison of hydroxyapatite and polymethylmethacrylate cements for use with verte-

broplasty. *AJNR Am J Neuroradiol* 2002;23(10): 1647-1651.

85. Higgins KB, Harten RD, Langrana NA, Reiter MF: Biomechanical effects of unipedicular vertebroplasty on intact vertebrae. *Spine (Phila Pa 1976)* 2003;28(14):1540-1548.
86. Steinmann J, Tingey CT, Cruz G, Dai Q: Biomechanical comparison of unipedicular versus bipedicular kyphoplasty. *Spine (Phila Pa 1976)* 2005; 30(2):201-205.
87. Kayanja MM, Schlenk R, Togawa D, Ferrara L, Lieberman I: The biomechanics of 1, 2, and 3 levels of vertebral augmentation with polymethylmethacrylate in multilevel spinal segments. *Spine (Phila Pa 1976)* 2006;31(7):769-774.
88. Vishnubhotla S: *A Biomechanical Evaluation of Dynamic Stabilization Systems*. Toledo, OH, University of Toledo. Thesis.
89. Rampersaud YR, Annand N, Dekutoski MB: Use of minimally invasive surgical techniques in the management of thoracolumbar trauma: Current concepts. *Spine (Phila Pa 1976)* 2006;31 (11, Suppl)S96-S104.
90. Verlaan JJ, Diekerhof CH, Buskens E, et al: Surgical treatment of traumatic fractures of the thoracic and lumbar spine: A systematic review of the literature on techniques, complications, and outcome. *Spine (Phila Pa 1976)* 2004;29(7):803-814.

CHAPTER 13
Classification of Spinal Injury

Kris Radcliff, MD Worawat Limthongkul, MD Lawrence Delasotta, MD, MPH
Jeffrey Moore, BS Alan M. Levine, MD Alexander R. Vaccaro, MD, PhD

Introduction

An ideal spine classification system distinguishes stable versus unstable injuries, guides clinical decision-making, and has high reproducibility and reliability. A stable spine protects the spinal cord under normal physiologic load.[1] For both the cervical and thoracolumbar spine, White and Panjabi[1,2] proposed a checklist of items, composed of clinical, radiographic, and neurologic parameters able to assess stability.

Several goals exist for the use of such a classification system: predicting an outcome of a particular injury, assisting the physician in treatment decision-making, and standardizing nomenclature for scientific communication. Classification systems are based on mechanistic considerations,[2-6] radiologic description of fracture patterns,[6-12] and injury prognosis.[13-15] The factor that complicates the development of a comprehensive spinal injury classification system is the significant anatomic differences between the major regions of the spine.

The initial spine trauma classification systems were based upon radiographic criteria. CT and MRI provide greater detail about disease that is incorporated into modern classification systems. CT provides excellent spine resolution of bony spine injuries, but may not indicate subtle instability or ligamentous damage. MRI provides visualization of the ligament and neural elements; however, MRI may be highly sensitive but not specific for spinal ligamentous injury, compared to intraoperative findings.[16] Modern classification systems become more accurate with improved imaging modalities.

Upper Cervical Spine Injuries

The upper cervical spine (occiput to C2) has unique anatomic and mechanical features. Predictable injury patterns are based on the mechanism of injury. A comprehensive classification system to group upper cervical spine injuries is nonexistent. Instead, a mechanism of injury is gathered from the history to determine the appropriate classification scheme.

The occipital-cervical junction has both ligamentous and bony components. Axial loading may result in injury to the occipital condyles. The most commonly cited classification for injuries to the occipital condyles is that of Anderson and Montesano,[7] which encompasses three types. The first is an impaction-type fracture, the second is a basilar skull–type fracture, and the third is an avulsion-type fracture (**Figure 1**). These injuries are usually stable, and managed conservatively. The third type of injury may be associated with an unstable atlanto-occipital dislocation. Management is rarely altered by these classifications.

Dr. Limthongkul or an immediate family member is a member of a speakers' bureau or has made paid presentations on behalf of Cerapedics; and has received nonincome support (such as equipment or services), commercially derived honoraria, or other non-research-related funding (such as paid travel) from Medtronic. Dr. Levine is deceased. At the time this chapter was written Dr. Levine or an immediate family member had received royalties from Elsevier and US Spine; was a member of a speakers' bureau or had made paid presentations on behalf of Accuray; served as a paid consultant to or was an employee of US Spine; and had received research or institutional support from Accuray, Amgen Co., and Medtronic Sofamor Danek. Dr. Vaccaro or an immediate family member serves as a board member, owner, officer, or committee member of the North American Spine Society, American Spinal Injury Association, and the Cervical Spine Research Society; has received royalties from Aesculap/B.Braun, DePuy, a Johnson & Johnson company, Globus Medical, Medtronic Sofamor Danek, K2M, Stout Medical, Progressive Spinal Technology, and Applied Spinal Intellectual Properties; serves as a paid consultant to or is an employee of K2M; has received research or institutional support from AO North America, DePuy, a Johnson & Johnson company, Medtronic Sofamor Danek, and Stryker; and owns stock or stock options in Globus Medical, Disk Motion Technology, Progressive Spinal Technologies, Advanced Spinal Intellectual Properties, Computational Biodynamics, Stout Medical, Paradigm Spine, K2M, Replication Medica, Spinology, Spine Medica, Orthovita, Vertiflex, Small Bone Technologies, NeuCore, Crosscurrent, Syndicom, In Vivo, Flagship Surgical, Pearl Driver, Location Based Intelligence, and Gamma Spine. None of the following authors or any immediate family member has received anything of value from or owns stock in a commercial company or institution related directly or indirectly to the subject of this chapter: Dr. Radcliff, Dr. Delasotta, and Dr. Moore.

FIGURE 1

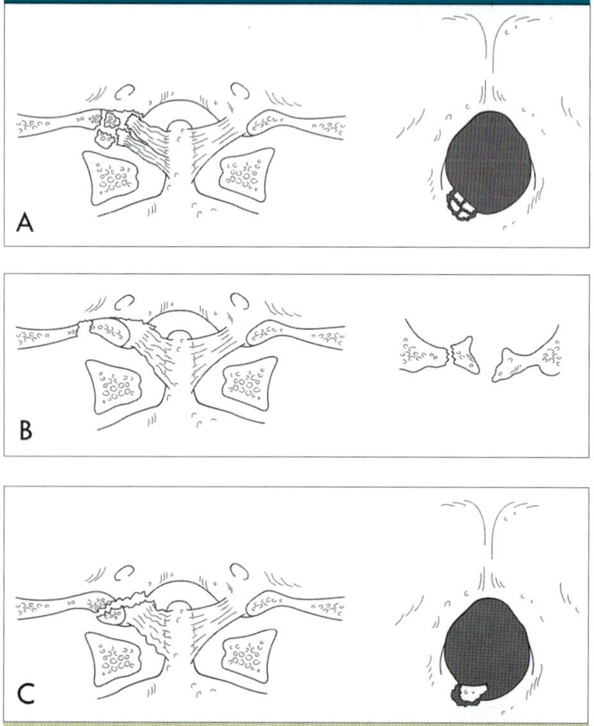

Figure 1 The classification of Anderson and Montesano describes three basic types of occipital condyle fractures. The first (**A**) is an impaction-type fracture, which is usually the result of an asymmetric axial load to the head; it may be associated with other lateral mass fractures in the upper cervical spine. The next type (**B**) is a basilar skull–type occipital condyle fracture. The final type (**C**) is an avulsion-type occipital condyle fracture, which may be the result of a distraction force applied through the alar and apical ligament complex. (Adapted with permission from Anderson P, Montesano P: Morphology and treatment of occipital condyle fractures. *Spine (Phila Pa 1976)* 1988;13(7):731.)

FIGURE 2

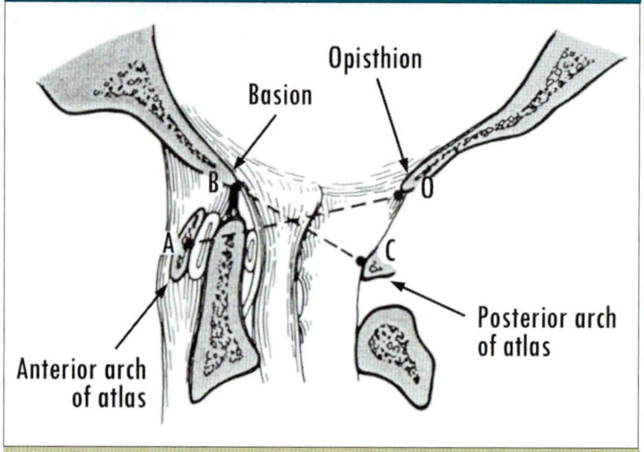

Figure 2 Powers' ratio: if BC/OA is greater than 1, then an anterior occipito-atlantal dislocation exists. Ratios less than 1 are normal except in posterior dislocations, associated fractures of the odontoid process or the ring of the atlas, and congenital anomalies of the foramen magnum. (Reproduced with permission from Jarrett PJ, Whitesides TE Jr: Injuries of the cervicocranium, in Browner BD, Jupiter JB, Levine AM, Trafton PG, eds: *Skeletal Trauma: Fractures, Dislocations, Ligamentous Injuries*. Philadelphia, PA, WB Saunders, 1992, p 668.)

Early atlanto-occipital dislocation classifications were based on radiographic reference lines of midline structures. If the ratio of two reference lines was greater than 1, a dislocation or significant subluxation was suspected (**Figure 2**).[17] Subsequently, Traynelis et al[18] used the direction and degree of displacement to define and categorize occipitocervical dislocations (**Figure 3**). CT is the current standard of care for screening cervical spine trauma patients. Recently, the normative anatomy of the craniocervical joints has been described based on CT scan as a criterion for evaluation of dislocation.[12,19-21] More recent classification systems have been proposed based on MRI evidence[10,22] of craniocervical ligament disruption and displacement of the craniocervical joints.

Four subtypes of atlas fractures have been described: (1) anterior and posterior isolated arch fractures, (2) lateral mass fractures, (3) burst-type fractures of the atlas,[6] and (4) isolated horizontal avulsion-type fractures.[23] These injuries are generally managed conservatively with external immobilization (**Figure 4**). Therefore, fracture classification of atlas fractures does not change fracture management.

Atlantoaxial instability is either due to rotatory (with or without involvement of the transverse ligament) or transverse ligament injuries. Fielding and Hawkins[24] classified rotatory atlantoaxial instability based on a series of 17 patients (**Figure 5**). In type I lesions, the transverse ligament and rotation around the dens are intact. Type II lesions represent mild insufficiency of the transverse ligament. Type III lesions are both transverse and secondary stabilizer ligament insufficiencies. Type IV lesions are a posterior shift of the lateral masses with a rotatory subluxation at the C1-C2 articulation. However, recent studies have questioned the classification and categorization of rotatory subluxation given the large range of normal C1-C2 motion.[11,25,26]

There is no formal classification of atlantoaxial instability following transverse ligament ruptures. However, two types of injury patterns are noted radiologically: (1) midsubstance ruptures through the ligament and (2) bony avulsions through the C1 lateral masses. The latter injury subtype is considered to heal more readily. The integrity of the

FIGURE 3

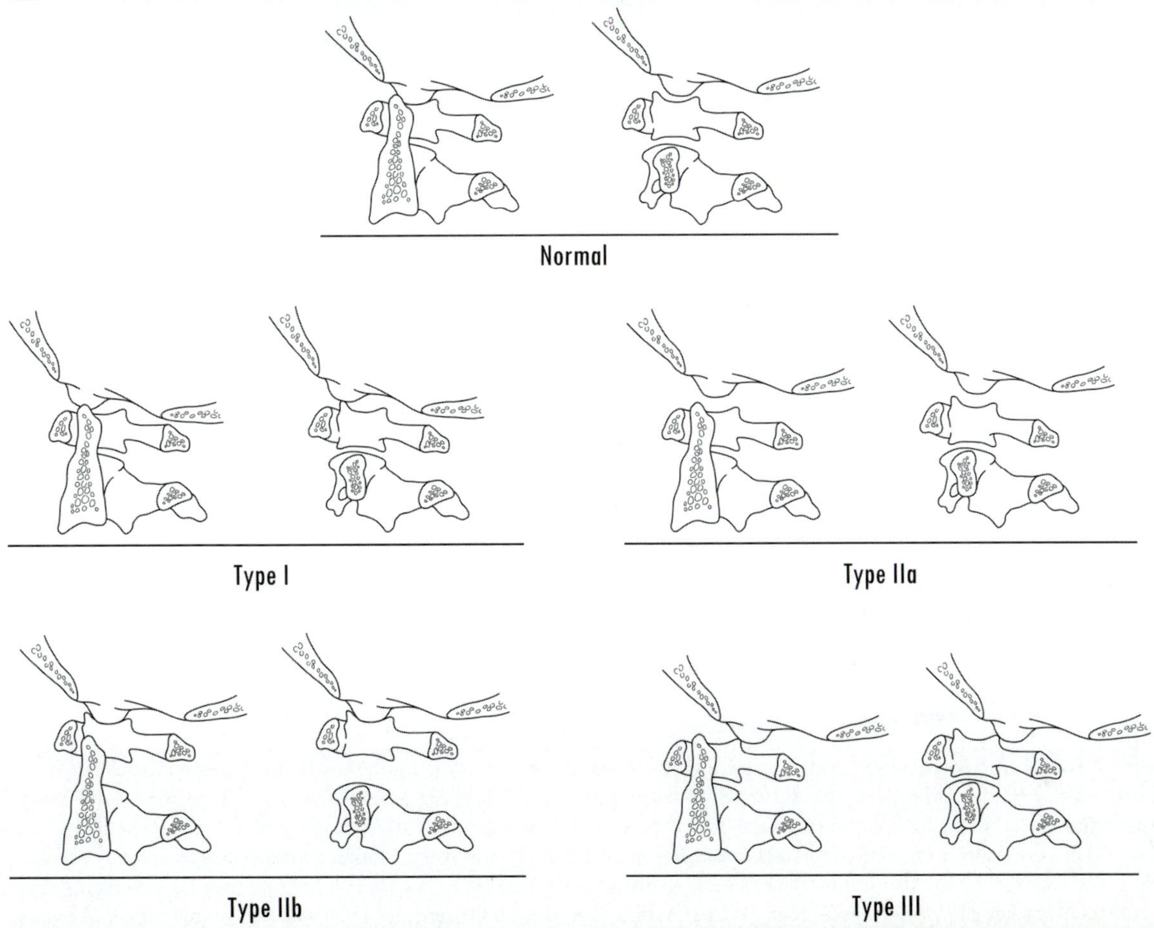

Figure 3 The classification of Traynelis et al[18] takes into account both the direction and level of upper cervical dislocation. Type I injuries (antero-occipital cervical dislocations) are more common than type III, but both are easily missed on routine radiographs. Type II injuries are distraction types, with type IIa occurring predominantly at the occipitoatlantal level and type IIb occurring at the atlantoaxial level. Not accounted for in this classification are double-level distraction injuries, which are uniformly fatal. Type III injuries, posterior atlanto-occipital dislocations, occur infrequently. (Reproduced from Levine AM: Classification of spinal injury, in Levine AM, Eismont FJ, Garfin SR, Zigler JE, eds: *Spine Trauma*. Philadelphia, PA, WB Saunders, 1998, pp 113-132.)

transverse ligament is evaluated by the atlanto-dens interval (ADI) on a lateral radiograph. The normal ADI is 3 mm or less in an adult and 3 to 5 mm in a child. An ADI of greater than 5 mm is pathologic and suggests ligamentous instability (**Figure 6**). A posterior ADI less than 14 mm also is associated with an increased risk for poor outcome in patients undergoing surgery for rheumatoid arthritis.

There are three main types of odontoid fractures, some of which have been subcategorized. The Anderson and D'Alonzo classification,[27] which consists of three types of dens fractures,[28-33] has been validated. The distinction between type II and type III fractures is important for fracture healing and management (**Figure 7**). Type II fractures are susceptible to nonunion. Important prognostic factors include age greater than 55 years, fracture displacement greater than 4 mm, fracture comminution, and smoking. Treatment recommendations for immobilization, osteosynthesis, or C1-C2 fusion are based on the risk factors for nonunion.

Traumatic spondylolisthesis of the axis, or hangman's fractures, are a well-known and classified entity. Levine and Edwards[23] modified the classification of Effendi et al[5] to produce the most widely used classification. Type I fractures are symmetric, minimally displaced, and stable. Type IA injuries are asymmetric fractures around the C1

FIGURE 4

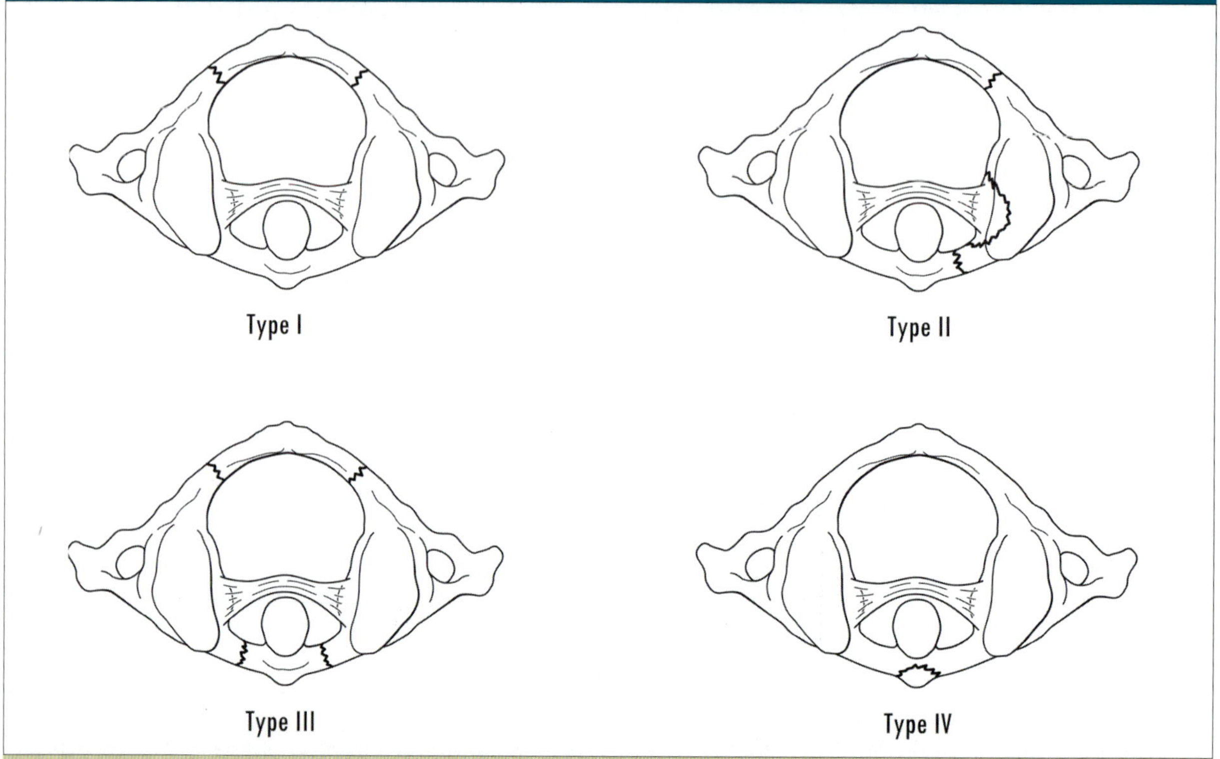

Figure 4 Four major types of fractures can occur at the level of the atlas. Type I, the most common, is a posterior arch fracture, which results from hyperextension and axial loading. It may be associated with other injuries caused by the same mechanism, such as traumatic spondylolisthesis. Type II, or lateral mass fracture, is the result of axial loading and lateral bending. There is usually a fracture line anterior and posterior to the lateral mass, causing asymmetric spreading. A second fracture line can also be present in the contralateral posterior arch. Type III, or a Jefferson fracture, is a burst fracture resulting from axial loading of C1. Two, three, four, or five fracture lines can be present, although most commonly there are four fracture lines—two in the anterior arch and two in the posterior arch. The final category, type IV, is an avulsion fracture of the anterior tubercle of the atlas. (Reproduced from Levine AM: Classification of spinal injury, in Levine AM, Eismont FJ, Garfin SR, Zigler JE, eds: *Spine Trauma*. Philadelphia, PA, WB Saunders, 1998, pp 113-132.)

FIGURE 5

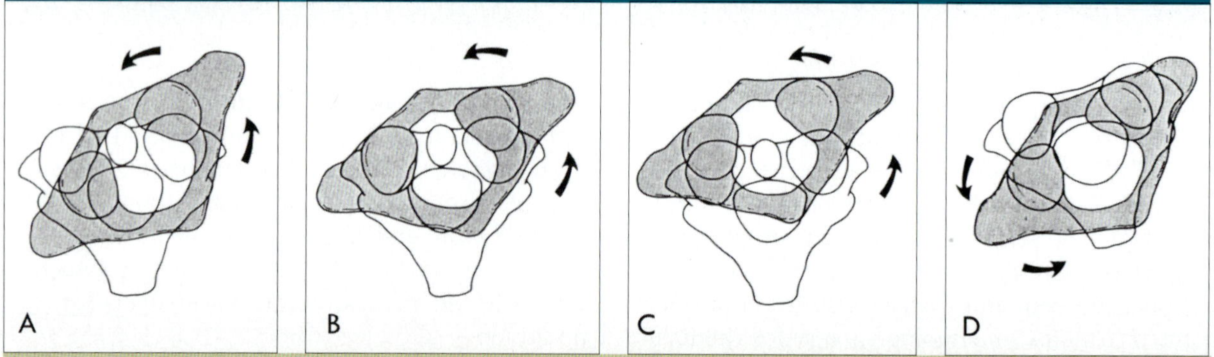

Figure 5 Four types of rotatory fixation as defined by Fielding and Hawkins:[24] **A,** type I: rotatory fixation with no anterior displacement and the odontoid as the pivot; **B,** type II: rotatory fixation with anterior displacement of 3 to 5 mm and one lateral articular process as the pivot; **C,** type III: rotatory fixation with anterior displacement of more than 5 mm; and **D,** type IV: rotatory fixation with posterior displacement. (Reproduced with permission from Jarrett PJ, Whitesides TE Jr: Injuries of the cervicocranium, in Browner BD, Jupiter JB, Levine AM, Trafton PG, eds: *Skeletal Trauma: Fractures, Dislocations, Ligamentous Injuries*. Philadelphia, PA, WB Saunders, 1992, p 676.)

FIGURE 6

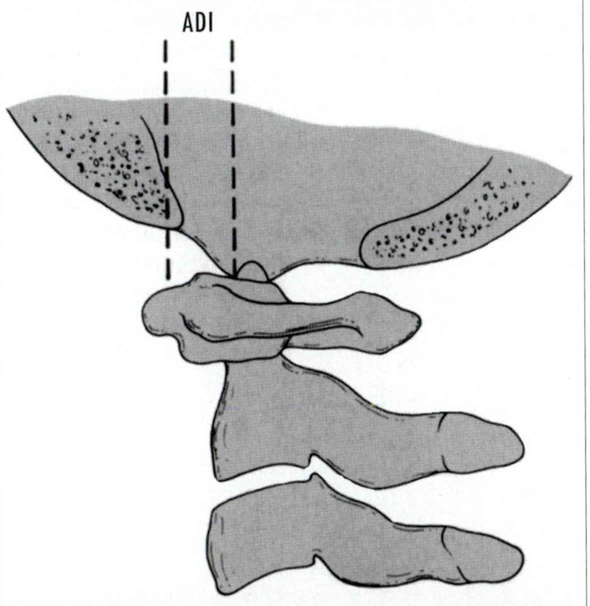

Figure 6 The atlanto-dens interval (ADI) is a method of determining the stability of the atlantoaxial segment. If the ADI is greater than 3 mm on flexion-extension radiographs in an adult, rupture of the transverse ligament is implied. However, in a child, an ADI of up to 5 mm may be normal. However, if the ADI exceeds 5 mm in an adult, both the transverse ligament and the accessory ligaments (facet capsules and alar and apical ligaments) are incompetent. (Reproduced with permission from Jarrett PJ, Whitesides TE Jr: Injuries of the cervicocranium, in Browner BD, Jupiter JB, Levine AM, Trafton PG, eds: *Skeletal Trauma: Fractures, Dislocations, Ligamentous Injuries*. Philadelphia, PA, WB Saunders, 1992, p 672.)

FIGURE 7

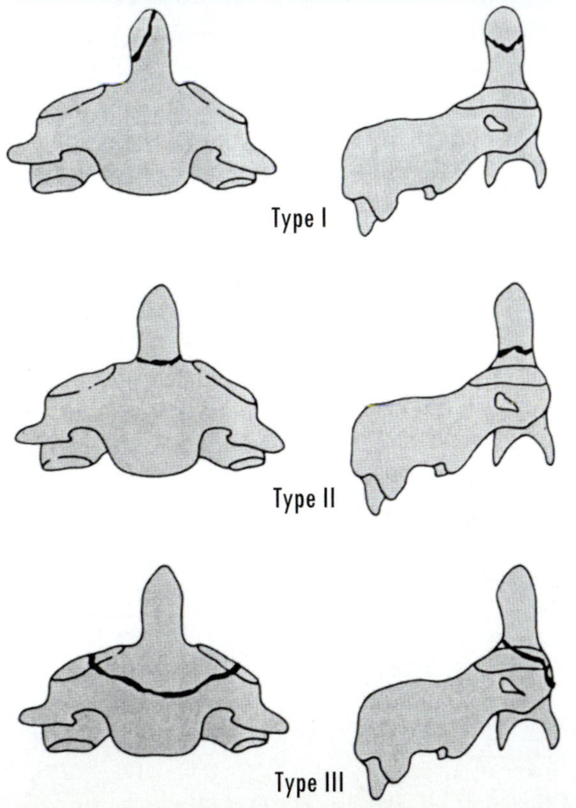

Figure 7 The most widely used classification of odontoid fractures is that published by Anderson and D'Alonzo. Type I is an oblique avulsion fracture through the tip of the dens. It is an infrequent fracture and its significance is uncertain, as some believe that there is no instability associated with it, whereas others think that it may represent an avulsion of the apical ligament from a distraction injury. Type II is a fracture at the junction of the odontoid process with the body of C2. Although not included in this classification, the amount and direction of displacement have significance for treatment and prognosis. Type III is usually an oblique fracture through the body of the axis. (Redrawn with permission from Anderson LD, D'Alonzo RT: Fractures of the odontoid process of the axis. *J Bone Joint Surg Am* 1974;56(8):1663-1674.)

ring, making them less visible on lateral radiographs. These fractures are stable, but can involve spinal cord compression and vertebral artery injury. Type II injuries are unstable, with more than 3 mm of displacement. These injuries show anterior displacement and angulation. Type IIA lesions are flexion-distraction injuries that require different treatment than type II injuries. Type IIA injuries include minimal translation, but greater than 15° of angulation. Type IIA injuries are important because they are considered to involve injury to the posterior disk anulus and therefore are unstable in traction. Type III injuries are associated with facet injuries at C2-C3 and require surgical intervention (**Figure 8**).

Lower Cervical Spine Injuries

There are several classifications for cervical spine injury in the segments from C3 to C7. Initial classifications were based on bony injury morphology and hypothesized mechanism of injury. Recent classifications now include the function of the ligamentous restraints and neurologic elements.

Axial loading injuries include compression fractures and burst fractures. Compression fractures of the lower cervical spine are similar to those of the thoracolumbar spine. Holdsworth[34,35] subcategorized compression fractures, although this classification may not be clinically useful since they are all managed conservatively. Burst fractures are axial loading injuries that involve the anterior and

FIGURE 8

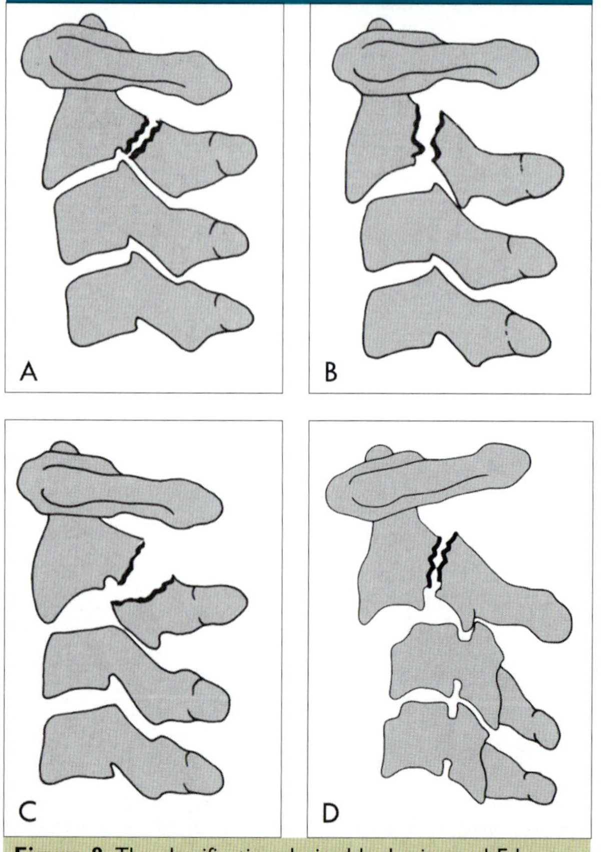

Figure 8 The classification devised by Levine and Edwards[23] for traumatic spondylolisthesis of the axis accounts for the majority of fractures of this type. **A,** The most common pattern is type I, which is characterized radiographically by a fracture through the neural arch with minimal translation (< 3 mm) and minimal angulation. Not pictured in the classification is the later addition of type IA, which has also been called atypical hangman's fracture. **B,** Type II fractures have significant angulation (> 3°) and translation (> 3 mm) and are much more unstable than type I fractures. **C,** Type IIA fractures are identified radiographically by an oblique fracture line with minimal translation but significant angulation. **D,** Type III axial fractures combine bilateral facet dislocation between C2 and C3 with a fracture of the neural arch of the axis. (Reproduced with permission from Jarrett PJ, Whitesides TE Jr: Injuries of the cervicocranium, in Browner BD, Jupiter JB, Levine AM, Trafton PG, eds: *Skeletal Trauma: Fractures, Dislocations, Ligamentous Injuries*. Philadelphia, PA, WB Saunders, 1992, p 683.)

TABLE 1

Sub-axial Cervical Spine Injury Classification System

Classification	Points
Morphology	
No abnormality	0
Compression (simple only)	1
Compression (burst)	2
Distraction (eg, facet perch, hyperextension)	3
Rotational/translational (eg, facet dislocation, unstable teardrop, or advanced stage flexion-compression injury)	4
Discoligamentous complex	
Intact	0
Indeterminate (eg, isolation interspinous widening, MRI signal change only)	1
Disrupted (eg, widening of anterior disk space, facet perch, or dislocation)	2
Neurologic involvement	
Intact	0
Nerve root injury	1
Complete cord injury	2
Incomplete cord injury	3
Continuous cord compression (neuro modifier in the setting of a neurologic deficit)	+1
Management	
Nonsurgical	≤ 3
Equivocal	4
Surgical	≥ 5

(Adapted with permission from Dvorak MF, Fisher CG, Fehlings MG, et al: The surgical approach to subaxial cervical spine injuries: An evidence-based algorithm based on the SLIC classification system. *Spine (Phila Pa 1976)* 2007;32(23):2620-2629.)

middle spinal columns. When axial loading forces are combined with a flexion vector, a teardrop fracture, also known as a triangular vertebral body fracture,[36] may occur. Allen et al[3] divided this injury into five stages of flexion-compression injury. Facet injuries may involve flexion distraction, translation, or rotation mechanisms of injury. The morphology of facet injuries includes fractures or dislocations of unilateral or bilateral facets. In dislocations, the inferior and superior articular facets remain intact, while the inferior articular process comes to rest anterior to the superior articular process.[37] In fractures, a process breaks off and vertebral translation occurs. Finally, extension injuries occur throughout the spine. Those occurring in the lower cervical spine are of two types: (1) those causing spinal cord injury without apparent fracture and (2) those in the spondylotic spine with anterior spinal column widening. Although minor injuries occur frequently, it is rare that anterior avulsions, clay-shoveler's fractures, or fractures of the transverse processes are of much clinical significance.

Recently, Vaccaro et al[38] proposed a comprehensive lower cervical spine fracture classification referred to as SLIC (Sub-axial Cervical Spine Injury Classification). It is based on subaxial spine injury, including morphology, discoligamentous complex integrity, and neurologic status. The system integrates a morphology component (compression, distraction, or translation/rotation) instead of the mechanistic classification previously described[39] because combined mechanisms of injury are so common (**Table 1**). In the SLIC system, the highest injury component determines the overall morphology score. For instance, a flexion-compression injury with interspinous widening is considered a distraction injury due to the separation of the posterior elements. The interrater reliability significantly improved relative to previous classifications.[38,40]

FIGURE 9

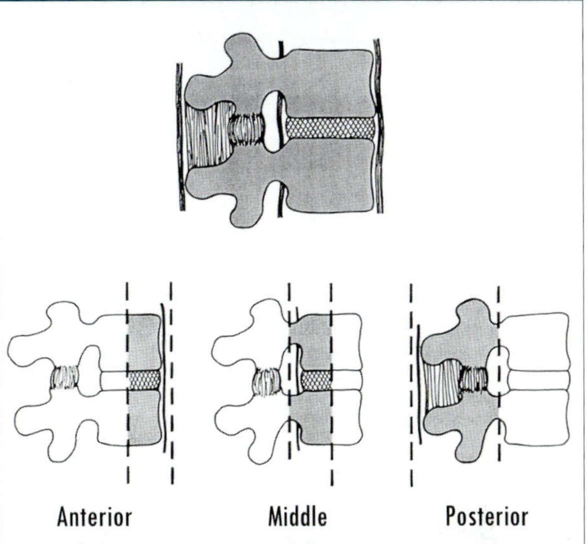

Figure 9 The three-column classification model of the spine proposed by Denis[8,41] represented an advance in thinking about spinal injuries over the previous two-column model. The concept of the middle column composed of the posterior longitudinal ligament, the posterior aspect of the anulus fibrosis, and the posterior portion of the vertebral body and disk, were added. (Reproduced with permission from Eismont FJ, Garfin SR, Abitbol JJ: Thoracic and upper lumbar spine injuries, in Browner BD, Jupiter JB, Levine AM, Trafton PG, eds: *Skeletal Trauma: Fractures, Dislocations, Ligamentous Injuries*. Philadelphia, PA, WB Saunders, 1992, p 744.)

FIGURE 10

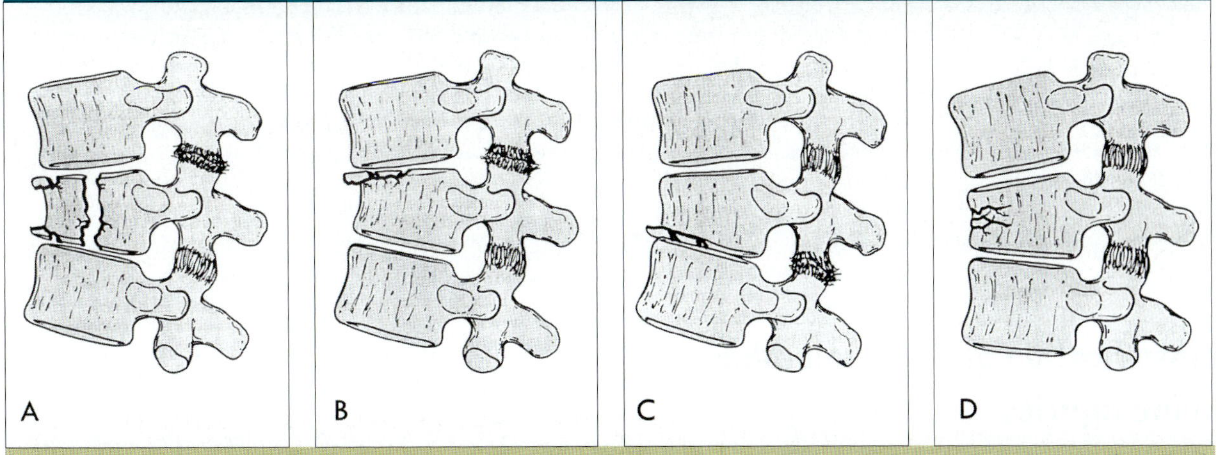

Figure 10 Although it has not been as widely used as the classification of burst fractures, Denis proposed a classification of compression fractures. The critical feature of all four types is that the posterior wall of the vertebral body is intact with the fracture line either involving the end plates or the anterior portion of the body. **A,** These fractures may involve both end plates, with or without a coronal plane fracture. **B,** The most common type involves fractures of the superior end plate alone. Nonetheless, isolated fracture of the inferior end plate can occur (**C**). **D,** The final pattern is a buckling fracture of the anterior cortex with both end plates intact. This type must be carefully differentiated from a minimally displaced flexion-distraction injury. (Reproduced with permission from Eismont FJ, Garfin SR, Abitbol JJ: Thoracic and upper lumbar spine injuries, in Browner BD, Jupiter JB, Levine AM, Trafton PG, eds: *Skeletal Trauma: Fractures, Dislocations, Ligamentous Injuries*. Philadelphia, PA, WB Saunders, 1992, p 746.)

FIGURE 11

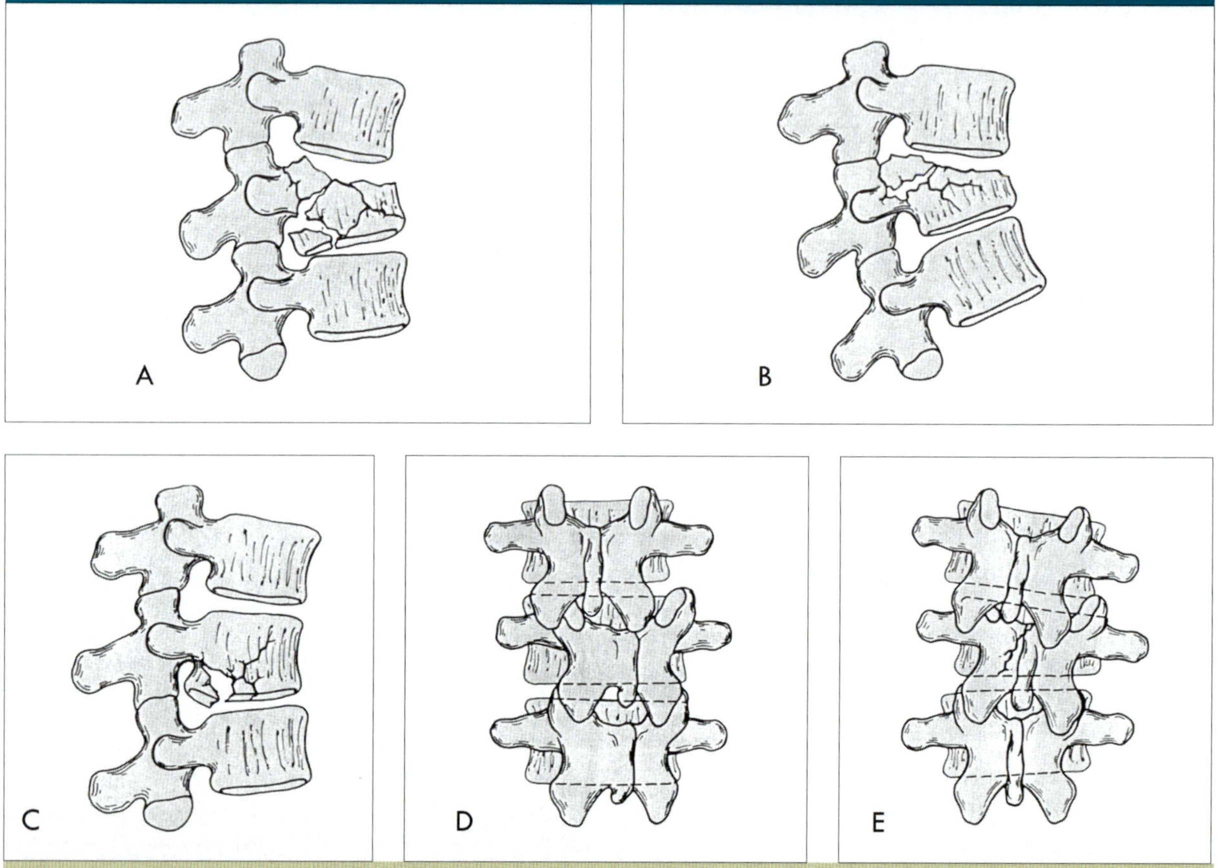

Figure 11 The Denis classification of burst fractures is used to describe the majority of injuries of this type and is helpful in subdividing the injuries according to differing treatment patterns. The common element is disruption of the posterior wall of the vertebral body in all cases. The type **A** fracture is predominantly an axial loading injury with minimal kyphosis. A comminution of both end plates occurs, and there may also be fractures in the posterior elements. Type **B** fractures tend to have more kyphosis and sparing of the posterior elements. Comminution of the superior end plate and upper portion of the vertebral body occur, with retropulsion of the posterosuperior portion into the canal. The first two types represent the vast majority of burst fractures. Type **C** fractures involve the inferior portion of the vertebral body and end plate with retropulsion of the posterior inferior corner of the body into the canal. These are extremely uncommon. The type **D** fracture is a combination of a type A fracture with rotation, which is best appreciated on an AP radiograph. This type must be carefully differentiated from a shear injury. Type **E** is a lateral burst fracture that results from a combination of axial loading and lateral bending, and is also best appreciated on AP radiograph. (Adapted with permission from Eismont FJ, Garfin SR, Abitbol JJ: Thoracic and upper lumbar spine injuries, in Browner BD, Jupiter JB, Levine AM, Trafton PG, eds: *Skeletal Trauma: Fractures, Dislocations, Ligamentous Injuries*. Philadelphia, PA, WB Saunders, 1992, p 753.)

Classification of Thoracolumbar Spine Injuries

Thoracolumbar Junction

The thoracolumbar junction (between T10 and L2) has unique anatomic and mechanical features that affect the mechanism, development, and prognosis of fractures. The majority of spine injuries in this location occur at the transition zone, where the chest lever arm and lower lumbar spine interact. The three types of thoracolumbar fractures described are compression, distraction, and shear injuries. There are considered to be three load-bearing columns of the thoracolumbar spine: anterior, middle, and posterior column.[8] Denis[41] hypothesized that the middle column was the critical element in spinal stability. Subsequent fracture classifications and descriptions are based on the consideration of three-column spinal stability (**Figure 9**).

Compression fractures are defined by their intact posterior wall (middle column), and are subdivided into four types.[8,41] The prognostic values

TABLE 2

Load-Sharing Classification

Classification	Points
Comminution/involvement	
Little = < 30% comminution on sagittal plane section CT	1
More = 30% to 60% communtion	2
Gross = > 60% comminution	3
Apposition of fragments	
Minimal = Minimal displacement on axial CT cut	1
Spread = At least 2-mm displacement of < 50% cross section of body	2
Wide = At least 2-mm displacement of > 50% cross section of body	3
Deformity Correction	
Little = Kyphotic correction ≤ 3° on lateral plain films	1
More = Kyphotic correction 4° to 9°	2
Most = Kyphotic correction ≥ 10°	3

(Adapted with permission from Parker JW, Lane JR, Karaikovic EE, Gaines RW: Successful short-segment instrumentation and fusion for thoracolumbar spine fractures: A consecutive 41/2-year series. *Spine (Phila Pa 1976)* 2000;25(9):1157-1169.)

FIGURE 12

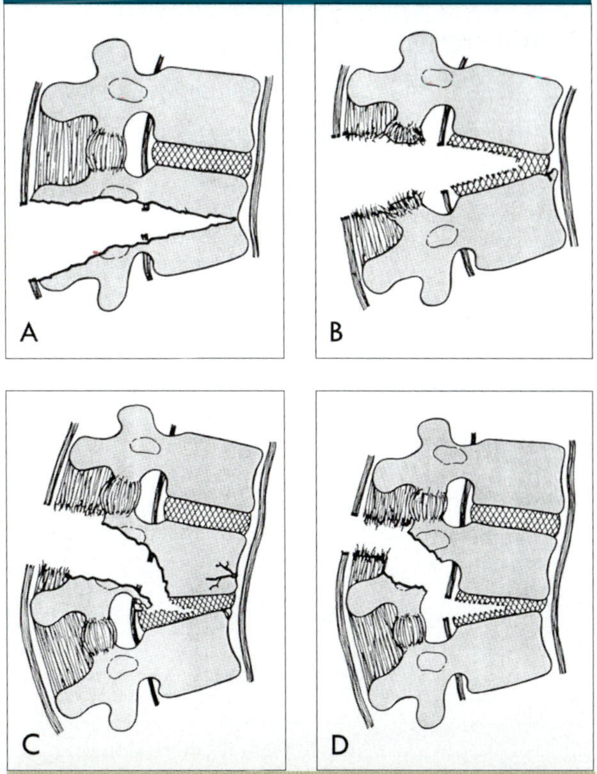

Figure 12 This group of drawings illustrates the Denis classification of flexion-distraction injuries, which is very helpful in subdividing injuries according to types requiring different treatment. These may occur through one level, completely through bone, traversing the spinous process, pedicles, and vertebral body (**A**), and are often called Chance fractures. The second type (**B**) occurs through two levels, completely through ligamentous structures, traversing the supraspinous and interspinous ligaments, joint capsules, ligamentum flavum, and disk, but does not involve the anterior longitudinal ligament. With displacement, this is a bilateral facet dislocation. The final two types involve either the posterior column, injured through ligamentous structures, and the middle column, injured through bone (**C**), or the posterior column through bone and the middle column through ligament and disk (**D**). (Reproduced with permission from Eismont FJ, Garfin SR, Abitbol JJ: Thoracic and upper lumbar spine injuries, in Browner BD, Jupiter JB, Levine AM, Trafton PG, eds: *Skeletal Trauma: Fractures, Dislocations, Ligamentous Injuries*. Philadelphia, PA, WB Saunders, 1992, p 754.)

of these subdivisions remain unclear (**Figure 10**). The classification of burst fractures, proposed by Denis,[8] is related to the prognosis and outcome of surgical reconstruction (**Figure 11**). Type A fractures involve comminution of both end plates, and constitute 40% of all burst fractures. They are generally due to axial compression that results in pedicle and posterior element comminution. Type B fractures involve the superior end plate and result from flexion with axial compression. Retropulsion into the spinal canal may result from the posterosuperior corner of the vertebral body. This fracture pattern constitutes 40% of burst fractures. Rare type C fractures occur at the inferior endplate. Comminution results from a flexion and compression mechanism. Type D fractures are shear force–related injuries, whereas type E fractures are lateral burst fractures—uncommon injury patterns. The load-sharing classification (**Table 2**) of thoracolumbar burst fractures correlates well with short-segment posterior instrumentation outcomes.[42] It was originally designed to assess vertebral body stability that bears axial loads associated with short-segment instrumentation following burst fracture. It incorporates fracture comminution, diastasis of fracture fragments, and angular deformity into a score range from 3 to 9. A score greater than or equal to 7 predicts a worse prognosis for short-segment posterior instrumentation.[43]

FIGURE 13

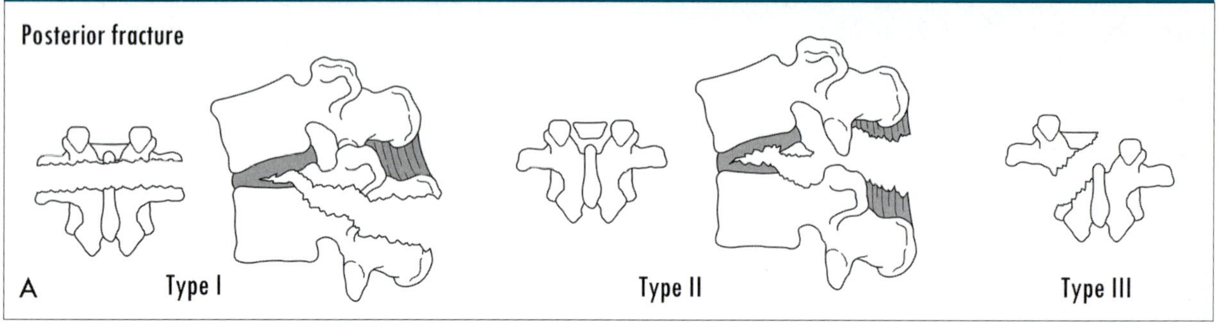

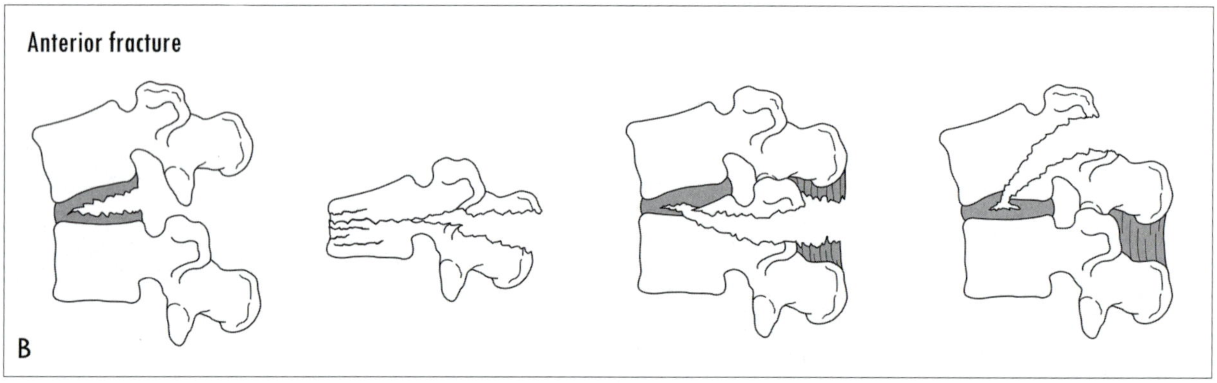

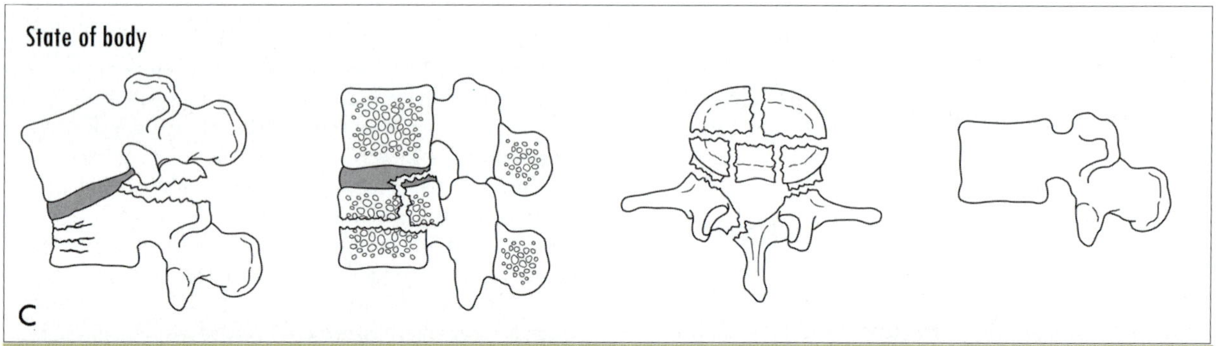

Figure 13 The classification of flexion-distraction injuries proposed by Gertzbein and Court-Brown allowed more precision in the description of these injuries. Each component of the injury, the posterior portion of the fracture, the anterior portion of the fracture, and the vertebral body, could be described by one of three choices. Its complexity, however, does not add significantly to our ability to understand or treat the injury but simply to our ability to describe it precisely. **A**, The posterior elements can be fractures through the pedicles, through ligamentous structures, or obliquely across, usually involving the pars on one side. **B**, The anterior portion of the injury can go through the disk, the vertebral body, or obliquely through the disk and body from either direction. **C**, The body can be wedged, comminuted, or intact. (Adapted with permission from Gertzbein SD, Court-Brown CM: Flexion-distraction injuries of the lumbar spine. *Clin Orthop Relat Res* 1988;227:52-60.)

Distraction injuries are subdivided to differentiate bony from ligamentous components. The Denis classification consists of four parts (**Figure 12**): (1) one level through bone, (2) one level through ligaments, (3) two levels with the middle column injured through bone, and (4) two levels with the middle column injured through ligament.[41] The classification of Gertzbein and Court-Brown[9] allows more precise definitions of anterior element, body, and posterior element injuries (**Figure 13**). The fracture-line route from posterior to anterior determines late stability of the injury. Thus, injuries considered to involve only bone have the best prognosis due to a high rate of healing. Injuries that involve posterior ligaments and anterior bone are functionally less stable. When the injury line goes through the interspinous ligament, facet capsule, and disk, a poor prognosis is

FIGURE 14

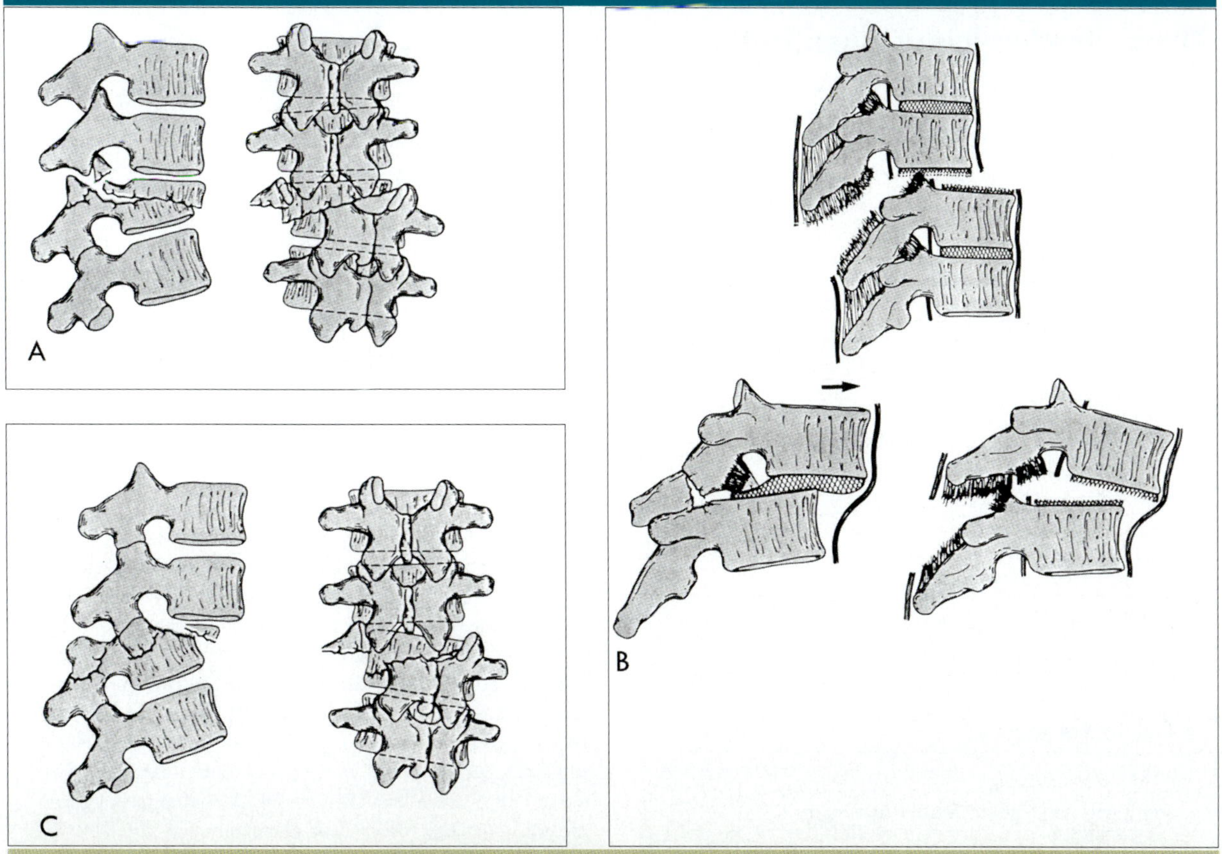

Figure 14 The Denis classification of fracture-dislocations describes a group of diverse injuries that most authors attribute to a shear mechanism. They are high, complex, and unstable, as the shear force is usually added to some other injury mechanism. Type **A** is a flexion-rotation injury, either occurring through the bone or through the disk. There is complete disruption of all three columns of the spine, usually with the anterior longitudinal ligament remaining as the only intact structure. Commonly, this is stripped off of the anterior portion of the vertebral body below. These injuries are usually associated with fractures of the superior facet of the more caudal vertebra. Type **B** is a shear injury. The type that produces anterior spondylolisthesis of the more cephalad vertebra usually fractures a facet, whereas that causing posterior listhesis of the more cephalad vertebra normally does not cause a fracture of the facet joint. Type **C** is a bilateral facet dislocation. This is a flexion-distraction injury but with the disruption of the anterior column in addition to the posterior and middle columns. This disruption through the anterior column may occur through either the anterior intervertebral disk or the anterior vertebral body. (Reproduced with permission from Eismont FJ, Garfin SR, Abitbol JJ: Thoracic and upper lumbar spine injuries, in Browner BD, Jupiter JB, Levine AM, Trafton PG, eds: *Skeletal Trauma: Fractures, Dislocations, Ligamentous Injuries*. Philadelphia, PA, WB Saunders, 1992, p 758.)

predicted. This injury causes severe translation with a high probability for neurologic deficit. Consequently, surgical reduction and stabilization are required.[44]

Shear injuries, or fracture-dislocations, are described in the thoracolumbar spine as well.[41] Denis noted three different types (**Figure 14**) based on mechanism of injury. These fractures are best identified by bidirectional translation, seen on AP and lateral radiographs. As a group, they represent the most complex and unstable injuries.[41]

Vaccaro et al created the Thoracolumbar Injury Classification and Scoring System (TLICS).[38] The TLICS was created in response to a need for a simple, standardized clinical tool. TLICS includes elements of morphology of bony injury (independent of mechanism), posterior ligamentous complex integrity, and neurologic status. Fractures are divided into compression, distraction, or shear/rotational morphologies. The integrity of the posterior ligamentous complex is assessed. Additionally, neurologic injury is included in the comprehensive scale.[38] This system correlates well with ligamentous injury extent, and assists in management decisions[45,46] (**Table 3**).

TABLE 3

Thoracolumbar Injury Classification System (TLICS)

Classification	Points
Morphology	
No abnormality	0
Compression (simple only)	1
Compression (burst)	2
Rotational/translational	3
Distraction	4
Posterior ligamentous complex status disrupted in tension, rotation, or translation	
Intact	0
Indeterminate/suspect	2
Injured	3
Neurologic involvement	
Intact	0
Nerve root injury	2
Complete cord/conus medullaris injury	2
Incomplete cord/conus medullaris injury	3
Cauda equina	3
Management	
Nonsurgical	≤ 3
Equivocal	4
Surgical	≥ 5

(Adapted from with permission from Vaccaro AR, Lehman RA Jr, Hurlbert RJ, et al: A new classification of thoracolumbar injuries: The importance of injury morphology, the integrity of the posterior ligamentous complex, and neurologic status. *Spine (Phila Pa 1976)* 2005;30(20):2325-2333.)

FIGURE 15

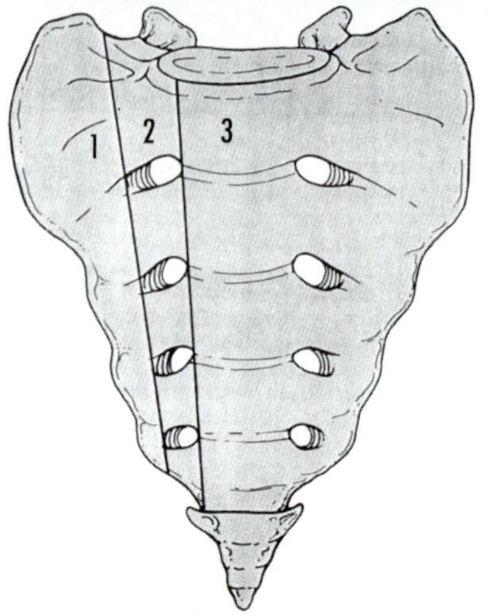

Figure 15 Denis et al classified 236 fractures of the sacrum into zones. Zone 1 was the region of the sacral ala, which comprised a group of 118 patients of whom 5.9% had neurologic deficit. Zone 2 was the region of the neuroforamina with the fracture line involving one or more foramina but exiting without involving the central neural canal. This group was composed of 81 patients of whom 24.4% had neurologic findings. The final group of patients had fractures in zone 3 with central neural canal involvement. This pattern was seen in only 21 patients, but the rate of neurologic deficit was extremely high (56.7%). (Redrawn from Denis F, Davis S, Comfort T: Sacral fractures: An important problem. Retrospective analysis of 236 cases. *Clin Orthop Relat Res* 1988;227:67-81.)

Non–Thoracolumbar Junction Fractures

The thoracolumbar junction is the most common site of injury. Rare injuries may occur to the adjacent thoracic or lower lumbar spine. Above the thoracolumbar junction, the thoracic spine is more stable because of the presence of the rib cage. Injuries to this region commonly involve high-energy mechanisms that result in translation or rotation. Below the thoracolumbar junction, the low lumbar spine (L3 to S1) is highly mobile, with a normal lordotic sagittal alignment. The injury patterns in the low lumbar spine exhibit different characteristics than the two other regions. Finally, the anatomic difference in neural tissue in the spinal canal among the thoracic, thoracolumbar, and low lumbar spine result in different prognostic outcomes for similar radiologic fracture patterns. The terminology of Ferguson and Allen et al[39] is commonly used to describe injuries to these anatomic locations, even though the neurologic tissue and biomechanics of injury are significantly different from the thoracolumbar junction.

Classification of Sacral Fractures

Vertical sacral fracture classifications by Denis[47] predict neurologic deficit (**Figure 15**). Zone 1 injuries through the ala are associated with a 5% incidence of neurologic deficit. Zone 2 injuries traverse the neuroforamen, involving at least one foramen, without sacral canal involvement. Neurologic deficit occurred in 28.4% of patients with a zone 2 injury. Finally, zone 3 fractures involve the sacral canal, and 56.7% of patients had neurologic deficit. Thus, the zone classification of Denis and the anatomic classification of the fracture line help to establish treatment protocols.

FIGURE 16

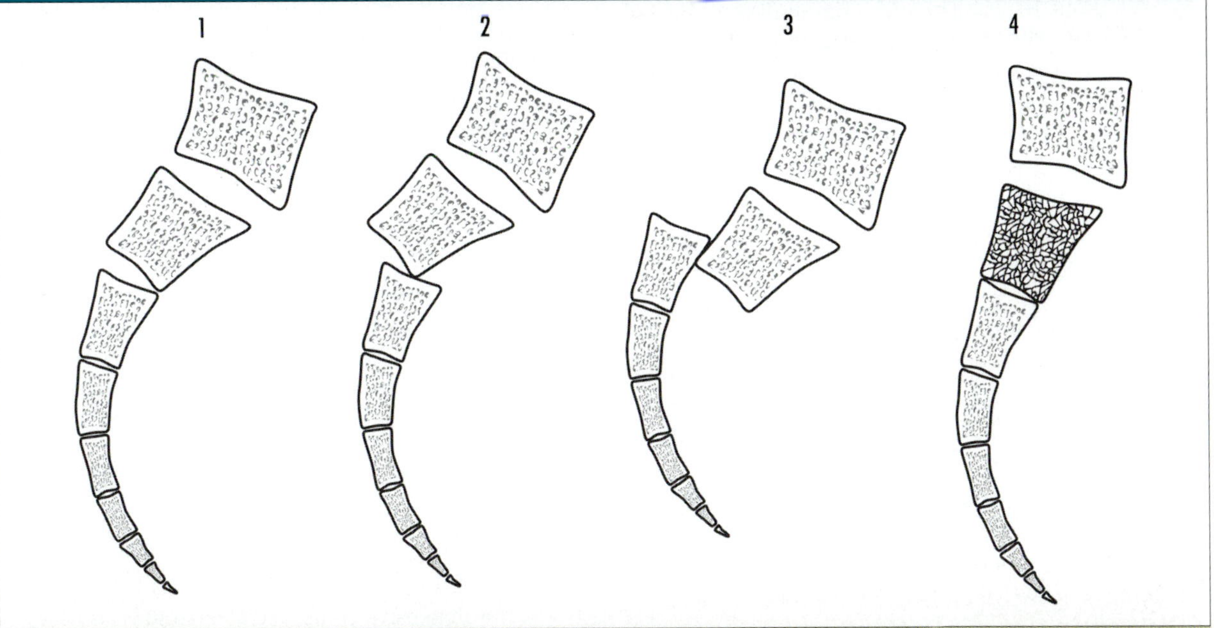

Figure 16 Subclassification of Denis zone 3 fractures as suggested by Strange-Vognsen and Lebech.[52] Type 1 fractures are flexion injuries with angulation and no translation. Type 2 fractures are combination flexion and translation injuries. Type 3 fractures are pure translation injuries in flexion or extension (flexion illustrated here). Type 4 fractures are axial loading injuries that result in comminuted fractures of the S1 and possibly S2 vertebral bodies. This classification is not mutually exclusive with that of Denis et al. (Adapted with permission from Schildhauer TA, Bellabarba C, Nork SE, Barei DP, Routt ML Jr, Chapman JR: Decompression and lumbopelvic fixation for sacral fracture-dislocations with spino-pelvic dissociation. *J Orthop Trauma* 2006;20(7):447-457.)

Notable subtypes of the Denis classification include sacral stress fractures in the sacral alae or vertebral body.[48] Such injuries occur in elderly women with osteoporosis due to normal physiologic stress on bone. These injuries can result in severe back pain.[49]

Another important subtype of sacral injury includes transverse fractures of the sacrum.[50,51] A transverse sacral fracture classification was proposed by Roy-Camille et al and modified by Strange-Vognsen and Lebech (**Figure 16**).[52,53] Multiple longitudinal and transverse sacral fractures may result in the axial skeleton becoming disconnected from the pelvis, termed spinopelvic dissociation.[54] Such injuries may result in severe cauda equina compression. Sacral laminectomy and segmental fixation is the best management option for this condition.[54]

Sacral fracture subtypes are not mutually exclusive. For instance, bilateral Denis type 3 vertical sacral fractures may occur with a horizontal (Strange-Vognsen) type 2 injury, creating an "H" type fracture.[55]

The Future of Spinal Classification Systems

A universally applicable spine injury classification system incorporates several different factors: regional anatomic differences, neurologic injury, mechanism of injury, and radiologic description. A universal classification system allows accurate communication between centers, to facilitate prognostic evaluations and to delineate treatment.

Look for future classification systems to include "host" factors related to spinal trauma injury. The Cierny-Mader classification of osteomyelitis[56,57] includes host factors relevant to the status of the disease. Relevant host factors in a spine classification may include patient age,[58] preexisting spinal stenosis,[55] spondyloarthropathy,[59] metastatic or infectious disease process, systemic medical conditions, and osteoporosis.[60] These factors demonstrate important survival and recovery predictions following spine trauma.

References

1. White AA III, Panjabi MM: *Clinical Biomechanics of the Spine*. Philadelphia, PA, JB Lippincott, 1978.
2. White AA III, Panjabi MM: The clinical biomechanics of the occipitoatlantoaxial complex. *Orthop Clin North Am* 1978;9(4):867-878.
3. Allen BL Jr, Ferguson RL, Lehmann TR, O'Brien RP: A mechanistic classification of closed, indirect fractures and dislocations of the lower cervical spine. *Spine (Phila Pa 1976)* 1982;7(1):1-27.
4. Bohler L: *The Treatment of Fractures*, ed 4. Baltimore, MD, W Wood, 1935.
5. Effendi B, Roy D, Cornish B, Dussault RG, Laurin CA: Fractures of the ring of the axis: A classification based on the analysis of 131 cases. *J Bone Joint Surg Br* 1981;63-B(3):319-327.
6. Jefferson G: Fracture of the atlas vertebra: Report of four cases and a review of those previously recorded. *Br J Surg* 1920;7:407-422.
7. Anderson PA, Montesano PX: Morphology and treatment of occipital condyle fractures. *Spine (Phila Pa 1976)* 1988;13(7):731-736.
8. Denis F: The three column spine and its significance in the classification of acute thoracolumbar spinal injuries. *Spine (Phila Pa 1976)* 1983;8(8): 817-831.
9. Gertzbein SD, Court-Brown CM: Flexion-distraction injuries of the lumbar spine: Mechanisms of injury and classification. *Clin Orthop Relat Res* 1988;227:52-60.
10. Gonzalez LF, Fiorella D, Crawford NR, et al: Vertical atlantoaxial distraction injuries: Radiological criteria and clinical implications. *J Neurosurg Spine* 2004;1(3):273-280.
11. Mönckeberg JE, Tomé CV, Matías A, Alonso A, Vásquez J, Zubieta JL: CT scan study of atlantoaxial rotatory mobility in asymptomatic adult subjects: A basis for better understanding C1-C2 rotatory fixation and subluxation. *Spine (Phila Pa 1976)* 2009;34(12):1292-1295.
12. Rojas CA, Bertozzi JC, Martinez CR, Whitlow J: Reassessment of the craniocervical junction: Normal values on CT. *AJNR Am J Neuroradiol* 2007; 28(9):1819-1823.
13. Lucas JT, Ducker TB: Motor classification of spinal cord injuries with mobility, morbidity and recovery indices. *Am Surg* 1979;45(3):151-158.
14. McAfee PC, Yuan HA, Fredrickson BE, Lubicky JP: The value of computed tomography in thoracolumbar fractures: An analysis of one hundred consecutive cases and a new classification. *J Bone Joint Surg Am* 1983;65(4):461-473.
15. McAfee PC, Yuan HA, Lasda NA: The unstable burst fracture. *Spine (Phila Pa 1976)* 1982;7(4): 365-373.
16. Rihn JA, Fisher C, Harrop J, Morrison W, Yang N, Vaccaro AR: Assessment of the posterior ligamentous complex following acute cervical spine trauma. *J Bone Joint Surg Am* 2010;92(3):583-589.
17. Powers B, Miller MD, Kramer RS, Martinez S, Gehweiler JA Jr: Traumatic anterior atlanto-occipital dislocation. *Neurosurgery* 1979;4(1): 12-17.
18. Traynelis VC, Marano GD, Dunker RO, Kaufman HH: Traumatic atlanto-occipital dislocation: Case report. *J Neurosurg* 1986;65(6):863-870.
19. Bellabarba C, Mirza SK, West GA, et al: Diagnosis and treatment of craniocervical dislocation in a series of 17 consecutive survivors during an 8-year period. *J Neurosurg Spine* 2006;4(6): 429-440.
20. Chang W, Alexander MT, Mirvis SE: Diagnostic determinants of craniocervical distraction injury in adults. *AJR Am J Roentgenol* 2009;192(1):52-58.
21. Radcliff KE, Ben-Galim P, Dreiangel N, et al: Comprehensive computed tomography assessment of the upper cervical anatomy: What is normal? *Spine J* 2010;10(3):219-229.
22. Horn EM, Feiz-Erfan I, Lekovic GP, Dickman CA, Sonntag VK, Theodore N: Survivors of occipitoatlantal dislocation injuries: Imaging and clinical correlates. *J Neurosurg Spine* 2007;6(2):113-120.
23. Levine AM, Edwards CC: Fractures of the atlas. *J Bone Joint Surg Am* 1991;73(5):680-691.
24. Fielding JW, Hawkins RJ: Atlanto-axial rotatory fixation: (Fixed rotatory subluxation of the atlanto-axial joint). *J Bone Joint Surg Am* 1977; 59(1):37-44.
25. Hicazi A, Acaroglu E, Alanay A, Yazici M, Surat A: Atlantoaxial rotatory fixation-subluxation revisited: A computed tomographic analysis of acute torticollis in pediatric patients. *Spine (Phila Pa 1976)* 2002;27(24):2771-2775.
26. Villas C, Arriagada C, Zubieta JL: Preliminary CT study of C1-C2 rotational mobility in normal subjects. *Eur Spine J* 1999;8(3):223-228.
27. Anderson LD, D'Alonzo RT: Fractures of the odontoid process of the axis. *J Bone Joint Surg Am* 1974;56(8):1663-1674.
28. Amyes EW, Anderson FM: Fracture of the odontoid process; report of sixty-three cases. *AMA Arch Surg* 1956;72(3):377-393.
29. Clark CR, White AA III: Fractures of the dens: A multicenter study. *J Bone Joint Surg Am* 1985; 67(9):1340-1348.
30. Lind B, Nordwall A, Sihlbom H: Odontoid fractures treated with halo-vest. *Spine (Phila Pa 1976)* 1987;12(2):173-177.
31. Maiman DJ, Larson SJ: Management of odontoid fractures. *Neurosurgery* 1982;11(4):471-476.

32. Ryan MD, Taylor TK: Odontoid fractures: A rational approach to treatment. *J Bone Joint Surg Br* 1982;64(4):416-421.
33. Southwick WO: Management of fractures of the dens (odontoid process). *J Bone Joint Surg Am* 1980;62(3):482-486.
34. Holdsworth F: Fractures, dislocations, and fracture-dislocations of the spine. *J Bone Joint Surg Am* 1970;52(8):1534-1551.
35. Holdsworth FW: Fractures, dislocations and fracture dislocations of the spine. *J Bone Joint Surg Br* 1963;45-B(1):6-20.
36. Lee C, Kim KS, Rogers LF: Triangular cervical vertebral body fractures: Diagnostic significance. *AJR Am J Roentgenol* 1982;138(6):1123-1132.
37. Taylor AR: The mechanism of injury to the spinal cord in the neck without damage to vertebral column. *J Bone Joint Surg Br* 1951;33-B(4):543-547.
38. Vaccaro AR, Lehman RA Jr, Hurlbert RJ, et al: A new classification of thoracolumbar injuries: The importance of injury morphology, the integrity of the posterior ligamentous complex, and neurologic status. *Spine (Phila Pa 1976)* 2005;30(20):2325-2333.
39. Ferguson RL, Allen BL Jr: A mechanistic classification of thoracolumbar spine fractures. *Clin Orthop Relat Res* 1984;189:77-88.
40. Dvorak MF, Fisher CG, Fehlings MG, et al: The surgical approach to subaxial cervical spine injuries: An evidence-based algorithm based on the SLIC classification system. *Spine (Phila Pa 1976)* 2007;32(23):2620-2629.
41. Denis F: Spinal instability as defined by the three-column spine concept in acute spinal trauma. *Clin Orthop Relat Res* 1984;189:65-76.
42. Parker JW, Lane JR, Karaikovic EE, Gaines RW: Successful short-segment instrumentation and fusion for thoracolumbar spine fractures: A consecutive 41/2-year series. *Spine (Phila Pa 1976)* 2000;25(9):1157-1170.
43. Dai LY, Jiang LS, Jiang SD: Conservative treatment of thoracolumbar burst fractures: A long-term follow-up results with special reference to the load sharing classification. *Spine (Phila Pa 1976)* 2008;33(23):2536-2544.
44. Levine AM, Bosse M, Edwards CC: Bilateral facet dislocations in the thoracolumbar spine. *Spine (Phila Pa 1976)* 1988;13(6):630-640.
45. Vaccaro AR, Rihn JA, Saravanja D, et al: Injury of the posterior ligamentous complex of the thoracolumbar spine: A prospective evaluation of the diagnostic accuracy of magnetic resonance imaging. *Spine (Phila Pa 1976)* 2009;34(23):E841-E847.
46. Schweitzer KM, Vaccaro AR, Harrop JS, et al: Interrater reliability of identifying indicators of posterior ligamentous complex disruption when plain films are indeterminate in thoracolumbar injuries. *J Orthop Sci* 2007;12(5):437-442.
47. Denis F, Davis S, Comfort T: Sacral fractures: An important problem. Retrospective analysis of 236 cases. *Clin Orthop Relat Res* 1988;227:67-81.
48. Lourie H: Spontaneous osteoporotic fracture of the sacrum: An unrecognized syndrome of the elderly. *JAMA* 1982;248(6):715-717.
49. Babayev M, Lachmann E, Nagler W: The controversy surrounding sacral insufficiency fractures: To ambulate or not to ambulate? *Am J Phys Med Rehabil* 2000;79(4):404-409.
50. Bonin JG: Sacral fractures and injuries to the cauda equina. *J Bone Joint Surg Br* 1945;27:113-127.
51. Carl A, Delman A, Engler G: Displaced transverse sacral fractures: A case report, review of the literature, and the CT scan as an aid in management. *Clin Orthop Relat Res* 1985;194:195-198.
52. Strange-Vognsen HH, Lebech A: An unusual type of fracture in the upper sacrum. *J Orthop Trauma* 1991;5(2):200-203.
53. Gibbons KJ, Soloniuk DS, Razack N: Neurological injury and patterns of sacral fractures. *J Neurosurg* 1990;72(6):889-893.
54. Schildhauer TA, Bellabarba C, Nork SE, Barei DP, Routt ML Jr, Chapman JR: Decompression and lumbopelvic fixation for sacral fracture-dislocations with spino-pelvic dissociation. *J Orthop Trauma* 2006;20(7):447-457.
55. Okada S, Maeda T, Ohkawa Y, et al: Does ossification of the posterior longitudinal ligament affect the neurological outcome after traumatic cervical cord injury? *Spine (Phila Pa 1976)* 2009;34(11):1148-1152.
56. Cierny G III, Mader JT, Penninck JJ: A clinical staging system for adult osteomyelitis. *Clin Orthop Relat Res* 2003;414:7-24.
57. Mader JT, Shirtliff M, Calhoun JH: Staging and staging application in osteomyelitis. *Clin Infect Dis* 1997;25(6):1303-1309.
58. Fassett DR, Harrop JS, Maltenfort M, et al: Mortality rates in geriatric patients with spinal cord injuries. *J Neurosurg Spine* 2007;7(3):277-281.
59. Whang PG, Goldberg G, Lawrence JP, et al: The management of spinal injuries in patients with ankylosing spondylitis or diffuse idiopathic skeletal hyperostosis: A comparison of treatment methods and clinical outcomes. *J Spinal Disord Tech* 2009;22(2):77-85.
60. Kim HS, Park SK, Joy H, Ryu JK, Kim SW, Ju CI: Bone cement augmentation of short segment fixation for unstable burst fracture in severe osteoporosis. *J Korean Neurosurg Soc* 2008;44(1):8-14.

CHAPTER 14
An Imaging Atlas of Spinal Injury

Stephen L. Gabriel Rothman, MD Jack E. Zigler, MD

Introduction

The diagnosis and ultimate treatment of the injured spine will often require numerous imaging studies. Although little has changed in what the imaging studies show, advances in technology have changed the way clinicians look at the neuroradiologic armamentarium. For generations, the primary imaging modality of choice has been a routine plain radiograph of the spine. Virtually all emergency departments have a suite of high-quality, state-of-the-art radiology machines and trained technologists. The immobilized patient with suspected spinal injuries is typically carefully positioned in the radiology suite for the appropriate plain radiographs of the injured portion of the spine. In some cases, this is problematic. The person with suspected spine injury needs to be moved very carefully by a trained team. Because of that, properly positioned radiographs are sometimes very difficult to perform. Supine patients with thick shoulders are particularly difficult to evaluate because the thickness of the shoulders attenuates the x-ray beam, obliterating the detail of the lower cervical spine. Furthermore, the more severely a patient is injured, the more likely it is that the radiological evaluation will be time-consuming for all involved staff.

For more than 25 years, CT was the most important secondary imaging modality. After evaluation of the routine plain radiographs, the patient is usually next sent for a CT scan for three possible reasons:

1. In instances where an obvious bony lesion was seen, CT would be performed for further evaluation of the fracture to determine the subtleties of the bony pathologic anatomy. The main purpose of CT would be to optimize the surgical or conservative treatment of the already diagnosed bony injury.
2. In cases where routine radiographs were of poor technical quality and adequate evaluation of a portion of the spine could not be made, CT would be performed to "clear" the obscured anatomic zone.
3. In patients for whom routine plain radiographs were thought to be normal but the index of suspicion for an occult spinal injury was high, CT would be performed as the benchmark for the diagnosis of difficult-to-see bony injury.

To some extent, this has changed over the last few years in two clinical situations: (1) the very severely traumatized patient with suspected injury to multiple body parts and systems, and 2) the patient brought in to the emergency facility immobilized with even the remote possibility of occult cervical injury.

Because of the general availability of very rapid, multidetector CT scanners, there has been a shift away from the routine radiographic evaluation of the cervical spine in favor of high-resolution CT scans. In many institutions, patients brought in to the hospital immobilized following suspected cervical spine trauma will not even stop to have plain radiographs of the cervical spine. Even if the clinical suspicion is relatively low for a bony spinal injury, when the patient is already lying supine and is restrained, he or she can be brought directly to the CT scanner. There is no need for flexion/extension movement of the patient's neck; indeed, there need not be any motion of the patient whatsoever. The current generation of CT scanners produces images so quickly that it actually takes longer to put the patient on the table than it does to generate the images. Once the axial CT scans are captured into the memory of the computer, appropriate multiplanar reformations are now done with ease. It has become the rule in many institutions to replace most, or even all, cervical radiographs with reformatted CT scans regardless of the level of concern for disruptive injury. Consequently, it is not surprising that the majority of CT scans done in the emergency department setting will be normal. It is felt at these

Dr. Rothman or an immediate family member owns stock or stock options in Johnson & Johnson. Dr. Zigler or an immediate family member serves as a board member, owner, officer, or committee member of Cervical Spine Research Society; has received royalties from Zimmer, K2M, and Osprey; serves as a paid consultant to or is an employee of Alphatec Spine and Synthes; owns stock or stock options in Flexuspine; and has received nonincome support (such as equipment or services), commercially derived honoraria, or other non-research-related funding (such as paid travel) from AO and Synthes.

institutions that the monetary and radiation exposure costs to those patients who turn out not to be injured is a reasonable trade-off in the long run, to allow the diagnosis of occult bony lesions that would otherwise be missed.

Patients with multiple injuries, including soft-tissue injuries of the chest, abdomen, and pelvis, are now primarily evaluated by CT. It is not unusual with a multisystem-injured patient to have a whole-body CT scan from the neck through the pelvis. The primary interest in these cases of blunt force abdominal or chest trauma is looking for rupture of an abdominal viscus, or pulmonary, cardiac, or vascular trauma. The display device of the CT scanner is set to optimize the image of bone, and films can be made of the spine in any projection. Many CT scanners can actually produce three-dimensional renderings of the spine or surface renderings of the spine that can be turned in three-dimensional space if the appropriate computer hardware is available.

Three thousand years ago, Ecclesiastes said "there was nothing new under the sun." This is fundamentally true with regard to CT scanning. The techniques used with the current fast scanners are no different from those used on the most primitive second-generation scanner built 25 years ago. Nearly all of the pathologic conditions that can be seen using the current multidetector CT scanners were also diagnosable on second- and third-generation scanners using reformation software developed as early as the late 1970s, when one of us (S.R.) began using the first reformation software to produce fairly primitive spinal images in a variety of clinical settings. With the advent of third-generation CT scanners later in the1980s, thin-section, reformatted CT became universally available. The only problem was that it required a significant amount of effort on the part of the CT technologists and a considerable amount of hardware to produce the reformations. The current generation scanners, with their readily available computer hardware, have trivialized the process of reformation. A significant time burden is no longer necessary to produce high-quality sagittal, coronal, or oblique images. Indeed, the standard of care requires reformatted CT for every evaluation of the spine whether due to trauma or not.

The Injured Spine as a Dynamic Functional Unit

It is preferable, when reviewing imaging studies of the injured spine, to think dynamically. A set of images, be they plain radiographs, CT scans, or magnetic resonance images, often allows one to derive the mechanism of injury from the specific pathologic patterns. In the cervical spine, most people use the classification system of Allen et al.[1] This system defines injuries by the vector of the dominant forces applied to the spine. These include compression, distraction, flexion, extension, rotation, and lateral bending. More often than not, there are combined forces acting in concert to deform the cervical spine during catastrophic injury, and the imaging pattern may be complex. Within this chapter, an attempt will be made to use this classification wherever possible.

The pattern of bony and soft-tissue injury often provides useful clinical information to help formulate the immediate treatment of the spine. Some patterns of injury leave certain structures intact. Some patterns characteristically cause instability. Instability does not mean hypermobility. A rigorous definition of stability has been provided by White and Panjabi.[2] It is therefore useful at this time to reiterate the system for defining instability. Assimilation of these clinical hints is critical for optimal patient care.

White and Panjabi created a point system in which different structural or physiologic injuries are assigned a point value.[2] Injury to either the anterior or posterior bony elements, rendering them nonfunctional, scores 2 points each. Relative sagittal plane translation of more than 3.5 mm is awarded 2 points. Relative sagittal plane rotation greater than 11 mm also gets 2 points. A positive stretch test is awarded 2 points. Spinal cord damage is rated at 2 points, with 1 point for nerve root injury. A total score of 5 points or more indicates instability.

It is also useful to use a three-column model of the spine when discussing the injury mechanism or treatment options.[3] The more rigorous the analysis, the more logical the treatment options can become. The motion segments are divided into anterior, middle, and posterior columns (**Figure 1**).

The anterior column includes the anterior longitudinal ligament as well as the anterior half of the vertebral bodies and the intervening disk. The middle column extends from the midportion of the vertebral body to include the posterior longitudinal ligament to the base of the pedicles. The posterior column includes the laminar arches, the ligamenta flava, and the posterior wall of the neural canal. The spine will be stable if two of the three compartments are intact. Injury to all three columns is unstable, by definition.

FIGURE 1

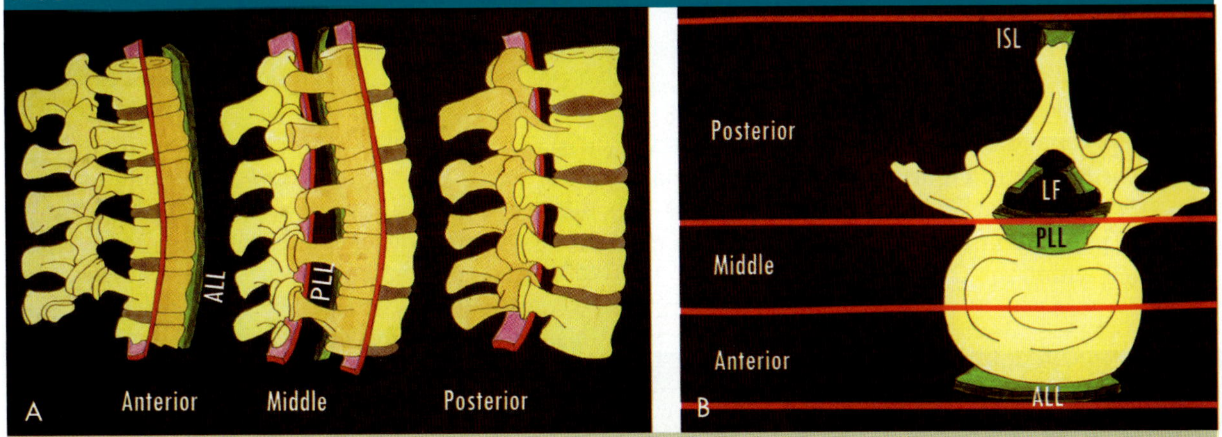

Figure 1 Sagittal (**A**) and axial (**B**) diagrams defining the anterior, middle, and posterior columns in the three-column spine concept of Denis[3]. ALL = anterior longitudinal ligament; PLL = posterior longitudinal ligament; ISL = interspinous ligament; LF = ligamentum flavum. (Courtesy of the late William Wilemon, MD.)

Imaging Techniques

Cervical Spine

Except for penetrating knife or bullet wounds, it is rare for a structural injury of the neck to occur from a direct blow to the cervical spine. It is far more likely that the spine is injured secondary to the head being put in motion with respect to the cervical spine. The head is so massive with respect to the cervical spine that the relative momentum of the moving head exceeds the ability of the spine's soft-tissue structures to overcome the inertia, causing the bones, joints, or cervical disks to fail. This may occur from a blow to the head where the head is quickly put in motion or the sudden application of significant deceleration forces to the body where the head continues moving. The classic example of this is the restrained driver whose car hits an immovable object. The body is restrained by the seat belt or steering wheel, but the head is free to follow Newton's law and just keeps on going.

It is useful to divide the cervical spine into two segments: the upper segment, the craniovertebral junction, which for our discussion will be defined as the base of the skull down through the C2-C3 disk; and the lower cervical spine, which we are defining as everything from the C2-C3 disk down to the C7-T1 disk. Injuries to these segments are radiographically diagnosed and often treated very differently. We begin our discussion at the craniovertebral junction.

Craniovertebral Junction

Figure 2 summarizes all the lesions of the craniocervical junction based on the vectors of the force being applied to the spine.

FIGURE 2

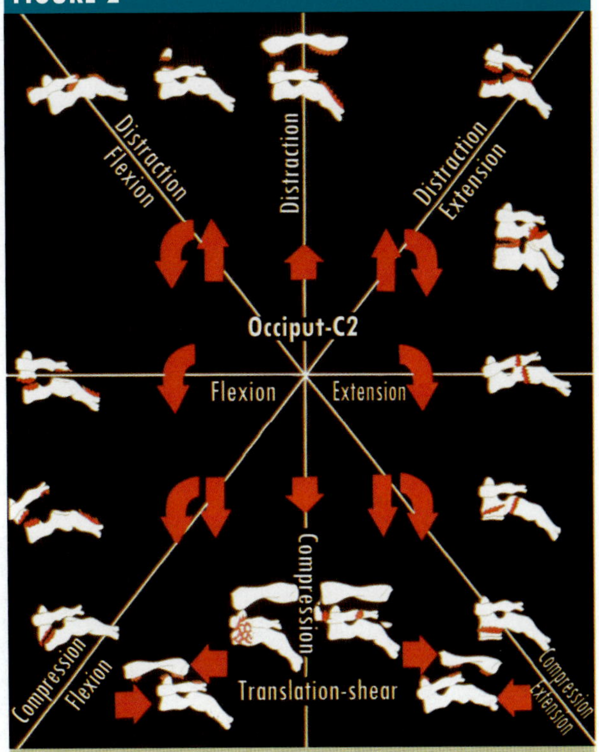

Figure 2 Injuries of the craniovertebral area as described by McAfee et al. (Courtesy of the late William Wilemon, MD.)

Injuries of the craniovertebral junction are relatively rare. There are several different types of basal skull fractures that may extend into the occipital condyles and cause joint injury.[4-6] These tend to be pain-producing injuries but are not biomechanically important. Disruptive injuries of the craniocervical joints, on the other hand, are devastating injuries. Typically, craniocervical subluxation occurs as a result of high-energy trauma in younger patients, who usually die from their injuries.[7,8] There are some lesions of these joints that do not lead to dislocation. The joint capsules can be partially torn. **Figure 3** is a very important axial view of C1. The C1 vertebra is intrinsically normal. There is no fracture here. The dens is well positioned within the C1 ring. The scan is very abnormal, however. The head is turned to the left (note the position of the mandible), and C1 is oriented normally. While many patients may be rotated when they are positioned in the scanner, they do not look like this. The C1 ring must rotate with the skull. There is never any rotation allowable at the normal occipitocervical articulation. Seeing the mandible rotated with respect to C1 is always abnormal and indicates severe injury to the joints at the base of the skull. Thin-section, reformatted CT scans of the base of the skull show bilateral subluxation of the occipital condyles in this patient (**Figure 4**). This is a distraction-rotation injury. The violent distraction has disrupted the joint capsules without a fracture. The rotation is identified by the abnormal position of the mandible with respect to the axial image of the C1 ring. Temporomandibular joint dislocation and/or mandibular ramus fractures could produce a similar image, but should be very clinically apparent and easily ruled out.

The classic compression lesion of the craniovertebral junction is due to a downward force vector of the skull upon the C1 ring, shattering it.[9,10] This is called the Jefferson fracture. Jefferson fractures may include one, two, three, or four separated fracture lines (**Figure 5**). The mechanism is similar in all cases. The occipital condyles are shaped like a pair of chisels facing away from each other. As the skull is forced down upon the neck, the outwardly sloping cranial facets force the superior articular processes of C1 apart. In the classic case, the C1 ring breaks in four places, two just anterior to the facet joints and two just behind them (**Figure 5,** *C*). The bony insertion of the transverse

FIGURE 3

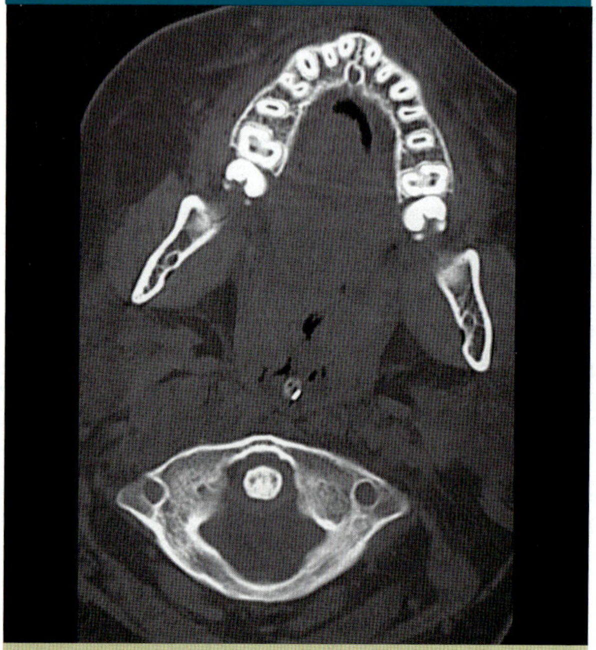

Figure 3 Axial CT scan of C1. The mandible is rotated approximately 10° from the plane of C1.

FIGURE 4

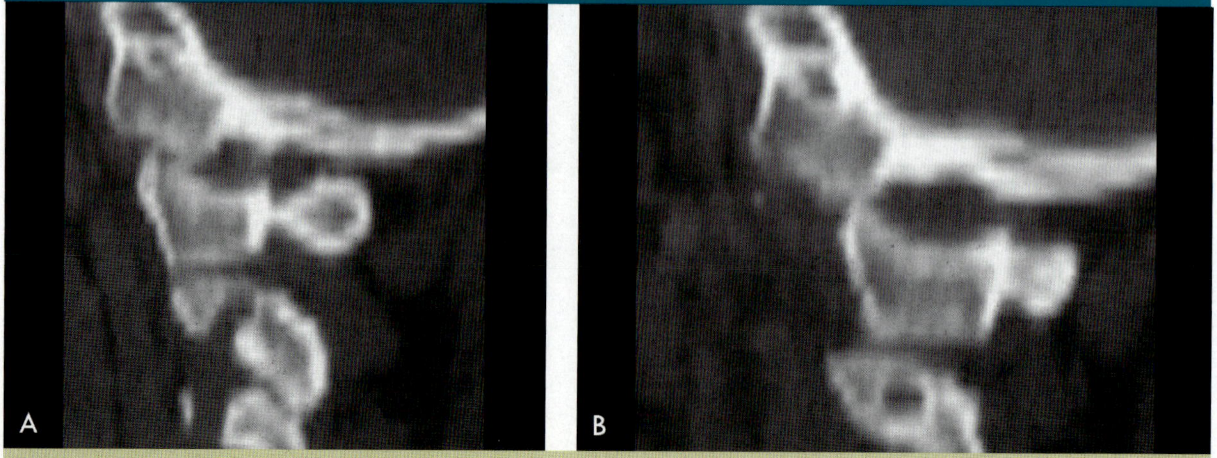

Figure 4 Sagittal reformatted CT scans of both occipital condyles and the lateral masses of C1. Subluxation is noted on one side (**A**) and dislocation on the other (**B**).

FIGURE 5

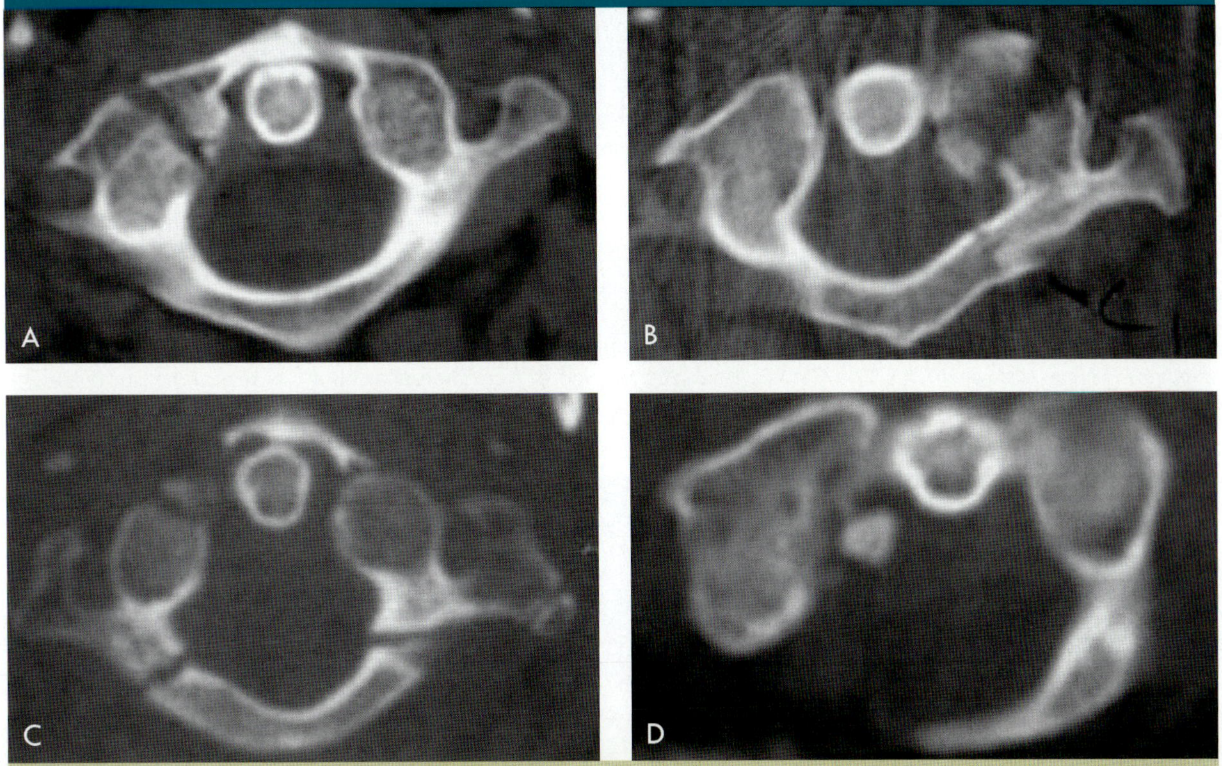

Figure 5 Axial CT images of Jefferson fractures. **A,** Single right-sided compression fracture of the neural ring through the articular process. **B,** Fractures of both anterior and posterior portions of the left side of the C1 neural arch. **C,** Four fractures of the neural ring: two of the anterior arch, and two of the posterior arch. **D,** Avulsion of the insertion of the transverse ligament.

ligament frequently becomes avulsed, and the transverse ligament loses its function (**Figure 5,** *D*). Often this is a self-decompressing injury, since the affected ring actually becomes wider than normal.

The diagnosis of Jefferson fracture is easy when lateral radiographs show the fracture lines or AP radiographs demonstrate widening of the C1 ring. When these findings are not present, the diagnosis may be very difficult. The lateral radiograph in **Figure 6** reveals a very subtle but important sign of Jefferson fracture. In this lateral view of the skull, there are no visible fractures. C1 appears oriented to the base of the skull. Look carefully at the tip of the dens and at the anterior atlantoaxial joint. The tip of the dens projects superior to a line drawn across the superior edges of the C1 ring. That is abnormal and indicates upward herniation of the dens through the ring. For that to occur, the ring of C1 must be broken, the transverse ligament traumatically avulsed or weakened by rheumatoid arthritis. The CT scan in this patient showed a subtle Jefferson fracture.

FIGURE 6

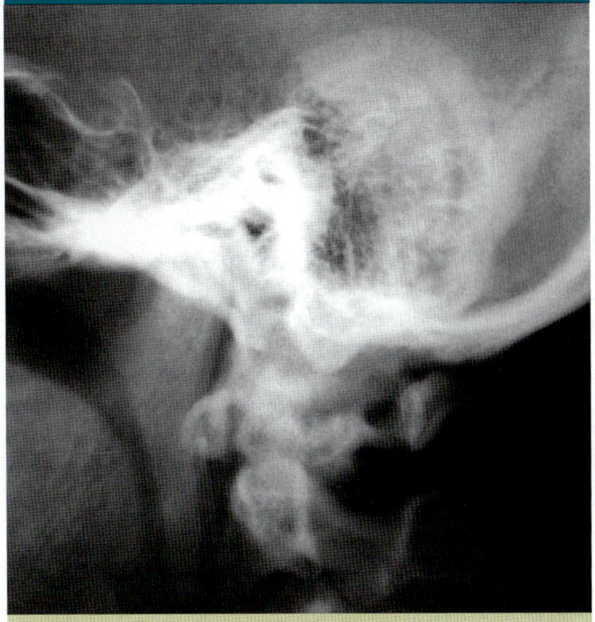

Figure 6 Lateral skull radiograph. Note slight upward herniation of the tip of the dens through the C1 ring.

FIGURE 7

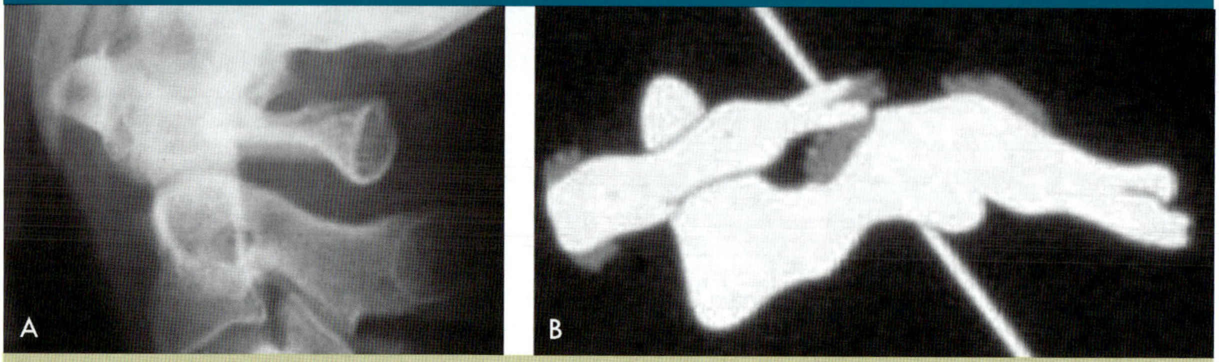

Figure 7 Flexion subluxation of C1 on C2: **A,** plain radiograph; and **B,** illustration. (Panel B is courtesy of the late William Wilemon, MD.)

FIGURE 8

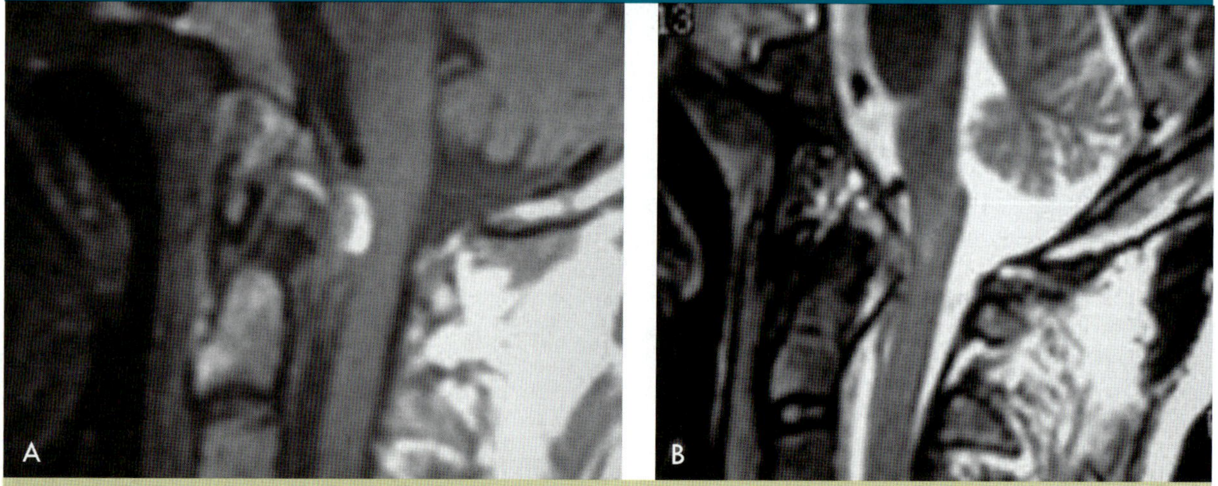

Figure 8 Sagittal T1-weighted (**A**) and T2-weighted (**B**) MRI scans of the craniovertebral junction showing rupture of the transverse ligament and anterior joint with acute hematoma.

Flexion subluxation of the cervical spine may tear the transverse ligament or more frequently avulse its attachment from the anterior arch of C1 (**Figure 7**). The posterior ligaments are also torn. These lesions are inherently unstable and will often present with devastating neurologic injury. The distance between the anterior arch of C1 and the dens should be less than 3 mm in adults and no more than 4 mm to 5 mm in children.[11,12]

T1-weighted MRI scans demonstrate acute hemorrhage in the torn transverse ligament (**Figure 8**). The blood is bright on T1 images and stands out clearly. The torn posterior longitudinal ligament, which attaches to the transverse ligament, is better seen on the T2-weighted images. This is due to the inherent contrast between the ligament and the bright cerebrospinal fluid. Fortunately, this patient was intact neurologically and the spinal cord appears intrinsically normal.

Fractures of the Dens

Fractures of the dens are very common.[13,14] In fact, they are the most common injuries in elderly people who suffer ground-level falls. They are also common in acceleration-deceleration injuries. Dens fractures are grouped into three types. Type 1 fractures, which are very rare, are essentially an avulsion of the tip of the dens. Type 2 fractures are a shearing fracture, which separates the dens from the body of C2; these are quite common. Type 3 fractures are much more complex lesions. In this type, the fracture line which separates the dens from the C2 body extends into the body of C2, and occasionally even into the C2-C3 disk space.

Figure 9 illustrates a type 1 dens fracture (perhaps a "type 1.5"). The fracture line does not traverse the base of the dens. Coronal CT is the procedure of choice for making the diagnosis. This is

FIGURE 9

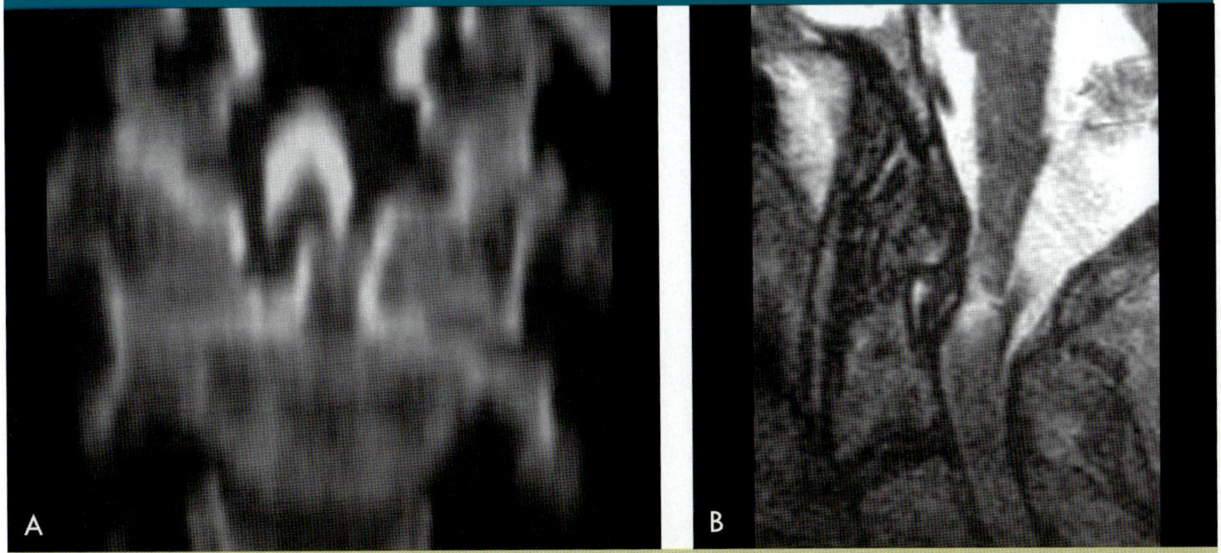

Figure 9 Type I dens fracture: **A,** coronal CT reformation demonstrating separation of the tip of the dens; **B,** sagittal T2-weighted MRI scan showing posterior displacement of the tip of the dens. Note also the hematoma of the spinal cord.

FIGURE 10

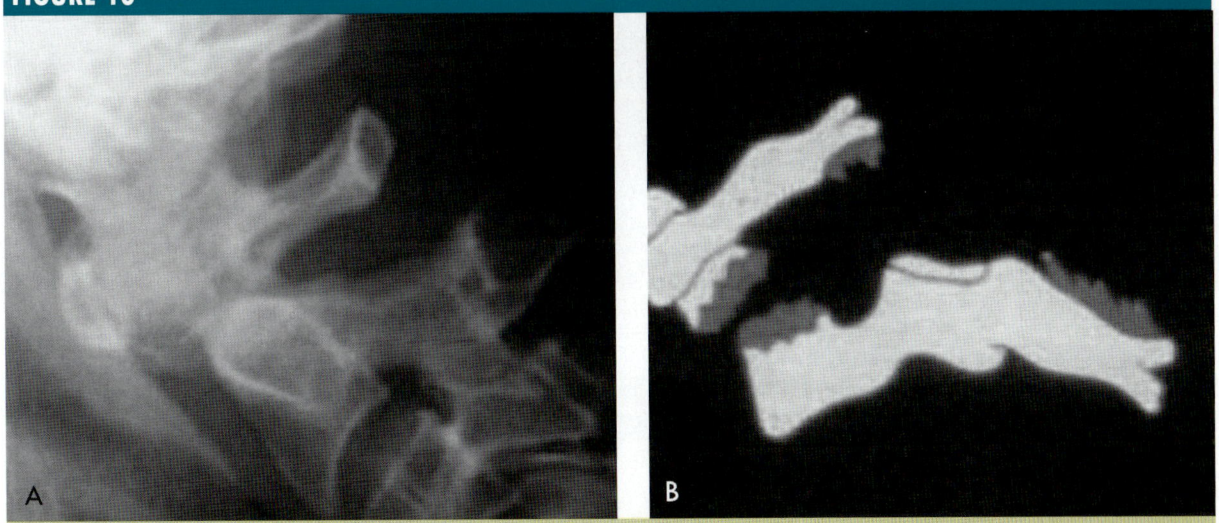

Figure 10 Hyperflexion fracture-dislocation of the dens: **A,** lateral radiograph; **B,** illustration of a similar injury. (Panel B is courtesy of the late William Wilemon, MD.)

an intrinsically unstable fracture that has, in this patient, caused anterior spinal cord injury.

Type 2 dens fractures occur from hyperflexion or hyperextension. The two different types are easily separable on any imaging study. When the head is projected into hyperflexion so that C2 fails, the transverse ligament forces the dens forward to the point that the base of the dens separates from the body of C2 (**Figure 10**). The transverse ligament, which is incredibly strong, maintains its integrity. If the forces are sufficient, C1 can dislocate forward upon C2. If this occurs, then the posterior ligamentous structures also fail.

Hyperextension type 2 dens fractures occur when violent hyperextension motion of the head causes the anterior arch of C1 to shear the dens from the body of C2 (**Figure 11**). The transverse ligament is intact but the posterior ligamentous structures fail. The spinal cord is usually injured by the posteriorly displaced odontoid tip.

FIGURE 11

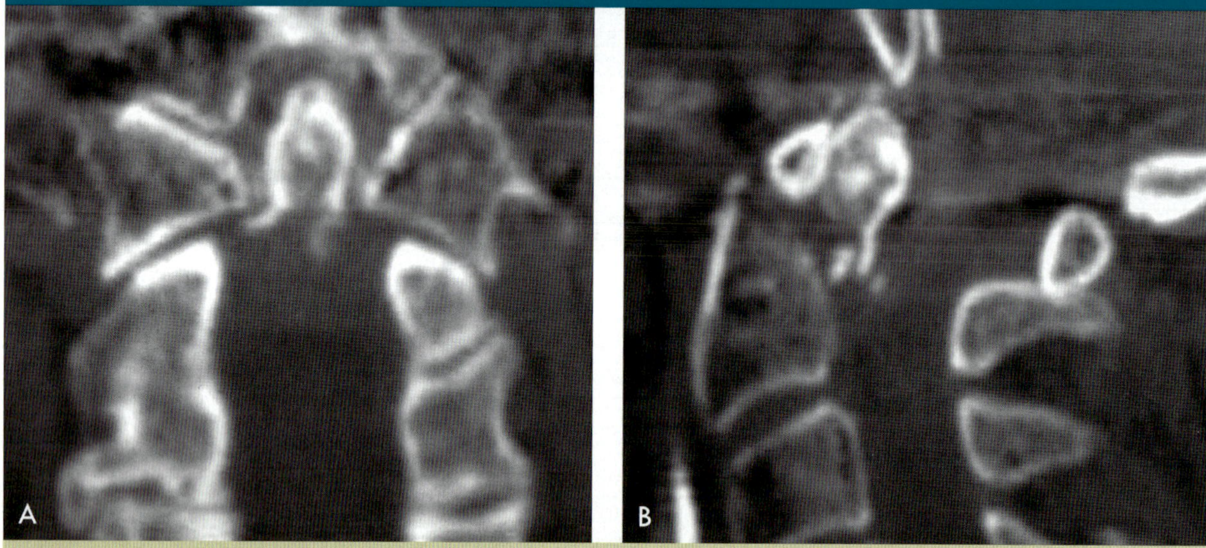

Figure 11 Hyperextension fracture-dislocation of C2: **A,** coronal; and **B,** sagittal CT reformation showing posterior displacement of the fragmented dens into the spinal canal.

FIGURE 12

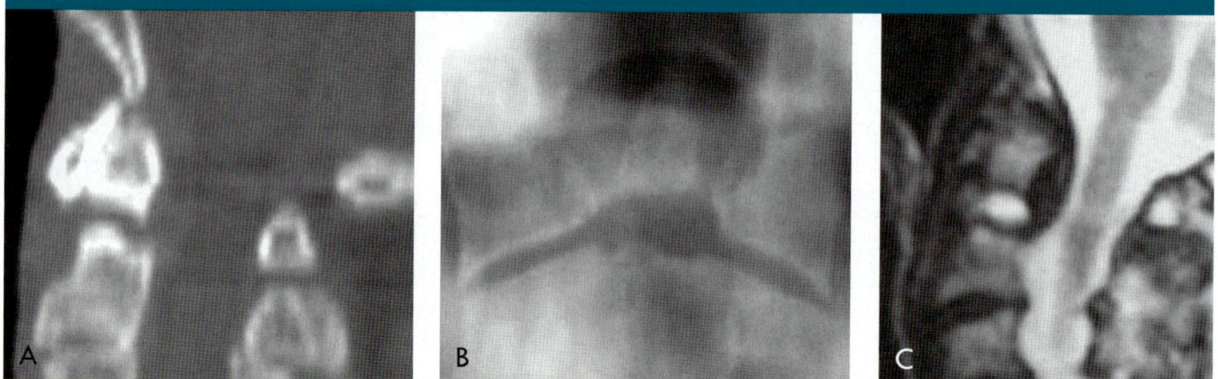

Figure 12 Pseudarthrosis of a previously ununited type 2 fracture of the base of the dens: sagittal (**A**) and coronal (**B**) CT reformations; **C,** sagittal T2-weighted MRI scan showing fluid in the pseudarthrosis.

These fractures will nearly always require immediate traction stabilization, followed by surgical fixation. The incidence of pseudarthrosis following nonsurgical treatment is disturbingly high due to both the intrinsic instability of the injury as well as the minimal bony contact between the dens and the body of C2. Even micromotion at this junction will often lead to fibrous union of the fragments.

Occasionally, in patients with no neurologic dysfunction, the diagnosis of dens fracture is not made immediately after injury. Many years may pass before symptoms of chronic neck pain or even signs of spinal cord compression occur, or the patient has an imaging study of the neck from some other unrelated matter. Routine radiographs and CT scans (**Figure 12,** *A* and *B*) will reveal a free-floating odontoid tip. The bony edges will be round and smooth. Note in **Figure 12,** *C* that fluid is often seen within the gap between the tip of the dens and the body of C2 on T2-weighted magnetic resonance images.

Type 3 dens fractures involve a large segment of the C2 vertebral body. They are oriented obliquely and often extend down to the C2-C3 disk space. There are broad fracture surfaces that tend to be apposed to one another and consequently bony union is the rule. As noted in the case in **Figure 13**, the fracture usually extends through one or both of the articular processes. This may lead to late arthritis in the C1-C2 articulation.

FIGURE 13

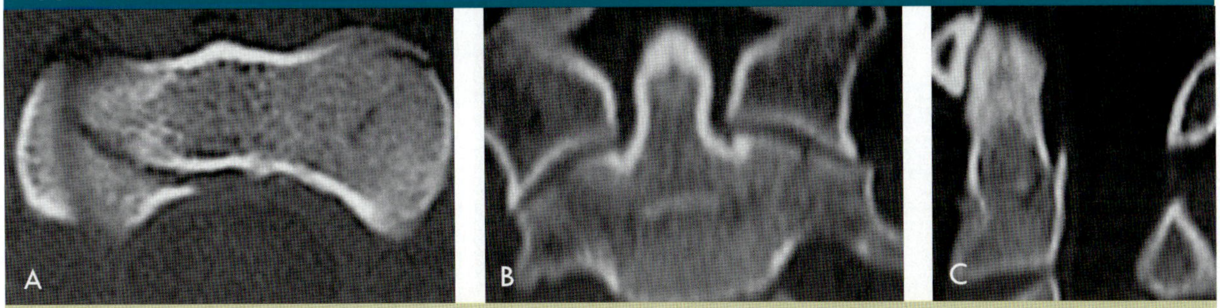

Figure 13 Axial (**A**), coronal (**B**), and sagittal (**C**) CT reformations of a type 3 dens fracture. The fracture extends obliquely through the C2 vertebra extending from the left articular process, sloping downward and forward through the body of the dens.

FIGURE 14

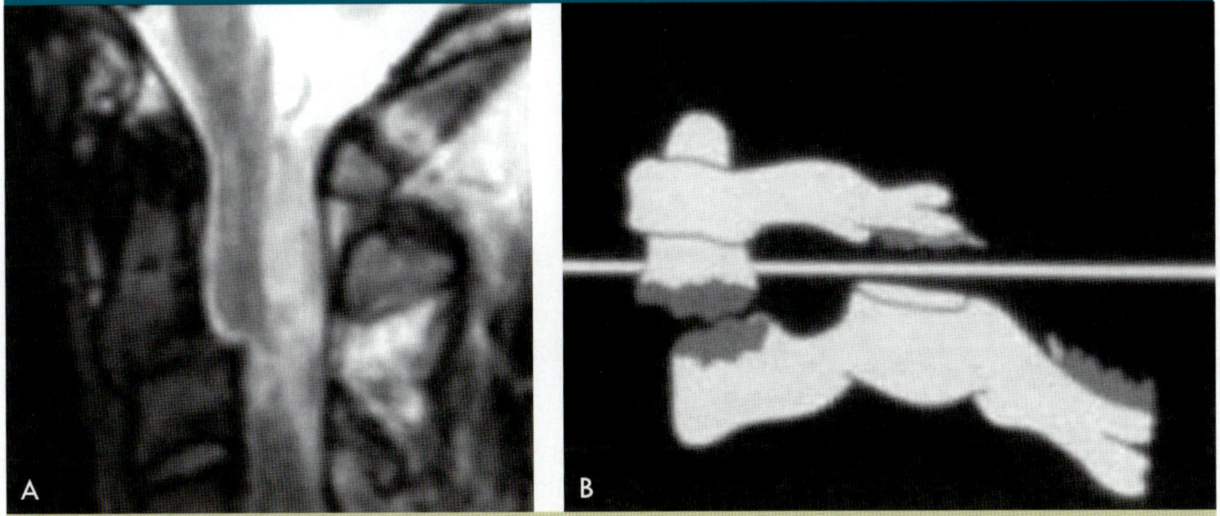

Figure 14 In this type 3 dens fracture variant, the fracture has sheared through the inferior end plate and the C2-C3 intervertebral disk: **A,** T2-weighted MRI scan; **B,** illustration. (Panel B is courtesy of the late William Wilemon, MD.)

The MRI scan in **Figure 14** demonstrates a variant of type 3 fracture in which the fracture line is nearly completely through the C2-C3 disk space. Note the transection of the spinal cord on the T2 MRI image.

Dens fractures are a common cause of C1-C2 subluxation but they are not the only cause. The second most common cause is demonstrated in **Figure 15**. This patient had these radiographs taken because he was involved in an automobile accident and had neck pain. One might think that this patent has a type 2 dens fracture from the accident. The lateral view shows obvious subluxation of C1 on C2. The AP radiograph shows that the bony edges of the free-floating dens are smooth and regular. The superior surface of the C2 body is smooth. This is clearly not a recent fracture. Is it really a fracture at all?

Os odontoidium is a common congenital malformation of C2.[15,16] It is caused by congenital failure of attachment of the tip of the dens, which arises embryologically from the occipital fourth somite (O4) to the peg of the dens, which is formed embryologically from the vertebral body of the first cervical somite. In the normal individual, the lower three-fourths of the C2 body arises from the symmetrically paired C2 somites. In many people, a line can be seen approximately 1 cm below the dens, which is the fetal remnant of the C1-C2 disk that disappears in the maturing fetus.

Figure 16, *A* is a diagram of the adult C2 vertebra with individual fetal segments depicted. In normal adults, one can usually see faint sclerotic bony fusion lines at the junction of the different ossification centers. **Figure 16,** *B* shows what

FIGURE 15

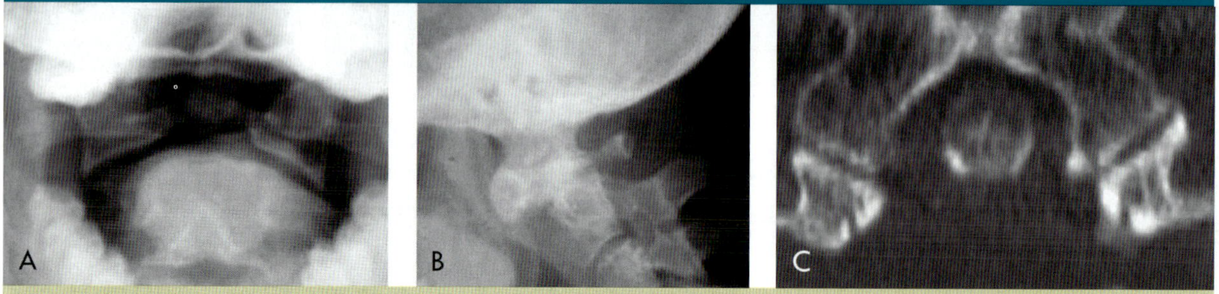

Figure 15 AP (**A**) and lateral (**B**) radiographs, and coronal CT reformation (**C**) of the same patient. There is a free-floating smooth ossicle between the lateral masses of C1. C1 has dislocated.

FIGURE 16

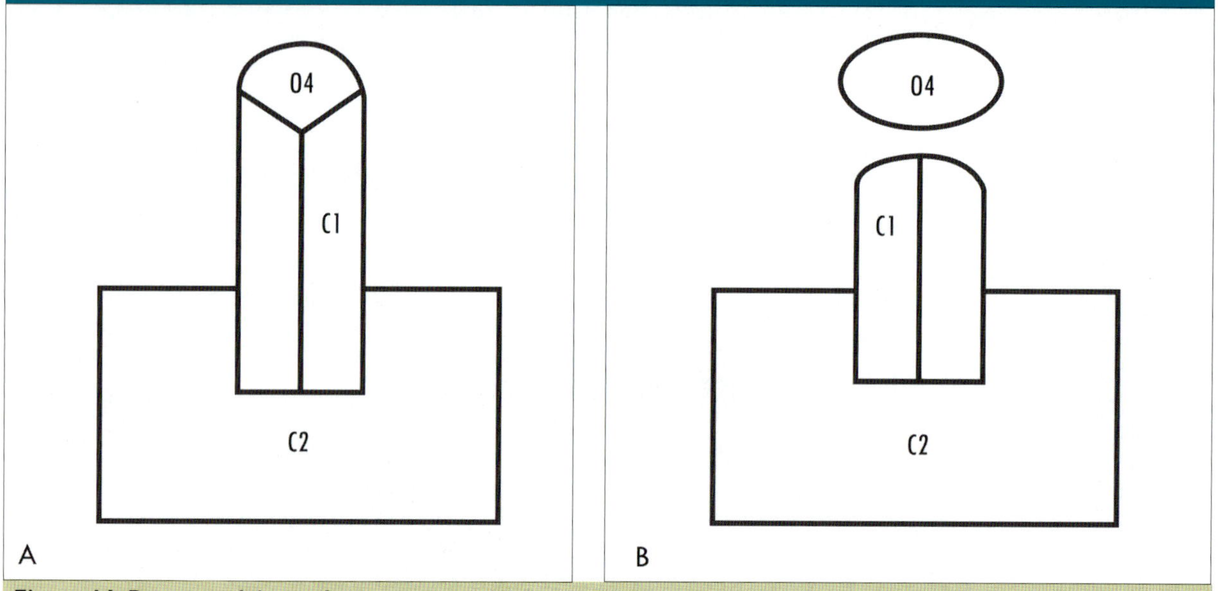

Figure 16 Diagrams of the ossification centers of the normal C2 vertebra (**A**) and the abnormal ossification centers in the os odontoidium anomaly (**B**). Note hyperplasia of the O4 segment and hypoplasia of the C1 portion of the dens.

occurs in the os odontoidium malformation. There is hypoplasia of the C1 segment of the dens and hyperplasia of the O4 segment with fibrous attachment of the two ossification centers. Note that the terminal ossicle in the patient shown in **Figures 14** and **15** does not have a central line of sclerotic bone. It cannot, therefore, be a fracture of the dens because the fusion plane between the two halves of C1 should be present. The correct diagnosis here is subluxing os odontoidium.

Hangman's Fracture

Hangman's fracture (**Figure 17**) is the name given to a bilateral fracture of the ring of C2. This type of fracture was the usual cause of death from judicial hanging using a submental knot. It is classically caused by traumatic hyperextension of the upper cervical spine, usually with associated distraction. The fracture occurs as the head is violently thrown backward so that the posterior arch of C2 fractures, and often, as in the diagram, so does the posterior arch of C1. This is a traumatic spondylolysis of the C2 ring.

The Spine Below C2

Figure 18 is a grade 1 compression-flexion injury with spinal cord contusion. The vertebral compression of the superior end plate of C4 is nearly impossible to diagnose on plain radiographs. Note the central cord lesion on the magnetic resonance image.

Figure 19 is a midsagittal CT reformation of a grade 2 flexion-compression fracture. Note

FIGURE 17

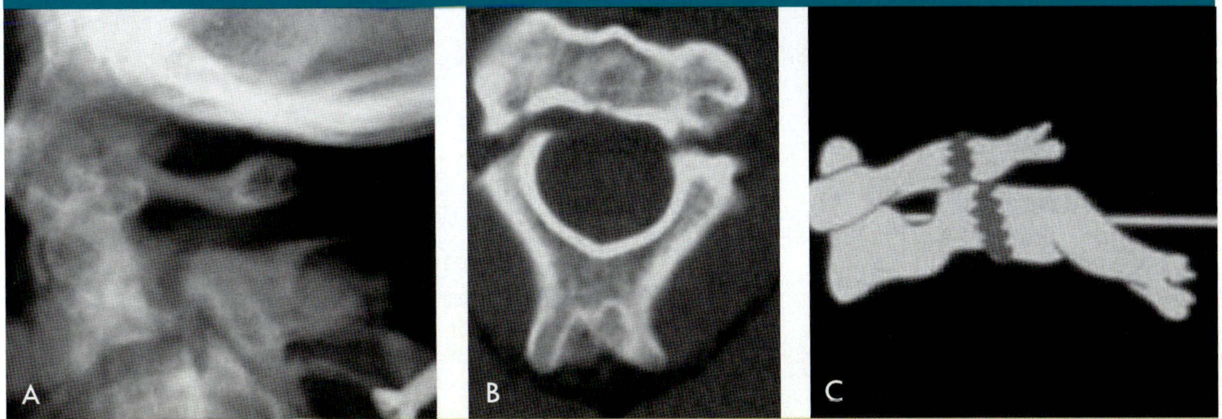

Figure 17 Hangman's fracture: lateral radiograph (**A**), axial CT scan (**B**), illustration (**C**). The fractures separate the posterior portion of the neural arch from the vertebral body. (Panel C is courtesy of the late William Wilemon, MD.)

FIGURE 18

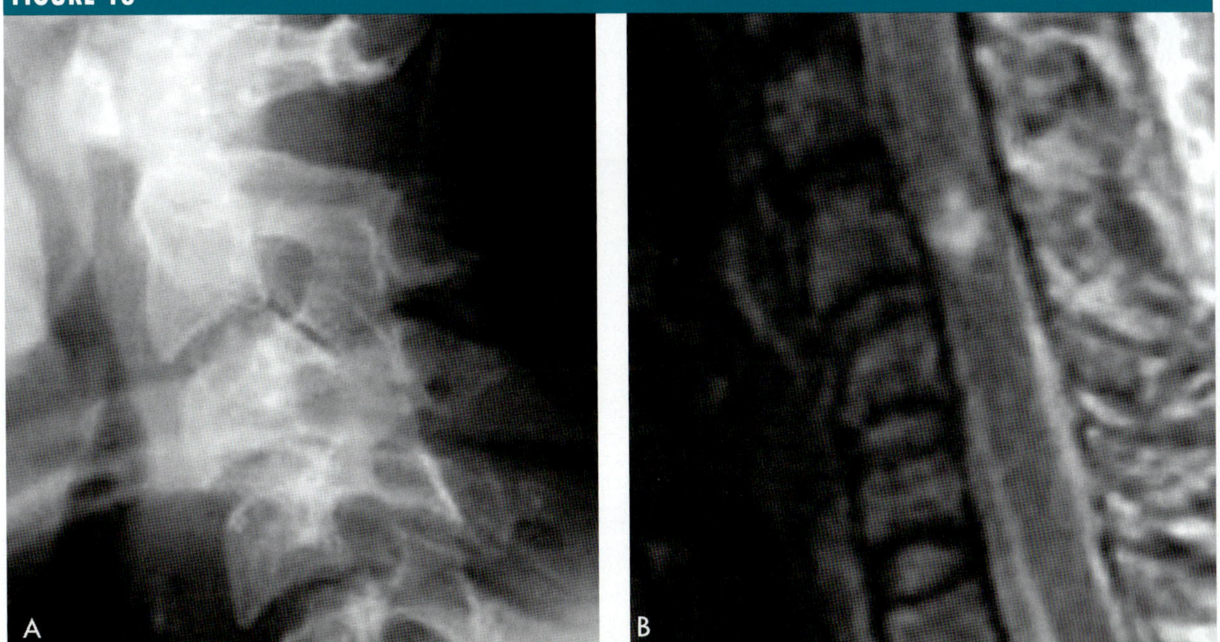

Figure 18 Grade I compression-flexion injury at C3-C4. Lateral radiograph (**A**) and midsagittal T2-weighted magnetic resonance image (**B**) of the same patient demonstrate little in the way of bony injury except for slight flattening of the anterior portion of the C4 body. Because of the narrowness of the spinal canal, there is a central cord contusion.

that more than 50% of the vertebral body is fractured. The middle and posterior columns are intact.

Compression Injuries

Compression fractures are caused by the application of direct axial load. With sufficient force, the neural ring explodes. A common pattern of bony injury due to axial compression of the spine with neither flexion nor extension is seen in **Figure 20**. Most often, the superior vertebral end plate is crushed because of the impacting force from the intervertebral disk. The vertebral body and the neural ring cleave due to outwardly expanding force on the vertebra. This type of fracture is common at the lumbosacral junction where it has been termed a crush-cleavage fracture. The cleavage force may actually be transmitted through the adjacent intervertebral disk and cleave the adjacent vertebra as we see here. The second fracture

FIGURE 19

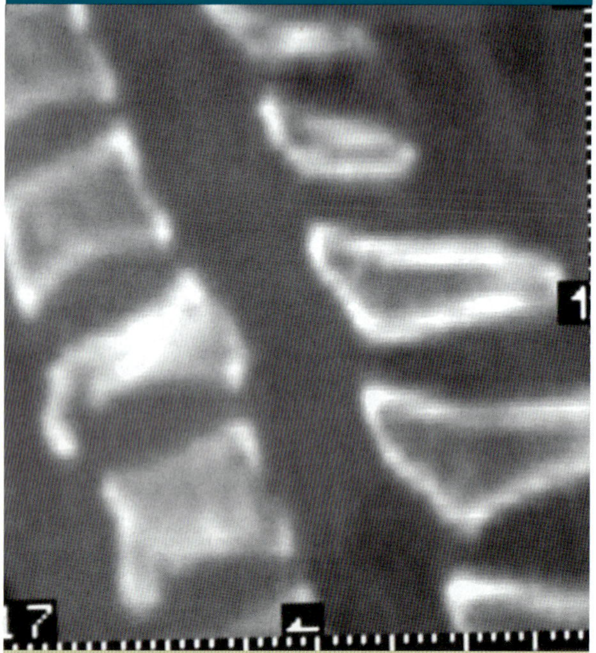

Figure 19 Flexion-compression fracture grade 2 midsagittal CT reformation showing loss of height of the vertebral body with sclerosis in the center of the body due to bony impaction.

FIGURE 20

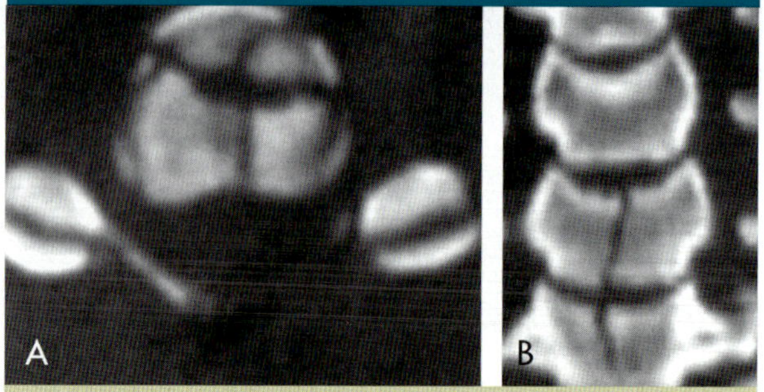

Figure 20 Cervical "burst" fracture (crush-cleavage): **A,** axial CT; and **B,** coronal reformation of a patient with a crush-cleavage fracture of C5. The axial view documents the fragmentation of the superior end plate, and the coronal reformation **(B)** show the extension of the cleavage portion of the fracture through the disk and down into the C6 vertebra.

FIGURE 21

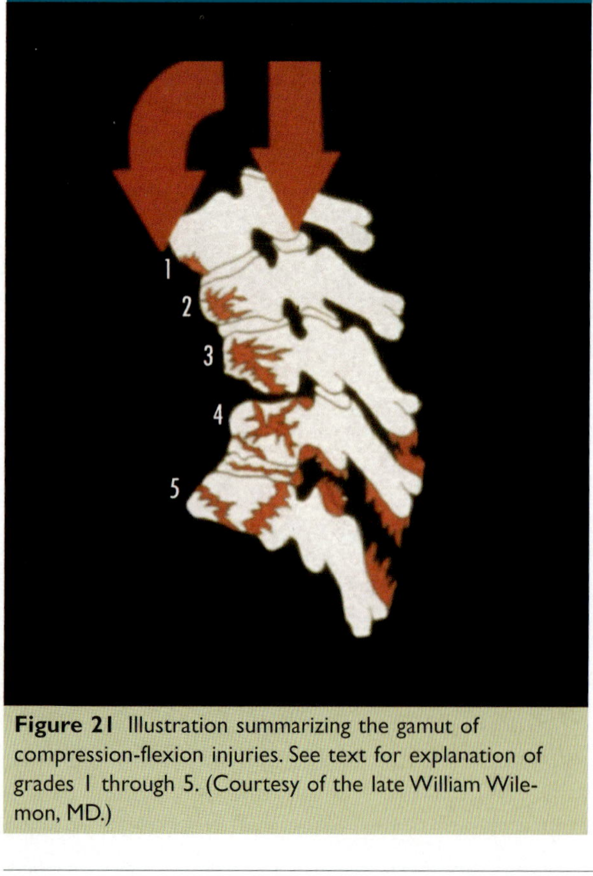

Figure 21 Illustration summarizing the gamut of compression-flexion injuries. See text for explanation of grades 1 through 5. (Courtesy of the late William Wilemon, MD.)

may be difficult or even impossible to see on plain radiographs.

Compression-Flexion Injuries

A summary of compression-flexion injuries is provided in **Figure 21**. Grade 1 fractures involve only the anterior portion of the vertebral end plate. Grade 2 fractures involve up to 50% of the anterior vertebra. Grade 3 fractures involve more than 50% of the vertebral body. Grade 4 fractures display comminution of the majority of the vertebral body with posterior ligamentous injury. Grade 5 lesions include all of the above, along with disruption of the facet joint capsules.

Grade 4 and 5 flexion-compression fractures are very unstable injuries and associated spinal cord injuries are common. **Figure 22** includes CT and MRI scans of two different patients with fractures of all three columns. There is central cleavage of the vertebral body and bilateral fractures of the neural arches. The spinal canal is compromised. The case shown in the MRI scan (**Figure 22,** *B*) shows comminution of the vertebral body with retropulsion of the posterior half of the body and spinal cord compression. Note the very long segment of cord swelling. It is clear from looking at these and similar cases why the level of neurologic injury may often extend two segments above a fracture.

Figure 23, *A* is a radiograph of a compression-flexion grade 5 fracture. The vertebral body is markedly comminuted. The interspinous distance between C5 and C6 is widened, indicating posterior ligamentous injury. The CT scans (**Figure 23,** *B* and *C*) are of a different patient with a similar

FIGURE 22

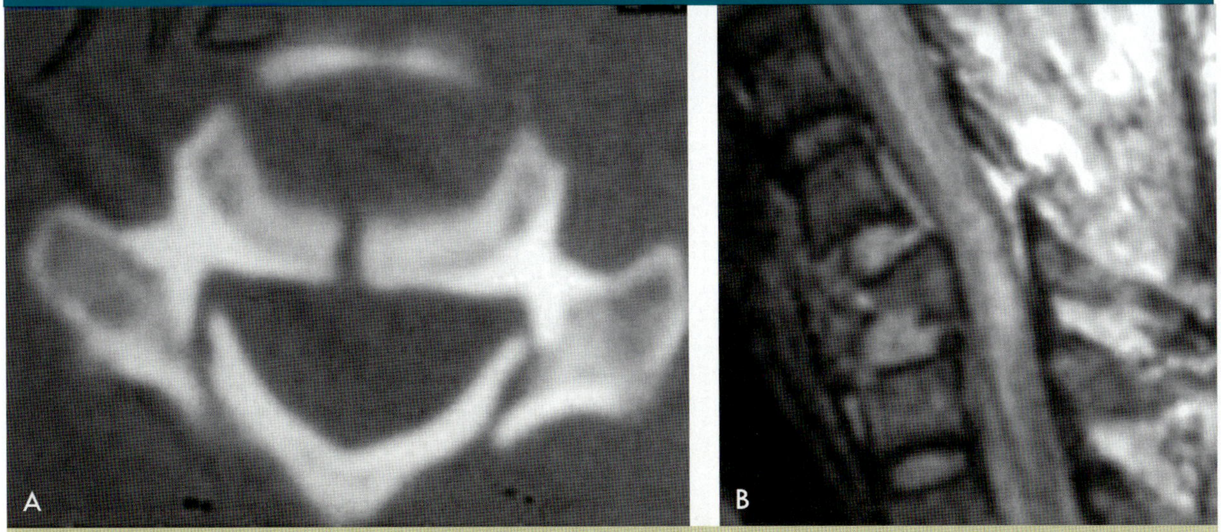

Figure 22 Unstable compression-flexion injury of the midcervical spine. **A,** Axial CT scan demonstrates compression of the vertebral body and bilateral laminar fractures. **B,** Sagittal T2-weighted MRI scan of a different patient depicts comminution of the vertebral body with retropulsion of a large bony fragment compressing an enlarged spinal cord. Note that the intrinsic cord swelling extends several segments from the bony lesion.

FIGURE 23

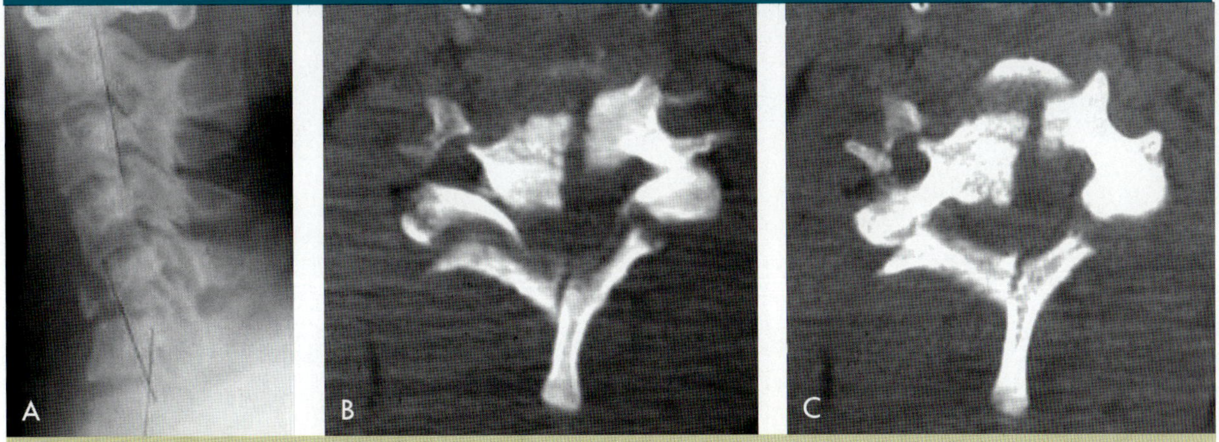

Figure 23 Compression-flexion injury: lateral radiograph (**A**) of one patient and axial CT scans (**B** and **C**) of another patient with hyperflexion-compression injuries. Note the very remarkable comminution of all three columns.

fracture. Note the very remarkable fragmentation of the vertebral body. Often, as in this case, there is a component of lateral bending or tilt that causes asymmetric crushing of the articular processes.

Hyperextension-Compression Injury

The mechanism of this injury is somewhat complex. The head is dramatically hyperextended, as depicted in **Figure 24**. A downward compressive force in combination with the hyperextension forces the vertebral body forward, usually shearing through the affected disk space. The MRI scan depicted here shows rupture of both the anterior and posterior longitudinal ligaments with compression of the cord between the forward migrating lamina of the upper vertebra and the superior end plate of the lower vertebral body. This is the usual mechanism of cord injury in most flexion fractures or dislocations. Note that the intervertebral disk is totally destroyed. A portion of the disk frequently migrates up behind the posterior longitudinal ligament, which is stripped away from the bone.

FIGURE 24

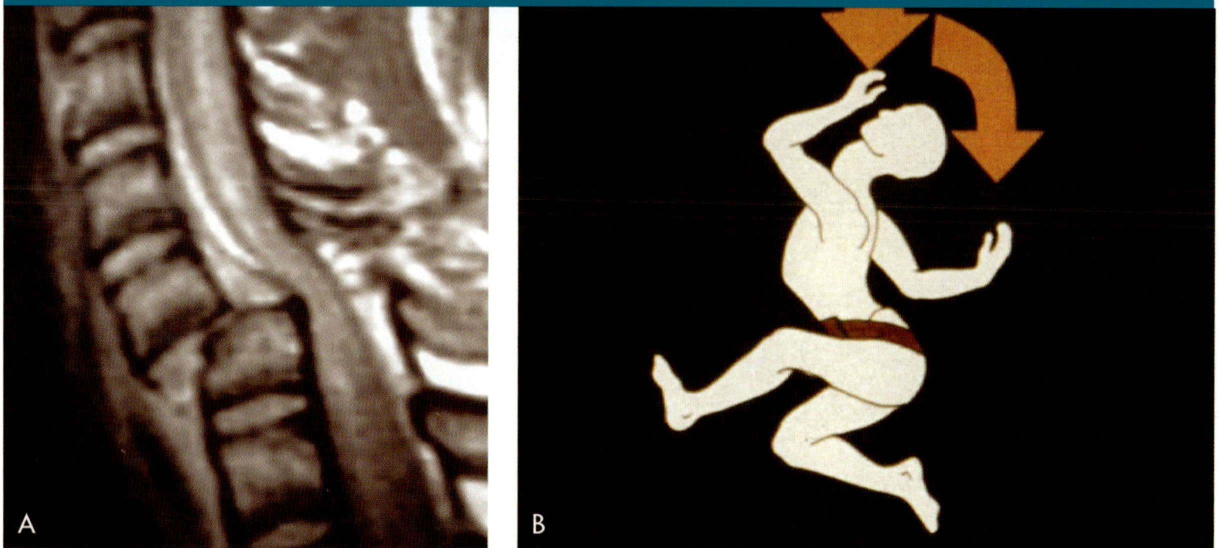

Figure 24 Hyperextension-compression injury. **A,** Midsagittal T2-weighted MRI scan shows laceration of the anterior longitudinal ligament and stripping of the posterior longitudinal ligament away from the upper vertebral body. **B,** Illustration depicting the mechanism of injury in hyperextension-compression. (Panel B is courtesy of the late William Wilemon, MD.)

FIGURE 25

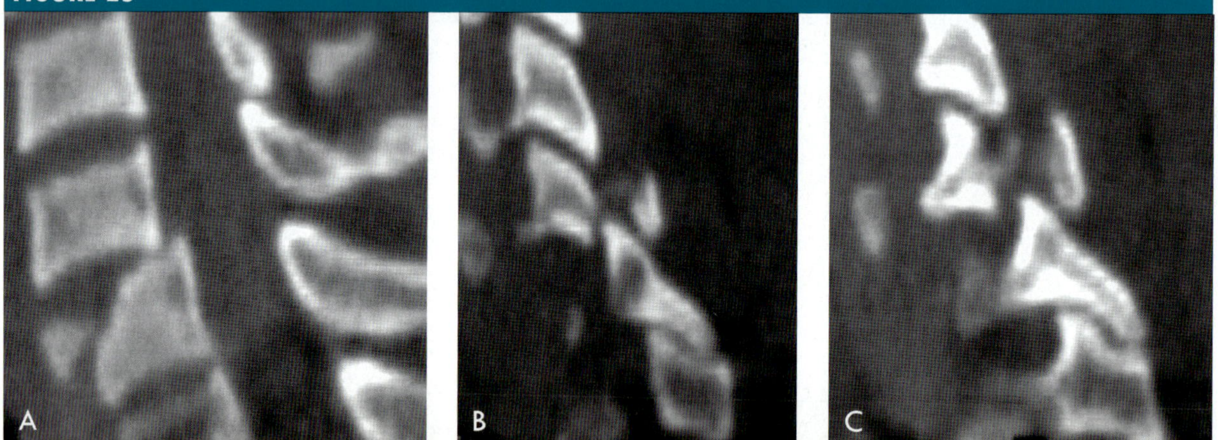

Figure 25 Hyperextension-compression injury: midsagittal (**A**) and lateral sagittal (**B** and **C**) CT reformations of a patient with hyperextension-compression. Note the anterior downward shearing of the lower vertebral body and fragmentation of the lateral mass and facet joints.

A CT scan of another patient with hyperextension-compression injury of the midcervical spine (**Figure 25**) shows the typical downward displaced bony fragment that has been cleaved from the C5 vertebra. This fragment remains attached to the anterior longitudinal ligament, which is ruptured just below. Note on the sagittal reformations you can see the compression fractures of the zygapophyseal joint.

Flexion-Distraction Injuries

Flexion-distraction injuries are very common in our mobile society. They are caused by violent forward motion of an individual where the head is flung upward and forward with forces that overwhelm the inertia of the soft tissues holding the head on. The typical injury occurs in restrained people in high-speed car accidents. When the automobile hits an immovable object, the entire body is flung forward. The trunk may be restrained by seat belts and shoulder harnesses, but the head is free to continue along its forward vector. If the forces are great enough, they may tear the ligamentous structures holding the various motion segments together. In these types of injuries, the bony trauma is much less severe than the soft-tissue trauma. Plain radiographs tend to be much less abnormal looking than in compression lesions. The radiograph in **Figure 26** demonstrates a common flexion-distraction injury of the lower cervical spine. There is traumatic spondylolysis of the C7 neural arch. The forward/upward vector has sheared the neural arch bilaterally. As the head recoils posteriorly, the bones have remained in alignment.

When the distracting forces are so dominant as to tear the joint capsules, the superior articular processes may dislocate. As the head and neck above the lesion recoil, the articular processes may realign and the radiographs look normal or nearly normal. Often, however, the facets do not realign properly. The superior articular processes may remain subluxed or even dislocated. When the superior articular process comes to lie anterior to the tip of the inferior articular process, the facets are said to be locked.

Figure 27 shows a typical flexion-distraction injury. The body of C5 is forward on C6. The zygapophyseal joint in **Figure 27,** *B* is subluxed; the superior articular process of C5 has slipped upward and forward but is still in apposition. The contralateral superior articular facet (**Figure 27,** *C*) is dislocated and locked anterior to the inferior articular processes. The tip of that process is also fractured by the recoiling superior process. This combination of abnormalities is very common.

Bilateral facet dislocation is depicted in **Figure 28**. The midsagittal view (**Figure 28,** *A*) demonstrates forward subluxation of C5 on C6. **Figure 28,** *B* is a more lateral sagittal view showing a locked facet. The axial view (**Figure 28,** *C*) is interesting as it shows two "naked" facets. The dislocated articular processes are seen to be separated one from the other.[17] **Figure 28,** *D* is a three-dimensional surface rendering of the CT data, which is a nice graphic representation of the

FIGURE 26

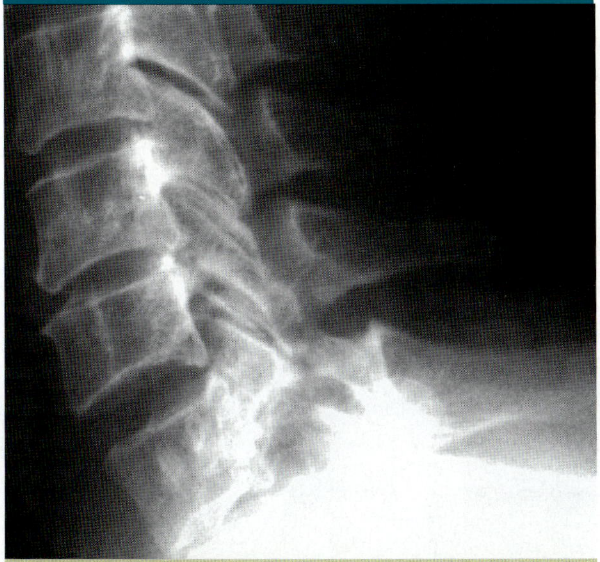

Figure 26 Flexion-distraction injury. Lateral radiograph demonstrates bilateral fractures of the neural arch of C7. These fractures commonly occur at the junction of the neck and the thoracic spine.

FIGURE 27

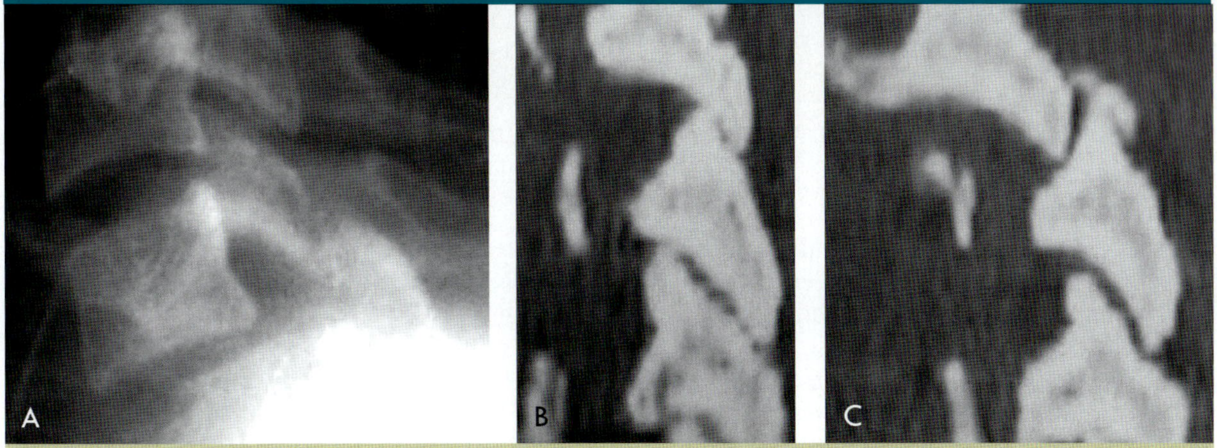

Figure 27 Flexion-distraction injury. Lateral radiograph (**A**) shows forward slippage of C5 on C6. No fractures are demonstrated. Bilateral lateral CT reformations through the articular processes (**B** and **C**) demonstrate 60% subluxation of the facet (**B**) and dislocation of the contralateral superior articular process (**C**).

FIGURE 28

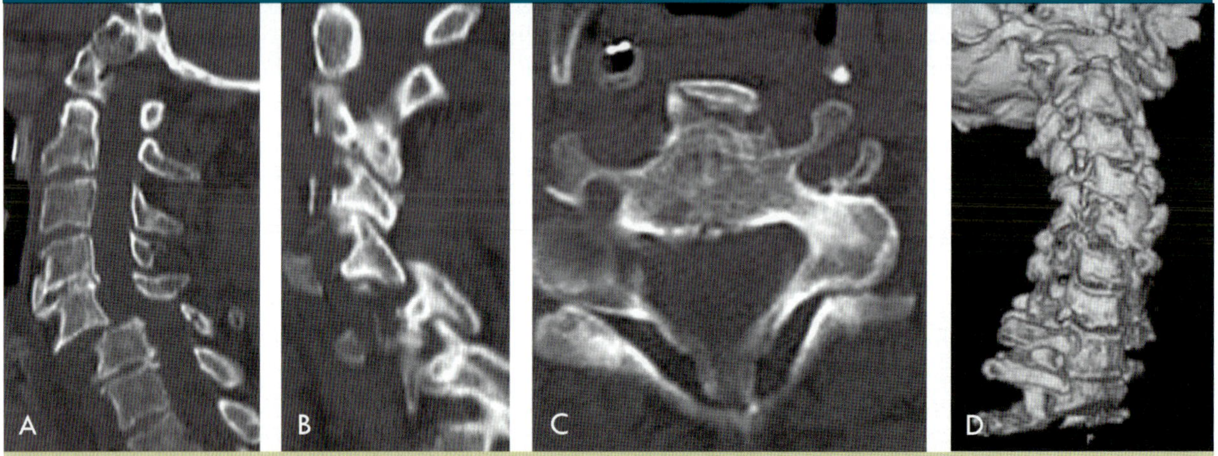

Figure 28 Flexion-distraction injury. Midsagittal (**A**) and lateral sagittal (**B**) CT reformations reveal subluxation of the vertebral body and dislocation of the articular process, with a "locked" facet. **C,** Axial CT scan demonstrates disarticulation of both facets. Two different neural arches are seen on the same axial CT slice, indicating the presence of subluxation even without the reformation. **D,** Three-dimensional surface rendering of the cervical spine reformatted from the axial CT data shows the abnormal position of the facet joints and vertebral body. (Courtesy of Diego Nunez, MD, New Haven, CT.)

FIGURE 29

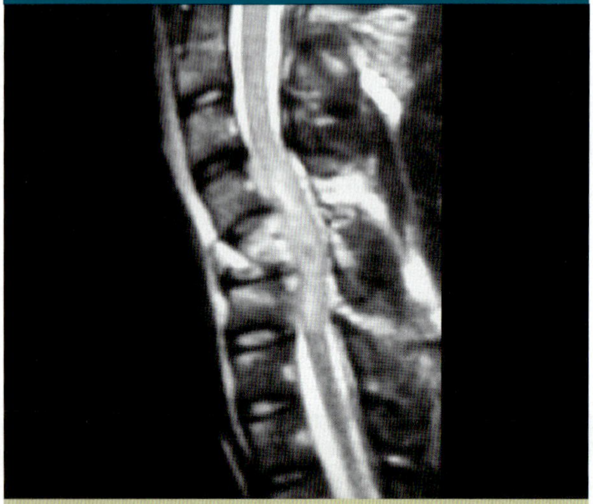

Figure 29 Flexion-distraction injury. Sagittal T2-weighted MRI scan showing dramatic fracture-dislocation of the vertebral body with spinal cord injury. The posterior ligaments are torn.

FIGURE 30

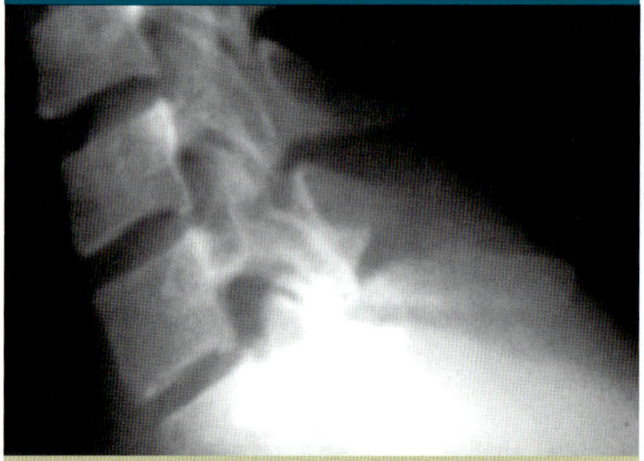

Figure 30 Flexion-distraction injury. Lateral radiograph showing avulsion of the spinous process of C7. Although it cannot be seen on the radiograph, the fracture line extended into the lamina.

axial data but rarely adds any useful diagnostic information. This view is useful to explain complex bony relationships to patient and their families.

The MRI scan of another patient with a flexion-distraction injury (**Figure 29**) shows even more violent distraction. There is dislocation of the vertebral body and fracture of the inferior end plate of C5. The spinal cord is dramatically swollen. The patient was devastated neurologically.

A common flexion-distraction injury that typically occurs at C7 is depicted in **Figure 30**. In this patient, the violent distraction has separated the body and most of the neural arch of C7 from the spinous process and the lamina. The interspinous ligaments are intact but the bone has broken.

A similar but less deforming avulsion of the tip of the transverse process of C7 (**Figure 31**) has been termed a clay shoveler's fracture. This is caused by violent contraction of the upper thoracic and posterior cervical muscles pulling off their attachment to the spinous process.

Severe trauma to the cervical spine may lead to multiple bone and joint lesions. The lateral radiograph in **Figure 32,** *A* was performed following severe trauma. The most obvious finding here is a hyperextension-compression fracture-dislocation at C5-C6. The C5 vertebral body is subluxed with avulsion of the anterior apophyseal ring. The C5-C6 disk is lacerated. There are also bilateral facet joint dislocations with locked facets. There is also a congenital anomaly at the craniocervical junction. Note the congenital failure of segmentation of C1-C2 with complete integration of the C1 ring into C2, as well as the round neural foramen of this anomalous pair of bones.

The treatment of choice for this type of injury is traction reduction of the locked facets at C5-C6. The lateral radiograph in **Figure 32,** *B* was performed during controlled cervical traction. Note that the traction has revealed a second occult hyperextension-distraction injury at C3-C4. The disk is lacerated and the facet joint capsules must be torn. The interspinous distance has widened dramatically with the traction. One can presume that the abnormally stabilized and congenitally fused C1-C2 bony pair predisposed the C3-C4 segment to additional stress during the hyperextension-distraction that caused the disk and ligamentous injury at C3-C4.

Hyperextension Injuries

Hyperextension injuries of the cervical spine frequently cause profound neurologic injury with little or no radiographic abnormality. The vertebral bodies are usually intact because they are generally fractured by flexion. Facet joint fractures, which do tend to occur with hyperextension, are often very difficult to see radiographically. The hockey player whose radiograph is shown in **Figure 33** was checked violently into the boards and developed the immediate onset of upper extremity weakness and abnormal sensation. The lateral

FIGURE 31

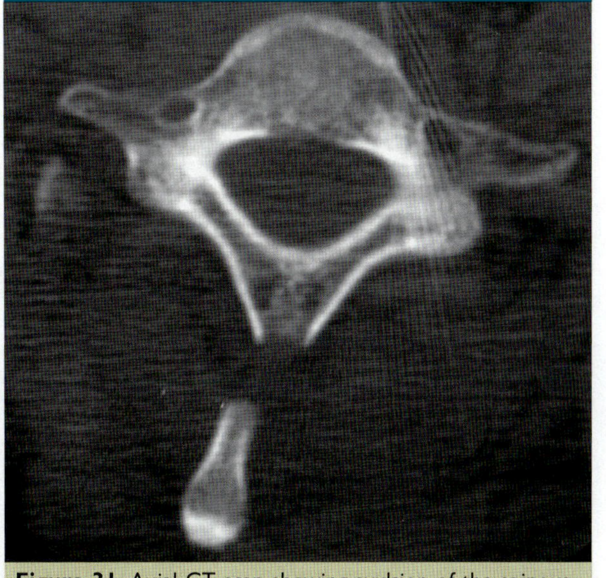

Figure 31 Axial CT scan showing avulsion of the spinous process of C7.

FIGURE 32

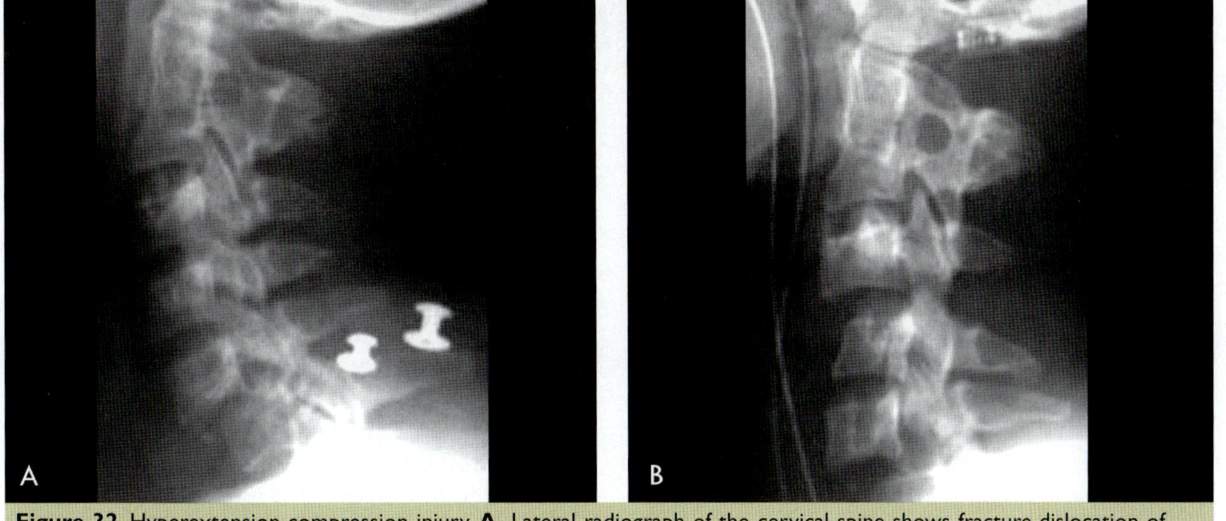

Figure 32 Hyperextension-compression injury. **A,** Lateral radiograph of the cervical spine shows fracture-dislocation of C5-C6. There is failure of segmentation of the C1-C2 level. **B,** Lateral radiograph during cervical traction reveals a second unstable level at C3-C4.

FIGURE 33

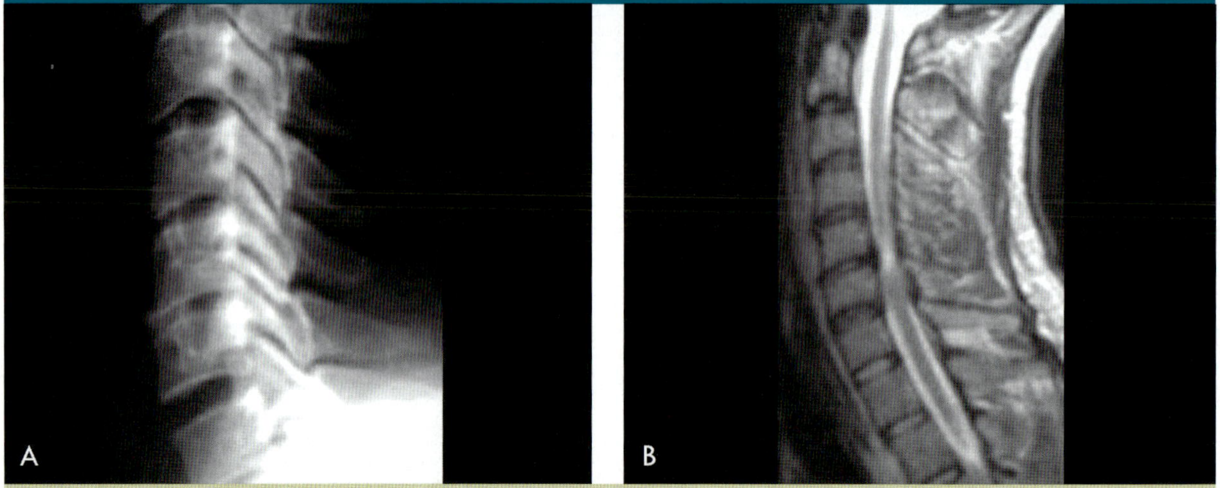

Figure 33 Hyperextension injury. Lateral radiograph (**A**) and midsagittal T2-weighted MRI scan (**B**) demonstrate no traumatic bone injury. The disk at C5-6 is degenerated and narrowed. Note the central cord contusion on the magnetic resonance image.

FIGURE 34

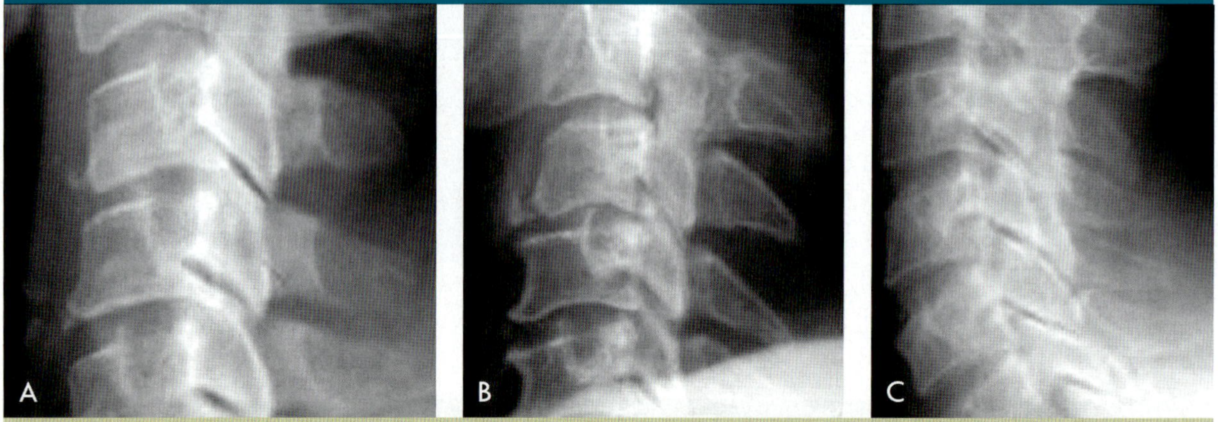

Figure 34 Lateral radiograph of patient **A** depicts avulsion of the anterior inferior apophysis of C3. Lateral radiograph of patient **B** shows avulsion of an anterior osteophyte. Lateral radiograph of the third patient (**C**) demonstrates a linear gas collection in the C4-5 disk indicating an annular fissure. Note, however, that the anterior portion of the disk space is wider than normal, indicating ligamentous injury.

radiograph (**Figure 33,** *A*) is normal except for a congenitally small spinal canal. The MRI scan (**Figure 33,** *B*) demonstrates the classic lesion of hyperextension, which is central cord contusion. These lesions are more common in the elderly,[18] where relatively minor trauma can cause severe neurologic injury with little or no radiographic evidence of injury.

The mechanism of injury in these cases is nearly always the same. The cord becomes compressed between the bulging disk and osteophyte of the upper vertebra and the lamina of the lower vertebra. There is generally no bony fracture or ligamentous tear. The cord injury occurs in the brief instant during which the hyperextension brings these structures in apposition. The only difference in the anatomy of the spine the instant after the contusion as compared to the instant before the contusion is the central cord lesion. Most of these patients will not benefit from decompression surgery.

Figure 34 depicts three different patients with hyperextension injuries and abnormal radiographs. In each case, the anterior longitudinal ligament is torn. In the first instance (**Figure 34,** *A*) there is avulsion of the anterior attachment of the disk and anterior longitudinal ligament to a normal vertebra. In the second case (**Figure 34,** *B*), there is

FIGURE 35

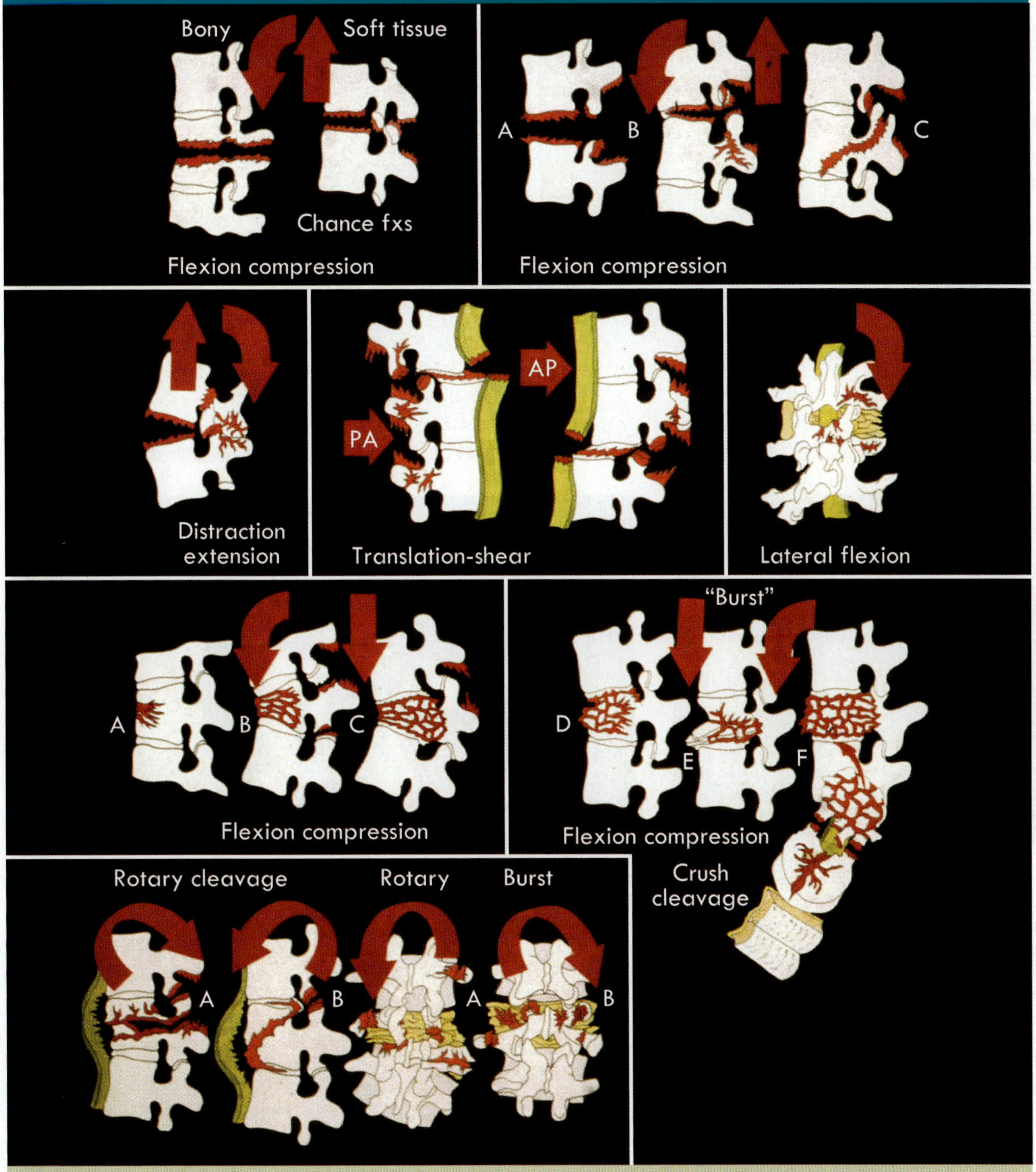

Figure 35 Categories of thoracolumbar injuries. fxs = fractures. (Courtesy of the late William Wilemon, MD.)

avulsion of an osteophyte from its attachment at the vertebral lip. The third radiograph (**Figure 34,** *C*) is really tricky. There is no obvious bony injury. The C4-5 disk space is widened and there is a linear fissure within the disk containing gas. This indicates a hypermobile disk with disk disease.

There are many variations on the themes presented above and many complicated injuries that occur due to complex vectors and different head positions. Using a logical approach to the various imaging studies, it should be possible for the astute observer to untangle even the most daunting injuries.

FIGURE 36

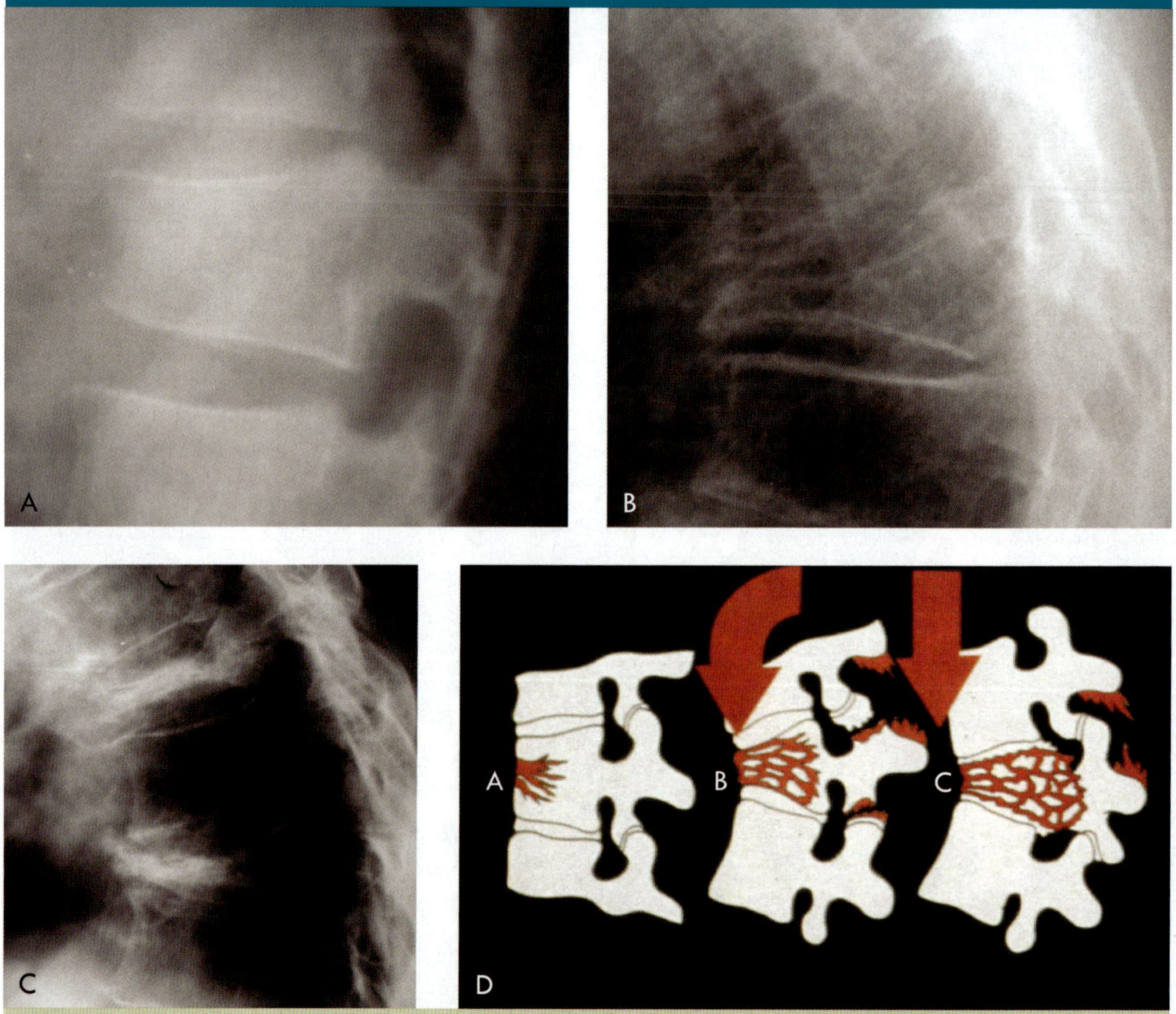

Figure 36 Compression fractures (flexion-compression). **A,** Lateral radiograph of an acute compression fracture. There is minimal loss of vertebral height with anterior cortical step-off. **B,** Lateral radiograph of another patient shows much more prominent vertebral compression. **C,** Lateral radiograph shows two vertebrae plana. The compressed vertebrae are densely sclerotic. **D,** Illustration of flexion-compression fractures according to Denis[3]. (Panel D is courtesy of the late William Wilemon, MD.)

Thoracic and Lumbar Spine

It is useful to categorize injuries of the thoracic and lumbar spines in a similar fashion, noting flexion or extension, distraction or compression tilt, rotation, and shear (**Figure 35**).[19]

Flexion-Compression

The most common fractures of the thoracic or lumbar spine are wedge compression fractures of the vertebral end plates. Within this group are those fractures that occur with minor trauma of everyday life, typically in older women with osteoporosis. This group may be caused by direct axial load or compression with some degree of flexion. These lesions are common in restrained automobile accident victims. **Figure 36,** *A* is a radiograph of a patient with an acute flexion-compression fracture. It is often difficult to distinguish an acute from a chronic compression fracture on plain radiographs. There are two telltale signs that are most useful, and both are seen here. In acute fractures, the anterior edge of the vertebra may have a subtle but sharp edge reflecting slight malalignment of the anterior cortex due to the injury. In chronic fractures, this edge smoothes out because of the healing. Acute fractures will often show a faint sclerotic line within the vertebral body itself. This line is formed because of the impaction of medullary bone at the fracture site. Within the zone of impaction, there is more bone than normal because of the compression of fragments from above and below the fracture line. Compression fractures tend to lose some height with time during the healing process. Vertebrae may become significantly wedged as seen in **Figure 36,** *B*. The end stage of the process, which by no means occurs in all or even the majority of patients, is "vertebra plana," near total loss of vertebral height (**Figure 36,** *C*). The residual bone may be densely sclerotic as seen in the two affected thoracic vertebrae here. **Figure 36,** *D* illustrates the Denis classification of these fractures.

Figure 37 shows a vertebra with impaction of both the superior and inferior end plates with little loss of height of the outer shell of the vertebra. For this pattern of fracture to occur, the intervertebral disk must be normal or nearly normal. The nucleus must be hydrated enough so that the intradiscal pressure exceeds the intraosseus pressure, collapsing the adjacent end plates. The hydrated nucleus behaves like a liquid in that it is deformable but not compressible. The disk will not herniate from axial load alone. The bony end plates will always fail before nuclear herniation.

In the acutely injured patient, CT is the procedure of choice. Axial scans show subtle cracks in the anterior cortex and medullary bone (**Figure 38,** *A* and *B*). They are easy to miss unless the slices are thin. MRI is the imaging procedure of choice for the evaluation of compression fractures of the spine because it will differentiate chronic from acute lesions. The MRI scans in **Figure 38,** *C* and *D* show a patient with numerous wedge compression fractures. Note that the disks at the involved segments are larger than normal. The intradiscal pressure being higher than the intraosseous pressure allows the disks to expand at the expense of the bony end plates. Chronic compression fractures show normal marrow signal

FIGURE 37

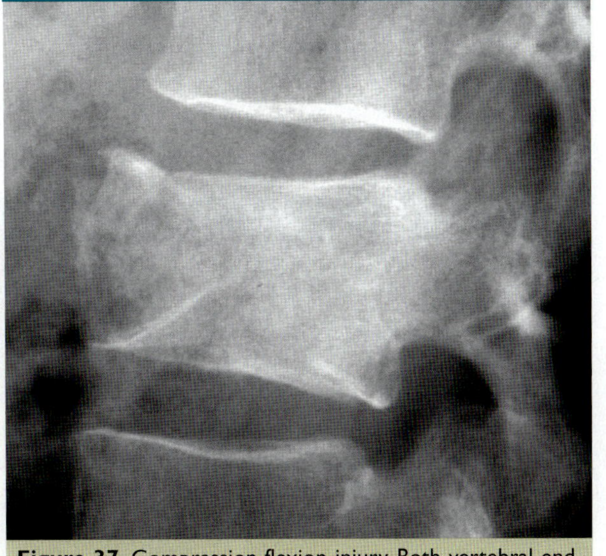

Figure 37 Compression-flexion injury. Both vertebral end plates are concave due to impaction fractures, yet the bony edges of the vertebra look relatively intact.

FIGURE 38

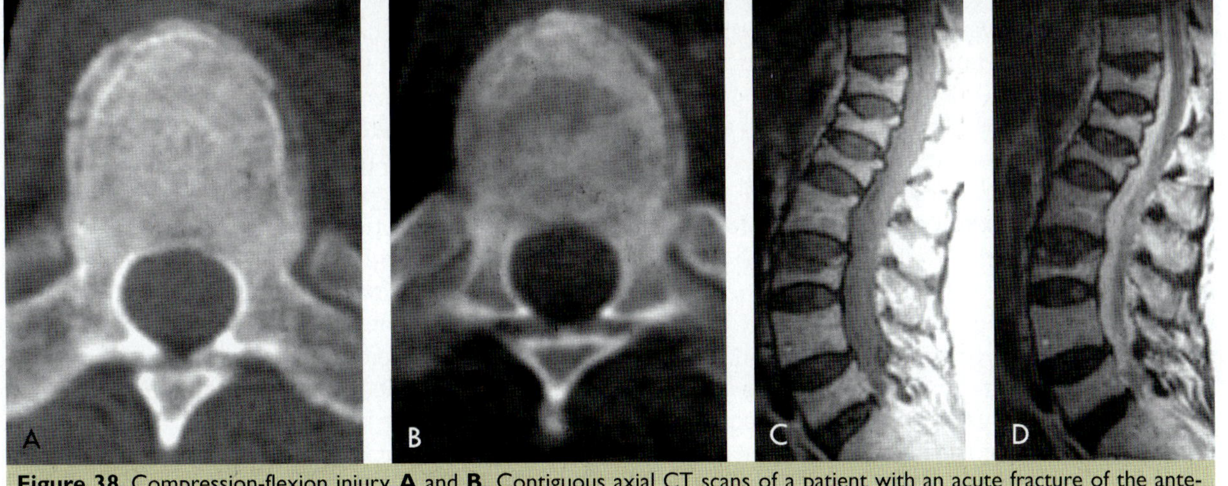

Figure 38 Compression-flexion injury. **A** and **B,** Contiguous axial CT scans of a patient with an acute fracture of the anterior portion of the vertebral body. Note the subtle linear cracks along the anterior rim of the vertebra. Reformations are often required to make the diagnosis because these fractures look similar to anterior bony osteophytes. Proton-density (**C**) and T2-weighted (**D**) MRI scans of another patient with multiple compression fractures of different ages. There is an evolving compression fracture of the superior end plate of L3 and old compression fractures of the other levels.

FIGURE 39

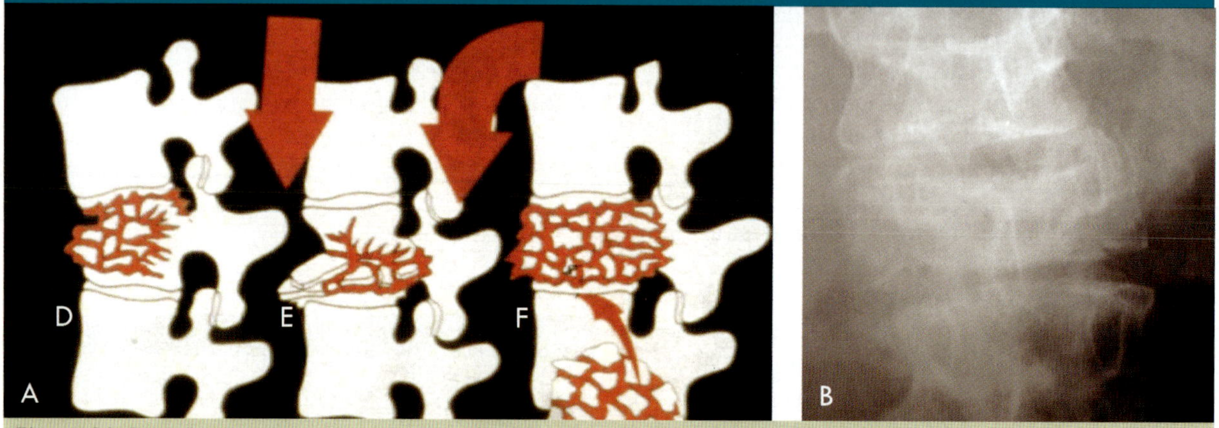

Figure 39 Burst fracture (axial load): **A,** illustration; **B,** AP radiograph. Note the widening of the interpedicular distance and generalized expansion of the vertebral body. (Panel A is courtesy of the late William Wilemon, MD.)

FIGURE 40

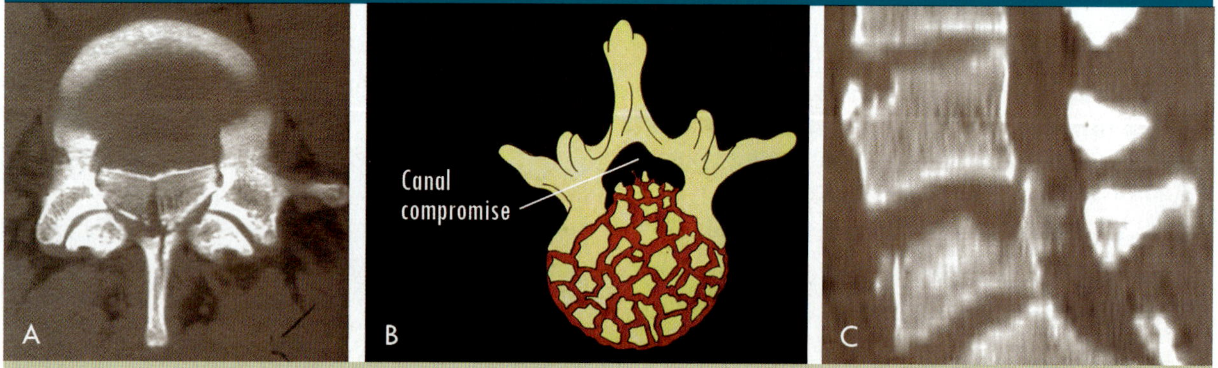

Figure 40 Burst fracture. **A,** Axial CT scan shows dramatic canal stenosis due to displacement of a large fragment of the posterior third of the vertebral body. **B,** Burst fracture illustration. **C,** Sagittal reformatted CT scan. (Panel B is courtesy of the late William Wilemon, MD.)

within the effected vertebra. Acute fractures will show zones of low signal on T1-weighted scans and bright signal on T2 and gradient echo images. Note in this case that all fractures are old except for the superior end plate of L3.

Fractures Due to Axial Load (Burst Fractures)

When axial load is the predominant force, a burst fracture occurs. The hallmark of the burst fracture is cleavage of the neural ring. The AP radiograph in **Figure 39,** *B* shows widening of the interpedicular distance. The entire vertebra appears wider than its mates. The greater the force, the more comminution. These three-column injuries are inherently unstable.

An interesting phenomenon—fragmentation of the superior end plate—may occur with burst fractures, as seen in **Figure 40**. The posterior longitudinal ligament remains intact even though the attached bone is shattered. In the depicted CT scans, there is a very large fragment of the posterior upper quadrant of the vertebral body that has separated and rotated into the spinal canal, causing significant canal compromise. It is remarkable that it is possible to acutely reduce this fragment of bone by distraction ligamentotaxis. For many years, the treatment of choice for acute burst fracture was indirect decompression by posterior distraction and fusion.

A very typical pattern of burst fracture is the crush-cleavage fracture.[20] The superior end-plate fragments and the posterior fragment may displace into the spinal canal. Extending down from the crushed end plate is a cleavage plane that separates the two halves of the vertebral body. There will be posterior extension of the fissure through the neural arch, usually through the lamina. Reduction of the fragment by ligamentotaxis can be

FIGURE 41

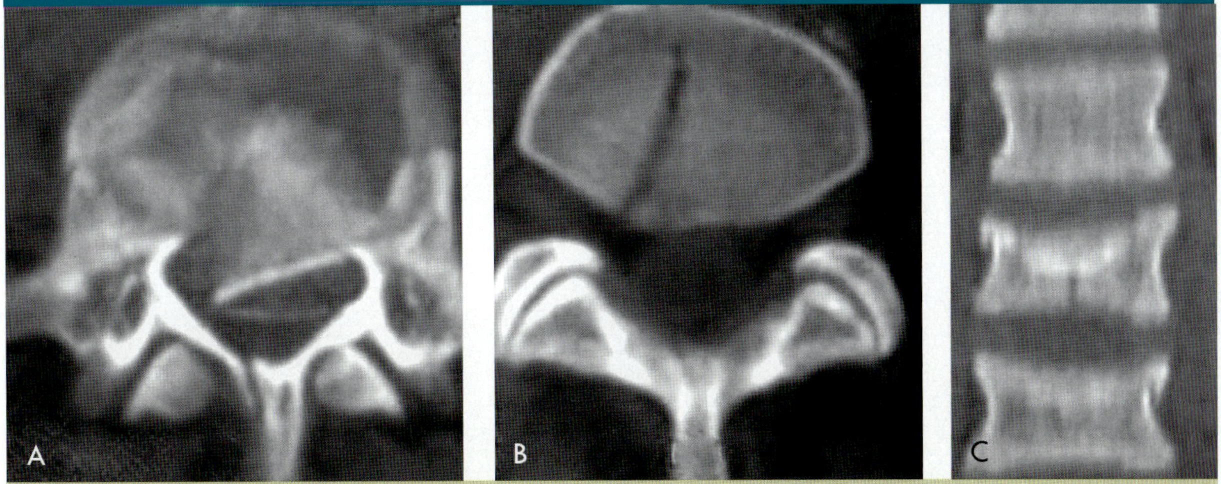

Figure 41 Burst fracture. **A,** Axial view through the superior end plate demonstrates the typical "crush" of the crush-cleavage fracture. **B,** Axial view through the lower third of the vertebra demonstrates the "cleavage." **C,** Coronal reformation shows the typical pattern of upper vertebral crush and lower vertebral cleavage.

FIGURE 42

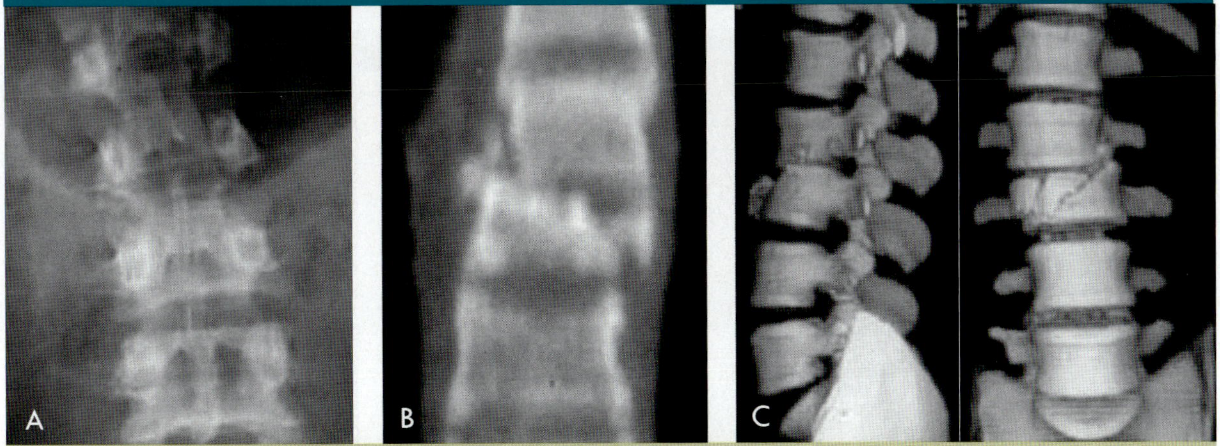

Figure 42 AP radiograph (**A**) and reformatted CT scan (**B**) of the same patient reveal a complex fracture in which there is a combination of compression, rotation, and lateral translation. **C,** Three-dimensional surface rendering of another patient. Compressive and rotatory forces are at work here, with lateral vertebral compression and comminution as well as rotatory displacement.

accomplished only if it is attempted within the first few days. Compare the axial views in the cases shown in **Figures 40** and **41**. Note that in the first instance, the posterior cortex of the displaced fragment has rotated 180° and is within the vertebral body. The second case (**Figure 41**) is more typical in that the posterior cortex is displaced posterocentrally within the neural canal. This case more clearly demonstrates how distraction force on the posterior longitudinal ligament can force this fragment back into the cavity in the vertebral body.

The forces that are applied to the spine in trauma may be complex. If there are rotatory vectors, then the fracture will be more complex. Depicted in **Figure 42** are two patients with flexion-compression-rotation fractures. Note the lateral offset of the two vertebral bodies. These fractures are very unstable and will almost always require stabilization.

Flexion-Distraction Fractures

Flexion-distraction fractures are very common in high-speed motor vehicle accidents when patients

FIGURE 43

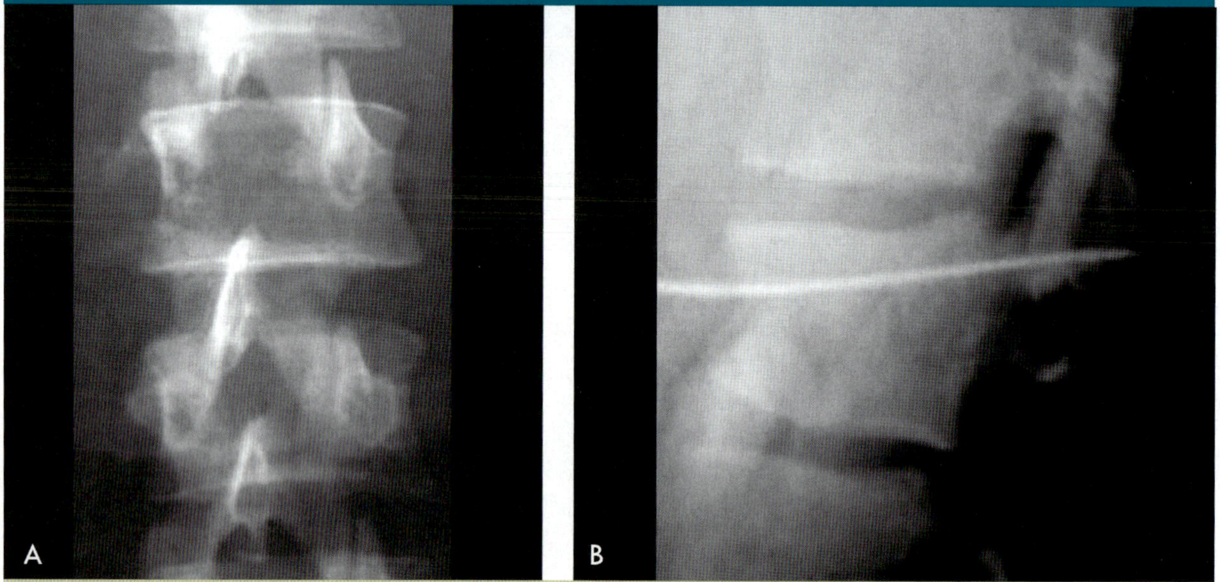

Figure 43 Bony Chance fracture (flexion-distraction injury). AP (**A**) and lateral (**B**) radiographs show the typical horizontal fracture line through the midbody, extending into the pedicles.

FIGURE 44

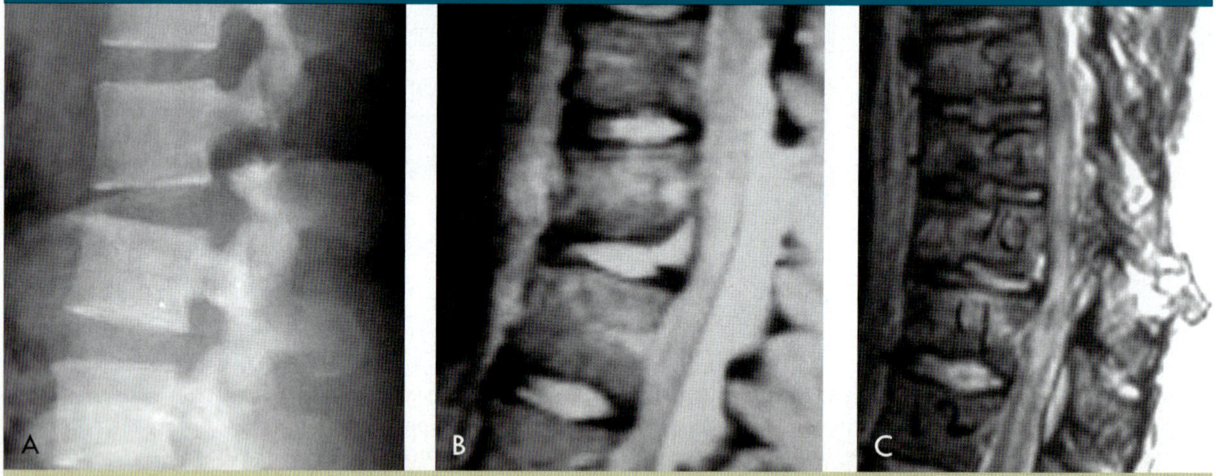

Figure 44 Bone and soft-tissue Chance fracture. Lateral radiograph (**A**) of a patient and midsagittal MRI scans (**B** and **C**) of a different patient reveal laceration of the intervertebral disk. The fracture extends superiorly into the vertebral body and cleaves off the posterior longitudinal ligament. The posterior interspinous ligaments are also sheared.

are restrained by lap seat belts. They are commonly known as Chance fractures.[21] The restrained lower torso remains relatively fixed to the seat of the car while the upper portion of the body is flung forward. If the forces are sufficient, the spine may be transected. There are three types of Chance fracture: those that traverse the bone from front to back, those that traverse disk and ligaments only, and those that go partially through bone and partially through the disk or ligaments. The patient in **Figure 43** has a bony Chance fracture. Note that there is a horizontal fracture line dividing the pedicles into upper and lower segments. The horizontal cleave is seen extending through the vertebral body on the lateral view.

Figure 44 demonstrates a Chance fracture that begins anteriorly through the intervertebral disk but extends upwardly through the bony neural arch separating it from the vertebral body. The two MRI scans are of another patient with a similar injury. Fluid is noted in the lacerated disk in **Figure 44,** *B*. Note that a small fragment of the pos-

FIGURE 45

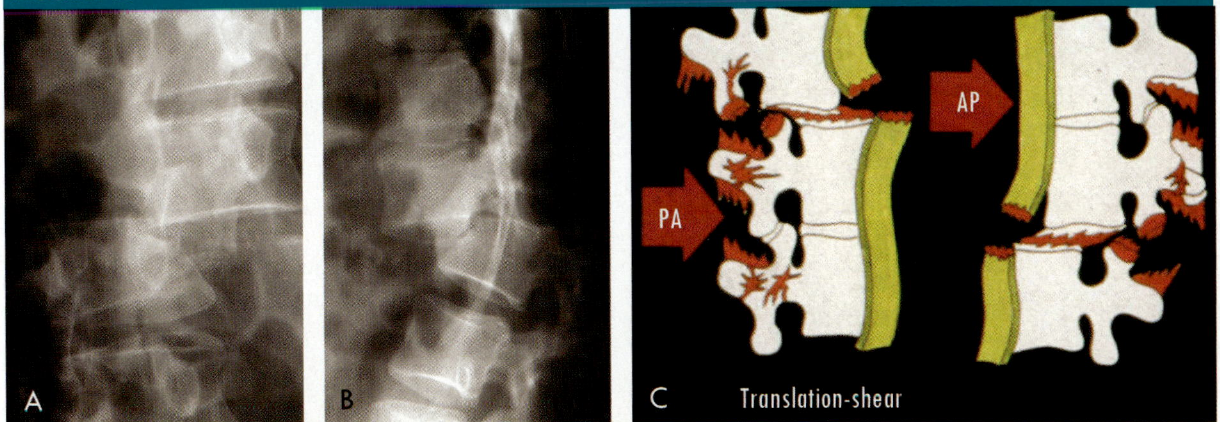

Figure 45 Translation injury. AP (**A**) and lateral (**B**) radiographs reveal dramatic offset of the upper half of the spine with respect to the lower half. There are no obvious bony fractures. **C,** Illustration of translation injury. (Panel C is courtesy of the late William Wilemon, MD.)

terior superior apophyseal ring has remained attached to the lower vertebra. **Figure 44,** *C* demonstrates the severe soft-tissue injury to the posterior ligaments. The transection is seen to extend from the lamina through the paraspinal ligaments and muscles.

Translation Fractures

Translation fractures are much less common than the ones described so far. They are the result of the application of shearing forces across the body, and are primarily disk and ligamentous transections. They are extremely unstable and require fixation. **Figure 45** shows such a fracture. AP and lateral radiographs show dramatic displacement of the upper half of the spine on the lower half. There is little in the way of bony injury. The cleavage force has transected the disk and all the interverebral ligaments.

The Role of Diagnostic Imaging in the Hurting But Not Seriously Injured Patient

Thus far, our discussion has concerned patients with definable anatomic injuries. Each has abnormalities on the imaging studies that were correlatable with their clinical presentation and symptoms. The majority of people who report back or neck pain following accidents have no definable anatomic lesion. What is the role of diagnostic imaging in the "hurting but not anatomically injured" patient? The answer to this question depends on the objective clinical signs and symptoms of the patient. Patients with cervical or lumbar radiculopathy will have objective motor and/or sensory findings. It is certainly appropriate that the evaluation of these patients include imaging studies. A common cause of postaccident arm or leg pain is irritation of nerve roots by some anatomic abnormality that was present within the spine but was not causing nerve irritation. In the legal vernacular, these lesions are termed preexisting conditions. In some of these patients with radiculopathy, surgical decompression or fusion will be determined to be the treatment of choice when correlating bony spurs or disk protrusions are found compressing nerves and the patients fail to improve on nonsurgical therapy. Radiographs and MRI or CT scans will demonstrate these neurocompressive lesions.

What about the patient with persistent postaccident axial back or neck pain? There is considerable controversy about the appropriate treatment. There may be little or no indication for performing MRI or CT if reconstructive surgery is not an immediate treatment option. What can one expect to see on these studies that will affect the treatment of back pain? **Figure 46** is an MRI scan on a typical patient with back pain following an automobile accident. The dark disk has obviously preceded the vehicular trauma. Is it responsible for ongoing symptoms?

The study reveals a degenerated L4-L5 disk that is dehydrated and bulging. There is a high-intensity zone within the posterior anulus. The likelihood that these abnormalities were caused by a recent accident is essentially zero.[22] It takes 2 to 3 years to darken a disk on MRI.[23] Furthermore, dark disks such as this are seen in a very large

FIGURE 46

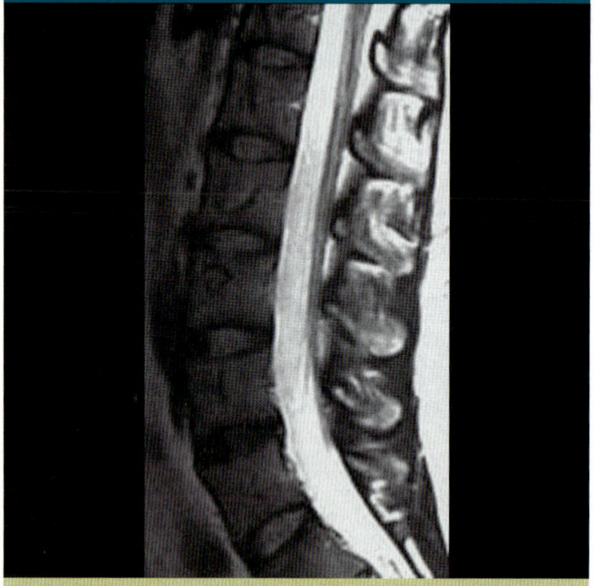

Figure 46 An MRI scan of a typical patient with back pain following an automobile accident.

percentage of the normal population.[24] Twenty percent of teenagers will have at least one abnormal disk on an MRI scan.[25,26] Consequently, we can never make the presumption that just because the accident caused the patient's pain, it also caused the abnormalities noted on the MRI scans.

The only way that one may appropriately make the diagnosis of acute disk injury is when the findings of acute disk herniation are present. An acute disk herniation can be distinguished from a chronic herniation using three criteria. (1) Acute disk herniations are brighter on MRI than the disks from which they come.[27,28] (2) If intravenous contrast agent is injected as part of the MRI study, the periphery of the extruded fragment will appear to enhance. In actual fact, a rim of inflammatory tissue surrounding the disk enhances. (3) Acute disk herniations will usually shrink dramatically on their own. Between 2 and 5 months, there will be fairly dramatic dehydration and resorption of the extruded fragment. This happens rarely with chronic disk herniations.

A high-intensity zone was also demonstrated on the scan in **Figure 46**. This finding is inappropriately called an annular tear. What we are seeing is abnormal tissue surrounding an annular fissure within the disk. In its position paper on definitions, the North American Spine Society and the American Society of Spine Radiology[29] cautioned against using the term annular tear because of the false presumption that these fissures were somehow due to trauma. High-intensity zones are clearly not due to trauma because annular fissures are found in all degenerated disks. High-intensity zones have been reported in up to 50% of abnormal disks in asymptomatic people.

A discussion of diskography as a diagnostic tool in the postinjury patient is beyond the scope of this chapter. The use of diskography remains somewhat controversial, although its use is becoming more main stream. There are geographic variations in the community acceptance of this modality. The experience of the diskographer and the relationship between surgical outcomes and the diskography findings all factor into the surgeon's decision making in considering this test result as just one piece in the diagnostic evaluation.

In summary, because all the abnormalities seen in the scans of people with back pain only (or with referred nonradicular pain) are also seen in large numbers of normal people and have never been proven to be caused by blunt force trauma, one can never presume that pain is coming from a disk noted to be abnormal on MRI or CT.

Conclusion

The proper analysis of the imaging studies done on the traumatized patient requires an understanding of the forces applied to the spine. The spine behaves in well-defined ways upon the application of disrupting forces. It is often possible to predict the types of injuries that will be present from the routine films even without the benefit of MRI or CT. The more one understands the biomechanics of trauma, the more likely that the surgical treatment will be appropriately conceived and executed.

Acknowledgment

Many of the figures in this chapter were drawn by the late William Wilemon, MD, a colleague, friend, artist, and orthopaedic surgeon.

References

1. Allen BL Jr, Ferguson RL, Lehmann TR, O'Brien RP: A mechanistic classification of closed, indirect fractures and dislocations of the lower cervical spine. *Spine (Phila Pa 1976)* 1982;7(1):1-27.
2. White AA, Panjabi MM, eds: *Clinical Biomechanics of the Spine*. Philadelphia, PA, JB Lippincott, 1978.
3. Denis F: The three column spine and its significance in the classification of acute thoracolumbar

spinal injuries. *Spine (Phila Pa 1976)* 1983;8(8): 817-831.

4. Noble ER, Smoker WR: The forgotten condyle: The appearance, morphology, and classification of occipital condyle fractures. *AJNR Am J Neuroradiol* 1996;17(3):507-513.
5. Clayman DA, Sykes CH, Vines FS: Occipital condyle fractures: Clinical presentation and radiologic detection. *AJNR Am J Neuroradiol* 1994;15(7): 1309-1315.
6. Montesano PX, Nelson EF: Occipital cranial injuries, in Levine AM, ed: *Orthopaedic Knowledge Update: Trauma.* Rosemont, IL, American Academy of Orthopaedic Surgeons, 1996, pp 311-315.
7. Gerlock AJ Jr, Mirfakhraee M, Benzel EC: Computed tomography of traumatic atlantooccipital dislocation. *Neurosurgery* 1983;13(3):316-319.
8. Zigler JE, Waters RL, Nelson RW, Capen DA, Perry J: Occipito-cervico-thoracic spine fusion in a patient with occipito-cervical dislocation and survival. *Spine (Phila Pa 1976)* 1986;11(6): 645-646.
9. Levine AM, Edwards CC: Fractures of the atlas. *J Bone Joint Surg Am* 1991;73(5):680-691.
10. Levine AM, Edwards CC: Traumatic lesions of the occipitoatlantoaxial complex. *Clin Orthop Relat Res* 1989;239:53-68.
11. Hinck VC, Hopkins CE: Measurement of the atlanto-dental interval in the adult. *Am J Roentgenl Radium Ther Nucl Med* 1960;84:945-951.
12. Locke GR, Gardner JI, Van Epps EP: Atlas-dens interval (ADI) in children: A survey based on 200 normal cervical spines. *Am J Roentgenl Radium Ther Nucl Med* 1966;97(1):135-140.
13. Anderson LD, D'Alonzo RT: Fractures of the odontoid process of the axis. *J Bone Joint Surg Am* 1974;56(8):1663-1674.
14. Blacksin MF, Lee HJ: Frequency and significance of fractures of the upper cervical spine detected by CT in patients with severe neck trauma. *AJR Am J Roentgenol* 1995;165(5):1201-1204.
15. Von Torklus D, Gehle W, eds: *The Upper Cervical Spine.* New York, NY, Grune & Stratton, 1972.
16. Rothman SLG, Chafetz NI: The radiological distinction between congenital os odontoidium and posttraumatic pseudarthrosis of the dens. Presented at *American Society of Neuroradiology Meeting.* Nashville, TN, May 3-7, 1994.
17. O'Callaghan JP, Ullrich CG, Yuan HA, Kiffer SA: CT of facet distraction flexion injuries of the thoracolumbar spine: The "naked" facet. *AJNR Am J Roentgenol* 1980;134(3):563-568.
18. Zigler JE, Capen DA, Rothman SL: Spinal disease in the aged. *Clin Orthop Relat Res* 1995;316: 70-79.
19. McAfee PC, Yuan HA, Fredrickson BE, Lubicky JP: The value of computed tomography in thoracolumbar fractures: An analysis of one hundred consecutive cases and a new classification. *J Bone Joint Surg Am* 1983;65(4):461-473.
20. Lindahl S, Willén J, Nordwall A, Irstam L: The crush-cleavage fracture: A "new" thoracolumbar unstable fracture. *Spine (Phila Pa 1976)* 1983;8(6): 559-569.
21. Chance GQ: Note on a type of flexion fracture of the spine. *Br J Radiol* 1948;21(249):452-453.
22. Quencer RM: The abnormal annulus fibrosus: Can we infer the acuteness of an annular injury? *AJNR Am J Neuroradiol* 2002;23(7):1069.
23. Erkintalo MO, Salminen JJ, Alanen AM, Paajanen HE, Kormano MJ: Development of degenerative changes in the lumbar intervertebral disk: Results of a prospective MR imaging study in adolescents with and without low-back pain. *Radiology* 1995; 196(2):529-533.
24. Stadnik TW, Lee RR, Coen HL, Neirynck EC, Buisseret TS, Osteaux MJ: Annular tears and disk herniation: Prevalence and contrast enhancement on MR images in the absence of low back pain or sciatica. *Radiology* 1998;206(1):49-55.
25. Tertti MO, Salminen JJ, Paajanen HE, Terho PH, Kormano MJ: Low-back pain and disk degeneration in children: A case-control MR imaging study. *Radiology* 1991;180(2):503-507.
26. Gibson MJ, Szypryt EP, Buckley JH, Worthington BS, Mulholland RC: Magnetic resonance imaging of adolescent disc herniation. *J Bone Joint Surg Br* 1987;69(5):699-703.
27. Czervionke LF: Lumbar intervertebral disc disease. *Neuroimaging Clin N Am* 1993;3:465-484.
28. Bundschuh CV: Imaging of the postoperative lumbosacral spine. *Neuroimaging Clin N Am* 1993; 3:499-516.
29. Fardon DF, Millette PC, Combined Task Forces of the North American Spine Society, American Society of Spine Radiology, American Society of Neuroradiology: Recommendations and classification of lumbar disc pathology: Recommendations of the combined task forces of the North American Spine Society, American Society of Spine Radiology and the Ameican Society of Neuoradiology. *Spine (Phila Pa 1976)* 2001;26(5):E93-E113.

CHAPTER 15

Surgical Approaches to the Cervical Spine

Scott H. Kitchel, MD

Key Points

- For anterior approaches, the surgeon must know the anatomy of the neck, including innervation of the pharynx, the larynx, and other local structures.
- Adequate studies must be obtained to define the pathology and the local anatomy, and the surgeon must review them preoperatively to select the optimal procedure and the proper approach.
- The surgeon must know the location of the vertebral arteries at the operative levels and be aware of vertebral artery anomalies.
- The surgeon must identify the correct levels and symptomatic side both preoperatively and intraoperatively.
- The surgeon should avoid cervical hyperextension during preoperative positioning for any patient with cervical stenosis.

Introduction

Surgical treatment of cervical spine disease requires an understanding of cervical anatomy, the disease process, and a comprehensive review of the imaging studies. Once the decision to undertake surgical treatment has been made, the importance of positioning and the appropriate surgical approach cannot be overemphasized. In this chapter, the current knowledge regarding surgical approaches to the cervical spine is presented. Many lesions of the cervical spine may be approached from more than one route. This chapter does not deal with indications for each approach, but rather summarizes the anatomy and technique for anterior, lateral, and posterior approaches to the cervical spine. The decision as to which approach is used must be individualized, depending on the surgical lesion as well as the expertise and experience of the operating surgeon. Whichever approach is chosen, the positioning and technique will have a major effect on the overall success of the surgical procedure.

Dr. Kitchel or an immediate family member has received royalties from SpineWave; is a member of a speakers' bureau or has made paid presentations on behalf of Nuvasive, Osteotech, and Stryker; serves as a paid consultant to or is an employee of Nuvasive, Osteotech, and SpineWave; and owns stock or stock options in Benvenue Medical, SpineWave, and Trans-1.

Posterior Approaches

History

Posterior approaches to the cervical spine were developed before other approaches.[1] Most authors believe this is because of the immediate accessibility of the posterior cervical structures.[2] Despite the apparent simplicity of the exposure, adequate positioning and technique are critical. Posterior approaches allow excellent exposure of the posterior elements of the cervical spine, including the spinous processes, laminae, and facet joints. The posterior spinal cord is also readily exposed, as well as the posterolateral corner of the cervical disks.[3]

Positioning

Positioning for posterior cervical approaches requires placing the patient in the prone position once the patient has been adequately anesthetized. This may be a formality in the patient with a lateral cervical disk herniation or of critical importance in a patient with unstable cervical fractures. I prefer that all patients to be positioned prone have placement of Gardner-Wells tongs or a Gardner head holder. This allows maintenance of accurate alignment of the cervical spine during turning.[1] A Stryker frame may still be used in patients with extreme instability or in whom combined anterior and posterior approaches are to be made in one surgical setting. However, because of the cumbersome nature of this device, it is not routinely recommended.

Once adequate anesthesia has been ensured, the tongs are applied. The patient is then log-rolled into the prone position using an attachment to the operating table appropriate to the tongs. Under routine conditions, four assistants are required to safely turn the patient, with the surgeon being responsible for stabilizing the head and neck. As soon as the patient is positioned, it is critical that

FIGURE 1

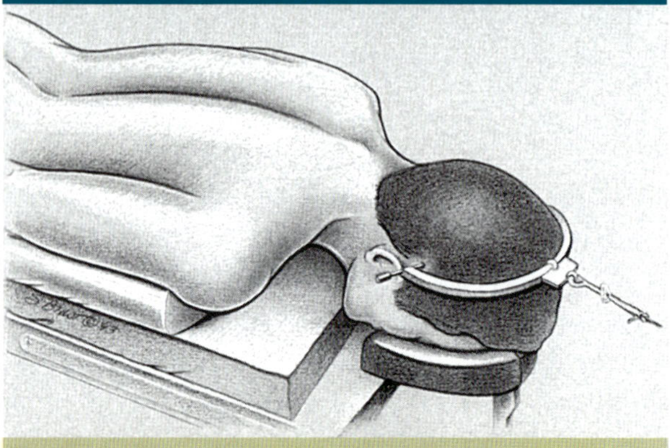

Figure 1 Appropriate prone positioning for posterior cervical approaches with rigid head immobilization. (Drawing by Susan E. Brust, MS, Tualatin, OR.)

pressure on the face and eyes be checked. The eyes must be kept free of any direct pressure from the frame, as prolonged pressure may result in intraocular damage or blindness.[2] Once the face and eyes have been checked, traction may be applied as needed.

The thorax is supported by chest rolls, which allow slight flexion of the hips. The knees are padded and also flexed. Equal pressure must be ensured and no direct contact with metal table parts is allowed. The table is then put into a reverse Trendelenburg position to raise the cervical spine to the surgeon's level. The neck is positioned in adequate flexion for exposure and to eliminate the skin folds. The amount of flexion is individualized to the pathologic findings. For improved radiographic visualization of the lower cervical spine, the shoulders may be taped in a depressed position or Boger straps may be placed on the wrists. In either case, the surgeon must bear in mind that excessive traction may cause stretching of the brachial plexus.

Many surgeons continue to perform posterior cervical approaches with the patient in the sitting position. This is particularly popular for posterior cervical foraminotomy and diskectomy. However, there have been several occurrences of air embolism related to this positioning.[4] As this may represent a fatal complication, I prefer the prone position for posterior cervical approaches.

Once adequate positioning (**Figure 1**) has been ensured and reconfirmed, the posterior cervical surface is prepared in a sterile fashion. Localization of the appropriate level is done through a combination of palpating anatomic landmarks and radiography. The occipital protuberance and prominent posterior spinous process of C2 are easily palpated. Similarly, the prominent spinous

FIGURE 2

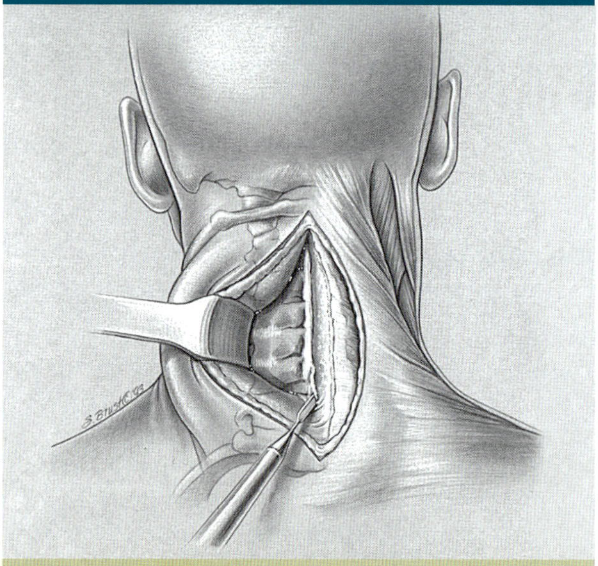

Figure 2 The midline muscular raphe in the posterior cervical spine. (Drawing by Susan E. Brust, MS, Tualatin, OR.)

processes at C7 and T1 are palpated. A needle may then be inserted into a spinous process and a lateral radiograph taken for localization.

Surgical Approach

The posterior skin approach is made in the midline, directly over the palpated spinous processes. The subcutaneous tissues are divided sharply to the level of the fascia. The electrocautery is then used to obtain hemostasis, and self-retaining retractors are placed. Following the plane of the deep cervical fascia, the ligamentum nuchae and supraspinous ligament are exposed with electrocautery. The incision continues down the median raphe to the level of the spinous processes. Care should be taken to stay in the median raphe (**Figure 2**) and to not cut any muscle, as this will lead to excessive blood loss and increased postoperative pain. Care is taken to not expose unnecessary levels, as this may result in spontaneous fusion.[2]

The tips of the spinous processes are then exposed with electrocautery, bearing in mind that these may be bifid in the midcervical region. The dissection is then carried in a subperiosteal plane down the spinous process and across the lamina to expose the facet joint. This may be performed using electrocautery or sharp dissection. Again, care is taken to not cut muscle. The self-retaining retractors are moved progressively to each deeper level.

The posterior elements of the cervical vertebrae are now exposed. Hemostasis is ensured with the

FIGURE 3

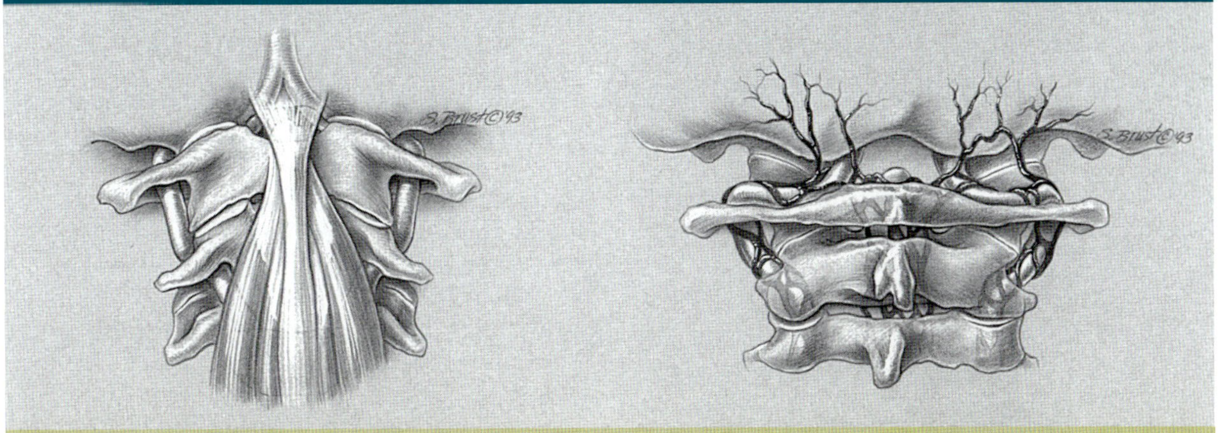

Figure 3 The posterior arch of C1 with the vertebral artery and vein passing through the groove. (Drawing by Susan E. Brust, MS, Tualatin, OR.)

electrocautery, and the surgeon is then ready to proceed with the specific procedure. The positioning and selection of retractors is individualized as to the procedure to be performed.

A few special comments are required regarding exposure of the occiput and posterior ring of C1. The exposure of the occiput is begun by palpation of the occipital protuberance. The median muscular raphe is also the key to this dissection.

The posterior arch of C1 lies in the interval between the occiput and the C2 spinous process. The posterior tubercle of C1 should be palpated and will generally be deep compared with both of these structures. Once the tubercle is palpated, the soft tissues should be dissected free with a sharp periosteal elevator. Once this is exposed, the dissection may be carried laterally along the bony ring. Caution must be exercised, as the ring may be thin and could be fractured by excessive pressure. The dura is also immediately vulnerable superior and inferior to the bony arch.[5] The lateral extent of the C1 arch exposure is limited by the passage of the vertebral artery over the arch of C1 as it enters the foramen magnum. The vertebral artery and vein pass through a groove in the posterior arch of C1 approximately 1.5 cm from the midline (**Figure 3**). The medial ridge of this groove is generally marked by the blue color of the vertebral vein. Through identifying this groove, damage to the vein and artery can be avoided. Exposure of the posterior arch of C1 more than 1.5 cm lateral to the midline is rarely necessary.[6] If this is indicated, then identification of the vertebral artery in the groove is critical.

If exposure of the posterior fossa dura is required, a direct approach through the foramen magnum is not suggested because of the anatomy of the vertebral artery.[7,8] Decompression of the foramen magnum and suboccipital bone is best facilitated by placement of two burr holes—one to the left and one to the right of the foramen magnum.[6] Bone may then be removed using rongeurs of various sizes to avoid the venous sinus in the midline. Suboccipital craniectomy, decompression of the foramen magnum, and occipitocervical fusions are all done using this technique.

Anterior Approach

History

Anterior surgical approaches to the cervical spine were pioneered in the early 1950s.[9] In 1955, Robinson and Smith[10] described the classic anterior cervical approach dissecting the plane between the trachea and carotid sheath. Southwick and Robinson[7] then expanded this approach to expose from C3 to T1. de Andrade and Macnab[11] are credited with extending the approach to the anterior occiput and skull base.

Ralph Cloward[3] must be recognized for his advancement of anterior cervical approaches, including the development of retractors and instruments. In 1981, Biller et al[12] described a new technique for improved anterior exposure of the skull base. Many other authors have advanced modifications of the original techniques, bringing us to our current knowledge of anterior cervical approaches.

Positioning

The patient is positioned supine for anterior cervical surgery. Transfer from the stretcher to the operating table should be accomplished carefully with

FIGURE 4

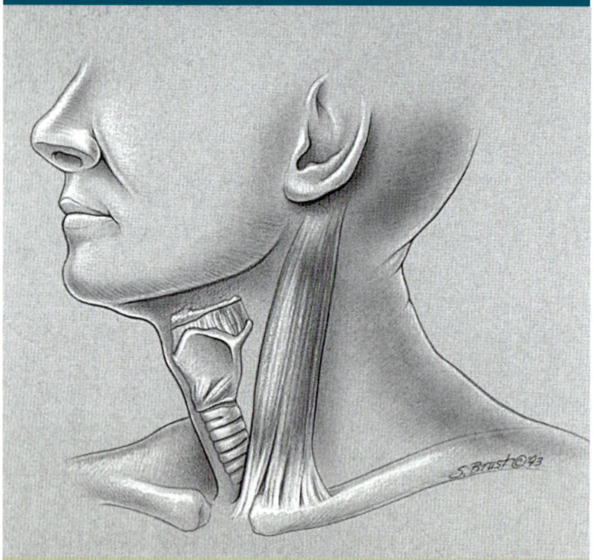

Figure 4 Anterior anatomic landmarks and appropriate skin incisions **[Au: Does figure show the incision marks? If not, please draw them on the figure]**. (Drawing by Susan E. Brust, MS, Tualatin, OR.)

appropriate precautions, especially in patients with unstable conditions. Stabilization of the head in a traction device or frame is the standard of care. This will facilitate exposure, avoid unwanted intraoperative movement, and allow distraction should this be required for bone grafting.[2]

The head must be extended adequately to allow exposure of the cervical spine. This degree of extension is individualized, depending on the patient's condition and the stiffness of the neck. This can be accomplished by carefully placing a rolled towel under the shoulders and allowing the head to gently extend to its limit. The head is then flexed slightly to allow the necessary amount of anterior clearance. Gently rotating the head away from the side of exposure will increase this access.

As with posterior positioning, if radiographic visualization of the lower cervical spine is needed, the shoulders may be taped in a depressed position. Alternatively, Boger straps may be used on the wrists. If either of these means of traction is used, care must be taken not to use excessive force, which would stretch the brachial plexus.[6]

Surgical Approach

Planning of the surgical approach requires palpating the anatomic landmarks and deciding which cervical levels must be exposed. Easily palpable landmarks include the sternocleidomastoid muscle, carotid artery, thyroid cartilage, cricoid cartilage, and clavicle (**Figure 4**). The thyroid cartilage is generally at the C3-C4 level and the cricoid cartilage lies over the C5-C6 level.

The first decision to be made is whether to make a right- or left-sided skin incision. There are two primary anatomic structures that must be considered in this decision. The first of these is the recurrent laryngeal nerve. Damage to this structure may cause permanent vocal cord paralysis and hoarseness. The left recurrent laryngeal nerve runs in the tracheoesophageal groove throughout the neck. In contrast to this, the right recurrent laryngeal nerve passes transversely from the carotid sheath to the medial musculovisceral column in a variable position between C6 and C7.

The second anatomic consideration is the entry of the thoracic duct into the jugular-subclavian vein junction on the left at the C7-T1 level. Identification of the thoracic duct is difficult.[7] Damage to this structure may result in chronic lymph drainage and possible chylothorax.[6]

Because of these two considerations, I recommend a left-sided approach for routine exposure from C3 to C7. At the cervicothoracic junction, the surgeon needs to balance the relative advantages of left-sided versus right-sided approaches, considering the thoracic duct and recurrent laryngeal nerve, respectively. Thoracic duct injuries, although bothersome, can usually be adequately treated, whereas recurrent laryngeal nerve injuries, especially if permanent, present a more disabling problem.

Once a decision has been made for a right- or left-sided incision and the patient positioned, the patient is sterilely prepared and draped. Location of the skin incision is critical for adequate exposure as well as for an acceptable cosmetic result. The landmarks are again palpated to select the correct level (**Figure 4**). The skin incision may be made longitudinally along the medial border of the sternocleidomastoid muscle or transversely in a skin crease from just lateral to the midline to the sternocleidomastoid. The transverse incision will yield a superior cosmetic result[2] and I prefer this technique. With lengthening of this incision, three vertebral bodies and four disk spaces may easily be exposed.[13]

Once the skin is incised, the subcutaneous fat is sharply incised to the level of the platysma muscle fibers. Hemostasis is ensured with electrocautery. Flaps superficial to the platysma muscle are then elevated superiorly and inferiorly. A self-retaining retractor is then placed. It is preferable to open the platysma muscle in line with its fibers over the medial border of the sternocleidomastoid. Care must be taken not to damage the underlying veins

FIGURE 5

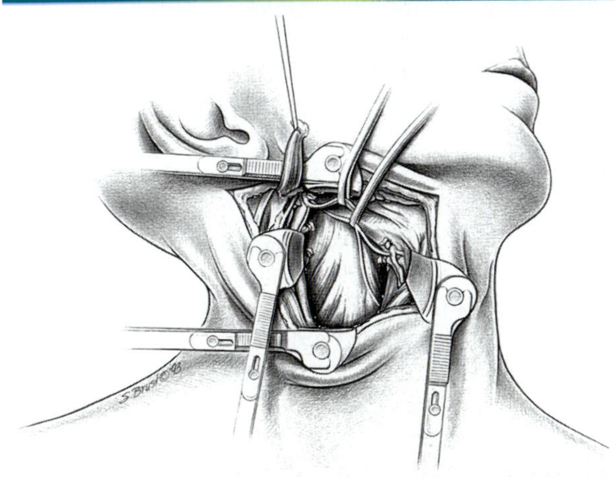

Figure 5 Anterior cervical exposure with retractors in place. (Drawing by Susan E. Brust, MS, Tualatin, OR.)

FIGURE 6

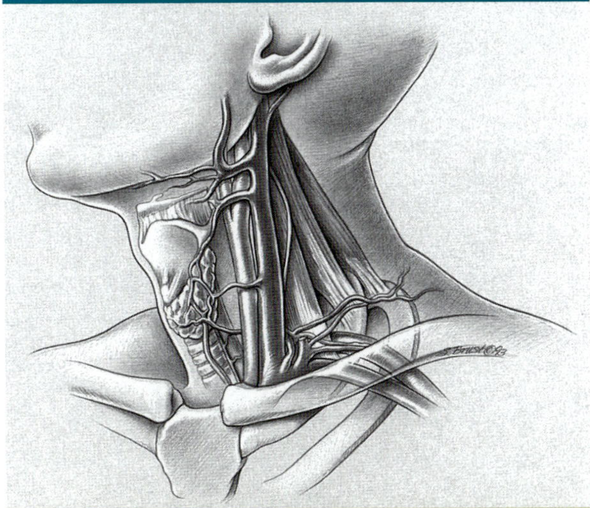

Figure 6 Anterior neurovascular structures encountered in dissection of the middle cervical fascia. (Drawing by Susan E. Brust, MS, Tualatin, OR.)

or sternocleidomastoid. The medial border of the sternocleidomastoid and the carotid sheath are the most important landmarks for the remainder of the approach. The sternocleidomastoid can be directly visualized and palpation carried down the middle cervical fascia just medial to the sternocleidomastoid.[14] The middle thyroid vein may be encountered in this interval between C4 and C6. If necessary, it may be ligated and divided. The carotid artery is palpated and dissection directed medial to it.

The carotid sheath is repeatedly palpated to ensure its protection.[15] Using blunt finger dissection, the anterior cervical bodies may then be palpated. The prevertebral fascia remains intact over the anterior cervical spine, with the trachea and esophagus retracted medially and the carotid sheath laterally. Blunt retractors are used exclusively at this point. Care should be taken to ensure that a transverse process is not being mistaken for the midline.

Once this has been confirmed, the prevertebral fascia is opened sharply in the midline. The more vascular area of this fascia is lateral[2] and the importance of starting at the midline cannot be overemphasized. With the fascia opened, the dissection continues laterally to elevate the longus colli muscle for safe retractor placement. At this point, the trachea and esophagus are retracted medially and the carotid sheath and sternocleidomastoid are retracted laterally. The surgeon must exercise caution as the dissection proceeds superficial to deep to maintain the same borders at each depth, ensuring adequate exposure for the surgical procedure.[14]

Self-retaining retractors may now be positioned within the wound to allow the surgery to proceed. Clawed blades are inserted under the flaps of the longus colli on both sides of the spine.[3] The self-retaining frame is then tightened. At this point, repeat inspection of the esophagus and trachea medially and the carotid sheath laterally is done to make sure they are not impinged on by the retractor. A blunt set of blades may then be placed longitudinally to increase vertical exposure (**Figure 5**). The planned surgical procedure may then be performed.

Depending on the level of the spine approached, several vessels and nerves may be encountered during the dissection down the middle cervical fascia[7] (**Figure 6**). In the more cephalad exposures, the digastric muscle, glossopharyngeal nerve, and hypoglossal nerve may be encountered. In most cephalad approaches, these may be retracted carefully cephalad. The paired superior laryngeal nerve and superior thyroid artery may be retracted caudad for C1-C3 approaches and cephalad for C4-C7 approaches. As previously mentioned, the middle thyroid vein may be ligated when necessary. The inferior thyroid vein and artery are retracted caudally for exposures at or above C7. Cephalad retraction of these structures is preferred for approaches at the cervicothoracic junction.

FIGURE 7

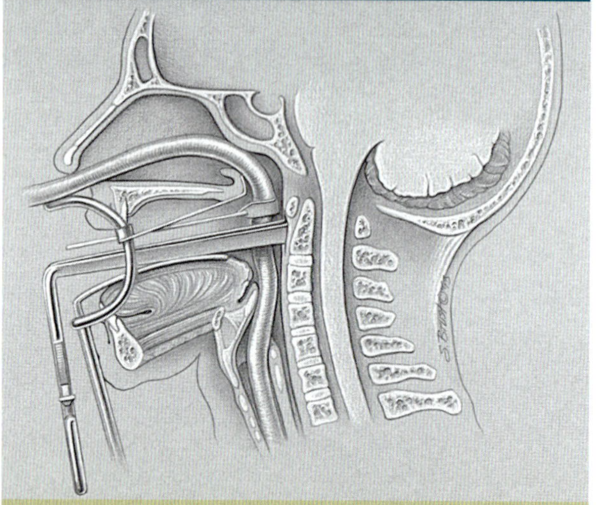

Figure 7 Lateral view of transoral retractors in position. (Drawing by Susan E. Brust, MS, Tualatin, OR.)

Other Anterior and Anterolateral Approaches

The Smith-Robinson anterior approach affords excellent visualization of the middle and lower cervical spine. However, it must be modified or other approaches may be needed for the upper cervical spine and the cervicothoracic junction. The remainder of this chapter deals with those other approaches by anatomic location.

Transoral Approach

History

Over the years many different anterior approaches to the craniocervical junction have been described. In 1962, Fang and Ong[16] described the transoral direct approach to the cervical spine. This has been the standard with which all other approaches to this region must be compared. In 1987, Archer et al[17] described their transmaxillary approach. However, this approach allows no exposure below the foramen magnum. Derome[18] presented his transbasal approach in 1988. Most observers believe it is too extensive for the craniocervical junction. James and Crockard[19] described an extended maxillotomy approach in 1991.

After reviewing all of the approaches, I believe that only the widely used transoral approach has withstood the test of time. This technique will be described in detail as will the lateral retropharyngeal approach to the upper cervical spine. The reader is directed to the references for descriptions of the other techniques.

Positioning

Positioning for transoral surgery requires immobilization of the head as well as adequate access to the mouth. Most surgeons prefer either the supine or lateral position. Compared with the sitting position, this decreases the drainage down via the esophagus into the stomach. Although the lateral position allows the surgeon to sit, I prefer the supine position because of the easier orientation to the anatomic structures.

The head may be immobilized with traction or in a table-mounted frame. Once anesthesia has been induced and the positioning is adequate, the mouth is cleaned out with oral chlorhexidine solution and a transoral retractor is placed (**Figure 7** and **8**). Great care must be taken not to impinge on the tongue and the lower teeth. The mouth is opened as far as possible and the soft palate is retracted with the curved palatal retractor. Another palatal retractor is used to retract the nasogastric and nasotracheal tubes into the tonsillar fauces.

Surgical Approach

The key anatomic landmark for palpation is the tubercle of the ring on C1.[16] Once this has been identified, the area is injected with epinephrine in a concentration of 1:200,000. This injection will create a plane between the pharynx and prevertebral tissues. A midline longitudinal incision is then made from the tubercle to the base of C2. In the midline, one should not encounter any bleeding.[3] The tissue can then be elevated in the plane between bone and the cervical mucosa laterally in each direction. An additional palatal retractor is now placed.

The insertion of the longus colli and the anterior longitudinal ligament into the tubercle of C1 (**Figure 8**) is divided with electrocautery. Electrocautery is additionally used to dissect free the C1 arch and C2 anterior body. The surgeon may then proceed with the indicated procedure.

Once the procedure is completed, the wound is copiously irrigated with antibiotic solution. The muscle and fascial layers are closed with one layer. The pharyngeal mucosa is then closed with absorbable sutures in a separate layer.

If further exposure is required, the mandibular-tongue-pharynx–splitting approach as described by Stauffer[20] may be used. A vertical incision is made from the center of the lower lip to the prominence of the chin, which is circumscribed, and the incision is then continued to the back of the chin. The mucous membrane is split and the mandible predrilled and cut in a step-cut fashion

FIGURE 8

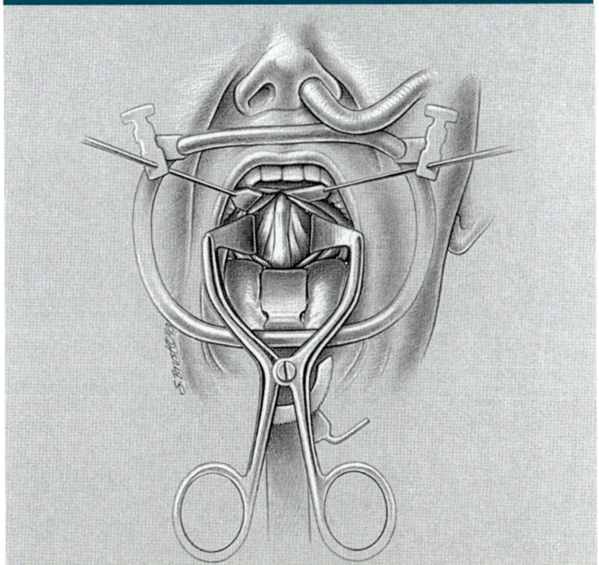

Figure 8 Location of the anterior longitudinal ligament and longus colli muscles in the transoral approach. (Drawing by Susan E. Brust, MS, Tualatin, OR.)

FIGURE 9

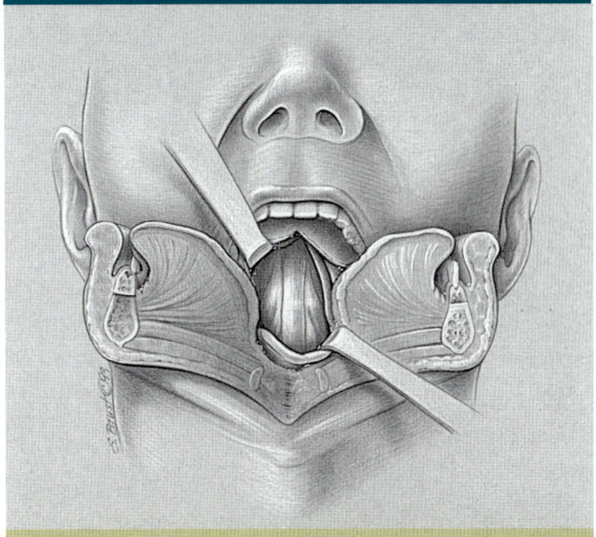

Figure 9 Splitting the mandible and tongue for the extended transoral approach. (Drawing by Susan E. Brust, MS, Tualatin, OR.)

to facilitate reapproximation. The tongue is split longitudinally through its central raphe (**Figure 9**). The halves of the mandible and tongue are retracted laterally on each side. The vertebral prominences are palpated in the midline and the mucosa is split in the middle, creating laterally based flaps. This allows anterior exposure from the clivus to C6.[20] Preoperative tracheostomy is required.

Anteromedial Retropharyngeal Approach to the Upper Cervical Spine

History

Because of the high risk of infection in transoral surgery, the anteromedial retropharyngeal approach to the upper cervical spine is preferred.[16,21] This approach really represents an extension and evolution of the Smith-Robinson anteromedial approach to the midcervical spine.[1,2,4,6,7,10,14,15,20,22-25] In 1973, Riley[14] described the extensile retropharyngeal approach using division of the stylohyoid and digastric tendons and dislocation of the ipsilateral temporomandibular joint. Southwick and Robinson[23] further modified this by using a transverse submandibular skin incision.

Positioning

Positioning considerations for this procedure are identical to those outlined in the discussion of anterior approaches.

Surgical Approach

A modified transverse submandibular incision is used[22] (**Figure 10**). This is made on the patient's right side if the surgeon is right-handed, allowing easier exposure.[22] This incision and the subsequent exposure are a logical cephalad extension of the traditional anterior Smith-Robinson incision. The dissection is carried sharply through the platysma muscle and flaps are mobilized in the subplatysmal plane of the superficial fascia.

The marginal mandibular branch of the facial nerve is found with a nerve stimulator and protected. By ligating the retromandibular vein and keeping the dissection deep and inferior to the internal jugular vein, the superficial branches of the fascial nerve are protected (**Figure 11**). The anterior border of the sternocleidomastoid is mobilized longitudinally by transecting the superficial layer of the deep cervical fascia. The carotid sheath is then palpated and the submandibular salivary gland is resected by suturing its duct. The jugulodigastric lymph nodes are resected if necessary.

The posterior bellies of the digastric and stylohyoid muscles are identified. The digastric tendon is divided and tagged for later repair. The hyoid and hypopharynx are then mobilized medially. This avoids exposure of the contaminated nasopharynx, hypopharynx, and esophagus.

The hypoglossal nerve is then identified with a nerve stimulator and mobilized from the base of the skull to the anterior border of the hypoglossal

FIGURE 10

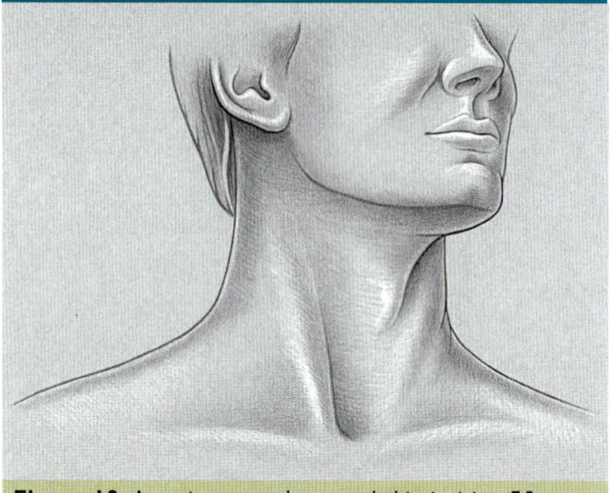

Figure 10 Anterior retropharyngeal skin incision **[Au: Please draw the incision marks on the figure]**. (Drawing by Susan E. Brust, MS, Tualatin, OR.)

FIGURE 11

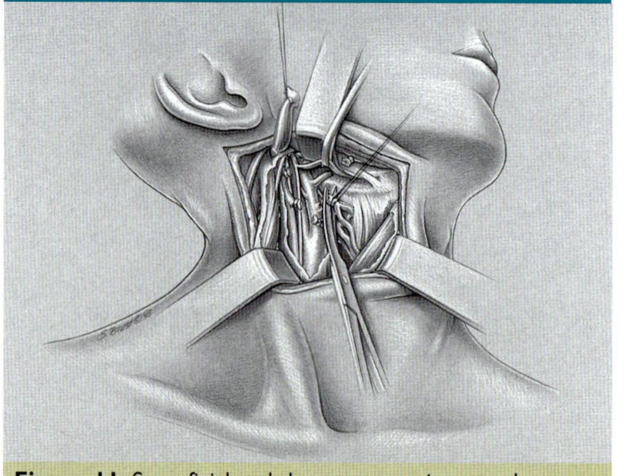

Figure 11 Superficial and deep anatomy in retropharyngeal dissection. (Drawing by Susan E. Brust, MS, Tualatin, OR.)

muscle (**Figure 11**). It is then retracted superiorly. The dissection may then proceed to the retropharyngeal space between the carotid sheath laterally and the larynx and pharynx anteromedially.

Beginning inferiorly, the superior thyroid artery and vein, lingual artery and vein, ascending pharyngeal artery and vein, and facial artery and vein are ligated to facilitate mobilization of the carotid sheath laterally. The superior laryngeal nerve is mobilized and protected. The alar and prevertebral fascia are transected longitudinally to expose the longus colli muscle. The midline then must be palpated and its position assured.

The longus colli muscle may then be detached from the anterior surface of C1 and C2. The C1 and C2 vertebrae are then exposed as indicated for the necessary procedure. With use of blunt handheld retractors, the surgery may then proceed.

Anterior Approach to the Cervicothoracic Junction

History

The lower cervical spine and cervicothoracic junction may be difficult to approach anteriorly in the patient with a short neck. This is often because of the position of the clavicle or deformity at the cervicothoracic junction secondary to trauma or bony destruction.

In many instances, the traditional anterior Smith-Robinson approach may suffice. However, if extended upper thoracic exposure is required, a modified supraclavicular approach or modified anterior approach as described by Kurz et al[26] may be indicated.

Positioning

For either the supraclavicular approach or the modified anterior approach, the patient is positioned supine as for a traditional anterior approach. The reader is referred to the earlier discussion of positioning for anterior approaches.

Surgical Approach

The supraclavicular approach begins with a transverse skin incision one fingerbreadth above the clavicle, which extends from just lateral to the midline to the posterior border of the sternocleidomastoid. The subcutaneous tissues are sharply incised and hemostasis is attained with electrocautery. The platysma is identified and split in line with the skin incision. The sternocleidomastoid must then be identified in its anterior and posterior margin. The external investing fascia is incised. A finger is then passed under the medial border of the sternocleidomastoid to free the veins deep to it. The clavicular head of the sternocleidomastoid is then divided lateral to medial. The divided ends are retracted cephalad and caudad. The middle cervical fascia is exposed in the floor of the incision (**Figure 12**). This fascia is then entered just lateral to the carotid sheath. Dissection is carried bluntly to the anterior surface of the anterior scalene muscle. At this point, the phrenic nerve is identified as it crosses the anterior scalene lateral to medial, cephalad to caudad. The phrenic nerve is retracted medially, the jugular vein is identified medially, and the carotid is palpated.

FIGURE 12

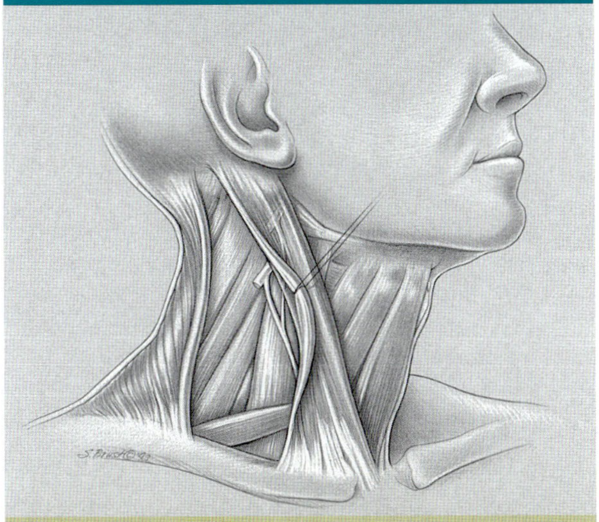

Figure 12 Supraclavicular approach anatomy. (Drawing by Susan E. Brust, MS, Tualatin, OR.)

FIGURE 13

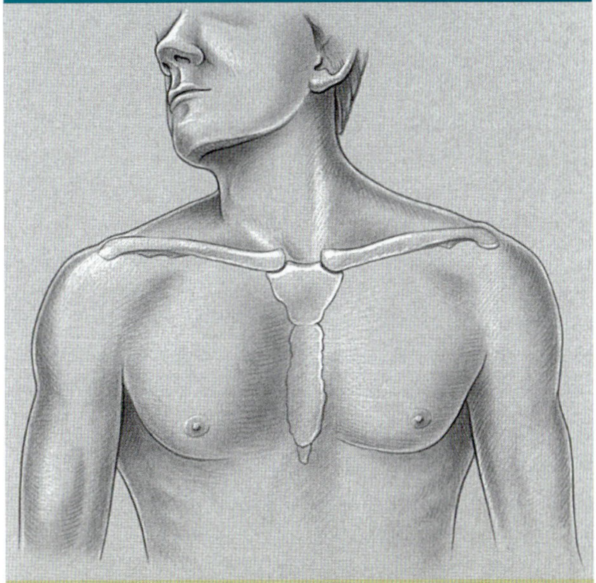

Figure 13 Anterior skin incision **[Au: Does figure show skin incision? If not, please draw it on the figure].** (Drawing by Susan E. Brust, MS, Tualatin, OR.)

The dissection is then carried medially along the anterior scalene and under the carotid sheath. The prevertebral fascia is followed to the spine and then to the midline. The prevertebral fascia may then be opened and retractors placed as discussed for other anterior approaches.

If even further caudad exposure is required, I recommend the modified anterior approach as described by Kurz et al.[26] The patient is positioned supine with neck extension. The skin incision (**Figure 13**) is left-sided and consists of a transverse and longitudinal limb. The longitudinal limb incision ends distally just past the manubriosternal junction. The transverse limb incision is carried 2 cm proximal and parallel to the left clavicle and extended laterally to the lateral border of the sternocleidomastoid muscle. The incision is carried through the skin and subcutaneous tissues, and the platysma is incised the length of the skin incision. Subcutaneous flaps are developed and the superficial anterior veins are ligated. The internal and external jugular veins, as well as the medial supraclavicular nerve, are retracted.

The manubrial and clavicular heads are elevated off their distal attachments and retracted laterally. The strap muscles are transected just below the clavicle and are elevated medially. The left half of the manubrium and the medial third of the clavicle are subperiosteally stripped. A Gigli saw is then used to cut the clavicle at the junction of its medial and middle thirds. The subclavian vein must be protected inferiorly and posteriorly to the clavicle.

The medial third of the clavicle is then disarticulated from the manubrium. In the proximal portion of the wound, a plane is found medial to the carotid sheath but lateral to the trachea and esophagus. This plane is followed to the prevertebral fascia. The prevertebral fascia is identified and blunt handheld retractors are placed to retract the trachea and esophagus medially and the carotid sheath laterally. The dissection may be carried caudad to T3 and cephalad to C5. Radiographic confirmation of the correct level is made and the procedure is performed.

Closure of this approach requires reapproximation of the strap muscles medially. The sternocleidomastoid is repaired to the clavicle periosteum. The subcutaneous tissues and skin are then closed in a routine fashion.

Summary

The keys to safe surgical exposure of the cervical spine are a thorough understanding of the anatomy and the pathology to be addressed. Once these issues have been resolved, then the appropriate approach may be selected, the patient safely positioned, and the correct level identified radiographically. Following routine surgical principles with these established techniques will yield gratifying results.

References

1. Murphy MJ, Southwick WO: Surgical approaches and techniques, in Cervical Spine Research Society Staff, eds: *The Cervical Spine*, ed 2. Philadelphia, PA, JB Lippincott, 1989.
2. Watkins RG, Dillin WH: Surgical approaches to the cervical spine, in Camins MB, O'Leary PF, eds: *Disorders of the Cervical Spine*. Baltimore, MD, Williams & Wilkins, 1992.
3. Cloward R: *Ruptured Cervical Intervertebral Discs*. Philadelphia, PA, Codman Signature Series, Codman & Shurteleff, 1974.
4. Shapiro HM, Drummond JC: Neurosurgical anesthesia and intracranial hypertension, in Jones DL, ed: *Anesthesia*. Philadelphia, PA, JB Lippincott, 1989.
5. Gumbs AA, Bloom ND, Bitan FD, Hanan SH: Open anterior approaches for lumbar spine procedures. *Am J Surg* 2007;194(1):98-102.
6. Robinson RA, Southwick WO: Surgical approaches to the cervical spine. *Instr Course Lect* 1960;17:229-330.
7. Southwick WO, Robinson RA: Surgical approaches to the vertebral bodies in the cervical and lumbar regions. *J Bone Joint Surg Am* 1957; 39(3):631-644.
8. Logue V: Compressive lesions at the foramen magnum, in Ruge D, Wiltse LL, eds: *Spinal Disorders: Diagnosis and Treatment*. Philadelphia, PA, Lea & Febiger, 1977, pp 249-273.
9. Maack RW, Spector JG: Anterior approaches to the cervical spine, in Bridwell KH, DeWald RL, eds: *The Textbook of Spinal Surgery*. Philadelphia, PA, JB Lippincott, 1991.
10. Robinson RA, Smith GW: Anterolateral cervical disc removal and interbody fusion for cervical disc syndrome. *Bull Johns Hopkins Hosp* 1955;96: 223-224.
11. de Andrade JR, Macnab I: Anterior occipitocervical fusion using an extra-pharyngeal exposure. *J Bone Joint Surg Am* 1969;51(8):1621-1626.
12. Biller HF, Shugar JM, Krespi YP: A new technique for wide-field exposure of the base of the skull. *Arch Otolaryngol* 1981;107(11):698-702.
13. Bailey RW, Badgley CE: Stabilization of the cervical spine by anterior fusion. *J Bone Joint Surg Am* 1960;42-A:565-594.
14. Riley LH Jr: Surgical approaches to the anterior structures of the cervical spine. *Clin Orthop Relat Res* 1973;91:16-20.
15. Robinson RA: *The Craft of Surgery*. Boston, MA, Little Brown, 1971.
16. Fang HS, Ong GB: Direct anterior approach to the upper cervical spine. *J Bone Joint Surg Am* 1962;44:1588-1604.
17. Archer DJ, Young S, Uttley D: Basilar aneurysms: A new transclival approach via maxillotomy. *J Neurosurg* 1987;67(1):54-58.
18. Derome PJ: The transbasal approach to tumors invading the base of the skull, in *Operative Neurosurgical Techniques*. Orlando, FL, Grune & Stratton, 1988, pp 619-633.
19. James D, Crockard HA: Surgical access to the base of skull and upper cervical spine by extended maxillotomy. *Neurosurgery* 1991;29(3): 411-416.
20. Stauffer ES: Mandibular splitting approach to the upper anterior vertebral canal, in Louis R, Weidner A, eds: *Cervical Spine*. New York, NY, Springer-Verlag, 1987.
21. Crockard A: Anterior approaches to the craniocervical junction, in Camins MB, O'Leary PF, eds: *Disorders of the Cervical Spine*. Baltimore, MD, Williams & Wilkins, 1992.
22. McAfee PC, Bohlman HH, Riley LH Jr, Robinson RA, Southwick WO, Nachlas NE: The anterior retropharyngeal approach to the upper part of the cervical spine. *J Bone Joint Surg Am* 1987;69(9): 1371-1383.
23. Southwick WO, Robinson RA: Recent advances in surgery of the cervical spine. *Surg Clin North Am* 1961;41:1661-1683.
24. Whitecloud TS, Kelley LA: Anterior and posterior approaches to the cervical spine, in Frymoyer JW, ed: *The Adult Spine*. New York, NY, Raven Press, 1991, pp 987-1013.
25. Khosla VK, Gupta SK, Sharma BS, Mathuriya SN: Anterior surgical approaches to the sub-axial cervical spine. *Neurol India* 2000;48(1):8-18.
26. Kurz LT, Pursel SE, Herkowitz HN: Modified anterior approach to the cervicothoracic junction. *Spine (Phila Pa 1976)* 1991;16(10 Suppl): S542-S547.

CHAPTER 16
Surgical Approaches to the Thoracic and Lumbar Spine

Scott H. Kitchel, MD

Key Points

- Thorough preoperative imaging and review of those studies will guide the selection of surgical technique and surgical approaches.
- Surgical approach must be tailored to the anatomy and surgical goals.
- The enthusiasm for new minimally invasive approaches for trauma must be tempered by the required experience for the surgeon and the lack of long-term outcomes in the literature.
- Adequate intraoperative imaging is a requirement for guiding the surgical approach and assessing decompression and stabilization.
- Combinations of anterior and posterior approaches may be appropriate for many cases of thoracolumbar spine trauma.

Thoracic Spine

The choice of surgical approach to the thoracic spine is generally determined by the site of the lesion to be addressed. There are three general approaches that may be chosen based on the structures to be exposed. The anterior transthoracic approaches allow access to the vertebral bodies, disk spaces, and pedicle on the side of the approach. They are best used for extensive resections, débridement of masses, or fusion of the vertebral bodies over multiple levels.[1] Posterolateral approaches access the transverse processes and ipsilateral pedicle, and provide limited access to the vertebral body.[2] They are best for simple biopsy or débridement. They may also be used for lateral disk excision. Posterior approaches expose the posterior elements and allow decompression of the spinal cord from posterior compressive lesions. They should not be considered for anterior compressive lesions or disk herniations.[3] They also provide access to the structures for posterior and posterolateral fusions.

Considerations in choosing a specific approach must include the purpose of the procedure, the spinal anatomy, and the location, size, level, and pathologic changes of the lesion to be treated. The patient must be positioned in a stable fashion for safety. The incision size must allow adequate illumination, visibility, and working room for any planned implants. Positioning and draping must be meticulous for the safety of the patient and the success of the planned procedure.

Recent advances in imaging and endoscopic techniques have popularized minimally invasive approaches for the treatment of thoracolumbar trauma. Whether this is done via an endoscopic approach, or with image guidance assistance, adequate exposure must be achieved to allow safe completion of an appropriate procedure that produces outcomes equivalent to or superior to outcomes of the comparable open procedure.[4-7]

Anterior Transthoracic Approaches

The thoracic spine from T2 to T12 may be safely exposed from a transthoracic approach. The safety of this approach was well described by Hodgson et al[8] from their work with tuberculous lesions in the 1950s. They reported excellent access to multiple vertebral bodies and a low mortality.

Transthoracic anterior approaches to the thoracic spine are indicated for resecting or débriding anterior lesions, including fractures, tumors, and infections.[1] They are also useful for correction of severe spinal deformity in scoliosis and kyphosis.[9,10] The major indication is for decompression of the spinal canal in conditions with anterior spinal cord compression. The approaches allow direct access to the vertebral bodies and disk spaces from T2 to T12.

The first consideration in transthoracic spinal surgery is whether to approach from the right or the left. In general, I prefer a left-sided approach because of the anatomy of the aorta and vena cava in the thoracic cavity. When approaching from the left and releasing the segmental vessels, the aorta

Dr. Kitchel or an immediate family member has received royalties from SpineWave; is a member of a speakers' bureau or has made paid presentations on behalf of Nuvasive, Osteotech, and Stryker; serves as a paid consultant to or is an employee of Nuvasive, Osteotech, and SpineWave; and owns stock or stock options in Benvenue Medical, SpineWave, and Trans-1.

FIGURE 1

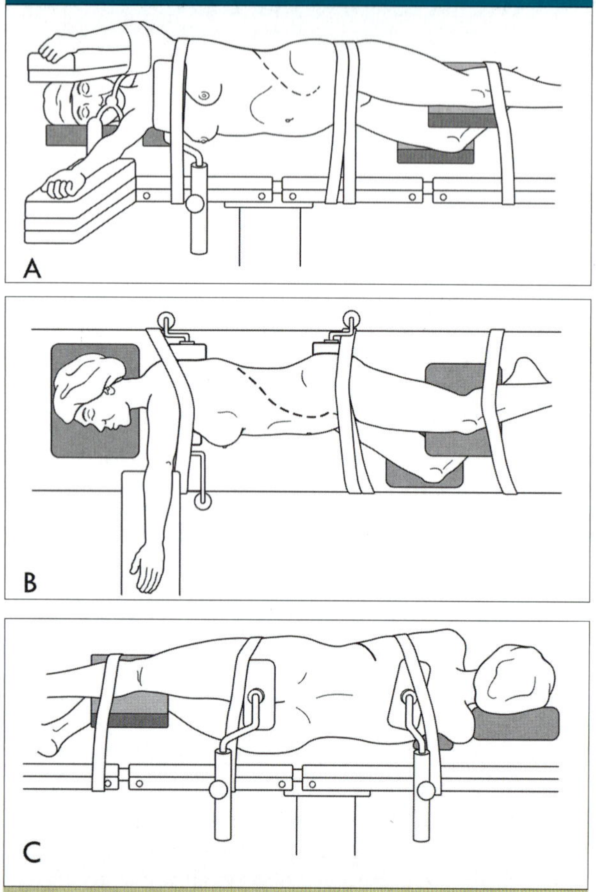

Figure 1 Lateral decubitus positioning for anterolateral approaches to the thoracic and lumbar spine. (Redrawn with permission from Kaneda K: Anterior surgical approach to the thoracolumbar, lumbar and lumbosacral spine, in Weinstein SL, Wiesel SW, eds: *The Lumbar Spine*. Philadelphia, PA, WB Saunders, 1990, p 976.)

will protect the more fragile vena cava from intraoperative trauma. The exception to this is the upper thoracic spine from T1 to T4. At these levels, I prefer a right-sided approach because of the aortic arch, common carotid artery, trachea, and esophagus. When performing anterior approaches for scoliosis, the approach should be made from the convex side of the curve.

The success of thoracoscopic techniques in the treatment of adolescent idiopathic scoliosis has led to enthusiasm for this procedure in thoracic spine trauma. Beisse et al[4] and Khoo et al[11] have shown that this approach is practical in experienced hands. Kim et al[5] address the steep learning curve for this procedure and suggest that the assistance of an experienced thoracoscopic surgeon and the willingness to convert to an open procedure is a requirement for this procedure. The practitioner must be convinced that he or she can complete a safe and thorough decompression via this technique before choosing it over the traditional open approach.[11]

Positioning

The importance of meticulous positioning for anterior thoracic approaches cannot be overemphasized. Patient safety, access to the spine, and adequate illumination will all directly follow from this step.

The patient should be positioned in a true lateral alignment (**Figure 1**). This allows surgeons to easily orient themselves to the anatomy at any time by leveling the bed. The operating table may be rotated as needed during various portions of the procedure. An axillary roll or pillow is used under the down axilla to prevent circulatory disturbance and protect the axillary nerve from compression.[12] Pillows should be placed under the lateral aspect of the down knee and between the knees to prevent pressure on the peroneal nerve. The head is placed on a pillow. Maintaining the torso in a true lateral position may be accomplished by the use of external pads anchored to the operative table or by the use of an air bag. I prefer to position the segment of the spine to be exposed over the break in the operative table. This offers the advantage of being able to extend the table to enhance exposure. Once adequate positioning is ensured, cloth tape is used to immobilize the pelvis and torso. The skin is protected over these areas by towels.

Upper Thoracic Approaches to T1-T4

As previously discussed, upper thoracic approaches to T1-T4 are generally made from the right side. The patient is positioned left side down with the right arm flexed as far cephalad as possible. This allows anterior retraction of the scapula.

The skin incision is made at the level of the fourth rib and carried medially and inferiorly around the angle of the scapula (**Figure 2**). The trapezius muscle is divided in line with the skin incision. Next, the latissimus dorsi is divided as far caudad as possible, the greater rhomboid is divided near the scapula, and the serratus anterior is divided at the caudalmost portion of the incision to protect the long thoracic nerve (**Figure 3**).

Once this has been accomplished, the scapula may be retracted anteriorly with a hook. Either the third or fourth rib may be removed. This decision must be based upon the cephalad and caudad extent of the lesion. At this point, self-retaining re-

FIGURE 2

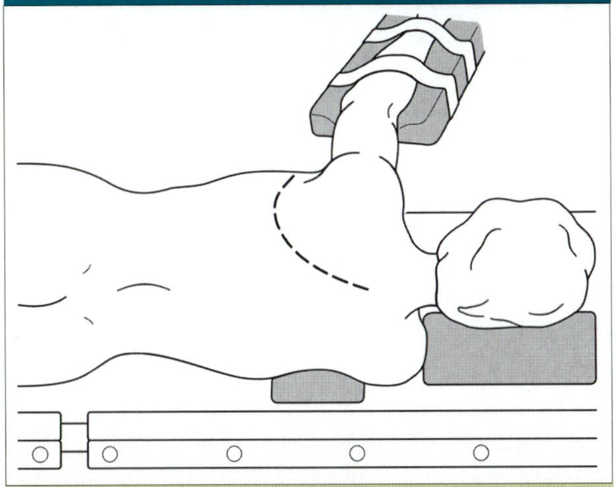

Figure 2 Position and skin incision for right-sided T1-T4 thoracotomy. (Redrawn with permission from Kaneda K: Surgical approaches to the thoracic and lumbar spine, in Weinstein SL, ed: *The Pediatric Spine: Principles and Practice*. New York, NY, Raven Press, 1994, p 1357.)

FIGURE 3

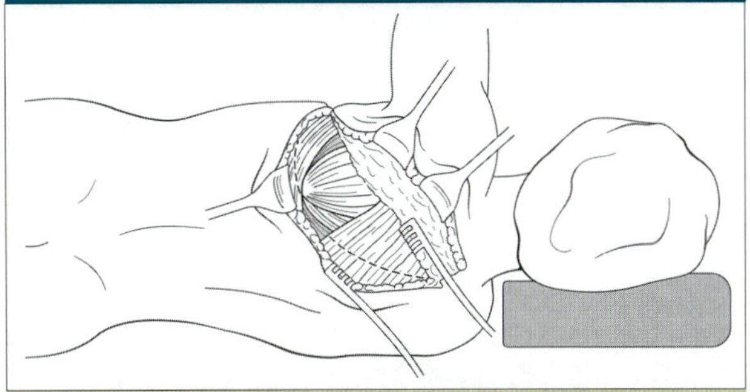

Figure 3 Muscular dissection for the upper thoracic approach. (Redrawn with permission from Kaneda K: Surgical approaches to the thoracic and lumbar spine, in Weinstein SL, ed: *The Pediatric Spine: Principles and Practice*. New York, NY, Raven Press, 1994, p 1357.)

tractors are applied. Meticulous hemostasis must be ensured through all muscular layers and costal vessels.

A decision now must be made between an extrapleural or transpleural approach. The extrapleural approach avoids contamination of the intrapleural cavity in case of infection or tumor; however, more time is taken with this dissection and the pleura may be torn incidentally. Because of this, in cases of spine trauma, I prefer a transpleural approach.

Once the appropriate rib has been selected, it is exposed subperiosteally with the use of electrocautery and periosteal elevators. Care must be taken to avoid injury to the neurovascular bundle in the subcostal groove on the inferior rib surface. The rib is removed from the costochondral junction anteriorly to the angle of the rib posteriorly with a rib cutter. The parietal pleura is then opened longitudinally, exercising caution to avoid any damage to the superior lobe of the lung. The adjacent ribs are then protected with moist packs, and a large self-retaining thoracotomy retractor is used to spread the incision. The lung is manually deflated.

At this point, adequate localization needs to be ensured. From within the chest, the lesion may be obvious. Counting the ribs from within the thoracic cavity may also be useful. If there is any indecision or uncertainty, a radiograph should be taken to ensure correct selection of the level.

The vertebral bodies are covered by the glistening parietal pleura. The intervertebral disks will appear as protrusions and the vertebrae feel concave between these disks. The aortic arch is closely applied to the anterior aspect of the vertebral bodies at the level of T4. Above this arise the subclavian artery, thoracic duct, and esophagus.

Further exposure is accomplished by an incision through the parietal pleura over the posterior rib and down onto the lateral vertebral body. The pleura is cleared by blunt dissection from lateral to midline. This may be accomplished over as many levels as necessary. The segmental vessels are ligated with metallic vascular clips in the midlateral region and transected to permit mobilization of the aorta. The appropriate vertebral bodies and disk spaces are then exposed and the procedure is performed.

When the spinal procedure is completed, the pleural cavity should be irrigated with warm antibiotic solution. The lung is reexpanded by forced ventilation and inspected for damage or air leaks. Chest tubes are inserted to evacuate blood and air. These are generally placed two levels below the rib resection and tunneled over the adjacent rib. One tube is normally directed cephalad to evacuate air and the other caudad to evacuate blood. A purse-string suture is placed around each tube and through the skin to maintain their position.

Closure is then accomplished by reapproximating the ribs with a mechanical rib approximator. Before this is tightened, heavy absorbable sutures are placed in a pericostal fashion around the rib, above and below it (**Figure 4**). The rib periosteum and intercostal muscles are approximated using running suture for airtight closure. The serratus anterior, latissimus dorsi, and rhomboids are approximated in separate layers. Then the trapezius is closed. The subcutaneous tissues and skin are

FIGURE 4

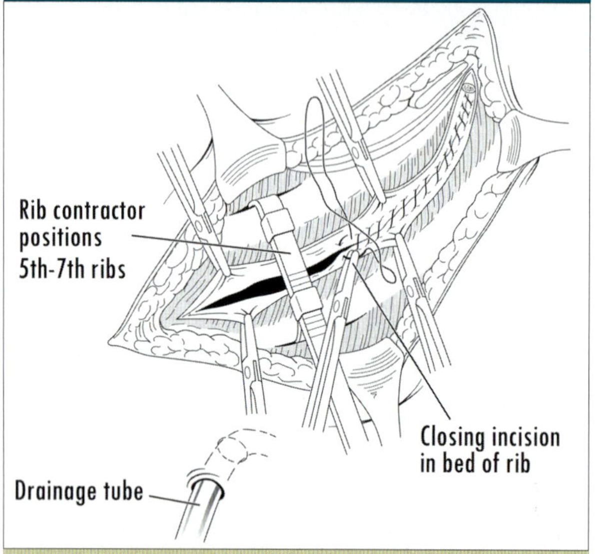

Figure 4 Reapproximation of the ribs with pericostal sutures. (Redrawn with permission from Johnson RM, Murphy MJ, Southwick WO: Surgical approaches to the thoracic spine, in Rothman RH, Simeone FA, eds: *The Spine*, ed 3. Philadelphia, PA, WB Saunders, 1992, p 1705.)

FIGURE 5

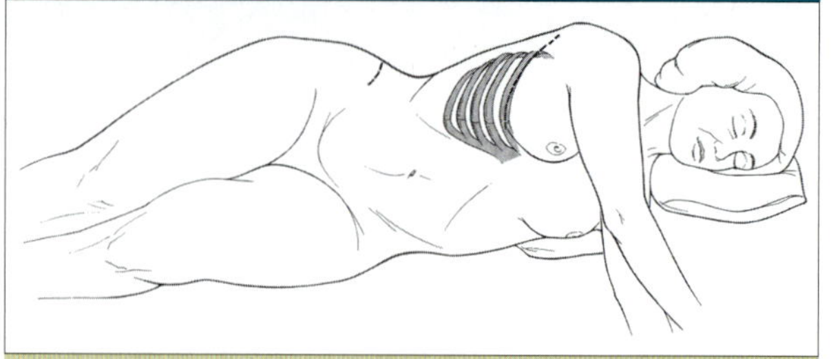

Figure 5 The skin incision placed two segments above the desired vertebra for transthoracic approaches. (Reproduced with permission from Eismont FJ, Garfin SR, Abitbol JJ: Thoracic and upper lumbar spine injuries, in Browner RB, Jupiter JB, Levine AM, Trafton PG, eds: *Skeletal Trauma: Principles and Practice*. Philadelphia, PA, WB Saunders, 1992, p 780.)

then approximated. The chest tubes are attached to water-seal constant suction and sterile dressings are applied.

Approaches from T5 to the Thoracolumbar Junction

Surgical approaches to these levels of the thoracic spine are generally made from the left. This is to allow the aorta to protect the friable vena cava. The patient is positioned left side up as described previously.

The level of the skin incision is based on the vertebral segment to be exposed. In general, the incision should be centered over the rib two levels cephalad to the desired vertebral body. The skin incision will run from the lateral border of the paravertebral muscles to a point as far anterior as necessary. The longer the incision, the more vertebral bodies that may be exposed (**Figure 5**). The serratus anterior muscle is divided using electrocautery. The rib to be resected is then selected. It is exposed subperiosteally with electrocautery and periosteal elevators. Care is taken to protect the neurovascular structures in the subcostal groove. The rib is removed from the costochondral junction anteriorly to the angle of the rib posteriorly with a rib cutter. The parietal pleura is then opened longitudinally to avoid damage to the lung. The remaining ribs are then protected with moist packs and a large self-retaining thoracotomy retractor is used to spread the incision. The lung is manually deflated.

At this point, adequate localization needs to be ensured. From within the chest, the lesion may be obvious. Counting the ribs from within the thoracic cavity may also be useful. If there is any indecision or uncertainty, a radiograph should be taken to ensure correct location.

The vertebral bodies are covered by the glistening parietal pleura. The intervertebral disk will appear as protrusions and the vertebrae will feel concave between the disks. The aorta is closely applied along the anterior vertebral bodies and the sympathetic trunk is visible more laterally (**Figure 6**).

The next step in the exposure is an incision through the parietal pleura over the posterior ribs and down onto the vertebral bodies. The pleura is cleared by blunt dissection from lateral to anterior. The segmental vessels are then ligated with metallic vascular clips and transected to allow mobilization of the aorta. The minimum number of vessels should be ligated to ensure preservation of spinal cord blood flow.[13] The vertebral bodies and disk spaces are then exposed and the procedure is performed.

When the surgical procedure is completed, the pleural cavity should be irrigated with warm antibiotic solution. The lung is reexpanded by forced ventilation and inspected for any damage or air leaks. Two chest tubes are inserted to evacuate blood and air. These are placed through skin incisions two segments below the incision and tunneled subcutaneously over the next cephalad rib. One tube is directed cephalad to evacuate air and one caudad to evacuate blood. A purse-string su-

FIGURE 6

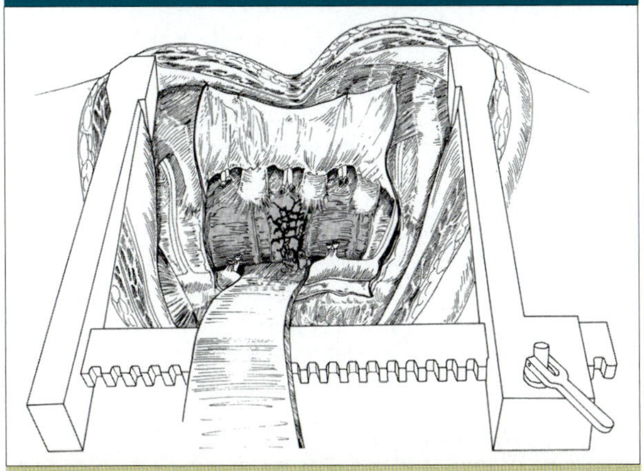

Figure 6 The relative positions of the aorta, thoracic segmental vessels, and sympathetic trunk. (Reproduced with permission from Eismont FJ, Garfin SR, Abitbol JJ: Thoracic and upper lumbar spine injuries, in Browner RB, Jupiter JB, Levine AM, Trafton PG, eds: *Skeletal Trauma: Principles and Practice*. Philadelphia, PA, WB Saunders, 1992, p 781.)

FIGURE 7

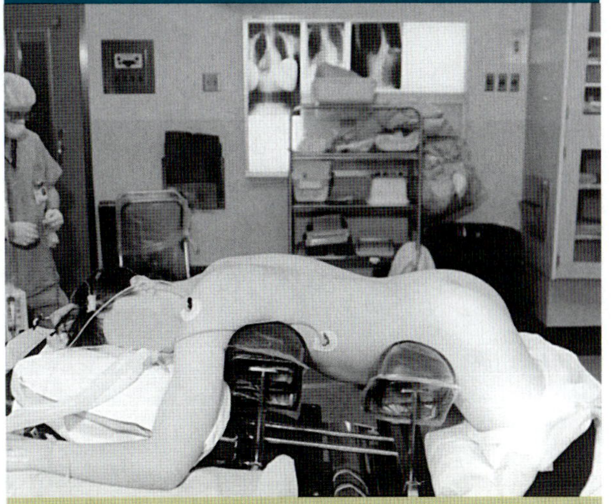

Figure 7 Patient positioning on the Relton-Hall frame. (Reproduced from Kitchel SH: Surgical approaches to the thoracic and lumbar spine, in Levine AM, Eismont FJ, Garfin SR, Zigler JE, eds: *Spine Trauma*. Philadelphia, PA, WB Saunders, 1998, pp 144-155.)

ture is placed around each tube and through the skin.

Closure is then accomplished by reapproximating the ribs with heavy absorbable pericostal sutures. The ribs are approximated with a mechanical clamp and these are tied. The rib periosteum and intercostal muscles are approximated using running suture for airtight closure. The serratus anterior is then closed in a separate layer. The subcutaneous tissues and skin are approximated. The chest tubes are attached to water-seal constant suction and sterile dressings are applied.

Posterolateral Approaches

The only posterolateral approach to the thoracic spine in use today is the costotransversectomy. This was first described by Menard[14] in 1894. In 1956, Seddon[15] augmented this exposure by incorporating a more lateral curvilinear incision, permitting more extensive exposure of the anterolateral vertebral bodies. Although rarely indicated in spinal trauma, this approach is discussed for its exposure of the transverse process, pedicle, and posterolateral vertebral body. Complications of these lateral extracavatary approaches have been nicely summarized by Resnick and Benzel.[16]

Positioning

In costotransversectomy approaches, the patient may be positioned either lateral or prone. The considerations for lateral positioning are identical to those discussed above for anterior transthoracic approaches. I prefer a prone position, primarily for easier direct access to the posterior structures.

Once adequate general anesthesia has been accomplished, the patient is rolled into the prone position on a Relton-Hall frame (**Figure 7**). This is adjusted to support the pelvis at the anterior iliac crests and the thorax at the level of the areolae. Care is taken to avoid compression of the lateral femoral cutaneous nerves caudally and the axillae must be free to ensure that no nerve damage occurs in the upper extremities. The hips and knees are flexed slightly and the knees padded. The head is maintained in a neutral position and the face protected.

Costotransversectomy

When the patient is positioned and draped, the anatomic landmarks must be palpated. The spinous processes should be identified along with the appropriate ribs and the paraspinal muscle mass. A longitudinal skin incision is centered over the level of the lesion and extended cephalad and caudad as necessary (**Figure 8**). The incision is made in the concavity just lateral to the paraspinal muscle mass. This is normally about 5 cm lateral to the midline (**Figure 9**).

The incision is carried sharply through subcutaneous tissues and hemostasis is ensured with electrocautery. The trapezius, latissimus dorsi, and lumbodorsal fascia are split in line with the skin incision. The paraspinal muscles are removed

FIGURE 8

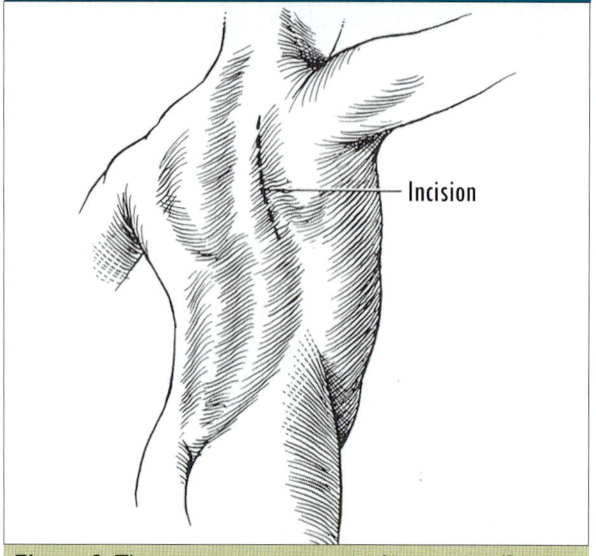

Figure 8 The costotransversectomy skin incision. (Redrawn with permission from Johnson RM, Murphy MJ, Southwick WO: Surgical approaches to the thoracic spine, in Rothman RH, Simeone FA, eds: *The Spine*, ed 3. Philadelphia, PA, WB Saunders, 1992, p 1715.)

FIGURE 9

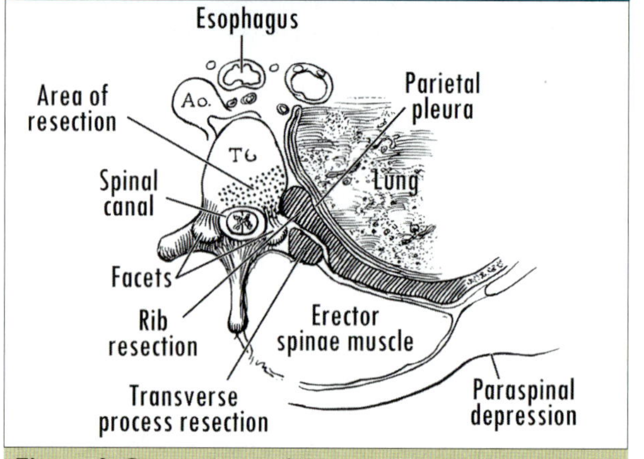

Figure 9 Cross section of the costotransversectomy approach. (Adapted with permission from Johnson RM, Murphy MJ, Southwick WO: Surgical approaches to the thoracic spine, in Rothman RH, Simeone FA, eds: *The Spine*, ed 3. Philadelphia, PA, WB Saunders, 1992, p 1716.)

sharply from their insertions on the ribs and the transverse processes and are retracted medially.

At this point, the correct level must be chosen. This can only be achieved by counting the ribs or, more reliably, by confirming the level with a radiograph. Once this has been achieved, the costotransverse ligaments are divided and the transverse process is resected at the junction with the lamina. The rib is then exposed in a subperiosteal dissection, leaving the intercostal neurovascular bundle and pleura intact. The rib is then transected and removed approximately 8 cm lateral to the vertebra. The costovertebral ligaments must be separated at the articulation of the rib to the vertebra.

Just anterior to the residual transverse process is the vertebral pedicle. Just above and below the pedicle lie the neural foramina with the exiting nerve roots. The dissection is then carried anteriorly in the extrapleural plane. The vertebral body and disk spaces are then exposed. The sympathetic trunk is raised in the plane with the pleura and protected. Once in this plane, the dissection can safely be extended cephalad and caudad. Should the pleura be violated, it is repaired immediately. As many transverse processes and rib bases are resected as are necessary for treatment of the lesion.

When the procedure is completed, the wound is filled with antibiotic irrigation and the lungs are inflated to check for air leaks. After this is done, the lumbodorsal fascia, paraspinal muscles, trapezius, and latissimus dorsi are repaired in separate layers. A suction drain is placed and the subcutaneous tissues and skin are closed.

The practicality of a dual tube technique for minimally invasive costotranversectomy has been demonstrated in a cadaver model;[17] however, this technique has gained widespread acceptance in the surgical community.

Posterior Approach

The direct posterior midline approach to the thoracic spine is the most common and is widely used. It was described independently by both Hibbs[18] and Albee[19] in 1911. In a straightforward approach, it allows access to the posterior elements for laminectomy, posterior internal fixation of the spine, and posterior or posterolateral fusion.

Positioning

In midline posterior approaches, the patient may be positioned either lateral or prone. The considerations for lateral positioning are identical to those discussed for anterior transthoracic approaches earlier in this chapter. I prefer a prone position, primarily for easier direct access to the posterior structures.

Once adequate general anesthesia has been accomplished, the patient is rolled into the prone position on a Relton-Hall frame (**Figure 7**). This is adjusted to support the pelvis at the anterior iliac crests and the thorax at the level of the areolae. Care is taken to avoid compression of the lateral femoral cutaneous nerves caudally, and the axillae must be free to ensure that no nerve damage occurs in the upper extremities. The hips and knees are flexed slightly and the knees padded. The head is maintained in a neutral position and the face is protected.

Posterior Midline Approach

When the patient is in a prone position and draped, the anatomic landmarks of the spinous processes are identified. A longitudinal midline incision is then made over the spinous processes over as many levels as are needed for exposure. The subcutaneous tissues are sharply divided to expose the thoracodorsal fascia and tips of the spinous processes. The fascia is split longitudinally over the spinous processes and the dissection is carried in a subperiosteal plane down the spinous processes across the lamina, exposing the base of the transverse processes. The entire transverse process and rib base may be exposed when necessary. In children and young adults, subperiosteal stripping may be accomplished with a Cobb elevator. However, in adults, the fascia and paraspinal muscles may be detached with the aid of electrocautery. The subperiosteal stripping should be done carefully to avoid damage to the neurovascular supply of the muscles or the muscles themselves.

After the surgical procedure is completed, the paraspinal muscles are reapproximated and the fascia is closed in separate layers. Generally, a suction drain is left deep to the fascia. The subcutaneous tissues and skin are then reapproximated. A sterile dressing is applied.

Minimally invasive procedures also have evolved at the thoracolumbar junction. Kim et al[5] have described a transdiaphragmatic thoracoscopic approach to these fractures. Rampersaud et al[7] nicely summarized the state of the art of these posterior procedures about the thoracolumbar junction. Pedicle screws may be placed safely at the thoracolumbar junction via several image-guided and tube-directed posterior approaches[20] with adequate training and experience.

Lumbosacral Spine

Surgical approaches to the lumbar spine have been developed and must be selected on the basis of the site of the lesion to be treated and the adjacent structures that need to be exposed. The general approaches to consider include the anterior, anterolateral, and posterior approaches. Anterior or anterolateral approaches achieve exposure of vertebral bodies, disk spaces, and the anterior spinal canal. Posterior approaches expose the posterior elements, transverse processes, and posterior spinal canal.

Considerations in choosing a specific approach must include the purpose of the planned procedure, the relevant anatomy, and the size, location, and extent of the lesion being treated. The patient must be positioned in a stable fashion for safety. The incision must allow adequate illumination, visualization, and working room. Positioning and draping must be meticulous for the safety of the patient and the success of the procedure.

Anterolateral Approaches

The thoracolumbar spine from T12 to the sacrum may be safely exposed from the anterolateral approach for treatment of trauma.[21] At the thoracolumbar junction, this requires a thoracoabdominal approach, and lower in the lumbar spine, a retroperitoneal approach.

This retroperitoneal approach is merely an extension of the flank incision used for lumbar sympathectomy. First described by Royle[22] in 1924, it was extended to expose the vertebral body by Francioli[23] in 1951. The thoracoabdominal approach is an extension of the thoracotomy, taking down the diaphragm to expose the lumbar spine. Both of these approaches are made from the left, to approach on the side of the aorta and to protect the vena cava.

Positioning

The patient is positioned in the lateral decubitus position for both the thoracoabdominal and retroperitoneal approaches. The reader is referred to the discussion on positioning for transthoracic approaches because the positioning is the same.

Thoracoabdominal Approach

The thoracoabdominal approach will give superior anterior exposure at the thoracolumbar junction in the treatment of trauma. Once the patient is positioned and draped, a curvilinear skin incision is made over the 10th rib, extending anteriorly and caudad (**Figure 10**). It may be extended variable distances anteriorly and caudad as needed for extensive exposure.

The subcutaneous tissues are divided with electrocautery and the latissimus dorsi and external abdominal oblique are divided. The periosteum of the 10th rib is incised and the rib is subperiosteally dissected free, taking care not to damage the neurovascular structures in the subcostal groove. The rib is then cut at the costochondral junction with a rib cutter and removed by cutting it posteriorly at its base. After the rib is removed, the pa-

FIGURE 10

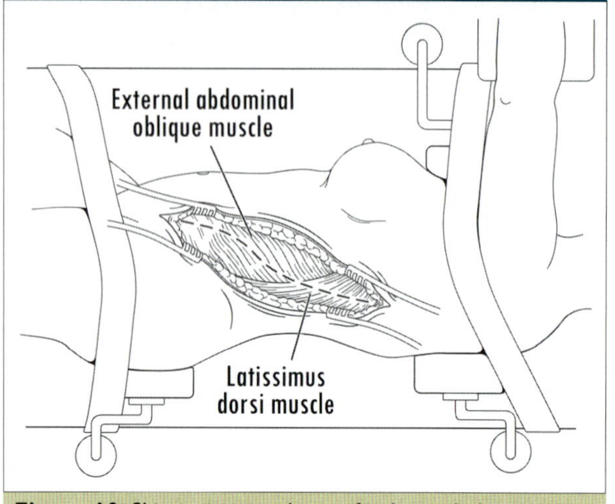

Figure 10 Skin incision and superficial muscle layers in thoracoabdominal approach. (Redrawn with permission from Kaneda K: Anterior surgical approach to the thoracolumbar, lumbar and lumbosacral spine, in Weinstein SL, Wiesel SW, eds: *The Lumbar Spine*. Philadelphia, PA, WB Saunders, 1990, p 977.)

FIGURE 11

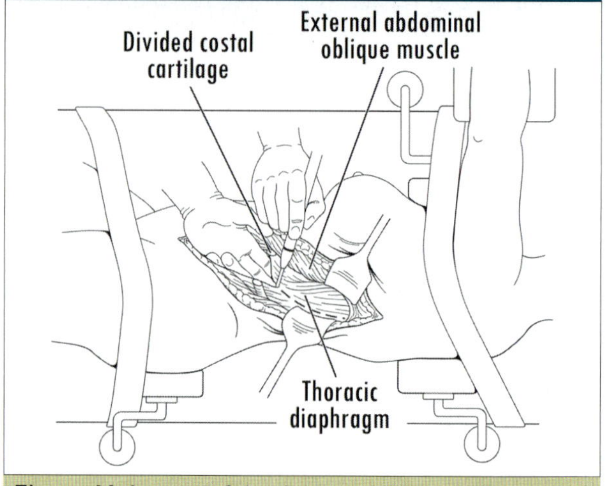

Figure 11 Incision of the thoracic diaphragm. (Redrawn with permission from Kaneda K: Anterior surgical approach to the thoracolumbar, lumbar and lumbosacral spine, in Weinstein SL, Wiesel SW, eds: *The Lumbar Spine*. Philadelphia, PA, WB Saunders, 1990, p 979.)

rietal pleura is opened along the bed of the resected rib.

Attention is then returned to the abdominal muscle layers. The external oblique, internal oblique, and transverse abdominal muscles are cut with the electrocautery in line with the skin incision. The peritoneum is bluntly dissected anteriorly and retracted medially. The diaphragm has then been exposed from both above and below. The diaphragm is then released from the thoracic side using electrocautery and leaving a 2-cm rim for reattachment (**Figure 11**).

When the diaphragm is released, the chest cavity and retroperitoneal spaces are connected. The lung is manually retracted cephalad and the peritoneal contents medially. The left diaphragmatic crus is dissected and the left psoas major is exposed. The kidney and ureter are retracted medially with the peritoneum. The psoas major is retracted posteriorly.

The vertebral bodies and disks are now exposed. A longitudinal incision is made over the parietal pleura along the lower thoracic vertebral bodies. This will expose the segmental vessels. These are ligated with metallic clips to allow mobilization of the aorta. The vertebral body may then be exposed. It is recommended that exposure be started over the relevant disk and the plane elevated posteriorly to the level of the transverse process deep to the pleura. This plane may extend cephalad or caudad as needed.

When the procedure has been completed, the psoas is allowed to fall back to its normal position. No suture is required. The parietal pleura is then closed over the vertebral column with a continuous suture. The diaphragm must be anatomically repaired with permanent suture. A chest tube is inserted through the chest wall to evacuate air and blood. The muscles of both the abdominal wall and thoracic wall must then be closed in layers. Following this, the subcutaneous tissues and skin are closed.

Retroperitoneal Approach to L2 and the Sacrum

This anterolateral approach will allow excellent visualization from the first subdiaphragmatic vertebra to the sacrum. The skin incision begins over the lateral half of the 12th rib and extends obliquely anterior and caudad to the lateral margin of the pectus fascia at the level of the anterior superior iliac spine. The external oblique muscle is divided parallel to its fibers. The inferior serratus posterior is transected in line with the incision. The internal oblique and transverse abdominal muscles are then opened in line with the incision (**Figure 12**).

The peritoneum is separated from the abdominal wall at the anterolateral incision under the 12th rib. The 12th rib may be resected if needed for bone graft or exposure. The kidney and ureter are retracted anteriorly and the psoas posteriorly. The dissection is carried bluntly onto the spine. The segmental vessels are identified and ligated as

FIGURE 12

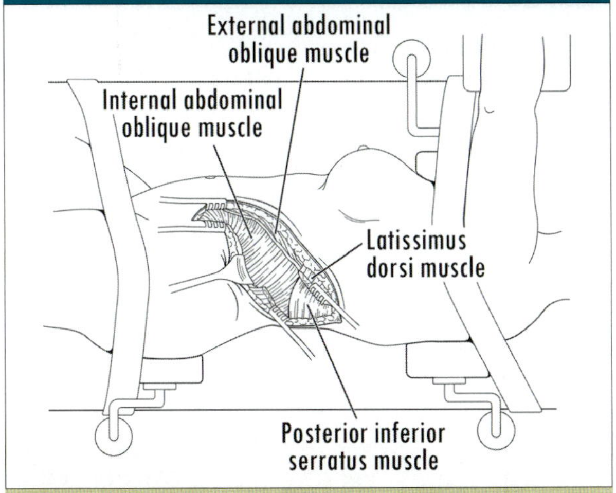

Figure 12 Retroperitoneal approach skin incision and superficial muscular layers. (Redrawn with permission from Kaneda K: Anterior surgical approach to the thoracolumbar, lumbar and lumbosacral spine, in Weinstein SL, Wiesel SW, eds: *The Lumbar Spine*. Philadelphia, PA, WB Saunders, 1990, p 982.)

FIGURE 13

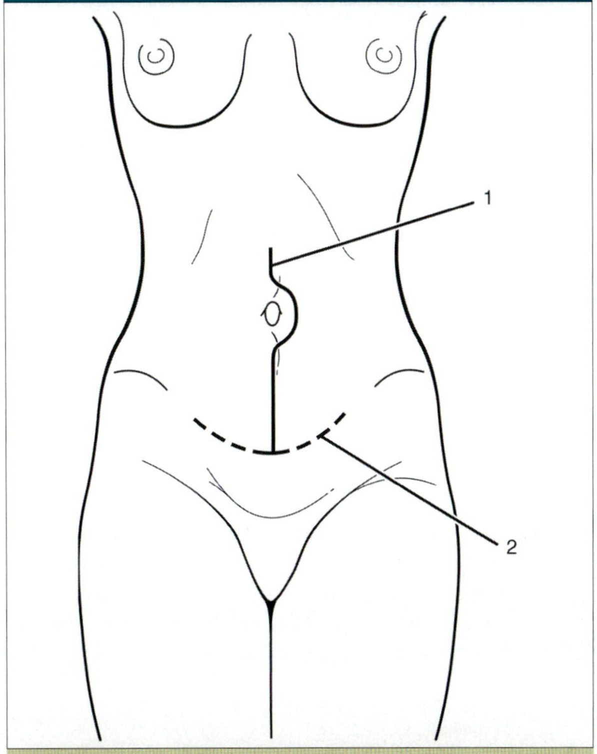

Figure 13 Skin incision for transperitoneal anterior approach. (Redrawn with permission from Kaneda K: Anterior surgical approach to the thoracolumbar, lumbar and lumbosacral spine, in Weinstein SL, Wiesel SW, eds: *The Lumbar Spine*. Philadelphia, PA, WB Saunders, 1990, p 984.)

necessary to mobilize the aorta and vena cava. The sympathetic trunk is retracted laterally.

Once the spinal procedure is completed, the psoas is allowed to fall back to its normal location. The muscles are repaired in individual layers and the subcutaneous tissues and then the skin are closed.

The surgeon is advised to exercise particular caution in this approach concerning two structures. First, the ureter must be identified and safely retracted anteriorly. Second, if the dissection is carried caudad to L3 or L4, the left iliac vein should be identified and protected before bone dissection is performed.

Extreme lateral percutaneous approaches as decribed by Ozgur et al,[24] augmented with real-time electromyographic monitoring, have been advocated for anterior decompression of lumbar fractures above L5. At this time, no long-term follow-up is available to evaluate this technique.

Anterior Transperitoneal Approaches

True anterior approaches to the lumbosacral spine are only indicated at the levels of L5 and the sacrum.[3,13]

In a true anterior approach, the patient is positioned supine. It is advantageous to place the lumbosacral junction over the break in the table so that the table may be extended if necessary. The skin incision is a median laparotomy incision curving around the navel on the left[25] (**Figure 13**). The anterior abdominal wall is divided on the linea alba. The peritoneum is incised longitudinally along the line of the skin incision. Self-retaining abdominal retractors are placed and the abdominal contents are packed upward. The parietal peritoneal layer is incised from 3 cm proximal to the aortic bifurcation to the sacral promontory (**Figure 14**). Care must be taken not to damage the superior hypogastric plexus, which provides sympathetic innervation of the urogenital system.

The fatty connective tissue that covers the retroperitoneal vessels is opened bluntly over the right common iliac artery. The right ureter passes over the right external iliac artery and must be identified and protected. The left peritoneum and subjacent vessels are moved as a unit (**Figure 15**). The middle sacral artery lies in front of the L5-S1 disk space and must be ligated. The approach has then given access from the L4-L5 disk to the sacrum.

Once the procedure has been completed, the parietal peritoneal layer is sutured with absorbable suture posteriorly. The packs are removed and the bowel contents and omentum are replaced. The anterior peritoneum is repaired, followed by clo-

FIGURE 14

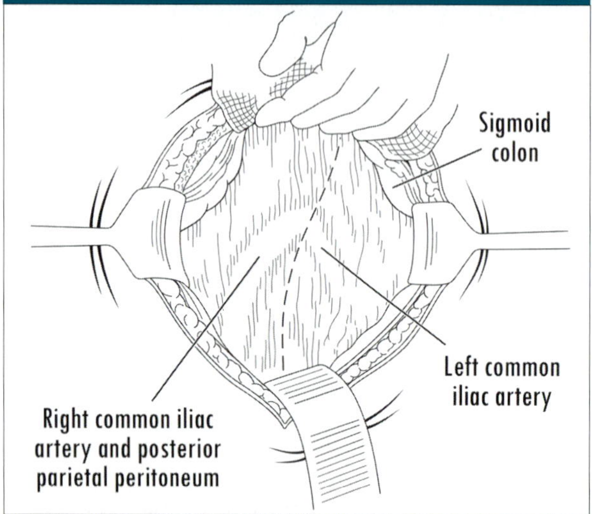

Figure 14 The posterior parietal peritoneal incision. (Redrawn with permission from Kaneda K: Anterior surgical approach to the thoracolumbar, lumbar and lumbosacral spine, in Weinstein SL, Wiesel SW, eds: *The Lumbar Spine*. Philadelphia, PA, WB Saunders, 1990, p 984.)

FIGURE 15

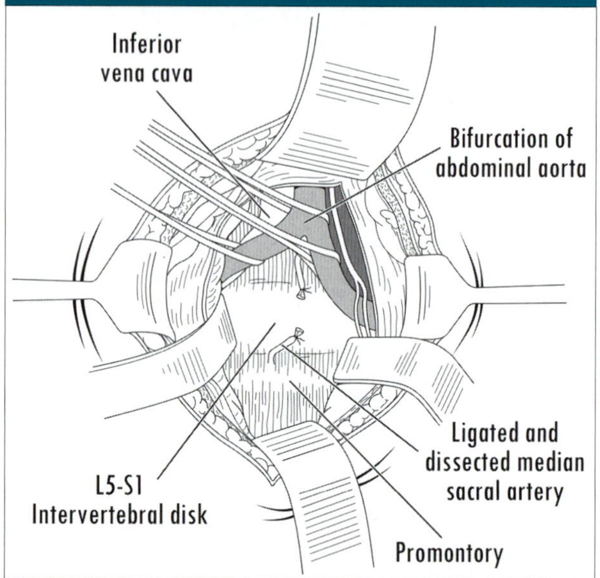

Figure 15 Exposure of the lumbosacral junction with the neurovascular structures retracted. (Redrawn with permission from Kaneda K: Anterior surgical approach to the thoracolumbar, lumbar and lumbosacral spine, in Weinstein SL, Wiesel SW, eds: *The Lumbar Spine*. Philadelphia, PA, WB Saunders, 1990, p 985.)

sure of the muscular layers, subcutaneous tissues, and skin.

Although this anterior approach offers excellent visualization of the anterior structures, the potential complications due to injury to ureters, vascular structures, and sympathetic innervation need to be considered. Damage to the superior hypogastric plexus in males may result in retrograde ejaculation.

Low Anterior Retroperitoneal Approach to L4 and the Sacrum

This approach is made using a minimally oblique incision on the left lower quadrant of the abdomen (**Figure 16**). The medial edge of the incision is the lateral edge of the rectus abdominis muscle. It is approximately two-thirds of the distance down from the umbilicus to the symphysis pubis. The external abdominal oblique muscle is split and the internal abdominal oblique muscle is cut. The transversus abdominis muscle is absent at the most caudad medial portion of the incision and it is cut at the more cephalad lateral aspect of the incision. The peritoneum is identified and pushed off the abdominal wall using lap sponges. The peritoneum is pushed off the psoas muscle and retracted medially. The ureter and iliac vessels are identified and the sacral promontory is easily seen. Self-retaining retractors such as the stable Bookwalter retractor are inserted taking care to adequately pad over the ureter and to be certain that the blades of the retractors are not compressing the great vessels. The iliac vessels are then mobilized from the spine to expose the L5-S1 disk space, and these vessels can then be gently retracted laterally using handheld vein retractors. Extensive anterior exposure of L5 and S1 can be obtained working in the crotch of the right- and left-sided vessels.

To gain access to the L4-5 interspace and the L4 vertebra, it is often necessary to mobilize the bifurcation of the distal aorta and inferior vena cava and to work between these vessels. Whether it is best to work between these vessels or lateral to them is dictated by the individual patient's local anatomy.

A word of caution must be added concerning this exposure. Unless the spine surgeon has extensive experience with this exposure, it is best performed by a general surgeon or vascular surgeon. Also, if the patient has significant aortofemoral vascular disease, another approach to the problem may be sought because mobilizing and retracting such diseased vessels may produce distal vascular occlusion.

Closure of the wound is performed in the standard layered fashion. The advantage of this exposure versus the transperitoneal exposure is that

FIGURE 16

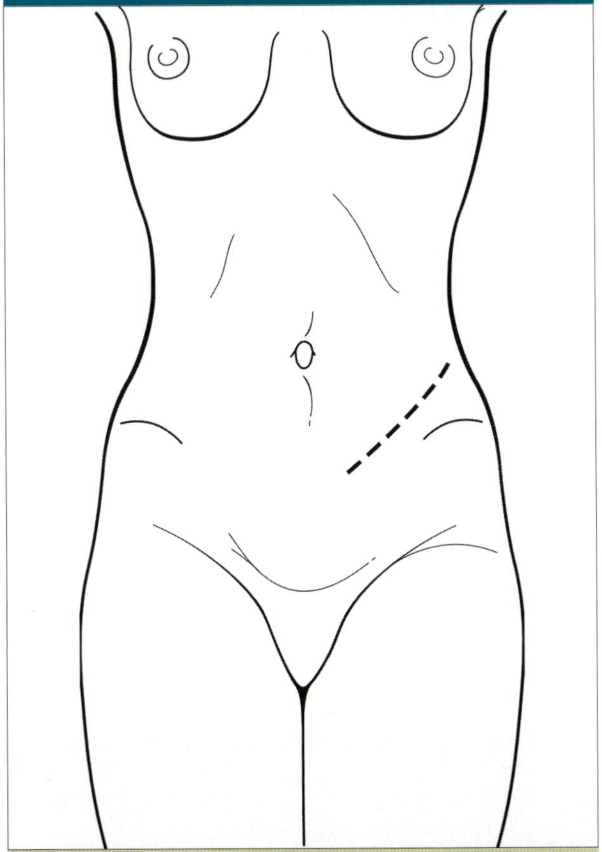

Figure 16 Skin incision for anterior retroperitoneal exposure of L4 to sacrum. (Reproduced from Kitchel SH: Surgical approaches to the thoracic and lumbar spine, in Levine AM, Eismont FJ, Garfin SR, Zigler JE, eds: *Spine Trauma.* Philadelphia, PA, WB Saunders, 1998, pp 144-155.)

FIGURE 17

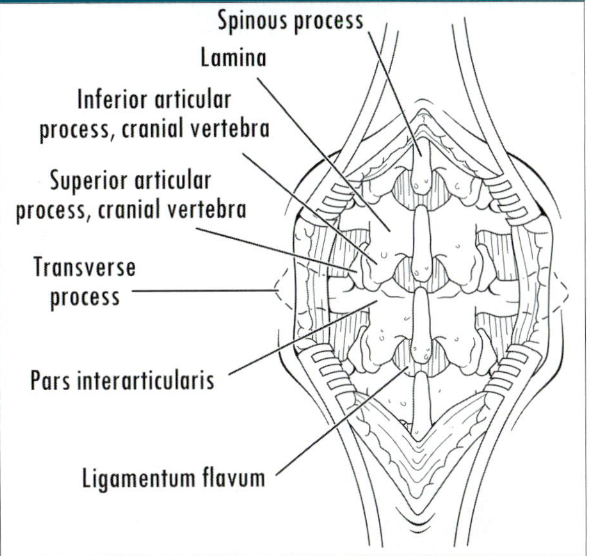

Figure 17 The posterior midline lumbar approach. (Reproduced from Kitchel SH: Surgical approaches to the thoracic and lumbar spine, in Levine AM, Eismont FJ, Garfin SR, Zigler JE, eds: *Spine Trauma.* Philadelphia, PA, WB Saunders, 1998, pp 144-155.)

retraction of the bowel is much easier and hence spine visualization is improved. The postoperative course is also easier as the ileus resolves more quickly with this approach.

Posterior Approaches

A posterior approach to the lumbosacral spine is most commonly used and allows excellent access to the posterior elements and spinal canal. It is indicated in the lumbosacral spine for posterior spinal canal decompression, posterior spinal instrumentation, and posterior or posterolateral fusion.

Many posterior approaches to the lumbar spine for trauma are done for placement of spinal instrumentation. In many cases, decompression may be indirect via spinal realignment or have been already accomplished via an anterior or anterolateral approach. In these instances, the consideration of percutaneous pedicle screw instrumentation must be considered. Although originally described for degenerative problems,[12] it has more recently been shown to be applicable in trauma.[6,26] Positioning is the same as for the open procedure, and image guidance via fluoroscopy or intraoperative CT is required for all devices.[6]

Positioning

Once adequate anesthesia has been induced, the patient is gently log-rolled and positioned prone on a spinal frame. The specific frame used is not as important as the concept of a well-padded, stable position that allows the abdomen to hang free. The free abdomen lowers abdominal pressure, which decreases retroperitoneal venous engorgement and thereby minimizes intraoperative blood loss. I prefer either a Relton-Hall frame or an Andrews frame (**Figure 7**).

Posterior Midline Approach

A posterior midline incision is made longitudinally along the palpable spinous processes. Sharp midline dissection is carried through the subcutaneous tissues to the lumbodorsal fascia. Hemostasis is ensured through use of electrocautery. The lumbodorsal fascia is identified in the midline where it merges with the supraspinous ligament. It is incised just lateral to the supraspinous ligament, and the paraspinal muscles are elevated subperiosteally off the spinous process (**Figure 17**). The bony

FIGURE 18

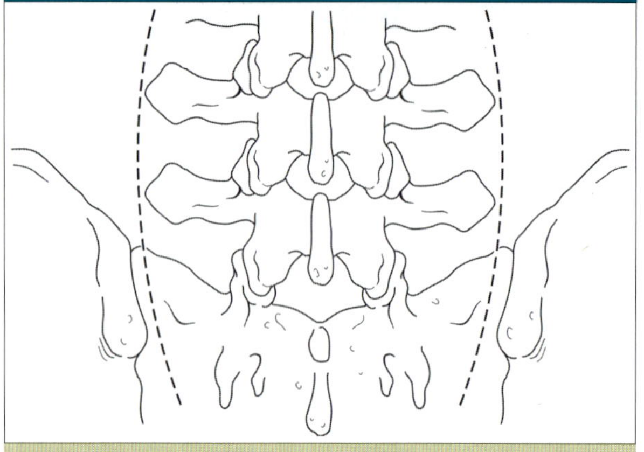

Figure 18 Skin incisions for posterolateral sacrospinalis-splitting incisions. (Redrawn with permission from Watkins R, ed: *Surgical Approaches to the Spine*. New York, NY, Springer Verlag, 1983.)

exposure continues laterally across the lamina to expose the capsule of the facet joint.

If fusion will not be performed, the capsule of the joint should be protected. If fusion is anticipated, the capsule is excised and the dissection continued laterally to expose the transverse process where it emerges from the lateral side anterior to the superior facet.

Once the procedure is completed, a suction drain is generally left deep to the muscular layer. The paraspinal muscles are reapproximated followed by the lumbodorsal fascia, subcutaneous tissues, and skin.

An alternative posterior approach may be employed for posterolateral fusion at the lumbosacral junction. The decision to employ this sacrospinalis-splitting incision requires that no work need be done in the spinal canal and no instrumentation employed. Patient positioning is identical to the midline posterior approach position. This approach has been popularized by Wiltse et al.[27] It provides direct access to the facet joints, transverse processes, and sacral ala.

After the patient is positioned, prepared, and draped, two parallel skin incisions are made approximately 3 cm lateral to the midline (**Figure 18**). Dissection is carried sharply through the subcutaneous tissues. Hemostasis is ensured with electrocautery. The lumbodorsal fascia and sacrospinalis are split in line with their fibers. Retractors are placed and the facet joints, transverse processes, and sacral alae are visualized.

When the procedure is completed, the wound is irrigated and the retractors are removed. The lumbodorsal fascia is closed, followed by closure of the subcutaneous tissues and skin.

This paraspinal approach may be made bilaterally for spinal fusion or unilaterally for lateral disk herniation.

Summary

The keys to safe surgical exposure of the thoracic and lumbar spine are a thorough understanding of the anatomy and the pathology to be addressed. Once these issues have been resolved, then the appropriate approach may be selected, the patient safely positioned, and the correct level identified radiographically. Following routine surgical principles with these established techniques will yield gratifying results.

References

1. Johnson RM, Murphy MJ, Southwick WD: Surgical approaches to the spine, in Rothman RH, Simeone FA, eds: *The Spine*, ed 3. Philadelphia, PA, WB Saunders, 1992.
2. Kostuck J: Surgical approaches to the thoracic and thoracolumbar spine, in Frymoyer JW, ed: *The Adult Spine: Principles and Practice*. New York, NY, Raven Press, 1991.
3. Kaneda K: Surgical approaches to the thoracic and thoracolumbar spine, in Weinstein SL, ed: *The Pediatric Spine: Principles and Practice*. New York, NY, Raven Press, 1994.
4. Beisse R, Mückley T, Schmidt MH, Hauschild M, Bühren V: Surgical technique and results of endoscopic anterior spinal canal decompression. *J Neurosurg Spine* 2005;2(2):128-136.
5. Kim DH, Jahng TA, Balabhadra RS, Potulski M, Beisse R: Thoracoscopic transdiaphragmatic approach to thoracolumbar junction fractures. *Spine J* 2004;4(3):317-328.
6. Maciejczak A, Barnas P, Dudziak P, Jagiełło-Bajer B, Litwora B, Sumara M: Posterior keyhole corpectomy with percutaneous pedicle screw stabilization in the surgical management of lumbar burst fractures. *Neurosurgery* 2007;60 (4, Suppl 2)232-242.
7. Rampersaud YR, Annand N, Dekutoski MB: Use of minimally invasive surgical techniques in the management of thoracolumbar trauma: Current concepts. *Spine (Phila Pa 1976)* 2006;31 (11, Suppl):S96-S104.
8. Hodgson AR, Stock FE, Fang HS, Ong GB: Anterior spinal fusion: The operative approach and pathological findings in 412 patients with Pott's disease of the spine. *Br J Surg* 1960;48:172-178.
9. Dwyer AF, Schafer MF: Anterior approach to sco-

liosis: Results of treatment in fifty-one cases. *J Bone Joint Surg Br* 1974;56(2):218-224.

10. Winter RB, Moe JH, Wang JF: Winter RB, Moe JH, Wang JF: Congenital kyphosis: Its natural history and treatment as observed in a study of one hundred and thirty patients. *J Bone Joint Surg Am* 1973;55(2):223-256.
11. Khoo LT, Beisse R, Potulski M: Thoracoscopic-assisted treatment of thoracic and lumbar fractures: A series of 371 consecutive cases. *Neurosurgery* 2002;51(5, Suppl)S104-S117.
12. Foley KT, Gupta SK, Justis JR, Sherman MC: Percutaneous pedicle screw fixation of the lumbar spine. *Neurosurg Focus* 2001;10(4):E10.
13. Gumbs AA, Bloom ND, Bitan FD, Hanan SH: Open anterior approaches for lumbar spine procedures. *Am J Surg* 2007;194(1):98-102.
14. Menard V: Cause de la paraplégie dans le mal de Pott. *Rev Orthop* 1894;5:47-64.
15. Seddon HJ: Pott's paraplegia, in Hollingsworth BL, ed: *Modern Trends in Orthopaedics*. London, United Kingdom, Butterworth, 1956.
16. Resnick DK, Benzel EC: Lateral extracavitary approach for thoracic and thoracolumbar spine trauma: Operative complications. *Neurosurgery* 1998; 43(4):796-803.
17. Musacchio M, Patel N, Bagan B, Deutsch H, Vaccaro AR, Ratliff J: Minimally invasive thoracolumbar costotransversectomy and corpectomy via a dual-tube technique: Evaluation in a cadaver model. *Surg Technol Int* 2007;16:221-225.
18. Hibbs RA: An operation for progressive spinal deformity. *NY State Med J* 1911;93:1013-1016.
19. Albee FH: Transplantation of a portion of the tibia into the spine for Pott's disease. *JAMA* 1911;57: 885-886.
20. Ringel F, Stoffel M, Stüer C, Meyer B: Minimally invasive transmuscular pedicle screw fixation of the thoracic and lumbar spine. *Neurosurgery* 2006;59(4 Suppl 2):ONS361-ONS367.
21. Robertson PA: Anterior approaches for thoracolumbar fractures. *ANZ J Surg* 2007;77 (Suppl 1):A54.
22. Royle ND: The treatment of spastic paralysis by sympathetic ramii-section. *Surg Gynecol Obstet* 1924;39:701-720.
23. Francioli P: Ways of approach in lumbar and lumbothoracic sympathectomies. *Helv Chir Acta* 1951;18(6):536-556.
24. Ozgur BM, Aryan HE, Pimenta L, Taylor WR: Extreme lateral interbody fusion (XLIF): A novel surgical approach for anterior lumbar interbody fusion. *Spine J* 2006;6(4):435-443.
25. Getty J, Kaneda K, Nakana N, et al: Surgical approaches, in Weinstein JS, Wiesel S, eds: *The Lumbar Spine*. Philadelphia, PA, WB Saunders, 1990.
26. Kaya RA, Aydin Y: Modified transpedicular approach for the surgical treatment of severe thoracolumbar or lumbar burst fractures. *Spine J* 2004; 4(2):208-217.
27. Wiltse LL, Bateman JG, Hutchinson RH, Nelson WE: The paraspinal sacrospinalis-splitting approach to the lumbar spine. *J Bone Joint Surg Am* 1968;50(5):919-926.

CHAPTER 17
Intraoperative Evaluation: Somatosensory-Evoked Potentials and Electromyography

Rob D. Dickerman, DO, PhD   Richard D. Guyer, MD

Key Points

- Intraoperative neurophysiologic monitoring can prevent neurologic injury during patient positioning and surgery.
- Somatosensory-evoked potentials (SSEPs) are intended to monitor dorsal column function and are most useful for intramedullary surgery or cases where spinal cord function may be affected during surgery.
- Hypotension negatively affects SSEPs and should be avoided at all times during spinal cord surgery.
- For SSEPs, an increase in latency of 10% of baseline value and/or a decrease in amplitude of more than 50% should be reason for intervention.
- Evoked electromyography through the pedicle can assist the surgeon in detecting a malpositioned pedicle screw or pedicle breach by the pedicle screw.

Introduction

Intraoperative neurophysiologic monitoring in spinal surgery is becoming increasingly popular, with its utilization spanning well beyond its initial realm of intramedullary spinal cord surgery. The obvious role for intraoperative neurophysiologic monitoring is to reduce the risk for injury to neural elements. There is substantial literature supporting risk reduction when using various forms of intraoperative monitoring.[1-7] Newer techniques have been developed that can assist the surgeon in the most routine approaches in spinal surgery. This chapter includes a review of the most recently published literature on neurophysiologic monitoring techniques and their clinical applications.

Dr. Dickerman or an immediate family member serves as a board member, owner, officer, or committee member of the North American Spine Society; has received royalties from Spinal USA and Osteomed; is a member of a speakers' bureau or has made paid presentations on behalf of Osteomed; serves as a paid consultant to or is an employee of Spinal USA and Osteomed; and owns stock or stock options in Vertiflex. Dr. Guyer or an immediate family member is a member of a speakers' bureau or has made paid presentations on behalf of DePuy, a Johnson & Johnson company and Synthes; and serves as a paid consultant to or is an employee of DePuy, a Johnson & Johnson company.

Somatosensory-Evoked Potentials

Somatosensory-evoked potentials (SSEPs) are used to assess dorsal column function within the spinal cord, not anterior column or motor function. The basis of SSEPs depends on an intact conducting pathway between the site of stimulation and the site of recording. Spinal cord function is assessed with SSEPs by monitoring changes in latency and amplitude, with the initial assumption that any changes in latency or amplitude may be detected early in the spinal cord injury milieu and thus be reversible. Intraoperative spinal cord injury most likely results from stretching or compression of vascular and/or neural structures leading to spinal cord ischemia or direct neural injury. Nash et al[3] introduced SSEP monitoring to mainstream spinal surgery over 30 years ago and it has been the most common form of monitoring to date. SSEPs may be recorded from the scalp (allowing for cortical and subcortical SSEP), epidural space, or interspinous ligament.[1,8,9] Obviously, cortical SSEPs traverse more neural synapses in their course and thus are more sensitive to depression by anesthetic agents. The most common technique is to record cortical responses after electrical stimulation of the posterior tibial or peroneal nerve. SSEPs have become a standard of care in certain spinal surgery procedures, although the intraoperative wake-up test remains comforting for most spine surgeons.

SSEP Monitoring

SSEP monitoring involves rapid computerized analysis on the millisecond level to delineate neural evoked potentials from other biologic/electrical potentials that may be detected. The inherent difficulty with SSEP monitoring in the operating theater lies with the numerous other biologic signals, including electrical equipment within the room such as electrocardiography (ECG), electroencephalography (EEG), and electromyography (EMG) equipment. Neural-evoked potentials are of significantly lower amplitude than all of the other aforementioned biologic devices. To consistently isolate the SSEP signals requires the utilization of signal-averaging techniques. Signal averaging takes the signal of interest and time-locks it to the stimulus while the background noise is random. The signal of interest is amplified, digitized, and successive trials are then averaged. Thus, with increasing trials, the random background noise will eventually approach zero, leaving the SSEP signal preserved and amplified. The ratio of signal-to-background noise increases in proportion to the square root of the number of trials. On average, it takes several hundred stimuli to extract the evoked potential waveform from the background noise. Today, the success rates for acquiring baseline SSEPs in the operating room approach 100%.[10-13]

Technique

The most common site for initial monitoring is a peripheral nerve in the lower extremity, usually the posterior tibial or peroneal nerve. The median nerve of the upper extremity may also be monitored concurrently as a "control" to help determine when a systemic factor for a drop in amplitude or an increase in latency may be occurring (ie, should a change occur in only lower extremity SSEPs, one may look at the upper extremity as a comparison to determine if this could be general anesthesia or a systemic factor). Stimulation electrodes may be subcutaneous needles or surface electrodes similar to EEG disk electrodes. Obviously, the subcutaneous electrodes provide more of a constant electrical impedance that is imperative during lengthy operations. The SSEP amplitude will increase as the stimulating intensity increases. Constant-current stimulators are used to deliver a constant stimulus, thus allowing for a change in impedance to be detected over time. Regarding unilateral versus bilateral stimulation, bilateral stimulation provides larger amplitudes and should be employed when SSEPs from unilateral stimulation are insufficient in amplitude. Bilateral stimulation may not detect a unilateral injury to the spinal cord. Thus, the technique that is preferred is alternating unilateral stimulation. Although peripheral nerve stimulation is the preferred technique, direct stimulation of the conus medullaris via an epidural catheter can be useful. This conus stimulation provides high-amplitude SSEPs and assists in detecting spinal injury in such cases as aortic cross-clamping that may lead to peripheral nerve ischemia.

Important relationships exist between sensory thresholds, rates of stimulation, and amplitudes. During anesthesia, SSEP amplitude increases linearly with increasing stimulus intensity until a threshold is reached at approximately 20 mA. Thus, for spinal cord monitoring, most use the higher stimulus intensities to maximize the opportunity for optimal recordings. The rate of stimulation also effects SSEP amplitude. Earlier studies have demonstrated a progressive decline in amplitude with increasing stimulus rates.[1] These studies concluded that a stimulus rate between 3.1 Hz and 5.1 Hz should be employed to optimize SSEP recordings.

Routine SSEPs monitoring spinal cord function typically involve the placement of recording electrodes along the ascending sensory pathway, in the skin, popliteal fossa, vertebral column, neck, and scalp. Cortical and subcortical SSEPs are recorded from scalp electrodes. Basic SSEP recordings plot amplitude over a time with particular attention to certain peaks. **Figure 1** demonstrates two superimposed cortical posterior tibial nerve SSEPs recorded during spinal surgery. The peaks used for intraoperative evaluation are positive peak 1 (P1) and negative peak 1 (N1). The latencies of these peaks and their interpeak amplitude (P1N1) are determined in each waveform and compared to baseline values.

As previously discussed, background noise can affect the ability to detect SSEPs, and several other physiologic factors contribute to alterations in amplitude and latency. The anesthesiologist plays an important role in spinal surgery, from the initial intubation, which with cervical instability may require a fiberoptic intubation, to final positioning, maintaining appropriate perfusion pressure for the spinal cord, temperature regulation, and oxygen saturation, and when monitoring, ensuring that volatile anesthetics do not interfere with SSEPs. Volatile anesthetics have been shown to significantly suppress cortical activity and thus abolish SSEPs.[14,15] Intravenous barbiturates, benzodiazepines, opioids, propofol, and muscle relaxants may all be used during SSEP monitoring without much effect on SSEP recordings.[16,17] An anesthesia study used a computerized target-controlled infusion device for propofol and intravenous applica-

FIGURE 1

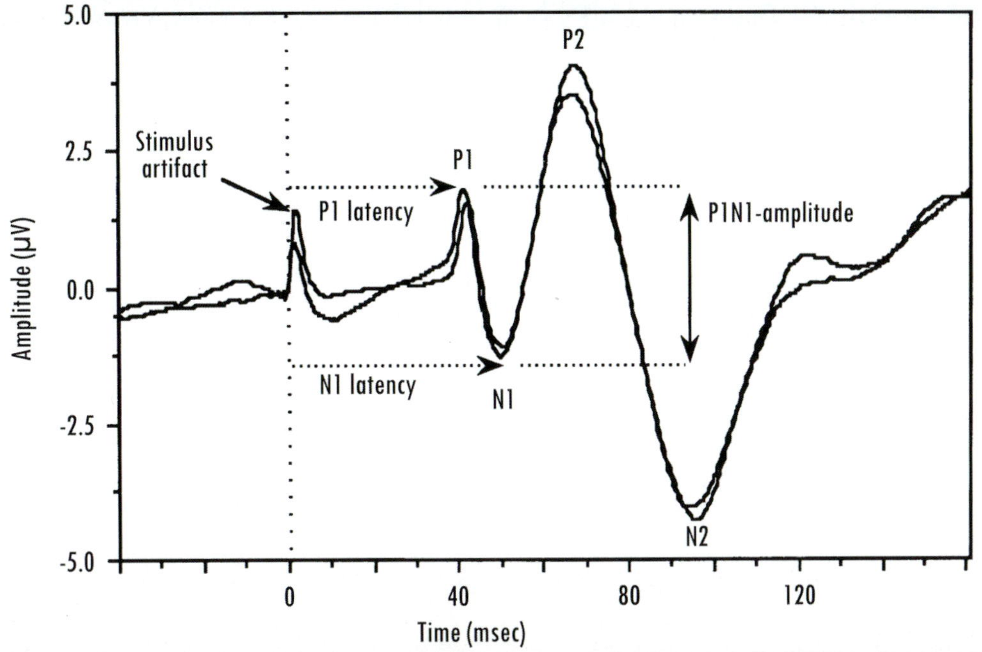

Figure 1 Somatosensory-evoked responses recorded during scoliosis surgery in a 20-year-old male patient. Anesthesia was alfentanil 2 µg/kg/min and 66% nitrous oxide. Total analysis time is 200 msec and 512 stimuli were averaged. The stimulus is applied 40 msec after the start of the sweep. This "mid-signal triggering" allows inspection of the baseline before the stimulus. (Reproduced with permission from Kalkman CJ: *Intraoperative Spinal Cord Function Monitoring With Somatosensory Evoked Potentials: Influence of Anesthetic and Physiologic Factors.* Amsterdam, The Netherlands, University of Amsterdam, 1990, Doctoral Thesis.)

tion of an opioid. Anesthesia was found to induce significant and consistent latencies of median (onset, N20, P25, and N35) and tibial (onset, P40, N50, and P60) SSEPs with mean variations of less than 6%.[18] The intraoperative SSEP amplitudes were less stable, with a relative standard deviation of 30% to 40%. The postoperative tibial SSEPs were not significantly changed in comparison to preoperative recordings. The authors conclude that by using a standardized anesthesia protocol with controlled application of sedatives and analgesics, the impact of anesthesia on preoperative SSEP can be predicted. Muscle relaxants do not affect SSEPs; however, some surgeons prefer concurrent monitoring with EMG and thus prohibit use of muscle relaxants. **Table 1** presents effects of commonly used anesthetics.[10,14-17,19-23] The anesthesiologist may need to use a body warmer to prevent any decreases in body temperature during the surgery. Hypothermia has been shown to decrease conduction velocities and increase synaptic delays in peripheral nerves.[24] Previous studies demonstrated that as nasopharyngeal temperature decreases, median nerve SSEP latencies increase in a linear fashion.[24] Based on these studies, most surgeons prefer having the extremities wrapped or covered, in addition to the core warming blanket, to prevent any discrepancies in core temperature and peripheral extremity temperature.

Hypotension negatively affects SSEPs and is one of the most important physiologic factors that the anesthesiologist must avoid during spinal surgery.[12,25] Hypotension leads to a decrease in spinal cord perfusion pressure and a subsequent deleterious ischemic cascade that may significantly permanently impair spinal cord function.[25] Cerebral autoregulation maintains spinal cord blood flow by regulating mean arterial pressures between 50 Hg and 150 mm Hg. Hypotension alone will not affect SSEPs; however, hypotension coupled with decreased oxygen saturation will decrease SSEP amplitudes and increase latencies. The possible irreversible effects of hypotension on spinal cord function require surgeons to communicate throughout the case with anesthesia and monitoring personnel to ensure that any changes in SSEPs

TABLE 1

Effects of Anesthetic Drugs on SSEPs in Order of Decreasing Effect of Amplitude of Primary Cortical SSEP Peaks

DRUG	AMPLITUDE	LATENCY
Halothane/enflurane/isoflurane[14,19]	↓↓↓ (dose-dependent)	↑↑
Nitrous oxide[20]	↓↓	=
Thiopental[17,21]	↓	↑
Midazolam[22]	↓	↑
Fentanyl/sufentanil/alfentanil/morphine[15,16]	↓=	=↑
Propofol[10]	=	↑
Muscle relaxants	=	=
Etomidate[23]	↑	↑↑

↑, moderate increase; ↑↑, marked increase; ↓, moderate decrease; ↓↓, marked decrease; =, no change.

(Reproduced from Kalkman CJ, Drummond JC: Intraoperative evaluation: Somatosensory evoked potentials and motor evoked potentials, in Levine AM, Eismont FJ, Garfin SR, Zigler JE: *Spine Trauma*. Philadelphia, PA, WB Saunders, 1998, pp 156-170.)

FIGURE 2

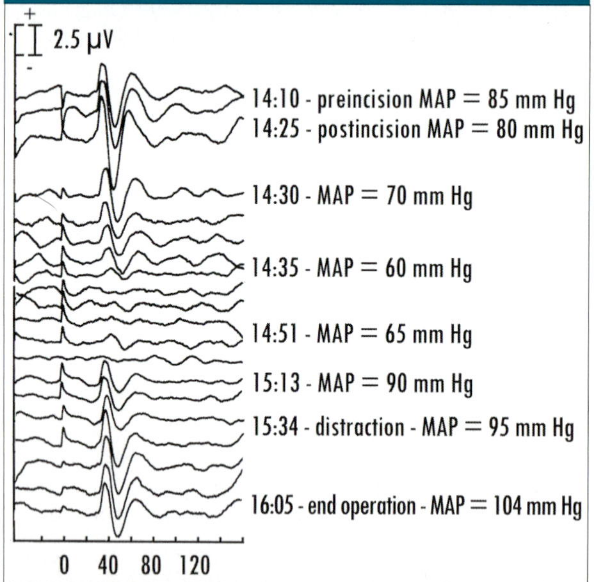

Figure 2 Loss of posterior tibial nerve SSEPs in a 14-year-old patient during institution of controlled hypotension after positioning in a Cotrel-Dubousset frame with 15 kg of traction. MAP = mean arterial pressure. (Reproduced from Kalkman CJ, Drummond JC: Intraoperative evaluation: Somatosensory evoked potentials and motor evoked potentials, in Levine AM, Eismont FJ, Garfin SR, Zigler JE: *Spine Trauma*. Philadelphia, PA, WB Saunders, 1998, pp 156-170.)

are not from hypotension and or ischemia. **Figure 2** demonstrates loss of posterior tibial nerve SSEPs during controlled hypotension.

SSEP Variability and Reliability

Consistent waveforms allow the monitoring personnel to report to the surgeon any changes that may occur during surgery. The consistent and reproducible waveforms, while important, may not be without variability. Determining when a waveform is a minor variability versus a pathologic sign is of utmost importance. To limit unnecessary and alarming interruptions during surgery, single waveforms are not used; instead, waveforms are averaged and compared over time. Obviously, special attention to detail in the waveforms is required during high-risk procedures, such as passing sublaminar wires or distraction. Absolute changes in amplitude and latency are the important parameters of intraoperative SSEP monitoring; the subsequent variability between successive recordings allows one to determine the magnitude of changes from baseline waveforms. Reliable monitoring requires consistent and reproducible SSEPs during the preoperative, intraoperative, and immediately postoperative time frames to ensure and protect spinal cord function. Variability within SSEPs is inherent due to the multiple other factors that may affect recordings. Variability can be reduced by eliminating frequencies that may affect collection of SSEP waveforms, such as by optimizing anesthetics, ensuring normal physiologic parameters of temperature, blood pressure, and saturation. In terms of anesthesia, the most widely accepted technique consists of premedicating with benzodiazepines, induction with barbiturates, and continuous infusion of fentanyl or sufentanil and nitrous oxide 50% to 66%. As stated previously, muscle relaxants do not affect SSEPs; however, recent literature supports simultaneous monitoring of EMG and SSEPs.[26,27]

Acquiring accurate recordings requires maximizing the SSEP signal-to-noise ratio in the preoperative period. One cannot underestimate the importance of baseline waveforms. The baseline waveforms will be used throughout the case for comparison and these waveforms may be affected preoperatively by a preexisting neurologic deficit. Patients with a preoperative spinal cord injury or neurologic deficit usually have low-amplitude potentials with "fatigue" of the response at higher stimulus frequencies. These patients typically respond to slower stimulation rates, 1.1 Hz to 2.1 Hz. **Figure 3** shows posterior tibial nerve SSEPs decreasing with increasing stimulus frequencies.

FIGURE 3

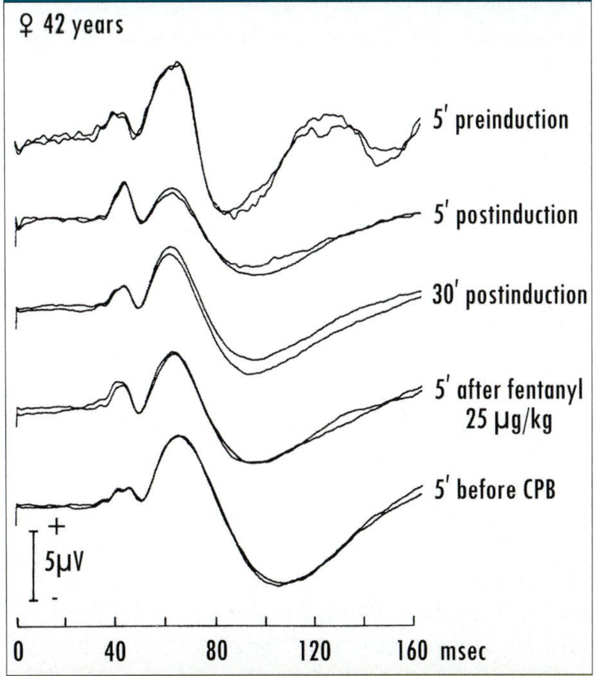

Figure 3 Posterior tibial nerve SSEPs before and during high-dose fentanyl (100 μg/kg) anesthesia. Note the minimal depression of P1N1 amplitude. CPB = cardiopulmonary bypass. The prime signs indicate minutes. (Reproduced with permission from Kalkman CJ, Leyssius AT, Bovill JG: Influence of high-dose opioid anaesthesia on posterior tibial nerve somatosensory cortical evoked potentials: Effects of fentanyl, sulfentanil and alfentanil. *J Cardiothorac Vasc Anesth* 1988;2(6):758-764.)

Pathologic Alerts

An increase in latency of the first cortical peak P1, occurring around 35 to 45 msec poststimulus by more than 3 msec or by 10% of baseline value and/or a decrease in the cortical P1N1 peak-to-peak amplitude of more than 50% should be reason for intervention.[24,28] The use of SSEPs for the prevention of neurologic injury is based on the assumption that significant changes in latency and amplitude will occur while spinal cord ischemia is still in a reversible stage. Immediate actions that may be taken include diminishing distraction, removal of instrumentation, and increasing mean arterial pressure. The surgeon should always consider both physiologic and nonphysiologic causes for alterations in SSEPs.

Inherent Limitations

As stated earlier, SSEPs only measure ascending sensory tracts—predominantly dorsal columns and to some extent dorsolateral columns. Thus, maintaining normal SSEPs throughout a surgery does not guarantee normal motor function. Selective injury to the anterior spinal cord may therefore go undetected, resulting in a false-negative result. Some surgeons argue the theory and need for SSEP monitoring during spinal cord surgery that requires splitting of the dorsal median fissure during surgery, thus temporarily losing SSEPs. The advances in intraoperative monitoring have led to an increase in utilization of intraoperative monitoring during spinal surgery.

Advances in SSEP Monitoring

Brau et al[29] studied patients for changes in SSEP and oxygen saturation (SaO_2) while undergoing anterior lumbar interbody fusion. Patients were considered to have abnormal SSEPs with any increase in latency and decrease in amplitude. Thirteen patients with exposure at L4-L5 had both loss of SSEP signals and loss of SaO_2 with exposure. All 13 patients had return to normal saturation and recovery of the SSEP signals within 15 minutes of removal of the retractors. Significant correlations ($P < 0.001$) were found in desaturation and loss of SSEPs. The study demonstrated that the majority (57%) of patients undergoing anterior lumbar interbody fusion at the L4-L5 level are subject to compression of the left iliac vessels enough to cause desaturation distally as measured by pulse oximetry. The vascular compromise, as well as the return to normal saturation, correlates with changes noted in SSEP soon after both deployment and removal of the retractors used for exposure. The authors concluded that a transient ischemic response leads to SSEP alterations and that failure of the SSEP signals to recover may be diagnostic of left iliac artery thrombosis. Although SSEPs are typically used only in the lower extremities, studies have demonstrated that SSEPs in upper and lower extremities may be of clinical utility. SSEPs were assessed in the upper and lower extremities during surgery to determine if vascular or neurologic injury may be going undetected with lower extremity monitoring only. The upper extremity SSEP monitoring detected changes in SSEPs revealing ischemia secondary to compression. Conclusions were that SSEP monitoring of the bilateral upper extremities should be considered during prolonged lumbar surgeries where vascular or neurologic compression/ischemia may occur in the upper extremities.

A study on 61 patients undergoing spinal cord surgery for tumors assessed the utility of SSEPs and EMG of the lower extremities and external anal and urethral sphincters during spinal cord surgery.[26] Lower extremity SSEPs were measured in 89% of the patients. Temporary neurologic deficits occurred in 4.9%, with permanent deficits in 1.6%. Electrically evoked EMG activity encountered during microsurgical dissection altered the surgical plan in 42% of the cases. The authors concluded that combined SSEP and EMG reliably and positively influenced decision making in the operating theater. Another study combining SSEP and transcranial electrical motor-evoked potential (tc-MEP) monitoring during anterior cervical spine surgery retrospectively analyzed 119 patients who underwent anterior cervical fusions.[30] Of the 119 patients, 6 neurophysiologic alerts occurred that prompted surgical or anesthesia adjustments. Three patients developed new motor weakness after surgery; one patient had tc-MEP–detected temporary right lower extremity weakness. Two patients developed neurologic deficits that were not detected; one patient developed quadriparesis postoperatively that was undetected due to excessive neuromuscular blockade, and the second patient developed transient C5-C6 nerve root compromise that was undetected secondary to poor baseline tc-MEPs. The results illustrated the potential utility of intraoperative SSEPs and tc-MEPs for detection of changes in spinal cord function related to patient positioning and hemodynamic effects during anterior cervical fusion.

SSEPs were also assessed with placement of 888 pedicle screws in 186 consecutive surgeries.[31] An acute or sustained loss of 50% in SSEP amplitude or an increase by 10% in latency from baseline was considered pathologic. No patients demonstrated changes in SSEPs during surgery, although five patients suffered postoperative radiculopathies. Malposition of the pedicle screws was verified by CT. All malpositioned screws were revised or removed without complications. The authors concluded that the use of SSEPs in evaluating pedicle screw placement during lumbar arthrodesis is of limited value.

Electromyography

As previously mentioned, SSEPs only detect sensory changes in the dorsal columns; thus pyramidal tract damage may go undetected. To monitor motor tracts, surgeons typically employ neurogenic motor-evoked potentials (MEPs) or transcranial MEPs (tc-MEPs).

Neurogenic MEPs monitor the motor tracts through needle electrodes placed in the lamina of the cervical spine. The transmitted signal is subsequently detected caudally as the stimulus descends through the corticospinal pathways. This system, while beneficial, is not as commonly employed as tc-MEPs. Transcranial MEPs use stimulation through the skull to depolarize cortical motor neurons, thus producing a descending volley in the corticospinal tracts, eventually through the peripheral nerve and into the muscle where it is detected. Levy[32] developed a system that recorded intraoperative MEPs with an electrical stimulation via electrodes through the cerebral cortex. The stimulator allows for detection of the transmitted signal in muscles of the upper or lower extremities. Newer technologies are now permitting the utilization of continuous free-running EMG throughout the surgery. This technique allows the surgeon to be notified if any changes occur during the entire case versus only during "critical" parts of the surgery.

Rationale for Both EMG and SSEP Monitoring

An outcome study retrospectively compared 66 patients who underwent neurosurgical intervention for lumbosacral lipomas with SSEP monitoring only versus 20 recent cases who underwent the same surgery with the addition of EMG monitoring intraoperatively.[5] Of the 66 retrospective cases, postoperative neurologic deficits occurred in 6% of the patients. The postoperative neurologic deficits were reduced to zero with the addition of intraoperative EMG monitoring. The authors went on to conclude that intraoperative multichannel EMG monitoring requires only minimal changes to anesthetic procedures and allows the surgeon to better identify the neural structures of complex malformations, reducing the risks of surgical damage and incomplete detethering.

Surgeons typically use SSEPs and tc-MEPs during intramedullary surgery for tumors. A study on the utilization of continuous free-running EMG with tc-MEP during intramedullary surgery on 13 patients found that continuous free-running EMG detected neurologic changes in 8 patients that may have been undetected otherwise.[33] There was only one false-positive report, leading the authors to conclude that continuous free-running EMG should be considered with intramedullary surgery.

We have a case that is very applicable to the benefits of simultaneous SSEP and tc-MEP monitoring. A patient with cervical myelopathy and instability was undergoing cervical laminectomy-decompression and posterior fusion with lateral mass screws. Baseline SSEPs were obtained after intubation and before positioning, and then repeated after being placed in the prone position. All SSEPs were normal. During the dissection out to the lateral masses, the neurophysiologists monitoring the case stated "all potentials are lost on the right extremity." We immediately checked anesthesia and monitoring leads and obtained fluoroscopic radiographs of the cervical spine; there were no changes. We abandoned the fusion part of the case and proceeded with emergent decompressive laminectomy. The patient was stabilized in a hard collar and extubated intact. The SSEP monitoring was incorrect! Our patient subsequently underwent anterior cervical stabilization without complications. We now routinely use SSEP and tc-MEP for myelopathic patients.

Pedicle screw stimulation via evoked EMG thresholds for < 11 mA are known to be associated with possible pedicle violation by the screw.[34] A study assessing the reliability of evoked EMG for thoracic pedicle screws demonstrated results consistent with lumbar evoked EMG studies that stimulation thresholds > 11 mA have a 97.5% negative predictive value, suggesting that cortical violation is highly unlikely. Although judgment of screw placement should not depend solely on stimulation thresholds, pedicle screw stimulation does provide rapid and useful intraoperative information on screw placement during procedures involving the use of thoracic pedicle screws.[34] In our own experience, we agree that evoked EMG through the pedicle screw provides reassurance to the surgeon; however, several technical notes are worth mentioning.[12] First, some surgeons probe the pedicle with the EMG probe before insertion of the pedicle screw to ensure the initial tap has not violated the cortex of the pedicle. The EMG probe is highly sensitive to surrounding soft-tissue conduction interference and should be protected from soft tissue by a plastic sleeve. Second, when the EMG probe travels through the pedicle into the vertebral body, the impedance values will increase significantly, possibly providing a false-negative value. Therefore, we recommend testing deep into the vertebral body initially (high value), and then slowly withdrawing the probe into the pedicle and circumferentially testing throughout the pedicle. Should all impedance values be > 12 mA, the surgeon can be reassured that the pedicle was not violated with the initial tap. When considering patient variability in impedance values, the surgeon must consider the bone density of each patient (eg, a postmenopausal female with osteopenia may have lower impedance values without violation of the pedicle due to the decreased bone mineral density). Lastly, should the surgeon prefer to bypass testing of the tap and go directly to testing the pedicle screw after it has been placed, we highly recommend using a plastic sleeve to prevent outside soft-tissue interference.

Intraoperative monitoring of tc-MEPs has been investigated recently as a means of preventing motor deficits associated with resection of intramedullary spinal cord tumors (IMSCTs).[35] A retrospective record review was conducted for 28 patients who underwent resection of an IMSCT using myogenic or muscle-recorded tc-MEPs. Of the 28 patients who underwent resection of an IMSCT using tc-MEPs, MEP changes occurred in 13 patients (46%). Impaired motor conduction was detected by changes in pattern and duration of the MEP waveform morphology and by an increase in voltage threshold. Alterations in morphology and reduction in duration of the MEP response persisted despite significant increases in stimulation voltage. In 12 patients, reductions in the complexity and/or loss of the tc-MEP waveform significantly correlated with motor grade loss in the immediate postoperative period ($P < 0.0001$), at discharge ($P < 0.001$), and at follow-up ($P < 0.001$). The decrease in the duration of the response correlated with motor grade loss immediately after surgery ($P < 0.001$), at discharge ($P < 0.0001$), and at follow-up ($P < 0.005$). The results support the application of distal muscle-recorded tc-MEPs to predict the occurrence and severity of postoperative motor deficits during resection of IMSCTs. Attention to such quantitative intraoperative monitoring data may help to minimize postoperative motor deficits by avoiding or correcting excessive spinal cord manipulation and modifying surgical technique during tumor resection.

Conclusions

This chapter provided an update on intraoperative neurophysiologic monitoring techniques and their role in spinal surgery. We offer six closing recommendations based on recent literature. (1) Intraoperative monitoring, possibly including SSEPs, EMG, and MEPs, should be performed with any of the following procedures: intramedullary spinal cord tumors, conus or cauda equina tumors, surgical rhizotomies for spasticity, and surgery for tethered cord. (2) Monitoring is mandatory whenever neurologic complications are expected on the basis of a known pathophysiologic mechanism. (3) MEP monitoring is reliable under general anesthesia and is essential for assessing the integrity of descending motor pathways from the cerebral cortex, brainstem, and especially the spinal cord. (4) SSEP monitoring is of value in assessing the functional integrity of sensory pathways leading from the peripheral nerve through the dorsal columns to the sensory cortex; however SSEPs cannot provide reliable information on the integrity of the motor system. (5) Evoked EMG to assess pedicle screw placement provides > 97% negative predictive value for reassurance to the surgeon. (6) Mapping of the corticospinal tract within the spinal cord, although safe and feasible, still lacks rigorous validation in terms of prognostic value and correlation with the postoperative neurologic outcome.

References

1. Nuwer MR, Dawson EC: Intraoperative evoked potential monitoring of the spinal cord: A restricted filter, scalp method during Harrington instrumentation for scoliosis. *Clin Orthop Relat Res* 1984;183:42-50.
2. Brown RH, Nash CL Jr, Berilla JA, Amaddio MD: Cortical evoked potential monitoring: A system for intraoperative monitoring of spinal cord function. *Spine (Phila Pa 1976)* 1984;9(3):256-261.
3. Nash CL Jr, Lorig RA, Schatzinger LA, Brown RH: Spinal cord monitoring during operative treatment of the spine. *Clin Orthop Relat Res* 1977;126:100-105.
4. Bieber E, Tolo V, Uematsu S: Spinal cord monitoring during posterior spinal instrumentation and fusion. *Clin Orthop Relat Res* 1988;229:121-124.
5. Valentini LG, Visintini S, Mendola C, et al: The role of intraoperative electromyographic monitoring in lumbosacral lipomas. *Neurosurgery* 2005;56(2, Suppl)315-323.
6. Meyer PR Jr, Cotler HB, Gireesan GT: Operative neurological complications resulting from thoracic and lumbar spine internal fixation. *Clin Orthop Relat Res* 1988;237:125-131.
7. Jones SC, Fernau R, Woeltjen BL: Use of somatosensory evoked potentials to detect peripheral ischemia and potential injury resulting from positioning of the surgical patient: Case reports and discussion. *Spine J* 2004;4(3):360-362.
8. York DH, Chabot RJ, Gaines RW: Response variability of somatosensory evoked potentials during scoliosis surgery. *Spine (Phila Pa 1976)* 1987;12(9):864-876.
9. Britt RH, Ryan TP: Use of a flexible epidural stimulating electrode for intraoperative monitoring of spinal somatosensory evoked potentials. *Spine (Phila Pa 1976)* 1986;11(4):348-351.
10. Kalkman CJ, ten Brink SA, Been HD, Bovill JG: Variability of somatosensory cortical evoked potentials during spinal surgery: Effects of anesthetic technique and high-pass digital filtering. *Spine (Phila Pa 1976)* 1991;16(8):924-929.
11. Bennett HL, Benson DR: Somatosensory evoked potentials for orthopaedic spine trauma. *J Orthop Trauma* 1989;3(1):11-18.
12. Whitaker C, Hisey M: Accuracy of percutaneous lumbar pedicle screws using plastic vs. metal dilation sleeves. *Spine J* 2005;5(Suppl):S120.
13. Lubicky JP, Spadaro JA, Yuan HA, Fredrickson BE, Henderson N: Variability of somatosensory cortical evoked potential monitoring during spinal surgery. *Spine (Phila Pa 1976)* 1989;14(8):790-798.
14. Wolfe DE, Drummond JC: Differential effects of isoflurane/nitrous oxide on posterior tibial somatosensory evoked responses of cortical and subcortical origin. *Anesth Analg* 1988;67(9):852-859.
15. Pathak KS, Brown RH, Cascorbi HF, Nash CL Jr: Effects of fentanyl and morphine on intraoperative somatosensory cortical-evoked potentials. *Anesth Analg* 1984;63(9):833-837.
16. Kalkman CJ, Leyssius AT, Bovill JG: Influence of high-dose opioid anesthesia on posterior tibial nerve somatosensory cortical evoked potentials: Effects of fentanyl, sufentanil, and alfentanil. *J Cardiothorac Anesth* 1988;2(6):758-764.
17. Drummond JC, Todd MM, U HS: The effect of high dose sodium thiopental on brain stem auditory and median nerve somatosensory evoked responses in humans. *Anesthesiology* 1985;63(3):249-254.
18. Strahm C, Min K, Boos N, Ruetsch Y, Curt A: Reliability of perioperative SSEP recordings in spine surgery. *Spinal Cord* 2003;41(9):483-489.

19. Peterson DO, Drummond JC, Todd MM: Effects of halothane, enflurane, isoflurane, and nitrous oxide on somatosensory evoked potentials in humans. *Anesthesiology* 1986;65(1):35-40.
20. Sloan TB, Koht A: Depression of cortical somatosensory evoked potentials by nitrous oxide. *Br J Anaesth* 1985;57(9):849-852.
21. McPherson RW, Sell B, Traystman RJ: Effects of thiopental, fentanyl, and etomidate on upper extremity somatosensory evoked potentials in humans. *Anesthesiology* 1986;65(6):584-589.
22. Sloan TB, Fugina ML, Toleikis JR: Effects of midazolam on median nerve somatosensory evoked potentials. *Br J Anaesth* 1990;64(5):590-593.
23. Kochs E, Treede RD, Schulte am Esch J: Increase in somatosensory evoked potentials during anesthesia induction with etomidate. *Anaesthesist* 1986;35(6):359-364.
24. van Rheineck Leyssius AT, Kalkman CJ, Bovill JG: Influence of moderate hypothermia on posterior tibial nerve somatosensory evoked potentials. *Anesth Analg* 1986;65(5):475-480.
25. Othman Z, Lenke LG, Bolon SM, Padberg A: Hypotension-induced loss of intraoperative monitoring data during surgical correction of scheuermann kyphosis: A case report. *Spine (Phila Pa 1976)* 2004;29(12):E258-E265.
26. Krassioukov AV, Sarjeant R, Arkia H, Fehlings MG: Multimodality intraoperative monitoring during complex lumbosacral procedures: Indications, techniques, and long-term follow-up review of 61 consecutive cases. *J Neurosurg Spine* 2004;1(3):243-253.
27. Paradiso G, Lee GY, Sarjeant R, Hoang L, Massicotte EM, Fehlings MG: Multimodality intraoperative neurophysiologic monitoring findings during surgery for adult tethered cord syndrome: Analysis of a series of 44 patients with long-term follow-up. *Spine (Phila Pa 1976)* 2006;31(18):2095-2102.
28. Forbes HJ, Allen PW, Waller CS, et al: Spinal cord monitoring in scoliosis surgery: Experience with 1168 cases. *J Bone Joint Surg Br* 1991;73(3):487-491.
29. Brau SA, Spoonamore MJ, Snyder L, et al: Nerve monitoring changes related to iliac artery compression during anterior lumbar spine surgery. *Spine J* 2003;3(5):351-355.
30. Bose B, Sestokas AK, Schwartz DM: Neurophysiological monitoring of spinal cord function during instrumented anterior cervical fusion. *Spine J* 2004;4(2):202-207.
31. Gundanna M, Eskenazi M, Bendo J, Spivak J, Moskovich R: Somatosensory evoked potential monitoring of lumbar pedicle screw placement for in situ posterior spinal fusion. *Spine J* 2003;3(5):370-376.
32. Levy WJ: Transcranial stimulation of the motor cortex to produce motor-evoked potentials. *Med Instrum* 1987;21(5):248-254.
33. Skinner SA, Nagib MM, Bergman TA, Maxwell RE, Msangi G: The initial use of free-running electromyography to detect early motor tract injury during resection of intramedullary spinal cord lesions. *Neurosurgery* 2005;56(2, Suppl):299-314.
34. Shi YB, Binette M, Martin WH, Pearson JM, Hart RA: Electrical stimulation for intraoperative evaluation of thoracic pedicle screw placement. *Spine (Phila Pa 1976)* 2003;28(6):595-601.
35. Quiñones-Hinojosa A, Lyon R, Zada G, et al: Changes in transcranial motor evoked potentials during intramedullary spinal cord tumor resection correlate with postoperative motor function. *Neurosurgery* 2005;56(5):982-993.

CHAPTER 18
Spinal Orthoses

Michael Vives, MD Steven R. Garfin, MD

Key Points

- Orthoses are external devices applied to the body to restrict motion in that particular body segment.
- Spinal orthoses are broadly categorized based on the region they are employed to immobilize: the cervical orthosis (CO), cervicothoracic orthosis (CTO), thoracolumbosacral orthosis (TLSO), lumbosacral orthosis (LSO), and sacroiliac orthosis (SIO).
- Improved flexural control of the cervical spine may be obtained by increasing the length of the orthosis (extending it onto the thorax) and increasing the rigidity of the connections between the proximal (submandibular and occipital) and distal (thoracic) rests.
- The halo vest provides the most rigid immobilization of the cervical spine of all the currently used orthoses. Proper application and maintenance are necessary to minimize complications.
- Most conventional TLSOs are more effective in limiting motion in the sagittal plane than in controlling rotation or lateral bending.

Dr. Vives or an immediate family member is a member of a speakers' bureau or has made paid presentations on behalf of Biomet and the Musculoskeletal Transplant Foundation; has received research or institutional support from DePuy, a Johnson & Johnson company, the Musculoskeletal Transplant Foundation, and Zimmer; and owns stock or stock options in Accelalox. Dr. Garfin or an immediate family member serves as a board member, owner, officer, or committee member of the Spine Arthroplasty Society; has received royalties from DePuy, a Johnson & Johnson company, and Lippincott; is a member of a speakers' bureau or has made paid presentations on behalf of DePuy, a Johnson & Johnson company; serves as a paid consultant to or is an employee of Applied Spine, Benvenue Medical, Cytonics Corp, DePuy, a Johnson & Johnson company, Disc Dynamics, EBI, Globus Medical, Magnifi Group, Nuvasive, SI Bone, Spinal Kinetics, SpineMark, SpineMedica, and Vertiflex; has received research or institutional support from AO North America, DePuy, a Johnson & Johnson company, EBI, Medtronic, and Synthes; and owns stock or stock options in Cytonics Corp, Orthovita, SI Bone, SpineMark, and SpineMedica.

Introduction

Throughout history, the majority of spinal injuries have been treated nonsurgically. Various forms of immobilization have been used in the management of spinal trauma for thousands of years. In his 1908 article, "The most ancient splints," Smith[1] described brace use in ancient Egypt more than 4,500 years ago. During the Middle Ages, body armor was worn by injured soldiers to help immobilize injuries to the axial skeleton. Early efforts at spinal bracing focused on treatment of spinal deformities, including Galen's chest-strapping method and Pare's leather-lined metal jacket, popular in the late 16th century.[2] Andry developed the "iron cross" in the early 18th century for cervical immobilization. This consisted of a straight metal upright with a cross and metal ring attached to the top for support of the head.[3] Spinal bracing continues to be a mainstay in the management of traumatic spinal disorders even today, during an age that has seen a proliferation of spinal implants and refined surgical techniques.

Orthoses are external devices applied to a segment of the body to restrict motion in that particular body segment.[4] As such, spinal orthoses can be broadly categorized based on the region they are employed to immobilize: the cervical orthosis (CO), cervicothoracic orthosis (CTO), thoracolumbosacral orthosis (TLSO), lumbosacral orthosis (LSO), and sacroiliac orthosis (SIO). Orthoses have various roles in the management of spine trauma patients including prehospital/provisional stabilization, postoperative adjunctive support, and as a definitive means of treatment. This chapter focuses on the biomechanics, laboratory studies, and clinical results of commonly used spinal orthoses in the management of spinal trauma.

Spinal orthoses have not been subject to the strict regulations and scrutiny applied to drugs and implantable devices. This is, in part, due to their designation as class I devices by the U.S. Food and Drug Administration. The currently available knowledge on these devices, therefore, is the product of observations of varying degrees of scientific merit. Additionally, many commercially available products do not have peer-reviewed data to support their purported effectiveness. Therefore, we have attempted to discuss the available

TABLE 1

Commonly Used Materials in the Fabrication of Orthoses

Material	Common Product Names, Tradenames
Ionomer	Surlyn thermoplastic
Olefin	Polypropylene
Polycarbonate	Lexan
Polyethylene	Vitrathene
Polyethylene foam	Plastazote, Aliplast
PVS (polyvinyl siloxane)	Kydex
Resins	Epoxy, polyester

data and review design features of various orthoses rather than make specific recommendations on the superiority of one commercial product versus another. In the text, various product names are mentioned. The manufacturers of these products and their locations are identified in an appendix at the end of this chapter.

Biomechanics and Biomaterials

Evolution in the understanding of complex spinal biomechanics has promoted advances in spinal bracing. In concept, the spine can be thought of as a series of semirigid bodies interconnected by viscoelastic linkages. Spinal kinematics involves motion in six degrees of freedom, with rotation about three axes and translation along the three coordinates.[5] For clinical considerations, testing (particularly involving human subjects) is typically confined to three planes of motion: flexion-extension, axial rotation, and lateral bending.

A variety of methods can be used to evaluate the efficacy of an orthosis. Standard radiography, typically using flexion-extension views, has been commonly employed. Cineradiography evaluates motion through the use of fluoroscopy with movie film. Goniometry uses external devices attached to the patient to measure spinal motion. Goniometry has been demonstrated to correlate fairly well with radiographic techniques[6] and avoids exposing patients to radiation. This advantage, however, is offset by some decreased accuracy and lack of information on motion at any individual segment. Recent technologic developments, such as electrogoniometry and advanced dynamic motion-analysis systems, offer the promise of improving on the methodologies of the past.[7,8]

Because bracing employs the application of external forces to control the position of the spine, orthotic design must account for regional variations of the surrounding anatomy. These include the chin and occiput, the vital soft-tissue structures of the anterior neck, the rigid thoracic rib cage, the compressible abdomen, and the bony pelvis at the base of the spine. The surrounding soft-tissue envelope has a substantial effect on the ability of an externally applied force to control spinal movement. Soft-tissue pressure measurements may be an objective method to assess the fit of a spinal orthosis. The role of soft-tissue pressure measurement as an index of applied corrective or stabilizing force, however, remains unclear.[9,10] The intervening soft-tissue envelope is also an area of potential complications, with problems ranging from skin breakdown, local pain, and decreased vital capacity, to increased lower extremity venous pressure.[11]

Along with our improved understanding of the biomechanics of spinal bracing, improvements in the materials available for brace manufacture have led to dramatic advancements in their design. Eighteenth century braces were generally constructed of leather, iron, and wood. Developments in Germany during the 19th and early 20th centuries led to many new brace designs, with paper cellulose and glue being added to wooden or iron frames.[3] Newer composite materials, polymer resins, and thermoplastics have generated a proliferation of commercially available orthoses that are lightweight and comfortable without sacrificing the stability afforded by the heavier, more cumbersome designs of the past. Commonly used materials in the fabrication of orthoses are listed in **Table 1**.

Beyond the advancements in our understanding of biomechanics and biomaterials, advances in computer engineering have led to innovative methods for customized production of orthoses with decreased time requirements. At our institutions, efforts to limit the length of inpatient admissions have necessitated a close working relationship between the treating physicians and the orthotists. A computerized database of key measurements that have been recorded over the years has allowed our orthotists to develop digitized models of various sizes and body types using computer-aided design/computer-aided manufacturing (CAD/CAM) technology. Using this approach, simple measurements at the sternal notch, xyphoid, and waist, along with linear measurements, can be performed and integrated with CAD/CAM technology to rapidly design a precision-fit orthosis in a fraction of the time needed for standard mold-based orthoses. Recent studies have evaluated this approach for bracing patients with idiopathic scoliosis. Braces comparable to those made using traditional mold techniques (in comfort and curve correction) could be produced in roughly one-third of the time previously required.[12,13]

Cervical Orthoses

Cervical orthoses can be divided into two general categories, soft and hard; hard orthoses are further divided into cervical and cervicothoracic braces. Soft collars provide little immobilization, but are often used in the treatment of whiplash-type injuries, where they may provide comfort and proprioceptive feedback to help "remind" a patient to voluntarily restrict motion. In a recent study using healthy subjects, the effect of soft and hard collars on both full active range of motion (ROM) and functional ROM during 15 activities of daily living (ADLs) was studied.[14] Rigid collars were found to be more restrictive of full, active ROM. For most ADLs, however, the motion recorded was not significantly different regardless of the device. The authors postulated that the soft collars function as proprioceptive guides, resulting in patients regulating their own ROM.

Rigid COs and CTOs come in several designs. All forms must be able to accommodate the vital soft-tissue structures in the neck, while simultaneously providing rigid immobilization of the mobile cervical spine. This is generally accomplished by firm seatings about the base of the skull and upper thorax, or cape of the neck and shoulders, connected by a rigid column. Most include an anterior opening to accommodate a tracheostomy tube. Examples of COs include the Philadelphia collar (**Figure 1**), the Miami J collar (**Figure 2**), the Aspen collar (**Figure 3**), and the Malibu collar (**Figure 4**).

The classic investigation of the effectiveness of various orthoses in immobilizing the cervical spine was performed by Johnson et al.[15] The methods of this study have often been emulated and the results frequently quoted since its publication in 1977. The authors evaluated a soft collar, Philadelphia collar, four-poster orthosis, sterno-occipital-mandibular immobilizer (SOMI), and a CTO. They used radiographs and overhead photographs taken at the extremes of motion in flexion-extension, rotation, and lateral bending. They

FIGURE 1

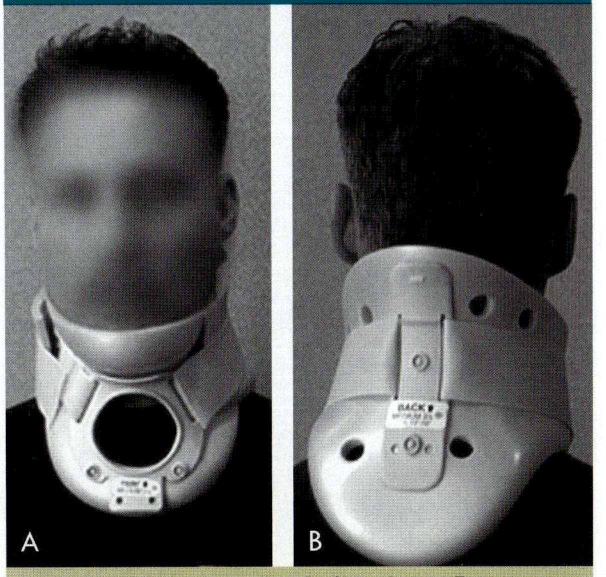

Figure 1 Philadelphia collar: **A,** frontal view; **B,** posterior view. Design includes anterior and posterior shells that are fastened with Velcro straps. The anterior hole can accommodate a tracheostomy tube.

quantified sagittal plane motion for each brace at every level of the cervical spine. As others had reported, they found that a soft collar offered no restriction of motion in any plane. They demonstrated that increasing the length of the orthosis (extending it onto the thorax) and increasing the rigidity of the connection improved the flexion control; however, lateral bending, total flexion, and extension were less controlled. They also demonstrated increased motion between the occiput and C1 in all the braces compared with the unbraced state. This paradoxical "snaking" motion has subsequently been described throughout the cervical and thoracolumbar spine.[16-18]

In 1997 Askins and Eismont[19] compared five commonly used COs in terms of their efficacy in restricting cervical motion. Goniometric and radiographic measurements found the NecLoc orthosis to be superior to the Miami J, Philadelphia, Aspen, and Stifneck orthoses in terms of flexion-extension, rotation, and lateral bending. The Miami J collar was also found to be superior to the Aspen and Philadelphia orthoses in extension and combined flexion-extension. Chin et al[20] demonstrated substantial motion in the upper cervical spine during mastication in patients immobilized in COs. The cervical spine appeared to go into compensatory extension from the act of jaw opening against the rigid chin support of the orthoses.[20]

FIGURE 2

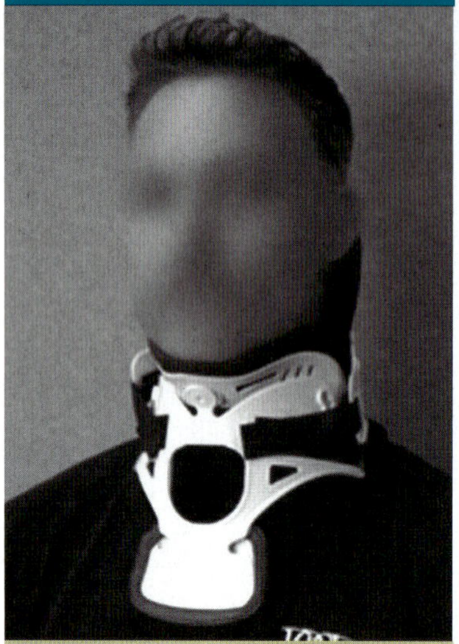

Figure 2 Miami J cervical orthosis. Design features include anterior and posterior shells with a soft lining that can be changed for hygiene purposes.

FIGURE 3

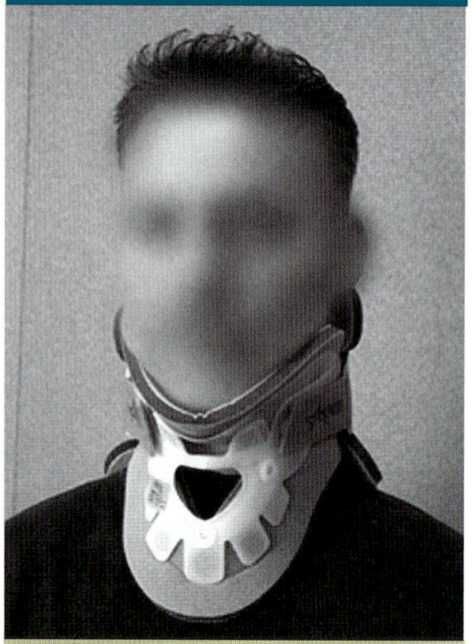

Figure 3 Aspen cervical collar. Patented tabs allow the collar to better conform to the patient when tightened.

FIGURE 4

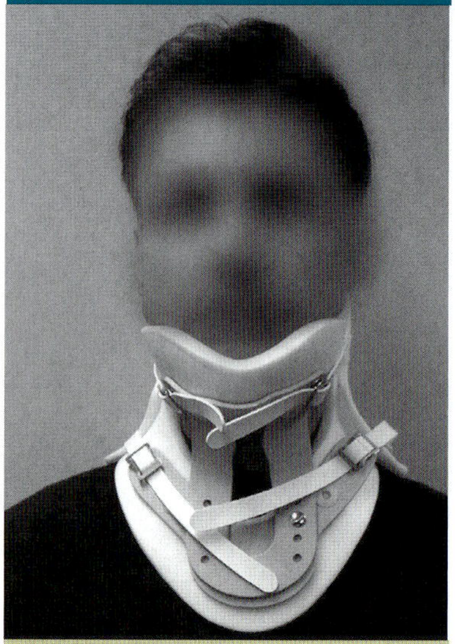

Figure 4 Malibu collar. Design features include tight-fitting chin and occipital rests and more anterior and posterior extension onto the thorax than the Philadelphia collar.

Known complications of COs include skin breakdown over bony prominences such as the sternum, mandible, and occiput. Skin breakdown is especially prevalent in multiple-trauma patients with prolonged recumbency and in patients with altered sensorium (**Figure 5**). One study reported orthosis-related decubiti in 38% of patients with associated severe closed head injuries.[21] Plaisier et al[22] compared the skin pressure associated with the use of the Stifneck, Philadelphia, Miami J, and Aspen collars in supine patients. They found that the Miami J and the Aspen collars produced the lowest chin and occiput pressures, both being below the mean capillary closing pressure.[22] Recently, increased intracranial pressure (ICP), as a consequence of rigid cervical orthotic immobilization, has been described. Hunt et al[23] studied the effects of rigid collar placement on ICP in head-injured patients. They found that rigid collars cause a small, but significant, increase in ICP, which may have deleterious effects in patients with severe head injuries and preexisting intracranial hypertension. They recommend early removal of rigid collars from head-injured patients, once cervical spine injury has been excluded. Because of limited availability or inexperienced caregivers, patients may receive ill-fitting orthoses. Using an electromagnetic tracking system, Bell et al[7] demonstrated that COs that are too large or too small permit excessive motion compared to properly fit collars.

FIGURE 5

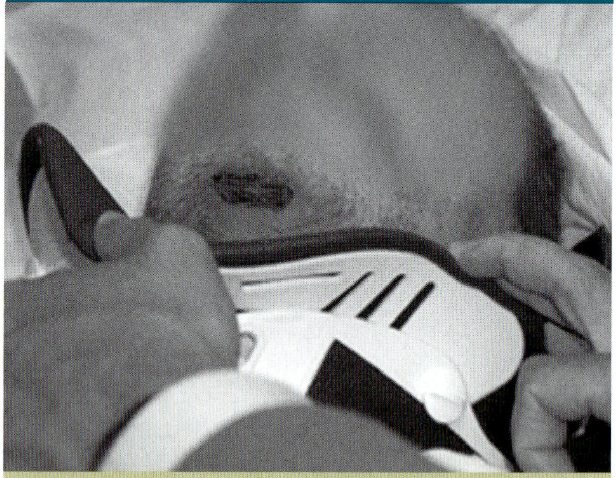

Figure 5 Polytrauma patient who developed skin breakdown in the submandibular region.

Methods for immobilizing the cervical spine of patients in the field have also been extensively studied. These include use of a cervical collar, a short board or sand-bag technique, or a combination of collar and short board. Cline et al[24] compared the Hare extrication collar (DynaMed/Galls, Lexington, KY), the Philadelphia collar, and their immobilization protocol, which consisted of a short board with forehead and chin straps. They concluded that the short board with straps pro-

FIGURE 6

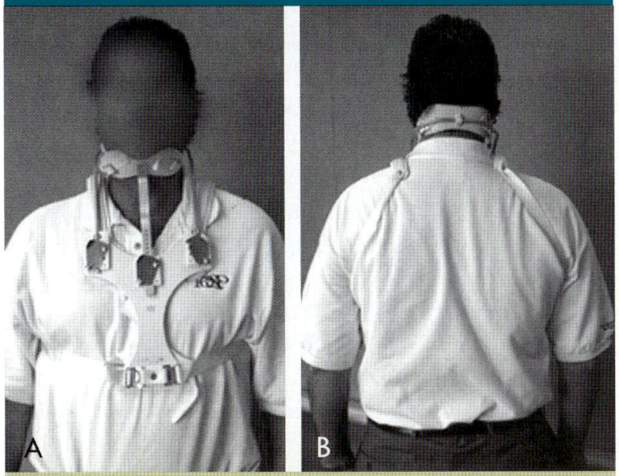

Figure 6 Sterno-occipito-mandibular immobilizer (SOMI): **A,** frontal view; **B,** posterior view. The three uprights that extend from the mandibular and occipital rests all connect anteriorly on the thoracic plate.

FIGURE 7

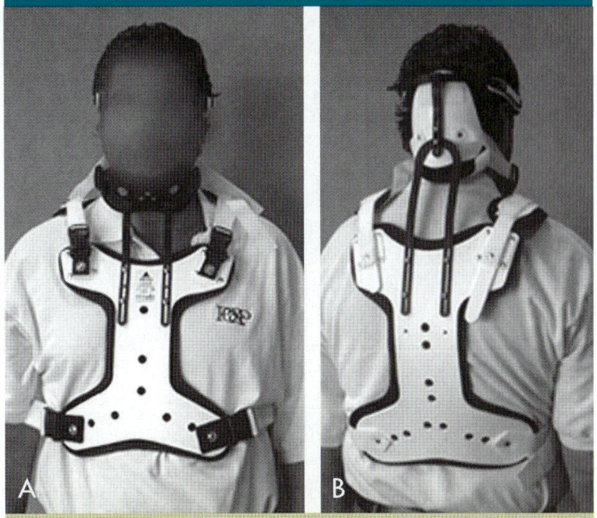

Figure 7 Minerva CTO: **A,** frontal view; **B,** posterior view. The padded U-shaped head band is attached to a large occipital flare that has a rigid connection to the posterior thoracic plate.

vided the best immobilization, and that the addition of a Philadelphia collar did not provide additional benefit. Podolsky et al[25] used goniometry to evaluate the immobilization provided by a soft collar, hard collar, Philadelphia collar, Hare extrication device, and their sand-bag technique (which used a board plus forehead tape). They found the sand-bag technique provided the most effective immobilization, but also applying a Philadelphia collar provided additional benefit.[25] Del Rossi et al[26] examined the effectiveness of various COs during the execution of spine-board transfer techniques. Ambu, Aspen, and Miami J collars all demonstrated similar effectiveness during log-roll and lift-and-slide maneuvers.[26]

Cervicothoracic Orthoses

The general design of CTOs involves occiput and chin supports attached to anterior and/or posterior thoracic plates. Examples include the SOMI (**Figure 6**), the Minerva brace (**Figure 7**), and the Yale brace (**Figure 8**). Compared with COs, these devices improve control in all planes of motion. This improved rigidity, however, comes at the expense of patient comfort. Patients with altered sensorium may be particularly at risk for skin issues at the chin and occiput as these orthoses tend to piston proximally when the head of the hospital bed is elevated. Some of the earlier authors distinguished between the two/four-poster designs and those with more extensive connections between the head and thoracic components.[15] The more recent, standardized classification system, however, categorizes the poster braces as CTOs along with the other designs. The traditional four-poster brace was shown to limit 79% of overall cervical flexion-extension, and to limit midcervical flexion to a comparable degree as the more rigid CTOs.[4,27] Due to their heavy design and high resting pressures on the chin and occiput,[6] this brace is less commonly used today.

FIGURE 8

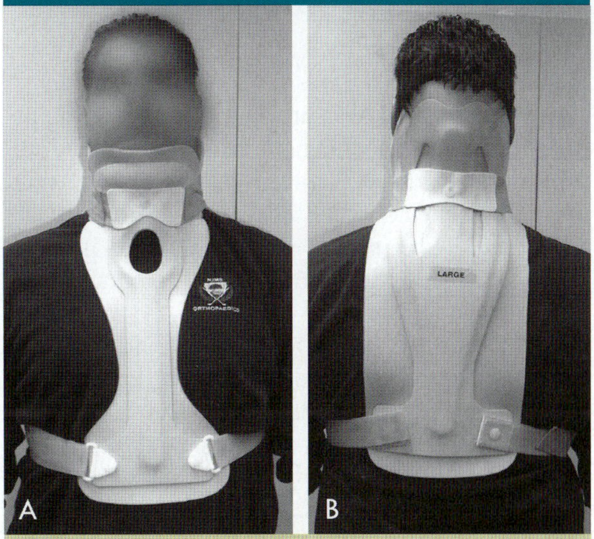

Figure 8 Yale brace: **A,** frontal view; **B,** posterior view. The head rest resembles a Philadelphia collar, from which the early version was originally adapted.

FIGURE 9

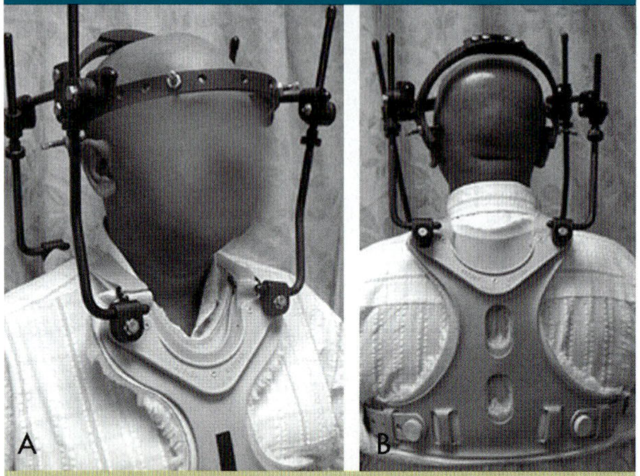

Figure 9 The Bremer halo vest (Bremer Halo Systems, DePuy Spine, Jacksonville, FL): **A,** frontal view; **B,** posterior view. This open-back crown design allows easier ring placement in the supine position.

The SOMI (**Figure 6**) consists of occipital and mandibular rests connected to a sternal plate by metal uprights. The sternal plate is secured to the thorax by padded metal "over-the-shoulder" straps and additional circumferential straps that cross in the back. Because there is no posterior thoracic plate, the occipital rests are supported by uprights from the sternal piece. This results in adequate control of flexion, but limited control of extension throughout the cervical spine.[15,27] These braces are fairly comfortable to patients, but also are associated with high resting pressures at the chin and occiput.[6]

The Minerva brace originally consisted of a heavy, custom, plaster jacket that created difficulties in maintaining patient hygiene and obtaining radiographs.[28] Later, the thermoplastic Minerva body jacket (TMBJ) was developed, which preserved the non-invasive nature of the original concept. Its lightweight, bivalved, Polyform shell allowed improved patient comfort and hygiene and interfered less with follow-up radiographs.[29] Donning this brace is rather complex, often requiring an orthotist for proper application. More recently, a prefabricated version of the Minerva body jacket has been developed, the Minerva CTO (**Figure 7**). Its design features a forehead band attached to a large occipital flare. Sharpe et al[30] reported that this orthosis limits overall sagittal plane motion by 79%, axial rotation by 88%, and lateral bending by 51%.

The original Yale brace (**Figure 8**) was designed as a modified Philadelphia collar with custom-molded anterior and posterior polypropylene thoracic extensions.[31] The modern version is prefabricated and usually made of Kydex. Although lighter and less cumbersome than most of the other CTOs, the Yale brace has similar efficacy in controlling motion. Johnson et al[32] reported that the Yale brace restricted 87% of overall flexion-extension, 75% of axial rotation, and 61% of lateral bending. Although CTOs have been shown to be fairly effective at limiting motion of the cervical spine, they should not be used to rigidly immobilize below the C7-T1 level despite their thoracic components. Most of the COs and CTOs are made of MRI-compatible materials to allow for advanced imaging if necessary.

The Halo Vest

The halo vest provides the most rigid immobilization of the cervical spine of all the currently used orthoses. The original version was inspired by a device used to treat facial fractures in pilots with overlying burns during World War II. Modified versions were used by Perry and Nickel to immobilize patients with polio who had undergone posterior cervical fusion.[33,34] The early halo devices consisted of a circumferential stainless steel ring with four pins for skull fixation. The ring was attached to a plaster jacket by upright posts.[35] Numerous improvements have been made to the various components of the halo vest, but the overall design principles remain the same. A ring is fixed to the skull with multiple pins. The ring is then attached to a vest by four connecting rods. Newer rings are made of composite materials, which have the beneficial properties of light weight, radiolucency, and compatibility with MRI. There does not appear to be a difference in fixation strength between newer radiolucent graphite rings and the earlier titanium ones.[36] Rings that are open posteriorly or have crown-type designs are currently popular. These designs allow for ease in placement because the head of the patient does not need to be passed through the ring. Additionally, since the patient is not lying on the back of the ring, there is less risk of cervical spine fracture displacement through ring manipulation or pin loosening from direct pressure.

Early halo vests were fashioned from heavy plaster of Paris. With the development of plastic technology, lightweight, easily applied vests of various sizes, based on chest circumference, have been fabricated (**Figure 9**). Adjustable supports and straps help customize the fit. The connecting rods are anodized to prevent seizing of the metal

FIGURE 10

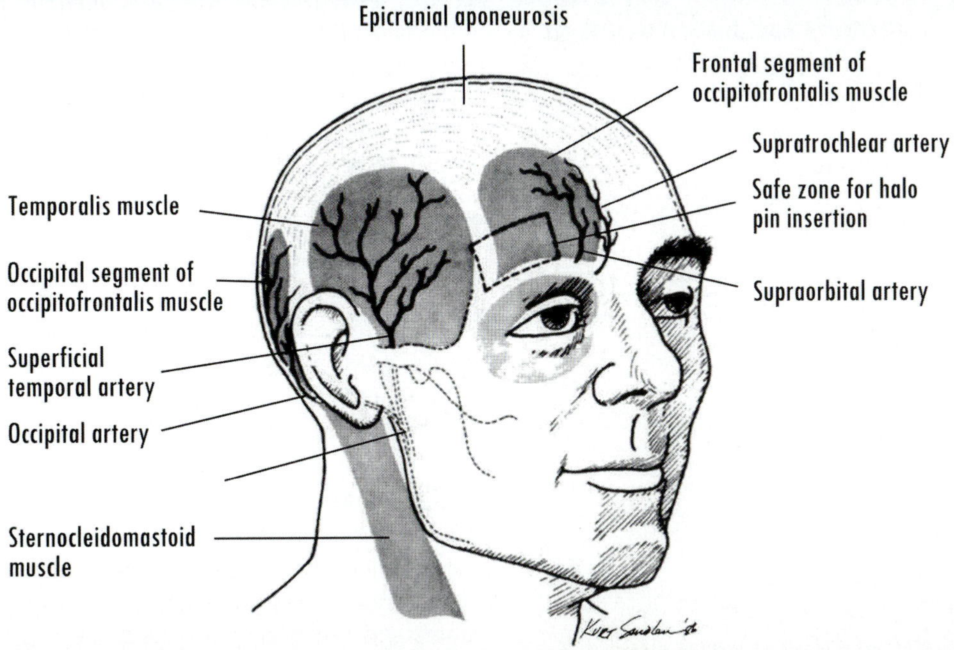

Figure 10 Diagram of the safe zone for placement of anterior halo-fixator pins. (Reproduced with permission from Ballock RT, Botte MJ, Garfin SR: Complications of halo immobilization, in Garfin SR, ed: *Complications of Spine Surgery*. Baltimore, MD, Williams & Wilkins, 1989, p 376.)

during tightening. The connecting rods in many designs are made of carbon fiber for their radiographic lucency, as well as for compatibility with MRI. Torque wrenches are included in the application sets to prevent overtightening of the bolts that connect the rods to the vest and the ring. Mirza et al[37] found that most commercially available vests provide comparable immobilization. Factors that they associated with decreased motion include decreasing the deformability of the vest, increasing vest snugness, and appropriate fit and application.[37]

Advancements have also been made in the field of halo pin materials and pin design. The popular pin composition at this time is stainless steel. Different pin-tip designs have been studied to determine which may provide the greatest resistance to shear forces at the pin-bone interface. Some systems have torque wrenches that break off at a set torque.[38] These wrenches are made to be low profile, allowing for ease of usage in cramped areas such as the posterior aspect of the skull.

Principles of Halo Application

A thorough understanding of pin insertion principles is essential, because many of the complications of halo fixation are related to inappropriate site selection or technique. Many years of clinical data have fine-tuned the optimal location of halo-pin placement. To minimize pin complications but maximize the rigidity of the halo-vest frame, two anterior and two posterior pins are usually placed. The standard position of the anterior pins is 1 cm superior to the orbital rim, over the lateral two-thirds of the orbit, below the level of the greatest circumference of the skull (**Figure 10**).[38] This is considered the *safe zone*. The skull thickness in this region averages approximately 2 mm for the outer cortical table and 3 mm for the intercalvarial space or inner diploe according to a cadaveric study.[39] Pins placed too medial may damage the supraorbital or supratrochlear nerves. Also, the frontal sinus has a varied position in the midline. The outer table of the frontal sinus is often thin, which can lead to perforation with medial pin placement. Laterally placed anterior pins, over the temporalis fossa, have been suggested to avoid unsightly scarring over the anterior forehead. At this location, however, the zygomatico-temporal nerve may be injured; this nerve provides sensation to the area over the temple. Pins in this location may traverse the temporalis muscle, which can cause irritation during mandibular motion (eg, eating). Additionally, in cadaveric studies, in this

TABLE 2

Procedure Summary for Application of the Halo Skeletal Fixator

1. Determine ring or crown size (hold ring or crown over head to visualize size)
2. Determine vest size (from chest circumference measurement)
3. Identify pin-site locations
4. Shave hair at posterior pin sites
5. Prepare pin sites with povidone-iodine solution
6. Apply local anesthesia
7. Advance sterile pins to level of skin
8. Have patient close eyes
9. Tighten pins at 2–in-lb increments in diagonal fashion
10. Tighten pins to 8–in-lb torque
11. Apply lock nuts to pins
12. Maintain cervical traction and raise patient trunk to 30°
13. Apply posterior portion of vest
14. Apply anterior portion of vest
15. Connect anterior and posterior portions of vest
16. Apply upright posts and attach ring to vest
17. Recheck fittings, screws, and nuts
18. Tape vest-removing tools to vest
19. Obtain cervical spine radiographs

(Adapted with permission from Botte MJ, Garfin SR, Byrne TP, Woo SL, Nickel VL: The halo skeletal fixator: Principles of application and maintenance. *Clin Orthop Relat Res* 1989;239: 12-18.)

region the skull has a thin outer and inner table with minimal cancellous diploe.[39]

Pin location for the posterior pins is less critical than for anterior pins. There are no neuromuscular structures at risk, and the skull has a nearly uniform thickness, with the thickest section being straight posterior. Direct posterior pin placement should be avoided, however, because the patient would lie on this pin when supine. The pins are usually placed diagonally opposite to the anterior pins, approximately 1 cm superior to the upper helix of the ear. Care should be taken to avoid any contact between the ring/pin and ear, while remaining inferior enough to the equator of the skull to prevent superior pin migration.[38]

Because the halo is not a static, unidirectional device, shear forces act at each of the pin sites. In a biomechanical study, Triggs et al[40] evaluated the transverse shear forces to failure of pins placed in decremental angles at 90°, 75°, and 60°. The load to deformity and failure were substantially higher for pins inserted perpendicular to the outer cortex of the skull as compared to 60°. To minimize the incidence of pin loosening, it is important to try to place pins as perpendicular to the skull as possible to provide the most strength at the pin-bone interface. As skull shapes differ, however, placing pins perpendicular to the tangent of the skull may be difficult.

Empiric observations led to early recommendations for pin-insertion torque of 6 in-lb. Cadaveric studies, however, have shown that pins inserted at up to 10 in-lb of pressure barely penetrate the outer table.[38] Biomechanical testing has demonstrated that 8 in-lb of insertional torque offers a more rigid pin-bone interface when compared to 6 in-lb.[41] Clinical trials in adults have borne this out, with reduced pin-site loosening, as well as less infection at the pin sites.[38]

Application of the halo apparatus should proceed in a stepwise fashion (**Table 2**). After ring application, with the cervical spine protected by manual traction, the patient's trunk can be elevated 30° for vest placement. The posterior portion of the vest is applied and connected to the halo, followed by the anterior portion. Alternative methods include log-rolling the patient, although it may be difficult to maintain cervical alignment. A recent cadaveric study demonstrated significant motion in C1-C2 instability models during application.[8] In instances of a "stable" fracture pattern, or following surgical stabilization, the patient can be instructed to sit upright, and the vest can be applied. All the vest locking bolts are then tightened to 28 in-lb of torque preset on the screwdriver. After application of the halo vest is complete, cervical spine alignment should be confirmed radiographically.

Baum et al[42] have documented an immediate 2– to 4–in-lb drop in pin fixation purchase following vest placement. The pins should therefore be retightened 24 to 48 hours after placement. A commonly used pin-care regimen consists of daily cleansing with diluted hydrogen peroxide (50:50 with water) on a cotton swab. Patients should be followed at predetermined intervals for reinspection of the pin sites, confirmation of the tightness of the connections, and reimaging of the injury.

Biomechanical Analysis

Although the halo is the most rigid external form of cervical immobilization, some motion and force transmission to the cervical elements does occur. In early studies, the halo device was reported to permit only 4% of flexion-extension, 4% of lateral bending, and 1% of rotational motion of the normal native cervical spine.[15] However, follow-up studies have shown that such significant immobilization is not routinely accomplished. One study has demonstrated up to 51° of motion with halo immobilization.[18] Segmentally, the greatest motion was observed at the occiput-C1 level (11.5°). The least motion was observed at C2-C3 (6.7°). When flexion was observed at one segment of the spine, extension was observed at another level, a phenomenon known as "snaking." Motion of the cervical spine was observed with patient position changes from supine to prone or from supine to sitting. However, there was no increased motion at the level of injury. In contrast, Anderson et al[43] reported greater than 3° of angulation and 1 mm of translation at the fracture site in 77% of the patients evaluated.

Other studies have examined the directional force generated by the halo device. Maximal forces appear to be exerted in the medial-lateral plane. However, in daily activities, anterior-posterior and vertical forces are much larger. This was confirmed by Lind et al,[18] who observed no horizontal motion in the halo device. They reported significant differences in distractive forces between the supine and upright positions, which they attributed to the added weight of the head. Distractive forces were particularly increased with shoulder shrugging, arm elevation, and deep breathing—although no patient experienced any discomfort. These distractive forces were most elevated in patients with tight-fitting vests. It was noted that the halo vest can be elevated by the sternum and the scapulae. They recommended that there be at least 30 mm of space between the sternum and the vest to prevent gross motion of the vest with daily activities. A vest called the 4PAD (AME/Orthofix, Richardson, TX) has been designed to minimize these forces by using four separate pads strategically placed on the thorax to provide snug fit without elevation from the scapulae.[44] It has not, however, had significant clinical usage. Patients should be cautioned regarding activities that involve substantial twisting and bending, as these tend to transmit undesirable forces to the cervical spine through the halo.

Complications

Although clinical studies have demonstrated the efficacy of the halo device, complications with its use are, unfortunately, not infrequent. Awareness of the most commonly seen complications can help minimize their severity and avoid catastrophic sequelae.

Pin loosening has been identified as one of the most common problems with the halo device.[45] In two large studies, pin loosening was observed in 36% and 60% of patients.[46,47] The hypothesized decrease in compressive pin forces with time was confirmed in a biomechanical study using instrumented halos in three patients. Pin-force values at the time of halo vest application and at subsequent clinical visits were compared by Fleming et al.[48] They measured an 83% drop in torque pressure by the time of halo removal. The authors posited the mechanism of pin loosening was via bone resorption at the pin tip. To help decrease loss of purchase, the pins may be retightened to 8 in-lb of torque as long as resistance is met on the first few turns of the pin and there are no signs of infection. If no resistance is met, then a new pin should be placed in another position. The old pin should be kept in place until the new pin has been rigidly placed, to keep the correct orientation of the ring on the skull.

Halo-pin infection rates have been reported to occur in approximately 20% of cases.[46,47] If drainage and erythema continue at a pin site even with aggressive pin care, bacterial cultures should be obtained and appropriate oral antibiotics started. If cellulitis persists, or an abscess forms, the pin should be removed and placed in another position. The patient may require incision and drainage of the abscess with parenteral antibiotics.[46]

Skull and dural penetration by a halo pin is a rare complication. This is often related to patient falls. Clinically, the patient may experience a headache, malaise, or visual disturbances if symptomatic pin penetration has occurred. Radiographs taken tangential to the skull may demonstrate whether pin perforation of the inner table has occurred. Although CT scans may demonstrate inner table perforation in severe cases, artifact may impair the ability to discern marginal perforations. Clear cerebrospinal fluid leakage from the pin site is a definitive sign that dural puncture has occurred. In these circumstances, a new pin should be placed in another region and the old pin removed.[47] Elevation of the head decreases intracerebral pressure and facilitates spontaneous closure of the dural tear. These tears usually heal in 4 to 5 days. If the tear does not heal or an infection is suspected (subdural abscess), formal surgical intervention may be necessary.[49]

Falls leading to such complications may be due to impairment of balance.[50] Using three-dimensional motion analysis, Ohnishi et al[51] evaluated the effects of a halo vest on gait. They found that use of a halo vest increases stride time, shortens stride length, and restricts motion between the shoulder girdle and trunk, between the trunk and pelvis, and decreases motion at the hip.[51]

Patients may report difficulty with swallowing during halo immobilization. Deglutition dysfunction leading to aspiration has been reported.[52] Many instances of swallowing difficulty are a result of the cervical spine's immobilization in the extended position. Morishima et al[53]performed a study in which patients were immobilized in various degrees of sagittal alignment using a noninvasive halo. Radiographic, electromyographic, and video fluoroscopic evaluations were performed. In hyperextension, several changes were noted in pharyngeal transit time, hyoid initial position and movement, suprahyoid muscle function, and laryngeal penetration.[53] Efforts to flex the cervical spine, while maintaining cervical reduction, may assist in dysphagia resolution.[46]

Pressure sores have been reported in 4% to 11% of patients during halo immobilization.[46] These sores frequently develop underneath the vest, or cast vest, secondary to pressure against prominent bony surfaces or due to insufficient padding or incorrect sizing of the vest. Principles of pressure-sore prevention include frequent turning, adequate vest padding, and routine skin inspections. Pressure sores are more prevalent in patient populations using a cast vest, rather than the padded prefabricated plastic vest. This is especially important in patients with neurologic deficits who may not have normal sensation over their trunk. Alternative strategies to halo immobilization, such as rigid internal fixation, should be considered in this patient population (spinal cord injury). In severe cases, pressure-sore treatment may require split-thickness skin grafting and/or employing rotational muscle flaps for coverage.[44]

Recently, concerns have been raised about the use of halo immobilization in elderly patients. Some studies have reported significantly higher complication rates and mortality in elderly patients treated with halo immobilization compared with other treatments and compared with halo immobilization in younger patients.[54-57] Because of these concerns, some have suggested that surgical treatment (especially for displaced type II odontoid fractures) should be strongly considered in elderly patients. Other studies have cited that although complications are common, most are minor with no increased risk for pneumonia or mortality.[58,59]

Pediatric Halo Considerations

Children and infants have been successfully treated with halo immobilization following both unstable cervical injuries and congenital abnormalities.[60,61] Because the skull is thinner and more pliable in children than in adults, the recommended pin torque pressure in children is 2 in-lb to 5 in-lb.[60] A multiple, low-torque pin-insertion technique is recommended to achieve maximal stability in infants and children younger than 3 years of age.[62]

In young children up to 12 years of age, pins can be inserted at 2 in-lb of torque pressure under general anesthesia. Halo pins should be placed under the largest diameter of the skull, taking care to avoid the frontal sinus and temporal regions. A CT scan of the head may be beneficial to identify the location of suture lines and bone fragments (in congenital cases) before placement of the halo. To prevent skull deformity in the presence of open suture lines and fontanelles, vigilant care must be taken to symmetrically distribute pressure on the skull through the halo pins.

A custom-made ring and vest are often required due to sizing issues in this age group. Once the halo is placed, the vest is applied in normal fashion and connected to the halo. Children require the same pin care as adults. Baum et al[42] observed that children have a higher rate of pin loosening than adults. Children with halo fixators should have close parental supervision and frequent medical follow-up.

Lumbar, Thoracolumbar, and Sacral Orthoses

Sacroiliac orthoses (SIOs), lumbosacral orthoses (LSOs), and thoracolumbosacral orthoses (TLSOs) are available in flexible and rigid variations. The flexible versions have similar designs compared to their rigid counterparts, but provide only mild immobilization. SIOs generally encircle the pelvis, spanning the tops of the iliac crests to the trochanters. These may provide relief in traumatic postpartum separation of the sacroiliac joints. LSOs extend from the pelvis to the xiphoid anteriorly and the inferior angle of the scapula posteriorly. TLSOs extend higher, generally to the midscapular level.

FIGURE 11

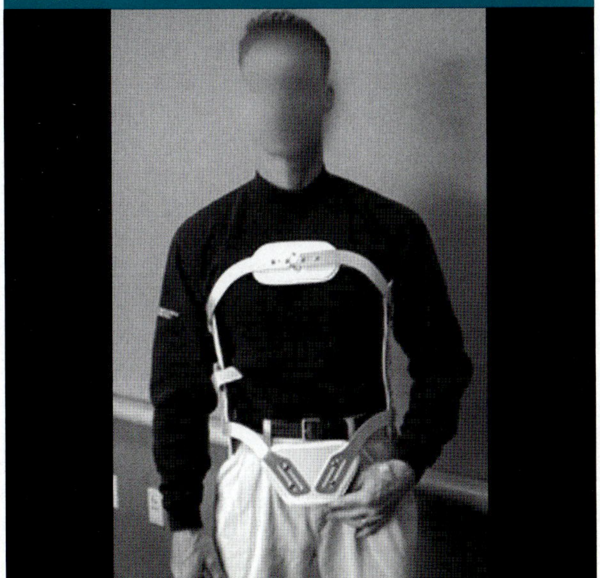

Figure 11 Jewett brace. The anterior pads rest on the sternum and pubic symphysis. The posterior pad crosses the upper lumbar spine. The design attempts to provide extension with three-point fixation.

FIGURE 12

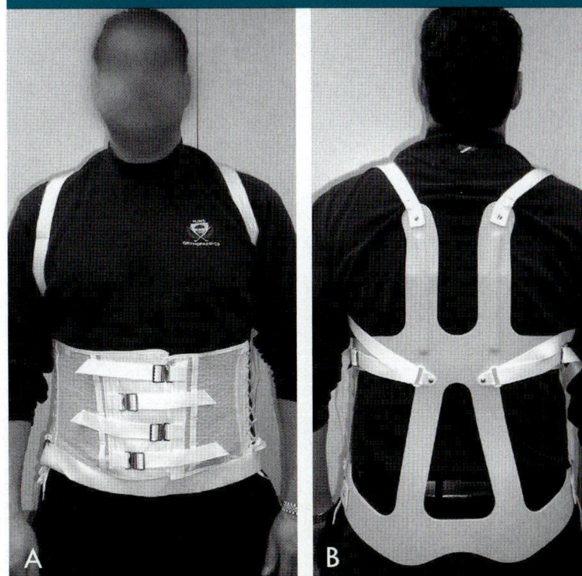

Figure 12 Knight-Taylor orthosis: **A,** frontal view; **B,** posterior view. Control of thoracic sagittal plane motion is achieved through axillary straps attached to posterior thoracic uprights.

Most conventional TLSOs are more effective in limiting motion in the sagittal plane than in controlling rotation or lateral bending. The Jewett hyperextension brace is a commonly prescribed noncustom-molded TLSO brace (**Figure 11**). It applies three-point fixation to the torso through anterior pads on the symphysis pubis and sternum and a posterior pad midway between the anterior pads. This arrangement of forces places the spine in slight extension. Similar to cervical collars, this brace is best in controlling motion in the flexion-extension plane, and less effective in controlling lateral bending and rotation. The Knight-Taylor brace (**Figure 12**) is another commonly used TLSO, and can be prefabricated or custom-molded. It has a corset-style front for abdominal compression and lateral and posterior uprights attached to over-the shoulder straps for thoracic control. Prefabricated TLSOs often consist of clamshell-style braces that can be ordered to measurements, and usually are fabricated out of 1/8- to 3/16-in low-density polyethylene with a full 1/4-in foam liner. The anterior and posterior shells are fastened in place with three Velcro closures per side. Some manufacturers include pneumatic bladders in the abdominal and/or lumbar areas to help customize the fit and accommodate volume changes. Prefabricated "customizable" TLSOs are also commercially available with apron-style fronts that can be adjusted with Velcro straps and telescoping sternal pads (**Figure 13**). These braces provide good control in all three planes, but once again, the major restriction is in the flexion-extension plane. Body habitus is an important consideration when attempting to use a

FIGURE 13

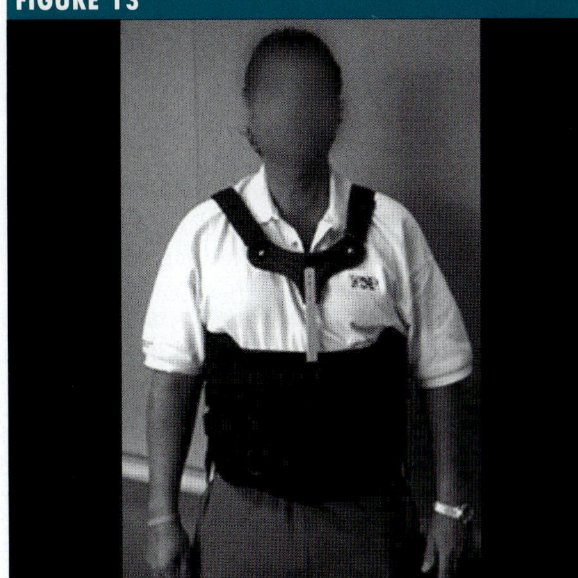

Figure 13 Prefabricated "customizable" TLSO. This particular design (Orthomerica, Orlando, FL) has an apron-style front with a telescoping sternal pad to help customize the fit.

FIGURE 14

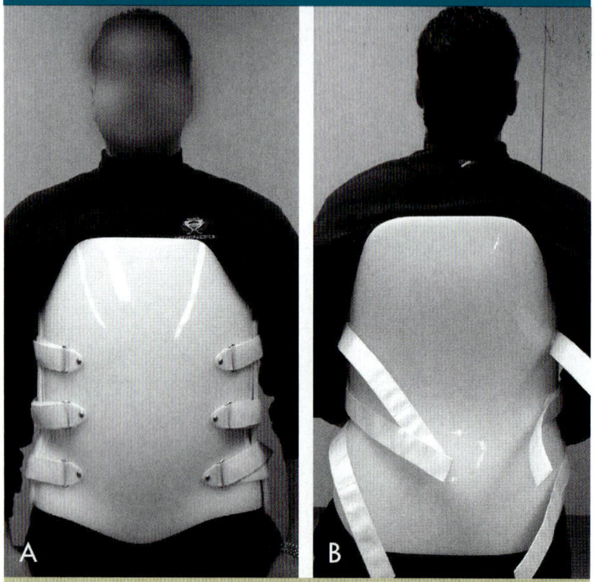

Figure 14 Custom-molded TLSO: **A,** frontal view; **B,** posterior view. This bivalve design is made from a plaster cast of the patient.

prefabricated orthosis. In an obese patient, a pendulous abdomen may prevent the anterior panel from making adequate contact with the sternum or pubic symphysis. For optimal control in all three planes in an unstable injury or challenging body habitus, a fully custom-molded TLSO (**Figure 14**) should be used. These are often formed from high-temperature thermoplastic that is custom-fitted from a plaster cast formed from the patient, or from computer-aided designs from body measurements at key points. When immobilization proximal to T5 is required, a cervical extension should be included.[63] If rigid immobilization distal to L4 is needed, a thigh cuff should be added to the orthosis to control pelvic motion.[64,65]

In comparison to COs, relatively few studies have been performed to scientifically evaluate the ability of external orthoses to immobilize the thoracolumbosacral spine. The earliest data on motion restriction with lumbar external supports was reported by Brown and Norton.[64] They evaluated three rigid LSOs, one flexible LSO, and a TLSO. Kirschner wires were inserted into the spinous processes of volunteers. The angles between the wires were measured to determine the amount of motion. Radiographic evaluation was also performed. Of note, they reported increased motion across the lumbosacral junction in all of the braces. Increased motion at L4-L5 was also noted while the volunteers were sitting. Compared with the unbraced state, all of the braces resulted in some flexion at L4-L5 and L5-S1 while standing. Lumsden and Morris[66] reported similar findings when they studied lumbosacral rotational motion in individuals wearing either a chairback brace or LSO corset. Volunteers had Steinmann pins placed in their posterior superior iliac spines. Motion was determined by radiographs and measurement of pin rotation. In each case, they found the braces increased motion at the lumbosacral level.[66] Fidler and Plasmans[65] used radiographs to compare the effect on lumbosacral motion of a corset, a brace, and a plaster jacket with and without a thigh cuff. They found the custom-molded plaster jacket to provide the best immobilization at the L1-L3 level. To improve immobilization at the L4-S1 levels, they recommended adding a thigh cuff to the orthosis.

Vander Kooi et al[67] evaluated the stabilization provided by a TLSO using video fluoroscopy. They assessed dynamic motion of the L3-L5 vertebral bodies under four conditions: unbraced, with a custom-fitted TLSO, with the TLSO and thigh extender at 0°, and again at 15°. They found that the TLSO reduced both the total L3-L5 range of motion and the intervertebral motion at each individual segment. Total rotation at L3 (with respect to the horizontal) was reduced from 70° without a brace to 50° with a TLSO. Addition of a thigh extension provided additional reduction to 10°. There was no significant difference between having the thigh extender at 0° or 15°.

Specific indications for TLSOs are less well defined than for COs. Bracing for compression fractures of the thoracolumbar spine is not tolerated well by the elderly. Treatment in these patients usually consists of early mobilization, close follow-up, and, in some cases, percutaneous cement augmentation procedures. A soft binder or corset may provide support and symptomatic relief. The cruciform anterior spinal hyperextension (CASH) brace (**Figure 15**) is another lightweight alternative that may be reasonably tolerated. In younger patients, however, anterior column fractures are often the result of greater energy than their osteoporotic counterparts, and therefore a more cautious approach is often favored. These patients are commonly treated with a Jewett or Knight-Taylor brace. However, the need for rigid bracing of these fractures is still a matter of debate. Ohana et al[68] retrospectively reviewed the outcome of 129 young patients with mild compression fractures who were treated with or without a Jewett hyperextension brace. They found that one-column fractures of the thoracolumbar spine with as much as 30% compression can be safely treated without

FIGURE 15

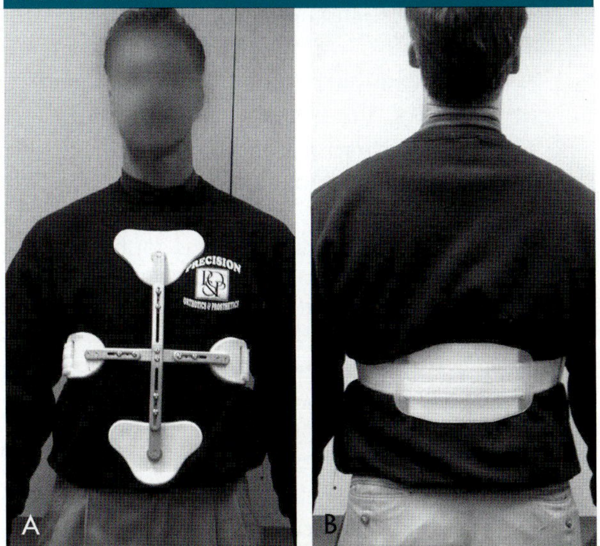

Figure 15 CASH brace: **A,** frontal view; **B,** posterior view. The lightweight design is better tolerated by elderly patients compared with bulkier braces.

FIGURE 16

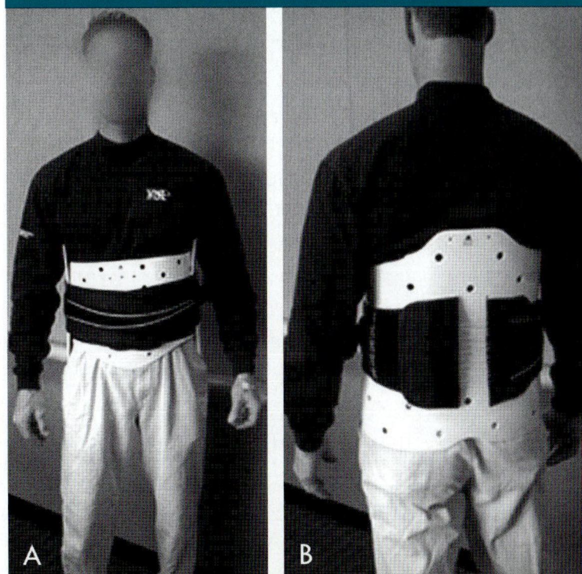

Figure 16 Prefabricated LSO: **A,** frontal view; **B,** posterior view. This design (California Compression Jacket, Orthomerica, Orlando, FL) has a "rip cord" used to adjust the snugness of the fit.

bracing, instead prescribing early ambulation, hyperextension exercises, and close follow-up.[68]

Burst fractures comprise another common entity in the spectrum of thoracolumbar injuries. Historically, neurologically intact patients with burst fractures were treated with bed rest for 4 to 12 weeks, followed by progressive mobilization. Today, controversy exists as to which injuries require surgical stabilization and which can be treated with bracing and early mobilization. Neurologic deficit is often an indication for surgical management. Other fairly well-accepted criteria for surgery, rather than bracing, include canal compromise of 50% or more, kyphotic deformity of greater than 30°, posterior column involvement, or tensile failure of the posterior ligamentous structures. Chow et al[69] retrospectively studied functional outcomes in 24 patients treated with hyperextension body casts and/or Jewett hyperextension braces for thoracolumbar burst fractures. None of these patients had posterior column fractures, significant kyphosis, or neurologic deficit. Patients were initially treated with bed rest and log-roll precautions until the predictable ileus and abdominal distension resolved 2 to 3 days later. At that point, patients were casted or braced and progressively mobilized. Patients were followed for a minimum of 1 year. They concluded that hyperextension casting or bracing with early mobilization reduced hospital time, avoided costs and risks of surgery, and allowed patients a relatively early return to work. Additionally, the authors mentioned that patients treated nonsurgically tended to experience moderate back pain up to a year after the injury, and that this pain eventually diminished over time.[69] A prospective, randomized study compared surgical versus nonsurgical treatment of stable thoracolumbar burst fractures without neurologic deficit.[70] Forty-seven consecutive patients were randomized to one of the two treatment groups; nonsurgical treatment employed either a body cast or a TLSO.[70] The authors found that surgical treatment of patients with such injuries provided no major long-term advantage compared with nonsurgical treatment.

More recently, the need for bracing in stable burst fractures without posterior ligamentous involvement has been questioned, after a systematic review of the literature found little evidence to support their use.[71] An interim analysis of a multicenter randomized clinical equivalence trial was recently published. This study found no difference between treatment with a TLSO and no orthosis at 3 months as measured with Roland Morris Disability Questionnaires for patients with AO type A3 bursts.[72] The study's authors, however, acknowledge that the influence of a brace on 1- and 2-year outcomes or on pain control and function remains to be determined.

LSOs (**Figure 16**) are often prescribed after arthrodesis for degenerative conditions of the lower lumbar spine. As discussed above, several studies demonstrate little or no immobilizing effect from wearing LSOs, and possibly an increase in L4-L5, L5-S1 motion after application of these orthoses. The point continues to be debated. Post–lumbar-fusion bracing is felt by some to help relieve pain and decrease the risk of pseudarthrosis and fixation failure, and is, therefore, prescribed by some surgeons for up to 12 weeks postoperatively. Others believe that LSOs do little to immobilize the lumbar spine beyond the stabilization provided by rigid surgical fixation.[73] Rohlmann et al[74] evaluated the effect of a brace with regard to loads on internal spinal fixation devices. Implant loads were measured using telemeterized fixators in six patients for several positions and activities, including sitting, standing, walking, bending forward, and lifting an extended leg in a supine position. They found that none of the braces tested were able to markedly reduce the loads on the fixators. They observed that higher fixator loads were often observed while wearing a brace. A more common role for postoperative bracing in the spinal trauma setting is as an adjuvant to posterior stabilization for unstable burst fractures. A TLSO is often prescribed when short-segment pedicle screw constructs have been used in the presence of anterior column structural insufficiency.

Summary

Spinal orthoses are commonly prescribed for the management of spinal injuries. There are many different types commercially available. The scientific evidence to document their effectiveness is variable. Despite the potential for complications, the halo remains the most rigid of external cervical immobilizers. A thorough appreciation of the biomechanics of spinal orthoses and their potential complications can help maximize their utility and minimize associated morbidity when treating spinal injuries.

Acknowledgment

The orthoses in the photographs were supplied by Precision Orthotics and Prosthetics, Linden, NJ. The models wearing the braces are Paul Goodman, CO, and David Sussman, CPO, both of Precision Orthotics and Prosthetics. We greatly appreciate their contribution to this chapter.

References

1. Smith GE: The most ancient splints. *BMJ* 1908;1: 732-734.
2. Peltier LF: *Orthopedics: A History and Iconography*. San Francisco, CA, Norman Publishing, 1993.
3. Edwards JW: *Orthopaedic Appliances Atlas*. St. Louis, MO, American Academy of Orthopaedic Surgeons, 1952.
4. The Committee on Prosthetics and Orthotics, American Academy of Orthopaedic Surgeons: *Atlas of Orthotics: Biomechanical Principles and Application*. St. Louis, MO, CV Mosby, 1975.
5. White AA, Panjabi MM: Physical properties and functional biomechanics of the spine, in White AA, Panjabi MM, eds: *Clinical Biomechanics of the Spine*, ed 2. Philadelphia, PA, JB Lippincott, 1990.
6. Fisher SV, Bowar JF, Awad EA, Gullickson G Jr: Cervical orthoses effect on cervical spine motion: Roentgenographic and goniometric method of study. *Arch Phys Med Rehabil* 1977;58(3):109-115.
7. Bell KM, Frazier EC, Shively CM, et al: Assessing range of motion to evaluate the adverse effects of ill-fitting cervical orthoses. *Spine J* 2009;9(3): 225-231.
8. DiPaola CP, Sawers A, Conrad BP, et al: Comparing cervical spine motion with different halo devices in a cadaveric cervical instability model. *Spine (Phila Pa 1976)* 2009;34(2):149-155.
9. Chase AP, Bader DL, Houghton GR: The biomechanical effectiveness of the Boston brace in the management of adolescent idiopathic scoliosis. *Spine (Phila Pa 1976)* 1989;14(6):636-642.
10. Willner S: Effect of the Boston thoracic brace on the frontal and sagittal curves of the spine. *Acta Orthop Scand* 1984;55(4):457-460.
11. Sypert GW: External spinal orthotics. *Neurosurgery* 1987;20(4):642-649.
12. Wong MS, Cheng JC, Wong MW, So SF: A work study of the CAD/CAM method and conventional manual method in the fabrication of spinal orthoses for patients with adolescent idiopathic scoliosis. *Prosthet Orthot Int* 2005;29(1):93-104.
13. Cottalorda J, Kohler R, Garin C, Genevois P, Lecante C, Berge B: Orthoses for mild scoliosis: A prospective study comparing traditional plaster mold manufacturing with fast, noncontact, 3-dimensional acquisition. *Spine (Phila Pa 1976)* 2005;30(4):399-405.
14. Miller CP, Bible JE, Jegede KA, Whang PG, Grauer JN: Soft and rigid collars provide similar restriction in cervical range of motion during fifteen activities of daily living. *Spine (Phila Pa 1976)* 2010;35(13):1271-1278.
15. Johnson RM, Hart DL, Simmons EF, Ramsby GR, Southwick WO: Cervical orthoses: A study comparing their effectiveness in restricting cervical

motion in normal subjects. *J Bone Joint Surg Am* 1977;59(3):332-339.

16. Colachis SC Jr, Strohm BR: Radiographic studies of cervical spine motion in normal subjects: Flexion and hyperextension. *Arch Phys Med Rehabil* 1965;46(11):753-760.
17. Hartman JT, Palumbo F, Hill BJ: Cineradiography of the braced normal cervical spine: A comparative study of five commonly used cervical orthoses. *Clin Orthop Relat Res* 1975;109:97-102.
18. Lind B, Sihlbom H, Nordwall A: Forces and motions across the neck in patients treated with halo-vest. *Spine (Phila Pa 1976)* 1988;13(2): 162-167.
19. Askins V, Eismont FJ: Efficacy of five cervical orthoses in restricting cervical motion: A comparison study. *Spine (Phila Pa 1976)* 1997;22(11): 1193-1198.
20. Chin KR, Auerbach JD, Adams SB Jr, Sodl JF, Riew KD: Mastication causing segmental spinal motion in common cervical orthoses. *Spine (Phila Pa 1976)* 2006;31(4):430-434.
21. Chendrasekhar A, Moorman DW, Timberlake GA: An evaluation of the effects of semirigid cervical collars in patients with severe closed head injury. *Am Surg* 1998;64(7):604-606.
22. Plaisier B, Gabram SG, Schwartz RJ, Jacobs LM: Prospective evaluation of craniofacial pressure in four different cervical orthoses. *J Trauma* 1994; 37(5):714-720.
23. Hunt K, Hallworth S, Smith M: The effects of rigid collar placement on intracranial and cerebral perfusion pressures. *Anaesthesia* 2001;56(6): 511-513.
24. Cline JR, Scheidel E, Bigsby EF: A comparison of methods of cervical immobilization used in patient extrication and transport. *J Trauma* 1985; 25(7):649-653.
25. Podolsky S, Baraff LJ, Simon RR, Hoffman JR, Larmon B, Ablon W: Efficacy of cervical spine immobilization methods. *J Trauma* 1983;23(6): 461-465.
26. Del Rossi G, Heffernan TP, Horodyski M, Rechtine GR: The effectiveness of extrication collars tested during the execution of spine-board transfer techniques. *Spine J* 2004;4(6):619-623.
27. Johnson RM, Owen JR, Hart DL, Callahan RA: Cervical orthoses: A guide to their selection and use. *Clin Orthop Relat Res* 1981;154:34-45.
28. Benzel EC, Larson SJ, Kerk JJ, et al: The thermoplastic Minerva body jacket: A clinical comparison with other cervical spine splinting techniques. *J Spinal Disord* 1992;5(3):311-319.
29. Millington PJ, Ellingsen JM, Hauswirth BE, Fabian PJ: Thermoplastic Minerva body jacket–A practical alternative to current methods of cervical spine stabilization: A clinical report. *Phys Ther* 1987;67(2):223-225.
30. Sharpe KP, Rao S, Ziogas A: Evaluation of the effectiveness of the Minerva cervicothoracic orthosis. *Spine (Phila Pa 1976)* 1995;20(13):1475-1479.
31. Zeleznik R, Chapin W, Hart D, Smith H, Southwick WO, Zito M: Yale cervical orthosis: Fabrication. *Phys Ther* 1978;58(7):861-864.
32. Johnson RM, Hart DL, Owen JR, Lerner E, Chapin W, Zeleznik R: The Yale cervical orthosis: An evaluation of its effectiveness in restricting cervical motion in normal subjects and a comparison with other cervical orthoses. *Phys Ther* 1978; 58(7):865-871.
33. Perry J, Nickel VL: Total cervicalspine fusion for neck paralysis. *J Bone Joint Surg Am* 1959;41(1): 37-60.
34. Botte MJ, Garfin SR, Byrne TP, Woo SL, Nickel VL: The halo skeletal fixator: Principles of application and maintenance. *Clin Orthop Relat Res* 1989;239:12-18.
35. Botte MJ, Byrne TP, Abrams RA, Garfin SR: Halo skeletal fixation: Techniques of application and prevention of complications. *J Am Acad Orthop Surg* 1996;4(1):44-53.
36. Lerman JA, Haynes RJ: Open versus closed halo rings: Comparison of fixation strengths. *Spine (Phila Pa 1976)* 2001;26(19):2102-2104.
37. Mirza SK, Moquin RR, Anderson PA, Tencer AF, Steinmann J, Varnau D: Stabilizing properties of the halo apparatus. *Spine (Phila Pa 1976)* 1997; 22(7):727-733.
38. Botte MJ, Byrne TP, Garfin SR: Application of the halo device for immobilization of the cervical spine utilizing an increased torque pressure. *J Bone Joint Surg Am* 1987;69(5):750-752.
39. Garfin SR, Botte MJ, Centeno RS, Nickel VL: Osteology of the skull as it affects halo pin placement. *Spine (Phila Pa 1976)* 1985;10(8):696-698.
40. Triggs KJ, Ballock RT, Lee TQ, Woo SL, Garfin SR: The effect of angled insertion on halo pin fixation. *Spine (Phila Pa 1976)* 1989;14(8): 781-783.
41. Garfin SR, Lee TQ, Roux RD, et al: Structural behavior of the halo orthosis pin-bone interface: Biomechanical evaluation of standard and newly designed stainless steel halo fixation pins. *Spine (Phila Pa 1976)* 1986;11(10):977-981.
42. Baum JA, Hanley EN Jr, Pullekines J: Comparison of halo complications in adults and children. *Spine (Phila Pa 1976)* 1989;14(3):251-252.
43. Anderson PA, Budorick TE, Easton KB, Henley MB, Salciccioli GG: Failure of halo vest to prevent in vivo motion in patients with injured cervical spines. *Spine (Phila Pa 1976)* 1991;16(10, Suppl) S501-S505.

44. Fukui Y, Krag M, Huston D, Ambrose T, Vaccaro AR: Halovest dynamic loads: full crossover comparison of three vest types. *Spine (Phila Pa 1976)* 2002;27(3):241-249.

45. Glaser JA, Whitehill R, Stamp WG, Jane JA: Complications associated with the halo-vest: A review of 245 cases. *J Neurosurg* 1986;65(6):762-769.

46. Lind B, Sihlbom H, Nordwall A: Halo-vest treatment of unstable traumatic cervical spine injuries. *Spine (Phila Pa 1976)* 1988;13(4):425-432.

47. Garfin SR, Botte MJ, Waters RL, Nickel VL: Complications in the use of the halo fixation device. *J Bone Joint Surg Am* 1986;68(3):320-325.

48. Fleming BC, Krag MH, Huston DR, Sugihara S: Pin loosening in a halo-vest orthosis: A biomechanical study. *Spine (Phila Pa 1976)* 2000;25(11): 1325-1331.

49. Garfin SR, Botte MJ, Triggs KJ, Nickel VL: Subdural abscess associated with halo-pin traction. *J Bone Joint Surg Am* 1988;70(9):1338-1340.

50. Richardson JK, Ross AD, Riley B, Rhodes RL: Halo vest effect on balance. *Arch Phys Med Rehabil* 2000;81(3):255-257.

51. Ohnishi K, Miyamoto K, Kato T, Shimizu K: Effects of wearing halo vest on gait: Three-dimensional analysis in healthy subjects. *Spine (Phila Pa 1976)* 2005;30(7):750-755.

52. Kelly PM, Beregin D, Cunningham U, Higgins T, Poynton AR, Walsh MG: Deglutition dysfunction in cervical orthosis. *J Bone Joint Surg Br* 2002; 84-B(Suppl 1):2-3.

53. Morishima N, Ohota K, Miura Y: The influences of Halo-vest fixation and cervical hyperextension on swallowing in healthy volunteers. *Spine (Phila Pa 1976)* 2005;30(7):E179-E182.

54. Majercik S, Tashjian RZ, Biffl WL, Harrington DT, Cioffi WG: Halo vest immobilization in the elderly: A death sentence? *J Trauma* 2005;59(2): 350-358.

55. Tashjian RZ, Majercik S, Biffl WL, Palumbo MA, Cioffi WG: Halo-vest immobilization increases early morbidity and mortality in elderly odontoid fractures. *J Trauma* 2006;60(1):199-203.

56. Lögters T, Hoppe S, Linhart W, et al: On the problem of halo vest treatment in the elderly: Results of a retrospective analysis. *Unfallchirurg* 2006;109(4):306-312.

57. Taitsman LA, Altman DT, Hecht AC, Pedlow FX: Complications of cervical halo-vest orthoses in elderly patients. *Orthopedics* 2008;31(5):446.

58. van Middendorp JJ, Slooff WB, Nellestein WR, Oner FC: Incidence of and risk factors for complications associated with halo-vest immobilization: A prospective, descriptive cohort study of 239 patients. *J Bone Joint Surg Am* 2009;91(1): 71-79.

59. Daentzer D, Flörkemeier T: Conservative treatment of upper cervical spine injuries with the halo vest: An appropriate option for all patients independent of their age? *J Neurosurg Spine* 2009; 10(6):543-550.

60. Kopits SE, Steingass MH: Experience with the "halo-cast" in small children. *Surg Clin North Am* 1970;50(4):935-943.

61. Osenbach RK, Menezes AH: Pediatric spinal cord and vertebral column injury. *Neurosurgery* 1992; 30(3):385-390.

62. Mubarak SJ, Camp JF, Vuletich W, Wenger DR, Garfin SR: Halo application in the infant. *J Pediatr Orthop* 1989;9(5):612-614.

63. White AA, Panjabi MM: *Clinical Biomechanics of the Spine*. Toronto, Ontario, Canada, JB Lippincott, 1978.

64. Brown T, Norton PL: The immobilizing efficiency of back braces: Their effect on the posture and motion of the lumbosacral spine. *J Bone Joint Surg Am* 1957;39(1):111-139.

65. Fidler MW, Plasmans CM: The effect of four types of support on the segmental mobility of the lumbosacral spine. *J Bone Joint Surg Am* 1983;65(7): 943-947.

66. Lumsden RM II, Morris JM: An in vivo study of axial rotation and immoblization at the lumbosacral joint. *J Bone Joint Surg Am* 1968;50(8): 1591-1602.

67. Vander Kooi D, Abad G, Basford JR, Maus TP, Yaszemski MJ, Kaufman KR: Lumbar spine stabilization with a thoracolumbosacral orthosis: Evaluation with video fluoroscopy. *Spine (Phila Pa 1976)* 2004;29(1):100-104.

68. Ohana N, Sheinis D, Rath E, Sasson A, Atar D: Is there a need for lumbar orthosis in mild compression fractures of the thoracolumbar spine? A retrospective study comparing the radiographic results between early ambulation with and without lumbar orthosis. *J Spinal Disord* 2000;13(4): 305-308.

69. Chow GH, Nelson BJ, Gebhard JS, Brugman JL, Brown CW, Donaldson DH: Functional outcome of thoracolumbar burst fractures managed with hyperextension casting or bracing and early mobilization. *Spine (Phila Pa 1976)* 1996;21(18): 2170-2175.

70. Wood K, Buttermann G, Mehbod A, et al: Operative compared with nonoperative treatment of a thoracolumbar burst fracture without neurological deficit: A prospective, randomized study. *J Bone Joint Surg Am* 2003;85-A(5):773-781.

71. Giele BM, Wiertsema SH, Beelen A, et al: No evidence for the effectiveness of bracing in patients with thoracolumbar fractures. *Acta Orthop* 2009; 80(2):226-232.

72. Bailey CS, Dvorak MF, Thomas KC, et al: Comparison of thoracolumbosacral orthosis and no orthosis for the treatment of thoracolumbar burst fractures: Interim analysis of a multicenter randomized clinical equivalence trial. *J Neurosurg Spine* 2009;11(3):295-303.

73. Connolly PJ, Grob D: Bracing of patients after fusion for degenerative problems of the lumbar spine—yes or no? *Spine (Phila Pa 1976)* 1998; 23(12):1426-1428.

74. Rohlmann A, Bergmann G, Graichen F, Neff G: Braces do not reduce loads on internal spinal fixation devices. *Clin Biomech (Bristol, Avon)* 1999; 14(2):97-102.

Appendix

Manufacturers for the Orthoses Named in This Chapter

Product Name	Manufacturer, Location
Cervical and Cervicothoracic Orthoses	
NecLoc	Jerome Medical, Moorestown, NJ
Miami J	Jerome Medical, Moorestown, NJ
Aspen	Aspen Medical Products, Irvine, CA
Malibu	Seattle Systems, Paulsbo, WA
Stifneck	Laerdal Medical Corporation, Wappingers Falls, NY
Philadelphia Collar	Philadelphia Collar Co, Philadelphia, PA
SOMI	Zinco Industries, Pasadena, CA
Ambu	Ambu, Ballerup, Denmark
Minerva (TMBJ)[a]	Seattle Systems, Paulsbo, WA
Minerva (CTO)	Seattle Systems, Paulsbo, WA
Yale	Orthomedics, Brea, CA
Thoracolumbosacral Orthoses	
Jewett	Florida Brace Corp, Winter Park, FL
Knight-Taylor	Orthomerica, Orlando, FL
Cruciform anterior spinal hyperextension (CASH)	Seattle Systems, Paulsbo, WA

[a]TMBJ = thermoplastic Minerva body jacket.

CHAPTER 19
Occipitocervical Trauma

Jonathan G. Roper, MD Daveed D. Frazier, MD Frank J. Eismont, MD

Key Points

- Occipitocervical dislocation is rare in the hospital, but is present in 5% to 12% of traffic fatalities, especially pedestrians struck by cars.
- In patients with occipitocervical dislocations, initial traction can produce severe overdistraction and increased paralysis or death. Initial placement in a halo vest is the safest stabilization.
- Most of the patients with occipitocervical dislocation who come to the emergency department have some degree of spinal cord dysfunction and also have associated cranial nerve palsies.
- Treatment of occipitocervical dislocation always requires a posterior occiput-C2 fusion using autogenous bone graft and this is best supplemented with rod/screw or plate/screw instrumentation.
- Occipital condyle fractures may require occiput-C1 fusion if the fracture compromises the alar ligaments and produces occipitocervical instability.

Introduction

Injuries to the craniocervical junction are commonly seen in the coroner's office, but are seen only rarely in the emergency department. In a postmortem study of 112 victims of trauma, Bucholz and Burkhead[1] found that 9 (8%) had atlanto-occipital dislocations. In a similar study of 50 consecutive fatal craniospinal injuries, Davis et al[2] found that six of the victims (12%) had head-on-neck dislocations. Alker et al,[3] in a review of 146 fatalities from traffic accidents, found occipitoatlantal dislocations in 8 victims (5%). In this and in most series, this injury occurs most commonly in pedestrians struck by cars.

In contrast, only 2 of Bohlman's 300 hospitalized patients with cervical fractures or dislocation or both had occipitocervical dislocations (0.67% incidence), and both patients died after a short period of time.[4] Similarly, Clark et al[5] reviewed 236 patients seen at their hospital and found only 2 occipitocervical dislocations (0.85% incidence), with both patients dying as a result of the injury.

Occipitocervical instability is also seen as the result of certain diseases of the spine,[6] including ankylosing spondylitis[7] and rheumatoid arthritis,[8,9] but these patients have a chronic history of progressive symptoms. This chapter is limited to those patients affected by acute traumatic occipitocervical instability.

There are now many case reports and small series of patients with occipitoatlantal dislocations surviving long enough to be treated.[4,5,10-28] Many of these patients survive over a long term. With the skills and availability of emergency medical services continually improving, it is probable that a higher percentage of patients with this injury will survive long enough to be seen in our emergency departments. Although many will not survive because of the intrinsic nature of the injury, it is important that this injury be promptly recognized and properly treated to maximize the number of patients surviving with this injury and to minimize their neurologic deficit. Govender et al[29] reported four patients who had sustained traumatic dislocation of the atlanto-occipital joint. One patient, who was neurologically intact, was successfully treated nonsurgically. The remaining three recovered neurologically after an occipitocervical fusion.[29]

Normal Anatomy

The occipitocervical junction has been thoroughly studied from both the anatomic and radiographic viewpoints. The bony constraints are limited to the convex occipital condyles articulating with the congruent concave superior lateral masses of the atlas. These joints are flatter and less restrictive in children than in adults, and hence children younger than 12 years of age have increased joint mobility[30,31] and are more predisposed to injury at this level. Another bony constraint is the posterior arch of the atlas, which provides a limit to

Dr. Roper or an immediate family member owns stock or stock options in NuVasive. Dr. Frazier or an immediate family member owns stock or stock options in NuVasive, Orthovita, and Spineology. Dr. Eismont or an immediate family member has received royalties from Alphatec Spine; serves as a paid consultant to Alphatec Spine; and owns stock or stock options in Alphatec Spine.

FIGURE 1

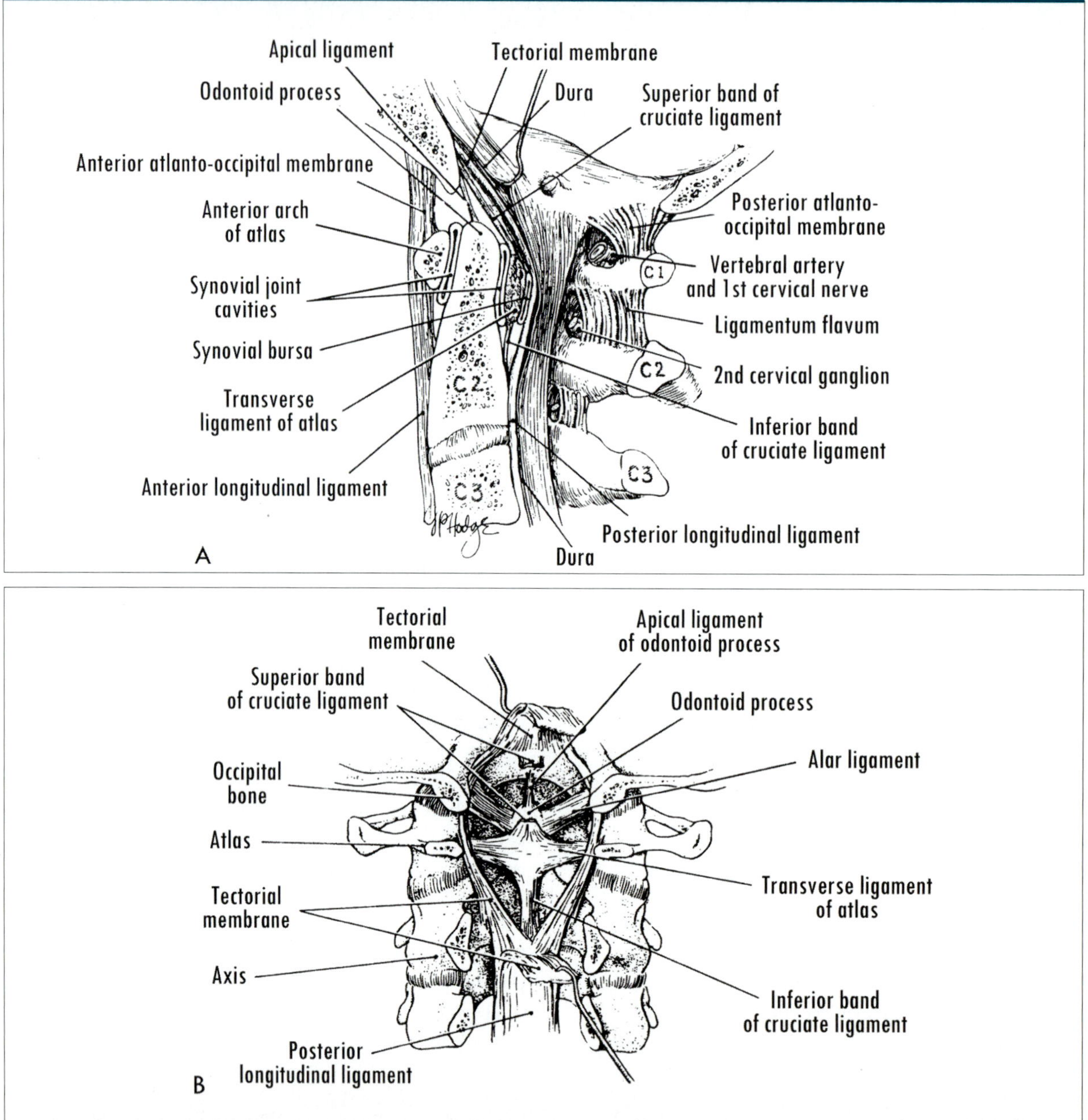

Figure 1 **A,** A midsagittal section through the craniocervical junction. This shows the appropriate relationship of the basion or anterior aspect of the foramen magnum to the ring of C1 and the odontoid process and nicely illustrates the ligaments at the occipitocervical junction. **B,** A coronal section demonstrating the ligaments at the craniocervical junction. Note especially the alar ligaments and the tectorial membrane. (Reproduced with permission from Martel W: The occipito-atlanto-axial joints in rheumatoid arthritis and ankylosing spondylitis. *Am J Roentgenol Radium Ther Nucl Med* 1961;86:223-240.)

occiput-C1 (C0-C1) extension when it abuts against the base of the skull.[32]

There are many ligamentous constraints,[32] but the most formidable are the paired alar ligaments coursing from the superolateral aspect of the odontoid process to the medial aspects of the occipital condyles. The tectorial membrane, which is a superior continuation of the posterior longitudinal ligament, is also very important. Lesser ligamentous restraints include the anterior and posterior atlanto-occipital membrane, the C0-C1 articular joint capsules, and the insignificant apical ligament extending from the tip of the odontoid to the basion (**Figure 1**).

FIGURE 2

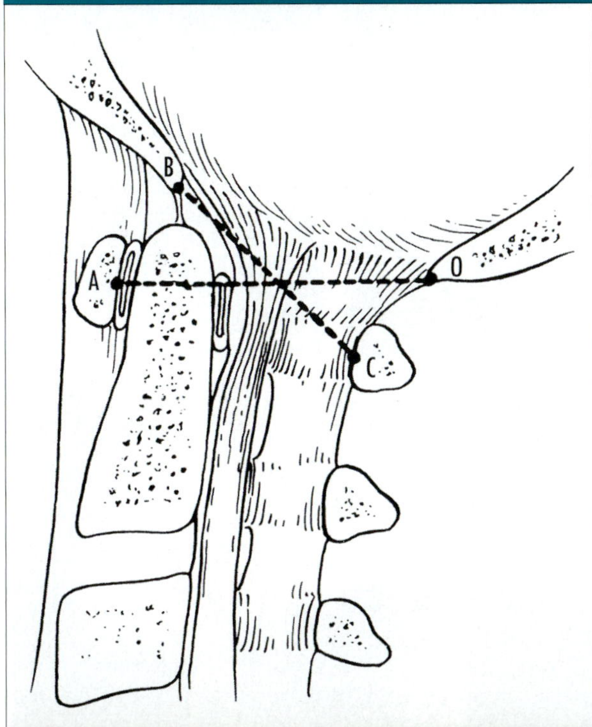

Figure 2 This drawing represents a midsagittal section through the craniocervical junction. B = basion; O = opisthion; A = anterior arch of atlas; C = posterior arch of atlas. The ratio BC/OA should always equal 1 or less. If it is greater than 1, the patient most likely has an anterior occipitocervical subluxation dislocation. (Reproduced with permission from Powers B, Miller MD, Kramer RS, Martinez S, Gehweiler JA Jr: Traumatic anterior atlanto-occipital dislocation. *Neurosurgery* 1979;4(1):12-17.)

FIGURE 3

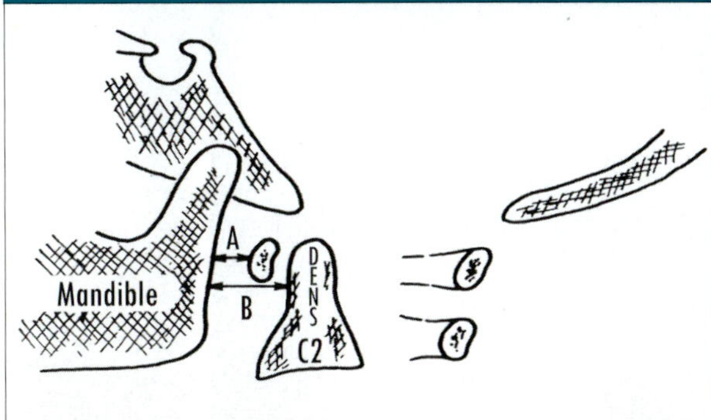

Figure 3 This drawing shows the normal relationship of the posterior ramus of the mandible in relation to the anterior ring of C1 and the dens. Radiographs were taken of 23 normal patients, and distance A averaged 2 mm with a range from –10 mm to +9 mm. The average for distance B was 10 mm, with a range from 2 to 17 mm. Distances significantly greater than these averages denote anterior occipitocervical dislocation, and distances significantly smaller indicate likely posterior occipitocervical dislocation. All radiographs must be done with the patient's mouth closed. (Reproduced with permission from Dublin AB, Marks WM, Weinstock D, Newton TH: Traumatic dislocation of the atlanto-occipital articulation [AOA] with short-term survival: With a radiographic method of measuring the AOA. *J Neurosurg* 1980;52(4):541-546.)

The motion available at the occipitocervical junction is 21° extension, 3° flexion, 7° rotation to each side, and 5° lateral bending to each side.[32,33]

Radiographic Evaluation

Many articles have been written concerning the radiographic assessment of the upper cervical spine and the normal ligamentous and osseous constraints.[9,27,31,34-42] The lateral radiograph should show the basion over the posterior aspect of the odontoid process. It is often stated that the distance from the basion to the top of the odontoid process should be 5 mm or less, but this is not always true. Greater distances are frequently seen in the normal population. In the original study of Wholey et al,[41] the average distance in normal patients was 5 mm, but distances up to 10 mm were observed in infants.

The Powers ratio[38,43] is also useful for assessing occipitocervical alignment (**Figure 2**). Lines are drawn from the opisthion to the anterior arch of the atlas (line OA) and from the basion to the posterior arch of the atlas (line BC). The ratio of distances BC/OA should be 1.0 or less. If the ratio exceeds 1.0, there is probably an anterior occipitoatlantal dislocation. Unfortunately, this ratio will not be helpful in diagnosing the much less common occipitoatlantal posterior dislocation or pure distraction injuries.

Occipitoatlantal dislocation can also be suspected if the posterior ramus of the mandible is too far posterior and overlying the anterior aspect of the C2 vertebra, indicating a posterior occipitoatlantal dislocation. If the posterior ramus of the mandible is too far anterior to the C2 vertebra, this would be consistent with an anterior occipitoatlantal dislocation (**Figures 3** and **4**).[13]

Although seldom indicated in acute cervical injuries, flexion-extension cervical radiographs should reveal C0-C1 translation of 1 mm or less. Translation greater than 1 mm indicates occipitoatlantal instability.[42]

On a lateral radiograph, a line drawn down the sphenoid ridge from the posterior aspect of the sella turcica to the basion should always pass just posterior to the posterior aspect of the dens and

FIGURE 4

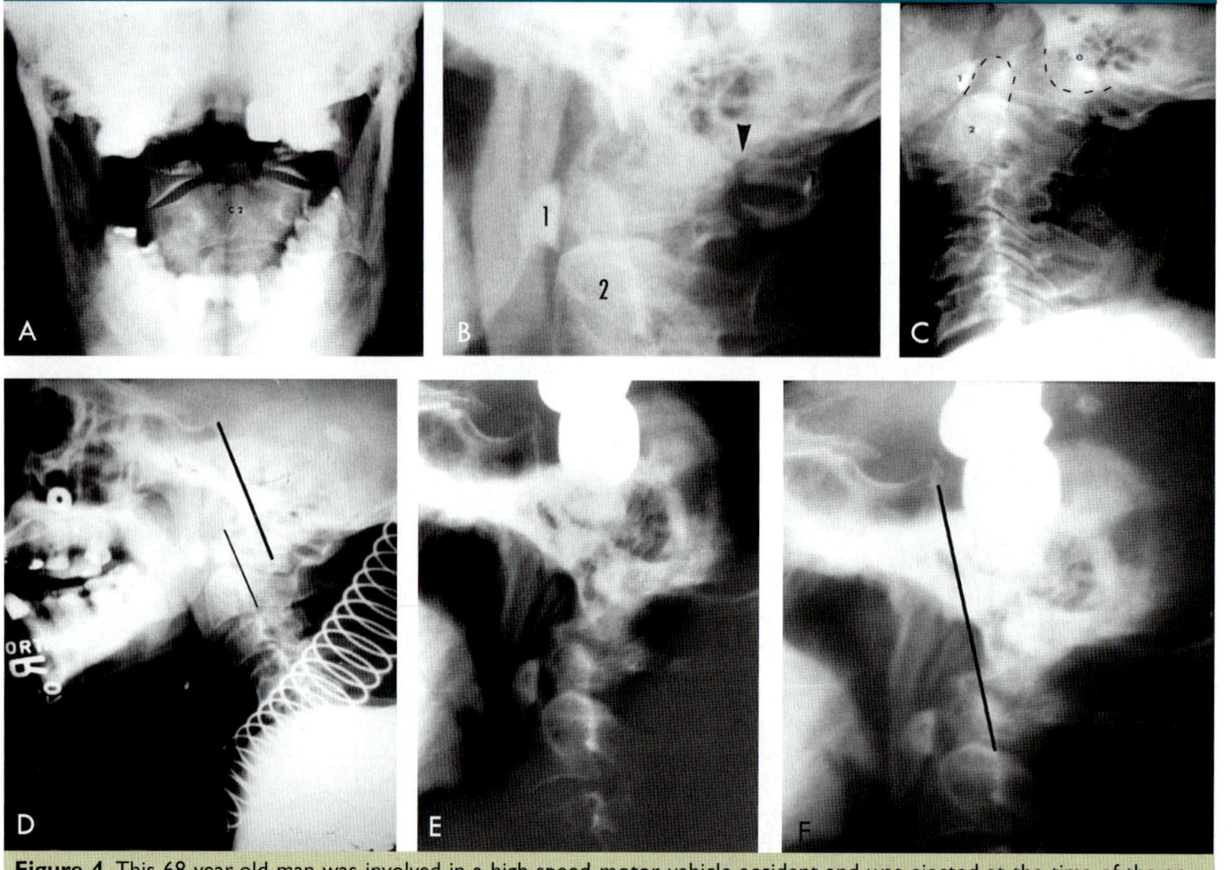

Figure 4 This 68-year-old man was involved in a high-speed motor vehicle accident and was ejected at the time of the accident. He reported neck pain and had a fracture of his femur. He was initially neurologically normal and was placed in a soft cervical collar and his femur was immobilized. **A,** AP radiograph of the upper cervical spine looks relatively normal. **B,** Cone-down lateral radiograph of the upper cervical spine reveals a fracture of the posterior arch of C1 (arrowhead). It also appears that his basion is slightly more posterior than normal. There is significant soft-tissue swelling in the retropharyngeal space at C1 and C2. **C,** At 10 days after injury, the dotted lines mark occipital condyles and the odontoid process. It is apparent that his head is posteriorly displaced on the atlas. At this time, he was in a soft cervical collar. He was experiencing problems with hypertension and paroxysmal atrial tachycardia and respiratory distress associated with a spastic quadriparesis. His head-on-neck dislocation was diagnosed at this time, and he was placed in skull tong traction of 4.6 kg. **D,** Lateral radiograph also shows a posterior dislocation. The thick dark line demonstrates Wackenheim's line extending from the posterior sella turcica down the clivus and over the basion. This line should normally be tangential to the posterior aspect of the odontoid. In this case, there is almost 2 cm of posterior subluxation. It can also be noted that the posterior aspect of the ramus of the mandible significantly overlaps the anterior arch of the atlas, which, according to Dublin's criteria, also denotes posterior occipitocervical dislocation. **E,** Lateral radiograph of the upper cervical spine shows that the occiput is correctly located over the atlas and odontoid but that there is moderate overdistraction. At this time, the weight was reduced to 2.3 kg of traction. The patient's quadriparesis resolved over several hours and his spasticity subsided over approximately 6 weeks. **F,** Wackenheim's line is now drawn and is almost perfectly tangential to the posterior aspect of the odontoid as it would normally be seen. This shows that the posterior occipital subluxation has been corrected. (Reproduced with permission from Eismont FJ, Tay KB: Injuries of the upper cervical spine, in Herkowitz HN, Garfin SR, Eismont FJ, Bell GR, Balderston RA, eds: *The Spine*, ed 5. Philadelphia, PA, Elsevier, 2006, pp 1081-1083 and with permission from Eismont FJ, Bohlman HH: Posterior atlanto-occipital dislocation with fractures of the atlas and odontoid process. *J Bone Joint Surg Am* 1978;60(3):397-399. Other figure elements are from Eismont FJ, Frazier DD: Craniocervical trauma, in Levine AM, Eismont FJ, Garfin SF, Zigler JE, eds: *Spine Trauma*. Philadelphia, PA, WB Saunders, 1998, pp 196-208.)

FIGURE 4 *(CONTINUED)*

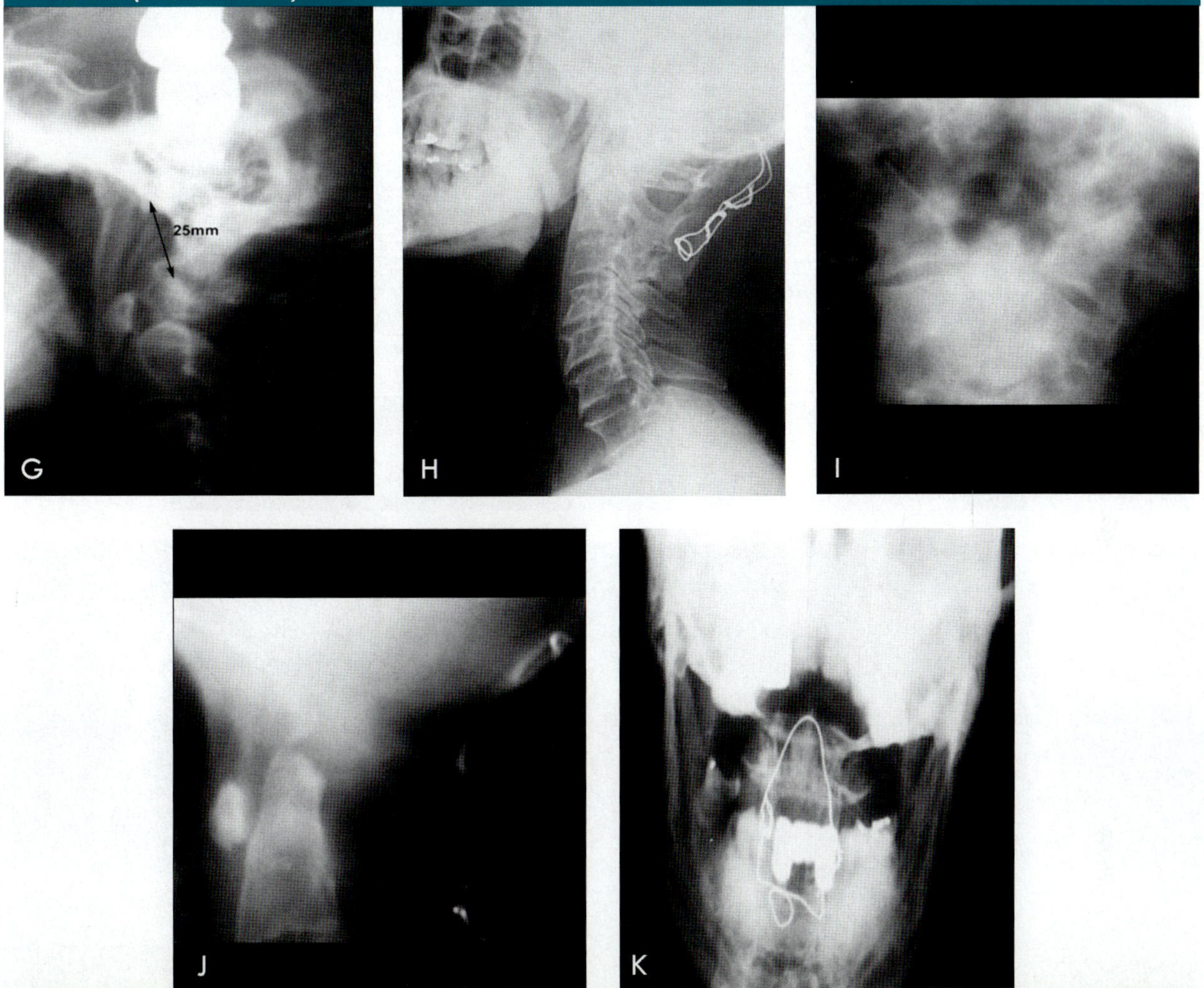

Figure 4 *(continued)* **G,** This measurement from the basion to the tip of the odontoid measures 25 mm. This line of Harris should normally be 12 mm or less. Hence, this line demonstrates the overdistraction that is present. **H,** At 6 weeks after injury, a halo and body cast was applied to immobilize the patient's head on his neck. Twelve weeks after injury a posterior fusion from the occiput to C3 was performed with iliac crest bone graft wired in place. This lateral tomogram made 10 weeks after fusion demonstrates avulsion of the apex of the odontoid process, which is a type I odontoid fracture. This probably includes the bone attachment of the alar ligaments. This film also shows that the relationship of the basion to the odontoid has been restored to normal and also shows that the posterior laminar line is now again normal. There is also spontaneous fusion anteriorly extending from the basion down to the anterior arch of C1. **I,** AP tomogram obtained 10 months after fusion reveals that the tip of the odontoid process is avulsed and is a type I odontoid fracture. The occipital condyles are again congruous. **J,** Lateral radiograph obtained 11 months after the original injury shows a solid posterior occiput to C3 fusion with good alignment of the occipitocervical junction. **K,** AP radiograph 14 months after injury shows normal alignment of the occipitocervical junction has been maintained. (Reproduced with permission from Eismont FJ, Tay KB: Injuries of the upper cervical spine, in Herkowitz HN, Garfin SR, Eismont FJ, Bell GR, Balderston RA, eds: *The Spine*, ed 5. Philadelphia, PA, Elsevier, 2006, pp 1081-1083 and with permission from Eismont FJ, Bohlman HH: Posterior atlanto-occipital dislocation with fractures of the atlas and odontoid process. *J Bone Joint Surg Am* 1978;60(3):397-399. Other figure elements are from Eismont FJ, Frazier DD: Craniocervical trauma, in Levine AM, Eismont FJ, Garfin SF, Zigler JE, eds: *Spine Trauma*. Philadelphia, PA, WB Saunders, 1998, pp 196-208.)

FIGURE 5

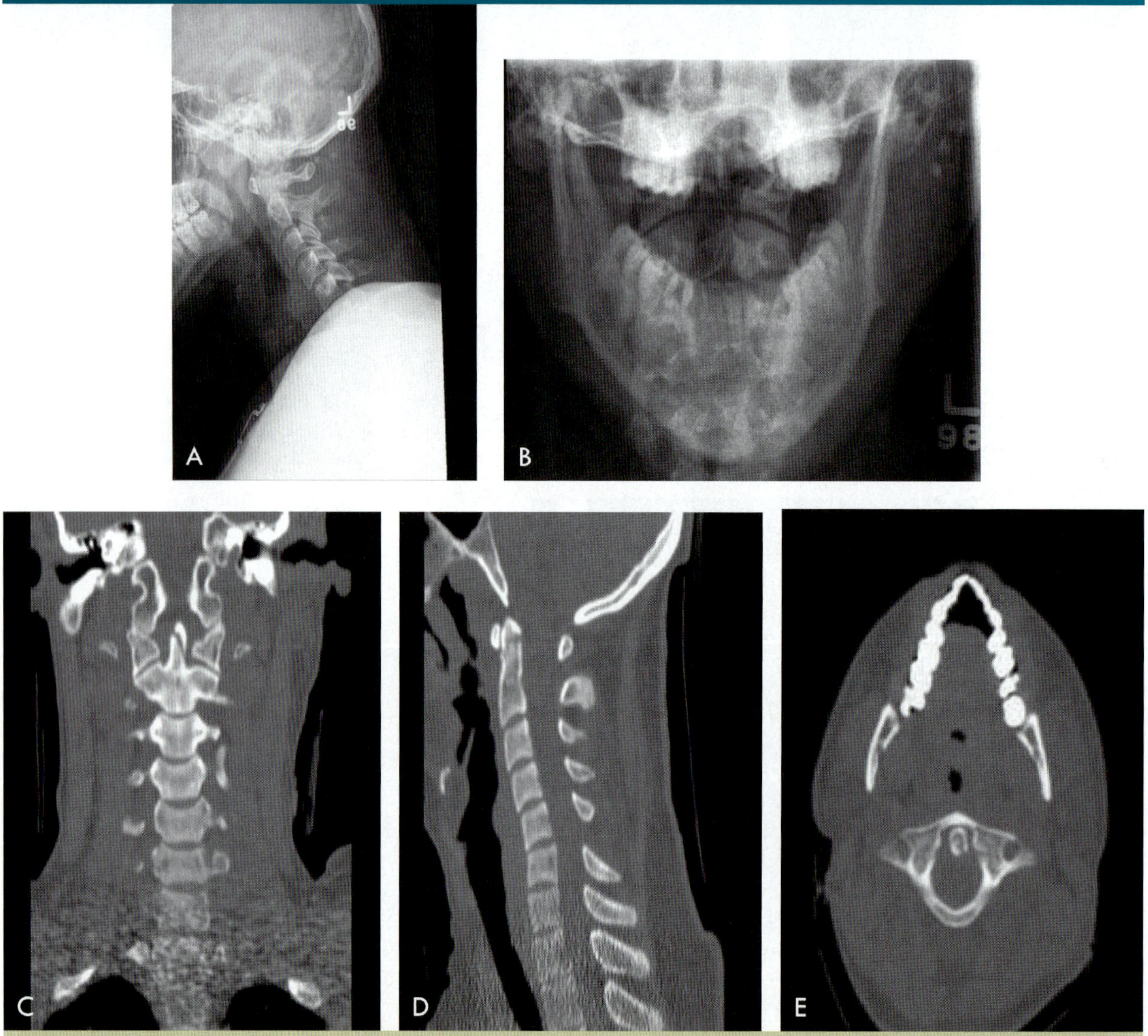

Figure 5 This 18-year-old boy was involved in a motor vehicle accident and was not wearing his seat belt. He was neurologically normal and complained only of neck pain. **A,** Lateral radiograph shows minimally increased soft-tissue swelling in the upper retropharyngeal area. **B,** Open-mouth odontoid view does not show any abnormality. **C,** Coronal reconstructed CT scan shows an oblique fracture of the tip of the odontoid consistent with a type I fracture. This is minimally displaced. Presumably, this is a fracture as a result of traction on the left alar ligament at the time of injury. **D,** This midsagittal reconstructed CT scan confirms the type I odontoid fracture. The alignment of the upper cervical spine looks normal. The patient has a coincidental C5-C6 facet subluxation and facet injury. **E,** This transverse CT image confirms the oblique type I odontoid fracture. This patient was treated surgically for the C5-C6 facet subluxation and instability. He was immobilized in a rigid cervical collar for 8 weeks and the odontoid fracture healed with no residual occipitocervical instability.

should actually be tangential to the dens and just touching it. This line is called Wackenheim's line (**Figure 4**). If this line is more posterior to the dens, it indicates a posterior occipital displacement (**Figure 4,** *D*). If this line is anterior and cuts through the odontoid or is anterior to the odontoid, it indicates an anterior occipital displacement.

The lateral radiograph should show a smooth, gently curved line posteriorly from the opisthion to the inner aspect of the lamina of the atlas, the axis, and the more caudal cervical vertebrae. Any sharp deviation of this line at the C0-C1 level could signify an occipitoatlantal dislocation.

A retropharyngeal space exceeding 5 mm measured anterior to C3 is seen with most upper cer-

FIGURE 6

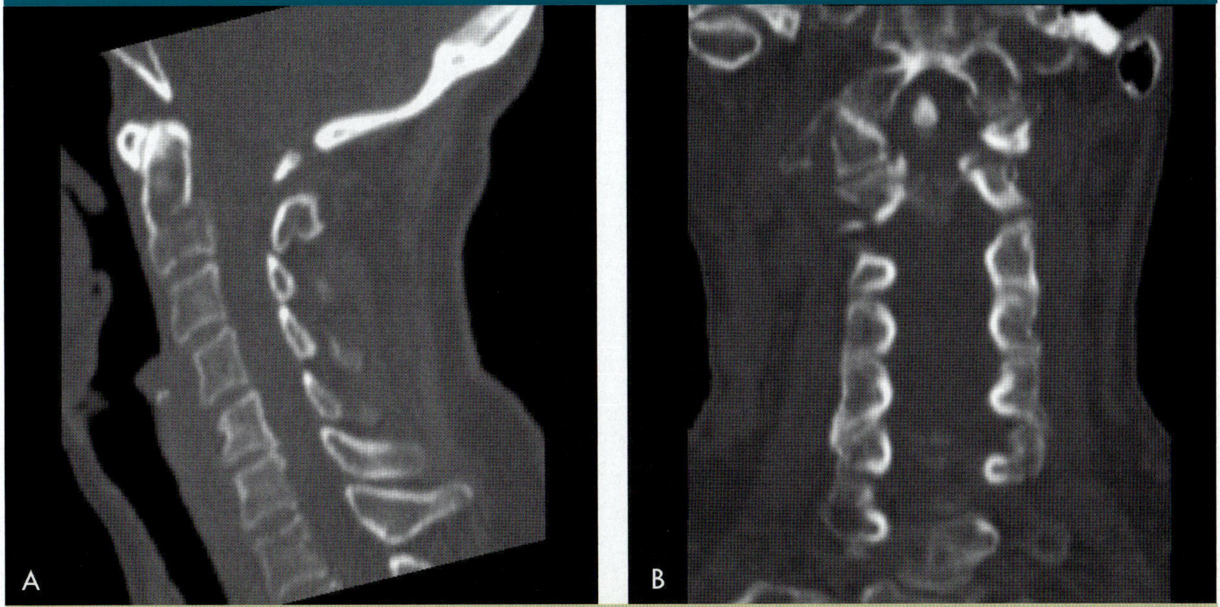

Figure 6 This patient fell from a golf cart, sustaining these injuries of the upper cervical spine. She was neurologically normal, with the exception of sustained clonus that persisted for 4 days following her injury. **A,** This midsagittal reconstructed CT scan shows a severely comminuted type III odontoid fracture. **B,** This coronal reconstructed CT scan shows that there is an impaction fracture of the occipital condyle on the left side. This would be regarded as a type I impacted occipital condyle fracture according to the classification system of Anderson and Montesano. The patient was initially immobilized in a halo vest. Her clonus resolved over 4 days. At 8 weeks, the CT scan as well as flexion and extension radiographs showed good healing of the fractures and no residual instability.

vical spine injuries, and occipitoatlantal injuries are no exception. Many of these patients will have marked retropharyngeal swelling (**Figure 4**, *B*). In many of the postmortem studies, free air is seen in the retropharyngeal space as a result of concomitant rupture of the posterior pharyngeal wall.

CT scans[34] with sagittal and coronal reconstruction are usually diagnostic.

Fractures may be seen with occipitoatlantal dislocations and the most typical would be avulsion fractures related to the alar ligaments. This could be from the superolateral portion of the odontoid process as described by Anderson and D'Alonzo[44] as type I odontoid fractures (**Figures 4** and **5**). They considered it to be an uncommon fracture but of no clinical significance. Most would now agree that this fracture could very well be associated with severe and life-threatening occipitocervical instability, and Scott et al[39] have correctly emphasized the significance of this type I odontoid fracture. The other associated fracture can be an avulsion fracture of the medial aspect of the occipital condyle (**Figures 6** and **7**). Anderson and Montesano[10] classified this as their type III occipital condyle fracture and recognized its association with head-on-neck dislocations.

There can also be midsubstance tears to the alar ligaments. This can be seen on special MRI images if this is clinically suspected (**Figure 7**).

Any widening or asymmetry of the occipitoatlantal joints should also alert the clinician to probable head-on-neck instability (**Figure 8**). Kaufman et al[36] have reviewed this joint in children on cross-table lateral skull radiographs and found that a joint space of 4.5 mm or less is normal and that a joint space of 5 mm or more suggests occipitocervical distraction or dislocation injury.

Osteoligamentous injury at the craniocervical junction can present on a spectrum from simple sprain or fracture up to atlanto-occipital dislocation. This is often associated with local damage to neurovascular structures, especially the vertebral arteries. Reddy et al[45] used Doppler flow velocities of the vertebral artery as it courses in its most vulnerable location. The tortuous path of the vertebral artery at the V3 segment starts between the transverse process foramen of the atlas, then courses behind the superior facet in the arterial groove before penetrating the atlanto-occipital membrane. High-velocity trauma with a rapid deceleration can stretch the vertebral artery, causing intimal damage, dissection, and thrombosis. They

FIGURE 7

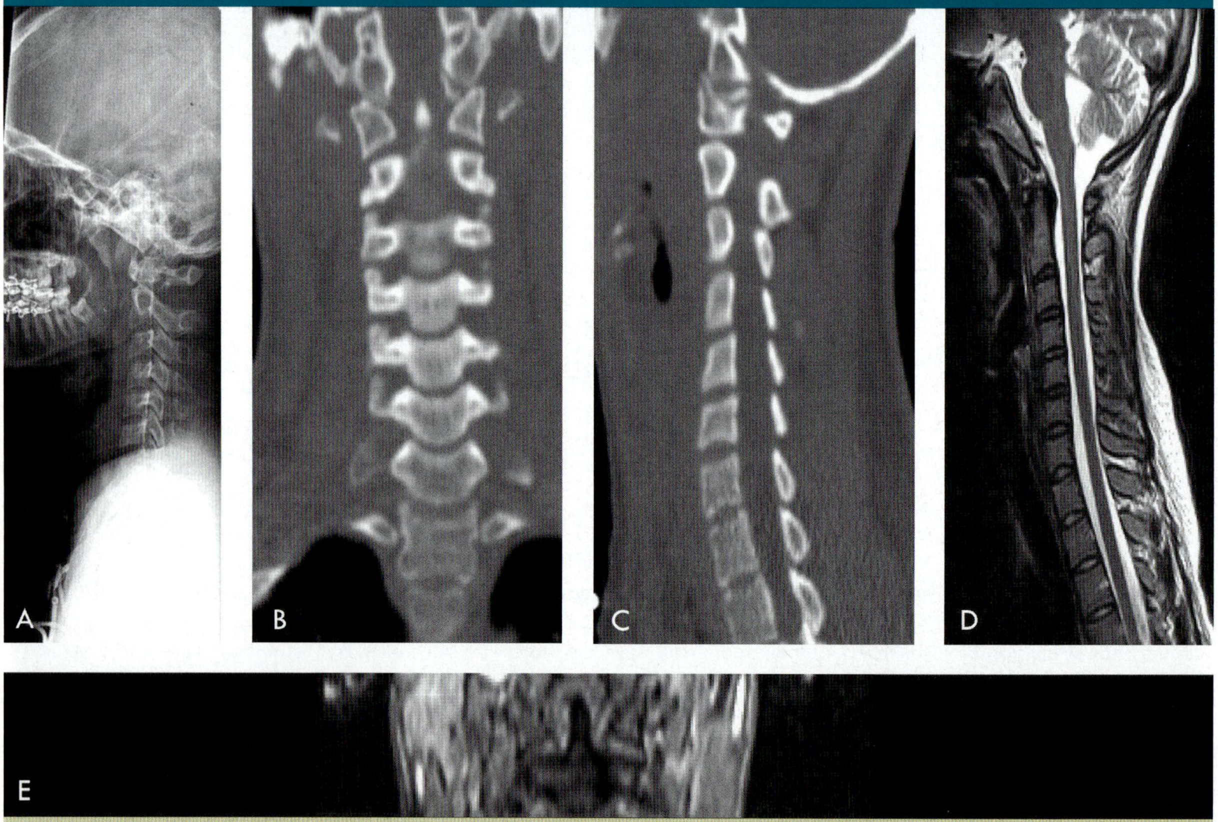

Figure 7 This patient was involved in a motor vehicle accident and reported upper cervical spine pain. She was neurologically normal. **A,** Lateral radiograph shows increased soft-tissue swelling in the upper cervical spine retropharyngeal area. The alignment of the spine appears normal. **B,** Coronal reconstructed CT scan shows a fracture of the medial aspect of the left occipital condyle, which is minimally displaced. It is difficult to tell whether this is an impaction fracture of the occipital condyle or whether it is an avulsion due to tension on the alar ligament. **C,** Left sagittal reconstructed CT scan shows the minimally displaced occipital condyle fracture. The retropharyngeal soft-tissue swelling can again be seen. **D,** Midsagittal T2-weighted MRI scan shows that there is adequate room for the spinal cord at this level. **E,** Coronal magnetic resonance image through the odontoid and through the alar ligaments bilaterally. The alar ligament on the left side (the same side as the occipital condyle fracture) is clearly intact. On the right side, there is no cut that shows the alar ligament attaching to the odontoid. Presumably, the alar ligament has been avulsed from the right side of the odontoid. This patient remained neurologically normal. She was immobilized in a rigid cervical collar for 8 weeks. The flexion and extension radiographs at that time showed that the spine was stable at the occipitocervical junction. She was allowed to gradually resume her normal activities.

evaluated 33 patients with injuries at the craniocervical junction and found that patients with severe trauma revealed mean flow-velocity values of 19 cm/s (in 22 cases) and flow void (4 cases). They found flows in a control population to be 24 to 42 cm/s. In the four cases with a flow void, a four-vessel cerebral angiography revealed dissection of the vertebral artery. They recommend V3 segment Doppler Studies of the vertebral arteries in patients with head and neck trauma, as well as in intubated polytrauma patients with suspected craniocervical involvement.[45]

Pathology of Occipitocervical Subluxation and Dislocation

The pathologic findings in these head-on-neck dislocations have been accurately described in the literature and are a combination of clinical findings of those who survived this injury and gross pathologic findings of those who did not survive.[1-3,46,47]

Many of the gross anatomy dissections reveal disruption of all occipitocervical ligaments, as would be expected (**Figure 9**). The injury may

FIGURE 8

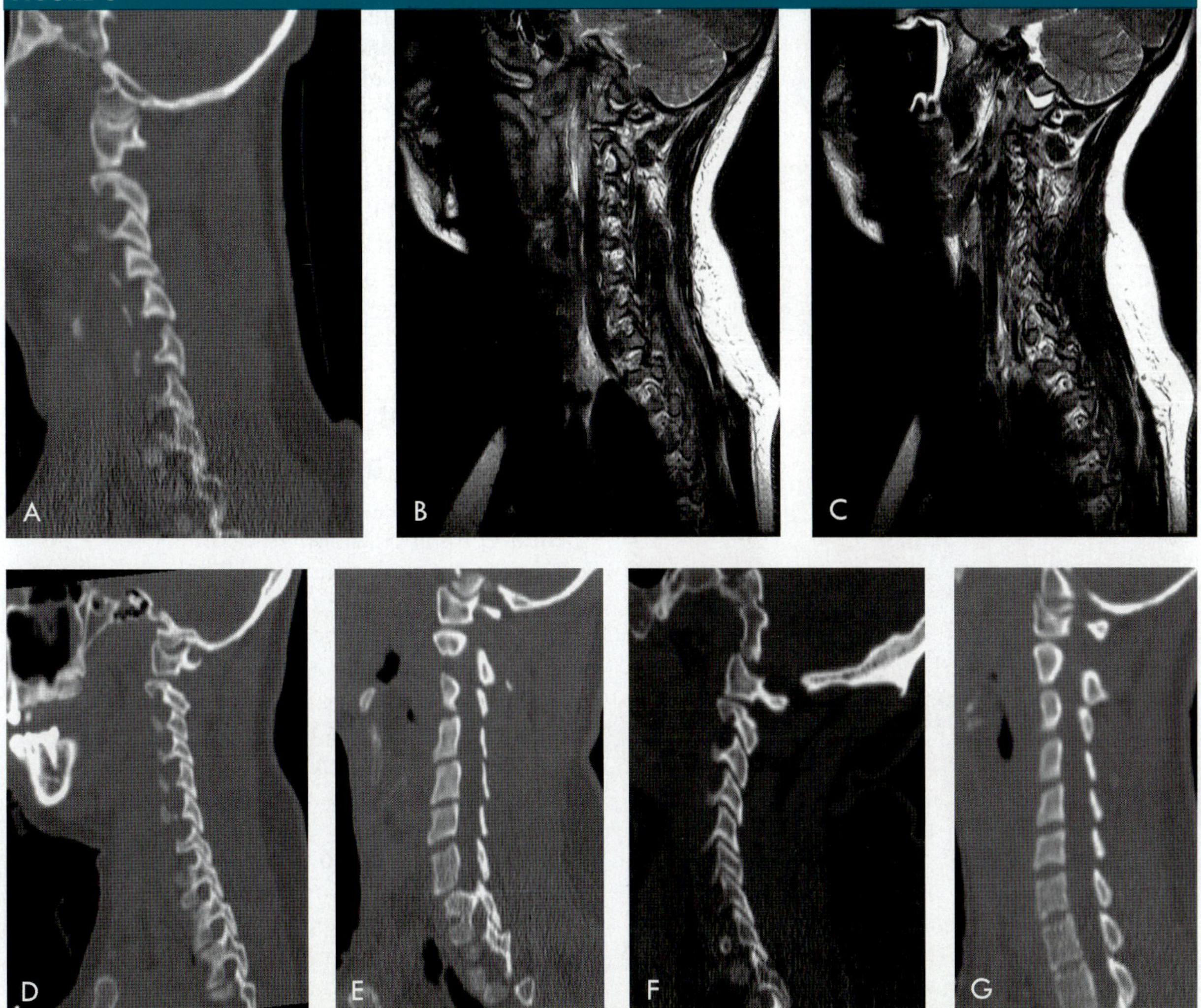

Figure 8 This figure demonstrates the different types of occipitoatlantal joint disruption seen in five different patients. With the exception of **A,** all these abnormalities are consistent with significant occipitocervical instability. Missing these simple findings on the imaging studies could cause significant neurologic deterioration or even death. **A,** Sagittal reconstructed CT scan shows the normal relationship of the occipital condyle to the lateral mass of C1. **B,** Sagittal T2-weighted MRI scan shows that there is increased fluid in the occiput-C1 joint. **C,** Sagittal T2-weighted MRI scan shows an even greater amount of fluid in the occiput-C1 joint. **D,** Sagittal reconstructed CT scan shows asymmetry of the occiput-C1 joint. **E,** Reconstructed CT scan shows fracture lines in the base of the skull adjacent to the occipital condyle. **F,** Sagittal reconstructed CT scan shows gross joint asymmetry. **G,** Sagittal reconstructed CT scan illustrating a fracture of the occipital condyle.

be limited to soft tissue or it may involve bone avulsion, as with the alar ligament attachments, or it may involve occipital condyle fractures.

The extent of neural and vascular damage varies from normal to complete disruption. The neural tissue at this level includes the brainstem with its respiratory and cardiovascular centers, the nuclei and tracts of various cranial nerves, and all sensory and motor tracts, including the very prominent decussation of the corticospinal tracts. In surviving patients it is common to see respiratory and cardiovascular instability,[48] cranial nerve palsies (Collet-Sicard syndrome),[49] and various degrees of sensorimotor impairment[14,15] (**Figures 4, 10** and **11**). Those patients with incomplete motor paralysis can have very bizarre clinical pictures depending on which part of the pyramidal decussation is involved.[50] This can include weak arms and normal legs, weak legs and normal arms, and even weakness in one arm and the contralateral leg, hence the term "cruciate" paralysis.[51]

FIGURE 9

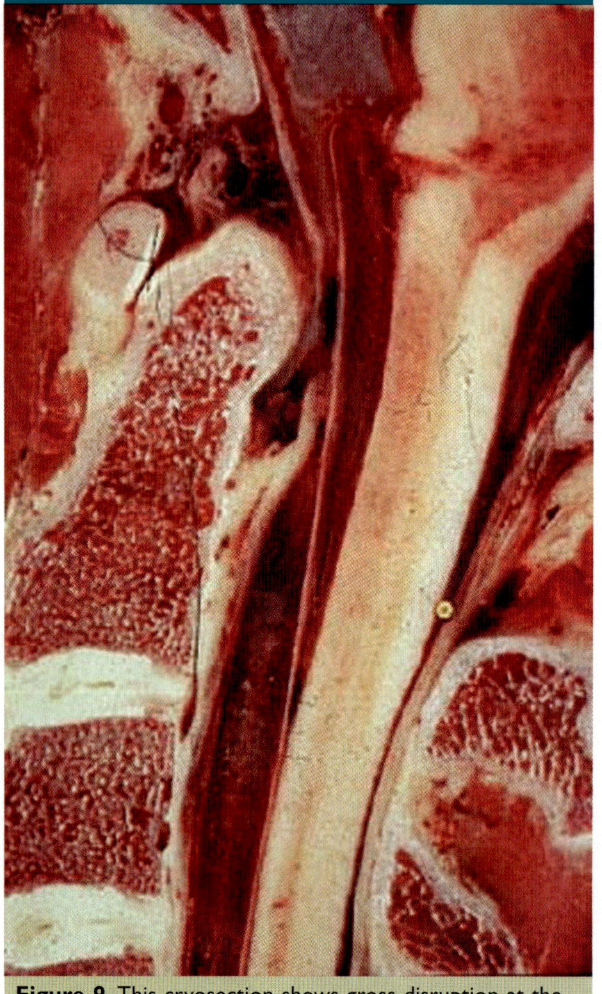

Figure 9 This cryosection shows gross disruption at the cranial cervical junction. Specimen radiographs had only shown a slight atlantoaxial asymmetry. There is a subluxation and anterior rotation of the atlas, and the anterior atlanto-occipital membrane, the apical ligament, the cruciate ligament, and the tectorial membrane are ruptured. Note the avulsion of the ligamentum flavum from the lamina of C2. (Reproduced with permission from Wolfgang Rauschning, MD, PhD, at www.spineuniverse.com.)

Classification of Occipitocervical Subluxation and Dislocation

Based on a review of the literature and a personal case, Traynelis et al[24] developed a classification system for occipitocervical subluxation and dislocation (**Figure 12**). The systems graded type I through III. Type I involves anterior displacement of the occiput with respect to the atlas. Type II is a longitudinal distraction injury with separation of the occiput from the atlas. Type III, which is quite rare, involves posterior displacement of the occiput with respect to the atlas.[24] This classification helps to provide some rationale for treatment. In a type II injury, primarily a longitudinal distraction injury in which good alignment is maintained, initial traction would not be indicated because it could lead to a progressive neurologic deficit. However, in type I or type III injuries, 5 lb of traction might be indicated to realign the bone structures and decompress the brainstem or spinal cord. Eismont and Bohlman[14] reported a type III dislocation where placement of longitudinal traction led to significant improvement of quadriparesis over several hours.

Treatment of Occipitoatlantal Dislocations and Subluxations

As with all injuries, treatment begins with assessment and immobilization at the injury scene. All patients with major trauma, and especially those with a neurologic deficit, should be suspected of having an occipitocervical injury. Initial management should consist of maintaining an adequate airway according to the ABC (airway, breathing, circulation) protocol of trauma and immobilizing the cervical spine in a neutral position. In the emergency department, once this injury is suspected, the ideal initial treatment is application of a halo vest (**Figures 10** and **11**). If tong traction is applied, no more than 5 lb should be used and a radiograph should be taken immediately because these injuries are very easily overdistracted (**Figure 4**). If the patient is a child, care should be taken to use the split-mattress technique described by Herzenberg et al[52] to maintain normal alignment and avoid forced forward flexion of the head.

If a patient with this injury requires intubation, it is recommended that this be nasotracheal rather than orotracheal. It is also recommended that the head and neck be stabilized in a neutral position to minimize the risk of neurologic injury.[53]

This injury can occasionally be treated with 3 months of halo-vest immobilization provided the initial ligamentous and bone injury is relatively limited and stable.[29] After 3 months of immobilization, flexion and extension radiographs can be done to assess stability, and a delayed occipitocervical fusion can then be performed if needed. One case was successfully treated with 3 weeks of traction after reduction with traction, but this is certainly uncommon.[11]

Because this is normally an extremely unstable injury, a posterior occipitocervical fusion is usually indicated[14,15,17,20] (**Figures 4, 10, 11** and **13**). A

FIGURE 10

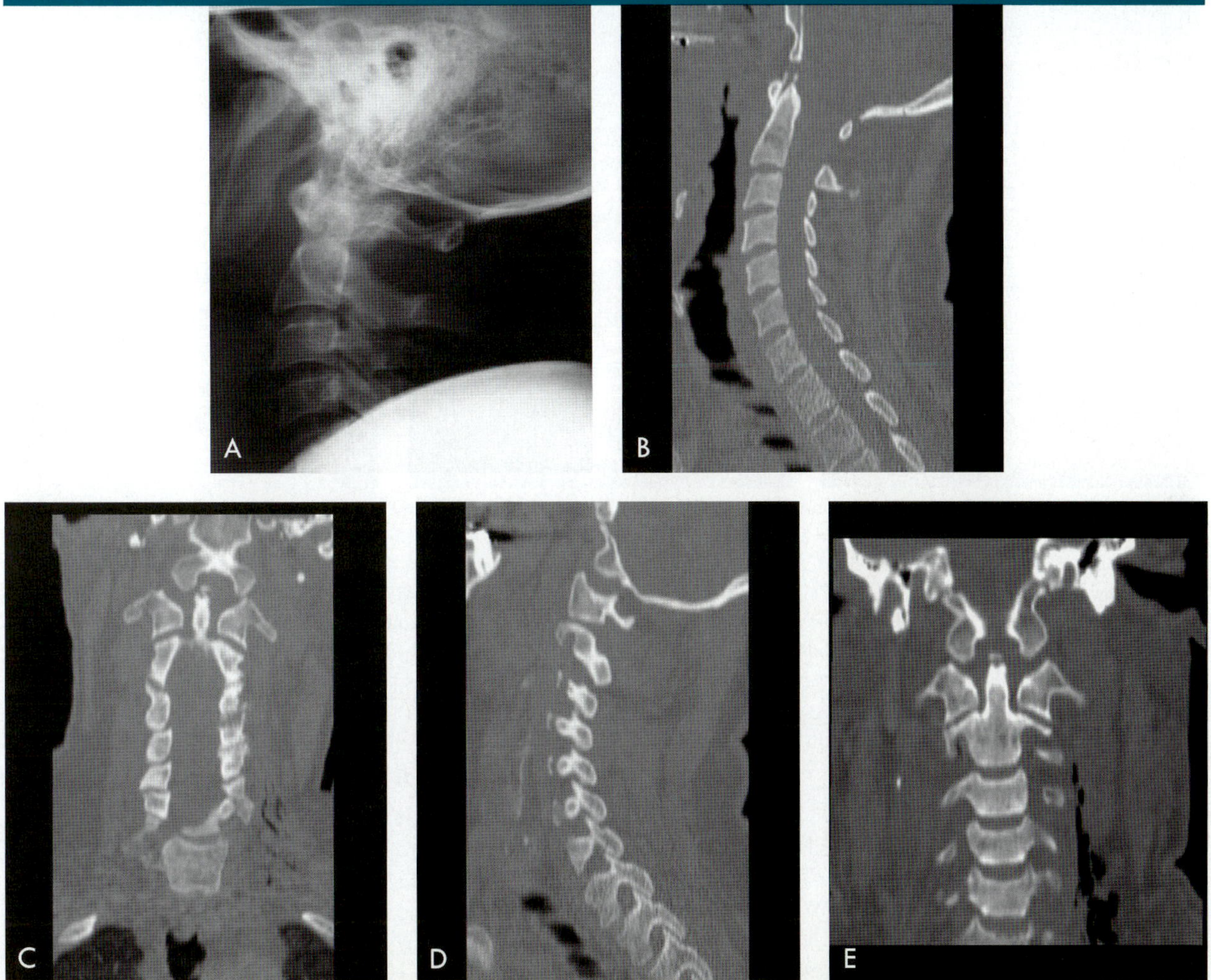

Figure 10 This elderly gentleman was involved in a motor vehicle accident and sustained pulmonary contusions and an upper cervical spine injury. He had cranial nerve VI palsies with dysconjugate gaze, as well as cranial nerve IX and X dysfunction with dysphagia and cranial nerve XII dysfunction with lateral tongue deviation. He did not have any signs of myelopathy and his strength in all four extremities was normal. **A,** Lateral radiograph of the cervical spine shows grossly normal alignment and moderately severe retropharyngeal soft-tissue swelling. **B,** Midline sagittal reconstructed CT scan shows grossly normal alignment. **C,** Coronal reconstructed CT scan shows gross displacement of the occipital condyles from the C1 lateral masses. The spine is displaced approximately 1 cm to the right in relation to the skull. There is also an apparent fracture of the tip of the odontoid. **D,** Right sagittal reconstructed CT scan shows marked widening of the joint space at the level of the occipital condyle and the lateral mass of the atlas. **E,** In the emergency department, the patient was placed in a halo vest and his spine was reduced under fluoroscopic control. This coronal reconstructed CT scan shows good reduction of the occipitocervical joint. The patient was intubated because of his pulmonary contusion. Approximately 12 hours after arrival in the emergency department, the patient was taken to surgery. He was turned to the prone position while in the halo vest and the posterior aspect of the halo vest was removed and a posterior reduction and fusion was performed.

fusion from the occiput to the atlas is theoretically adequate treatment (**Figure 13**), but this is most often not realistic because of other associated injuries to the upper cervical spine and because a fusion just from the occiput to the atlas usually is not biomechanically solid enough to stabilize this severe injury. A fusion from the occiput to the axis is most often necessary. Of the seven patients surgically treated by one of us (F.J.E.),[14,20] a fusion to a lower level was necessary in six patients because of associated injuries. The timing of surgery should be individualized, and it is normally performed as soon as the patient is medically stable enough to tolerate it.

The technique of posterior occipitocervical fusion depends on the surgeon's preference. Each

FIGURE 10 ***(CONTINUED)***

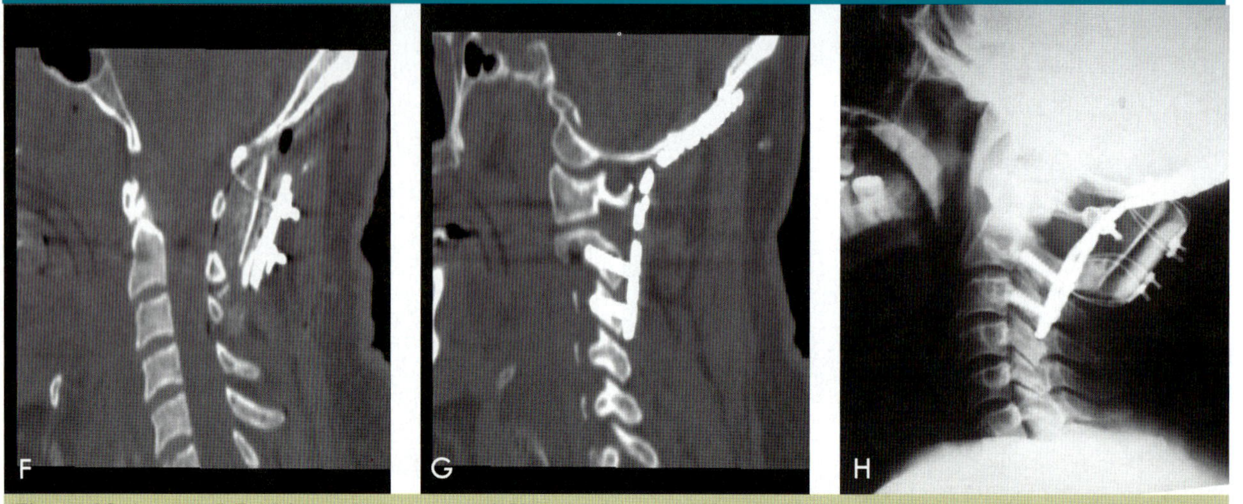

Figure 10 *(continued)* **F,** Midsagittal reconstructed CT scan shows positioning of the structural autograft bone from occiput to C2 supplemented with allograft bone and cables. **G,** Screws were placed at the level of the skull and screws were placed at the level of the C2 pedicles and the C3 lateral masses. Bilateral plates were used. Supplemental cables were placed around the lamina of C1 and around the plates on each side. Following the surgery, the patient was removed from his halo vest and mobilized in a rigid cervical collar. **H,** A follow-up radiograph at 6 months demonstrates good alignment and a solid occiput-C3 fusion. He required supplemental stomach peg feeding for approximately 3 months before he was able to swallow without aspiration. His sixth cranial nerve palsy also resolved at approximately 6 months after the injury.

technique gives predictably good results when performed as outlined by the author. In the past, some authors have recommended posterior wiring with or without a rod. At this time, most surgeons would recommend posterior screw/rod constructs or posterior plates and screws with autogenous bone graft. We present each of these techniques below.

Surgical Setup

We recommend that these patients be placed in a halo vest and the spine be reduced before surgery. The injuries are unstable and these patients are therefore intubated fiberoptically with a nasotracheal tube. Intubation is done with the patient awake and the patient is kept awake until transfer to the prone position on the surgical table and the patient has been neurologically assessed in this new position. Once positioning is complete, a lateral radiograph is taken to ensure adequate alignment of the occipitocervical junction.[54] We currently use fluoroscopy to assess our reduction before incision. The fluoroscopy machine is then prepped into the operative field. Intraoperative somatosensory-evoked potential monitoring and motor-evoked responses are used to assess the physiologic status of the spinal cord during the procedure.

Occipitocervical Wiring Technique

A posterior midline incision is made from the midocciput to just below the level to be fused. Subperiosteal dissection is used to expose the squamous portion of the occipital bone, the foramen magnum, the posterior ring of C1, and the spinous processes, laminae, and facets of the lower vertebrae to be fused. Care is taken to preserve all ligaments and joint capsules below the level of the fusion.

Wertheim and Bohlman[55] described a triple wiring technique which avoids passage of intracranial wires. Their technique is a modification of a technique originally described by Robinson and Southwick.[56] In the modified procedure, a high-speed burr is used to make a trough on either side of the external occipital protuberance. Care is taken to avoid the transverse and superior sagittal sinuses cephalad to the protuberance. A towel clip is then used to make a hole through the outer table and a titanium cable is looped through this hole and around the bony ridge. A second cable is passed around the arch of the atlas. A third cable is passed through a drill hole in the base of the spinous process of the axis or under the C2 lamina. Two curved corticocancellous struts taken from the posterior iliac crest are prepared with three drill holes equal distances apart. The occiput is decorticated and the grafts are anchored in

FIGURE 11

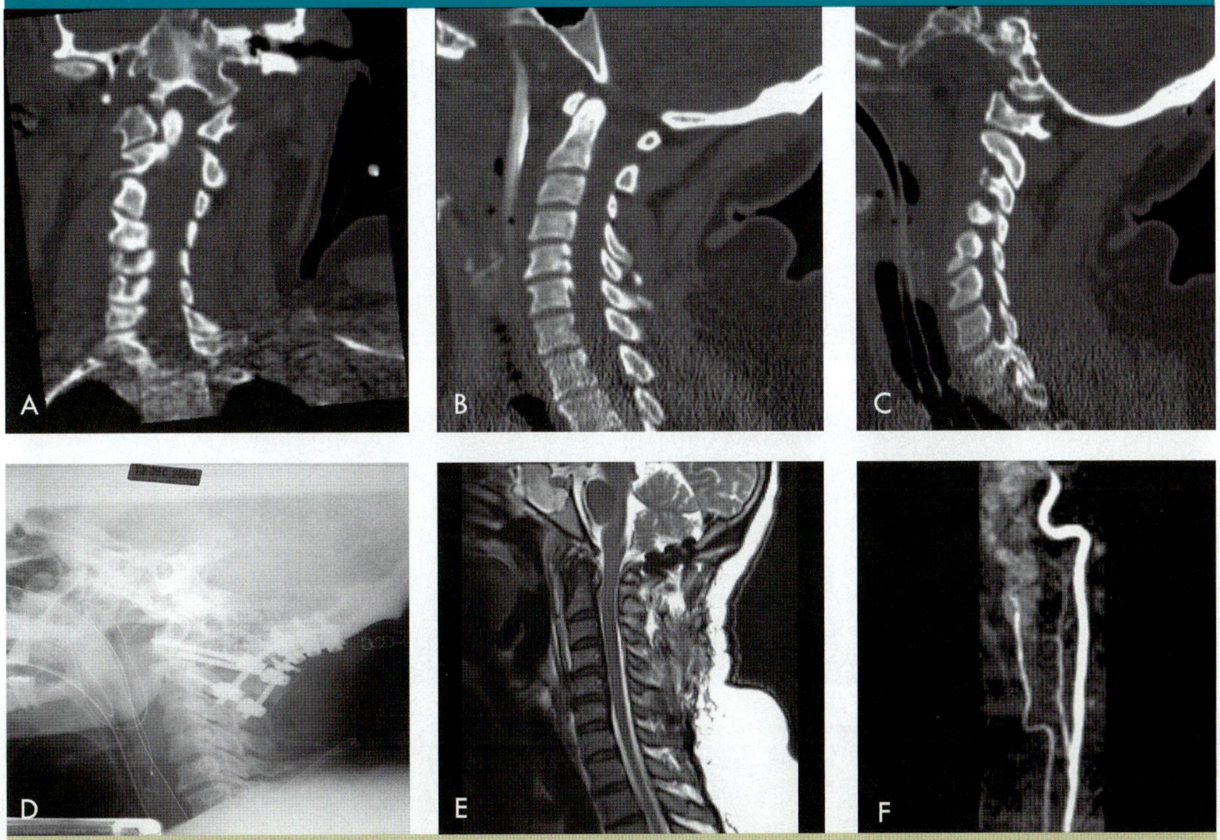

Figure 11 This 44-year-old female pedestrian was struck by a truck. She had a severe Brown-Séquard syndrome with severe right-sided paralysis and multiple cranial nerve palsies. Because of a history of a previous bullet wound to the buttock, the patient did not have an MRI scan at the time of admission. **A,** Coronal reconstructed CT scan shows severe occiput-C1 instability and the spine is subluxed approximately 1 cm to the right of the base of the skull. There is gross disruption of the occipitoatlantal joints. **B,** Midline sagittal reconstructed CT scan shows normal alignment in this plane. **C,** Right sagittal reconstructed CT scan shows the distracted occipitoatlantal joint. **D,** The patient had been stabilized in a halo vest in the emergency department. She was taken to surgery emergently, and the occipital cervical reduction and instrumentation and fusion was performed using C2 pedicle screws and C1 lateral mass screws. **E,** Postoperatively, it was decided that because the previous gunshot wound was old and her paralysis was significant, MRI could be performed. This midsagittal T2-weighted MRI scan shows that there is adequate room for the spinal cord, although she does have a congenitally narrow spinal canal from the C1 level down to the inferior C5 level. **F,** Magnetic resonance angiography was also performed and showed that the patient's vertebral arteries were normal bilaterally. The patient's halo vest was removed postoperatively and she was immobilized in a rigid cervical collar for 3 months following the surgery. She had a slow improvement in her neurologic function and a solid occiput-C2 fusion at 4 months postoperatively. (Courtesy of Allan Levi, MD, PhD, Department of Neurological Surgery, University of Miami Miller School of Medicine, Miami, FL.)

FIGURE 12

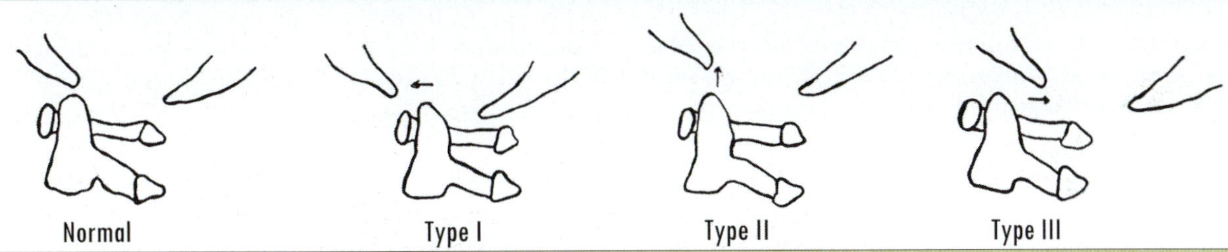

Figure 12 These drawings represent the classification system of Traynelis et al describing occipitocervical subluxation and dislocation. (Redrawn from Traynelis VC, Marano GD, Dunker RO, Kaufman HH: Traumatic atlanto-occipital dislocation: Case report. *J Neurosurg* 1986;65(6):863-870.)

FIGURE 13

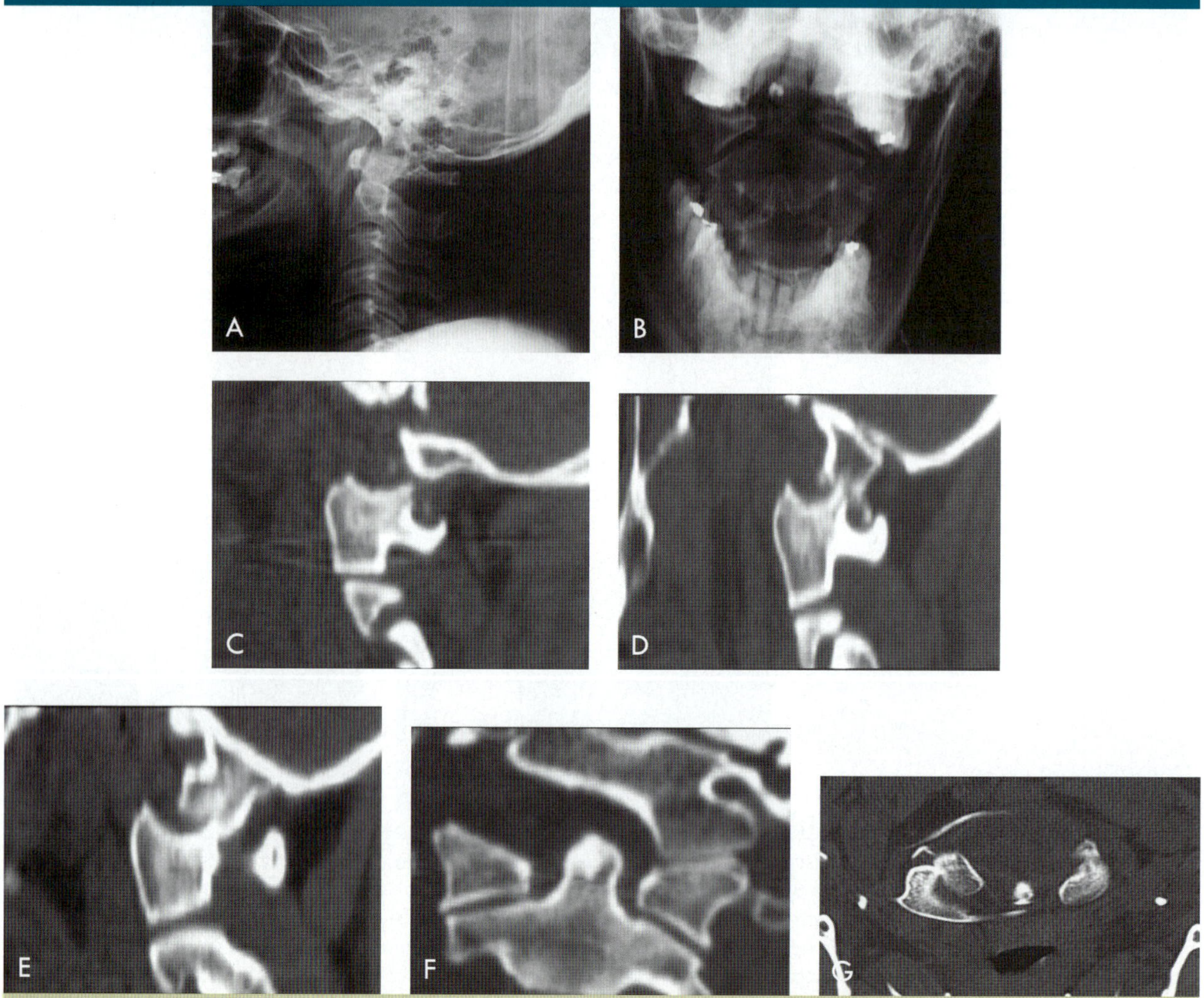

Figure 13 This patient, who was injured when his car struck a tree, had an immediate onset of pain in his upper cervical spine and with radiation to the back of his head. **A,** Lateral radiograph shows normal alignment of the upper cervical spine and the occipitocervical junction. There is no abnormal soft-tissue swelling. The basion appears to be directly over the tip of the odontoid and is less than 1 cm from the tip. Wackenheim's line is not drawn here, but the bony line down the clivus and the posterior aspect of the basion appears to be tangential to the posterior aspect of the odontoid. **B,** Open-mouth view of the odontoid is abnormal. The patient's right lateral mass of C1 appears smaller than the lateral mass of C1 on the left side. There is also some asymmetry, with the distance from the lateral mass of C1 to the odontoid being shorter on the right side than on the left side. **C,** Parasagittal CT reconstruction shows that his occipital condyle on the right side is posterior to the lateral mass of C1. **D,** This image is slightly more medial than that in **C** and shows that the occipital condyle is impacted into the posterior aspect of the posterior lip of the right lateral mass of C1. **E,** This view is even more medial, and again shows the occipital condyle to be posteriorly displaced and impacted into the posterior lip of the lateral mass of C1. **F,** Coronal reconstruction of the CT scan shows that the left-sided occipitoatlantal joint is normal. On the right side, the occipital condyle is posterior to the lateral mass of C1; hence, it is not seen on this view. **G,** Transverse axial image shows the abnormal appearance of the right-sided occipitoatlantal joint. (Reproduced with permission from Eismont FJ, Tay KB: Injuries of the upper cervical spine, in Herkowitz HN, Garfin SR, Eismont FJ, Bell GR, Balderston RA, eds: *The Spine*. Philadelphia, PA, Elsevier, 2006, pp 1084-1086.)

place on both sides of the spine by the cables. Additional cancellous bone graft is packed between the grafts. After meticulous hemostasis is obtained, the wound is closed in layers.[55] In the series described by Wertheim and Bohlman,[55] all 13 of their patients developed a solid fusion using this combination of bone grafting and halo immobilization.

In the past, the technique described by Robinson and Southwick[56] in 1960 has been used rou-

FIGURE 13 *(CONTINUED)*

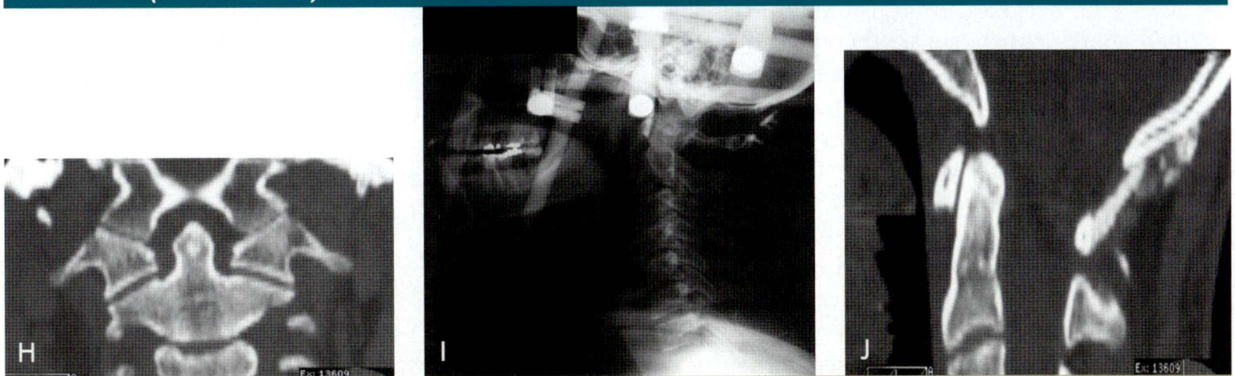

Figure 13 *(continued)* **H,** The patient was initially placed in skull-tong traction, but the occipitoatlantal dislocation could not be reduced. The patient was therefore taken to surgery. At the time of surgery, with a combination of skull-tong traction and manual manipulation with a cable passed under the posterior arch of C1, the occiput-C1 dislocation was reduced with an audible "clunk." Fusion was performed using titanium cables to fasten autograft bone to the base of the skull posteriorly and to the posterior arch of C1. This postoperative coronal CT reconstruction shows complete reduction of the occipitoatlantal joint bilaterally. **I,** Lateral radiograph shows the bone graft and cables in place. Because rigid internal fixation was not used, the patient was immobilized in a halo vest postoperatively. **J,** Midsagittal reconstructed CT scan shows the bone graft healing at 3 months from the time of surgery. (Reproduced with permission from Eismont FJ, Tay KB: Injuries of the upper cervical spine, in Herkowitz HN, Garfin SR, Eismont FJ, Bell GR, Balderston RA, eds: *The Spine*. Philadelphia, PA, Elsevier, 2006, pp 1084-1086.)

FIGURE 14

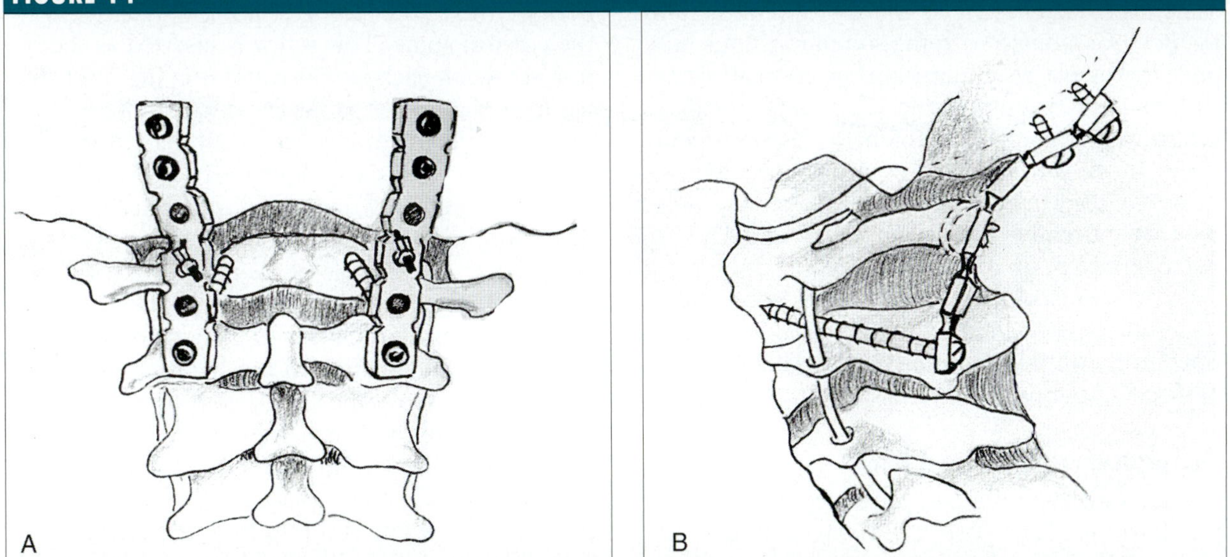

Figure 14 These drawings represent AP (**A**) and lateral (**B**) views of the occipital cervical plating technique using C1-C2 transarticular screws and titanium reconstruction plates with bicortical skull screws. Because the transarticular C1-C2 screw is the most critical in terms of its positioning, the C1-C2 transarticular screw is always the first screw to be placed in this construct. The path would initially be drilled and tapped. A plate would then be bent to accommodate the local anatomy. The plate must fit flush against the skull, fit against the posterior ach of C1, and fit the contour of the posterior arch of C2. The C1-C2 transarticular screw is then placed through the plate and tightened to within two turns of its final position. The plate is then held against the skull, and two or three screws are then placed into the skull on each side. These lateral screws in the skull are always bicortical. A cable is also usually passed under the posterior arch of C1 and passed around the plate and then tightened. The distal tip of the C1-C2 transarticular screw should be just to the anterior cortex of C1. It can also protrude slightly through the anterior cortex, but it should be kept in mind that the internal carotid artery lies within a few millimeters of the usual anterior exit point for these screws. (Reproduced from Eismont FJ, Frazier DD: Craniocervical trauma, in Levine AM, Eismont FJ, Garfin SF, Zigler JE, eds: *Spine Trauma*. Philadelphia, PA, WB Saunders, 1998, pp 196-208.)

tinely by one of us (F.J.E.) and has been reported by Starr et al[57]. The exposure is the same as described above. Burr holes are then placed on each side in the occiput 1 cm lateral to midline and 1 cm posterior to the foramen magnum. A Woodson elevator is passed through the burr hole toward the foramen magnum to separate the dura from the skull. A titanium cable is then placed in the burr hole and brought out through the foramen magnum, and one cable is passed on each side of the skull. A third and fourth cable are passed under the posterior arch of the atlas on each side, and a fifth and sixth cable are placed under the lamina of the axis, one on each side. The same type of thick corticocancellous iliac bone graft is obtained. Drill holes are placed in the bone graft at the cephalad and caudad end. The occipital cable is placed through the cephalad drill hole and secured to itself, the cable under C2 is placed through the caudad drill hole and secured to itself, and the cable under the posterior arch of C1 is passed over the graft and secured to itself on each side. If the patient's iliac crest bone is soft, then a cortical allograft plate of bone is used in the exact same fashion as described above to give structural support. Combined with the soft autogenous bone graft that is placed underneath the cortical plate, this construct is quite stable. All patients in this group were immobilized in a halo vest postoperatively. In the series of Starr et al,[57] all 20 patients achieved a stable occipitocervical fusion and only one patient required revision surgery one day postoperatively for a fractured graft.

When either of these techniques is used, the patient should be immobilized in a halo vest postoperatively until the fusion is solid. This will usually occur at approximately 3 months.

Occipitocervical Rod and Wire

Several authors in the past have recommended a modification of the posterior wiring technique in which a 4- to 5-mm threaded Steinmann pin (or contoured rod) is wired to the occiput and the spinal laminae to be fused. In this technique, two burr holes are drilled in the occiput 10 mm posterior to the foramen magnum. The dura is carefully dissected from the inner table of the occiput. Titanium cables are passed into the occipital burr holes and are brought out through the foramen magnum. Sublaminar or facet cables are passed inferiorly at the levels to be fused. The rod or pin is then contoured to the lordotic curve of the occipitocervical junction and fixed to the previously passed cables. If sublaminar cables are used, they are positioned at the most lateral aspect of the laminae to provide the maximal surface for bony fusion. The occiput, facet joints, and posterior elements of the vertebrae to be fused are decorticated. A corticocancellous graft is then placed and the wound is closed in the standard fashion.[36,58-62]

Occipitocervical Plating Technique and Screw/Rod Technique

The surgical approach for the plating technique is the same as that for the occipitocervical wiring technique. Once the exposure is complete, the plate used is contoured to fit the occipitocervical junction with the head in neutral (**Figures 14** and **15**). The plate can either be a standard reconstruction plate, which is available with hole separations of 8 mm or 12 mm, or a specially designed cervical plate. The reconstruction plates are always easily available and are relatively inexpensive. We will more commonly use rod/screw constructs as the poly-axial screw affords more flexibility in screw starting point.

These constructs (**Figure 16**) are designed around a transarticular C1-C2 screw on each side because this is the strongest point of fixation in the cervical spine. This screw is inserted as the first screw on each side because it is the most difficult to place and has the most stringent requirements for the starting point location and screw orientation. This transarticular C1-C2 screw placement was originally developed to provide stable fixation of the atlantoaxial joint from a posterior approach.[63] The pedicle of C2 is palpated with a blunt elevator to clearly define its borders. The C1-C2 joint is identified with a Penfield elevator, and a small Steinmann pin can be inserted into the atlas just above the C1-C2 joint to safely retract the greater occipital nerve on each side and provide visualization into the C1-C2 joint. The starting point for screw placement of the C1-C2 transarticular screw is 3 mm to 5 mm above the C2-C3 facet joint, and it should be as medial as possible and still remain within the C2 pedicle. A lateral C-arm fluoroscopy image is used to help guide the placement of the screw, and the surgeon aims exactly straight ahead (no medial or lateral angulation) toward the anterior arch of C1. The hole is drilled with a 2.5-mm bit and tapped in the appropriate fashion.[19,64,65] A CT scan obtained preoperatively will aid in defining the C1-C2 anatomy, and sagittal reconstruction through the C1 and C2 lateral masses is necessary to assess the course of the screws. This is especially important because in about 10% to 15% of patients, the location of the vertebral artery or the size of the C2

FIGURE 15

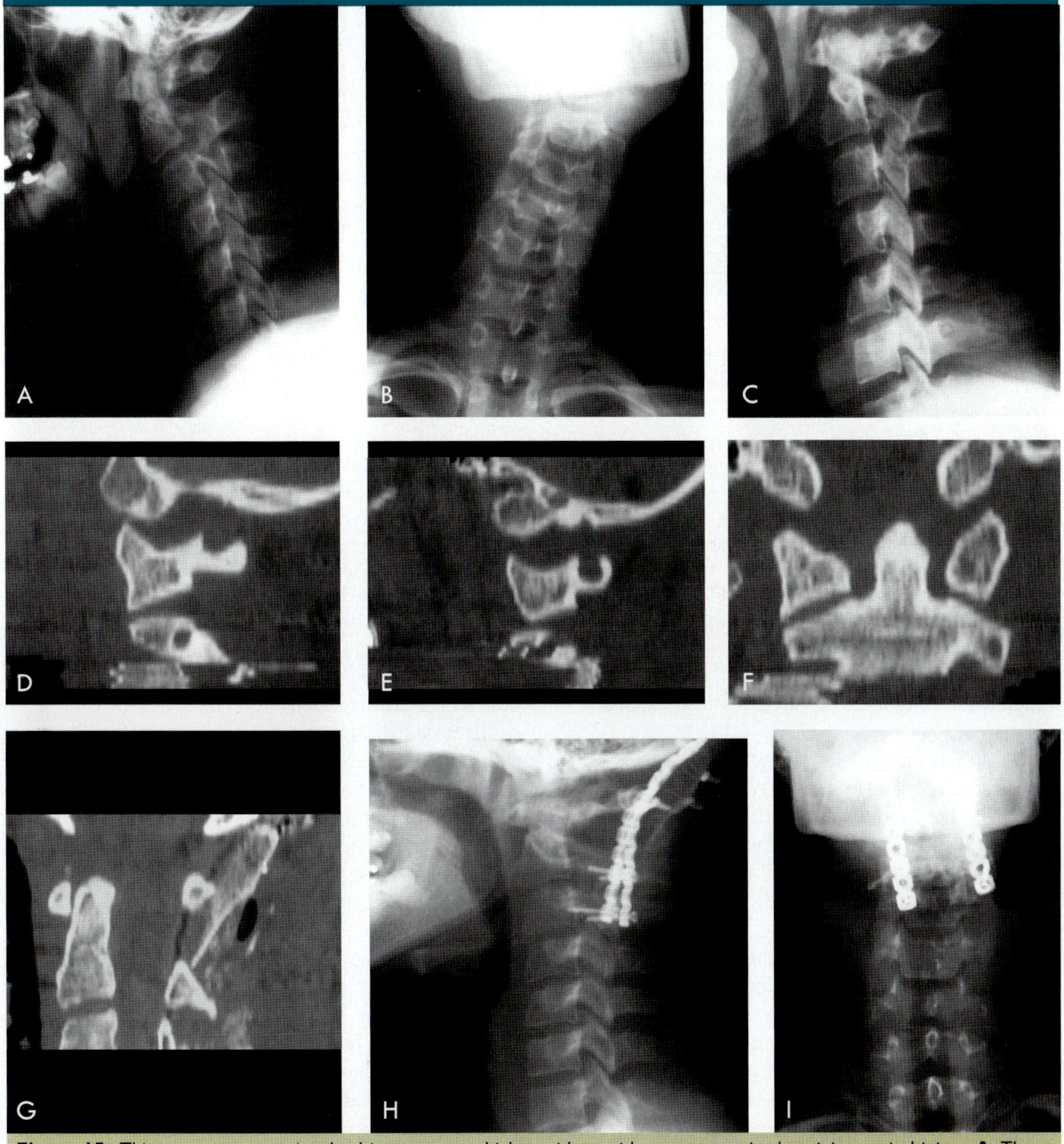

Figure 15 This young man was involved in a motor vehicle accident with an unrecognized occipitocervical injury. **A,** The patient at the time of his original presentation to the emergency department had a tremendous amount of soft-tissue swelling at the C3 level. No injury was diagnosed at this time and the patient was sent out of the emergency department in a collar. **B,** AP radiograph when the patient returned to the emergency department 10 days later shows severe torticollis. **C,** In 5 lb of traction, it can be seen that the patient's head is separating from his cervical spine. **D** and **E,** The CT scan reconstruction shows that the occipital condyles are distracted from the C1 lateral masses. On each side, it can also be seen that the course of the vertebral artery precludes usual positioning for placement of C1-C2 transarticular screws. **F,** This coronal CT reconstruction again shows the C1-C2 distraction. **G,** Postoperatively, the large central bone graft can be seen extending from the base of the skull posteriorly down to the C2 spinous process and lamina. This type of structural graft is essential with or without the use of plates and screws. **H** and **I,** Lateral and AP radiographs taken approximately 2 years after stabilization of the cervical spine reveal maintenance of good alignment and a solid posterior fusion from occiput to C3. (Reproduced from Eismont FJ, Frazier DD: Craniocervical trauma, in Levine AM, Eismont FJ, Garfin SF, Zigler JE, eds: *Spine Trauma*. Philadelphia, PA, WB Saunders, 1998, pp 196-208.)

FIGURE 16

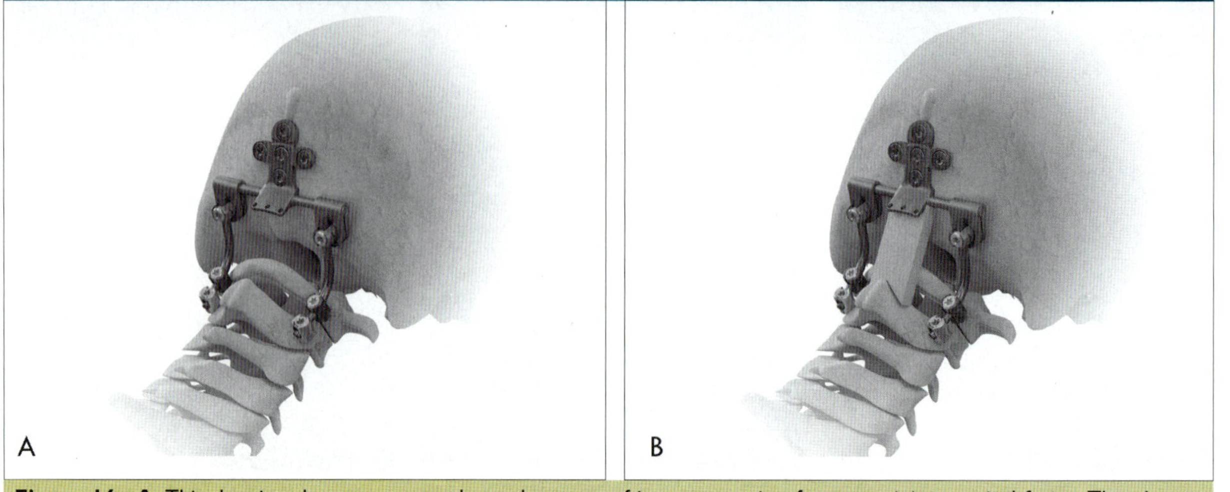

Figure 16 **A,** This drawing shows a commonly used pattern of instrumentation for an occipito-cervical fusion. The plate on the skull utilizes midline and para-midline screws to obtain the best occipital fixation. This construct shows bilateral C1 screws placed into the center of each of the lateral masses of C1 and bilateral C2 screws which can either be in the C2 pedicles or through the pedicles and into the C2 vertebral body. An alternative to the separate screws into C1 and C2 would be the use of bilateral C1-2 transarticular screws. **B,** This drawing shows the use of a bone graft from the occiput to the C2 posterior elements. The graft can be an autograft or an allograft plus BMP. There must be good contact between the graft and the patient's occipital bone and C2 posterior element bone in order to promote the development of a solid occiput-C2 fusion. Please note that posterior cervical screws are not FDA approved and this represents an off-label use.

pedicle precludes the use of C1-C2 transarticular screws.

If C1-C2 transarticular screws cannot be used, then adequate fixation can be obtained using bilateral C2 pedicle screws and using either C1 lateral mass screws or C1 sublaminar cables (**Figure 11**). The C1 lateral mass screws are placed beneath the C1 lamina in the middle of the lateral mass. If bicortical screw fixation is used, it should be noted that the internal carotid artery is normally only a few millimeters away from the anterior C1 exit point.

If the fusion is to extend below C2, the lateral mass screws at the lower levels are placed at this time. See chapter 27 on Cervical Facet Fractures and Dislocations for details concerning placement of lateral mass screws from C3 to C7.

The occipital screws are then placed in a bicortical fashion. Two or three screws can usually be placed into the occiput on each side. It is not uncommon for cerebrospinal fluid leakage to occur during placement of these screws, but simple insertion of the screw of the appropriate length appropriately seals the hole and prevents postoperative spinal fluid leakage. Using a drill guide with an accurate depth stop and gradually increasing the drill depth by 2-mm increments can often prevent this dural penetration from occurring. The placement of occipital screws in other locations has been optimized through the study of cadaver skulls.[66,67] Although we do not use screws above the superior nuchal line, recent studies have shown that placing unicortical screws above the superior nuchal line may be performed safely.[67] Concern about intracranial venous sinus violation has prevented us from using this technique. Many clinicians advocate use of a central occipital plate with fixed adaptation to cervical screws and rods. We have used both the lateral and the central screw placement techniques and found them equally effective; however, central screws are better with biomechanical testing.

Several authors have described a technique of open reduction and direct internal fixation with atlanto-occipital transarticular screws.[68,69] Direct screw fixation was performed using a cannulated screw system to reduce the atlanto-occipital dislocation. The C1 posterior arch was exposed laterally to visualize the junction where the arch joined the C1 lateral mass. The entry point is made with a high-speed drill while retracting the exiting C2 nerve caudally. Under fluoroscopic guidance, an end-threaded, 1.5-mm–diameter Kirschner wire was drilled through the center of the occipital condyles. The tip is directed below the edge of the clivus and dorsal to the basion. This positioning avoids the hypoglossal canals, which are in the anterolateral and cephalad portions of the condyles. The cranial trajectory is approximately 45°, with a 0° position relative to the sagittal plane.[69] This fixation technique has been used in combination with transarticular fixation of the atlantoaxial joint[68] or in isolation.[69]

Although the plates and screws give a rigid fixation of the occiput to the cervical spine, the technique is not complete without adding a central fusion (**Figures 10** and **15**). This is done using the same techniques described above using cables to fix autologous corticocancellous bone grafts to the skull and to the cervical spine. The reader is referred to the previous discussion for details.

Postoperatively, the patient is immobilized in a rigid cervical collar (**Figure 11**). If the fixation of the spine has been suboptimal, the patient is immobilized using a halo vest until the fusion is solid. The main difference between the simple wiring techniques and those techniques using internal fixation is that a halo vest is always needed after simple cable techniques, and a rigid cervical collar will usually suffice after using rigid internal fixation techniques.

Results of Treatment

The results of treatment depend on the severity of the initial injury and on the emergency and early hospital treatment. One of us (F.J.E.) has treated seven patients with this injury.[14,20] The one patient who had an initial complete paralysis at the brainstem level died after 4 days. Of the two patients who had an incomplete quadriplegia, one recovered to normal function and one improved from 0 to 1 of 5 muscle strength and being respirator-dependent acutely to 2 to 4 of 5 muscle strength and being ventilator-free after 8 years; however, she is still a wheelchair ambulator. One patient had myelopathy, and he improved moderately. One patient who had normal spinal cord function had cranial nerve deficits with severe dysphagia and visual problems caused by a sixth cranial nerve palsy that improved over 6 months. Two patients were neurologically normal and remained normal at final follow-up.

Complications

In our experience, complications during the evaluation and treatment of these life-threatening injuries can occur in the following phases of patient care: time of injury, surgical approach, perioperative, and late complications. Initially, complications can arise from undiagnosed comorbid conditions that occurred at the time of injury. Unrecognized global instability can be exacerbated by the application of even small amounts of traction.[14] Vertebral artery occlusion can be difficult to diagnose in the unconscious/intubated patient.[45] Torina et al[70] performed a retrospective review of 632 patients and found a 13% incidence of vertebral artery thrombosis. They concluded that the absence of neurologic symptoms in a patient with cervical spine fracture does not preclude vertebral artery thrombosis. Unrecognized cranial nerve dysfunction can lead to aspiration with subsequent pneumonia.[49] Pseudomeningocele formation, although uncommon, can be a cause of morbidity in survivors of atlanto-occipital dislocation.[71] Posttraumatic syringomyelia is increasingly seen to be a cause of delayed morbidity after craniocervical trauma. This insidious and late appearance makes diagnosis and treatment more difficult.[71] The "presyrinx state" of spinal cord thickening with increased signal on the T2-weighted images is important because it may indicate the development of syringomyelia with associated clinical deterioration.[72]

Second, complications can be a result of the surgical approach and fixation. As mentioned previously, extreme care must be used while positioning the patient to ensure that the head is maintained in a neutral position. We always apply a halo vest when the diagnosis is initially made and this facilitates turning the patient to the prone position for surgical stabilization. A wake-up test is normally performed after prone positioning to ensure there has been no loss of neurologic function. Dural tears and spinal fluid leaks commonly occur as a result of this particular injury.[20,73] In addition, injury to the vertebral artery can occur with transarticular screw placement across the atlantoaxial joint. Gluf et al[74] reported on 191 adult patients in whom at least one C1-C2 transarticular screw was placed. Complications occurred in 32 patients. Most were minor; however, five (3%) had vertebral artery injury. One bilateral injury resulted in death.[74]

Postoperatively, these patients can develop any or all of the common medical problems including postoperative wound infection. A retrospective survey of 850 spinal procedures was conducted to determine risk factors for postoperative spinal infection. Wimmer et al[75,76] evaluated patients following 574 posterior and 276 anterior procedures. A postoperative infection was evident in 22 of 850 procedures (19 early/3 late infections, 4 superficial/18 deep infections). Most infections (21 of 22) occurred with posterior instrumentation. Risk factors included extended preoperative hospitalization ($P < 0.04$), high blood loss ($P < 0.01$), and prolonged operation time ($P < 0.001$). Diabetes, corticosteroid therapy, previous spinal surgery, obesity, chronic infection, and smoking were also found to play a role. Their results suggest that extended prophylaxis should be considered in posterior instrumentation, especially when risk factors are apparent.[75,76]

Lastly, late complications can occur. Nonunions are rare;[77] more common is associated degeneration and instability of adjacent segments in the cervical spine. Matsunaga et al[78] performed a biomechanical analysis of buckling alignment to assess for preoperative prediction of subaxial subluxation after occipitocervical fusion. The subjects were 25 patients with rheumatoid atlantoaxial dislocation and 15 patients with nonrheumatoid atlantoaxial dislocation who underwent occipitocervical fusion. They found five segments of nonfused vertebrae had subluxation after surgery in the rheumatoid group, and no subluxation was encountered in the nonrheumatoid group. They concluded that in patients with rheumatoid arthritis, segments that show abnormal buckling before surgery are likely to develop subluxation after occipitocervical fusion.[78] Matsunaga et al[79,80] followed 16 patients with rheumatoid arthritis with myelopathy who underwent occipitocervical fusion with a rectangular rod for more than 10 years. He found that subaxial subluxation developed in 31% of patients after surgery. Only one patient had symptoms from the adjacent level degeneration during greater than 10 years of observation.[79,80] Kraus et al[81] found similar results, with postoperative subluxation seen in 6% of patients who underwent atlantoaxial fusion and 36% after occipitocervical fusion. Matsunaga et al[82] also looked at the significance of the occipitoaxial angle and its association with swan-neck deformity and subaxial subluxation. They followed 38 patients for more than 5 years. They measured the angle between McGregor's line and the inferior surface of C2 in healthy volunteers and in patients who had occipitocervical fusion. Matsunaga and associates found that because subaxial subluxation often occurred within 1 year, it was likely that mechanical forces were the driving force because natural inflammatory process could not present this early. This study found that if the occiput-C2 angle was fixed within two standard deviations of the measured value for volunteers, subaxial subluxation occurred after surgery in only one patient. Of patients in whom the occiput-C2 angle was fixed at a position of more than 30° from normal, swan-neck malalignment occurred after surgery. In addition, they found that 34% of patients experienced subaxial subluxation after surgery. The site of subluxation was most commonly seen at C4-C5, and the majority was seen 3 years postoperatively. They found that 86% of the patients who experienced subaxial subluxation were fused in flexion, in which the anteversion of the occipital bone against the axis was excessive (minus position). They concluded that the position of fixation of the occipital bone and axis is crucial to prevent swan-neck deformity and subaxial subluxation; accordingly, they recommend an intraoperative radiograph before fusion.[82]

Occipital Condyle Fractures

Occipital condyle fractures were first described in an article by Sir Charles Bell[83] in 1817 in which he described a patient who suddenly dropped dead as he turned his head to thank his doctor while leaving the hospital. The death was caused by compression of the medulla oblongata from a fractured occipital condyle. Since then, there has been abundant literature on this entity. Alker et al[84] saw only 3 cases in 258 traffic accident deaths. The reported incidence of occipital condyle fractures has increased more recently. Bloom et al[85] reported 9 cases among 55 cases of severe head and cervical injuries. The routine use of high-resolution helical CT scans has made the diagnosis easier to obtain.[85-93] Occipital condyle fractures have been described and categorized by Anderson and Montesano[10] (**Figure 17**). Their type I fracture is an impacted occipital condyle fracture occurring as a result of axial loading of the skull on the atlas (**Figures 6** and **7**). This may be associated with an incompetent alar ligament on the side of the fracture, but stability is provided by the contralateral alar ligament and the tectorial membrane.

Their type II fracture is an occipital condyle fracture associated with a basilar skull fracture (**Figure 8,** *E*). The mechanism is a direct blow to the skull. Stability is provided by the alar ligaments, which remain intact, and a normal tectorial membrane.

Their type III fracture is an avulsion fracture of the occipital condyle by the alar ligament (**Figure 18**). This may occur as a result of rotation or lateral bending or both. Once this injury has occurred, the tectorial membrane and the contralateral alar ligaments are loaded and if these also are weakened, significant occipitocervical instability may occur.

The treatment of type I and type II occipital condyle fractures is immobilization in a rigid col-

FIGURE 17

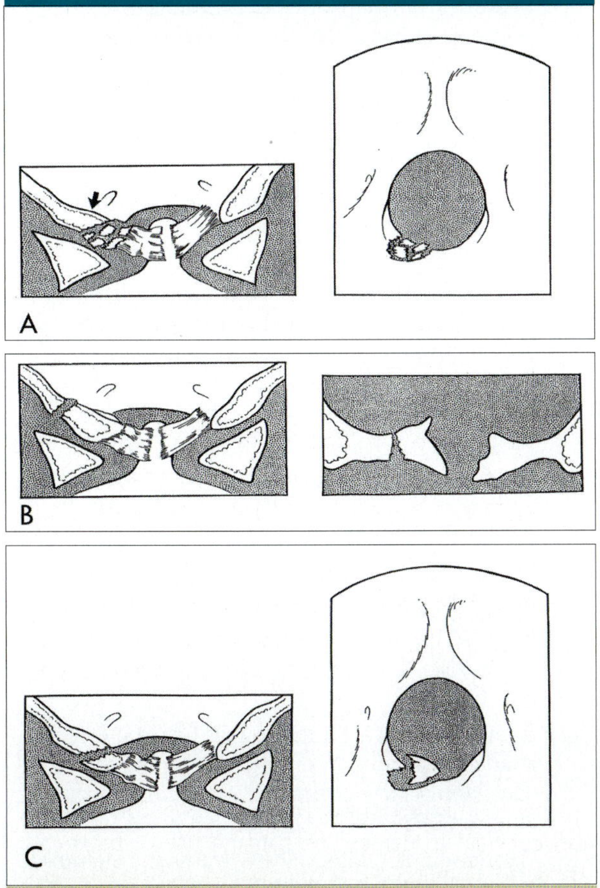

Figure 17 These figures illustrate the best available classification for fractures involving the occipital condyles. **A,** This is an impacted occipital condyle fracture. In most cases, this would be a stable injury and can be treated with a collar. **B,** This occipital condyle fracture is associated with a basilar skull fracture. In most cases this would be stable. **C,** This condyle fracture destabilizes the origin of the alar ligament and may be associated with significant occipitocervical instability. (Reproduced with permission from Anderson PA, Montesano PX: Morphology and treatment of occipital condyle fractures. *Spine (Phila Pa 1976)* 1988;13(7): 731-736.)

FIGURE 18

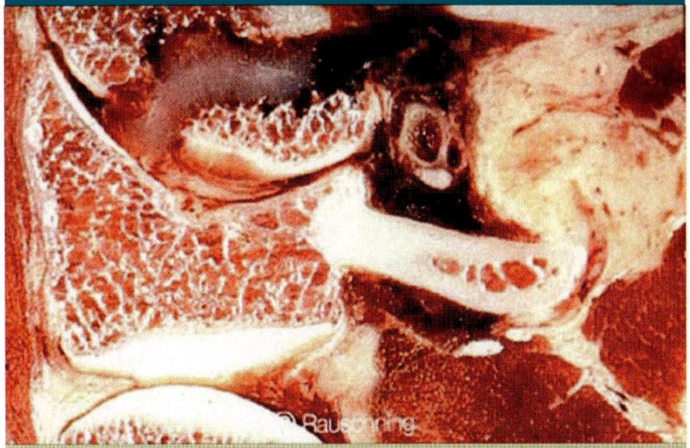

Figure 18 This is an occipital condyle fracture as seen on cryosectioning. The fragment was avulsed by the (intact) alar ligament. On plain radiographs, this fracture was barely visible and was only detected at second-look evaluation. The avulsed fragment is displaced posteriorly and medially; embedding medium fills the wide fracture gap. Note the torn posterior joint capsule and muscle ruptures under the posterior arch of the atlas. The vertebral artery and the underlying C1 nerve are surrounded by wide venous sinuses. In the atlantoaxial joint, the posterior meniscoid and the joint capsule are torn, pulling the C2 nerve into the joint space. (Reproduced with permission from Wolfgang Rauschning, MD, PhD at www.spineuniverse.com.)

lar for 6 to 8 weeks. The treatment of a type III fracture of the occipital condyle can range from immobilization in a rigid collar for 8 to 12 weeks, to halo immobilization, to posterior occipitocervical fusion if enough of the remaining bony and ligamentous restraints have been injured.

There have been many reports that highlight the associated nerve palsies that often accompany this injury. The occipital condyles are in close relationship to the hypoglossal canal (less than 0.5 mm), and this contains the cranial nerve XII and the jugular foramen (less than 1 cm), which includes cranial nerves IX, X, and XI.[94] Occipital condyles also have a close anatomic relationship to the brainstem and vascular structures.[92] Most patients seen after this injury have lower cranial nerve dysfunction, as lesions in the brainstem and vessels rarely survive.[49,93,95-97]

The most common palsy seen is that of cranial nerve XII, the hypoglossal nerve. Patients may report a peculiar sensation affecting one side of the tongue,[98] or they may find it difficult to speak or have difficulty with mastication. Posttraumatic hypoglossal nerve palsy can result from an insult anywhere along its anatomic pathway from the medulla oblongata to the tongue; however, with occipital condyle fractures, they often stem from disruption of the hypoglossal canal.[99-102] Others have postulated a traction-type injury.[103,104] Recovery after posttraumatic hypoglossal nerve palsy is variable. The vast majority of cases continue to have some residual deficit,[98] although complete recovery is possible.[103]

Occipital condyle fractures can also be associated with Wallenberg syndrome. This syndrome consists of a Horner sign, hemiparesis, cerebellar ataxia, and crossed hemianesthesia. Miyazaki et al[105] described a case in which a violent direct axial load hit the right anterior part of the head, forcing the occipital condyle toward the atlas. This produced a comminuted triangle-shaped fracture with the right occipital condyle at its base and the right jugular foramen at its apex (type I fracture). This palsy occurred at the time of injury; however, most appear later, probably because of fragment migration and callus formation.[105]

Summary

The most important aspect of medical care for a patient with occipitocervical instability is the emergency and early hospital treatment. Recognition and prompt immobilization are essential to successful treatment. It is important to assess the patient for comorbid conditions such as cranial nerve palsies or vertebral artery thrombosis. Most patients with occipitocervical subluxation or dislocation who survive will require a posterior occipitocervical fusion. Of those patients with type I or type II occipital condyle fractures, rigid collar immobilization usually will achieve a satisfactory result.

References

1. Bucholz RW, Burkhead WZ: The pathological anatomy of fatal atlanto-occipital dislocations. *J Bone Joint Surg Am* 1979;61(2):248-250.
2. Davis D, Bohlman H, Walker AE, Fisher R, Robinson R: The pathological findings in fatal craniospinal injuries. *J Neurosurg* 1971;34(5): 603-613.
3. Alker GJ, Oh YS, Leslie EV, Lehotay J, Panaro VA, Eschner EG: Postmortem radiology of head neck injuries in fatal traffic accidents. *Radiology* 1975; 114(3):611-617.
4. Bohlman HH: Acute fractures and dislocations of the cervical spine: An analysis of three hundred hospitalized patients and review of the literature. *J Bone Joint Surg Am* 1979;61(8):1119-1142.
5. Clark CR, Igram CM, el-Khoury GY, Ehara S: Radiographic evaluation of cervical spine injuries. *Spine (Phila Pa 1976)* 1988;13(7):742-747.
6. Englander O: Non-traumatic occipito-atlanto-axial dislocation. *Br J Radiol* 1942;15:341-345.
7. Hunter T: The spinal complications of ankylosing spondylitis. *Semin Arthritis Rheum* 1989;19(3): 172-182.
8. Redlund-Johnell I: Atlanto-occipital dislocation in rheumatoid arthritis. *Acta Radiol Diagn (Stockh)* 1984;25(3):165-168.
9. Martel W: The occipito-atlanto-axial joints in rheumatoid arthritis and ankylosing spondylitis. *Am J Roentgenol Radium Ther Nucl Med* 1961;86: 223-240.
10. Anderson PA, Montesano PX: Morphology and treatment of occipital condyle fractures. *Spine (Phila Pa 1976)* 1988;13(7):731-736.
11. Banna M, Stevenson GW, Tumiel A: Unilateral atlanto-occipital dislocation complicating an anomaly of the atlas: A case report. *J Bone Joint Surg Am* 1983;65(5):685-687.
12. Bools JC, Rose BS: Traumatic atlantooccipital dislocation: Two cases with survival. *AJNR Am J Neuroradiol* 1986;7(5):901-904.
13. Dublin AB, Marks WM, Weinstock D, Newton TH: Traumatic dislocation of the atlanto-occipital articulation (AOA) with short-term survival: With a radiographic method of measuring the AOA. *J Neurosurg* 1980;52(4):541-546.
14. Eismont FJ, Bohlman HH: Posterior atlanto-occipital dislocation with fractures of the atlas and odontoid process. *J Bone Joint Surg Am* 1978; 60(3):397-399.
15. Evarts CM: Traumatic occipito-atlantal dislocation. *J Bone Joint Surg Am* 1970;52(8):1653-1660.
16. Fruin AH, Pirotte TP: Traumatic atlantooccipital dislocation: Case report. *J Neurosurg* 1977;46(5): 663-666.
17. Georgopoulos G, Pizzutillo PD, Lee MS: Occipito-atlantal instability in children: A report of five cases and review of the literature. *J Bone Joint Surg Am* 1987;69(3):429-436.
18. Gabrielson TO, Maxwell JA: Traumatic atlanto-occipital dislocation; with case report of a patient who survived. *Am J Roentgenol Radium Ther Nucl Med* 1966;97(3):624-629.
19. Grob D, Dvorak J, Panjabi MM, Antinnes JA: The role of plate and screw fixation in occipitocervical fusion in rheumatoid arthritis. *Spine (Phila Pa 1976)* 1994;19(22):2545-2551.
20. Montane I, Eismont FJ, Green BA: Traumatic occipitoatlantal dislocation. *Spine (Phila Pa 1976)* 1991;16(2):112-116.
21. Page CP, Story JL, Wissinger JP, Branch CL: Traumatic atlantooccipital dislocation: Case report. *J Neurosurg* 1973;39(3):394-397.
22. Pang D, Wilberger JE Jr: Traumatic atlanto-occipital dislocation with survival: Case report and review. *Neurosurgery* 1980;7(5):503-508.
23. Rockswold GL, Seljeskog EL: Traumatic atlantocranial dislocation with survival. *Minn Med* 1979;62(3):151-152, 154.
24. Traynelis VC, Marano GD, Dunker RO, Kaufman HH: Traumatic atlanto-occipital dislocation: Case report. *J Neurosurg* 1986;65(6):863-870.
25. Van den Bout AH, Dommisse GF: Traumatic atlantooccipital dislocation. *Spine (Phila Pa 1976)* 1986;11(2):174-176.
26. Watridge CB, Orrison WW, Arnold H, Woods GA: Lateral atlantooccipital dislocation: Case re-

port. *Neurosurgery* 1985;17(2):345-347.

27. Woodring JH, Selke AC Jr, Duff DE: Traumatic atlantooccipital dislocation with survival. *AJR Am J Roentgenol* 1981;137(1):21-24.
28. Ide C, Nisolle JF, Misson N, et al: Unusual occipitoatlantal fracture dissociation with no neurological impairmen: Case report. *J Neurosurg* 1998; 88(4):773-776.
29. Govender S, Vlok GJ, Fisher-Jeffes N, Du Preez CP: Traumatic dislocation of the atlanto-occipital joint. *J Bone Joint Surg Br* 2003;85(6):875-878.
30. Apple JS, Kirks DR, Merten DF, Martinez S: Cervical spine fractures and dislocations in children. *Pediatr Radiol* 1987;17(1):45-49.
31. Cattell HS, Filtzer DL: Pseudosubluxation and other normal variations in the cervical spine in children: A study of one hundred and sixty children. *J Bone Joint Surg Am* 1965;47(7):1295-1309.
32. Werne S: Studies in spontaneous atlas dislocation. *Acta Orthop Scand Suppl* 1957;23:1-150.
33. Panjabi M, Dvorak J, Duranceau J, et al: Three-dimensional movements of the upper cervical spine. *Spine (Phila Pa 1976)* 1988;13(7):726-730.
34. Gerlock AJ Jr, Mirfakhraee M, Benzel EC: Computed tomography of traumatic atlantooccipital dislocation. *Neurosurgery* 1983;13(3):316-319.
35. Grobovschek M, Scheibelbrandner W: Atlanto-occipital dislocation. *Neuroradiology* 1983;25(3): 173-174.
36. Kaufman RA, Carroll CD, Buncher CR: Atlantooccipital junction: Standards for measurement in normal children. *AJNR Am J Neuroradiol* 1987; 8(6):995-999.
37. Lee C, Woodring JH, Goldstein SJ, Daniel TL, Young AB, Tibbs PA: Evaluation of traumatic atlantooccipital dislocations. *AJNR Am J Neuroradiol* 1987;8(1):19-26.
38. Putnam WE, Stratton FT, Rohr RJ, Stitzell W, Roat G: Traumatic atlanto-occipital dislocations: Value of the Powers ratio in diagnosis. *J Am Osteopath Assoc* 1986;86(12):798-804.
39. Scott EW, Haid RW Jr, Peace D: Type I fractures of the odontoid process: Implications for atlanto-occipital instability. Case report. *J Neurosurg* 1990; 72(3):488-492.
40. Shapiro R, Youngberg AS, Rothman SL: The differential diagnosis of traumatic lesions of the occipito-atlanto-axial segment. *Radiol Clin North Am* 1973;11(3):505-526.
41. Wholey MH, Bruwer AJ, Baker HL Jr: The lateral roentgenogram of the neck; with comments on the atlanto-odontoid-basion relationship. *Radiology* 1958;71(3):350-356.
42. Wiesel SW, Rothman RH: Occipitoatlantal hypermobility. *Spine (Phila Pa 1976)* 1979;4(3):187-191.
43. Powers B, Miller MD, Kramer RS, Martinez S, Gehweiler JA Jr: Traumatic anterior atlanto-occipital dislocation. *Neurosurgery* 1979;4(1): 12-17.
44. Anderson LD, D'Alonzo RT: Fractures of the odontoid process of the axis. *J Bone Joint Surg Am* 1974;56(8):1663-1674.
45. Reddy M, Reddy B, Schöggl A, Saringer W, Matula Ch: The complexity of trauma to the cranio-cervical junction: Correlation of clinical presentation with Doppler flow velocities in the V3-segment of the vertebral arteries. *Acta Neurochir (Wien)* 2002;144(6):575-580.
46. Shkrum MJ, Green RN, Nowak ES: Upper cervical trauma in motor vehicle collisions. *J Forensic Sci* 1989;34(2):381-390.
47. Tepper SL, Fligner CL, Reay DT: Atlanto-occipital disarticulation: Accident characteristics. *Am J Forensic Med Pathol* 1990;11(3):193-197.
48. Lesoin F, Blondel M, Dhellemmes P, Thomas CE, Viaud C, Jomin M: Post-traumatic atlanto-occipital dislocation revealed by sudden cardiopulmonary arrest. *Lancet* 1982;2(8295):447-448.
49. Hashimoto T, Watanabe O, Takase M, Koniyama J, Kobota M: Collet-Sicard syndrome after minor head trauma. *Neurosurgery* 1988;23(3):367-370.
50. Bell HS: Paralysis of both arms from injury of the upper portion of the pyramidal decussation: "Cruciate paralysis". *J Neurosurg* 1970;33(4): 376-380.
51. Nielsen JM: *A Textbook of Clinical Neurology*, ed 3. New York, NY, Paul B. Hoeber, Inc, 1951.
52. Herzenberg JE, Hensinger RN, Dedrick DK, Phillips WA: Emergency transport and positioning of young children who have an injury of the cervical spine: The standard backboard may be hazardous. *J Bone Joint Surg Am* 1989;71(1):15-22.
53. Bivins HG, Ford S, Bezmalinovic Z, Price HM, Williams JL: The effect of axial traction during orotracheal intubation of the trauma victim with an unstable cervical spine. *Ann Emerg Med* 1988; 17(1):25-29.
54. Smith MD: Occipital cervical fusion. *Techn Orthop* 1994;9(1):37-42.
55. Wertheim SB, Bohlman HH: Occipitocervical fusion: Indications, technique, and long-term results in thirteen patients. *J Bone Joint Surg Am* 1987; 69(6):833-836.
56. Robinson RA, Southwick WO: Surgical approaches to the cervical spine. *Instr Course Lect* 1960;17:299-330.
57. Starr J, Eismont FJ, Scuderi G: Posterior occipitocervical fusion for non-rheumatoid instability. Presented at the *Annual Meeting of the Cervical Spine Research Society*. Desert Springs, CA, December 1992.

58. Fehlings MG, Errico T, Cooper P, Benjamin V, DiBartolo T: Occipitocervical fusion with a five-millimeter malleable rod and segmental fixation. *Neurosurgery* 1993;32(2):198-208.
59. Ashraf J, Crockard HA, Ransford AO, Stevens JM: Transoral decompression and posterior stabilisation in Morquio's disease. *Arch Dis Child* 1991; 66(11):1318-1321.
60. Ransford AO, Crockard HA, Pozo JL, Thomas NP, Nelson IW: Craniocervical instability treated by contoured loop fixation. *J Bone Joint Surg Br* 1986; 68(2):173-177.
61. Sakou T, Kawaida H, Morizono Y, Matsunaga S, Fielding JW: Occipitoatlantoaxial fusion utilizing a rectangular rod. *Clin Orthop Relat Res* 1989;239: 136-144.
62. Sonntag VK, Dickman CA: Craniocervical stabilization. *Clin Neurosurg* 1993;40:243-272.
63. Grob D, Magerl F: Surgical stabilization of C1 and C2 fractures. *Orthopade* 1987;16(1):46-54.
64. Grob D, Dvorak J, Panjabi M, Froehlich M, Hayek J: Posterior occipitocervical fusion: A preliminary report of a new technique. *Spine (Phila Pa 1976)* 1991;16(3, Suppl):S17-S24.
65. Grob D, Jeanneret B, Aebi M, Markwalder TM: Atlanto-axial fusion with transarticular screw fixation. *J Bone Joint Surg Br* 1991;73(6):972-976.
66. Ebraheim NA, Lu J, Biyani A, Brown JA, Yeasting RA: An anatomic study of the thickness of the occipital bone: Implications for occipitocervical instrumentation. *Spine (Phila Pa 1976)* 1996; 21(15):1725-1730.
67. Zipnick RI, Merola AA, Gorup J, et al: Occipital morphology: An anatomic guide to internal fixation. *Spine (Phila Pa 1976)* 1996;21(15): 1719-1730.
68. Grob D: Transarticular screw fixation for atlanto-occipital dislocation. *Spine (Phila Pa 1976)* 2001; 26(6):703-707.
69. Feiz-Erfan I, Gonzalez LF, Dickman CA: Atlantooccipital transarticular screw fixation for the treatment of traumatic occipitoatlantal dislocation: Technical note. *J Neurosurg Spine* 2005;2(3): 381-385.
70. Torina PJ, Flanders AE, Carrino JA, et al: Incidence of vertebral artery thrombosis in cervical spine trauma: Correlation with severity of spinal cord injury. *AJNR Am J Neuroradiol* 2005;26(10): 2645-2651.
71. Reed CM, Campbell SE, Beall DP, Bui JS, Stefko RM: Atlanto-occipital dislocation with traumatic pseudomeningocele formation and post-traumatic syringomyelia. *Spine (Phila Pa 1976)* 2005;30(5): E128-E133.
72. Fischbein NJ, Dillon WP, Cobbs C, Weinstein PR: The "presyrinx" state: A reversible myelopathic condition that may precede syringomyelia. *AJNR Am J Neuroradiol* 1999;20(1):7-20.
73. Eismont FJ, Wiesel SW, Rothman RH: Treatment of dural tears associated with spinal surgery. *J Bone Joint Surg Am* 1981;63(7):1132-1136.
74. Gluf WM, Schmidt MH, Apfelbaum RI: Atlantoaxial transarticular screw fixation: A review of surgical indications, fusion rate, complications, and lessons learned in 191 adult patients. *J Neurosurg Spine* 2005;2(2):155-163.
75. Wimmer C, Gluch H, Franzreb M, Ogon M: Predisposing factors for infection in spine surgery: A survey of 850 spinal procedures. *J Spinal Disord* 1998;11(2):124-128.
76. Wimmer C, Nogler M, Frischhut B: Influence of antibiotics on infection in spinal surgery: A prospective study of 110 patients. *J Spinal Disord* 1998;11(6):498-500.
77. Gluf WM, Brockmeyer DL: Atlantoaxial transarticular screw fixation: A review of surgical indications, fusion rate, complications, and lessons learned in 67 pediatric patients. *J Neurosurg Spine* 2005;2(2):164-169.
78. Matsunaga S, Sakou T, Sunahara N, Oonishi T, Maeda S, Nakanisi K: Biomechanical analysis of buckling alignment of the cervical spine: Predictive value for subaxial subluxation after occipitocervical fusion. *Spine (Phila Pa 1976)* 1997;22(7): 765-771.
79. Mori T, Matsunaga S, Sunahara N, Sakou T: 3- to 11-year followup of occipitocervical fusion for rheumatoid arthritis. *Clin Orthop Relat Res* 1998; 351:169-179.
80. Matsunaga S, Ijiri K, Koga H: Results of a longer than 10-year follow-up of patients with rheumatoid arthritis treated by occipitocervical fusion. *Spine (Phila Pa 1976)* 2000;25(14):1749-1753.
81. Kraus DR, Peppelman WC, Agarwal AK, DeLeeuw HW, Donaldson WF III: Incidence of subaxial subluxation in patients with generalized rheumatoid arthritis who have had previous occipital cervical fusions. *Spine (Phila Pa 1976)* 1991; 16(10, Suppl):S486-S489.
82. Matsunaga S, Onishi T, Sakou T: Significance of occipitoaxial angle in subaxial lesion after occipitocervical fusion. *Spine (Phila Pa 1976)* 2001; 26(2):161-165.
83. Bell C: Surgical observation. *Middlesex Hosp J* 1817;4:469-470.
84. Alker GJ Jr, Oh YS, Leslie EV: High cervical spine and craniocervical junction injuries in fatal traffic accidents: A radiological study. *Orthop Clin North Am* 1978;9(4):1003-1010.
85. Bloom AI, Neeman Z, Slasky BS, et al: Fracture of the occipital condyles and associated craniocervi-

cal ligament injury: Incidence, CT imaging and implications. *Clin Radiol* 1997;52(3):198-202.

86. Bloom AI, Neeman Z, Floman Y, Gomori J, Bar-Ziv J: Occipital condyle fracture and ligament injury: Imaging by CT. *Pediatr Radiol* 1996; 26(11):786-790.
87. Clayman DA, Sykes CH, Vines FS: Occipital condyle fractures: Clinical presentation and radiologic detection. *AJNR Am J Neuroradiol* 1994;15(7): 1309-1315.
88. Young WF, Rosenwasser RH, Getch C, Jallo J: Diagnosis and management of occipital condyle fractures. *Neurosurgery* 1994;34(2):257-261.
89. Blacksin MF, Lee HJ: Frequency and significance of fractures of the upper cervical spine detected by CT in patients with severe neck trauma. *AJR Am J Roentgenol* 1995;165(5):1201-1204.
90. Link TM, Schuierer G, Hufendiek A, Horch C, Peters PE: Substantial head trauma: Value of routine CT examination of the cervicocranium. *Radiology* 1995;196(3):741-745.
91. Wasserberg J, Bartlett RJ: Occipital condyle fractures diagnosed by high-definition CT and coronal reconstructions. *Neuroradiology* 1995;37(5): 370-373.
92. Noble ER, Smoker WR: The forgotten condyle: The appearance, morphology, and classification of occipital condyle fractures. *AJNR Am J Neuroradiol* 1996;17(3):507-513.
93. Bozboga M, Unal F, Hepgul K, Izgi N, Turantan MI, Turker K: Fracture of the occipital condyle: Case report. *Spine (Phila Pa 1976)* 1992;17(9): 1119-1121.
94. Cirak B, Akpinar G, Palaoglu S: Traumatic occipital condyle fractures. *Neurosurg Rev* 2000;23(3): 161-164.
95. Bolender N, Cromwell LD, Wendling L: Fracture of the occipital condyle. *AJR Am J Roentgenol* 1978;131(4):729-731.
96. Dickman CA, Papadopoulos SM, Sonntag VK, Spetzler RF, Rekate HL, Drabier J: Traumatic occipitoatlantal dislocations. *J Spinal Disord* 1993; 6(4):300-313.
97. Desai SS, Coumas JM, Danylevich A, Hayes E, Dunn EJ: Fracture of the occipital condyle: Case report and review of the literature. *J Trauma* 1990;30(2):240-241.
98. Kaushik V, Kelly G, Richards SD, Saeed SR: Isolated unilateral hypoglossal nerve palsy after minor head trauma. *Clin Neurol Neurosurg* 2002; 105(1):42-47.
99. Castling B, Hicks K: Traumatic isolated unilateral hypoglossal nerve palsy—case report and review of the literature. *Br J Oral Maxillofac Surg* 1995; 33(3):171-173.
100. Demisch S, Lindner A, Beck R, Zierz S: The forgotten condyle: Delayed hypoglossal nerve palsy caused by fracture of the occipital condyle. *Clin Neurol Neurosurg* 1998;100(1):44-45.
101. Massaro F, Lanotte M: Fracture of the occipital condyle. *Injury* 1993;24(6):419-420.
102. Orbay T, Aykol S, Seçkin Z, Ergün R: Late hypoglossal nerve palsy following fracture of the occipital condyle. *Surg Neurol* 1989;31(5):402-404.
103. Brennan RJ, Shirley JP, Compton JS: Bilateral hypoglossal nerve palsies following head injury. *J Emerg Med* 1993;11(2):167-168.
104. Dukes IK, Bannerjee SK: Hypoglossal nerve palsy following hyperextension neck injury. *Injury* 1993;24(2):133-134.
105. Miyazaki C, Katsume M, Yamazaki T, Aoki K, Kuroki T, Takasu N: Unusual occipital condyle fracture with multiple nerve palsies and Wallenberg syndrome. *Clin Neurol Neurosurg* 2000; 102(4):255-258.

CHAPTER 20
Fractures of the Atlas

Kris Radcliff, MD Lauren R. Maher, BA Joseph Hong, BS Rebecca Stinsman, BS
Alan M. Levine, MD Alexander R. Vaccaro, MD, PhD

Introduction

Atlas fractures account for 2% to 13% of all cervical spine injuries and approximately 1.3% of all spine fractures.[1] Atlas fractures are rarely associated with neurologic injury.[2] However, the most serious implications and problems with treatment have not remained with the fracture itself, but rather with injuries associated with the atlas fracture.

Fractures of the atlas were initally described in 1822, when Sir Astley Cooper, in a treatise on dislocations and fractures of the joints, described the first case.[3] Between 1822 and 1920, a period of almost 100 years, only 46 cases were subsequently reported. This prompted Geoffrey Jefferson to publish his noted report "Fracture of the Atlas Vertebra," in which he reviewed his experience of four cases as well as the 46 cases that had been previously reported in the literature. He very astutely analyzed the fracture and contributed a great deal to our knowledge of this injury.[4,5]

Pathoanatomy

The atlas is distinct from the other cervical vertebrae in that its vertebral body is actually functionally absorbed into the structure of the axis (dens). Instead of a vertebral body, the atlas has a very thick anterior arch that connects the two lateral masses (**Figure 1**). The lateral masses of the atlas form an articulation with the occipital condyles and the facet joints of C2. The occiput-C1 joints are positioned obliquely in the coronal plane, with the result that compressive forces from the skull are directed radially outward into the C1 ring. The weakest portions of the C1 ring are at the junctions of the anterior and posterior arches with the lateral masses.

The vertebral arteries course proximally from C2 and enter the C1 foramen transversarium before crossing along the posterior arch of the atlas. The groove on the atlas for the vertebral artery lies just behind the lateral mass and thins the posterior arch at that location. The vertebral artery may be injured in association with C1 fractures. Occasionally accessory foramina are present through which the vertebral artery may course. In 15% of patients in one study, the vertebral artery groove may have bony walls called a ponticulus posticus.[6] The vertebral artery may be endangered if a surgeon attempts to place a C1 lateral mass screw through the posterior arch of C1 if a ponticulus posticus is present (**Figure 2**).

The primary ligamentous stabilizers of the C1-C2 articulation are the cruciate ligament, the transverse ligament, and the alar ligaments. Because no disk is present between the occiput and C1 or C1-C2, the local anatomic relationships are maintained by the substantial ligamentous structures in the upper cervical region (**Figure 3**). The cruciate ligament is the main ligamentous structure in the occiput-C1-C2 complex. The ascending branch attaches to the basion at the anterior edge of the foramen magnum and the descending

Dr. Levine is deceased. At the time this chapter was written, Dr. Levine or an immediate family member had received royalties from Elsevier and US Spine; was a member of a speakers' bureau or had made paid presentations on behalf of Accuray; served as a paid consultant to or was an employee of US Spine; and had received research or institutional support from Accuray, Amgen, and Medtronic Sofamor Danek. Dr. Vaccaro or an immediate family member serves as a board member, owner, officer, or committee member of the North American Spine Society, American Spinal Injury Association, and the Cervical Spine Research Society; has received royalties from Aesculap/B.Braun, DePuy, a Johnson & Johnson company, Globus Medical, Medtronic Sofamor Danek, K2M, Stout Medical, Progressive Spinal Technology, and Applied Spinal Intellectual Properties; serves as a paid consultant to or is an employee of K2M; has received research or institutional support from AO North America, DePuy, a Johnson & Johnson company, Medtronic Sofamor Danek, and Stryker; and owns stock or stock options in Globus Medical, Disk Motion Technology, Progressive Spinal Technologies, Advanced Spinal Intellectual Properties, Computational Biodynamics, Stout Medical, Paradigm Spine, K2M, Replication Medica, Spinology, SpineMedica, Orthovita, Vertiflex, Small Bone Technologies, NeuCore, CrossCurrent, Syndicom, In Vivo, Flagship Surgical, Pearl Diver, Location Based Intelligence, and Gamma Spine. None of the following authors or any immediate family member has received anything of value from or owns stock in a commercial company or institution related directly or indirectly to the subject of this chapter: Dr. Radcliff, Ms. Maher, Mr. Hong, and Ms. Stinsman.

FIGURE 1

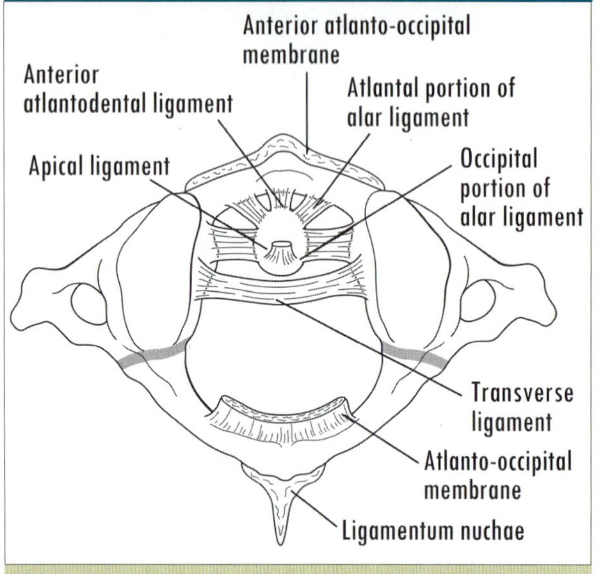

Figure 1 This drawing of the atlas demonstrates many of the features that distinguish it from other cervical levels. Its articulations with the atlas and the occiput lie in the anterior third of the ring. A relatively thin area of the ring lies just posterior to the joint surface (cross-hatching) as the vertebral artery passes across the superior surface of the ring at that point. The occipital membrane is in fact a thinned-out portion of the ligamentum flavum. All of the primary ligamentous structures, however, are also attached to the anterior third of the ring, leaving the posterior portion of the ring isolated structurally from the more significant anterior portion. Even the anterior portion of the ring (residual body) is relatively thinner than the more anterolateral portions containing the joints and the ligamentous attachments. (Redrawn with permission from Dvorak J, Panjabi MM: Functional anatomy of the alar ligaments. *Spine (Phila Pa 1976)* 1987;12(2):183-189.)

FIGURE 2

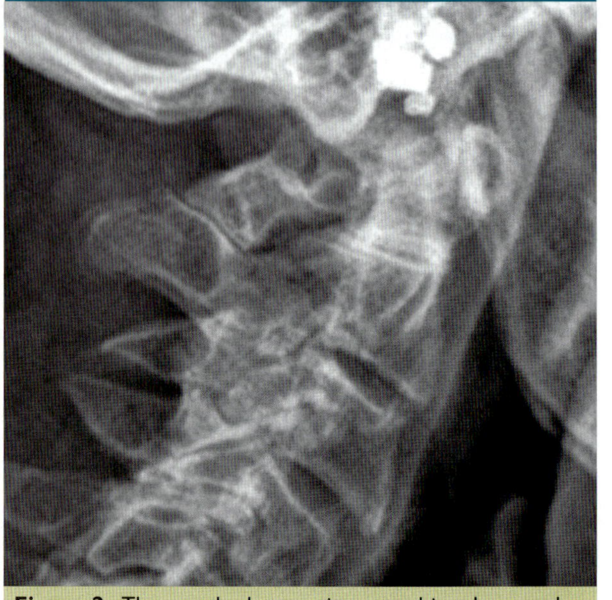

Figure 2 The vertebral artery is encased in a bony arch on the posterior rostral aspect of C1 (ponticulus posticus). The vertebral artery may be injured if a surgeon attempts to place a screw through the posterior arch of C1.

branch to the body of C2.[7] The transverse ligament (transverse atlantal ligament [TAL]) extends from one condyle of the atlas to the opposite condyle of the atlas and is apposed to the posterior margin of the dens. The transverse ligament is chiefly responsible for preventing anterior subluxation of C1 on C2.

Secondary stabilizers include the anterior longitudinal ligament, apical ligaments, and alar ligaments. The anterior longitudinal ligament attaches to the anterior margin of the body of C2 and anterior ring of C1. The stability of the occipital-C1 joint is also dependent on ligamentous attachments between the dens and the skull. The alar and apical ligaments are attached to the superior border of the dens and course obliquely to the medial surfaces of the occipital condyles. The apical ligaments connect the tip of the dens to the anterior edge of the foramen magnum. Dvorak et al[8] demonstrated that the alar ligaments contribute to limited axial rotation to the opposite side. Transection of one alar ligament results in a 30% increase in axial rotation in the other direction.

Posterior ligamentous stabilizers include the ligamentum flavum, posterior atlanto-occipital membrane, and posterior atlantoaxial membrane. The posterior atlanto-occipital membrane attaches to the posterior border of the ring of C1 and the posterior border of the foramen magnum. The posterior atlantoaxial membrane attaches from the skully to the posterior border of the ring of C1 and courses down to the posterior ring of C2. The ligamentum flavum is markedly attenuated in the upper cervical spine and begins between C2 and C3.

Equally important for stability in the upper cervical spine are the various muscular attachments. The longus colli (the superior oblique portion) attaches to the anterior and inferior margin of the arch of C1. In addition, the rectus capitis lateralis traverses from the anterior border of the transverse process of C1 to the lateral surface of the occiput. The rectus capitis medialis runs from the transverse process in a medial direction toward the anterior border of the foramen magnum. At a deeper level, the rectus capitis posterior minor traverses from the posterior border of the ring of

FIGURE 3

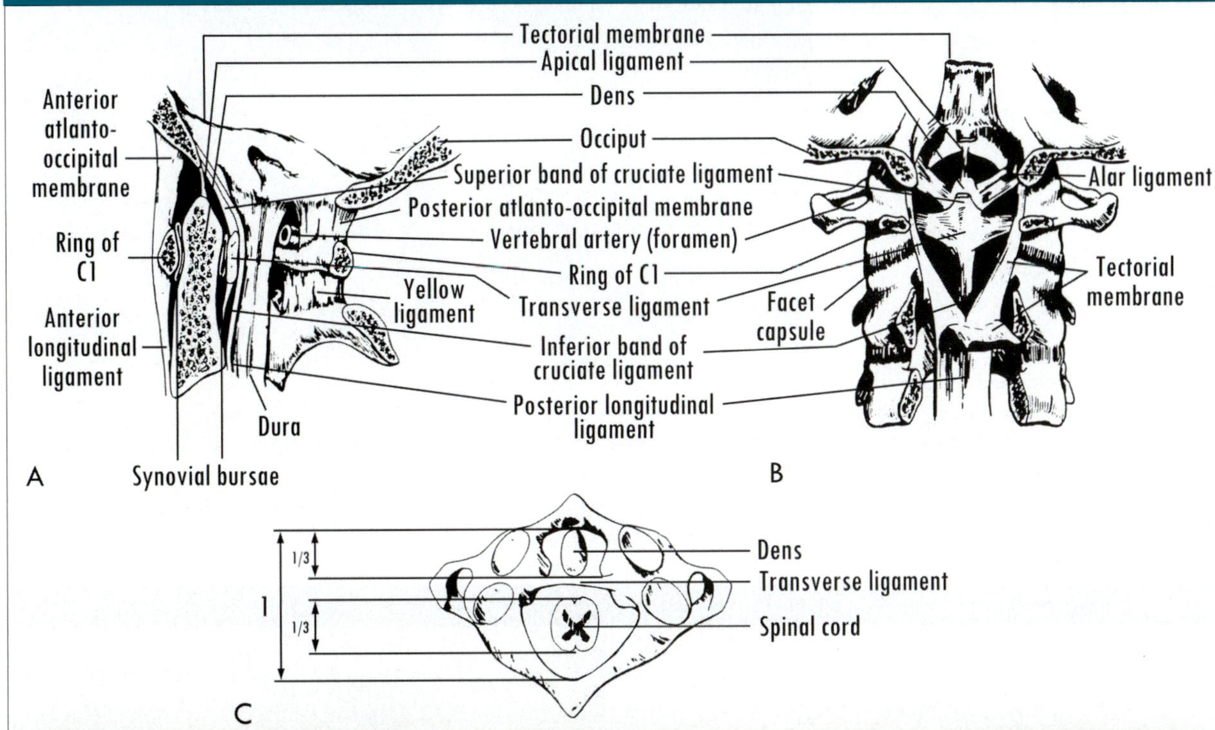

Figure 3 Lateral (**A**) and coronal (**B**) views of the upper cervical spine demonstrate the vertical attachments of the occiput and atlas to C1. These include the anterior and posterior atlanto-occipital membrane as well as the posterior longitudinal ligaments, anterior longitudinal ligament, and the ligamentum flavum. Some of the ligamentous attachments run from the dens (C2) to the occiput, stabilizing but bypassing C1 (cruciate, alar, and apical ligaments). The axial view (**C**) shows Steel's "rule of thirds of structures" within the ring of C1. (Reproduced with permission from White AA III, Panjabi MM, eds: *Clinical Biomechanics of the Spine*. Philadelphia, PA, JB Lippincott, 1988, p 134.)

C1 to the occiput. Similarly, the superior oblique muscle traverses from the lateral aspect of the ring of the atlas to the posterior surface of the skull, and the inferior oblique muscle courses from C2 obliquely to the lateral aspect of the C1 ring.

Classification and Mechanisms of Injury

The classification of fractures of the atlas is often predicated on the anatomic location of the fracture fragments and the amount of displacement. The basic injury patterns are (1) posterior arch fracture, (2) lateral mass fracture, (3) burst injury (the eponymous Jefferson fracture), (4) avulsion fracture from the anterior arch of C1, (5) transverse process fracture, (6) anterior arch fracture, and (7) comminuted unilateral intra-articular lateral mass fracture.[9]

The most common injury is the posterior arch fracture (**Figure 4**). Posterior arch fractures generally occur through the weakest portion of the posterior arch at the area of the junction of the posterior arch and the lateral masses. The most vulnerable location is the area where the vertebral artery courses over the top of the posterior arch, where the bone is most thin.[10-12] Fractures of the posterior arch of C1 have been thought to be the result of a hyperextension mechanism. This has been described as a hyperextension injury resulting from a bending moment to the posterior arch of C1 between the occiput and the ring of C2.[13,14] There is a very high association with other injuries known to result from hyperextension, such as C2 anterior avulsion fractures and type I traumatic spondylolisthesis of the axis.

The second type of injury is a fracture involving the lateral mass (**Figure 5**). Depending on the number of fracture lines, these have been called variously two-part or three-part fractures of the ring of C1.[2,10,15,16] These fractures can either enter the lateral mass in an intra-articular position or occur posterior to the lateral mass. Thus the treatment is the same whether the injury has two parts (fractures anterior and posterior to the lateral mass on one side) or three parts (with an additional contralateral posterior arch fracture). The displace-

FIGURE 4

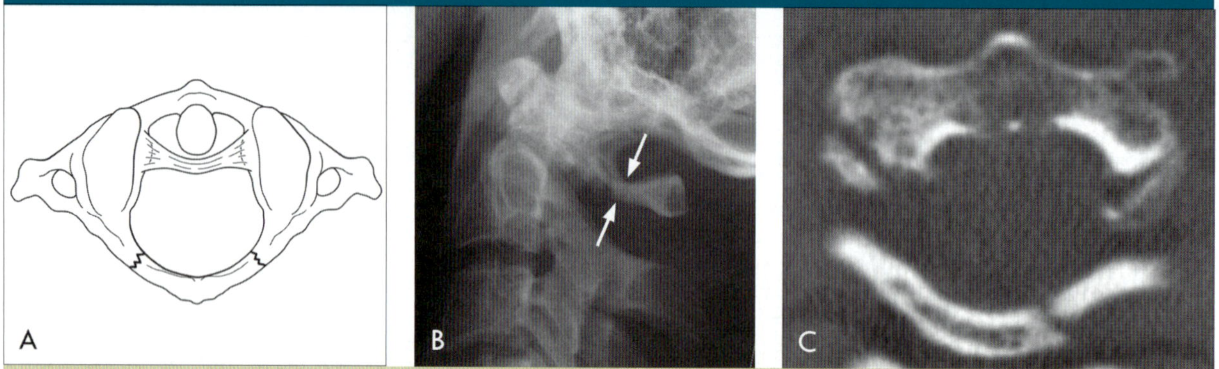

Figure 4 Posterior arch fracture. Both the drawing (**A**) and the lateral radiograph (**B,** arrows) show the position of the posterior arch fracture. Often, on the lateral view, the fracture is difficult to visualize as it may be so close to the posterior edge of the facet as to be obscured by the overlying structures. In that case, the only evidence of fracture may be an angular deformity of the orientation of the posterior arch. **C,** Axial CT scan demonstrates a displaced posterior arch C1 fracture. (**A** and **B** are reproduced from Levine AM: Fractures of the atlas, in Levine AM, Eismont FJ, Garfin SR, Zigler JE, eds: *Spine Trauma.* Philadelphia, PA, WB Saunders, 1998, pp 209-226.)

FIGURE 5

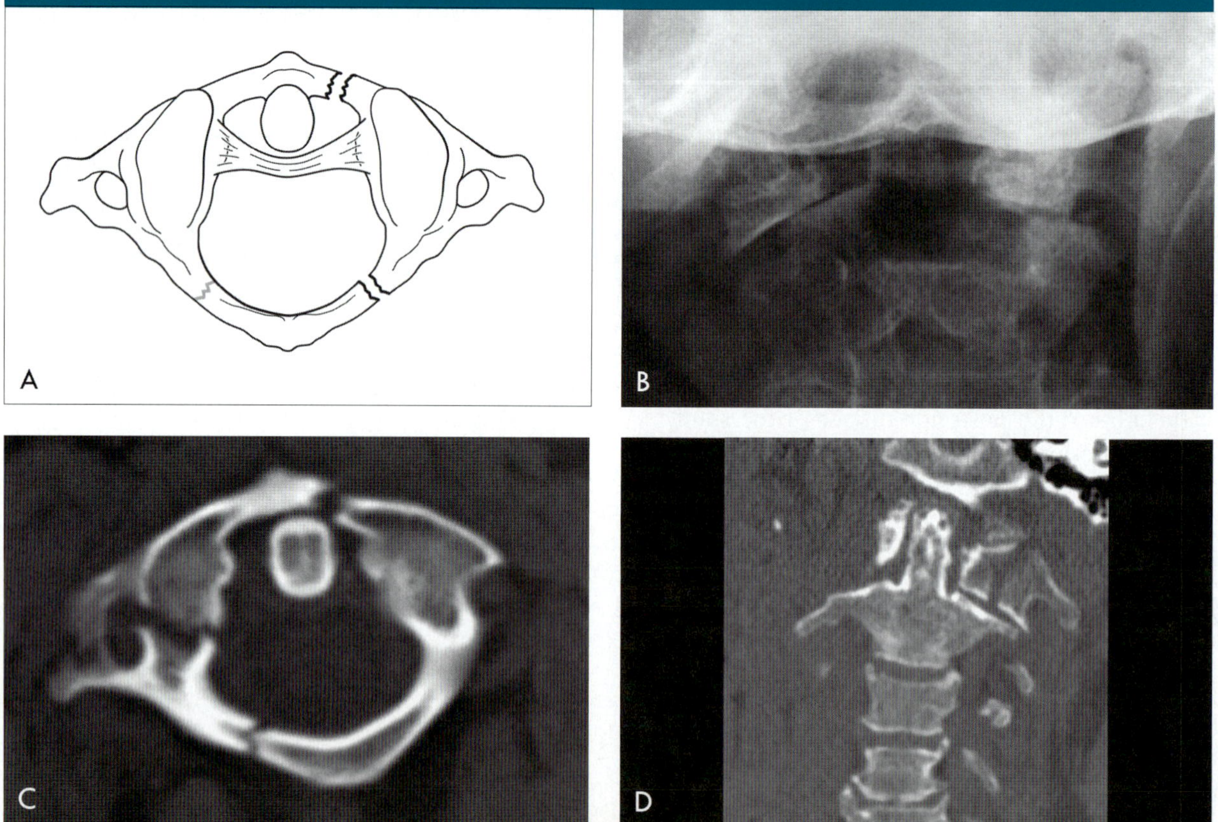

Figure 5 Lateral mass fracture. This injury consists of one fracture just anterior to the joint surface and one just posterior to the surface (**A**), which in some cases may extend into the joint. A third fracture may also be present in the contralateral posterior arch. **B,** The typical finding on the open-mouth view is displacement of only one lateral mass of the C1 (with reference to C2) joint surface, whereas the other side has a normal anatomic relationship. In the extreme situation, one lateral mass may actually be displaced from its position between the occipital condyle and the lateral mass of C2. **C,** The lateral mass fracture can also be intra-articular in the coronal plane, as demonstrated on this axial CT scan. **D,** A sagittal plane intra-articular lateral mass fracture may also develop, resulting in subluxation of the occipital condyle into the fracture site. (**A** and **B** are reproduced from Levine AM: Fractures of the atlas, in Levine AM, Eismont FJ, Garfin SR, Zigler JE, eds: *Spine Trauma.* Philadelphia, PA, WB Saunders, 1998, pp 209-226.)

ment of the fracture fragment is apparently unrelated to direct disruption of the TAL. The main risk associated with this injury is late-onset posttraumatic arthritis and pain.[16] A subtype of lateral mass fractures is an intra-articular fracture of the lateral mass with a sagittal fracture component. Subluxation of the occipital condyle into the fracture gap may result with secondary lateral displacement of the fracture. Subsidence and settling in such a scenario may lead to a "torticollis" appearance and loss of motion.[17]

A four-part fracture involving the lateral masses and arches is called a Jefferson fracture.[4,5,18-25] This involves a four-part fracture to the ring. The typical fracture pattern involves two fractures in the anterior arch and two fractures in the posterior arch (**Figure 6**), but it may occasionally consist of only one central fracture in the anterior arch. A Jefferson fracture usually results from direct axial compression of the occiput directly downward on the arch of C1.[2,26] A Jefferson fracture typically results in a symmetric displacement of the lateral masses, whereas in the lateral mass fracture it is asymmetric only on the injured side. Significant variability can be present in the displacement of Jefferson fractures (**Figure 7**). Due to the oblique orientation of the lateral masses, the compression force displaces the articular masses laterally. The result is a rupture of the weak atlantal ring due to the tensile forces, usually at the site of attachment of the anterior and posterior arches to the lateral masses.[4] Neurologic deficit is rare secondary to a Jefferson fracture because of the outward displacement of the lateral masses away from the spinal cord.

The fourth type of fracture is an anterior arch fracture of C1. There are two types of anterior arch fractures of C1. One subtype is a horizontal fracture of the anterior arch of C1 (**Figure 8**). The typical pattern of injury is a transverse split in a horizontal direction through the anterior tubercle of C1. This is considered an avulsion fracture.[27-29] The mechanism is hyperextension resulting in an avulsion fracture of the insertion of the superior oblique portion of the longus colli. The key feature of this fracture is that the inner cortex of the C1 ring remains intact while the outer cortex is disrupted. The second subtype of anterior arch fractures occurs in the sagittal plane. These fractures breach the outer and inner cortices of C1, typically adjacent to the dens (**Figure 8,** *C*). These fractures typically occur from a bending or hyperflexion moment.

The final type of injury is the transverse process fracture of the atlas, which can be either unilateral or bilateral (**Figure 9**).[30] The mechanism of injury occurs from a forced lateral flexion injury resulting in a contralateral avulsion fracture. This is an exceedingly rare injury, and insufficient clinical and experimental data exist to confirm the hypothesized mechanism of injury.

Combination Fractures and Associated Injuries

About 43% of all C1 fractures are associated with C2 fractures.[31] Gleizes et al[32] found 31 of 784 patients had combined C1-C2 injuries. In the original description of combined C1-C2 fractures, Jefferson[4] et al reported that 19 of the 46 cases had combination fractures of C1 and C2.[33] The cause of combined atlantoaxial fractures varies per age group. In young adults, in whom these types of fractures are rare, combined atlantoaxial fractures are usually a result of motor vehicle accidents. In the elderly, the incidence of combined atlantoaxial fractures is much higher. The combined fracture is usually the result of a fall.[31] The difference in occurrence between young adults and the elderly is probably also due to brittleness of bones as a result of osteoporosis and other age-related diseases in the elderly.

The four most prevalent combination fractures reported are C1–type II odontoid fractures (both stable and unstable), C1–type III odontoid fractures, C1–hangman's fractures (stable and unstable) and C1–miscellaneous axis fractures including multiple ring fractures, lateral mass fractures, and other fractures of C2. C1–type II odontoid and C1–type III odontoid fractures have been reported in a range of 5% to 53% of all cases of C1 fractures, depending on the literature.[34] The least common type of combined atlantoaxial fractures are C1–hangman's fractures.[33]

Combined atlantoaxial fractures are associated with a higher rate of neurologic deficit, morbidity, and mortality. Of the original series, Jefferson[4] reported that 11 of 19 patients had significant neurologic injuries, with increased morbidity and mortality for the combined injury group. Dickman et al[34] report a 0% incidence of neurologic deficits in isolated atlas fractures and a 2% incidence of neurologic deficits in isolated axis fractures, but a 12% incidence of neurologic deficits in combined C1-C2 fractures.

The most commonly associated fracture with a Jefferson fracture is a posteriorly displaced type II odontoid fracture.[2,12,35-38] Odontoid fractures can either be associated with a posterior C1 arch fracture or with a Jefferson fracture. Additionally, pos-

FIGURE 6

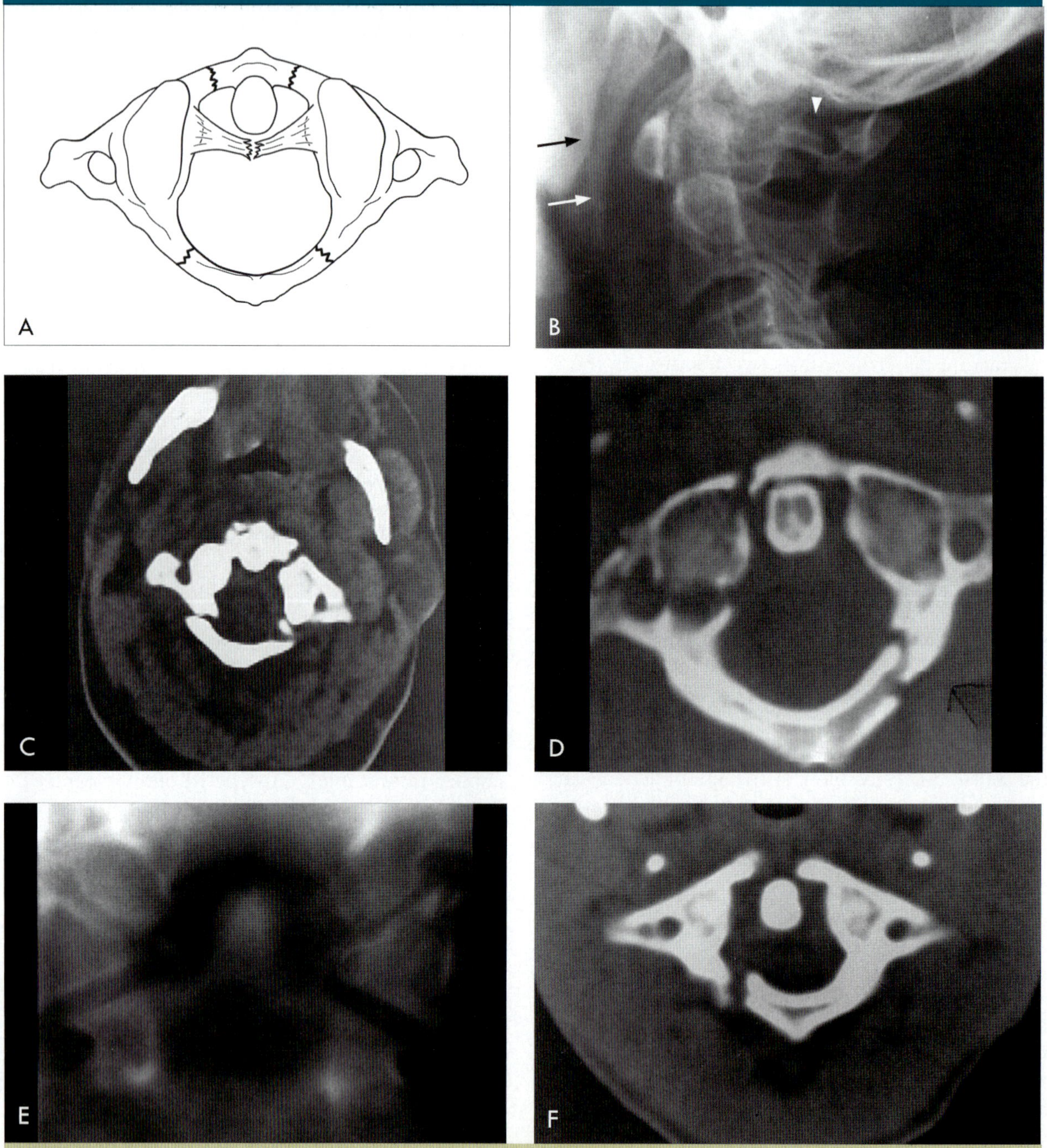

Figure 6 Jefferson or burst fracture. This injury can have a number of various patterns, but the classic injury is described as a four-part fracture with two fractures in the anterior ring and two in the posterior portion (**A**). The lateral radiograph in this patient with a four-part fracture (**B**) simply shows a posterior arch fracture (arrowhead), but there is a greatly increased anterior soft-tissue shadow (arrows) at the C1-C2 level. The CT scan (**C**) shows the four-part fracture pattern with symmetrical displacement. Although some lateral mass fractures have a three-part pattern (two in the posterior arch and one in the anterior arch), this CT scan shows a three-part injury (**D**), and the open-mouth view (**E**) shows symmetrical spreading of the lateral masses. The difference between the two injuries is the variation in the ligamentous disruption that is associated with the injury. The three-part Jefferson fracture has symmetrical ligamentous disruption, whereas the lateral mass fracture has asymmetrical disruption; for the same total amount of spreading of the lateral masses, the true lateral mass fracture may be more unstable. **F,** Two-part injuries are seen with one fracture in the anterior arch and one in the posterior arch, usually more in the midline of each arch than is seen in the four- and three-part fractures. (Reproduced from Levine AM: Fractures of the atlas, in Levine AM, Eismont FJ, Garfin SR, Zigler JE, eds: *Spine Trauma*. Philadelphia, PA, WB Saunders, 1998, pp 209-226.)

FIGURE 7

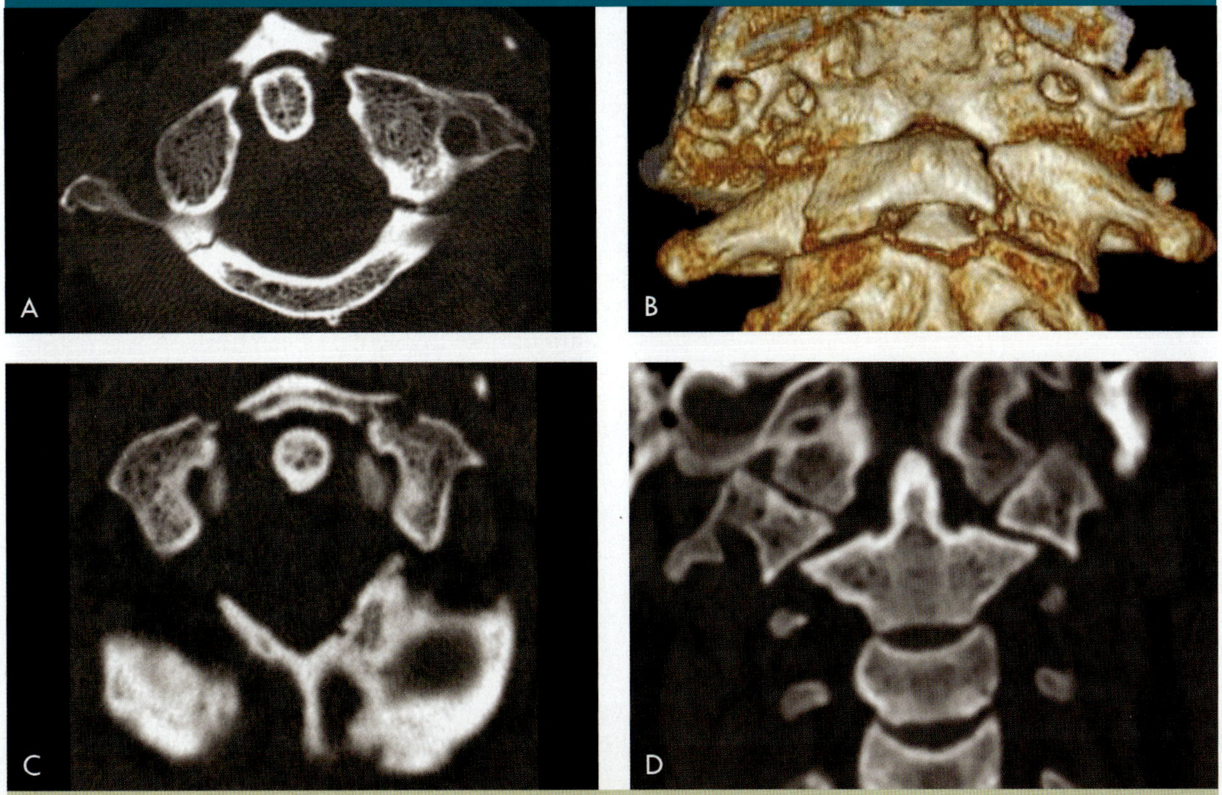

Figure 7 A, Axial CT scan demonstrating a minimally displaced Jefferson fracture of C1, characterized by two fractures of the anterior arch and two fractures of the posterior arches. **B,** Frontal view of a three-dimensional image of a minimally displaced Jefferson fracture of C1, characterized by two fractures of the anterior arch and two fractures of the posterior arch (not visible in this view). Minimal overhang of the lateral masses of C1 over C2 is present. **C,** Axial CT scan demonstrating a displaced Jefferson fracture of C1. **D,** Coronal CT scan demonstrating a severely displaced Jefferson fracture of C1 with significant overhang of the lateral masses of C1 on C2.

FIGURE 8

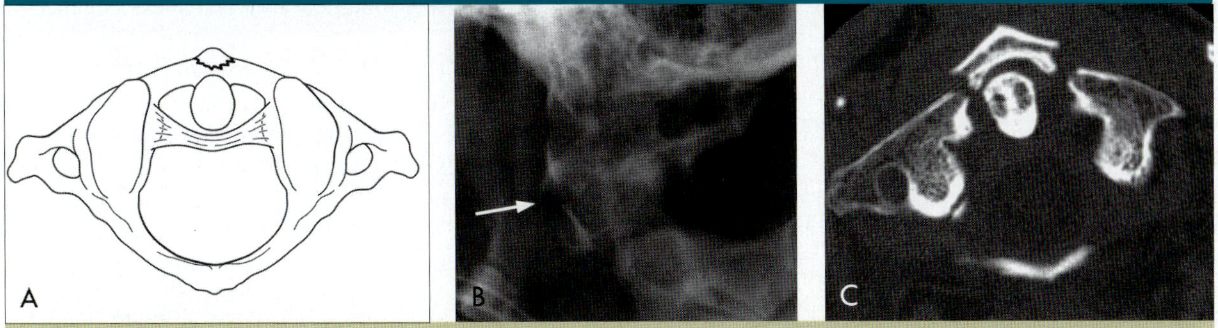

Figure 8 A, The drawing shows the minimal involvement of the structure of C1. The anterior avulsion fracture from the tubercle of C1 is a stable injury and looks worse on the lateral radiograph (**B,** arrow) than it manifests clinically. **C,** A displaced anterior arch may also occur from a bending moment. (**A** and **B** are reproduced from Levine AM: Fractures of the atlas, in Levine AM, Eismont FJ, Garfin SR, Zigler JE, eds: *Spine Trauma*. Philadelphia, PA, WB Saunders, 1998, pp 209-226.)

FIGURE 9

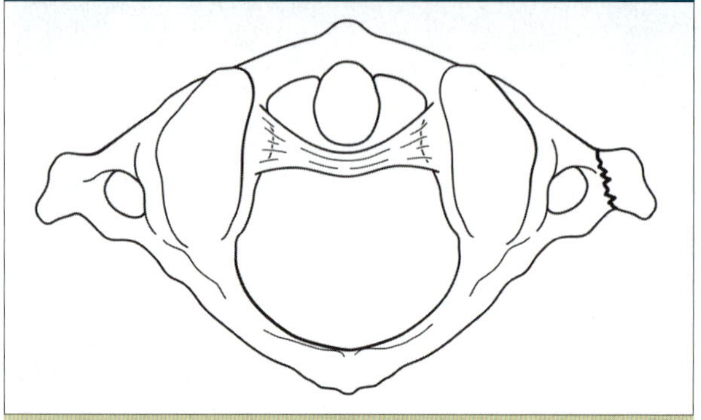

Figure 9 Transverse process fracture. This fracture may be seen as either a unilateral or bilateral injury and is almost always discovered as an incidental finding on the CT scan while investigating another injury in the upper cervical spine. (Reproduced from Levine AM: Fractures of the atlas, in Levine AM, Eismont FJ, Garfin SR, Zigler JE, eds: *Spine Trauma*. Philadelphia, PA, WB Saunders, 1998, pp 209-226.)

terior arch fractures may be associated with other hyperextension or axial-loading injuries in the lower cervical spine.[39] These may include laminar fractures in the lower cervical spine. The lateral mass fractures with asymmetric lateral bending and axial loading are frequently associated with unilateral facet fractures or pillar fractures, located more distally in the cervical spine. Jefferson fractures, which are axial-loading injuries, are frequently associated with burst fractures of the lower cervical spine.

Clinical Presentation and Radiologic Evaluation

Patients typically report nonspecific symptoms, including suboccipital pain, headaches, and a stiff neck.[11,19] Jefferson fractures are generally not associated with neurologic deficits.

The presence of a neurologic deficit should prompt work-up for a possible vascular injury. There have been several reports of vascular injury in the setting of a Jefferson fracture,[40,41] including posterior inferior cerebellar artery (PICA) territory infarction,[42] basilar artery occlusion, and locked-in syndrome.[43-46] Proposed treatment of such injuries with thrombolysis has been described.[47] It is important to recognize a vertebral artery occlusion preoperatively to appropriately plan surgical fixation techniques to avoid endangering the remaining vertebral artery. Alternative techniques may be indicated with a lower risk of vertebral artery injury such as translaminar or short pars screw fixation at C2.

Imaging Work-up

An injury to C1 is frequently recognized on a lateral cervical radiograph or a CT cervical spine taken at the time of admission and evaluation. Certain radiographic features help to determine whether a patient has an isolated posterior arch fracture, a more complicated ring fracture, or a combination of injuries. Patients with isolated posterior arch fractures commonly have evidence of an abnormality only on lateral plain radiography, which shows a defect in the posterior arch with either of the following: (1) a clearly visible defect, or (2) an abnormal orientation of the posterior arch. An open-mouth odontoid view[48,49] or coronal CT scan through the midpoint of the C1 lateral masses will help delineate the presence of lateral mass fractures or a Jefferson fracture, as the displacement of the lateral masses will be evident (**Figure 10**). Such fracture resolution is now provided by routine CT imaging. Horizontal or anterior avulsion fractures are most frequently seen on the lateral radiograph or sagittal CT, whereas transverse process fractures are seen on the open-mouth radiograph or axial CT. According to Spence et al,[52] when the combined overhang of the lateral masses of the atlas extends more than 6.9 mm beyond the lateral masses of C2, the TAL can be expected to be disrupted. However, in a clinical series of 39 patients, Dickman et al[53] claimed that the 7-mm criterion on open-mouth radiographs would have detected only 39% of atlas fractures with disrupted TALs. After correction for magnification on standard radiography technique, a criterion of 8.1 mm has also been recommended as diagnostic of transverse ligament injury.[54]

Currently the use of CT scan[55] with three-dimensional reconstructions is the standard screening tool for cervical spine trauma. For combined injuries of the upper cervical spine, such as dens and atlas fractures, three-dimensional reconstructions in the sagittal, coronal, and axial planes are required for accurate visualization. Furthermore, in the case of hyperlordosis, the orientation of the axial plane may affect the accuracy of measurements.[56] The presence of a severe neurologic deficit, or injury to the vertebral groove, transverse foramen, or the ponticulus posticus should prompt CT or MRI angiography to evaluate vertebral artery injury.

Treatment

The major goal of treatment of atlas fractures is to achieve patient comfort and protect the spine from

FIGURE 10

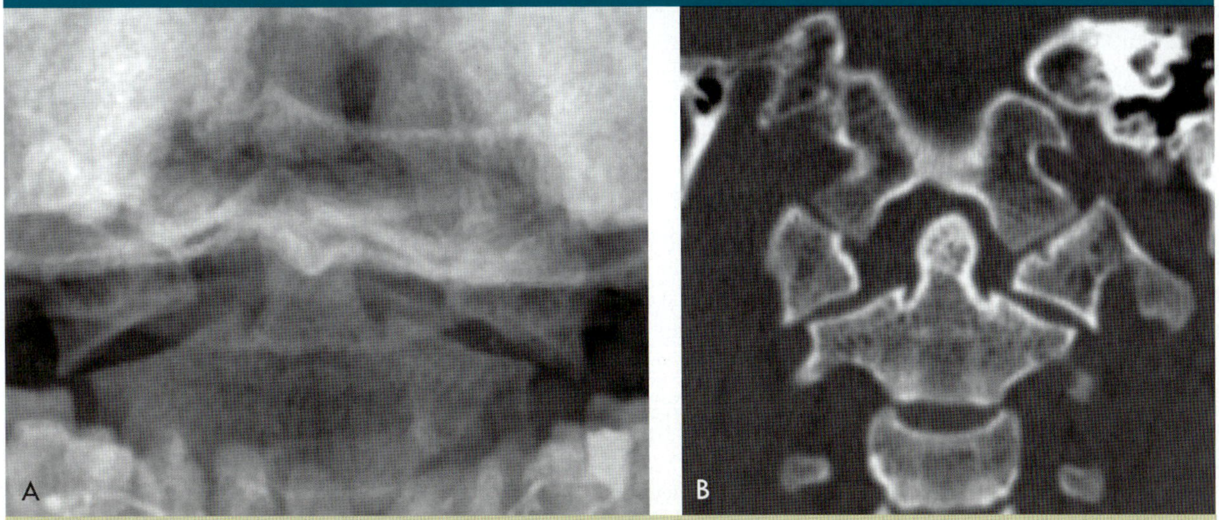

Figure 10 A, Open-mouth odontoid radiograph view demonstrates significant lateral overhang of C1 on C2. **B,** Coronal CT scan demonstrates similar lateral overhang of C1 on C2.

further injury until union of the atlas occurs. In most patients, approximately 2 to 3 months are usually required until callus is evident at the junction sites.

Isolated anterior and posterior arch fractures may be treated nonsurgically in a cervical orthosis. Displaced lateral mass fractures may be treated with a cervical orthosis or with traction for reduction and then halo immobilization. Finally, patients with avulsion fractures of either the anterior portion of the ring or the transverse processes are most frequently treated in a symptomatic fashion with collar immobilization. The incidence of these fractures is so small that long-term follow-up and results are currently not available.

Treatment options for Jefferson fractures include collar or halo immobilization,[57,58] internal fixation (osteosynthesis), or C1-C2 fusion. Nondisplaced Jefferson fractures may be managed with a collar or halo immobilization for 3 months after injury. Jefferson fractures with more than 8.1 mm overhang of the lateral masses on odontoid view are considered to be unstable. Unstable fractures have a worse prognosis with nonsurgical treatment. However, based on a series of 39 patients, Dickman et al[53] have identified late instability in 5 of 23 patients with intact TALs initially treated nonsurgically. They did not identify instability in any of the 16 patients with disruption treated operatively. The authors concluded that timely recognition of an unstable atlas fracture may avoid the additional morbidity incurred through an occipital fusion.

The recent trend in management of all types of atlas fractures is collar immobilization and immediate mobilization. The long-term consequences of lack of fracture reduction and joint congruity are unclear at this time. Closed reduction and immobilization has the theoretical advantage of maintaining occiput-C1 and C1-C2 rotation. Closed reduction requires the use of prolonged traction for reduction of the lateral masses through ligamentotaxis.[59] Traction should continue until early fracture healing is achieved. These treatments are intended to minimize the risk of atlantoaxial instability or atlantal nonunion. Levine and Edwards[2] have claimed successful fracture union in 96% of 34 patients with no late instability.

If external immobilization with a halo vest is chosen as the method of treatment, the goal of treatment should be maintenance of alignment, not reduction of deformity. It is impossible to achieve a reduction of this fracture by use of a halo vest. The position of the halo with reference to the vest should be such that the neck is maximally straightened and lengthened in a resting position to prevent a significant axial compression force from being applied to the fracture while the patient is upright. For patients with significantly displaced Jefferson fractures or lateral mass fractures (7 mm to 10 mm of total displacement), rupture of the transverse ligament should be suspected. As demonstrated by Segal et al,[16] nonunion of these injuries is more common than nondisplaced fractures. In addition, as the displacement becomes more significant, joint incongruity can become an important factor. Axial traction is necessary to maintain fracture reduction. Halo immobilization alone is sufficient. As demonstrated by Han et al[19] and Zimmerman et al,[25] immediate immobilization in a halo vest does not achieve or maintain reduction of the lateral masses. Even with short-term traction in a halo vest for reduction, upon removal of the traction and placement in a halo vest, the fracture slips back to its original position. Because the primary mechanism of injury in these fractures is either axial loading or axial loading and lateral bending, axial traction is required to achieve reduction. Thus, constant axial traction is necessary for the reduction of the injury. Patients with significant displacement can have axial traction applied through a halo ring, initially with 10 lb of traction and up to 40 lb as necessary to achieve full reduction of the ring on open-mouth view. It is imperative that traction reduction occur in a monitored setting under the immediate direct supervision of an experienced physician. Complete symmetry of the C1-C2 lateral masses is the goal. Once the fracture has been fully reduced and the fragments brought in contact, approximately 4 to 6 weeks must pass before preliminary healing of the fracture is sufficient to allow immobilization of the patient in a halo vest without subsequent loss of reduction. The degree of healing can be assessed periodically by removing the traction from the halo and allowing the patient to lie in a supine position for 1 hour, after which an open-mouth radiograph is taken. If the reduction is maintained, then the patient can be mobilized in a halo vest, and if the reduction is lost, the traction can be replaced and the reduction regained and held until it is possible to remove the traction weight without loss of reduction. Immobilization in a halo vest for an additional 6 weeks will bring the total immobilization period to approximately 3 months.

Possible surgical indications include prevention of subsequent degeneration due to malalignment and avoidance of the complications of immobilization.

There are five surgical treatment options for treatment of an unstable Jefferson fracture. The goals of surgical treatment are a more anatomic reconstruction, earlier mobilization, and prevention of degenerative change.

C1 osteosynthesis with lateral mass screws has been proposed as an option for the treatment of a displaced Jefferson fracture. Böhm et al[60] have reported a case series of 8 patients with C1 fractures treated with posterior bilateral lateral mass screws and fracture reduction with a crosslink. C1 osteosynthesis via anterior lateral mass screws have been described by Ruf et al[61] in a series of six cases of unstable Jefferson fractures. They implanted a steel plate or connecting bar between the screws. However, transoral approaches involve significant dysphagia and wound complications for the patients. This procedure has the obvious advantage of preservation of partial C1-C2 motion as documented in their series. No C1-C2 instability was observed on follow-up flexion-extension radiographs. Additionally, there is a significant possibility of injury to the internal carotid artery or hypoglossal nerve from an anterior approach.[62]

C1-C2 posterior cervical fusion may be accomplished using the Magerl technique (C1-C2 transarticular screws) (**Figure 11**).[63,64] Transarticular screws are particularly dangerous to place if there is significant C1-C2 rotation.[65] It may also be difficult to place transarticular screws safely if the lateral masses are significantly laterally displaced as the trajectory of screw insertion beginning at the C2 pars may place the vertebral artery at risk of injury. Preoperative traction reduction is essential before either technique, because this technique will not result in direct reduction of the displaced Jefferson fracture fragments.[63,66]

C1-C2 posterior fusion may also be accomplished with C1 lateral mass and C2 fixation. Either C2 pedicle screws[67,68] or C2 isthmus screws[69] have been described for distal fixation. This technique affords segmental fixation and is associated with reduced risk to the vertebral artery in the case of residual rotatory subluxation of C1 on C2. Furthermore, the technique allows the possibility for transverse axial compression via a cross-link and reduction of the lateral diastasis of C1 on C2. Additionally, segmental C1-C2 fixation allows for distraction instrumentation that may partially reduce basilar invagination secondary to a displaced C1 fracture.[68]

Anterior C1-C2 fixation may also be accomplished using transarticular process screw fixation. Several variations of this technique have been described, including screws placed into the C2 vertebral body aiming proximally and screws placed into the C1 lateral masses aiming distally. The problem with an anterior fixation strategy is the inability to perform grafting between C1 and C2. This may require in some patients adjuvant posterior instrumentation and grafting.[70] Anterior C1-C2 osteosynthesis using an atlantoaxial reduction plate is another theoretical possibility.

Often, the treatment of the patient is determined not by the atlas fracture but rather by the

FIGURE 11

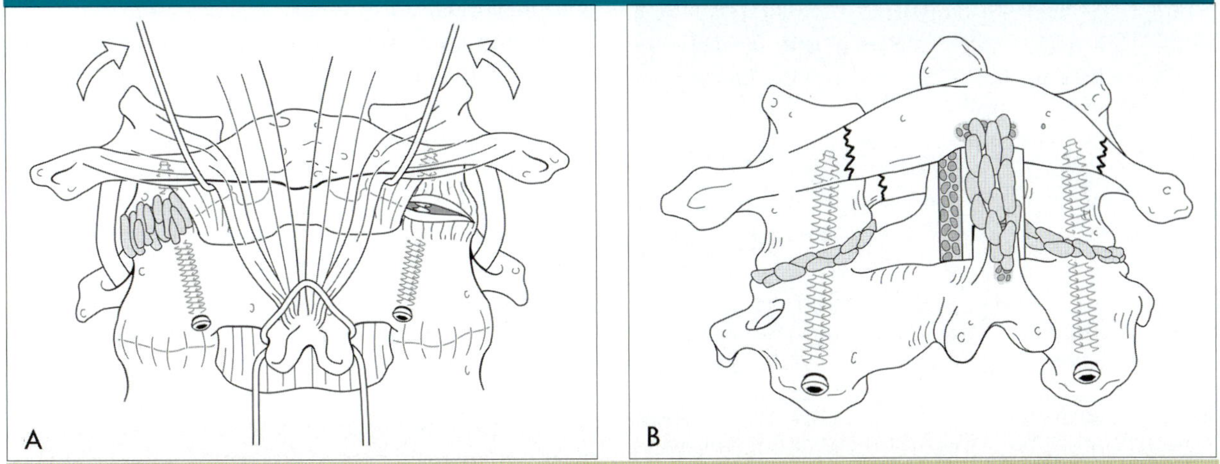

Figure 11 An alternative method for the treatment of a widely displaced lateral mass or Jefferson fracture is the transarticular C1-C2 screw fixation. The reduction of the fracture is initially obtained with halo traction. Generally, about 30 to 35 lb of traction is necessary to achieve an anatomic reduction that will make placement of the screws relatively straightforward. Anatomical reduction is necessary to reduce the risk of vertebral artery injury. Further reduction is not possible once the surgical stabilization has begun. A biplanar image is used. The only variation in the standard technique is that the joints are fully exposed **(A)** so that the cartilage can be curetted out for fusion, and no fixation of bone graft is possible between the fractured arch of C1 and the lamina of C2. Grafting is done directly into the joints and also as an onlay from C1 to C2 **(B)** so that as healing occurs, a solid arthrodesis will also occur. With satisfactory screw fixation, either the halo vest can be continued postoperatively or collar immobilization can be employed. (Reproduced from Levine AM: Fractures of the atlas, in Levine AM, Eismont FJ, Garfin SR, Zigler JE, eds: *Spine Trauma*. Philadelphia, PA, WB Saunders, 1998, pp 209-226.)

concurrent injury. The treatment of a dens fracture associated with a C1 fracture is dictated by the degree of displacement of the dens fracture. A nondisplaced fracture may be managed appropriately with a collar, halo vest, or an odontoid screw. A displaced fracture should be treated with a posterior C1-C2 arthrodesis. Similarly, a posterior arch fracture combined with a traumatic spondylolisthesis of the axis may be treated according to the displacement of the axis. Hadley[33] compiled 48 articles detailing treatment methods for various C1-C2 combined fractures. Particular techniques may be more appropriate for specific injury patterns. For treatment of combined C1 and type II odontoid fractures, successful treatment options include semirigid immobilization (collar), rigid immobilization such as a halo, anterior odontoid screw fixation, posterior fusion with and without instrumentation, and other methods of surgical stabilization and fusion. For combined C1 and type II odontoid fractures that are considered to be unstable (with an atlanto-dens interval ≥ 5 mm), external immobilization alone has a high failure rate; surgical reduction, fixation, and fusion is suggested for these cases. For combined C1 and type III odontoid fractures, halo immobilization is a successful method of treatment of most patients.

Results of Treatment and Complications

Atlas fractures commonly heal without considerable morbidity or late sequelae. Isolated arch fractures usually proceed to union and patients remain symptom-free in the long term. In the group of patients with posterior arch fractures combined with other associated injuries, any residual symptoms are most commonly related to the other injury. For patients with lateral mass and Jefferson fractures, the data on overall results are relatively clear. For patients treated in a halo vest with minimally displaced fractures, there is little tendency toward increased displacement during treatment. In the setting of significant fracture displacement, traction has been successful in achieving fracture alignment long term. In one series, mean total displacement was reduced from 12.3 mm to 3.9 mm at final follow-up.[2] All of these patients subsequently underwent flexion-extension radiographs with no demonstrated instability. Another case series of 34 patients demonstrated at average 4.5-year follow-up that approximately 80% of patients had residual neck pain, but none needed secondary arthrodesis. Nonunion occurred in 17% of patients.[71] Initial fracture displacement was considered to be predic-

FIGURE 12

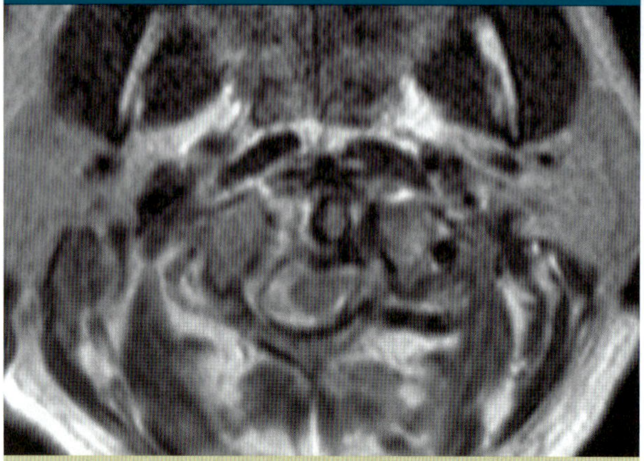

Figure 12 Axial MRI through C1 lateral masses demonstrating an avulsed transverse atlantal ligament from right C1 lateral mass. This avulsion may be associated with chronic atlantodental instability.

tive of late sequelae. Reduction of the articular alignment may be important in avoiding late degenerative changes in the joint. Secondary progressive dural compression and myelopathy are possible with nonunion, particularly in cases in which the fracture fragment directly impinges on the dural sac. Complications in the treatment of these injuries are relatively rare. Interestingly, the injury may be complicated by direct trauma to the greater occipital nerve.[72] Especially in older individuals, who are placed in a Yale brace or Philadelphia collar, the numbness over the occiput from greater occipital nerve injury can result in a decubitus ulcer over the occiput. Prior to application of a brace, the occipital sensation should be checked; if it is absent, halo-vest management should be considered.

C1-C2 instability has been rarely reported after the conservative treatment of unstable Jefferson fractures. Damage to the ligamentous stabilizers such as the facet capsules and cruciate ligamentous complex may result in late instability (**Figure 12**). Dynamic flexion and extension radiographs are recommended after treatment for evaluation of C1-C2 stability after conservative treatment of Jefferson fractures. Further drawbacks of halo-vest immobilization include considerable patient discomfort and potential infectious complications, particularly in elderly patients.[73] Complications of halo-vest use for treatment are well documented and include loosening pins, bone erosion, skull perforation, and cerebrospinal fluid leaks. Appropriate care of the halo vest and torquing of the pins is critical for minimizing treatment complications.

Incongruent C0-C1 or C1-C2 joints may in the future restrict motion and have been reported to cause considerable residual neck pain.[16] Application of a halo vest after a short period of axial traction has repeatedly failed to maintain the initially achieved reduction, leading to an incongruence of the C0-C1 and the C1-C2 joints. Although the incidence is poorly documented because of the lack of long-term follow-up of this patient population, degenerative changes of incongruent joint surfaces are possible in both the occipitoatlantal and atlantoaxial joints. Asymmetric degenerative changes may be expected with lateral mass fractures, whereas bilateral degenerative changes may be expected in Jefferson fractures. Early manifestations are pain with head rotation and occasionally on cervical flexion and extension. Late radiographic evidence of sclerosis and loss of joint space has been documented. If increased symptoms occur, occipitocervical fusion may provide a solution to the pain.

In conclusion, atlas fractures span a spectrum of injury and instability from trivial to significant. Treatment should be directed at appropriate goals, and more long-term follow-up is necessary in studying the implications of lateral mass and Jefferson fractures and their effect on long-term discomfort related to articular congruity.

References

1. An HS: Cervical spine trauma. *Spine (Phila Pa 1976)* 1998;23(24):2713-2729.
2. Levine AM, Edwards CC: Fractures of the atlas. *J Bone Joint Surg Am* 1991;73(5):680-691.
3. Cooper A: *A Treatise on Dislocations, and on Fractures of the Joints*. London, United Kingdom, Longman, Hurst Rees, Orme Browne, E. Cox & Son, 1822, p 542.
4. Jefferson G: Fracture of the atlas vertebra: Report of four cases and a review of those previously reported. *Br J Surg* 1920;7:407-422.
5. Jefferson G: Remarks on fractures of the first cervical vertebra. *BMJ* 1927;2:153-157.
6. Young JP, Young PH, Ackermann MJ, Anderson PA, Riew KD: The ponticulus posticus: Implications for screw insertion into the first cervical lateral mass. *J Bone Joint Surg Am* 2005;87(11):2495-2498.
7. Horn EM, Feiz-Erfan I, Lekovic GP, Dickman CA, Sonntag VK, Theodore N: Survivors of occipitoatlantal dislocation injuries: Imaging and clinical correlates. *J Neurosurg Spine* 2007;6(2):113-120.

8. Dvorak J, Panjabi MM, Gerber M, Wichmann W: CT-functional diagnostics of the rotatory instability of upper cervical spine: 1. An experimental study on cadavers. *Spine (Phila Pa 1976)* 1987;12(3):197-205.
9. Levine AM, Edwards CC: Traumatic lesions of the occipitoatlantoaxial complex. *Clin Orthop Relat Res* 1989;239:53-68.
10. Levine AM, Edwards CC: Treatment of injuries in the C1-C2 complex. *Orthop Clin North Am* 1986;17(1):31-44.
11. Sherk HH, Nicholson JT: Fractures of the atlas. *J Bone Joint Surg Am* 1970;52(5):1017-1024.
12. Sherk HH: Fractures of the atlas and odontoid process. *Orthop Clin North Am* 1978;9(4):973-984.
13. White AA III, Panjabi MM: The clinical biomechanics of the occipitoatlantoaxial complex. *Orthop Clin North Am* 1978;9(4):867-878.
14. White AA III, Panjabi MM, eds: *Clinical Biomechanics of the Spine*. Philadelphia, PA, JB Lippincott, 1991.
15. Hays MB, Alker GJ Jr: Fractures of the atlas vertebra: The two-part burst fracture of Jefferson. *Spine (Phila Pa 1976)* 1988;13(6):601-603.
16. Segal LS, Grimm JO, Stauffer ES: Non-union of fractures of the atlas. *J Bone Joint Surg Am* 1987;69(9):1423-1434.
17. Clyburn TA, Lionberger DR, Tullos HS: Bilateral fracture of the transverse process of the atlas. *J Bone Joint Surg Am* 1982;64(6):948.
18. Hamilton AR: Injuries of the atlantoaxial joint. *J Bone Joint Surg Br* 1951;33-B(3):434-435.
19. Han SY, Witten DM, Mussleman JP: Jefferson fracture of the atlas: Report of six cases. *J Neurosurg* 1976;44(3):368-371.
20. Hentzer L, Schalimtzek M: Fractures and subluxations of the atlas and axis: A follow-up study of 20 patients. *Acta Orthop Scand* 1971;42(3):251-258.
21. Hinchey JJ, Bickel WH: Fracture of the atlas. *Ann Surg* 1945;121(6):826-832.
22. Marlin AE, Williams GR, Lee JF: Jefferson fractures in children: Case report. *J Neurosurg* 1983;58(2):277-279.
23. Mixter SJ, Osgood RB: Traumatic lesions of the atlas and axis. *Ann Surg* 1910;51(2):193-207.
24. Pierce DS, Barr JS: Fractures and dislocations at the base of the skull and upper cervical spine, in Clark CR, Ducker TB, eds: *The Cervical Spine*. Philadelphia, PA, JB Lippincott, 1983, pp 196-206.
25. Zimmerman E, Grant J, Vise WM, Yashon D, Hunt WE: Treatment of Jefferson fracture with a halo apparatus: Report of two cases. *J Neurosurg* 1976;44(3):372-375.
26. Kesterson L, Benzel E, Orrison W, Coleman J: Evaluation and treatment of atlas burst fractures (Jefferson fractures). *J Neurosurg* 1991;75(2):213-220.
27. Jevtich V: Horizontal fracture of the anterior arch of the atlas: Case report. *J Bone Joint Surg Am* 1986;68(7):1094-1095.
28. Proubasta IR, Sancho RN, Alonso JR, Palacio AH: Horizontal fracture of the anterior arch of the atlas: Report of two cases and review of the literature. *Spine (Phila Pa 1976)* 1987;12(6):615-618.
29. Stewart GC Jr, Gehweiler JA Jr, Laib RH, Martinez S: Horizontal fracture of the anterior arch of the atlas. *Radiology* 1977;122(2):349-352.
30. Bransford R, Falicov A, Nguyen Q, Chapman J: Unilateral C-1 lateral mass sagittal split fracture: An unstable Jefferson fracture variant. *J Neurosurg Spine* 2009;10(5):466-473.
31. Guiot B, Fessler RG: Complex atlantoaxial fractures. *J Neurosurg* 1999;91(2 Suppl):139-143.
32. Gleizes V, Jacquot FP, Signoret F, Feron JM: Combined injuries in the upper cervical spine: Clinical and epidemiological data over a 14-year period. *Eur Spine J* 2000;9(5):386-392.
33. Hadley MN: Management of combination fractures of the atlas and axis in adults. *Neurosurgery* 2002;50(3 Suppl):S140-S147.
34. Dickman CA, Hadley MN, Browner C, Sonntag VK: Neurosurgical management of acute atlas-axis combination fractures: A review of 25 cases. *J Neurosurg* 1989;70(1):45-49.
35. Bailey DK: The normal cervical spine in infants and children. *Radiology* 1952;59(5):712-719.
36. Hadley MN, Dickman CA, Browner CM, Sonntag VK: Acute traumatic atlas fractures: Management and long term outcome. *Neurosurgery* 1988;23(1):31-35.
37. Levine AM, Fischgrund J, Edwards C: Fractures of the C1-C2 complex: Concurrent spinal injuries. *J Orthop Trauma* 1993;7(2):172.
38. Lipson SJ: Fractures of the atlas associated with fractures of the odontoid process and transverse ligament ruptures. *J Bone Joint Surg Am* 1977;59(7):940-943.
39. Korres SD, Kosmides A, Andreakos K, Kavadias K, Lupassis G: Fracture de Jefferson avec dislocation occipito-cervicale. *Eur J Orthop Surg Traumatol* 1991;1(2):77-79.
40. Muratsu H, Doita M, Yanagi T, et al: Cerebellar infarction resulting from vertebral artery occlusion associated with a Jefferson fracture. *J Spinal Disord Tech* 2005;18(3):293-296.
41. Weller SJ, Rossitch E Jr, Malek AM: Detection of vertebral artery injury after cervical spine trauma

using magnetic resonance angiography. *J Trauma* 1999;46(4):660-666.

42. Walsh GS, Cusimano MD: Vertebral artery injury associated with a Jefferson fracture. *Can J Neurol Sci* 1995;22(4):308-311.
43. Ashley WW Jr, Rivet D, Cross DT III, Santiago P: Development of a giant cervical vertebral artery pseudoaneurysm after a traumatic C1 fracture: Case illustration. *Surg Neurol* 2006;66(1):80-81.
44. Peltier J, Toussaint P, Page C, et al: Dissection of the vertebral artery complicating Jefferson fracture. *Eur J Orthop Surg Traumatol* 2004;14(4): 230-233.
45. Schoeggl A, Reddy M, Bavinzski G: A lateral mass fracture of C1 associated with left vertebral artery and mid-basilar artery occlusion. *J Neurotrauma* 2001;18(7):737-741.
46. Siegel M, Alberts R: Unusual sign of a Jefferson fracture: A case report. *Spine (Phila Pa 1976)* 1992;17(5):605-607.
47. Sugrue PA, Hage ZA, Surdell DL, Foroohar M, Liu J, Bendok BR: Basilar artery occlusion following C1 lateral mass fracture managed by mechanical and pharmacological thrombolysis. *Neurocrit Care* 2009;11(2):255-260.
48. Flournoy JG, Cone RO, Saldana JA, Jones MD: Jefferson fracture: Presentation of a new diagnostic sign. *Radiology* 1980;134(1):88.
49. Harris JH Jr: Acute injuries of the spine. *Semin Roentgenol* 1978;13(1):53-68.
50. Penning L: Prevertebral hematoma in cervical spine injury: Incidence and etiologic significance. *AJR Am J Roentgenol* 1981;136(3):553-561.
51. Templeton PA, Young JW, Mirvis SE, Buddemeyer EU: The value of retropharyngeal soft tissue measurements in trauma of the adult cervical spine: Cervical spine soft tissue measurements. *Skeletal Radiol* 1987;16(2):98-104.
52. Spence KF Jr, Decker S, Sell KW: Bursting atlantal fracture associated with rupture of the transverse ligament. *J Bone Joint Surg Am* 1970;52(3): 543-549.
53. Dickman CA, Greene KA, Sonntag VK: Injuries involving the transverse atlantal ligament: Classification and treatment guidelines based upon experience with 39 injuries. *Neurosurgery* 1996;38(1): 44-50.
54. Heller JG, Viroslav S, Hudson T: Jefferson fractures: The role of magnification artifact in assessing transverse ligament integrity. *J Spinal Disord* 1993;6(5):392-396.
55. Baumgarten M, Mouradian W, Boger D, Watkins R: Computed axial tomography in C1-C2 trauma. *Spine (Phila Pa 1976)* 1985;10(3):187-192.
56. Radcliff KE, Ben-Galim P, Dreiangel N, et al: Comprehensive computed tomography assessment of the upper cervical anatomy: What is normal? *Spine J* 2010;10(3):219-229.
57. Haus BM, Harris MB: Case report: nonoperative treatment of an unstable Jefferson fracture using a cervical collar. *Clin Orthop Relat Res* 2008;466(5): 1257-1261.
58. Lee TT, Green BA, Petrin DR: Treatment of stable burst fracture of the atlas (Jefferson fracture) with rigid cervical collar. *Spine (Phila Pa 1976)* 1998; 23(18):1963-1967.
59. Kontautas E, Ambrozaitis KV, Kalesinskas RJ, Spakauskas B: Management of acute traumatic atlas fractures. *J Spinal Disord Tech* 2005;18(5): 402-405.
60. Böhm H, Kayser R, El Saghir H, Heyde CE: Direct osteosynthesis of instable Gehweiler Type III atlas fractures: Presentation of a dorsoventral osteosynthesis of instable atlas fractures while maintaining function. *Unfallchirurg* 2006;109(9):754-760.
61. Ruf M, Melcher R, Harms J: Transoral reduction and osteosynthesis C1 as a function-preserving option in the treatment of unstable Jefferson fractures. *Spine (Phila Pa 1976)* 2004;29(7):823-827.
62. Hong JT, Lee SW, Son BC, Sung JH, Kim IS, Park CK: Hypoglossal nerve palsy after posterior screw placement on the C-1 lateral mass: Case report. *J Neurosurg Spine* 2006;5(1):83-85.
63. McGuire RA Jr, Harkey HL: Primary treatment of unstable Jefferson's fractures. *J Spinal Disord* 1995; 8(3):233-236.
64. Hein C, Richter HP, Rath SA: Atlantoaxial screw fixation for the treatment of isolated and combined unstable Jefferson fractures—experiences with 8 patients. *Acta Neurochir (Wien)* 2002; 144(11):1187-1192.
65. Paramore CG, Dickman CA, Sonntag VK: The anatomical suitability of the C1-2 complex for transarticular screw fixation. *J Neurosurg* 1996; 85(2):221-224.
66. Schären S, Jeanneret B: Atlas fractures. *Orthopade* 1999;28(5):385-393.
67. Tan J, Li L, Sun G, et al: C1 lateral mass-C2 pedicle screws and crosslink compression fixation for unstable atlas fracture. *Spine (Phila Pa 1976)* 2009; 34(23):2505-2509.
68. Ames CP, Acosta F, Nottmeier E: Novel treatment of basilar invagination resulting from an untreated C-1 fracture associated with transverse ligament avulsion: Case report and description of surgical technique. *J Neurosurg Spine* 2005;2(1):83-87.
69. Tessitore E, Momjian A, Payer M: Posterior reduction and fixation of an unstable Jefferson fracture with C1 lateral mass screws, C2 isthmus screws, and crosslink fixation: Technical case report. *Neurosurgery* 2008;63(1, Suppl 1):E100-E101.

70. Guo X, Ni B, Wang M, Wang J, Li S, Zhou F: Bilateral atlas laminar hook combined with transarticular screw fixation for an unstable bursting atlantal fracture. *Arch Orthop Trauma Surg* 2009; 129(9):1203-1209.

71. Levine AM: Avulsion of the transverse ligament associated with fracture of the atlas: A case report. *Orthopedics* 1983;6:1467-1471.

72. Zielinski CJ, Gunther SF, Deeb Z: Cranial-nerve palsies complicating Jefferson fracture: A case report. *J Bone Joint Surg Am* 1982;64(9):1382-1384.

73. Fowler JL, Sandhu A, Fraser RD: A review of fractures of the atlas vertebra. *J Spinal Disord* 1990; 3(1):19-24.

CHAPTER 21
Odontoid Fractures

Travis G. Maak, MD   Jonathan N. Grauer, MD   Alexander R. Vaccaro, MD, PhD

Introduction

In the adult population, odontoid fractures account for 9% to 15% of cervical spine fractures.[1-3] These injuries usually result from low-energy impact such as falls in the elderly or high-energy impact such as motor vehicle accidents in the young and middle-aged.[4-6] Moreover, odontoid fractures are the most common individual cervical spine fracture for people over 70 years of age and represent the majority of spine fractures for those over 80 years of age.[7] The identification, classification, and treatment of odontoid fractures remain controversial and are evolving along with fixation techniques.

Anatomy

Osseous Structure

The osseous anatomy of the upper cervical spine is unique and allows the high degree of motion normally seen in this region. C1, also known as the atlas, is a ring that articulates with the occiput above and C2, or axis, below. This C2 articulation occurs via facet joints and the odontoid, which extends into the arch of C1 and articulates with the anterior portion of the C1 ring (**Figure 1**). The C1-C2 (atlantoaxial) articulation allows for significant mobility while maintaining stability.[8,9] In fact, this articulation accounts for 50% of total cervical spine axial rotation.[9-11]

In 1968, Steel[12] coined the "rule of thirds," noting that at the level of C1, approximately one-third of the ring is occupied by the odontoid process, one-third by the spinal cord, and one-third by "free" space. It has since been documented that this "free" space is composed of cerebrospinal fluid, thecal tissues, and vascular tissues.[13] The C1-C2 sagittal diameter available for the spinal cord at this level ranges from 14.2 mm to 15.8 mm, while the spinal cord diameter in this region is approximately 8 mm.[14-17] This large diameter difference accounts for the relatively low incidence of spinal cord injuries at this level.[18,19]

Heller et al[20] documented such variable morphology of the odontoid process in an anatomic analysis of 120 axis vertebrae. The mean odontoid minimum anteroposterior diameter was 6.2 mm but ranged widely, from 2.8 mm to 8.7 mm. The mean minimum transverse diameter was 4.5 mm and had an even larger range. Men generally had larger dimensions than women by approximately 10%, and no race differences were identified.

Musculoligamentous Support

The occiput-C2 complex facilitates movement of the head relative to the spine. A unique aspect of this anatomic region is the large degree of motion that is normally present while maintaining stability.[21] In fact, nearly 50% of cervical flexion-extension and rotation occur in this region.[22,23] Because the bony anatomy allows such large motion, much of the stability of this region is provided by the ligamentous and muscular anatomy (**Figure 1**).[24]

The alar and transverse ligaments play key roles in stabilizing this upper cervical region due to the absence of intervertebral disks and the presence of horizontally aligned facets at the occipitoatlantal

---

Dr. Grauer or an immediate family member is a member of a speakers' bureau or has made paid presentations on behalf of Stryker; serves as a paid consultant to or is an employee of Alphatech Spine, DePuy, a Johnson & Johnson company, Smith & Nephew, and Stryker; and has received research or institutional support from Stryker and Medtronic Sofamor Danek. Dr. Vaccaro or an immediate family member serves as a board member, owner, officer, or committee member of the North American Spine Society, American Spinal Injury Association, and the Cervical Spine Research Society; has received royalties from Aesculap/B.Braun, DePuy, a Johnson & Johnson company, Globus Medical, Medtronic Sofamor Danek, K2M, Stout Medical, Progressive Spinal Technology, and Applied Spinal Intellectual Properties; serves as a paid consultant to or is an employee of K2M; has received research or institutional support from AO North America, DePuy, a Johnson & Johnson company, Medtronic Sofamor Danek, and Stryker; and owns stock or stock options in Globus Medical, Disk Motion Technology, Progressive Spinal Technologies, Advanced Spinal Intellectual Properties, Computational Biodynamics, Stout Medical, Paradigm Spine, K2M, Replication Medica, Spinology, Spine Medica, Orthovita, Vertiflex, Small Bone Technologies, NeuCore, Crosscurrent, Syndicom, In Vivo, Flagship Surgical, Pearl Driver, Location Based Intelligence, and Gamma Spine. Neither Dr. Maak nor any immediate family member has received anything of value from or owns stock in a commercial company or institution related directly or indirectly to the subject of this chapter.

FIGURE 1

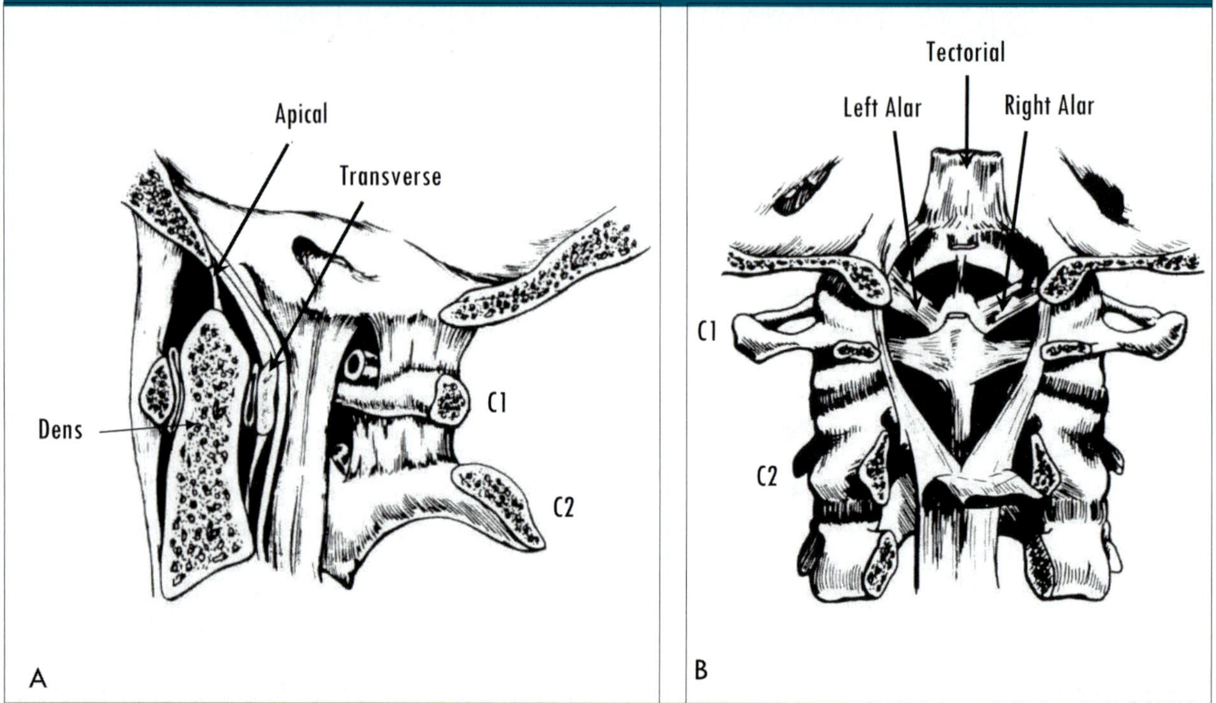

Figure 1 Osseous and ligamentous anatomy. **A,** The C2 articulation extends into the arch of C1 and articulates with the anterior portion of the C1 ring. The transverse ligament extends from the lateral mass of C1 around the posterior surface of the middle and upper third of the dens to insert onto the contralateral lateral mass. **B,** The alar ligaments arise from the medial aspect of the occipital condyles and lateral masses of the atlas, respectively, and insert broadly along the lateral portion of the odontoid. (Reproduced with permission from White AA, Panjabi MM: *Clinical Biomechanics of the Spine*, ed 2. Philadelphia, PA, Lippincott, 1990.)

region.[21,25-29] The transverse ligament is a well-defined band of connective tissue that holds the odontoid process of C2 against the anterior ring of the atlas. This ligament extends from the lateral mass of C1 around the posterior surface of the middle and upper third of the dens to insert onto the contralateral lateral mass.[30] The transverse ligament is the principal and most crucial of the ligamentous components of the atlantoaxial complex.[23,31,32]

The alar ligaments consist of two different parts—the occipito alar and atlanto alar ligaments. These ligaments arise from the medial aspect of the occipital condyles and lateral masses of the atlas, respectively. They insert broadly along the lateral portion of the odontoid. The alar ligaments restrict contralateral rotation and lateral bending of the atlas on the axis.[28,29] Paired accessory ligaments exist as ligamentous bands that originate contiguous with the transverse ligament and insert immediately onto the odontoid process directly above its base medial to the respective apophyseal articulations.[33] Together with the alar ligaments, the accessory and apical ligaments function as secondary stabilizers of the atlanto-dens complex.[28,29] Other contributing ligaments include the tectorial membrane, which is an extension of the posterior longitudinal ligament, anterior longitudinal ligament, posterior occipitoatlantal and atlantoaxial membranes, ligamentum flava, and nuchal ligament. The tectorial membrane functions as a primary flexion and extension limiter. It is aided in this role by the other contributing ligaments, with anterior ligaments providing stability during extension and posterior ligaments providing stability during flexion.[31]

The primary function of the occipito-atlanto-axial ligamentous complex is to protect the spinal cord by restricting the motions within well-defined limits.[21] Rupture of the alar and transverse ligaments may occur without associated vertebral fracture, and may result in instability of the upper cervical spine.[21,23,34,35]

Other surgically relevant anatomy includes the suboccipital triangle, which is bounded by the superior oblique, inferior oblique, and rectus capitis posterior major. The floor of the triangle is established by the posterior occipitoatlantal mem-

FIGURE 2

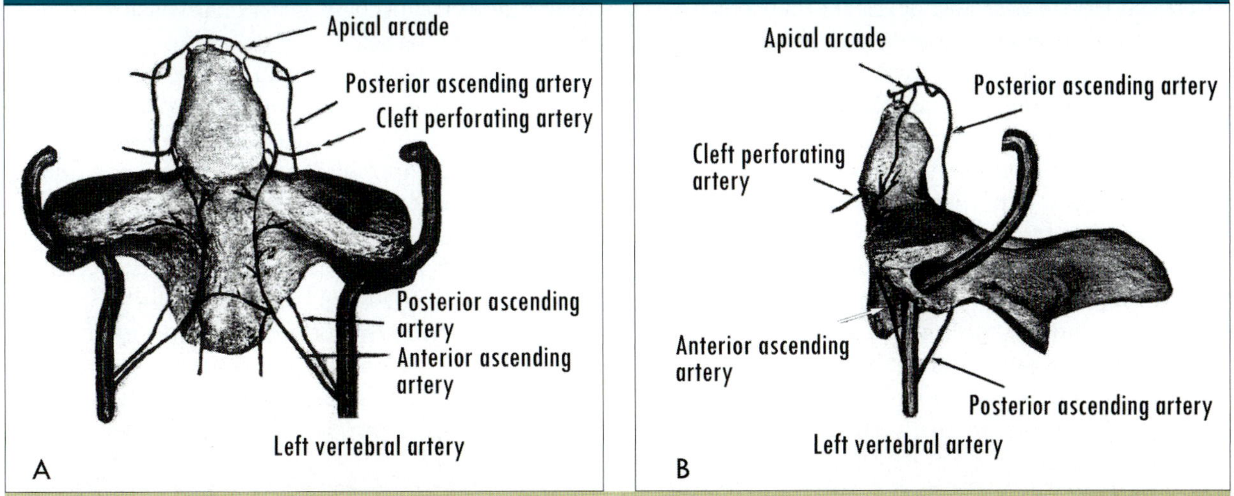

Figure 2 Lateral (**A**) and posteroanterior (**B**) figures demonstrating the vascular supply to the odontoid process. (Reproduced with permission from Schiff DC, Parke WW: The arterial supply of the odontoid process. *J Bone Joint Surg Am* 1973;55(7):1450-1456.)

brane and the posterior arch of the atlas, and the roof is established by the greater occipital nerve and occipital artery. The vertebral artery and suboccipital nerve are contained within this triangular space.

Vascularity

There have been several studies evaluating the vascular supply to the atlantoaxial region.[33,36,37] The odontoid, which has the most tenuous blood supply, receives contributions from three primary feeders: the anterior ascending artery, the posterior ascending artery, and the cleft perforating artery.[37] The anterior ascending arteries originate from the anteromedial surface of the respective vertebral arteries. They then run from the foramen between C2 and C3, course through the longus colli muscle, anastomose at the midaxis, and finally perforate the anterior of the axis (**Figure 2**, *A*). Like the anterior ascending arteries, the posterior ascending arteries also arise from the vertebral arteries. They then run through a groove formed by the junction of the axis body and pedicle, after which they perforate the anterior aspect of the axis and branch medially to the posterior longitudinal ligament (**Figure 2**, *B*). The posterior ascending arteries then anastomose with the anterior ascending arteries to unite the anterior and posterior vascular supplies. This anastomosis occurs in an apical arcade through which they contribute to the formation of a vascular network at the tip of the odontoid and the alar ligaments.[38] The cleft perforators are small vessels that originate from the extracranial portion of the internal carotid artery. They anastomose with the anterior ascending arteries at the middle of the axis, as well as proximally where they aid in supplying the lateral aspect of the odontoid process.[37]

Horizontal arteries have also been noted to contribute to the odontoid vascular arcade.[38] These horizontal arteries consist of four anterior and two posterior arteries that run on each side of the anterior aspect of the atlas. The superoanterior horizontal arteries anastomose with each other as well as with the apical vascular network, and the inferoanterior horizontal arteries anastomose with the ipsilateral anterior ascending artery. The posterior horizontal arteries arise from the ascending pharyngeal artery and merge with the apical vascular network. An intraosseous anastomosis also exists within the odontoid process, which connects arteries entering from the odontoid base with those entering from the apex.

In addition to odontoid process vascular feeders, the internal carotid and vertebral arteries course through the odontoid region and are important to consider in any upper cervical spine surgery. The internal carotid artery courses rostrally in an anterolateral direction to enter the base of the skull through the canalis caroticus. The vertebral artery courses through the cervical vertebrae and passes through the foramina transversaria before running over the posterior lamina of the atlas. It then enters the skull through the foramen magnum. The anatomic course of the vertebral arteries has many variants that can produce surgical complications if not previously identified. Thus, it is crucial to consider and delineate their course before surgical intervention in the odontoid region.

Overall, an extensive vascular network surrounds the odontoid. However, there is a relative watershed area around the base of the odontoid, which has been hypothesized to contribute to nonunions at this site.[33,39,40] Not only may there be a relatively decreased normal vascular supply, but the supply may be further compromised secondary to traumatic disruption.[39,41]

Nonetheless, other studies have shown that the vascular supply to the odontoid process was not eliminated in acute fractures and nonunion. Vertebral angiograms demonstrated that, while the posterior and anterior ascending arteries may have been damaged due to trauma, vascular supply was maintained to the odontoid process.[38,42] Thus, the high incidence of nonunion, especially with fractures at the base of the odontoid, is likely multifactorial and may be related to the interposition of soft tissues and lack of stability at the site of the fracture.[43,44]

Embryology

The embryology of the axis vertebra, including the fusion of ossification centers at varied time points, can be a source of confusion. For this reason, an appreciation of the difference between normal development and pathology is important.

The axis forms from five primary ossification centers that arise during the third to fifth months of fetal development. These ossification centers include the centrum, two posterior elements, and two centers that will eventually develop into the odontoid process. The two primary ossification centers of the odontoid generally fuse 3 to 4 months following birth. The centrum and posterior elements usually fuse at approximately 3 years of age to form the vertebral body and posterior arch.[45]

The vertebral body and odontoid are the last to fuse.[45] Until this occurs, a cartilaginous region, termed the dentocentral synchondrosis, separates the two odontoid centers from the vertebral centrum. It is crucial to recognize the potential remnants of an incompletely closed dentocentral synchondrosis as these may masquerade as a physeal fracture in infants and children.[45] The fusion of the odontoid to the rest of the C2 vertebra does not begin until approximately 3 years of age. These ossification centers begin complete fusion between years 3 and 6.[46] By the age of 6 years, fusion is generally complete and only a small sclerotic line in the body of C2 remains visible on radiographic images.[46]

Secondary ossification centers are found at the inferior end plate of C2 (ring apophysis) and at the proximal end of the dens (ossiculum terminale). The ring apophysis generally appears during adolescence and fuses to the vertebral body between 13 and 15 years of age.[45] The ossiculum terminale appears at approximately 8 to 10 years and fuses with the dens between 10 and 13 years of age.[45,46] During this period, it is important to consider that the V-shaped appearance of the cartilage between the ossiculum and the body of the odontoid process can be misconstrued as a potential C1 fracture.

Another relatively common developmental factor that can be misinterpreted as evidence of trauma is congenital variation of C1 and C2.[45,47] One of the more common lesions is hypoplasia of the dens, which may occur in many of the skeletal dysplasias, as well as disorders such as Down syndrome.[48,49] Ossification variations and synchondroses should not be confused with traumatic disruption of the ring.

Classification

The classification of odontoid fractures has evolved over the last 3 decades. Schatzker et al[33] initially classified odontoid fractures as high or low depending on where the fractures were in relation to the accessory ligaments. In this cohort, high fractures were associated with considerable displacement and relative instability, while low fractures were nondisplaced and rarely moved with voluntary head motion. This classification system was never widely adopted.

Anderson and D'Alonzo proposed the most widely accepted classification system for odontoid fractures in the 1970s (**Figure 3**).[50] Type I fractures were described to be near the tip of the odontoid process, above the transverse ligament, and are infrequently encountered. Type II fractures occur at the base of the odontoid, between the level of the transverse ligament and the C2 vertebral body, and are the most common type of odontoid fracture.[51] Type III fractures extend into the vertebral body.

As with any classification system, the Anderson and D'Alonzo classification does help guide treatment. Type I fractures are generally thought to occur by avulsion of the apical and/or alar ligaments and to be relatively stable. These can generally be treated with collar immobilization. None-

FIGURE 3

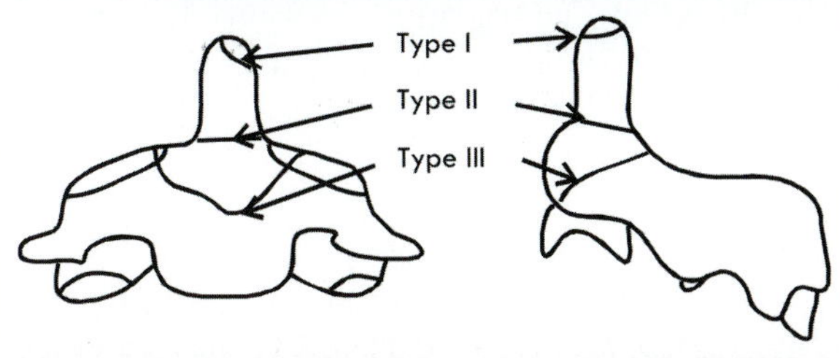

Figure 3 Anderson and D'Alonzo classification. Type I fractures are near the tip of the odontoid process, above the transverse ligament. Type II fractures occur at the base of the odontoid, between the level of the transverse ligament and the C2 vertebral body. Type III fractures extend into the vertebral body. (Reproduced with permission from Grauer JN, Shafi B, Hilibrand AS, et al: Proposal of a modified, treatment-oriented classification of odontoid fractures. *Spine J* 2005;5(2):123-129. Http://www.sciencedirect.com/science/journal/15299430.)

theless, this fracture type may also herald an inherently unstable occipital-cervical dislocation, particularly if bilateral type I odontoid fractures or a contralateral occipital condyle fracture is present. If this diagnosis is made, more aggressive treatment is warranted. Type II fractures are less stable and their treatment is more controversial. Immobilization options may include a collar,[1,50] halo,[3] or anterior[52] or posterior[53-56] internal fixation. Increased patient age, extent and direction of fracture displacement, delay in diagnosis, and fracture comminution have all been shown to negatively influence union rates.[1,2,50] Type III fractures are relatively stable unless significantly displaced and can generally be treated with collar immobilization.

This crucial treatment decision has been complicated by difficulty in precisely defining when a type II fracture extends inferiorly enough to be considered a type III fracture. Many authors refer to such intermediate fractures as "shallow" or "high" type III fractures. These injuries thus fall into a gray zone between type II and type III fractures for which some authors suggest fixation.[1,55] Nonetheless, this ambiguity leads to confusion in the literature.

To address this limitation, more precise definitions for distinguishing type II fractures from type III fractures have been suggested.[56] Type II fractures were defined as fractures located at the inferior aspect of the anterior C1 ring with no extension into the superior articular facets of C2. Thus, oblique fractures in the anterior/posterior plane with mild C2 vertebral body extension and no C2 facet involvement remained type II fractures. However, if the fracture extended into at least one of the superior articular facets of C2, the fracture was classified as a type III fracture.

A second limitation of the Anderson and D'Alonzo description of type II fractures is a lack of distinction between fractures, which have a broad range of different morphologies and associated management considerations. For example, fracture-line obliquity, displacement, and comminution clearly affect management recommendations. This is highlighted by the different types of fracture stabilization that are now advocated for different subpopulations of odontoid fractures.

To address this limitation, Hadley et al[57] introduced a type IIA fracture subclass defined as a type II fracture complicated by an additional chip-fracture fragment at the anterior or posterior aspect of the base of the odontoid. This subclass (representing 5% of type II odontoid fractures) was observed to progress to nonunion regardless of initial fracture displacement, age, or neurologic status. Consequently, consideration for surgical intervention for such injuries was recommended.

Nonetheless, there is still a wide array of fracture patterns that are classified as type II fractures. For this reason, Grauer et al[56] proposed a treatment-oriented type II subtype classification system consisting of type IIA, IIB, and IIC fractures (**Figure 4**). Type IIA was defined as a minimally or nondisplaced type II fracture with no comminution. These fractures are generally managed with external immobilization or, rarely, anterior screw osteosynthesis or a posterior C1-C2 fusion. Type IIB is a displaced fracture extending from anterior-superior to posterior-inferior or a transverse fracture. These fractures are amenable to anterior screw fixation following fracture reduction, assuming adequate bone density. Type IIC is a displaced fracture line extending from anterior-inferior to posterior-superior or a fracture with significant comminution. These fractures are generally managed with posterior atlantoaxial stabilization.

Mechanism of Injury

Odontoid fractures usually result from low-energy impact, such as falls in the elderly, or high-velocity impact, such as motor vehicle accidents in the young and middle-aged.[4-6,11] Several studies have looked at the actual forces associated with inducing these injuries.

In 1912, Fritzsche noted that the alar and apical ligaments became tight at the extremes of

FIGURE 4

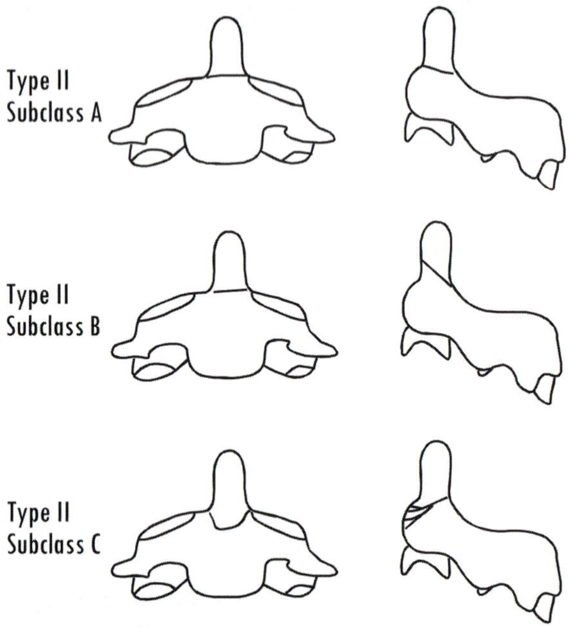

Figure 4 Proposed modification of type II odontoid fractures including types IIA, IIB, and IIC. Type IIA is a minimally or nondisplaced type II fracture with no comminution, type IIB is a displaced fracture extending from anterior-superior to posterior-inferior or a transverse fracture, and type IIC is a fracture line extending from anterior-inferior to posterior-superior or a fracture with significant comminution. (Reproduced with permission from Grauer JN, Shafi B, Hilibrand AS, et al: Proposal of a modified, treatment-oriented classification of odontoid fractures. *Spine J* 2005; 5(2):123-129. Http://www.sciencedirect.com/science/journal/15299430.)

flexion, extension, and rotation of the head.[58] It was thus postulated that any impact on the head that forced it into an extreme position may result in avulsion of the dens and subsequent odontoid fracture. However, a review of the literature suggested that odontoid fractures are not the result of a simple shear or avulsion, but rather may be produced by a combination of forces with added displacement due to shearing.[33]

Flexion, extension, lateral bending, and rotation-extension have also been tested but have not produced odontoid fractures observed clinically.[11,59] Thus, while a multifactorial mechanism is most likely responsible for the various odontoid fractures seen clinically, the primary force for these fractures is generally agreed to be hyperextension or hyperflexion of the cervical spine.

Presentation

In children and young adults, odontoid fractures are associated with high-velocity accidents, as noted above. This population has a high incidence of concomitant injuries. In fact, odontoid injuries may be missed because the patient is unconscious and/or has distracting injuries.[40,60] On the other hand, in the elderly, the mechanism of injury is more often low-velocity falls. There may be altered mental status or other reasons why symptoms related to an odontoid fracture are not recognized or conveyed.

If the patient can effectively communicate, however, the most common complaint is poorly localized high posterior cervical pain, which may radiate in the distribution of the greater occipital nerve.[33] Other common complaints include paravertebral muscle spasm, tenderness, and limited neck motion.

The frequency of associated neurologic injury is variable among multiple studies, ranging from 2% to 27%.[61-65] When present, however, it may be catastrophic because of the high level of spinal cord injury.[66] Neurologic loss may range from tetraplegia with respiratory center involvement to occipital neuralgia due to greater occipital nerve involvement. Other neurologic presentations may include Brown-Séquard syndrome, upper extremity monoplegia, hemiparesis, and quadriparesis.[39,61] Less specific symptoms may also exist, including generalized upper extremity motor and sensory weakness, fecal and urinary incontinence, dysphagia, and spastic paresis.[40,43,50]

A high suspicion must be maintained for other contiguous or noncontiguous spine fractures once an odontoid fracture is identified. In 1927, Jefferson[67] initially described upper cervical spine injuries to be highly associated with odontoid fractures. Since this time, multiple other associated cervical spine fractures have been documented.[19] In fact, noncontiguous spine fractures associated with odontoid fractures have a reported incidence of up to 20%.[19,33,63,68]

Imaging

In the workup of an acute cervical spine injury, most clinicians recommend three views of the cervical spine including AP, cross-table lateral, and open-mouth odontoid cervical radiographs.[69,70] Some centers additionally obtain oblique images. If a chronic injury is believed to exist, flexion/extension views may be obtained as well. Plain radiographs, however, have limitations in terms of their sensitivity in the upper cervical spine and cervicothoracic junction, where injuries commonly occur.[71]

CT is performed if a high index of suspicion for a fracture exists, if a bony injury is identified or suspected on plain radiographs, or if the patient has an altered mental status or distracting injury.[69,70,72] Sagittal and coronal reformats are important to evaluate for transverse fractures, which can be missed on axial imaging, and to better define fractures if identified. Data have suggested that if a cervical CT is obtained, further plain radiographic imaging is not required.[73] In fact, recent data suggest that CT imaging should be used to obtain rapid, efficient cervical spine evaluation and negates the need for plain radiographic imaging.[74]

MRI may be considered if there is a neurologic deficit. In this setting, MRI can help define cord changes. Additionally, information can be obtained about potential ligamentous injury at and around an injury of interest.

In addition, it is important that the rest of the spine be evaluated when any spinal fracture is identified. This is generally advocated due to an approximately 34% risk of noncontiguous spine fractures.[75] This can be done with plain radiographs. However, reformats from a chest/abdomen/pelvis CT are often possible as these scans may be independently indicated in the evaluation of a trauma patient.

Pediatrics

Although cervical spine injury is relatively uncommon in children, the cervical region from the occiput to the second cervical vertebrae is the most commonly injured region of the spine and is at particular risk in children under 10 years of age.[76-81] The relatively large head and shorter neck of the young child places the fulcrum and concentration of forces within this region of the cervical spine.[82] Furthermore, at this age, this region is inherently more unstable due to an increased ligamentous laxity, underdeveloped musculature, horizontal facet orientations, and relatively smaller condyles.[83] Thus, while fractures and dislocations are relatively rare in this age group, when they occur, the upper cervical spine is more often involved than the lower.[84-87] These injuries have been most often associated with motor vehicle accidents, falls on the head, and obstetric trauma.[84,87-89]

Odontoid fractures generally occur at the level of the physis between the odontoid and centrum and represent the equivalent of a type II odontoid fracture.[80,90] Anterior displacement of the atlas and odontoid may also occur.[58,87,90-92] Primary treatment includes reduction through gentle traction and concurrent head extension. External immobilization can then generally be achieved with a halo vest.[92] As with any pediatric halo, more pins with less torque should be used than are used with an adult halo.

When these physeal fractures are nondisplaced, they may be difficult to diagnose radiographically.[80] Seimon[93] described children's reports of pain when moving from a sitting to a lying position and with neck extension, but absence of pain when fully upright. The differential including odontoid fracture should also include pseudosubluxation,[80,94] the normal anterior angulation of the odontoid,[87] odontoid hypoplasia, and os odontoideum,[95,96] because each of these may also be associated with atlantoaxial instability in a spine-injured child.

Os Odontoideum

Os odontoideum was first described by Giacomini in 1886 and has been further characterized as an anomaly of the second cervical vertebrae that can be identified radiologically by a small, round, or oval corticated ossicle separated from the base of the odontoid. Below this ossicle is a shortened odontoid process extending from the vertebral body of the axis.[97] Hypertrophy of the anterior arch and hypoplasia of the posterior arch of the atlas may also be present.[95,98]

While this anomaly has been well described, the etiology remains unclear. Etiologic hypotheses currently include developmental, congenital, and traumatic causes. Developmental abnormalities include failure of the odontoid process to fuse with the body of the axis or the ossiculum terminale to fuse with the main odontoid process. A congenital etiology is supported by evidence of familial os odontoideum and other related deformities including Klippel-Feil syndrome, myelodysplasia, epiphyseal dysplasia, and Down syndrome.[99-102] Traumatic causes have been suggested by Fielding et al,[95] who associated os odontoideum with fracture nonunion. This association arose from a comparison of pre- and posttraumatic radiographic examinations of patients with os odontoideum. The study suggested that fracture of the proximal odontoid process and subsequent contracture of the alar ligaments may increase the potential for nonunion. The proximal odontoid fracture fragment may then remodel to become an os odontoideum. Other studies have been conducted that substantiate this potential etiology.[103,104] Nevertheless, further studies are required to more fully establish these theories.

As described previously, the stability of the atlantoaxial articulation depends on the integrity of the odontoid process and the associated ligaments. If either the odontoid process or the ligaments are disrupted, atlantoaxial instability may result. This disruption may be due to traumatic or atraumatic causes. Nevertheless, the previously noted large area available for the spinal cord in this region allows most patients with atlantoaxial instability to remain asymptomatic. This includes patients with os odontoideum.

Much controversy currently exists regarding the appropriate management of asymptomatic patients with os odontoideum and ranges from prophylactic fusion to observation.[101,105,106] One series of five patients treated conservatively documented no neurologic deficits after more than 1 year of follow-up.[105] Another series of 37 cases found no significant difference in outcome among asymptomatic patients when comparing conservative treatment with posterior fusion.[107] Thus, given the potential morbidity and lack of significant benefit of atlantoaxial fusion in asymptomatic patients, observation may be most appropriate in the asymptomatic patient if there is not excessive movement on dynamic flexion/extension films.

Excessive movement in the atlantoaxial region can be evaluated by analyzing the following: (1) the space available for the spinal cord (SAC), which has been related to development of cervical myelopathy; (2) the Instability Index, or the change in SAC from flexion to extension; and (3) the sagittal plane rotation angle, or the difference of atlantoaxial angle between flexion and extension.[106,108] In patients with os odontoideum, the SAC is measured from the upper posterior margin of the body of the axis to the posterior arch of the atlas while in flexion.[109] However, if canal stenosis exists, the SAC may be defined by the distance from the os odontoideum to the posterior arch of the atlas.[107] A SAC between 11 mm and 13 mm has been associated with progressive myelopathy.[106,107] An Instability Index of greater than 40% and a sagittal plane rotation angle of greater than 20° have also been associated with an increased risk of developing neuropathy.[106]

If one or more of these criteria exist, or if neurologic symptoms occur secondary to atlantoaxial instability related to an os odontoideum, surgery is indicated.[107] In this event, posterior atlantoaxial fusion has been widely accepted, and different techniques have been suggested.[95,110-112] One must be cautious of potential neurologic complications with such intervention,[111] and if atlantoaxial fusion is impossible, occipitocervical fusion may be appropriately considered with or without resection of the posterior atlantal arch.[105,109,111,113]

Treatment Considerations

Certainly, there are many different types of odontoid fractures, as noted in the classification section above. Each type of fracture has specific treatment options and considerations that will be reviewed below. However, it is important to note that there are general treatment principles that must be respected. Many variables can alter the management of a specific injury.

Importantly, medical comorbidities must be considered when developing a treatment plan. It has previously been noted that the population sustaining odontoid fractures is gradually increasing in age. Whether this is due to better prevention in younger populations, increased incidence in older populations, or a mere reflection of the general population aging as a whole is difficult to delineate. Nonetheless, the older patient population is generally associated with decreased bone density, are less optimized for surgical intervention, and do not well tolerate halo immobilization.

Increased mortality rates have been noted in the elderly population.[4,6,7,114,115] Individual concomitant medical illnesses such as diabetes mellitus, rheumatoid arthritis, coronary artery disease, and hypertension have not been directly associated with increased mortality, although comparative data are limited in this area.[116]

Treatment Options and Outcomes

In the treatment of odontoid fractures, a variety of treatment options exist, ranging from cervical collar immobilization to advanced internal fixation techniques. These treatment modalities are reviewed in the following sections.

External Immobilization

Type I odontoid fractures are rare, but are generally treated with collar immobilization when encountered. The caveat to this rule, as noted above, is that an occipital-cervical dislocation should be ruled out. This potential injury can be effectively imaged using sagittal reformatted CT to assess the congruency of the facets/occipital condyles and/or MRI to assess for edema at the occipital-cervical junction.[117] If these findings are noted, a posterior occipital-cervical fusion is generally performed.[83,118-120] If neurologically intact, however, halo-vest immobilization with close monitoring may be considered.[121]

Most type III odontoid fractures can be treated with collar immobilization; however, halo-vest immobilization may also be considered.[19,51,64,66,122] The exception to this is a type III fracture associated with anterior displacement, which may require internal fixation to achieve stability and prevent further displacement.[61] In addition, many fractures that have previously been termed "shallow type III" may act functionally more like type II odontoid fractures and require internal stabilization.[123]

Type II odontoid fractures are, in general, less stable and associated with lower union rates than type I and type III odontoid fractures. Treatment of these injuries is less well defined. External immobilization with a cervical collar has led to inconsistent results.[66,68] The associated nonunion rate is believed to be due to instability of this fracture pattern. As previously noted, decreased vascularity at the watershed region of the base of the odontoid has also been proposed as a factor in nonunion,[42] but the validity of this hypothesis has been questioned.[43,44] Consequently, many clinicians have recommended greater immobilization of these injuries.[68] A halo vest may be considered, but this treatment modality is still associated with a significant nonunion rate in several series, ranging from 26% to 80%.[6,18,63,65,66,123-126]

Several factors appear to be associated with an increased incidence of nonunion for type II odontoid fractures. These include posterior fracture displacement, displacement greater than 4 to 6 mm, greater than 10° of angulation, fracture comminution, fracture malalignment during follow-up, delayed treatment, and patients older than 40 to 65 years of age (**Table 1**).[18,19,39,61,127-132]

The increased incidence of type II odontoid fracture nonunion in elderly patients treated with external immobilization[68,115,133,134] is particularly concerning as epidemiological and retrospective case-control studies have shown a high prevalence of this fracture pattern in this population.[6,7,114,115] Moreover, multiple studies have documented higher rates of complications with halo immobilization in this population (in the range of 26%), including poor reduction maintenance, pneumonia, wound infection, cerebral spinal fluid leakage, and even death.[124] Thus, some studies have suggested primary internal fixation in elderly patients.[68,115,133,134]

If a nonunion does result from external immobilization, dynamic radiographs are appropriately considered to assess the amount of movement at the nonunion site. If there is significant movement and/or symptoms, surgical intervention should be considered. If there is not significant movement and/or symptoms in the younger population, surgical stabilization may still be considered to prevent potential catastrophic decline with a traumatic event. In the elderly population, however, this may be deemed to be an acceptable risk when weighed against the potential morbidity of surgical intervention.

Posterior Odontoid Stabilization

In situations where external immobilization is believed to be insufficient, intolerable, or ineffective, surgical intervention may be considered. This treatment may also be warranted if other considerations come into play such as with the polytrauma patient or with a neurologic deficit.

Several posterior techniques have been described for stabilization of odontoid fractures. The common goal is to achieve a solid C1-C2 fusion. The primary disadvantages of these techniques are the morbidity associated with posterior cervical approaches and the loss of rotational motion after fusion of this cervical level.[135] Techniques have gradually evolved from wire constructs to more stable screw constructs.

Gallie[53] described the first posterior C1-C2 wiring technique. This technique used a single central wire placed in a sublaminar position under the ring of C1 and around the C2 spinous process. The wire provides stability and serves to secure a structural autograft in place. Brooks and Jenkins[54] later devised an alternative wiring technique using bilateral sublaminar C1-C2 wires with two structural autograft blocks (one on each side) (**Figure 5**). When compared biomechanically, the Brooks construct is 2.5 times more stable than the Gallie consruct.[136]

Posterior wiring has proven to afford simple and effective internal fixation of odontoid fractures achieving fusion rates of 80% to 100%,[39,64,137] compared with 68% for nonsurgical treatment of type II fractures.[61] However, most of these series have been in combination with halo bracing, while fusion rates as low as 20% have been described without this adjuvant stabilization.[138] Further disadvantages of this procedure include the risk of spinal cord injury with passage of the sublaminar wires and inability to use these techniques with concurrent C1 arch fractures.

An alternative method of C1-C2 stabilization is that of transarticular, or Magerl, screws (**Figure 5**).[55] After open posterior exposure of the upper cervical spine, screws are placed in a percuta-

TABLE 1

Studies on Conservatively Treated Type II Fractures of the Odontoid Process[a]

	Nonunion/Numbers of Patients Treated Conservatively						
Author(s)	**Level of Evidence**	**Total**	**Collar**	**Minerva or SOMI**	**Skull Traction**	**Halo Vest**	**Factors Associated With Type II Fracture NonUnion**
Anderson and D'Alonzo[50]	III	8/22	-	-	8/22	-	-
Clark and White[61]	II	11/41	3/3	-	1/3	7/35	> 5-mm displacement in any direction > 10° of angulation
Dunn and Seljeskog[66]	III	19/59	-	-	NR	-	> 2 mm of posterior displacement Age > 65 years Delay > 7 days
Ekong et al[62]	II	6/12	-	-	-	6/12	> 4-6 mm displacement in any direction Age > 55 years
Govender et al[42]	II	50/109	-	50/109	-	-	Age > 40 years > 4 mm displacement Posterior displacement
Greene et al[127]	III	25/88	NR/5	NR/9	-	NR/81	> 6-mm displacement in any direction
Hadley et al[18]	III	8/31	1/2	2/6	-	5/23	-
Hadley et al[19]	III	19/68	NR/2	NR/8	-	NR/65	> 6-mm displacement in any direction
Hanigan et al[4]	III	3/6	2/5	-	-	1/1	-
Hanssen and Cabanela[63]	III	3/15	1/2	0/3	-	2/10	Posterior displacement
Koivikko et al[128]	III	37/69	-	-	-	37/69	> 1-mm fracture gap > 5-mm posterior displacement Delay >4 days > 2-mm posterior redisplacement
Lennarson et al[116]	III	11/33	-	-	-	11/33	Age > 50 years
Maiman and Larson[64]	III	15/15	-	8/8	6/6	1/1	-
Müller et al[115]	III	4/41	4/19	0/1	-	0/21	-
Pepin et al[6]	III	7/13	NR	-	NR	1/3	-
Polin et al[129]	III	12/34	7/15	-	-	5/19	Age > 40 years
Ryan and Taylor[130]	III	27/35	-	-	-	27/35	Posterior displacement
Schweigel[65]	III	7/42	NR	NR	NR	3/20	> 4-mm displacement in any direction
Seljeskog[131]	III	2/27	-	-	1/12	1/15	-

TABLE 1 *(CONTINUED)*

Studies on Conservatively Treated Type II Fractures of the Odontoid Process[a]

Author(s)	Level of Evidence	Nonunion/Numbers of Patients Treated Conservatively: Total	Collar	Minerva or SOMI	Skull Traction	Halo Vest	Factors Associated With Type II Fracture NonUnion
Stoney et al[132]	II	4/22	-	-	-	4/22	> 3-mm posterior displacement > 20° angulation Delay > 3 days
Ziai and Hurlbert[68]	III	8/39	NR/15	NR/2	-	NR/17	Age > 65 years
Total		**286/821 (34.8%)**	**18/46 (39.1%)**	**60/127 (47.2%)**	**16/43 (37.2%)**	**123/319 (38.6%)**	

[a]Total values and percentages include only completely reported data and exclude all non-reported (NR) values.
SOMI = Sternal Occipital Mandibular Immobilizer.
(Adapted with permission from Maak TG, Grauer JN: Contemporary management of odontoid injuries. *Spine (Phila Pa 1976)* 2006;11 (11 Suppl):S53-S61.)

FIGURE 5

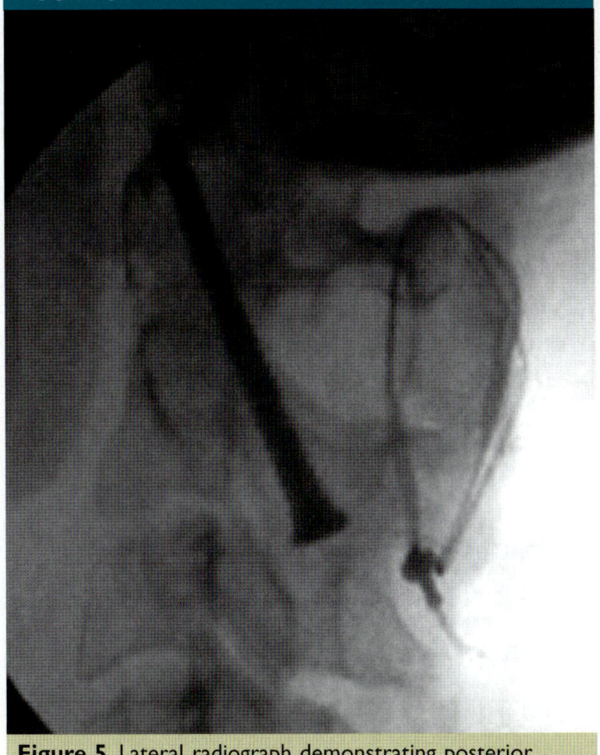

Figure 5 Lateral radiograph demonstrating posterior transarticular (Magerl) screws with Brooks-Jenkins posterior wiring.

neous fashion along the isthmus of C2 and into the C1 lateral mass. The percutaneous screw placement allows for an appropriate screw trajectory, which would not be afforded from the open exposure. In its early description, this technique was combined with adjunctive posterior wiring fixation; however, not all screw constructs have implemented such wiring. Notably, absence of posterior wiring in this construct is associated with increased flexion and extension motion, but has been accepted by many.[139]

Biomechanically, Magerl screw constructs have been shown to have a tenfold increased rotational stiffness and similar lateral bending stiffness to that of posterior wiring techniques.[140,141] The increased stability has led most clinicians to treat these patients with a postoperative collar, as opposed to a halo. Using this protocol, fusion rates have been reported to approach 100%.[55,142-144] Nonetheless, there are clearly limitations to this technique. These limitations include the required reduction of C1 on C2 before screw placement, risk of vertebral artery injury, and potential bleeding from dissection surrounding the C2 pedicle.[145] If transarticular screws are considered, the preoperative CT scan should be evaluated to make sure that an appropriate and safe screw trajectory exists. This evaluation can be achieved by looking at the parasagittal CT images. It is critical to evaluate the path of the vertebral arteries as described previously, specifically the presence of any anatomic

FIGURE 6

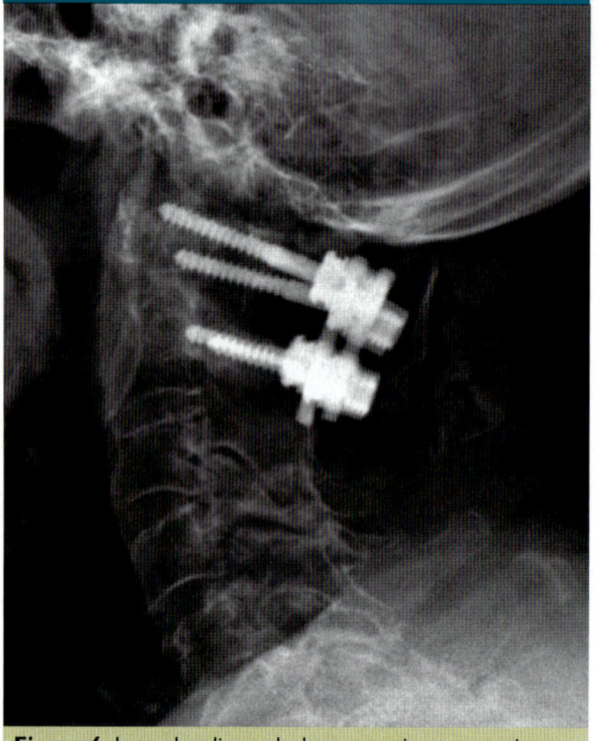

Figure 6 Lateral radiograph demonstrating a posterior C1-C2 polyaxial screw and rod (Harms) fixation for an odontoid nonunion.

FIGURE 7

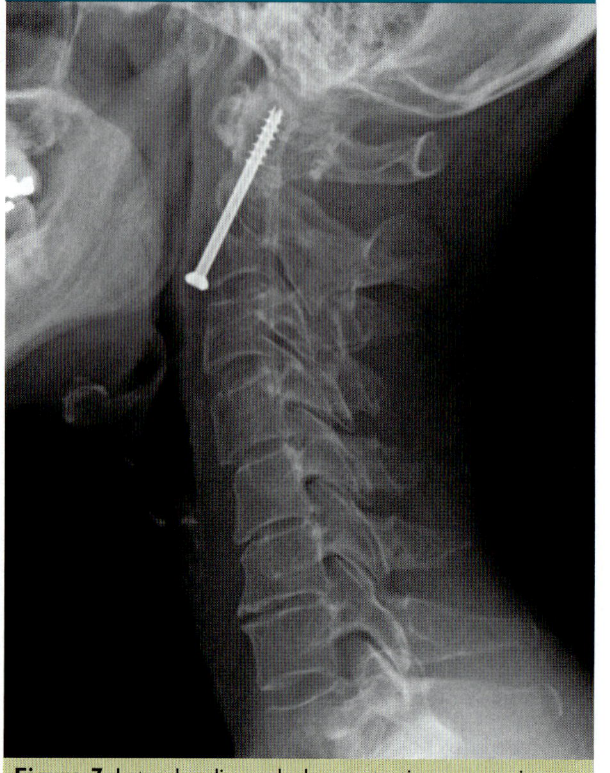

Figure 7 Lateral radiograph demonstrating an anterior odontoid screw for a displaced type II fracture.

variants, because these may be injured when using this fixation method.

To avoid the limitations of transarticular fixation, an alternate technique for screw fixation has been described and popularized by Harms using posterior C1 lateral mass and C2 pars polyaxial screws (**Figure 6**).[145] Once the screws are placed, the reduction of C1 relative to C2 can be adjusted if necessary before securing the screws with a short rod construct. This technique produced 100% fusion of all 37 patients at 1 year and had no neurologic, vascular, or implant complications. Biomechanical comparison of this technique to bilateral C1-C2 transarticular screws with different wiring techniques demonstrated significantly decreased motion in lateral bending and axial rotation with both the Harms and transarticular screw constructs.[146] Moreover, no significant difference was documented between the transarticular and Harms methods.

Posterior fixation constructs as described above can also be extended up the occiput or down to the subaxial spine if necessary. This may be considered to address concomitant injuries or if there is difficulty with securing fixation points.

Anterior Odontoid Fixation

The need for C1-C2 fusion is common to all posterior techniques for odontoid stabilization. Unfortunately, this requirement eliminates approximately 50% of cervical rotation.[135] This led to the development of alternative stabilization techniques for type II odontoid fractures, namely direct osteosynthesis with anterior screw fixation (**Figure 7**).[51,135] Full preservation of C1-C2 motion using this technique, however, has been questioned.[147]

Direct anterior odontoid fixation was first described by Böhler[51] in 1982, and investigators have further refined this technique. The fracture may be reduced preoperatively or intraoperatively. A standard low cervical approach is made around the C5-C6 level. The prevertebral plane is then developed, allowing access to the C2-3 disk space. The entry site for the screw, which is placed across the fracture, is at the anterior-inferior corner of the C2 end plate (through the anterior portion of the C2-3 disk space) and is crucial to the success of this procedure. Specifically designed retractors and biplanar fluoroscopy are helpful for this process.

In its initial description, two odontoid screws were advocated. However, studies have shown no significant difference between the biomechanical stability[126] or union rates[148] of one or two screws. Moreover, it is often technically not possible to safely place two screws, such as when the medullary cavity of the dens is extremely small.[148,149] Accordingly, a single screw is recommended by most clinicians for this procedure.

There are several distinct advantages to using an anterior odontoid screw as opposed to posterior C1-C2 fixation techniques. As already noted, the C1-C2 motion can potentially be spared. Moreover, the anterior approach is less traumatic than posterior approaches and this technique does not require bone graft harvest, thus decreasing postoperative morbidity. This method can also be considered with concomitant C1 ring fractures, assuming the transverse ligament is intact. Multiple clinical studies have documented odontoid fracture fusion rates that ranged from 83% to 100% following anterior screw placement for the appropriately selected patient.[51,52,123,142,150]

There are, nonetheless, clear reasons not to use anterior odontoid fixation. One such reason is fracture geometry. This method is only appropriate for reducible type II fractures of the correct obliquity to allow compression across the fracture site and avoid displacement with lag screw fixation (type IIA injuries described above by Grauer et al[56]). In addition, this fixation should not be used in the setting of osteoporotic bone, pathologic fracture, or nonunions where fracture healing and/or fixation will be impaired. Thus, in the elderly population in which osteoporosis is prevalent, posterior fusion may be better considered. Patients with cervical or thoracic kyphosis and short, thick necks may also not allow the appropriate trajectory for screw placement.

Treatment Summary

Odontoid fractures continue to pose a clinical challenge. We are generally seeing fractures in older patients with increased medical comorbidities and decreased bone density. Many type I and type III fractures can be treated with simple collar immobilization. Type II fractures continue to pose the greatest controversy. Certainly, there have been advances in the types of fixation options available today. However, there is no consensus as to the best treatment for different fracture patterns and patient populations.

The lack of consensus on this topic potentially reflects the reality that there is not yet any single ideal solution for this clinical problem. For this reason, no definitive conclusion can be drawn for treatment of this fracture type. This was highlighted by a study questioning 35 experienced spinal surgeons regarding treatment of specific spinal injuries.[151] Although there was a high degree of commonality in management for most injuries, a case of a type II odontoid fracture would have been treated anteriorly by 50% and posteriorly by 50% of those questioned. The results of ongoing and future studies will hopefully help direct better treatment decisions regarding odontoid fractures.

References

1. Subach BR, Morone MA, Haid RW Jr, McLaughlin MR, Rodts GR, Comey CH: Management of acute odontoid fractures with single-screw anterior fixation. *Neurosurgery* 1999;45(4):812-820.
2. Lee PC, Chun SY, Leong JC: Experience of posterior surgery in atlanto-axial instability. *Spine (Phila Pa 1976)* 1984;9(3):231-239.
3. Vaccaro AR, Madigan L, Ehrler DM: Contemporary management of adult cervical odontoid fractures. *Orthopedics* 2000;23(10):1109-1115.
4. Hanigan WC, Powell FC, Elwood PW, Henderson JP: Odontoid fractures in elderly patients. *J Neurosurg* 1993;78(1):32-35.
5. Marchesi DG: Management of odontoid fractures. *Orthopedics* 1997;20(10):911-916.
6. Pepin JW, Bourne RB, Hawkins RJ: Odontoid fractures, with special reference to the elderly patient. *Clin Orthop Relat Res* 1985;193:178-183.
7. Ryan MD, Henderson JJ: The epidemiology of fractures and fracture-dislocations of the cervical spine. *Injury* 1992;23(1):38-40.
8. Rogers MA, Crockard HA, Moskovich R, et al: Nystagmus and joint position sensation: Their importance in posterior occipitocervical fusion in rheumatoid arthritis. *Spine (Phila Pa 1976)* 1994; 19(1):16-20.
9. Puttlitz CM, Melcher RP, Kleinstueck FS, Harms J, Bradford DS, Lotz JC: Stability analysis of craniovertebral junction fixation techniques. *J Bone Joint Surg Am* 2004;86(3):561-568.
10. Panjabi M, Dvorak J, Duranceau J, et al: Three-dimensional movements of the upper cervical spine. *Spine (Phila Pa 1976)* 1988;13(7):726-730.
11. Mouradian WH, Fietti VG Jr, Cochran GV, Fielding JW, Young J: Fractures of the odontoid: A laboratory and clinical study of mechanisms. *Orthop Clin North Am* 1978;9(4):985-1001.
12. Steel HH: Anatomical and mechanical considerations of the atlanto-axial articulations. *J Bone Joint Surg Am* 1968;50A:1481-1482.

13. Jauregui N, Lincoln T, Mubarak S, Garfin S: Surgically related upper cervical spine canal anatomy in children. *Spine (Phila Pa 1976)* 1993;18(14): 1939-1944.
14. Nordqvist L: The sagittal diameter of the spinal cord and subarachnoid space in different age groups: A toentgenographic post-morten study. *Acta Radiol Diagn (Stockh)* 1964;Suppl 227:1-96.
15. Inoue H, Ohmori K, Takatsu T, Teramoto T, Ishida Y, Suzuki K: Morphological analysis of the cervical spinal canal, dural tube and spinal cord in normal individuals using CT myelography. *Neuroradiology* 1996;38(2):148-151.
16. Thijssen HO, Keyser A, Horstink MW, Meijer E: Morphology of the cervical spinal cord on computed myelography. *Neuroradiology* 1979;18(2): 57-62.
17. Kameyama T, Hashizume Y, Sobue G: Morphologic features of the normal human cadaveric spinal cord. *Spine (Phila Pa 1976)* 1996;21(11): 1285-1290.
18. Hadley MN, Browner C, Sonntag VK: Axis fractures: A comprehensive review of management and treatment in 107 cases. *Neurosurgery* 1985; 17(2):281-290.
19. Hadley MN, Dickman CA, Browner CM, Sonntag VK: Acute axis fractures: A review of 229 cases. *J Neurosurg* 1989;71(5 Pt 1):642-647.
20. Heller JG, Alson MD, Schaffler MB, Garfin SR: Quantitative internal dens morphology. *Spine (Phila Pa 1976)* 1992;17(8):861-866.
21. White AA, Panjabi MM: *Clinical Biomechanics of the Spine*, ed 2. Philadelphia, PA, Lippincott, 1990.
22. Penning L, Wilmink JT: Rotation of the cervical spine: A CT study in normal subjects. *Spine (Phila Pa 1976)* 1987;12(8):732-738.
23. Fielding JW, Cochran GB, Lawsing JF III, Hohl M: Tears of the transverse ligament of the atlas: A clinical and biomechanical study. *J Bone Joint Surg Am* 1974;56(8):1683-1691.
24. Sun PP, Poffenbarger GJ, Durham S, Zimmerman RA: Spectrum of occipitoatlantoaxial injury in young children. *J Neurosurg* 2000;93(1 Suppl): 28-39.
25. Dvorak J, Froehlich D, Penning L, Baumgartner H, Panjabi MM: Functional radiographic diagnosis of the cervical spine: Flexion/extension. *Spine (Phila Pa 1976)* 1988;13(7):748-755.
26. Giguère JF, St-Vil D, Turmel A, et al: Airbags and children: A spectrum of C-spine injuries. *J Pediatr Surg* 1998;33(6):811-816.
27. Dvorak J, Hayek J, Zehnder R: CT-functional diagnostics of the rotatory instability of the upper cervical spine: Part 2. An evaluation on healthy adults and patients with suspected instability. *Spine (Phila Pa 1976)* 1987;12(8):726-731.
28. Dvorak J, Panjabi MM: Functional anatomy of the alar ligaments. *Spine (Phila Pa 1976)* 1987;12(2): 183-189.
29. Dvorak J, Schneider E, Saldinger P, Rahn B: Biomechanics of the craniocervical region: The alar and transverse ligaments. *J Orthop Res* 1988;6(3): 452-461.
30. Panjabi MM, Oxland TR, Parks EH: Quantitative anatomy of cervical spine ligaments: Part I. Upper cervical spine. *J Spinal Disord* 1991;4(3):270-276.
31. Driscoll DR: Anatomical and biomechanical characteristics of upper cervical ligamentous structures: A review. *J Manipulative Physiol Ther* 1987; 10(3):107-110.
32. Heller JG, Amrani J, Hutton WC: Transverse ligament failure: A biomechanical study. *J Spinal Disord* 1993;6(2):162-165.
33. Schatzker J, Rorabeck CH, Waddell JP: Fractures of the dens (odontoid process): An analysis of thirty-seven cases. *J Bone Joint Surg Br* 1971;53(3): 392-405.
34. Dickman CA, Hadley MN, Pappas CT, Sonntag VK, Geisler FH: Cruciate paralysis: A clinical and radiographic analysis of injuries to the cervicomedullary junction. *J Neurosurg* 1990;73(6):850-858.
35. Dunbar HS, Ray BS: Chronic atlanto-axial dislocations with late neurologic manifestations. *Surg Gynecol Obstet* 1961;113:757-762.
36. Schatzker J, Rorabeck CH, Waddell JP: Nonunion of the odontoid process: An experimental investigation. *Clin Orthop Relat Res* 1975;108: 127-137.
37. Schiff DC, Parke WW: The arterial supply of the odontoid process. *J Bone Joint Surg Am* 1973; 55(7):1450-1456.
38. Althoff B, Goldie IF: The arterial supply of the odontoid process of the axis. *Acta Orthop Scand* 1977;48(6):622-629.
39. Apuzzo ML, Heiden JS, Weiss MH, Ackerson TT, Harvey JP, Kurze T: Acute fractures of the odontoid process: An analysis of 45 cases. *J Neurosurg* 1978;48(1):85-91.
40. Southwick WO: Management of fractures of the dens (odontoid process). *J Bone Joint Surg Am* 1980;62(3):482-486.
41. Montesano PX, Anderson PA, Schlehr F, Thalgott JS, Lowrey G: Odontoid fractures treated by anterior odontoid screw fixation. *Spine (Phila Pa 1976)* 1991;16(3, Suppl):S33-S37.
42. Govender S, Maharaj JF, Haffajee MR: Fractures of the odontoid process. *J Bone Joint Surg Br* 2000; 82(8):1143-1147.
43. Crockard HA, Heilman AE, Stevens JM: Progressive myelopathy secondary to odontoid fractures:

Clinical, radiological, and surgical features. *J Neurosurg* 1993;78(4):579-586.

44. Moskovich R, Crockard HA: Myelopathy due to hypertrophic nonunion of the dens: Case report. *J Trauma* 1990;30(2):222-225.
45. Ogden JA: Radiology of postnatal skeletal development: XII. The second cervical vertebra. *Skeletal Radiol* 1984;12(3):169-177.
46. Bailey DK: The normal cervical spine in infants and children. *Radiology* 1952;59(5):712-719.
47. Ogden JA, Murphy MJ, Southwick WO, Ogden DA: Radiology of postnatal skeletal development: XIII. C1-C2 interrelationships. *Skeletal Radiol* 1986;15(6):433-438.
48. Gillman EL: Congenital absence of the odontoid process of the axis; report of a case. *J Bone Joint Surg Am* 1959;41-A(2):345-348.
49. Martel W, Uyham R, Stimson CW: Subluxation of the atlas causing spinal cord compression in a case of Down's syndrome with a "manifestation of an occipital vertebra". *Radiology* 1969;93(4): 839-840.
50. Anderson LD, D'Alonzo RT: Fractures of the odontoid process of the axis. *J Bone Joint Surg Am* 1974;56(8):1663-1674.
51. Böhler J: Anterior stabilization for acute fractures and non-unions of the dens. *J Bone Joint Surg Am* 1982;64(1):18-27.
52. Geisler FH, Cheng C, Poka A, Brumback RJ: Anterior screw fixation of posteriorly displaced type II odontoid fractures. *Neurosurgery* 1989;25(1): 30-38.
53. Gallie WE: Fractures and dislocations of the cervical spine. *Am J Surg* 1939;46(3):495-499.
54. Brooks AL, Jenkins EB: Atlanto-axial arthrodesis by the wedge compression method. *J Bone Joint Surg Am* 1978;60(3):279-284.
55. Jeanneret B, Magerl F: Primary posterior fusion C1/2 in odontoid fractures: Indications, technique, and results of transarticular screw fixation. *J Spinal Disord* 1992;5(4):464-475.
56. Grauer JN, Shafi B, Hilibrand AS, et al: Proposal of a modified, treatment-oriented classification of odontoid fractures. *Spine J* 2005;5(2):123-129.
57. Hadley MN, Browner CM, Liu SS, Sonntag VK: New subtype of acute odontoid fractures (type IIA). *Neurosurgery* 1988;22(1 Pt 1):67-71.
58. Blockey NJ, Purser DW: Fractures of the odontoid process of the axis. *J Bone Joint Surg Br* 1956; 38(4):794-817.
59. Althoff B: Fracture of the odontoid process: An experimental and clinical study. *Acta Orthop Scand Suppl* 1979;177:1-95.
60. Marar BC, Tay CK: Fracture of the odontoid process. *Aust N Z J Surg* 1976;46(3):231-236.
61. Clark CR, White AA III: Fractures of the dens: A multicenter study. *J Bone Joint Surg Am* 1985; 67(9):1340-1348.
62. Ekong CE, Schwartz ML, Tator CH, Rowed DW, Edmonds VE: Odontoid fracture: Management with early mobilization using the halo device. *Neurosurgery* 1981;9(6):631-637.
63. Hanssen AD, Cabanela ME: Fractures of the dens in adult patients. *J Trauma* 1987;27(8):928-934.
64. Maiman DJ, Larson SJ: Management of odontoid fractures. *Neurosurgery* 1982;11(4):471-476.
65. Schweigel JF: Management of the fractured odontoid with halo-thoracic bracing. *Spine (Phila Pa 1976)* 1987;12(9):838-839.
66. Dunn ME, Seljeskog EL: Experience in the management of odontoid process injuries: An analysis of 128 cases. *Neurosurgery* 1986;18(3):306-310.
67. Jefferson G: Remarks on fractures of the first cervical vertebra. *Br Med J* 1927;2(3473):153-157.
68. Ziai WC, Hurlbert RJ: A six year review of odontoid fractures: The emerging role of surgical intervention. *Can J Neurol Sci* 2000;27(4):297-301.
69. Pasquale M, Fabian TC: Practice management guidelines for trauma from the Eastern Association for the Surgery of Trauma. *J Trauma* 1998; 44(6):941-957.
70. Keats TE, Dalinka MK, Alazraki N, et al: Cervical spine trauma: American College of Radiology. ACR Appropriateness Criteria. *Radiology* 2000; 215 Suppl:243-246.
71. Shaffer MA, Doris PE: Limitation of the cross table lateral view in detecting cervical spine injuries: A retrospective analysis. *Ann Emerg Med* 1981;10(10):508-513.
72. Castillo M, Mukherji SK: Vertical fractures of the dens. *AJNR Am J Neuroradiol* 1996;17(9): 1627-1630.
73. Diaz JJ Jr, Gillman C, Morris JA Jr, May AK, Carrillo YM, Guy J: Are five-view plain films of the cervical spine unreliable? A prospective evaluation in blunt trauma patients with altered mental status. *J Trauma* 2003;55(4):658-664.
74. Sanchez B, Waxman K, Jones T, Conner S, Chung R, Becerra S: Cervical spine clearance in blunt trauma: Evaluation of a computed tomography-based protocol. *J Trauma* 2005;59(1):179-183.
75. Green RA, Saifuddin A: Whole spine MRI in the assessment of acute vertebral body trauma. *Skeletal Radiol* 2004;33(3):129-135.
76. Hadley MN, Zabramski JM, Browner CM, Rekate H, Sonntag VK: Pediatric spinal trauma: Review of 122 cases of spinal cord and vertebral column injuries. *J Neurosurg* 1988;68(1):18-24.
77. Hamilton MG, Myles ST: Pediatric spinal injury: Review of 174 hospital admissions. *J Neurosurg* 1992;77(5):700-704.

78. Hill SA, Miller CA, Kosnik EJ, Hunt WE: Pediatric neck injuries: A clinical study. *J Neurosurg* 1984;60(4):700-706.
79. McGrory BJ, Klassen RA, Chao EY, Staeheli JW, Weaver AL: Acute fractures and dislocations of the cervical spine in children and adolescents. *J Bone Joint Surg Am* 1993;75(7):988-995.
80. Cattell HS, Filtzer DL: Pseudosubluxation and other normal variations in the cervical spine in children: A study of one hundred and sixty children. *J Bone Joint Surg Am* 1965;47(7):1295-1309.
81. Fesmire FM, Luten RC: The pediatric cervical spine: Developmental anatomy and clinical aspects. *J Emerg Med* 1989;7(2):133-142.
82. Tepper SL, Fligner CL, Reay DT: Atlanto-occipital disarticulation: Accident characteristics. *Am J Forensic Med Pathol* 1990;11(3):193-197.
83. Hosono N, Yonenobu K, Kawagoe K, Hirayama N, Ono K: Traumatic anterior atlanto-occipital dislocation: A case report with survival. *Spine (Phila Pa 1976)* 1993;18(6):786-790.
84. Anderson JM, Schutt AH: Spinal injury in children: A review of 156 cases seen from 1950 through 1978. *Mayo Clin Proc* 1980;55(8):499-504.
85. Henrys P, Lyne ED, Lifton C, Salciccioli G: Clinical review of cervical spine injuries in children. *Clin Orthop Relat Res* 1977;129:172-176.
86. Stauffer ES, Mazur JM: Cervical spine injuries in children. *Pediatr Ann* 1982;11(6):502-511.
87. Sherk HH, Schut L, Lane JM: Fractures and dislocations of the cervical spine in children. *Orthop Clin North Am* 1976;7(3):593-604.
88. Gaufin LM, Goodman SJ: Cervical spine injuries in infants: Problems in management. *J Neurosurg* 1975;42(2):179-184.
89. Pennecot GF, Leonard P, Peyrot Des Gachons S, Hardy JR, Pouliquen JC: Traumatic ligamentous instability of the cervical spine in children. *J Pediatr Orthop* 1984;4(3):339-345.
90. Griffiths SC: Fracture of odontoid process in children. *J Pediatr Surg* 1972;7(6):680-683.
91. Bhattacharyya SK: Fracture and displacement of the odontoid process in a child. *J Bone Joint Surg Am* 1974;56(5):1071-1072.
92. Ewald FC: Fracture of the odontoid process in a seventeen-month-old infant treated with a halo: A case report and discussion of the injury under the age of three. *J Bone Joint Surg Am* 1971;53(8):1636-1640.
93. Seimon LP: Fracture of the odontoid process in young children. *J Bone Joint Surg Am* 1977;59(7):943-948.
94. Swischuk LE: Anterior displacement of C2 in children: Physiologic or pathologic. *Radiology* 1977;122(3):759-763.
95. Fielding JW, Hensinger RN, Hawkins RJ: Os Odontoideum. *J Bone Joint Surg Am* 1980;62(3):376-383.
96. Juhl M, Seerup KK: Os odontoideum: A cause of atlanto-axial instability. *Acta Orthop Scand* 1983;54(1):113-118.
97. Teng MM, Shoung HM, Chang CY, Guo WY, Tiu CM, Chang T: CT and myelogram findings of os odontoideum. *Comput Med Imaging Graph* 1989;13(2):179-184.
98. Holt RG, Helms CA, Munk PL, Gillespy T III: Hypertrophy of C-1 anterior arch: Useful sign to distinguish os odontoideum from acute dens fracture. *Radiology* 1989;173(1):207-209.
99. Kirlew KA, Hathout GM, Reiter SD, Gold RH: Os odontoideum in identical twins: Perspectives on etiology. *Skeletal Radiol* 1993;22(7):525-527.
100. Sherk HH, Dawoud S: Congenital os odontoideum with Klippel-Feil anomaly and fatal atlanto-axial instability: Report of a case. *Spine (Phila Pa 1976)* 1981;6(1):42-45.
101. Morgan MK, Onofrio BM, Bender CE: Familial os odontoideum: Case report. *J Neurosurg* 1989;70(4):636-639.
102. Saltzman CL, Hensinger RN, Blane CE, Phillips WA: Familial cervical dysplasia. *J Bone Joint Surg Am* 1991;73(2):163-171.
103. Hukuda S, Ota H, Okabe N, Tazima K: Traumatic atlantoaxial dislocation causing os odontoideum in infants. *Spine (Phila Pa 1976)* 1980;5(3):207-210.
104. Schuler TC, Kurz L, Thompson DE, Zemenick G, Hensinger RN, Herkowitz HN: Natural history of os odontoideum. *J Pediatr Orthop* 1991;11(2):222-225.
105. Dai L, Yuan W, Ni B, Jia L: Os odontoideum: Etiology, diagnosis, and management. *Surg Neurol* 2000;53(2):106-109.
106. Watanabe M, Toyama Y, Fujimura Y: Atlantoaxial instability in os odontoideum with myelopathy. *Spine (Phila Pa 1976)* 1996;21(12):1435-1439.
107. Spierings EL, Braakman R: The management of os odontoideum: Analysis of 37 cases. *J Bone Joint Surg Br* 1982;64(4):422-428.
108. Abe H, Tsuru M, Mitsumori K: Atlanto-axial dislocation—instability index and indications for surgery (author's transl). *No Shinkei Geka* 1976;4(1):57-72.
109. Shirasaki N, Okada K, Oka S, Hosono N, Yonenobu K, Ono K: Os odontoideum with posterior atlantoaxial instability. *Spine (Phila Pa 1976)* 1991;16(7):706-715.
110. Marcotte P, Dickman CA, Sonntag VK, Karahalios DG, Drabier J: Posterior atlantoaxial facet screw fixation. *J Neurosurg* 1993;79(2):234-237.

111. Smith MD, Phillips WA, Hensinger RN: Fusion of the upper cervical spine in children and adolescents: An analysis of 17 patients. *Spine (Phila Pa 1976)* 1991;16(7):695-701.

112. Stillerman CB, Wilson JA: Atlanto-axial stabilization with posterior transarticular screw fixation: Technical description and report of 22 cases. *Neurosurgery* 1993;32(6):948-955.

113. Koop SE, Winter RB, Lonstein JE: The surgical treatment of instability of the upper part of the cervical spine in children and adolescents. *J Bone Joint Surg Am* 1984;66(3):403-411.

114. Bednar DA, Parikh J, Hummel J: Management of type II odontoid process fractures in geriatric patients; a prospective study of sequential cohorts with attention to survivorship. *J Spinal Disord* 1995;8(2):166-169.

115. Müller EJ, Wick M, Russe O, Muhr G: Management of odontoid fractures in the elderly. *Eur Spine J* 1999;8(5):360-365.

116. Lennarson PJ, Mostafavi H, Traynelis VC, Walters BC: Management of type II dens fractures: A case-control study. *Spine (Phila Pa 1976)* 2000;25(10):1234-1237.

117. Govender S, Vlok GJ, Fisher-Jeffes N, Du Preez CP: Traumatic dislocation of the atlanto-occipital joint. *J Bone Joint Surg Br* 2003;85(6):875-878.

118. Grob D: Transarticular screw fixation for atlanto-occipital dislocation. *Spine (Phila Pa 1976)* 2001;26(6):703-707.

119. Sponseller PD, Cass JR: Atlanto-occipital fusion for dislocation in children with neurologic preservation: A case report. *Spine (Phila Pa 1976)* 1997;22(3):344-347.

120. Bundschuh CV, Alley JB, Ross M, Porter IS, Gudeman SK: Magnetic resonance imaging of suspected atlanto-occipital dislocation: Two case reports. *Spine (Phila Pa 1976)* 1992;17(2):245-248.

121. Papadopoulos SM, Dickman CA, Sonntag VK, Rekate HL, Spetzler RF: Traumatic atlantooccipital dislocation with survival. *Neurosurgery* 1991;28(4):574-579.

122. Fujii E, Kobayashi K, Hirabayashi K: Treatment in fractures of the odontoid process. *Spine (Phila Pa 1976)* 1988;13(6):604-609.

123. Aebi M, Etter C, Coscia M: Fractures of the odontoid process: Treatment with anterior screw fixation. *Spine (Phila Pa 1976)* 1989;14(10):1065-1070.

124. Glaser JA, Whitehill R, Stamp WG, Jane JA: Complications associated with the halo-vest: A review of 245 cases. *J Neurosurg* 1986;65(6):762-769.

125. Lesoin F, Autricque A, Franz K, Villette L, Jomin M: Transcervical approach and screw fixation for upper cervical spine pathology. *Surg Neurol* 1987;27(5):459-465.

126. Sasso R, Doherty BJ, Crawford MJ, Heggeness MH: Biomechanics of odontoid fracture fixation: Comparison of the one- and two-screw technique. *Spine (Phila Pa 1976)* 1993;18(14):1950-1953.

127. Greene KA, Dickman CA, Marciano FF, Drabier JB, Hadley MN, Sonntag VK: Acute axis fractures: Analysis of management and outcome in 340 consecutive cases. *Spine (Phila Pa 1976)* 1997;22(16):1843-1852.

128. Koivikko MP, Kiuru MJ, Koskinen SK, Myllynen P, Santavirta S, Kivisaari L: Factors associated with nonunion in conservatively-treated type-II fractures of the odontoid process. *J Bone Joint Surg Br* 2004;86(8):1146-1151.

129. Polin RS, Szabo T, Bogaev CA, Replogle RE, Jane JA: Nonoperative management of Types II and III odontoid fractures: The Philadelphia collar versus the halo vest. *Neurosurgery* 1996;38(3):450-457.

130. Ryan MD, Taylor TK: Odontoid fractures in the elderly. *J Spinal Disord* 1993;6(5):397-401.

131. Seljeskog EL: Non-operative management of acute upper cervical injuries. *Acta Neurochir (Wien)* 1978;41(1-3):87-100.

132. Stoney J, O'Brien J, Wilde P: Treatment of type-two odontoid fractures in halothoracic vests. *J Bone Joint Surg Br* 1998;80(3):452-455.

133. Garfin SR, Botte MJ, Waters RL, Nickel VL: Complications in the use of the halo fixation device. *J Bone Joint Surg Am* 1986;68(3):320-325.

134. Lind B, Nordwall A, Sihlbom H: Odontoid fractures treated with halo-vest. *Spine (Phila Pa 1976)* 1987;12(2):173-177.

135. Apfelbaum RI, Lonser RR, Veres R, Casey A: Direct anterior screw fixation for recent and remote odontoid fractures. *J Neurosurg* 2000;93(2, Suppl) 227-236.

136. Hanley EN Jr, Harvell JC Jr: Immediate postoperative stability of the atlantoaxial articulation: A biomechanical study comparing simple midline wiring, and the Gallie and Brooks procedures. *J Spinal Disord* 1992;5(3):306-310.

137. Sherk HH, Snyder B: Posterior fusions of the upper cervical spine: Indications, techniques, and prognosis. *Orthop Clin North Am* 1978;9(4):1091-1099.

138. Fried LC: Atlanto-axial fracture-dislocations: Failure of posterior C.1 to C.2 fusion. *J Bone Joint Surg Br* 1973;55(3):490-496.

139. Henriques T, Cunningham BW, Olerud C, et al: Biomechanical comparison of five different atlantoaxial posterior fixation techniques. *Spine (Phila Pa 1976)* 2000;25(22):2877-2883.

140. Montesano PX, Juach EC, Anderson PA, Benson DR, Hanson PB: Biomechanics of cervical spine internal fixation. *Spine (Phila Pa 1976)* 1991;16 (3, Suppl)S10-S16.

141. Grob D, Crisco JJ III, Panjabi MM, Wang P, Dvorak J: Biomechanical evaluation of four different posterior atlantoaxial fixation techniques. *Spine (Phila Pa 1976)* 1992;17(5):480-490.

142. Dickman CA, Foley KT, Sonntag VK, Smith MM: Cannulated screws for odontoid screw fixation and atlantoaxial transarticular screw fixation: Technical note. *J Neurosurg* 1995;83(6): 1095-1100.

143. Dickman CA, Sonntag VK: Posterior C1-C2 transarticular screw fixation for atlantoaxial arthrodesis. *Neurosurgery* 1998;43(2):275-281.

144. Coyne TJ, Fehlings MG, Wallace MC, Bernstein M, Tator CH: C1-C2 posterior cervical fusion: Long-term evaluation of results and efficacy. *Neurosurgery* 1995;37(4):688-693.

145. Harms J, Melcher RP: Posterior C1-C2 fusion with polyaxial screw and rod fixation. *Spine (Phila Pa 1976)* 2001;26(22):2467-2471.

146. Melcher RP, Puttlitz CM, Kleinstueck FS, Lotz JC, Harms J, Bradford DS: Biomechanical testing of posterior atlantoaxial fixation techniques. *Spine (Phila Pa 1976)* 2002;27(22):2435-2440.

147. Jeanneret B, Vernet O, Frei S, Magerl F: Atlantoaxial mobility after screw fixation of the odontoid: A computed tomographic study. *J Spinal Disord* 1991;4(2):203-211.

148. Jenkins JD, Coric D, Branch CL Jr: A clinical comparison of one- and two-screw odontoid fixation. *J Neurosurg* 1998;89(3):366-370.

149. Schaffler MB, Alson MD, Heller JG, Garfin SR: Morphology of the dens: A quantitative study. *Spine (Phila Pa 1976)* 1992;17(7):738-743.

150. Esses SI, Bednar DA: Screw fixation of odontoid fractures and nonunions. *Spine (Phila Pa 1976)* 1991;16(10, Suppl)S483-S485.

151. Grauer JN, Vaccaro AR, Beiner JM, et al: Similarities and differences in the treatment of spine trauma between surgical specialties and location of practice. *Spine (Phila Pa 1976)* 2004;29(6): 685-696.

CHAPTER 22
Atlantoaxial Rotatory Deformities

Bradford L. Currier, MD Christopher Frank Wagener, MD

Introduction

The first reported case of atlantoaxial rotatory deformity (AARD) was described by Sir Charles Bell in 1830.[1] His patient suffered a dislocation of the atlas as a result of a deep ulcer involving the posterior pharynx that "destroyed the transverse ligament." Since that time, numerous names have been given to the condition, including rotatory dislocation of the atlas,[2] maladie de Grisel,[3] nontraumatic dislocation of the atlantoaxial joint,[4] spontaneous hyperaemic dislocation of the atlas,[5] and atlantoaxial rotatory fixation,[6] to name a few. Although all of these disorders share certain radiographic and clinical features, the names proposed often represented an attempt to describe a subset of the condition or were offered to help describe the suspected pathophysiology. Reviewing the anatomy and biomechanics of the upper cervical spine will help to understand this interesting spectrum of disorders.

Anatomy

The occipital condyles sit in the cup-shaped superior articular facets of the atlas. The orientation of the joints allows a large degree of rotation in the sagittal plane (flexion and extension) but only about 5° of rotation to each side.[7] The inferior articular facets of the atlas and the superior facets of the axis are slightly convex. The geometry of these joints allows a great deal of motion at the expense of stability.[8] In addition to the facet joints, a synovial cavity exists between the anterior arch of the atlas and the dens and another between the dens and the transverse ligament. The C1-C2 synovial joints may be isolated structures or have intercommunications.[9] Approximately 50% of the rotation of the cervical spine occurs at the C1-C2 joint.[8] In a cadaver study performed by Dvorak et al,[7] 32° of rotation in each direction was possible when all ligamentous structures were intact. In a CT evaluation of normal adults, the mean rotation at C1-C2 was approximately 43° (range, 32° to 50°).[10] On the basis of these data and the CT evaluation of 43 patients with suspected rotatory instability, Dvorak et al[10] concluded that more than 8° of rotation at C0-C1 or 56° at C1-C2, or a right-left difference of more than 5° at C0-C1 or 8° at C1-C2 represents hypermobility. Approximately 65° of rotation is required for complete atlantoaxial rotatory dislocation.[9,11,12] Only minimal flexion, extension, and lateral bending occur at the atlantoaxial level.

The ligamentous structures of the occipital-atlantoaxial complex have been studied extensively (**Figure 1**).[13] The cruciform ligament consists of the transverse ligament running horizontally and the longitudinal fasciculi oriented vertically. The transverse ligament arises from the medial aspect of each lateral mass of the atlas and passes behind the dens, which acts as a pivot point during rotation. The transverse ligament holds the dens in place and maintains the space available for the spinal cord behind the dens, especially during flexion.

The alar ligaments consist of two portions: one part extends between the sides of the dens and the occipital condyles, and the other portion connects the dens with the lateral masses of the atlas (**Figure 2**).[14,15] The alar ligaments are the primary restraints to axial rotation and side bending in the C0-C1-C2 complex, and accessory support is provided by the tectorial membrane, accessory atlantoaxial ligaments, and joint capsules.[14]

The capsular ligaments are loose coverings of the C1-C2 facet joints that contain synovial fluid and function mechanically to limit rotation.[16] The greater occipital nerves are located in close approximation to the C1-C2 capsules on each side.

Steel[17] demonstrated that the internal diameter of the ring of the atlas is approximately 3 cm; the spinal cord and odontoid are each about 1 cm in

Dr. Currier or an immediate family member serves as a board member, owner, officer, or committee member of the Cervical Spine Research Society, the North American Spine Society, the Lumbar Spine Research Society, and the Council for Value in Spine Surgery; and has received royalties from DePuy, a Johnson & Johnson company and Stryker. Dr. Wagener or an immediate family member is a member of a speakers' bureau or has made paid presentations on behalf of Synthes, Globus Medical, Lanx, and Opus; serves as a paid consultant to or is an employee of Amgen Co, Lanx, Globus Medical, Synthes, and Opus Medical; serves as an unpaid consultant to Opus Medical; and owns stock or stock options in Amgen Co.

FIGURE 1

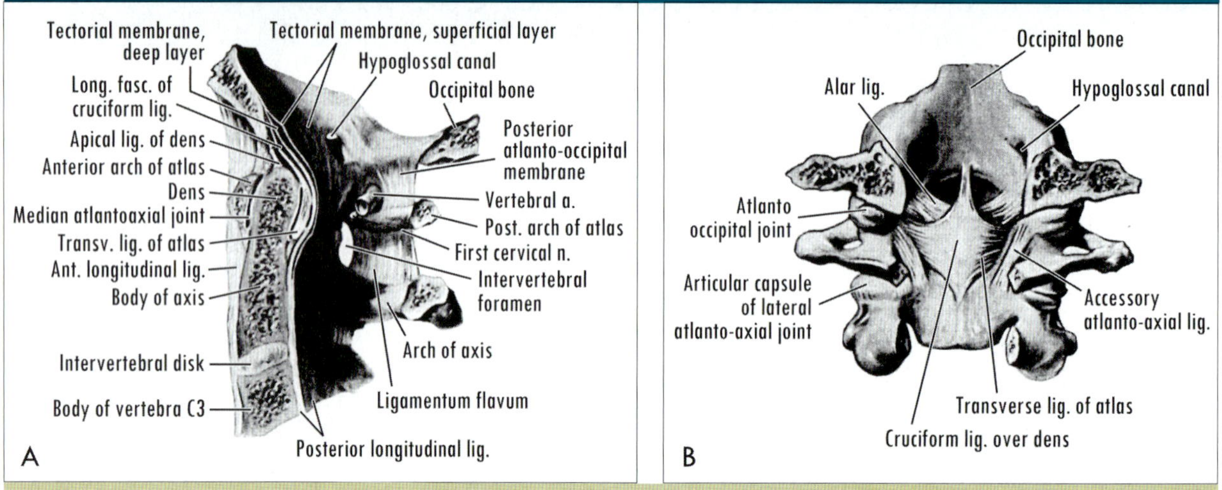

Figure 1 **A,** Upper cervical spine and skull in median longitudinal section. **B,** Upper cervical spine and skull viewed from the posterior aspect after removal of the arches, the tectorial membrane, and posterior longitudinal ligament. (Reproduced with permission from Hollinshead WH: *Anatomy for Surgeons: The Back and Limbs*, ed 3. Philadelphia, PA, Harper & Row, 1982, vol 3.)

FIGURE 2

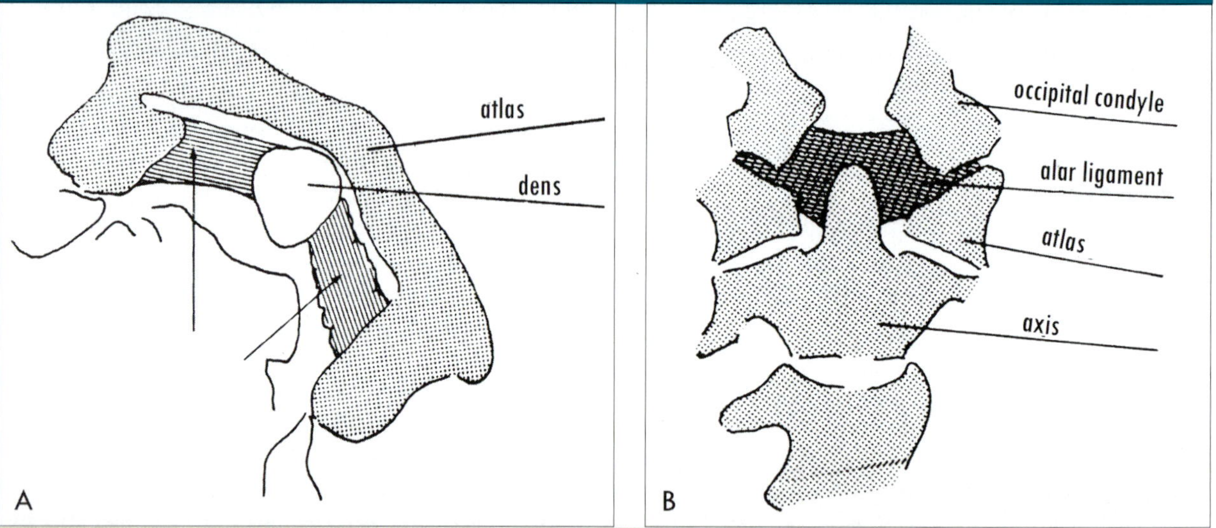

Figure 2 Alar ligaments. **A,** Axial view with rotation of head to the left. **B,** Coronal view. (Reproduced with permission from Dvorak J, Panjabi MM: Functional anatomy of the alar ligaments. *Spine (Phila Pa 1976)* 1987;12(2):183-189.)

diameter. Thus, there is approximately 1 cm of "free space." This concept has become known as Steel's "rule of thirds," and it suggests that anterior displacement of the atlas on the axis exceeding 1 cm can damage the cord.[17,18] The canal can also be narrowed by rotation. The dens is the pivot point for C1-C2 rotation. It is located centrally in the coronal plane, but it is eccentrically placed in the sagittal plane. During rotation, the ring of C1 swings across the vertebral foramen of C2, narrowing the spinal canal.[8,9] Coutts[9] noted that an average-sized canal will be narrowed to 7 mm when C1 is rotated on C2 to the point of complete dislocation (65°). He also recognized that when the transverse ligament is incompetent, allowing anterior shift of the atlas, less rotation is required to lead to significant canal compromise. Fielding and Reddy[19] estimated that the combination of 7 mm of anterior atlantal shift and 50° of rotation would lead to fatal cord compression.

Normally, the space between the odontoid and the anterior ring of C1 is small. This distance,

FIGURE 3

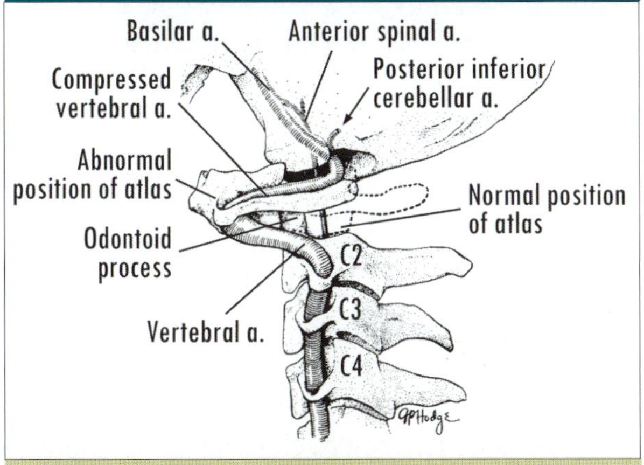

Figure 3 Lateral view of occipitocervical complex demonstrates compression of vertebral artery by atlantoaxial dislocation. The artery may be compressed at the C1 intervertebral foramen or the point at which the occipital condyle slides over the groove in the C1 lamina. (Reproduced with permission from Schneider RC, Crosby EC: Vascular insufficiency of brain stem and spinal cord in spinal trauma. *Neurology* 1959;9:643-656.)

FIGURE 4

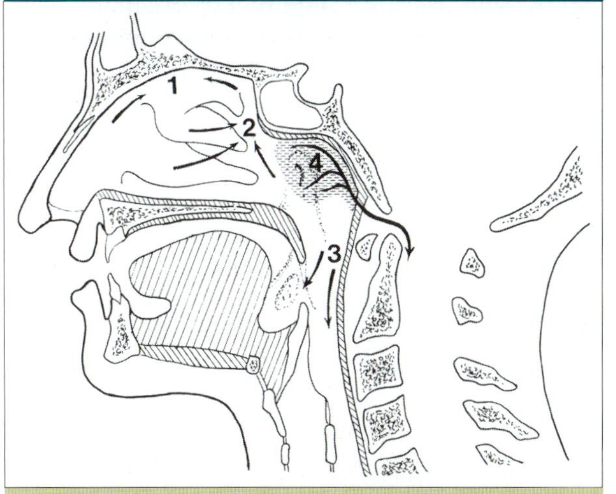

Figure 4 Venous drainage of the nasal cavity, nasopharynx, and oral pharynx. Drainage from the upper lateral wall of the nasal cavity goes into the orbital veins through the anterior and posterior ethmoidal veins (1), whereas drainage from the lower lateral nasal wall and the nasal septum goes to the pterygoid plexus, deep in the face, through tributaries of the sphenopalatine veins (2). The oropharynx drains into tonsilar tributaries of the maxillary veins and the posterior pharyngeal plexus (3). The posterior nasopharyngeal region (cross-hatched area [4]) drains by way of the pharyngovertebral veins through the pharyngobasilar fascia and anterior atlantooccipital membrane to communicate with periodontoidal plexus and epidural veins. (Reproduced with permission from Parke WW, Rothman RH, Brown MD: The pharyngovertebral veins: An anatomical rationale for Grisel's syndrome. *J Bone Joint Surg Am* 1984;66(4):568-574.)

called the atlantodental interval (ADI), measures up to 3 mm in adults[17,20] and 4 mm[17,21] or 4.5 mm[22] in children. Locke et al[21] described a normal, asymptomatic child with an ADI of 5 mm.

The vertebral arteries assume a tortuous course between the atlas and axis but are tethered in the foramina transversaria of each vertebra. Normal rotation does not impair the circulation in these vessels, but excessive atlantoaxial displacement, especially anteriorly, may compromise blood flow. Fielding[6,8] and Schneider and Crosby[23] speculated that such vascular compromise could lead to brainstem or cerebellar infarction and death (**Figure 3**). The combination of anterior displacement and excessive rotation can cause neurologic changes secondary to direct compression and vascular compromise.[6]

A direct connection between the lymphatic drainage of the pharynx and the upper cervical spine was described in the 1930s,[4,9] but the anatomic details of the connections were not understood. Parke et al[24] performed injection studies of the valveless epidural sinuses of human perinatal cadavers. They demonstrated retrograde filling of a series of veins that had numerous lymphatic anastomoses and appeared to drain the posterosuperior pharyngeal region. They called these the pharyngovertebral veins (**Figure 4; area 4 of diagram**).

Biomechanics

The primary restraint to anterior atlantoaxial subluxation is the transverse ligament. In a biomechanical study, Fielding et al[20] demonstrated that the ADI never exceeded 3 mm in adults before rupture of the transverse ligament. After rupture of the transverse ligament, the ADI measured 3 to 5 mm. They found that the alar ligaments are secondary restraints to forward displacement of the atlas, and when the ADI measured 10 to 12 mm, all restraints, including the alar ligaments, were ruptured. The tensile strength of the transverse ligament is greater than that of the alar ligaments.[15,20] Fielding et al[20] found that if the transverse ligament is ruptured, the alar ligaments are inadequate to prevent further significant displacement when a force similar to that which caused transverse ligament rupture is applied.

The primary function of the alar ligaments is to prevent excessive rotation (**Figure 2**). The secondary restraints to rotation include the tectorial membrane, the accessory atlantoaxial ligaments, and the joint capsules (**Figure 1**).[14] Each alar ligament primarily limits rotation to the opposite side, but the ligaments do not work independently. Transection of either ligament results in a significant increase in rotation to both sides.[25] To allow a wide range of rotation, the alar ligaments must be lax in neutral rotation.[11,17,26,27] The laxity of the alar ligaments necessary for rotation is taken up when the occiput and atlas move anteriorly relative to the odontoid a distance equal to the transverse diameter of the dens. The alar ligaments, therefore, cannot function as secondary restraints to further anterior C1-C2 translation until all of the "free space" of the spinal canal at C1 has been occupied by the dens.[17] Coutts[9] found that the alar ligaments become taut and limit rotation beyond 45°. If the head is tilted laterally, however, the distance between the occipital condyle and the dens is diminished and the alar ligament is relaxed, and rotation can continue up to 65°.[9,28]

Goel et al[11] showed that very small loads are required to produce large degrees of rotation at C0-C2; this finding suggests that the neck muscles are the primary stabilizers in the physiologic range of motion. Axial torque increases after the first 20° of rotation until the point of maximal resistance, which corresponds to complete rotatory dislocation of C1-C2. Up until the point of dislocation, Goel et al[11] found that both capsular ligaments and the alar ligament on the side opposite the rotation were only mildly stretched and spontaneous reduction occurred after release of the rotational load. If the specimens were loaded well beyond that point, alar ligament avulsion and C1-C2 capsular ligament rupture occurred and spontaneous reduction did not occur. The transverse ligament and C0-C1 capsular ligaments did not rupture even with maximal rotational loading.

Lateral flexion of the head is coupled with rotation of C2 such that the spinous process of C2 is deviated to the side opposite the direction of head tilt. This conjoined motion occurs as a result of the coronally oblique contour of the articular processes between C2 and C3. During lateral flexion, the inferior facet on the concave side glides downward and backward, whereas the facet on the convex side slides upward and forward, producing rotation as well as tilt.[8] Werne[26] found that when the head is tilted to one side, the opposite alar ligament becomes taut. With further attempts at lateral bending, the dens rotates and thereby tightens the other alar ligament. Motion is inhibited only after both alar ligaments are tight. These findings were confirmed by Panjabi et al,[27] who also demonstrated that the alar ligaments limit flexion at both the C0-C1 joints and the C1-C2 joints. The alar ligaments are most taut and therefore most at risk of rupture when the head is rotated and flexed.[15]

The capsular ligaments have a secondary role in preventing excessive atlantoaxial rotation and lateral tilt. Disruption of the capsular ligaments alone should not lead to rotational dislocation.[16]

Classification

A spectrum of disorders can be considered AARD. They may be classified anatomically by the degree of rotation or subluxation, clinically by the duration of disease or response to treatment, by the degree of kinematic impedance,[29] or by the cause of the condition.

Corner[2] suggested an anatomic classification of rotatory deformities. The term atlantoaxial dislocation should be reserved for the infrequent occurrence of complete dislocation of the C1-C2 facet joints.[2,30-33] The more common situation involves a temporary or permanent rotational deformity of the C1-C2 joints within their physiologic range of motion. Fielding and Hawkins[6] recommended that the term atlantoaxial rotatory displacement be used to describe the condition, rather than terms such as atlantoaxial rotatory subluxation, dislocation, or instability. The joints are not truly subluxed or dislocated, and unless there is concomitant transverse ligament laxity, there is no instability.

In 1931, Berkheiser and Seidler[4] provided the first anatomic classification scheme for "nontraumatic dislocations" that developed after upper respiratory tract infections. They described three deformity patterns: anterior unilateral, anterior bilateral, and posterior unilateral. They noted that the odontoid serves as the axis of rotation, with symmetric subluxation of both atlantoaxial facet joints. When the atlantal facet of the intact joint, which is rotating posteriorly, reaches its full excursion, it serves as the pivot point for further anterior subluxation of the opposite side.

Fielding and Hawkins[6] expanded on this concept and recognized the importance of transverse ligament integrity. Based on their series of 17 patients, they described four types of deformities (**Figure 5**). Type I was the most common pattern, occurring in eight of their cases. The transverse ligament was intact, and the fixed C1-C2 rotation was symmetric and within the normal range of rotation for the C1-C2 joints. As described by Berkheiser and Seidler,[4] the dens had acted as the

FIGURE 5

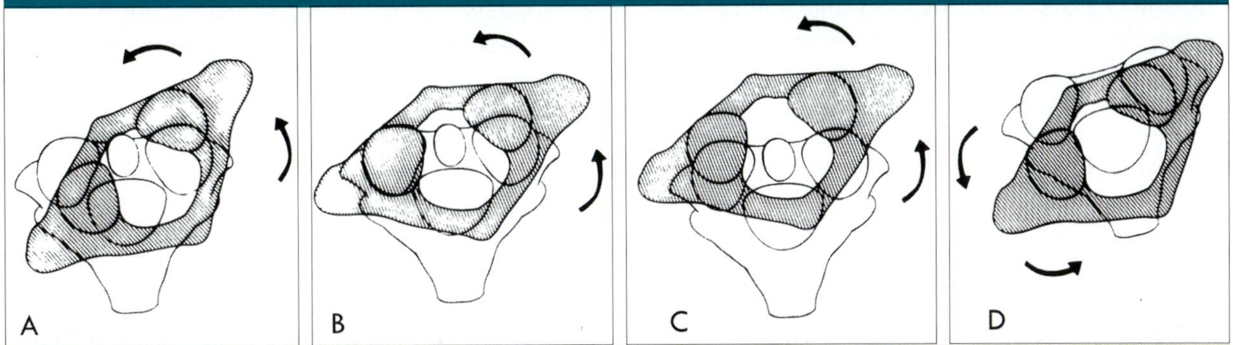

Figure 5 Four types of rotatory fixation: **A,** type I: rotatory fixation with no anterior displacement and the odontoid acting as the pivot; **B,** type II: rotatory fixation with anterior displacement of 3 to 5 mm, one lateral articular process acting as the pivot; **C,** type III: rotatory fixation with anterior displacement of more than 5 mm; and **D,** type IV: rotatory fixation with posterior displacement. (Reproduced with permission from Fielding JW, Hawkins RJ: Atlanto-axial rotatory fixation. (Fixed rotatory subluxation of the atlanto-axial joint.) *J Bone Joint Surg Am* 1977;59(1):37-44.)

axis of rotation in those cases. Type II deformities occurred in five patients and were identified by mild deficiency of the transverse ligament with an ADI of 3 mm to 5 mm. In these cases, the intact joint acted as the pivot point for anterior unilateral displacement of the opposite side. The amount of fixed rotation exceeded the normal excursion of the C1-C2 complex. The distinction between type I and type II deformities may not always represent deficiency of the transverse ligament in the pediatric age group because the ADI may be as great as 4 mm[17,21] or 4.5 mm[22] in normal children. Three patients in the Fielding and Hawkins series had a type III deformity, in which the ADI was more than 5 mm, a finding suggesting deficiency of the transverse ligament and the secondary ligamentous stabilizers.[6,20] Both lateral masses were displaced anteriorly, and one side was rotated further forward than the other. The type IV lesion was described as a posterior shift of one or both lateral masses of the atlas.

Posterior dislocation of C1 relative to C2 without odontoid fracture or C1 anterior arch deficiency is a rare phenomenon but has been reported in the literature (**Figure 6**).[34-37] Berkheiser and Seidler[4] had described a unilateral posterior deformity but stated that "a bilateral posterior dislocation is impossible because of the approximation of the odontoid process to the posterior surface of the anterior arch of the atlas." In the one case reported by Fielding and Hawkins,[6] the patient was a 68-year-old woman whose dens was absent from inflammatory erosion caused by rheumatoid arthritis.

FIGURE 6

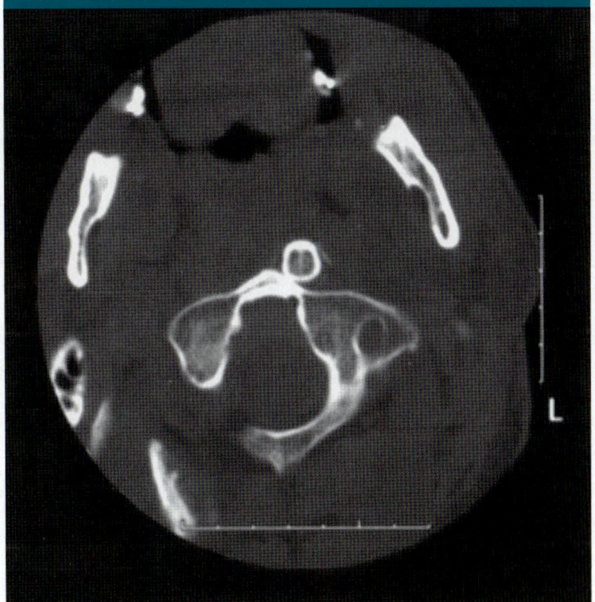

Figure 6 Axial CT showing posterior dislocation of the atlas without fracture of its anterior arch or odontoid. The patient was successfully treated with closed reduction and halo immobilization. He was neurologically intact. (Reproduced with permission from Neumann U, Urbanski H, Riedel K: Posterior atlantoaxial dislocation without fracture of the odontoid: A case report. *J Bone Joint Surg Am* 2003; 85(7):1343-1346.)

Rotatory deformities may be classified on the basis of the clinical course of the disease. Fielding and Hawkins[6] introduced the term atlantoaxial rotatory fixation to describe the condition in which the deformity is fixed and refractory to nonsurgical management. Patients with fixation may have C1-C2 facet joints that are dislocated or held within the normal range of motion and may or may not have laxity of the transverse ligament. Rotatory fixation may follow an infection or trauma or have other causes. Fielding and Hawkins[6] stated that "the importance of recognizing atlanto-axial rotatory fixation lies in the fact that it may indicate a compromised atlanto-axial complex with the potential to cause neural damage or even death."

Pang and Li,[29] in the only prospective study of the clinical manifestation, diagnosis, management and outcome of children with atlantoaxial rotatory fixation, classified patients quantitatively based on motion impedance assessed by abnormal C1-C2 rotational dynamics on CT. The severity of the pathologic condition can be assessed objectively using a dynamic motion curve, as it may relate to damage within the articulating surfaces themselves. Delay in treatment strongly correlated with severity (ie, "stickiness" or limited motion) because it likely relates to damage within the articulating facets.[29]

The importance of the classification schemes lies in the increasing risk of spinal instability with potential neurologic compromise and the higher likelihood of recurrent deformity with the more severe types. In the Fielding and Hawkins series,[6] a type III fixation caused the only fatality, and the patient with a type IV lesion had a neurologic deficit. Phillips and Hensinger[38] reported on a series of children with AARD. Eight of their patients had a type I deformity, and 14 had a type II lesion. None of the patients had either type III or type IV patterns. All five of the children who had a recurrence of their deformity had a type II subluxation. A minority of patients in the series described above[6,38] were involved in major trauma; most developed AARD following minor trauma or an upper respiratory infection, or it occurred spontaneously. When the deformity occurs following major trauma, the condition is potentially more unstable, associated fractures may occur, and the treatment and prognosis are different.[9,30-32,39,40]

Etiology

The cause of AARD is generally either an infection or a traumatic event, but the condition may also arise spontaneously or in association with other conditions such as rheumatoid disease. Isolated case reports have documented rotatory deformities caused by ankylosing spondylitis,[41] metastatic tumor,[42] generalized ligamentous laxity,[43,44] eosinophilic granuloma,[44] and by deformities following a suboccipital craniotomy and C1-C3 laminectomy[45] and various other nondestabilizing procedures about the head and neck.[46,47] AARD should be differentiated from the congenital variant by the associated anatomic abnormalities, irreducible nature, and time/age of diagnosis.

The cause in the case described by Bell[1] was a severe local infection. Many other physicians reported cases of AARD after infectious processes in the 100 years between Bell's report and Grisel's article in 1930.[48,49] Desfosses[3] published a case report in the same year and called the condition "maladie de Grisel"; the eponym "Grisel's syndrome" has been in common usage since then. Jones[5] noted that the infection did not need to be in the nasopharyngeal region, as suggested by Grisel. This fact has been confirmed by many authors who have described cases resulting from a wide variety of conditions, including upper respiratory infection, sinusitis, tonsillitis, otitis media, parotiditis, mastoiditis, acute rheumatic fever, and many others.[4,44,46,47,49-52]

The first reported case of traumatic atlantoaxial rotatory dislocation was described by Buisson in 1852. A 16-year-old boy sustained a fatal neck injury when a cart fell on him. The autopsy revealed a complete anterior dislocation of the right atlantoaxial joint, which narrowed the spinal canal by 50%.[2] In 1907, Corner[2] brought attention to Buisson's case and described 17 others previously reported in the literature; he added 2 cases of his own. Some of the cases were diagnosed clinically without the benefit of radiographs because radiography was not introduced until 1896, but eight of the cases were confirmed to be dislocations by autopsy. Corner noted that an injury of less severity could cause a rotatory subluxation, which would be distinguished from a dislocation only in the "quantity of its symptoms, not in their quality." He correctly surmised that subluxation ("displacement") would prove to be more common than dislocation.

Pathophysiology

The pathophysiology of AARD is not well defined; there is a paucity of pathologic information because the vast majority of patients survive the condition. Rotatory deformities have been documented in all age groups, from infancy to the seventh decade of life. There is a clear predilection for children and young adults regardless of cause.[6,38,46] In Corner's review of the literature,[2] traumatic C1-C2 rotatory dislocation was more common in adults than children, but he included many cases with associated upper cervical fractures. Isolated rotatory dislocation is an unusual injury in children and is very rare in adults.[2,30-33] Atlantoaxial rotatory displacement resulting from minor trauma is also much more common in children.[6,38] There must be strong radiographic evidence and appropriate history to confirm the traumatic etiology of the diagnosis.

In two large reviews of the literature from the 1940s, more than three-fourths of the patients with Grisel's syndrome were younger than 13 years of age.[46,52] In 1969, Keuter[53] noted that the incidence of the condition in adults was increasing relative to that in children. Between 1981 and 1989, 11 patients with Grisel's syndrome were described in the North American literature; their average age was 17.5 years.[51] The widespread use of antibiotics for childhood infections may be responsible for the shift in age distribution.[51] The disease still primarily affects individuals younger than 30 years of age, in contrast to vertebral osteomyelitis, which is much more common in elderly persons.[54]

Parke et al[24] noted that the age distribution may be partly explained by the fact that the peripharyngeal lymphoid tissue is hypertrophic in childhood. The adenoids are especially prone to inflammation in children and are located in the area drained by the pharyngovertebral venous plexus (**Figure 4**). This venous system provides an anatomic rationale for Grisel's syndrome because it allows a hematogenous route for peripharyngeal septic exudates to enter the periodontoidal venous plexus and suboccipital epidural sinuses. Parke et al suggested that surgical trauma may enhance the transport of inflammatory products into the pharyngeal vertebral plexus; this possibility would explain the cases of Grisel's syndrome that occur after procedures such as tonsillectomy, adenoidectomy, or mastoidectomy. Positioning of the patient for these procedures may also be a factor.[46,47,55,56] Because upper respiratory tract infections are so much more common than Grisel's syndrome, Parke et al[24] theorized that affected children must have an anatomic predisposition to instability.

The upper cervical spine joints are much more mobile in children than adults, and this trait is manifested by a greater ADI[17,21,22] and subaxial pseudosubluxation.[57] Kawabe et al[58] found that the facets of the axis in children are more steeply inclined in the coronal plane and are more curved in the sagittal plane than those of adults. Children with the greatest mobility would presumably be at higher risk for rotatory deformities.

There are many theories concerning the pathologic changes that occur as a result of periodontoidal inflammation and lead to the development and fixation of rotatory deformities. Wittek[59] suggested that an effusion develops in the C1-C2 joints that stretches the facet capsules, and this stretching leads to excessive laxity. Coutts[9] implicated infolded inflammatory synovial fringes as the mechanism preventing reduction of the displaced joints. Grisel[48] believed that muscle spasm was primarily responsible for the displacement. Jones[5] theorized that decalcification of the bone adjacent to the ligamentous attachments occurs secondary to inflammatory hyperemia and leads to ligamentous laxity. He claimed that the infection need not be in the nasopharyngeal region, as suggested by Grisel, and that any infection leading to hyperemia of the base of the skull could lead to the disorder. Hess et al[55] suggested that reduction in the early stages of the disease is prevented by a combination of factors, including muscle spasms. Fielding and Hawkins[6] concluded that a combination of swollen capsular and synovial tissues and muscle spasm is responsible for blocking reduction in the early stages. If the deformity is not reduced, ligament and capsular contractures can occur, leading to atlantoaxial rotatory fixation. Wortzman and Dewar[60] proved that muscle spasm alone is not the mechanism that prevents reduction of rotatory displacement. They described four patients who underwent infiltration of local anesthetic into the C1-C2 joints. The patients experienced pain relief with reduced muscle spasm and thus improvement in range of motion, but radiographs showed persistent C1-C2 rotatory deformity.

Kawabe et al[58] provided more information on the synovial fringes described by Coutts.[9] They identified meniscus-like synovial folds at the occipitoatlantal and lateral atlantoaxial joints in infant cadavers but not in adults (**Figure 7**). Inflammation, infolding, or rupture of the folds into the joints was cited as the explanation for rotatory fixation. Atrophy of the synovial folds with advancing age may be another explanation for the age distribution of AARD.

Infolding of the synovial folds into the C1-C2 joints in association with muscle spasm and subsequent ligamentous contracture could also be the mechanism for persistent displacement in cases of traumatic AARD. Wortzman and Dewar[60] thought that tearing and invagination of the capsular ligaments of the atlantoaxial joints were the mechanism in traumatic cases of C1-C2 rotatory deformity. Traumatic articular cartilage damage or facet fracture may also block reduction of the joints.[6] Locking of the facet joints may explain the fixation in cases of complete dislocation.[2,30-33] Rotatory hypermobility or instability may occur after trauma

FIGURE 7

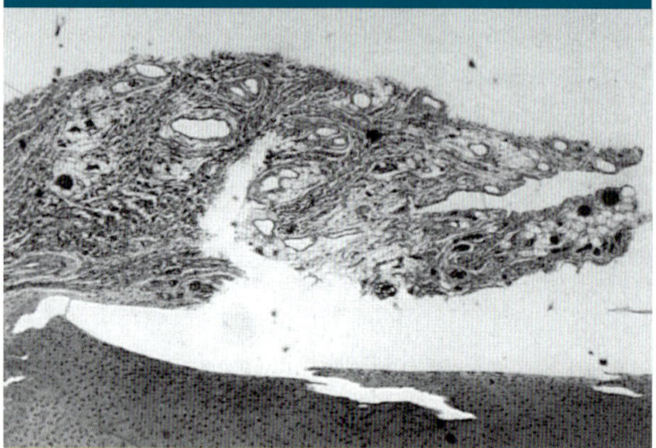

Figure 7 High-power view of a meniscus-like synovial fold found attached to the capsule of the lateral atlantoaxial joint in a 2-year-old girl. Note the rich blood supply. (Reproduced with permission from Kawabe N, Hirotani H, Tanaka O: Pathomechanism of atlantoaxial rotatory fixation in children. *J Pediatr Orthop* 1989;9(5):569-574.)

from irreversible stretching or rupture of the alar ligaments.[7] Morphologic changes within the joint itself may be an indication of the duration of the dislocation.

In long-standing cases of atlantoaxial rotatory fixation, the C0-C1 articulation may become hypermobile and rotate in the opposite direction from the C1-C2 deformity; this change would allow for clinical improvement of the torticollis. Ono et al[33] believed that children younger than 10 years of age have excessive C0-C1 hypermobility, which may explain some cases of atlantoaxial rotatory fixation. In these children, attempts at reduction only increase the C0-C1 counterrotation and do not alter the C1-C2 deformity.

Compensatory motion at the C0-C1 articulation secondary to atlantoaxial rotatory fixation may also contribute to delay in diagnosis. While normal physiologic axial rotation in children rarely exceeds ± 3°,[61] chronic fixation longer than 3 months has been associated with motion increases averaging greater than 30°, aiding the child in righting his or her forward visual axis. The subaxial cervical elements may also contribute to this rotational compensation.[29]

Clinical Findings

The typical patient with AARD is a child or young adult who presents with torticollis after minor trauma or an upper respiratory tract infection. The patient's head is rotated away from the anteriorly displaced C1-C2 joint and tilted toward the involved side, "like a bird with his head cocked listening for a worm."[60] He or she may be able to increase the deformity actively but cannot overcome the torticollis beyond the neutral position. Attempts to correct the deformity are painful.[2,4,6,38,48] The sternocleidomastoid on the side opposite the tilt may be in spasm, as if attempting to correct the deformity.[6,38,48] Over time, this may progress to actual contracture. On palpation, the C2 spinous process may be prominent and deviated to the side to which the chin is pointed, as a result of the lateral tilt of the head[2,6,8] or possibly from counterrotation of C2 in an attempt to realign the head.[46,62] This phenomenon is known as Sudeck's sign,[56] although it was described by Corner in 1907,[2] who also pointed out that the prominence of the C2 spinous process is due to flexion and forward displacement of the head. Before the advent of radiography, examination of the pharynx was an important part of the assessment. Corner noted that two prominences in the pharynx can be identified. The transverse process of the anteriorly rotated atlas can be palpated on one side and the lateral mass of the axis may be prominent on the other side if the corresponding lateral mass of the atlas is rotated posteriorly.

Neurologic involvement is fortunately uncommon. Although the condition is uncommon in older patients, they may be predisposed to neurologic compromise. Fielding and Hawkins[6] and Wilson et al[52] each reported only one patient with a neural deficit, and both patients were older than 60 years of age. Occipital neuralgia may occur because the greater occipital nerve runs in close proximity to the C1-C2 facet capsule.[4,6,16]

In long-standing cases of atlantoaxial rotatory fixation, facial flattening may occur. This feature was noted on presentation in 7 of 17 patients in the series of Fielding and Hawkins,[6] 6 of 10 in the Pang and Li[29] series, and 6 of 13 in the series of Crossman et al.[63]

With time, the torticollis may eventually resolve despite the persistence of the C1-C2 rotatory deformity. This phenomenon was first described by Wortzman and Dewar,[60] who noted that the radiologic abnormality returned to normal in only 1 of 23 cases. They thought that the improvement in head position was due to compensation in the lower cervical spine. More recently, the compensatory rotation has been shown to occur primarily at the occipitoatlantal joint.[6,33,64] Adults have less capacity for C0-C1 counterrotation and therefore may have persistent deformity.[33]

Goddard et al[30] described an association of atlantoaxial rotatory fixation with a fractured clavicle. The injuries all occurred from a fall onto the

FIGURE 8

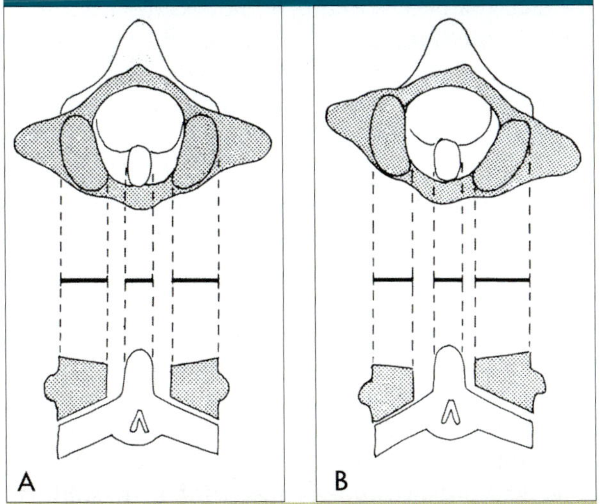

Figure 8 Atlantoaxial joint, demonstrating view seen on CT scan compared with open-mouth odontoid radiograph. **A,** Neutral position. **B,** Rotation to right. With rotation, findings on the open-mouth view include apparent approximation of the left atlantal articular mass to the odontoid, increase in width of the left atlantal articular mass, decreased width of the right atlantal articular mass, and a widened left and narrowed right atlantoaxial joint due to slope of joints in sagittal plane. (Reproduced with permission from Wortzman G, Dewar FP: Rotory fixation of the atlantoaxial joint: Rotational atlantoaxial subluxation. *Radiology* 1968;90(3):479-487.)

FIGURE 9

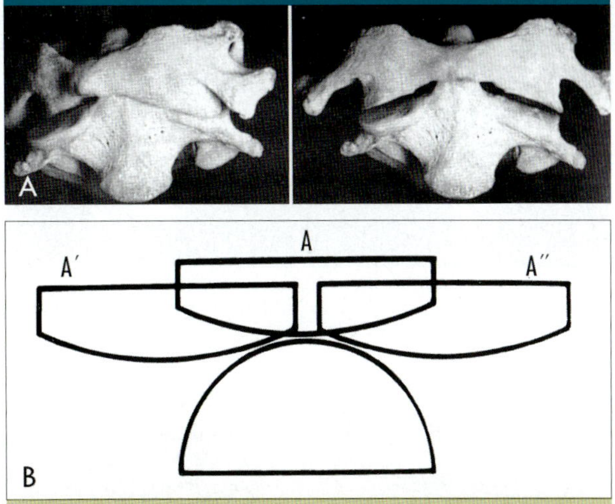

Figure 9 Apparent decrease in atlantoaxial joint space during rotation. **A,** Decreased joint space is shown on left, and neutral position is shown on right. **B,** One atlantoaxial joint as seen from side. The lower figure represents the convex superior facet of the axis, while the upper figure represents the corresponding inferior facet of the atlas. A represents neutral, and A' and A" represent positions of rotation. (Reproduced with permission from Fielding JW: Cineroentgenography of the normal cervical spine. *J Bone Joint Surg Am* 1957;39(6):1280-1288.)

shoulder. Attention may have been directed at the clavicle fracture, leading to delayed recognition and treatment of the cervical deformity with resultant fixation.

Diagnostic Evaluation

Plain Radiography

Plain radiographs are difficult to interpret because of the rotation and tilt of the C0-C1-C2 complex. Just 10 years after the introduction of radiography, Corner[2] noted the typical findings on a lateral radiograph. Because of C1-C2 rotation, "the two lateral masses of the atlas ... are seen laterally *en échelon*, obscuring the odontoid process." The two sides of the posterior arch of C1 are not superimposed on a lateral projection because of the tilt of C1.[4,6] The transverse ligament may be incompetent, leading to a widened ADI. It is difficult to measure the ADI on plain radiographs; lateral tomograms[6] or CT scans[65] are often necessary to assess this critical factor. The ADI normally measures up to 3 mm in adults[17,20] and 4 mm[17,21] or 4.5 mm[22] in children.

On the AP open-mouth projection, the lateral mass of the atlas that is rotated anteriorly appears wider and closer to the midline than its counterpart on the opposite side (**Figure 8**).[6,60] Unfortunately, the odontoid–lateral mass relationship is frequently asymmetric in normal individuals.[66,67] The C1-C2 joint spaces appear asymmetric, often leading to a narrow joint space on one side and a widened space on the opposite side.[4,6,60] Occasionally, the facet joint on one side may be totally obscured from apparent overlapping.[4,6] The change in height of the atlantoaxial facet joints is due to the convex shape of the opposing joint surfaces. In neutral, the convex inferior facet of the atlas sits on the summit of the convex superior facet of the axis. With rotation, the facets articulate at their periphery, causing the atlas to assume a lower position; this leads to apparent narrowing or overlap of the joint (**Figure 9**). The width of each joint space is dependent on whether one or both joints are subluxed. The spinous process of the axis may be rotated away from the side of the anteriorly displaced C1-C2 facet joint (Sudeck's sign).[2,56]

Sullivan[46] noted that unilateral posterior displacement of C1-C2 is also possible, in which case the C2 spinous process is rotated toward the

FIGURE 10

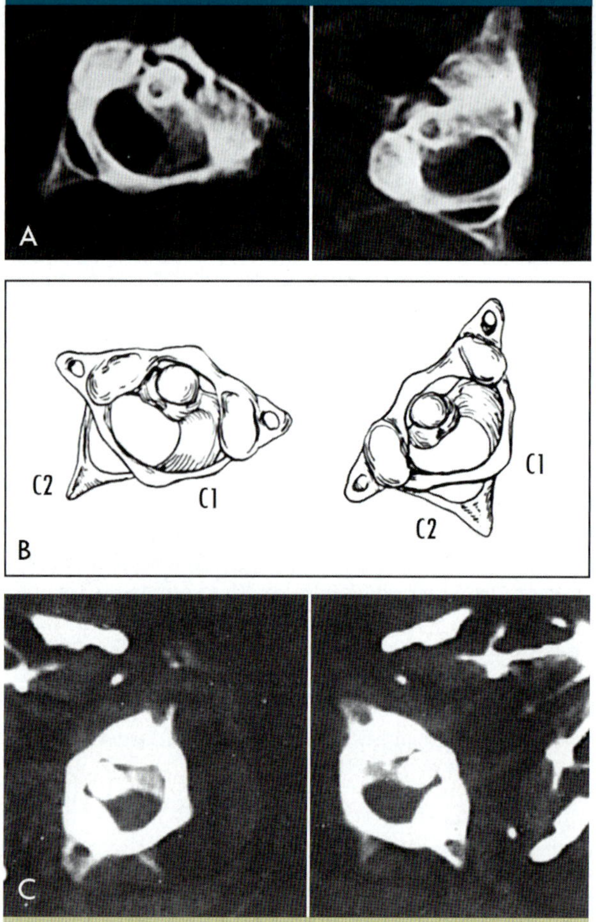

Figure 10 Dynamic CT evaluation of the atlantoaxial joint. **A,** CT scan obtained on maximal head rotation with face turned to the right (upper left). Maximal rotation with face turned to the left (upper right). Note that relative positions of C1 and C2 remain unchanged, a finding demonstrating fixation of rotational deformity. **B,** Diagrammatic representations of the CT scans. **C,** Dynamic CT scans of a normal patient: left, maximal rotation with face turned to the left; right, maximum rotation with face turned to the right. Note that the relative positions of C1 and C2 change with rotation. (Reproduced with permission from Rinaldi I, Mullins WJ Jr, Delaney WF, Fitzer PM, Tornberg DN: Computerized tomographic demonstration of rotational atlanto-axial fixation: Case report. *J Neurosurg* 1979;50(1): 115-119.)

involved side. In contrast, when a normal individual rotates the head, the axis does not rotate until approximately 50% of the normal rotation of the neck has occurred. Beyond that point, C2 will normally rotate in the same direction as the occiput and atlas, placing the C2 spinous process on the side opposite the chin. Ironically, lateral flexion of the head causes more rotation of C2 than pure rotation of the head. Because of coupled motion, the spinous process of the axis is rotated to the side opposite the direction of head tilt and tilted in the same direction.[8] Torticollis from any cause generally involves both rotation and head tilt, and therefore the axis will often be rotated in one direction and tilted in the other.[6]

AP tomograms may demonstrate that the two lateral masses of the atlas are in different planes, and this finding leads to the false impression that one lateral mass is absent.[6]

Wortzman and Dewar[60] recommended obtaining an AP open-mouth view with 10° to 15° of rotation to each side. They claimed that the radiologic criteria for diagnosis of atlantoaxial rotatory displacement is "persistent asymmetry of the odontoid in its relation to the articular masses of the atlas, with this asymmetry not being correctable by rotation." Two studies have demonstrated, however, that normal individuals may have asymmetric dens–C1 lateral mass relationships that do not correct with rotation.[66,67] Because the technique is not always reliable, it should be used only if better studies are not available.

Cineradiography

Cineradiography in the lateral projection has been shown to be one of the best procedures for demonstrating atlantoaxial rotatory fixation.[6,8] The atlas and axis are shown to move as a unit during attempted rotation. Since the advent of CT, this procedure has been performed infrequently.

Computed Tomography

CT may be helpful for differentiating cellulitis from an abscess in cases of Grisel's syndrome.[4] The alar and transverse ligaments can be visualized by CT, and thus it provides some information on the integrity of these structures.[7,68] Plain CT scanning is an excellent means of demonstrating abnormal C1-C2 relationships.[4,7,33,38,65,69] Unless the C1-C2 facet joints are dislocated, however, the rotational deformity seen on a static CT scan may represent simple head rotation in a normal individual because the joints are held within the physiologic range in most cases of AARD. Rinaldi et al[69] were the first to recommend dynamic CT for the diagnosis of atlantoaxial rotatory fixation. Their case report, published in 1979, clearly showed rotational displacement of the atlantoaxial joint that did not change with head rotation to either side (**Figure 10**). Many authors have confirmed that obtaining a CT scan in maximal head rotation to the left and maximal rotation to the right is the best means of demonstrating the condi-

FIGURE 11

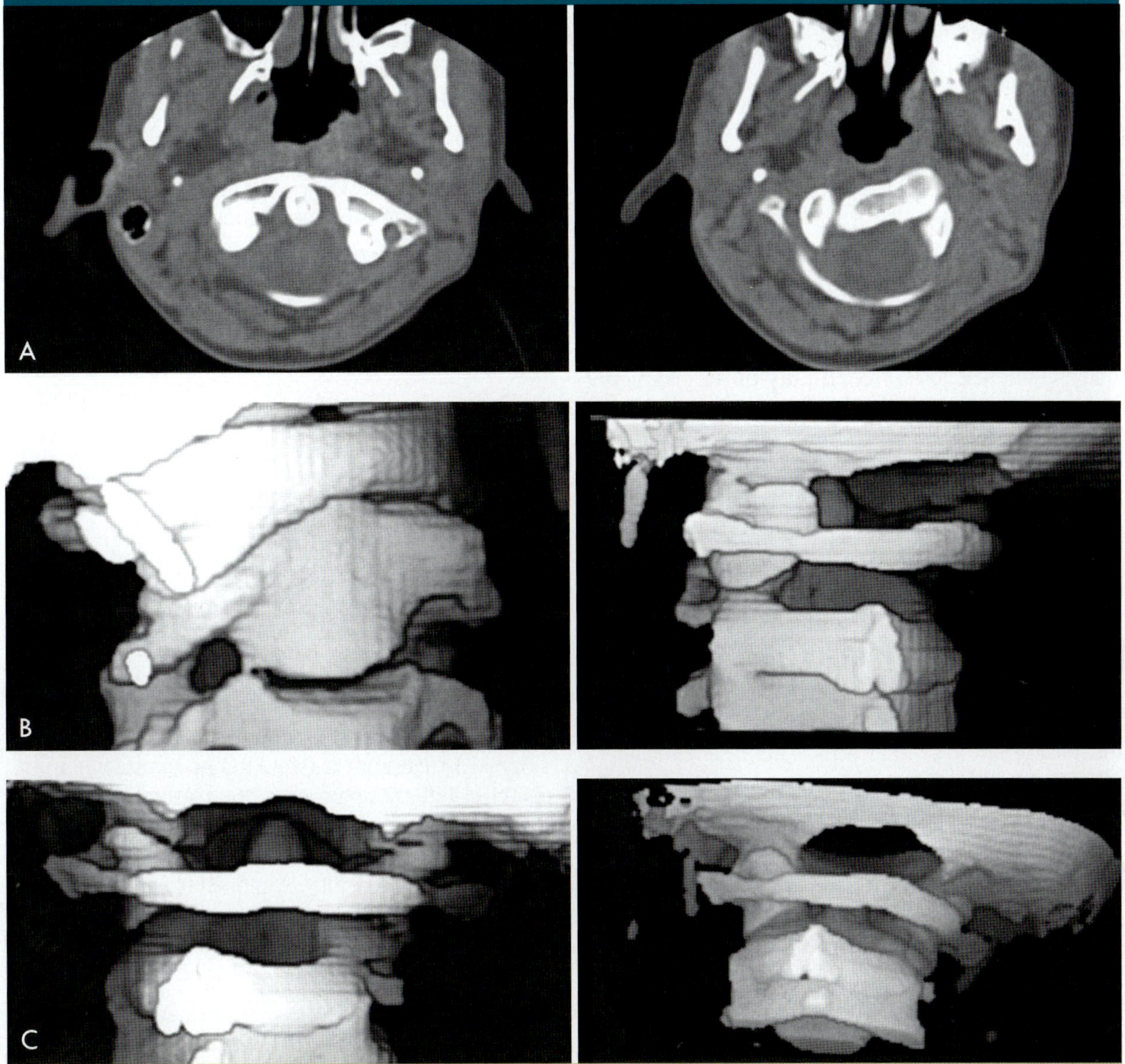

Figure 11 A 9-year-old girl with AARD. Profuse bleeding developed 24 hours after a tonsillectomy, and repeated attempts at intubation were made. Postoperatively, she reported painful torticollis. **A,** Plain CT scans demonstrate posterior displacement of the left atlantoaxial joint and anterior displacement of the right atlantoaxial joint. **B** and **C,** Three-dimensional CT scans demonstrate rotational displacement clearly but do not provide any additional information. (Reproduced from Currier BL: Atlantoaxial rotatory deformities, in Levine AM, Eismont FJ, Garfin SR, Zigler JE, eds: *Spine Trauma.* Philadelphia, PA, WB Saunders, 1998, pp 249-267.)

tion.[7,33,38,64,70] CT may also be used to demonstrate compensatory C0-C1 rotation or the unusual occurrence of simultaneous subluxation of both C0-C1 and C1-C2 joints.[33,64,65] The latter condition can be diagnosed with certainty only if the CT scan is obtained shortly after injury or onset of the condition because compensatory C0-C1 rotation leading to some pseudoreduction is common.[33] Three-dimensional CT scans are capable of demonstrating the static deformity very clearly (**Figure 11**), but the expense of the examination is rarely justified. Three-dimensional CT has the same limitations as two-dimensional static CT in that normal head rotation cannot be differentiated from a fixed deformity. All patients with suspected AARD and no fracture or instability should undergo dynamic CT scan of the cervical spine to rule out fixed rotation between C1 and C2.[29,71]

Magnetic Resonance Imaging

Dickman et al[72] reported success with direct visualization of the transverse ligament with MRI. They evaluated 20 normal subjects and 14 patients with various upper cervical spine problems using gradient-echo MRI pulse sequences. They had pathologic correlation in one case of transverse ligament disruption and one patient with a normal ligament. The authors concluded that the MRI characteristics of a torn transverse ligament are similar to the findings of a torn cruciate ligament in the knee. The normal ligament has a homogeneous low-signal intensity on gradient-echo images, whereas loss of continuity of the ligament with regions of high-signal intensity characterize a tear.[72] Although MRI is useful in evaluation of the anatomic structures of the C0-C1-C2 complex, to date there are limited studies with regard to high-signal changes within these ligaments and their sensitivity and specificity with regard to injury, age, or spinal degeneration.[73]

Differential Diagnosis

A wide variety of conditions can cause torticollis (**Table 1**). A careful history, physical examination, and radiographic evaluation are necessary to differentiate AARDs from other nondystonic (**Table 1**) and dystonic (**Table 2**) causes.[6,38,74-78]

Natural History

The natural history of AARD is poorly documented because most reports and series in the literature describe patients who underwent some form of treatment. Some patients have a benign course with rapid, spontaneous resolution of symptoms.[33,60] Alternatively, some patients continue to have symptomatic torticollis, a condition designated atlantoaxial rotatory fixation by Fielding and Hawkins.[6] In a group of 17 patients they described who had this condition, 2 refused operation and were followed for 8 years; these patients allowed a limited understanding of the natural history of refractory cases. The condition was unchanged in one of the children with persistent torticollis and facial flattening. The other child was asymptomatic, with a functional range of motion and no clinical deformity; however, the radiographic deformity persisted.

Persistent radiographic deformity despite clinical improvement has been described by others.[33,60] Ono et al[33] found that the clinical improvement in such cases resulted from compensatory C0-C1 rotation and documented that the phenomenon is relatively common. They described 13 children younger than 13 years of age with AARD who were treated conservatively. Five of the children had clinical and radiographic reduction, three seemed to have reduction but had persistent C1-C2 rotatory deformity with compensatory C0-C1 rotation, and the remaining five children had some degree of compensatory rotation but still had radiographic and clinical AARD. Ono et al also described one case of atlantoaxial rotatory fixation in an adult who exhibited only 10° of C0-C1 counterrotation, and they suggested that the degree of compensatory rotation possible is an age-related phenomenon.

Treatment

Conservative management is the initial treatment of AARD, although the ultimate regimen is often dictated by the time to diagnosis. The importance of timely diagnosis and initiation of treatment cannot be understated. The goals of treatment are to restore normal pain-free range of motion, prevent or reverse neurologic compromise, and restore spinal stability. The treatment options include symptomatic care, immobilization, traction, manipulation/closed reduction maneuvers, and surgery. In patients with AARD as a result of a nonviral infectious process, the treatment regimen must also include eradication of the infection. Close follow-up of patients is essential because recurrence of deformity,[38] ligamentous laxity,[6] or potentially unstable counterrotation of the occiput[33,64,65] may occur. Most patients will respond to conservative care.

Immobilization and Traction

Most cases of AARD that occur spontaneously following minor injury or an upper respiratory infection can be managed with immobilization and traction. This can be augmented with analgesics and muscle relaxants. Phillips and Hensinger[38] devised a protocol based on the time from the onset of symptoms to presentation. If the deformity has been present for less than 1 week, they advise immobilization in a soft collar and bed rest for 1 week. If the deformity does not reduce, then they advise hospitalization and the institution of traction. If the deformity has been present for more than 1 week but less than 1 month, they advise in-hospital traction followed by immobilization. If the patient presents more than 1 month after the onset of symptoms, they recommend attempting traction for up to 3 weeks; however, if no reduction is achieved, then arthrodesis should

TABLE 1

Nondystonic Causes of Torticollis

I. Congenital	II. Acquired
A. Malformation 1. Malformation of cervical spine a. C1-C2 articular anomalies b. Absence or laxity of transverse ligament c. Klippel-Feil syndrome ± Sprengel's deformity d. Spina bifida e. Other syndromes associated with cervical spine abnormalities 2. Absence or hypertrophy of cervical musculature 3. Malformation of central nervous system a. Arnold-Chiari malformation	A. Cervical musculoskeletal abnormalities 1. Atlantoaxial rotatory dislocation a. Trauma b. Infection Osteomyelitis Nasopharyngeal infection c. Ligamentous laxity d. Erosive e. Spontaneous 2. Atlantoaxial anterior subluxation a. Trauma b. Infection c. Eosinophilic granuloma d. Ligamentous laxity 3. C2-C3 rotatory dislocation a. Trauma b. Infection c. Spontaneous 4. Other bony abnormalities a. Fracture of clavicle or scapula b. Neoplasms of cervical spine Osteoid osteoma 5. Infection a. Nasopharyngeal infection b. Epidemic myalgia c. Osteomyelitis Cervical spine Rib 6. Traumatic soft-tissue injury to neck
B. Deformation (congenital postural torticollis) 1. Uterine abnormality 2. Oligohydramnios 3. Fetal crowding a. Large fetus b. Multiple fetuses	B. Neurologic abnormalities 1. Cervical spine cord lesions a. Syringomyelia b. Spinal cord tumors 2. Intracranial lesions a. Posterior fossa tumors b. Syringobulbia c. Colloid cyst of third ventricle 3. Peripheral nerve lesions a. Tumor of cranial nerve XI
C. Congenital muscular torticollis	C. Miscellaneous 1. Ocular torticollis Diplopia Congenital nystagmus Spasmus nutans 2. Sandifer's syndrome 3. Benign paroxysmal torticollis 4. Vestibular torticollis 5. Neuromuscular disorder 6. Psychological Munchausen's syndrome Hysteria

(Modified with permission from Suchowersky O, Calne DB: Non-dystonic causes of torticollis. *Adv Neurol* 1988;50:501-508.)

TABLE 2

Dystonic Causes of Torticollis

I. Primary (spasmodic torticollis)

II. Secondary
- A. Iatrogenic (neuroleptics, dopamine agonists)
- B. Metabolic defects (Wilson's disease, gangliosidosis)
- C. Degenerative central nervous system diseases (Parkinson's disease, progressive supranuclear palsy, Huntington's disease)
- D. Other central nervous system disorders (arteriovenous malformation, tumor, encephalitis)
- E. Trauma (closed head injury, neck trauma)

(Reproduced from Currier BL: Atlantoaxial rotatory deformities, in Levine AM, Eismont FJ, Garfin SR, Zigler JE, eds: *Spine Trauma.* Philadelphia, PA, WB Saunders, 1998, pp 249-267.)

be considered for symptomatic patients. After reduction, they advise immobilization to allow the stretched and edematous ligaments to heal. Although nontraumatic AARDs are much more common in children, the same principles of treatment used in children apply to adults.[79]

Head-halter traction has been in use since at least 1931[4] and may be effective in early cases. Fielding and Hawkins[6] advised skeletal skull traction in cases of rotatory fixation. The weight used is dependent on the age of the patient. They advised using about 3.5 kg in young children and up to 6.8 kg in adults. The weight may be increased in increments of 0.5 kg to 0.9 kg every 3 to 4 days until correction is achieved, or up to an arbitrary limit of 6.8 kg in children and 9.1 kg in adults.

Wetzel and La Rocca[49] devised a protocol of postreduction immobilization based on the classification scheme of Fielding and Hawkins[6] and on a study of cervical orthoses by Johnson et al.[80] They recommended a cervical collar for type I deformities, a Philadelphia collar or sternal occipitomental immobilizer for type II lesions, and a halo vest for type III lesions. Halos may be applied even in infants if a low-torque, multiple-pin technique is used.[81]

Fielding and Hawkins[6] advised immobilization for 3 months after reduction. Other authors recommend a period of 6 to 8 weeks[49] or until the patient has full pain-free range of motion.[38] After immobilization, flexion and extension radiographs should be obtained to rule out instability.

Weisskopf et al[82] describe their treatment algorithm for fixed AARD to include an initial closed reduction in all patients. Successful reduction is maintained in a halo body jacket for 8 to 12 weeks. Open reduction is performed for failure of closed reduction of the dislocation/subluxation.

Manipulation

The role of manipulation in the management of nontraumatic AARDs is limited. Subach et al[83] described the degenerative changes and joint incongruence found on preoperative CT scans associated with fixed or long-standing dislocations, indicating that manipulation alone would be insufficient in treatment and fusion would be required. Contrary to Fielding and Hawkins,[6] who did not recommend the procedure for fixed deformities "because of the inherent dangers," Weisskopf et al[82] recommended attempts at closed reduction initially for all patients. Phillips and Hensinger[38] noted that the best candidates for manipulation are patients with torticollis of recent onset, but the procedure is riskier than reduction by bed rest or traction. If manipulation is elected, they recommended continuous neurologic monitoring.

Numerous authors have described manipulation in cases of acute traumatic AARD.[2,28,31,32,84,85] Levine and Edwards[85] recommend performing the manipulation with the patient awake using topical anesthetic in the posterior pharynx. Gentle traction is applied through a halo ring and the skull and C1 are derotated. They note that the reduction is often accompanied by an audible pop and can be confirmed by palpation of the ring of C1 through the mouth. The spine may be immobilized in a halo vest if no fractures are present and the reduction is stable.[85] If the lateral mass of C1 reduces but snaps back into a subluxed or dislocated position, the deformity is considered unstable and surgical intervention is required (Alan M. Levine, MD, personal communication, 1995).

Sullivan[46] described a procedure for manipulation under anesthesia of AARD cases caused by inflammatory conditions about the neck. "The neck is hyperextended, its tilt and rotation exaggerated and as traction is applied to the head with countertraction to the shoulders, the head is slowly rotated toward the midline." He gave credit to Walton[86] for devising the method of reduction, although Walton's technique did not involve traction and was described for unilateral facet dislocations in the subaxial spine. Sullivan noted that the method was not always successful and could be dangerous in inexperienced hands or in the presence of a fracture or avulsion of the transverse ligament.

More recently, Jeszenszky et al[87] described a closed transoral method for reducing atlantoaxial subluxation/dislocations. The spinous process of the axis is stabilized with one hand while the index finger of the other hand applies pressure in counterrotation to the dislocation on the lateral mass of the atlas through the posterior wall of the pharynx (**Figure 12**). This maneuver was employed when others failed and was successful in reducing AARD with a delay in treatment up to 4 months.[82]

Fielding and Hawkins[6] described a 65-year-old woman in whom type III AARD developed when she yawned and twisted her neck. She was placed in traction, and after 10 days she turned her head in the direction of the deformity and died suddenly. An autopsy revealed that the cord was crushed from C1 as it displaced forward and rotated across the canal. On the basis of this case, Fielding et al[6,19] cautioned against increasing the deformity because it may increase rotation with further narrowing of the canal.

FIGURE 12

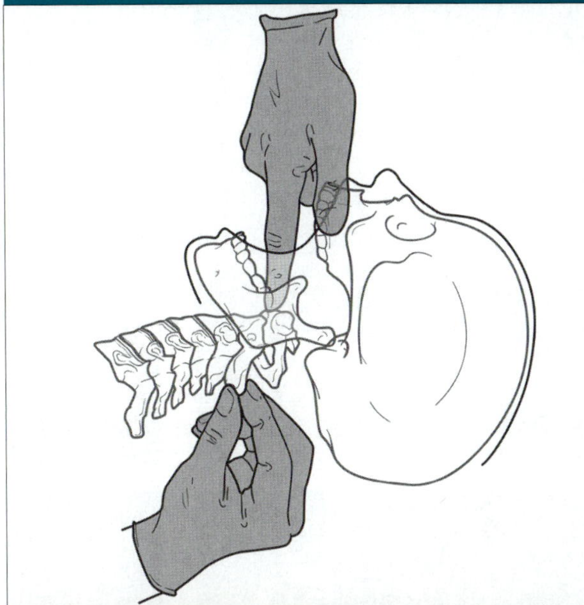

Figure 12 Schematic of transoral closed reduction according to Jeszenszky et al. The spinous process of the axis is locked by one hand while the index finger of the other hand presses in counter rotation to the dislocation on the lateral mass of the atlas through the posterior wall of the pharynx.

Surgical Management

A surgical approach is advised for cases of AARD with spinal instability, for cases with neural involvement, when conservative measures fail to achieve or maintain reduction (**Figure 13**), or when patients are not compliant.[6,39,85] Reducing the deformity and temporarily stabilizing the C1-C2 joints, to preserve motion, has theoretical appeal but it is not commonly performed. For those patients with chronic/irreducible rotatory subluxation, joint incongruity may prevent any hope for near-normal C1-C2 kinematics. In addition, postoperative scarring in any open technique would likely decrease the chances of normal motion. Studies describing such techniques are limited. Crossman et al[63] used an extreme lateral approach to the anterior C1 facet, directly reducing the subluxation, followed by postoperative halo immobilization. The mean axial rotation postoperatively was 102° (range, 85° to 130°) compared to 138° (range, 110° to 160°) in the control group. Although the range of motion was improved compared with the postoperative assessment, it was significantly reduced compared with that of healthy children, indicating that some permanent damage to the articulation had occurred. An alternative approach was described by Weisskopf et al in 2005.[82] After review, for those patients who failed closed reduction of the dislocation/subluxation, open reduction is performed. A modified transoral approach is used followed by temporary fixation of C1-C2 using a Harms T-plate. These implants are removed at 3 months. Definitive fusion using the same device was used for cases with significant degenerative changes or incongruence of the atlantoaxial joint found on either the preoperative CT or identified intraoperatively. In the group of patients temporarily stabilized, 4 of 10 fused spontaneously (**Figure 14**).[82]

Harms and Melcher[88] treated a 25-year-old man with AARD with temporary posterior C1 lateral mass and C2 pars interarticularis polyaxial screws and rods. The instrumentation was removed after several months and the patient had documented restoration of C1-C2 motion on dynamic MRI examinations.[88] Although motion preservation is desirable, no technique of temporary internal fixation has proven to be reliable. Therefore, for most surgeons, when surgery is indicated, a posterior C1-C2 fusion is the procedure of choice. Ultimately, surgeon preference and experience dictate approach. Preoperative traction should be attempted to reduce the deformity. If traction is unsuccessful, however, in situ C1-C2 fusion may be performed.[6,30,38] Three factors should be considered when performing an in situ fusion. First, the passage of wires may be more dangerous because the canal will be narrowed with fixed atlantoaxial ro-

FIGURE 13

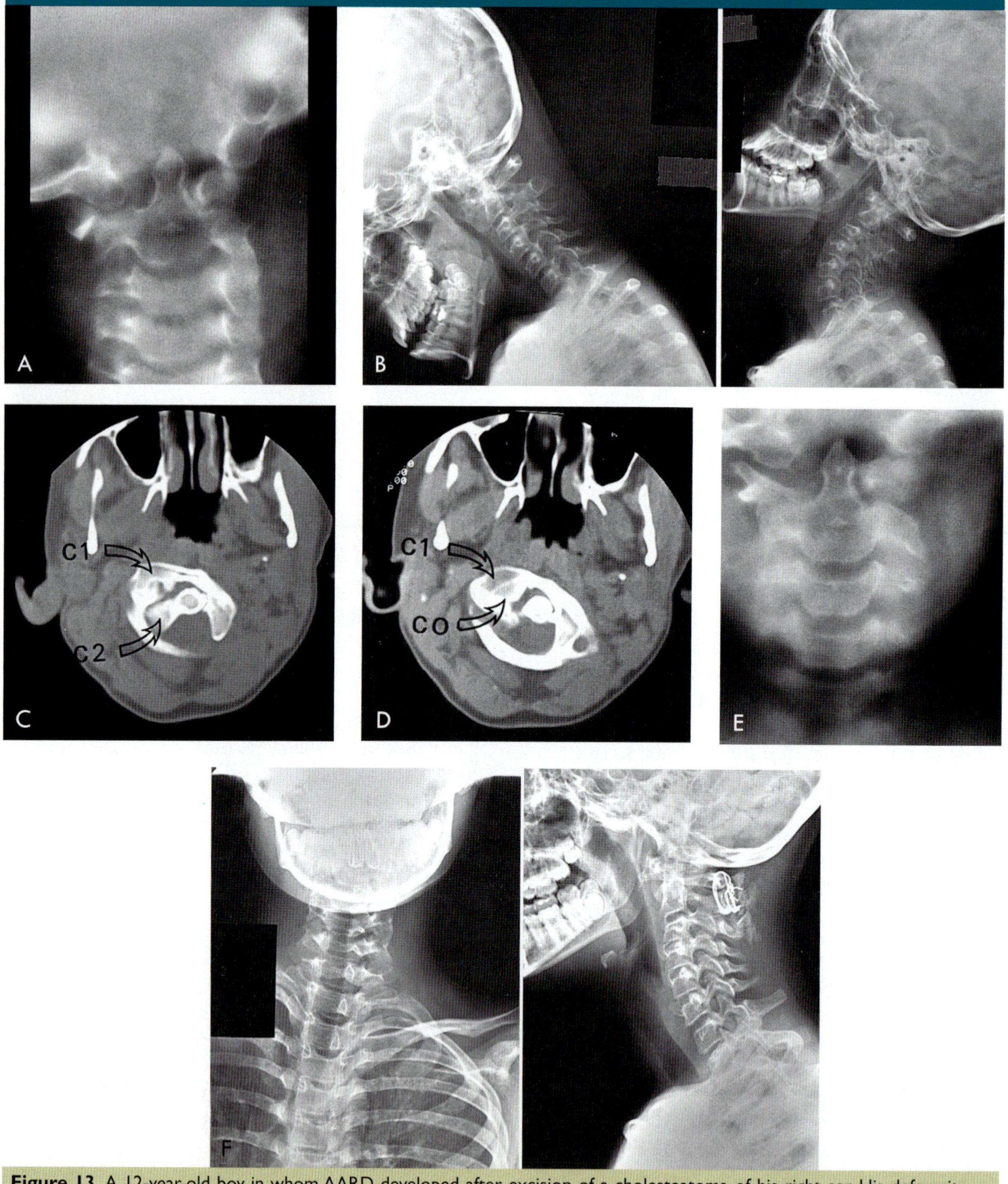

Figure 13 A 12-year-old boy in whom AARD developed after excision of a cholesteatoma of his right ear. His deformity was refractory to traction at home and 1 week of traction in the hospital. He presented 10 months after onset of torticollis. **A,** AP tomogram demonstrates complete dislocation of right atlantoaxial joint. **B,** Lateral flexion (left) and extension (right) radiographs demonstrate AARD with widened ADI. **C,** Static CT scan demonstrates dislocation of right atlantoaxial joint and asymmetric widening of the ADI. **D,** Static CT scan demonstrates subluxation of C0-C1 joints, presumably from compensatory counterrotation of the occiput. **E,** AP tomogram demonstrates partial reduction of C1-C2 joint after institution of skeletal traction. **F,** AP (left) and lateral (right) radiographs obtained 6 weeks after C1-C2 fusion. Fusion extended to C3 spontaneously. The patient had no complaints except neck stiffness and had marked improvement in torticollis. (Reproduced from Currier BL: Atlantoaxial rotatory deformities, in Levine AM, Eismont FJ, Garfin SR, Zigler JE, eds: *Spine Trauma.* Philadelphia, PA, WB Saunders, 1998, pp 249-267.)

FIGURE 14

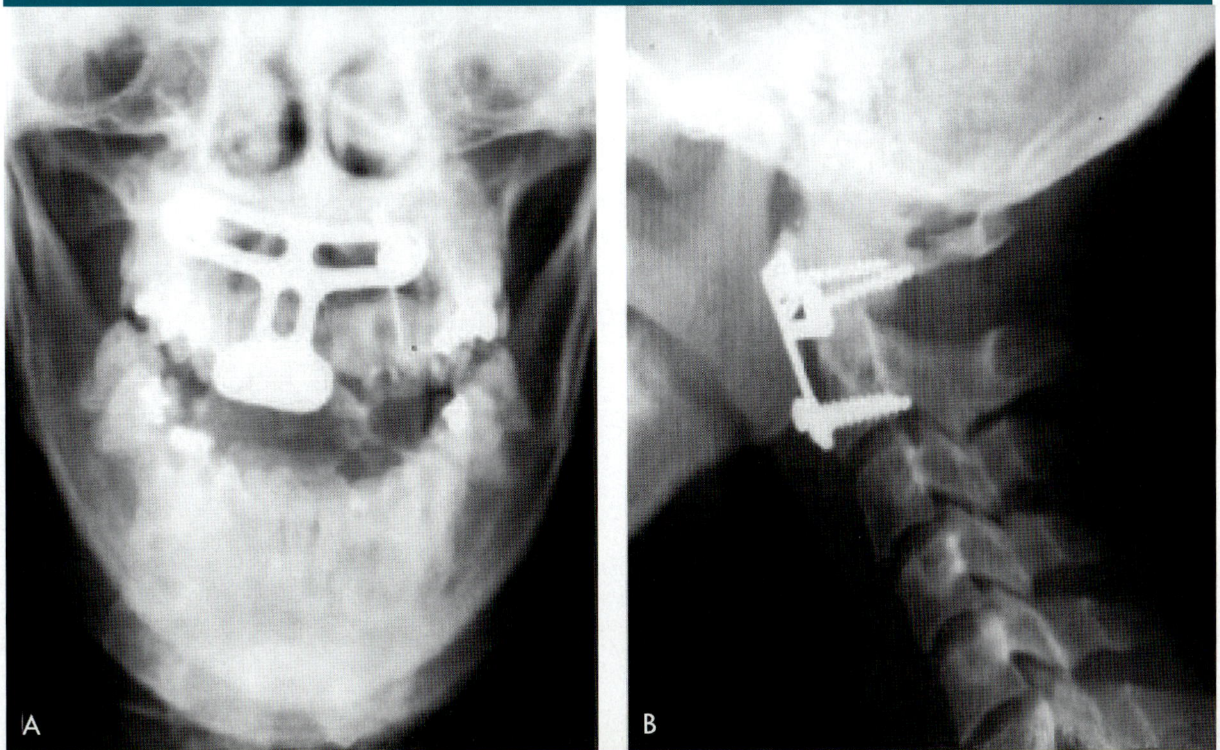

Figure 14 AP (**A**) and lateral (**B**) radiographs of the Harms T-plate used for temporary fixation of fixed AARD. Reduction and plate application is performed through a transoral approach. (Reproduced with permission from Weisskopf M, Naeve D, Ruf M, Harms J, Jeszenszky D: Therapeutic options and results following fixed atlantoaxial rotatory dislocations. *Eur Spine J* 2005;14(1):61-68.)

tation.[2] Second, the final clinical result, although acceptable, may not be as good as fusion after reduction.[30] Third, the improvement in torticollis is a consequence of compensatory C0-C1 rotation.[33] Conceivably, the nonphysiologic position of the C0-C1 joints may place the patient at some increased risk during future traumatic episodes, and the long-term effects of C0-C1 hypermobility are unknown. If a closed reduction is unsuccessful, open reduction is reasonable. A wire passed under the arch of C1 can be used to manually derotate the atlas. After the deformity is reduced, the wire may be used to maintain the alignment by incorporating it into a C1-C2 fusion. If the joint is fractured, an oblique wire is passed from the anteriorly displaced side of the C1 arch to the spinous process of C2.[85]

The type of posterior C1-C2 fusion performed is a matter of surgeon preference. In 1973, McGraw and Rusch[89] described a fusion method that is now commonly referred to as the Gallie technique. It consists of a rectangular corticocancellous iliac crest graft measuring 3 cm by 4 cm secured to the back of the C1 ring and lamina of C2 (with a notch for the C2 spinous process) with a loop of wire passing beneath the ring of C1, under the C2 spinous process, and around the graft (**Figure 15**). They reported excellent results in 14 of 15 patients treated with the technique and only one pseudarthrosis. Although Gallie is cred-

FIGURE 15

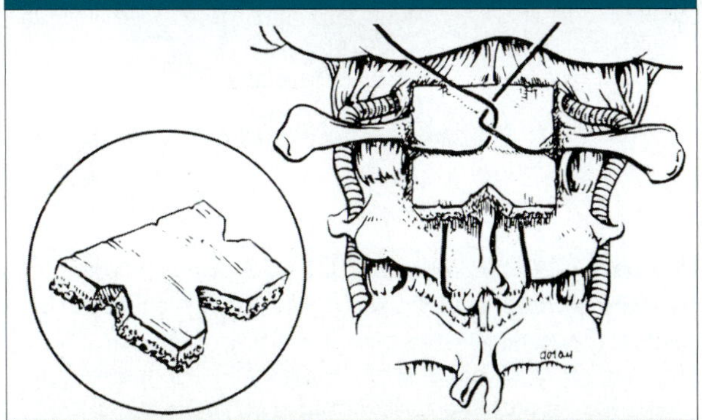

Figure 15 Gallie-type posterior C1-C2 fusion technique. (Reproduced with permission from McGraw RW, Rusch RM: Atlanto-axial arthrodesis. *J Bone Joint Surg Br* 1973; 55(3):482-489.)

FIGURE 16

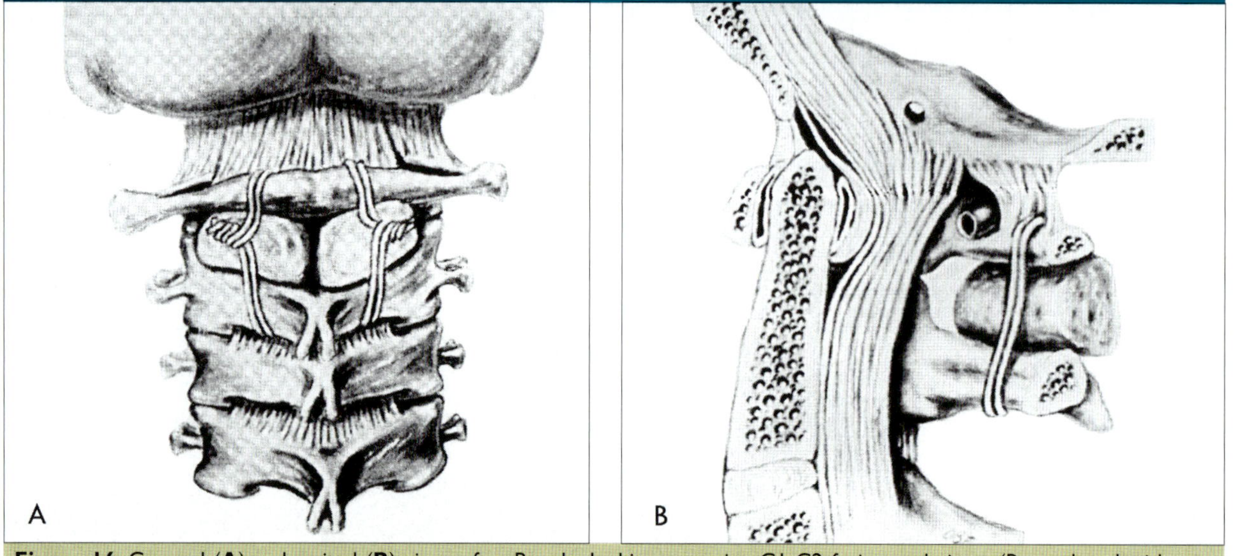

Figure 16 Coronal (**A**) and sagittal (**B**) views after Brooks-Jenkins posterior C1-C2 fusion technique. (Reproduced with permission from Brooks AL, Jenkins EB: Atlanto-axial arthrodesis by the wedge compression method. *J Bone Joint Surg Am* 1978;60(3):279-284.)

FIGURE 17

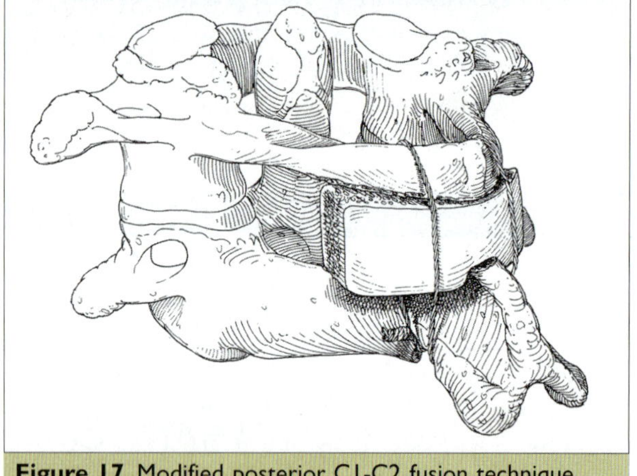

Figure 17 Modified posterior C1-C2 fusion technique combining elements of the Gallie and Brooks-Jenkins techniques. (Reproduced with permission from Dickman CA, Sonntag VK, Papadopoulos SM, Hadley MN: The interspinous method of posterior atlantoaxial arthrodesis. *J Neurosurg* 1991;74(2):190-198.)

ited with the original description of the technique, his frequently quoted 1939 article[90] describes basic principles of management of cervical spine trauma, including skeletal traction and fusion for subaxial dislocations and fracture-dislocations, but it does not mention atlantoaxial arthrodesis.

Brooks and Jenkins[91] described a wedge compression method of C1-C2 fusion in 1978. They recommended the use of two doubled 20-gauge wires passed beneath the arch of C1 and the lamina of C2 to secure two beveled, full-thickness iliac crest grafts in the interlaminar space (**Figure 16**). The reported advantage of the technique was the enhanced biomechanical stability in all planes conferred by the construct. They reported successful union in 12 (92%) of 13 patients treated by their technique.

Griswold et al[92] modified the Brooks-Jenkins technique slightly by securing each of the two grafts with two sublaminar wires. They reported a success rate in 96% by achieving a solid union in 30 patients. This rate was in contrast to the success rate of 60% in 10 patients treated by the Gallie method. Fielding et al[93] reported a success rate of 98% with the Gallie technique, however, suggesting that the difference in fusion rate between the techniques may not be significant. Griswold et al[92] claimed that the immediate added stability achieved with the modified Brooks-Jenkins construct allows the patient to be mobilized postoperatively with minimal external support. Fielding et al[93] placed their patients in postoperative traction for 6 weeks for the treatment of AARD but recognized that a halo cast may be a reasonable device to allow the patient to be ambulatory postoperatively. Dickman et al[94] described a modification of the Gallie technique that has some of the theoretical advantages of the Brooks-Jenkins wedge compression technique but does not require sublaminar wires at C2 (**Figure 17**). They had only 1 nonunion in 36 cases (97% union) treated for var-

FIGURE 18

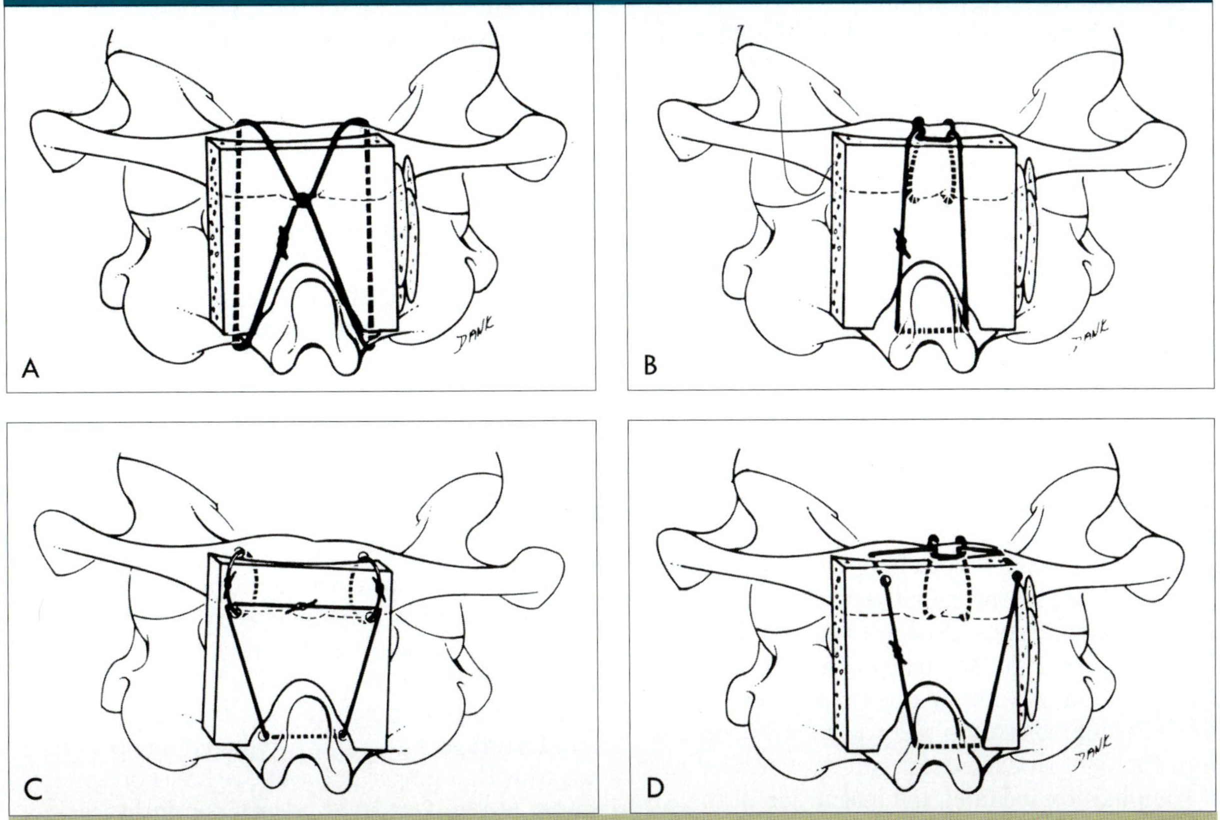

Figure 18 Different Gallie posterior C1-C2 fusion techniques. **A,** Wires passed under the lamina of the atlas and axis and secured over the graft. **B,** Wires passed through drill holes in the lamina of the atlas and through a hole in the base of the spinous process of the axis and through drill holes in the graft. **C,** Wire passed under the lamina of the atlas and through a hole in the spinous process of the axis and secured over the graft. **D,** Wire passed under the lamina of the atlas and through a hole in the spinous process of the axis and through drill holes in graft. (Reproduced with permission from Fielding JW, Hawkins RJ, Ratzan SA: Spine fusion for atlanto-axial instability. *J Bone Joint Surg Am* 1976;58(3):400-407.)

ious diagnoses (3 had transverse ligament tears, and there were no cases of AARD). All of their patients were managed in a halo for 3 months postoperatively.

It is generally understood that one difference between the Gallie and Brooks-Jenkins techniques is that the former involves a wire passing under or through the C2 spinous process, whereas the latter requires the passage of a sublaminar wire at C2. However, in the report by Fielding et al[93] of 46 patients who underwent a Gallie fusion, four different methods of performing the technique were described, one of which involved C2 sublaminar wires (**Figure 18**).

The choice of fusion technique is based on surgeon preference, but whatever method is chosen, the surgeon should follow the same postoperative regimen advised by the proponents to achieve a similar success rate.

If the posterior elements of C1 or C2 are deficient, the fusion may need to be extended to the occiput or to C3, respectively. Alternatively, rigid fixation of the atlas and axis may be used to maintain alignment and achieve a C1-C2 fusion.[88,95-104] These methods allow patients to be mobilized postoperatively without the need for a halo and the screws may also be used to achieve an open reduction. These techniques are now commonly used in C1-C2 fusions and they are discussed in more detail in chapter 24 on transverse ligament insufficiency.[88,95-105]

If reduction does not occur during positioning, the contracted C1-C2 joint may be released through the anterior or extreme lateral approach, followed by supplemental fixation or immobilization to maintain the correction.[63,87] Posterior soft-tissue release and manipulation with C1 lateral mass screws and C2 pedicle screws has also been used effectively to reduce the deformity. Rods or plates secured to the screws maintain the alignment.[88,97] C1-C2 transarticular screws are biomechanically sound, but the joints must be reduced before inserting the screws.

Although Fielding et al,[6,93] Griswold et al,[92] and Brooks and Jenkins[91] reported low complication rates, Smith et al[105] reported a high complication rate in patients who underwent upper cervical fusions for various diagnoses. Complications included loss of initial reduction in 14 of 47 patients, nonunions in 4 of 47, prolonged drainage or wound dehiscence from the iliac crest donor site in 7 of 46, and atelectasis and pneumonia in a patient who had a rib graft harvested. Neurologic problems were the most significant complications and were found to correlate with the preoperative neurologic status. Of 24 patients who were intact preoperatively, 4 had development of occipital neuralgias that resolved by 1 year postoperatively. Of nine patients with transient quadriparesis, eight did well but one had worsening with operation and died 2 weeks postoperatively. Of 13 patients with abnormal results of neurologic examinations preoperatively, 3 initially had worsening with operation, and at late follow-up one patient's condition was still worse than the preoperative condition. Factors that correlated with an increased risk of complication included the magnitude of the preoperative displacement, nonanatomic alignment of C1 on C2 (especially kyphosis), presence of genetically determined ligamentous laxity (Down syndrome or Ehlers-Danlos syndrome), and a history of cervical spine operation. Smith et al advised close scrutiny of the space available for the cord and suggested attempting to increase the space preoperatively through traction if possible. If the alignment of C1-C2 cannot be improved and the space available for the cord remains low, they suggested consideration of C1 decompression and occiput cervical fusion. They further cautioned against passage of sublaminar wires when the space available for the cord is small. The complication rate with current rigid fixation is quite low as long as preoperative planning and meticulous surgical technique are employed.[88,98,99]

Prognosis

The prognosis of patients with AARD is related to the duration of symptoms before institution of treatment, radiographic changes within the C1-C2 articulation, and the degree of laxity of the transverse ligament and the severity of associated fractures. Unfortunately, delay in diagnosis is common and adversely affects outcome.[82,83] In a study by Subach et al,[83] collar immobilization was successful as the only treatment modality in patients with symptoms occurring for 6 days, whereas the duration of symptoms for those patients requiring traction was 42 days. Age, sex, and cause of the subluxation were not found to be contributory. Recurrence of the deformity was also found to be related to the duration of symptoms. There is no large series of patients with AARD resulting from major trauma in the literature from which to base statements on prognosis for that patient subgroup. The study by Pang and Li[29] suggests that the more severe types of atlantoaxial rotatory subluxation were associated with severe trauma; less severe cases were associated with otolaryngologic procedures and nasopharangeal infections. In the series of Phillips and Hensinger[38] concerning "nontraumatic" AARD, 16 children were examined less than 1 month after the onset of symptoms, and all had reduction of the deformity either spontaneously or after a short period of traction. Three of the seven children who were seen more than 1 month after the onset of symptoms eventually required a fusion.

Recurrence of deformity in the series of Phillips and Hensinger[38] was much more common in the group with a longer delay to diagnosis or a more severe lesion. Recurrence developed in five patients with type II deformities (mild laxity of the transverse ligament), whereas none of the children with type I deformity had a recurrence (intact transverse ligament). The recurrences developed within 2 weeks in two children, within 2 months in two, and within 4 months in one. No specific cause for the recurrences was identified. The cause of the initial subluxation was trauma in two patients, upper respiratory tract infection in two, and unknown in one. The children with recurrences were rehospitalized and placed in traction. Reduction was achieved and maintained in three children, but the deformity in the other two could not be reduced and they underwent fusions.

Subach et al[83] reported similar findings in a retrospective review of 20 patients with atlantoaxial subluxation seen over a 7-year period. All patients reportedly had torticollis and neck pain, with decreased cervical motion for a mean of 11 days. The causes of the torticollis included infectious, postoperative, traumatic, and unknown etiologies. Of the 20 patients treated with conservative management, including closed reduction, cervical traction, and rigid immobilization, 6 failed requiring posterior fusion. The major determining factor in success of nonsurgical management was the duration of subluxation before initial reduction.

Neurologic deficits, vertebral artery compromise, and fatalities are fortunately uncommon, but all have been reported with AARD, especially in cases associated with transverse ligament laxity.[2,6]

In a study by Ishii et al,[106] acute and chronic patients with atlantoaxial subluxation were evaluated using three-dimensional CT reconstructions. A deformity in the C2 facet was associated with chronic dislocations (greater than 3 months) and correlated significantly with recurrent dislocations. In addition, greater than 20° of lateral inclination of the C1 facet indicated an irreducible subluxation.

Facial asymmetry has been found in 41% to 60% of patients with atlantoaxial rotatory deformity.[6,29,63] This is felt to be caused by persistent and asymmetric muscle pull on growing structures of the maxillofacial region. This can be troublesome from both a cosmetic and functional standpoint as dental malocclusion can occur.[63] Only one of five patients in the Fielding and Hawkins series who underwent a fusion was left with facial asymmetry.[6] Two patients refused operation and were treated conservatively; 8 years later, one remained unchanged and the other had no clinical deformity or facial asymmetry. Open reduction followed by halo application in the report by Crossman et al[63] resulted in cosmetic improvement in all patients with facial asymmetry.

Because 50% of cervical rotation occurs at the atlantoaxial joint, some loss of rotation occurs after C1-C2 fusion. Fielding et al[93] found that the restricted motion was less than expected and was age-dependent. Patients 20 years or younger lost an average of 13% rotation, those aged 20 to 40 years lost 25%, and those older than 40 years of age lost an average of 28%. Compensatory hypermobility of the C0-C1 articulation may be responsible for the minimal loss of motion after C1-C2 fusion. Persistent radiographic C1-C2 rotatory deformity occurs in a significant number of patients and is often associated with compensatory counterrotation of C0-C1.[33] The consequence of this laxity as it relates to a potential threat to the spinal cord is unknown. This phenomenon is described more completely in the following section. Ono et al[33] found that the clinical improvement in such cases resulted from compensatory C0-C1 rotation and documented that the phenomenon is relatively common.

Occipitoatlantal Rotatory Deformity

In 1958, Sullivan et al[107] described rotatory suboccipital dislocation "characterized by partial disengagement of one of the condyles of the occiput and its corresponding atlantal facet." They noted that the "child afflicted with this injury presents himself with torticollis that may or may not have been preceded by trivial trauma...[R]eduction occurs spontaneously."

A combination of occipitoatlantal deformity and AARD is rare. The injury was first reported by Washington in 1959,[108] and Fielding et al[65] described another case in 1978. Clark et al[64] reported a third case and documented through serial radiographs that the occipitoatlantal deformity was a compensatory phenomenon. In the first two cases and in a subsequent report by Altongy and Fielding,[109] the patients presented late and no radiographs had been taken at the onset of the condition to document whether the C0-C1 rotation was present initially. Conceivably, the C0-C1 deformity in all of these cases may have been compensatory. Because CT is rarely performed in cases of AARD in which the torticollis resolves, compensatory C0-C1 rotatory deformity may be underdiagnosed and patients with AARD who were presumed to have recovered may in fact still have AARD.[33]

Combined C0-C1 and C1-C2 rotatory deformities have been reported so rarely that no definite guidelines for treatment can be established. Fielding et al[65] and Clark et al[64] each treated one case with C0-C2 fusion. Clark et al[64] theorized that it would be safer to perform an in situ C0-C2 fusion than to attempt reduction of the deformity because traction could affect the more mobile occipitoatlantal joint instead of the fixed atlantoaxial complex "with potentially disastrous results." Fielding et al[65] performed C0-C2 fusion on one patient when it was suspected that both levels were injured primarily. In a subsequent report from the same institution,[109] the possibility that the C0-C1 subluxation was compensatory was considered, and the patient was treated with traction followed by C1-C2 fusion alone. The patient was immobilized in a halo vest for 6 weeks postoperatively to control the C0-C1 counterrotation and had an excellent clinical result. The advantage of preserving the normal flexion and extension motion of the C0-C1 joint must be weighed against the theoretical risk imposed by the preoperative traction necessary to realign the C1-C2 joints.

Ono et al[33] often ignored the interlocked atlas in cases of atlantoaxial rotatory fixation with compensatory C0-C1 counterrotation. They stated that "the physical appearance was usually well restored." Unfortunately, no long-term follow-up data were provided in their report.

Summary

AARDs represent a spectrum of disorders characterized by temporary or fixed rotation of C1 on C2. The degree of malrotation is generally within the range of physiologic motion of the joints and may be associated with compensatory counterrotation of C0-C1 or the subaxial spine. Conservative treatment is usually effective, but cases with a longer delay to diagnosis may be refractory to nonsurgical treatment. A variety of surgical options have been described, most commonly involving fusion of C1-C2. Other options, including open reduction with or without temporary internal fixation, have been used successfully in a small number of patients. Until larger series have been reported, C1-C2 fusion with contemporary techniques is advised when nonsurgical measures are unsuccessful.

References

1. Bell C: *The Nervous System of the Human Body: Embracing the Papers Delivered to the Royal Society on the Subject of Nerves.* London, United Kingdom, Longman & Company, 1830.
2. Corner EM: Rotary dislocations of the atlas. *Ann Surg* 1907;45(1):9-26.
3. Desfosses P: Un cas de maladie de Grisel: Torticolis naso-pharyngien par subluxation de l'atlas. *Presse Med* 1930;38:1179-1180.
4. Berkheiser EJ, Seidler F: Nontraumatic dislocations of the atlanto-axial joint. *JAMA* 1931;96: 517-523.
5. Jones RW: Spontaneous hyperæmic dislocation of the atlas. *Proc R Soc Med* 1932;25(4):586-590.
6. Fielding JW, Hawkins RJ: Atlanto-axial rotatory fixation. (Fixed rotatory subluxation of the atlanto-axial joint). *J Bone Joint Surg Am* 1977; 59(1):37-44.
7. Dvorak J, Panjabi M, Gerber M, Wichmann W: CT-functional diagnostics of the rotatory instability of upper cervical spine: 1. An experimental study on cadavers. *Spine (Phila Pa 1976)* 1987; 12(3):197-205.
8. Fielding JW: Cineroentgenography of the normal cervical spine. *J Bone Joint Surg Am* 1957;39(6): 1280-1288.
9. Coutts MB: Atlanto-epistropheal subluxations. *Arch Surg* 1934;29:297-311.
10. Dvorak J, Hayek J, Zehnder R: CT-functional diagnostics of the rotatory instability of the upper cervical spine: Part 2. An evaluation on healthy adults and patients with suspected instability. *Spine (Phila Pa 1976)* 1987;12(8):726-731.
11. Goel VK, Winterbottom JM, Schulte KR, et al: Ligamentous laxity across C0-C1-C2 complex: Axial torque-rotation characteristics until failure. *Spine (Phila Pa 1976)* 1990;15(10):990-996.
12. Mazzara JT, Fielding JW: Effect of C1-C2 rotation on canal size. *Clin Orthop Relat Res* 1988;237: 115-119.
13. Hollinshead WH: *Anatomy for Surgeons: The Back and Limbs,* ed 3. Philadelphia, PA, Harper & Row, 1982, vol 3.
14. Dvorak J, Panjabi MM: Functional anatomy of the alar ligaments. *Spine (Phila Pa 1976)* 1987;12(2): 183-189.
15. Dvorak J, Schneider E, Saldinger P, Rahn B: Biomechanics of the craniocervical region: The alar and transverse ligaments. *J Orthop Res* 1988;6(3): 452-461.
16. Crisco JJ III, Oda T, Panjabi MM, Bueff HU, Dvorák J, Grob D: Transections of the C1-C2 joint capsular ligaments in the cadaveric spine. *Spine (Phila Pa 1976)* 1991;16(10, Suppl): S474-S479.
17. Steel HH: Anatomical and mechanical considerations of the atlanto-axial articulations. *J Bone Joint Surg Am* 1968;50:1481-1482.
18. Spence KF Jr, Decker S, Sell KW: Bursting atlantal fracture associated with rupture of the transverse ligament. *J Bone Joint Surg Am* 1970;52(3): 543-549.
19. Fielding JW, Reddy K: Atlanto-axial rotatory deformity. *J Bone Joint Surg Am* 1969;51:1672-1673.
20. Fielding JW, Cochran GB, Lawsing JF III, Hohl M: Tears of the transverse ligament of the atlas: A clinical and biomechanical study. *J Bone Joint Surg Am* 1974;56(8):1683-1691.
21. Locke GR, Gardner JI, Van Epps EF: Atlas-dens interval (ADI) in children: A survey based on 200 normal cervical spines. *Am J Roentgenol Radium Ther Nucl Med* 1966;97(1):135-140.
22. Jackson H: The diagnosis of minimal atlanto-axial subluxation. *Br J Radiol* 1950;23(275):672-674.
23. Schneider RC, Crosby EC: Vascular insufficiency of brain stem and spinal cord in spinal trauma. *Neurology* 1959;9:643-656.
24. Parke WW, Rothman RH, Brown MD: The pharyngovertebral veins: An anatomical rationale for Grisel's syndrome. *J Bone Joint Surg Am* 1984; 66(4):568-574.
25. Panjabi M, Dvorak J, Crisco JJ III, Oda T, Wang P, Grob D: Effects of alar ligament transection on upper cervical spine rotation. *J Orthop Res* 1991; 9(4):584-593.
26. Werne S: Studies in spontaneous atlas dislocation. *Acta Orthop Scand Suppl* 1957;23:1-150.

27. Panjabi M, Dvorak J, Crisco J III, Oda T, Hilibrand A, Grob D: Flexion, extension, and lateral bending of the upper cervical spine in response to alar ligament transections. *J Spinal Disord* 1991;4(2):157-167.
28. Burkus JK, Deponte RJ: Chronic atlantoaxial rotatory fixation correction by cervical traction, manipulation, and bracing. *J Pediatr Orthop* 1986; 6(5):631-635.
29. Pang D, Li V: Atlantoaxial rotatory fixation: Part 3-a prospective study of the clinical manifestation, diagnosis, management, and outcome of children with alantoaxial rotatory fixation. *Neurosurgery* 2005;57(5):954-972.
30. Goddard NJ, Stabler J, Albert JS: Atlanto-axial rotatory fixation and fracture of the clavicle: An association and a classification. *J Bone Joint Surg Br* 1990;72(1):72-75.
31. Greeley PW: Bilateral (ninety degrees) rotatory dislocation of the atlas upon the axis. *J Bone Joint Surg* 1930;12:958-962.
32. Jones RN: Rotatory dislocation of both atlanto-axial joints. *J Bone Joint Surg Br* 1984;66(1):6-7.
33. Ono K, Yonenobu K, Fuji T, Okada K: Atlantoaxial rotatory fixation: Radiographic study of its mechanism. *Spine (Phila Pa 1976)* 1985;10(7): 602-608.
34. Jamshidi S, Dennis MW, Azzam C, Karim N: Traumatic posterior atlantoaxial dislocation without neurological deficit: Case report. *Neurosurgery* 1983;12(2):211-213.
35. Neumann U, Urbanski H, Riedel K: Posterior atlantoaxial dislocation without fracture of the odontoid: A case report. *J Bone Joint Surg Am* 2003;85(7):1343-1346.
36. Sud S, Chaturvedi S, Buxi TB, Singh S: Posterior atlantoaxial dislocation without associated fracture. *Skeletal Radiol* 2002;31(9):529-531.
37. Yoon DH, Yang KH, Kim KN, Oh SH: Posterior atlantoaxial dislocation without fracture: Case report. *J Neurosurg* 2003;98(1 Suppl):73-76.
38. Phillips WA, Hensinger RN: The management of rotatory atlanto-axial subluxation in children. *J Bone Joint Surg Am* 1989;71(5):664-668.
39. Moore KR, Frank EH: Traumatic atlantoaxial rotatory subluxation and dislocation. *Spine (Phila Pa 1976)* 1995;20(17):1928-1930.
40. Robertson PA, Swan HA: Traumatic bilateral rotatory facet dislocation of the atlas on the axis. *Spine (Phila Pa 1976)* 1992;17(10):1252-1254.
41. Leventhal MR, Maguire JK Jr, Christian CA: Atlantoaxial rotary subluxation in ankylosing spondylitis: A case report. *Spine (Phila Pa 1976)* 1990; 15(12):1374-1376.
42. White GM, Healy WL: Tumor-associated atlanto-axial rotatory fixation: A case report. *Spine (Phila Pa 1976)* 1987;12(4):406-408.
43. Wolf JW Jr, Kahler SG: Atlanto-axial rotatory fixation associated with the 18q- syndrome: Case report. *J Bone Joint Surg Am* 1980;62(2):295-297.
44. Marar BC, Balachandran N: Non-traumatic atlanto-axial dislocation in children. *Clin Orthop Relat Res* 1973;92:220-226.
45. Taddonio RF Jr, King AG: Atlantoaxial rotatory fixation after decompressive laminectomy: A case report. *Spine (Phila Pa 1976)* 1982;7(6):540-544.
46. Sullivan AW: Subluxation of the atlanto-axial joint, sequel to inflammatory processes of the neck. *J Pediatr* 1949;35(4):451-464.
47. Wilson BC, Jarvis BL, Haydon RC III: Nontraumatic subluxation of the atlantoaxial joint: Grisel's syndrome. *Ann Otol Rhinol Laryngol* 1987;96(6): 705-708.
48. Grisel P: Énucléation de l'atlas torticolis nasopharyngien. *Presse Med* 1930;38:50-54.
49. Wetzel FT, La Rocca H: Grisel's syndrome. *Clin Orthop Relat Res* 1989;240:141-152.
50. Bredenkamp JK, Maceri DR: Inflammatory torticollis in children. *Arch Otolaryngol Head Neck Surg* 1990;116(3):310-313.
51. Mathern GW, Batzdorf U: Grisel's syndrome: Cervical spine clinical, pathologic, and neurologic manifestations. *Clin Orthop Relat Res* 1989;244: 131-146.
52. Wilson MJ, Michele AA, Jacobson EW: Spontaneous dislocation of the atlanto-axial articulation, including a report of a case with quadriplegia. *J Bone Joint Surg Am* 1940;22:698-707.
53. Keuter EJ: Non-traumatic atlanto-axial dislocation associated with nasopharyngeal infections (Grisel's disease). *Acta Neurochir (Wien)* 1969;21(1):11-22.
54. Currier BL, Kim CW, Eismont FJ: Infections of the spine, in Herkowitz HN, Garfin SR, Eismont FJ, Bell GR, Balderston RA, eds: *The Spine*. Philadelphia, PA, WB Saunders Company, 2006, pp 1265-1316.
55. Hess JH, Bronstein IP, Abelson SM: Atlanto-axial dislocations: Unassociated with trauma and secondary to inflammatory foci in the neck. *Am J Dis Child* 1935;49:1137-1147.
56. Sudeck P: Torsion dislocation of atlas. *Deutsche Ztschr Chir* 1924;183:289.
57. Cattell HS, Filtzer DL: Pseudosubluxation and other normal variations in the cervical spine in children: A study of one hundred and sixty children. *J Bone Joint Surg Am* 1965;47(7):1295-1309.
58. Kawabe N, Hirotani H, Tanaka O: Pathomechanism of atlantoaxial rotatory fixation in children. *J Pediatr Orthop* 1989;9(5):569-574.

59. Wittek A: Ein fall von distensionsluxation im atlanto-epistropheal-gelenke. *München Med Wochenschr* 1908;55:1836-1837.

60. Wortzman G, Dewar FP: Rotary fixation of the atlantoaxial joint: Rotational atlantoaxial subluxation. *Radiology* 1968;90(3):479-487.

61. Pang D, Li V: Atlantoaxial rotatory fixation: Part 1—Biomechanics of normal rotation at the atlantoaxial joint in children. *Neurosurgery* 2004;55(3): 614-626.

62. Fielding JW: Selected observations of the cervical spine in the child. *Curr Pract Orthop Surg* 1973;5: 31-55.

63. Crossman JE, David K, Hayward R, Crockard HA: Open reduction of pediatric atlantoaxial rotatory fixation: Long-term outcome study with functional measurements. *J Neurosurg* 2004; 100(3, Suppl Spine):235-240.

64. Clark CR, Kathol MH, Walsh T, el-Khoury GY: Atlantoaxial rotatory fixation with compensatory counter occipitoatlantal subluxation: A case report. *Spine (Phila Pa 1976)* 1986;11(10): 1048-1050.

65. Fielding JW, Stillwell WT, Chynn KY, Spyropoulos EC: Use of computed tomography for the diagnosis of atlanto-axial rotatory fixation: A case report. *J Bone Joint Surg Am* 1978;60(8): 1102-1104.

66. Lee S, Joyce S, Seeger J: Asymmetry of the odontoid-lateral mass interspaces: A radiographic finding of questionable clinical significance. *Ann Emerg Med* 1986;15(10):1173-1176.

67. Paul LW, Moir WW: Non-pathologic variations in relationship of the upper cervical vertebrae. *Am J Roentgenol Radium Ther* 1949;62(4):519-524.

68. Daniels DL, Williams AL, Haughton VM: Computed tomography of the articulations and ligaments at the occipito-atlantoaxial region. *Radiology* 1983;146(3):709-716.

69. Rinaldi I, Mullins WJ Jr, Delaney WF, Fitzer PM, Tornberg DN: Computerized tomographic demonstration of rotational atlanto-axial fixation: Case report. *J Neurosurg* 1979;50(1):115-119.

70. Kowalski HM, Cohen WA, Cooper P, Wisoff JH: Pitfalls in the CT diagnosis of atlantoaxial rotary subluxation. *AJR Am J Roentgenol* 1987;149(3): 595-600.

71. Li V, Pang D: Atlanto-axial rotatory fixation, in Pang D, ed: *Disorders of the Pediatric Spine*. New York, NY, Raven Press, 1995, pp 531-553.

72. Dickman CA, Mamourian A, Sonntag VK, Drayer BP: Magnetic resonance imaging of the transverse atlantal ligament for the evaluation of atlantoaxial instability. *J Neurosurg* 1991;75(2): 221-227.

73. Vetti N, Kråkenes J, Eide GE, Rørvik J, Gilhus NE, Espeland A: MRI of the alar and transverse ligaments in whiplash-associated disorders (WAD) grades 1-2: High-signal changes by age, gender, event and time since trauma. *Neuroradiology* 2009;51(4):227-235.

74. Bredenkamp JK, Hoover LA, Berke GS, Shaw A: Congenital muscular torticollis: A spectrum of disease. *Arch Otolaryngol Head Neck Surg* 1990; 116(2):212-216.

75. Calne DB, Lang AE: Secondary dystonia. *Adv Neurol* 1988;50:9-33.

76. Marsden CD: The focal dystonias. *Semin Neurol* 1982;2:324-333.

77. Suchowersky O, Calne DB: Non-dystonic causes of torticollis. *Adv Neurol* 1988;50:501-508.

78. Truong DD, Dubinsky R, Hermanowicz N, Olson WL, Silverman B, Koller WC: Posttraumatic torticollis. *Arch Neurol* 1991;48(2):221-223.

79. Van Holsbeeck EM, MacKay NN: Diagnosis of acute atlanto-axial rotatory fixation. *J Bone Joint Surg Br* 1989;71(1):90-91.

80. Johnson RM, Hart DL, Simmons EF, Ramsby GR, Southwick WO: Cervical orthoses: A study comparing their effectiveness in restricting cervical motion in normal subjects. *J Bone Joint Surg Am* 1977;59(3):332-339.

81. Mubarak SJ, Camp JF, Vuletich W, Wenger DR, Garfin SR: Halo application in the infant. *J Pediatr Orthop* 1989;9(5):612-614.

82. Weisskopf M, Naeve D, Ruf M, Harms J, Jeszenszky D: Therapeutic options and results following fixed atlantoaxial rotatory dislocations. *Eur Spine J* 2005;14(1):61-68.

83. Subach BR, McLaughlin MR, Albright AL, Pollack IF: Current management of pediatric atlantoaxial rotatory subluxation. *Spine (Phila Pa 1976)* 1998; 23(20):2174-2179.

84. El-Khoury GY, Clark CR, Gravett AW: Acute traumatic rotatory atlanto-axial dislocation in children: A report of three cases. *J Bone Joint Surg Am* 1984;66(5):774-777.

85. Levine AM, Edwards CC: Treatment of injuries in the C1-C2 complex. *Orthop Clin North Am* 1986; 17(1):31-44.

86. Walton GL: Further observations on cervical dislocation and its reduction. *Boston Med Surg J* 1903;149:445-447.

87. Jeszenszky D, Willms R, Steigleder A, Jensen R, Rahman MA, Harms J: Closed reduction of C1-C2 rotary subluxations: A new method. Presented at the *14th Annual Meeting of the Cervical Spine Research Society*. Varese, Italy, Sept 17-19, 1998.

88. Harms J, Melcher RP: Posterior C1-C2 fusion with polyaxial screw and rod fixation. *Spine (Phila Pa 1976)* 2001;26(22):2467-2471.

89. McGraw RW, Rusch RM: Atlanto-axial arthrodesis. *J Bone Joint Surg Br* 1973;55(3):482-489.
90. Gallie WE: Fractures and dislocations of the cervical spine. *Am J Surg* 1939;46:495-499.
91. Brooks AL, Jenkins EB: Atlanto-axial arthrodesis by the wedge compression method. *J Bone Joint Surg Am* 1978;60(3):279-284.
92. Griswold DM, Albright JA, Schiffman E, Johnson R, Southwick W: Atlanto-axial fusion for instability. *J Bone Joint Surg Am* 1978;60(3):285-292.
93. Fielding JW, Hawkins RJ, Ratzan SA: Spine fusion for atlanto-axial instability. *J Bone Joint Surg Am* 1976;58(3):400-407.
94. Dickman CA, Sonntag VK, Papadopoulos SM, Hadley MN: The interspinous method of posterior atlantoaxial arthrodesis. *J Neurosurg* 1991;74(2): 190-198.
95. Barbour JR: Screw fixation and fractures of the odontoid process. *South Australian Clin* 1971;5: 20-28.
96. Currier BL, Yaszemski MJ: The use of C1 lateral mass fixation in the cervical spine. *Curr Opin Orthop* 2004;15(3):184-191.
97. Goel A, Desai KI, Muzumdar DP: Atlantoaxial fixation using plate and screw method: A report of 160 treated patients. *Neurosurgery* 2002;51(6): 1351-1357.
98. Goel A, Laheri V: Plate and screw fixation for atlanto-axial subluxation. *Acta Neurochir (Wien)* 1994;129(1-2):47-53.
99. Grob D, Jeanneret B, Aebi M, Markwalder TM: Atlanto-axial fusion with transarticular screw fixation. *J Bone Joint Surg Br* 1991;73(6):972-976.
100. Lu J, Ebraheim NA, Yang H, Heck BE, Yeasting RA: Anatomic considerations of anterior transarticular screw fixation for atlantoaxial instability. *Spine (Phila Pa 1976)* 1998;23(11):1229-1236.
101. Magerl F, Seeman PS: Stable posterior fusion of the atlas and axis by transarticular screw fixation, in Kehr P, Werdner PA, eds: *Cervical Spine*. Springer-Verlag, New York, NY, 1987, pp 322-327.
102. Reilly TM, Sasso RC, Hall PV: Atlantoaxial stabilization: Clinical comparison of posterior cervical wiring technique with transarticular screw fixation. *J Spinal Disord Tech* 2003;16(3):248-253.
103. Vaccaro AR, Ring D, Lee RS, Scuderi G, Garfin SR: Salvage anterior C1-C2 screw fixation and arthrodesis through the lateral approach in a patient with a symptomatic pseudoarthrosis. *Am J Orthop (Belle Mead NJ)* 1997;26(5):349-353.
104. Vaccaro AR, Lehman AP, Ahlgren BD, Garfin SR: Anterior C1-C2 screw fixation and bony fusion through an anterior retropharyngeal approach. *Orthopedics* 1999;22(12):1165-1170.
105. Smith MD, Phillips WA, Hensinger RN: Complications of fusion to the upper cervical spine. *Spine (Phila Pa 1976)* 1991;16(7):702-705.
106. Ishii K, Chiba K, Maruiwa H, Nakamura M, Matsumoto M, Toyama Y: Pathognomonic radiological signs for predicting prognosis in patients with chronic atlantoaxial rotatory fixation. *J Neurosurg Spine* 2006;5(5):385-391.
107. Sullivan CR, Bruwer AJ, Harris LE: Hypermobility of the cervical spine in children; a pitfall in the diagnosis of cervical dislocation. *Am J Surg* 1958; 95(4):636-640.
108. Washington ER: Non-traumatic atlanto-occipital and atlanto-axial dislocation; a case report. *J Bone Joint Surg Am* 1959;41(2):341-344.
109. Altongy JF, Fielding JW: Combined atlanto-axial and occipito-atlantal rotatory subluxation: A case report. *J Bone Joint Surg Am* 1990;72(6):923-926.

CHAPTER 23

Insufficiency of the Transverse Ligament

Mark A. Knaub, MD   Lawrence T. Kurz, MD   Harry N. Herkowitz, MD

Key Points

- The primary restraint to anterior translation of C1 on C2 is the transverse ligament.
- Congenital bony ankylosis of the cervical spine may impart increased stress on the transverse ligament, and sometimes lead to attenuation, or eventual rupture of the ligament.
- Acute rupture of the transverse ligament usually results from a high-energy injury.
- Stability of the C1-C2 articulation may be restored only by primary healing of the transverse ligament (in some children and with external immobilization) or surgical arthrodesis of C1-C2 (in most adults).
- C1-C2 transarticular screw fixation and direct polyaxial screw/rod fixation offer advantages over classic posterior C1-C2 wiring techniques.

Introduction

The mechanical integrity of the atlantoaxial joint is dependent upon both bony and ligamentous structures. Accordingly, atlantoaxial instability may arise from fracture, ligamentous disruption, or a combination of both. Insufficiency of the transverse ligament may arise from posttraumatic, congenital, infectious, arthritic, or inflammatory causes. Isolated traumatic disruptions of the ligament are relatively rare and may be accompanied by fractures of the atlantoaxial complex. A complete understanding of the complex anatomic relationships and the biomechanics of the atlantoaxial articulation is essential in evaluating and managing traumatic injuries to the transverse ligament. Knowledge of the radiographic appearance of the uninjured and injured upper cervical spine is also necessary when dealing with these injuries.

This chapter will focus on traumatic disruption of the transverse ligament. Other causes of transverse ligament insufficiency will be mentioned but not discussed in detail. Fractures of the upper cervical spine are covered in other chapters. A discussion of the anatomy and biomechanics of the atlantoaxial articulation will be followed by a description of the etiology of both traumatic and nontraumatic insufficiency of the transverse ligament. The radiographic evaluation of suspected C1-C2 injuries will then be reviewed. Finally, an in-depth discussion on the treatment of traumatic disruption of the transverse ligament is presented, including a detailed description of techniques for arthrodesis of the C1-C2 articulation. After reading this chapter, the clinician should have the tools necessary to effectively evaluate, diagnose, and treat patients with suspected traumatic atlantoaxial instability due to traumatic rupture of the transverse ligament.

Anatomy

The transverse ligament is a portion of the cruciform ligament, which represents only the middle of three layers that comprise the posterior occipitoatlantoaxial ligament complex. The most posterior portion of this complex is the tectorial membrane, which lies directly adjacent to the epidural space. This membrane is a continuation of the posterior longitudinal ligament that attaches to the anterior portion of the foramen magnum. The anterior layer of the occipitoatlantoaxial complex consists of the apical and alar ligaments. The alar ligaments are paired structures that attach to the posterolateral surface of the odontoid. They travel obliquely and attach to the medial aspects of the occipital condyles. The apical ligament runs from the tip of the odontoid process to the anterior edge of the foramen magnum. The transverse ligament is the horizontal portion of the cruciform ligament that attaches to the tubercles of the lateral masses of the atlas (C1). In doing so, the

Dr. Kurz or an immediate family member serves as a paid consultant to or is an employee of Stryker; and has received research or institutional support from Smith & Nephew and Apatech. Dr. Herkowitz or an immediate family member serves as a board member, owner, officer, or committee member of the American Board of Orthopaedic Surgery, Inc.; and has received royalties from Medtronic. Neither Dr. Knaub nor any immediate family member has received anything of value from or owns stock in a commercial company or institution related directly or indirectly to the subject of this chapter.

ligament passes posterior to the odontoid process, confining it to the articular notch on the posterior surface of the anterior arch of the atlas. The cruciform ligament also has ascending and descending components that run vertically and attach to the anterior edge of the foramen magnum and the body of C2, respectively.

The diameter of the ring of the atlas in the anterior-posterior plane is approximately 3 cm. The space within the ring can be divided into thirds, with each space containing specific structures. This has been referred to by many as Steel's "rule of thirds."[1] The odontoid process and the spinal cord each occupy approximately 1 cm of this space. The remainder of the anterior-posterior diameter is composed of "free space," which allows for a relatively large amount of anterior displacement of the C1 ring without adverse neurologic consequences. Subluxations greater than 1 cm may result in compression of the spinal cord. Translation associated with an odontoid fracture may not compromise the spinal cord because the odontoid process is typically tethered to the anterior ring of C1 by the transverse ligament. As a result, there is usually no encroachment on the space available for the cord within the C1 ring. However, spinal cord compression may occur in this setting when severe displacement results in kinking of the spinal cord between the posterior ring of the C1 arch and the body of C2. Congenital abnormalities that result in a hypoplastic or absent odontoid may also decrease the risk of spinal cord compression with upper cervical spine injuries,[2] likely due to the fact that less C1 ring volume is occupied by a rigid structure. Similarly, odontoid hypoplasia secondary to os odontoideum may also diminish the risk of spinal cord compression.

Biomechanics

The stability of the atlantoaxial complex is provided by both bony and ligamentous structures. Resistance to axial loading is provided by the bony architecture of the C1 and C2 facet joints. The horizontal orientation of these facet joints is optimal to resist axial loads but does little to restrain anterior or posterior translation of the atlas on the axis. While posterior translation of the C1 ring is limited by abutment of the anterior ring of C1 on the odontoid process, there is no bony resistance to anterior translation. The primary restraint to anterior translation of C1 on C2 is the transverse ligament. Secondary restraint is provided by the alar ligaments and the C1-C2 facet joint capsules. The alar ligaments also contribute to the rotational stability of the atlantoaxial articulation.[3]

The strength of the transverse ligament has been investigated. Spence et al[4] applied pure tensile loads to the transverse ligament via pins placed into the lateral masses of the atlas after the anterior and posterior arches were disrupted. The mean breaking strength of the transverse ligament in this cadaveric study was 58 kilopounds (range, 38-104). Fielding et al[5] used intact upper cervical spine specimens to assess the strength of the transverse ligament. To accomplish this, the C2 body was immobilized while an anteriorly directed force was applied to the intact, mobile, occiput-C1 segment. Under these loading conditions, the mean force necessary to rupture the ligament was 84 kilopounds. They also observed that the intact transverse ligament did not allow more than 3 mm of anterior translation of the atlas on the axis. Failure of the ligament usually occurred with 3 to 5 mm of translation. When failure of the ligament did occur, it did so abruptly in most cases. Seventy-five percent of failures occurred in the midsubstance of the ligament, while 25% occurred through avulsion of the tubercle of the lateral mass. No correlation could be found between the age of the patient at the time of death and the strength of the transverse ligament.

Anterior translation of C1 on C2 has been measured in asymptomatic volunteers. Jackson used flexion and extension lateral radiographs to examine the motion of the cervical spine in children and adults.[6] Maximum anterior translation of C1 on C2 was 2.5 mm in adults and 4.0 mm in children. These values are similar to those obtained in both experimental and clinical data presented by others.[5,7,8]

Etiology

Insufficiency of the transverse ligament may occur as a result of acute trauma, increased repetitive stress due to occipitalization of the atlas or congenital ankylosis of the cervical spine, or congenital absence or laxity of the ligament. The focus of this chapter will be on the acute traumatic causes but the other etiologies will be mentioned.

Congenital bony ankylosis of the cervical spine may impart increased stress on the transverse ligament and sometimes lead to attenuation, or eventual rupture of the ligament. The two most common situations in which this occurs are occipitalization of the atlas and Klippel-Feil syndrome. Occipitalization of the atlas represents partial or complete congenital ankylosis of the bony ring of C1 to the occiput. Ankylosis typically occurs between the anterior rim of the foramen magnum and the anterior arch of the atlas, although anterior/posterior fusions have been reported.[9] Normally, most of the flexion/extension of the upper cervical spine occurs at the occiput-C1 articulation. With occipitalization, no motion occurs between the occiput and the atlas. Therefore, excessive stress is transferred to the atlantoaxial joint and the transverse ligament during repetitive flexion and extension of the cervical spine. Gradual attenuation or rupture of the ligament may result in the late appearance of symptomatic atlantoaxial instability. Atlantoaxial instability is associated with occipitalization of the atlas in 39% to 54% of cases.[10-13] Patients with occipitalization also have a high rate of malpositioned or abnormally long odontoid processes. This may also contribute to the appearance of clinical symptoms in the setting of atlantoaxial instability.

Congenital ankylosis of C2-C3 may lead to the earlier appearance of symptoms and signs of spinal cord compression. This is especially true when it occurs in the setting of occipitalization of the atlas. Ankylosis of C2-C3 has been reported to occur in 47% to 68% of those patients with occipitalization.[12,14] In theory, the C1-C2 articulation is subjected to even greater repetitive stresses when the segments cranial and caudal to it are ankylosed. This could potentially lead to a higher than expected number of patients developing atlantoaxial instability with potential spinal cord compromise.

Congenital insufficiency of the transverse ligament may be seen in several disorders including Down syndrome and Morquio syndrome. It can also be idiopathic. The insufficiency may result from congenital absence or laxity of the transverse ligament. Up to 20% of patients with Down syndrome have evidence of atlantoaxial instability.[1,15] Most of these patients are asymptomatic, although several cases of neurologic compromise have been reported.[16,17] These patients typically present with neck pain, torticollis, or neurologic signs of spinal cord compression. Although recommendations for treatment of C1-C2 instability in Down syndrome patients range from simple limitation of activities to prophylactic atlantoaxial arthrodesis, there is no consensus.

Idiopathic anterior atlantoaxial instability occurs rarely in patients without any other abnormalities, and the diagnosis of "idiopathic" is one of exclusion. The patient should have no history of significant trauma, inflammatory disease, congenital abnormality, or infection. Although these cases may be truly "idiopathic," they may in fact represent the sequelae of an old, forgotten trauma.

The true incidence of traumatic rupture of the transverse ligament is unknown. As many of these injuries likely result in immediate death, most patients may not make it to the hospital for evaluation. Survival following acute traumatic rupture of the transverse ligament has been reported in the literature.[18-21] Dickman et al[18] reported on 39 patients with traumatic injury to the transverse ligament treated at their institution; 16 patients had isolated ligamentous tears of the ligament while the remainder had fractures of the lateral masses of C1 that resulted in insufficiency of the transverse ligament. Automobile accidents, automobile versus pedestrian accidents, and falls accounted for most of the 39 cases.

The incidence of severe head trauma associated with this injury is extremely high. Although patients exhibit a wide range of neurologic signs, there is no "typical" pattern of neurologic injury. Some patients have no neurologic deficit, whereas others exhibit severe unilateral weakness. However, because complete spinal cord injury at this level of the cord would be fatal, permanent quadriplegia is not seen with this injury pattern. In the series of Dickman et al,[18] one patient presented with complete C1 quadriplegia that resulted in death shortly after admission to the hospital. A second patient had "mild quadriparesis," while the remaining 37 patients had no neurologic injury. In the acute setting, the neck demonstrates severe muscle spasm and diminished range of motion. Other manifestations of this injury may include cardiac and respiratory abnormalities secondary to injury to their control centers in the upper cervical spine.

Because the vertebral arteries follow a tortuous course as they ascend through the mobile atlas and axis into the relatively fixed foramen magnum, excessive displacement of C1 on C2 may also result in their injury. Disruption of blood flow through the vertebral arteries may be secondary to transection of the artery, thrombosis of the vessel from an intimal tear, or from kinking of the vessel from persistent displacement. Manifestations include dizziness, syncope, or blurred vision.

The mechanism of injury seems to be related to shear forces along with a component of rotation. Rupture of the transverse ligament[5] has been produced experimentally by forced forward translation of C1 on C2. This results in shear stress on the transverse ligament. Anecdotal clinical experience also endorses the idea that anterior translation of C1 on C2 is the likely mechanism of

FIGURE 1

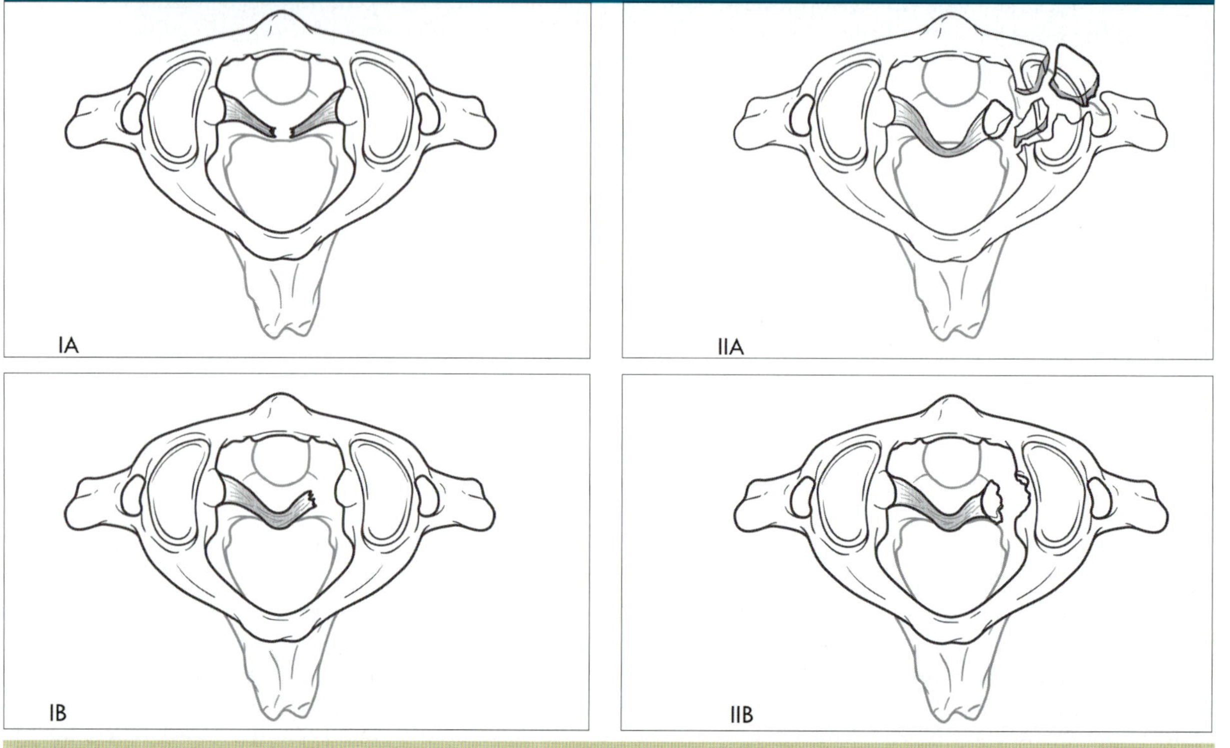

Figure 1 Classification system proposed by Dickman et al[18] for injuries of the transverse atlantal ligament. Type I injuries disrupt the ligament substance in its midportion (**IA**) or at its periosteal insertion (**IB**). Type II injuries disconnect the tubercle for insertion of the transverse ligament from the C1 lateral mass, involving a comminuted C1 lateral mass (**IIA**) or avulsion of the tubercle from the intact lateral mass (**IIB**).

injury. Speculation has arisen that the injury results from an anteriorly directed force to the back of the head, frequently with forced flexion. This speculation is supported by the findings that these patients often have an associated laceration over the occiput.[20,22]

Posttraumatic rupture of the transverse ligament has also been reported in children.[22-24] The anterior atlanto-dens interval (AADI) in these cases ranged from 7 to 15 mm. Any AADI greater than 5 mm in this situation puts the cord at risk for injury. Stiffness and pain in the neck may be the only clinical signs present after a significant head trauma, especially in the presence of normal neurologic function. Pennecot et al[22] reported a case in which the diagnosis was made 6.5 years after the injury. This delay in diagnosis brings to light the importance of obtaining prompt additional or follow-up imaging studies in a patient with neck pain following a significant trauma. Flexion and extension lateral radiographs taken after the resolution of muscle spasm, or an MRI study even before this resolution, will allow the diagnosis to be made.

Acute traumatic rupture of the transverse ligament may also be associated with burst fractures of the ring of C1 (Jefferson fractures).[4,25,26] This highly unstable situation may be inferred when the open-mouth odontoid radiograph shows bilateral lateral overhang of the lateral masses of C1, the sum of which exceeds 6.9 mm.[4] Recently, the reliability of this radiographic measurement has been questioned.[18] Transverse ligament injuries have also been found in conjunction with odontoid fractures. This injury pattern was found in 3 of 30 clinically stable patients with odontoid fractures treated at one institution.[27] The incidence may be higher in unstable patients. The report by Dickman et al[18] on transverse ligament injuries also included a group of 23 patients with tubercle avulsion fractures or injuries that disconnected the tubercle from the transverse ligament insertion on the lateral mass of C1. These bony injuries that rendered the transverse ligament functionally incompetent were classified and treated differently than pure ligament tears. Treatment, based on the classification system displayed in **Figure 1**, will be discussed later in this chapter.

FIGURE 2

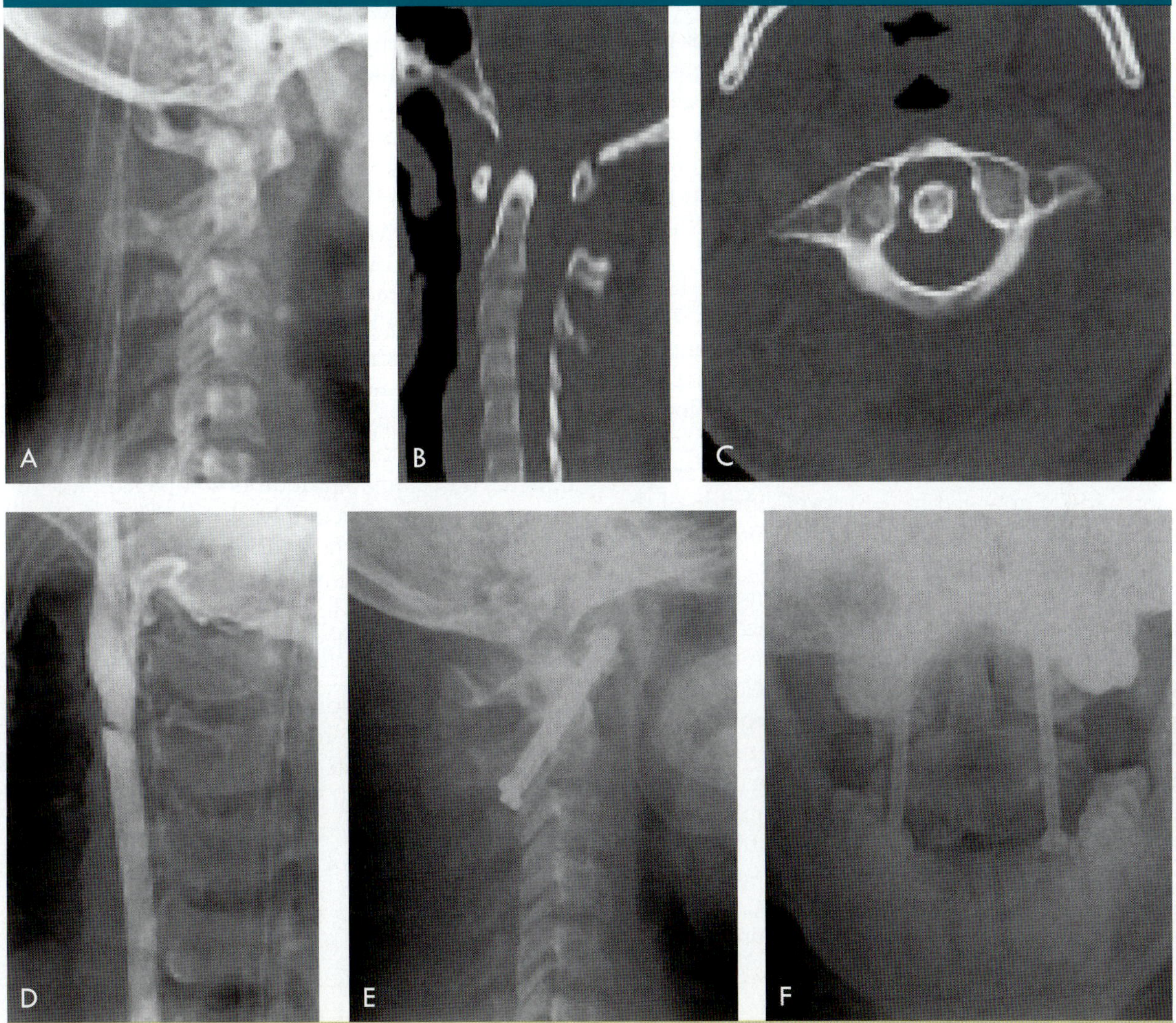

Figure 2 Lateral cervical spine radiograph (**A**) of a 20-year-old male who attempted suicide by hanging. Midline sagittal CT reconstruction (**B**) and axial CT (**C**) images before surgical intervention show an increased AADI. The patient was neurologically intact but sustained an injury to his common carotid artery (**D**) that required repair. After initial stabilization and carotid repair, the patient was taken to the operating room for posterior C1-C2 arthrodesis with bilateral transarticular screws. Postoperative lateral (**E**) and AP (**F**) radiographs show near complete reduction of C1 on C2 and adequate placement of the transarticular screws.

Radiographic Evaluation

The standard method for evaluation of transverse ligament ruptures is a lateral radiograph with the beam centered at the C2 level (**Figure 2,** *A*). The AADI in an adult should be no more than 3 mm, while the AADI in children should be ≤ 5 mm. Both the patient positioning during the radiograph and the body habitus of the patient play an important role in determining whether this injury will be detected on the lateral radiograph. Adult trauma patients are typically imaged in the supine position, on a rigid spine board, while wearing a cervical collar. This places the cervical spine in extension because of the relative small anterior-posterior diameter of the occiput compared to the chest. In a child, the larger diameter of the head relative to the chest places the cervical spine in relative flexion. In an awake, alert patient who is neurologically intact, the injury can be diagnosed by flexion-extension lateral radiographs. In the acute setting, patients may have significant protective paraspinal muscle spasms that inhibit motion, thereby limiting the efficacy of the test. On occasion, the paraspinal musculature can be injected with local anesthetic to overcome the protective muscle spasms. Alternatively, the patient may be immobilized in a rigid cervical orthosis for 7 to 10 days to allow the spasm to diminish. At that time adequate flexion-extension lateral radiographs can be obtained. In the obtunded or neurologically compromised patient, care must be taken to avoid compression of the neurologic structures while establishing the diagnosis. Flexion-extension radiographs should not be performed, and MRI should be obtained.

High-resolution CT scanning can also be useful in the evaluation of the transverse ligament. The mean density value of the transverse ligament is greater in its midportion than at its insertions into the atlas. This correlates well with the histologic structure of the transverse ligament, which demonstrates layers of collagen that are thicker and more closely arranged in the central portion of the ligament than laterally. The CT scan can easily differentiate between avulsion fractures of the ligament off the condyles of the lateral masses of C1, and midsubstance tears. Actual visualization of midsubstance tears of the ligament can be obtained with axial gradient-echo MRI scans angled parallel to the atlas.[18,28] The ligament's high degree of contrast with the surrounding structures permits its visualization in normal subjects. Tears of the ligament appear as a loss of anatomic continuity of the ligament containing regions of high signal intensity compared with the homogenous low signal intensity of the normal ligament. These MRI studies have also demonstrated avulsion fractures as well as midsubstance tears.

Treatment of Traumatic Disruption of the Transverse Ligament

The primary restraint to anterior translation of C1 on C2 is the transverse ligament. The secondary restraints, primarily the alar ligaments, are insufficient to prevent anterior translation of the atlas on the axis when the transverse ligament has been disrupted. Therefore, the goal of treatment of these injuries must be to restore the stability of the atlantoaxial articulation to its preinjury state. This can be accomplished only by primary healing of the transverse ligament or by surgical arthrodesis of C1 to C2.

Patients with neurologic symptoms or signs should be treated by primary posterior C1-C2 arthrodesis to provide immediate stability to the atlantoaxial articulation, thereby providing the best environment for neurologic recovery. In those patients without neurologic abnormalities, the age of the patient must be taken into consideration. Adults and children have different rates of transverse ligament healing when this injury is treated nonsurgically. Adults have limited healing potential and should therefore be treated with primary posterior C1-C2 arthrodesis if their AADI in flexion is greater than 4 mm. Children with transverse ligament injuries have a slightly higher chance of primary ligament healing when nonsurgical measures are employed. Good results may be obtained in some children when they are rigidly immobilized for 2 to 3 months. Careful observation is important in this group of patients to assess for increasing anterior displacement of C1 on C2, during external immobilization. When there is difficulty obtaining or maintaining reduction with rigid immobilization, posterior arthrodesis is required. After immobilization is completed, flexion-extension lateral radiographs should be performed to assess healing. If the AADI in flexion is found to be greater than 4 mm, adequate primary healing of the transverse ligament has not occurred and posterior arthrodesis should be performed.

Many techniques for arthrodesis of C1 to C2 have been described. Initial attempts at atlantoaxial arthrodesis consisted of wiring of the posterior arches of C1 and C2.[2,29-32] Variations (most notably the Brooks and Gallie techniques) in the course of the wire; the choice of hardware (cable versus wire); and the size, type, and positional placement of the bone graft have yielded fusion rates as high as 82%.[33] The efficacy of these techniques may be limited because of the need for rigid postoperative immobilization, many times in the form of a halo vest. Comparing different wiring techniques, biomechanical studies have shown that the Brooks technique is more effective in reducing motion between C1 and C2 than the Gallie technique.[34,35] The Brooks technique reduces axial rotation by 91% while the Gallie method does so by only 67%.[36] In addition, the Gallie technique fails to reduce lateral bending motion significantly.[37] Because these wiring/graft techniques restore the posterior tension band between C1 and C2 and provide a mechanical block to extension, flexion and extension motions are well controlled.[37] Other studies have demonstrated that both of these wiring techniques may result in significant graft displacement and wire loosening under repetitive loading conditions.[34,37] Finally, because posterior wiring techniques are dependent upon the integrity of the posterior arch of C1, they cannot be used in the setting of a traumatic disruption of the C1 ring.

In addressing some of the limitations of the other posterior wiring techniques, Magerl et al[38-40] developed a method of C1-C2 transarticular screw fixation that also used a midline posterior approach. This surgical technique is illustrated in **Figure 2**. Biomechanical studies have demonstrated that his method alone restricts axial rotation and lateral bending to a greater extent than the other posterior wiring techniques. However, they are less effective in limiting flexion and extension.[36,37,41,42] Gallie posterior wiring combined with transarticular screw fixation, often referred to as the Magerl-Gallie technique, theoretically adds the benefit of restoring the posterior tension band between C1 and C2. The efficacy of this combined technique manifested in greater motion reductions in destabilized cadaveric models.[34-37,43-45] Despite its biomechanical superiority over posterior wiring techniques, transarticular screws do have some drawbacks. Transarticular screws between C1 and C2 can be technically challenging to insert correctly. Errant technique has led to a significant incidence of neurovascular injury.[46-51] In addition, positioning of some patients, especially those with excessive thoracic kyphosis, may limit access to the C2 starting points without additional surgical exposure.

Magerl Transarticular Screw Technique

The patient is intubated and placed into the prone position with the head secured with Mayfield tongs and a Mayfield head holder attached to the operating table. The choice of operating table depends on surgeon preference and availability. The patient's chest and abdomen should be free of external compression. Traction with weights is usually not necessary. Biplanar fluoroscopic imaging is mandatory for this procedure. The recent availability of various image guidance systems may also prove helpful in the placement of C1-C2 transarticular screws. To aid in the actual insertion of the screws, the neck must be flexed as much as possible without causing displacement of C1 on C2. Prior to sterile preparation of the patient, lateral fluoroscopy should confirm reduction of any C1-C2 translation. A midline incision is made from the inion to the spinous process of C4. An incision of this length will require small stab wounds distally for percutaneous insertion of the guidewire, drill, tap, and screws. Alternatively, a long, midline posterior incision may be used. The occiput and the posterior arch of C1 are exposed as far lateral as possible without exposing the vertebral artery. The spinous processes, lamina, and articular processes of C2 and C3 are exposed subperiosteally without destroying the C2-C3 joint capsules. A small elevator is used to expose the cranial surface of the lamina and the isthmus of C2 bilaterally to the posterior capsule of the C1-C2 facet joints. If the venous plexus surrounding the greater occipital nerve is disrupted during the exposure, significant bleeding will occur. Hemostasis should be obtained and maintained with bipolar electrocautery and with thrombin-soaked gel foam. The greater occipital nerve and the surrounding vessels are retracted cephalad with a small elevator or a Kirschner wire inserted into the lateral mass of C1. If the ring of C1 is disrupted, exposure of the C1-C2 joints will allow for placement of bone graft into the joints after some of the articular cartilage is removed. If the posterior arch of C1 is intact, exposure of the C1-C2 articular facets is not necessary. As described by Gallie,[31] a sublaminar wire is passed under the ring of C1 and later used to stabilize the bone graft.

The reduction of the atlas on the axis is reassessed with lateral fluoroscopy. If C1 is still translated anteriorly on C2, reduction may be aided by gently pulling on the wire under the C1 arch and by carefully pushing on the spinous process of C2. Alternatively, a clamp may be used to pull posteriorly on the ring of C1 to assist in the reduction maneuver. Once exposure has been obtained and the reduction confirmed with lateral fluoroscopy, placement of the implants can begin. Both cannulated and solid screw systems are available and the choice depends largely on surgeon preference. The starting point for the guidewire or drill bit is located on the posterior surface of the C2 lamina, 3 mm cephalad and 2 mm lateral to the lower medial edge of the caudad articular process of C2. The cephalad/caudad angle is determined on the lateral fluoroscopic view. In this plane, the wire or drill bit should be aimed directly at the anterior arch of C1 (**Figure 2**, *E*). The correct trajectory of this screw is critical, as an incorrect trajectory may result in inadequate engagement of the C1 lateral mass and possibly injure the vertebral artery. As seen on the AP fluoroscopic view, the drill or guidewire should be directed strictly sagittal, with no medial or lateral angulation (**Figure 2**, *F*). The medial/lateral position of the starting point can be confirmed by directly palpating the medial edge of the C2 isthmus with a blunt dissector. By following these guidelines, the drill bit or guidewire should exit C2 at the posterior rim of the superior articular facet of C2 and enter the lateral mass of C1 in the middle or posterior third of the inferior articular facet of C1. The drill or guidewire should then exit the C1 lateral mass anteriorly,

FIGURE 3

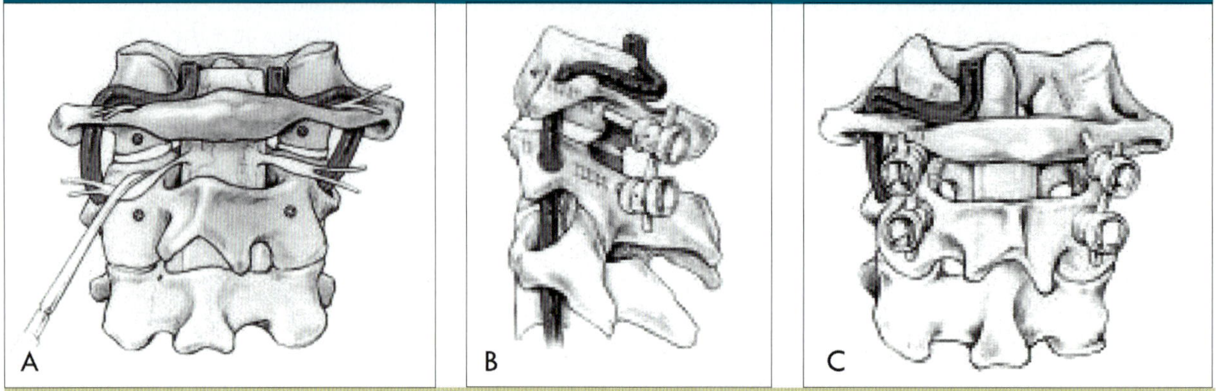

Figure 3 Illustration of the starting points for insertion of C1 lateral mass screws and C2 pedicle screws (**A**). Screw placement and orientation as seen in the lateral (**B**) and PA views (**C**). (Adapted with permission from Harms J, Melcher RP: Posterior C1-C2 fusion with polyaxial screw and rod fixation. *Spine (Phila Pa 1976)* 2001;26(22):2468-2469.)

immediately under the base of the skull. The depth of penetration of the drill bit or guidewire should be monitored closely with lateral fluoroscopy. The length of the screw is determined and the screw is placed after the tract has been tapped across the articular surfaces of the C1-C2 joint. The process is repeated on the contralateral side. After both screws have been placed, their position, length, and orientation are confirmed with biplanar fluoroscopy. Decortication of the posterior ring of C1 and the lamina of C2 is performed with a high-speed burr in preparation for bone grafting. A posterior wiring technique may then be employed to supplement the transarticular screw fixation by securing a bone graft with the previously placed C1 sublaminar wire.

An incompetent or fractured posterior arch of C1 precludes posterior wiring. In this situation, a direct arthrodesis of the C1-C2 facet joints should be performed. After exposure of the C2 isthmus bilaterally, the facet capsules of the C1-C2 joints are exposed by retracting the greater occipital nerve and its venous plexus cephalad with a Kirschner wire inserted into the C1 lateral mass. After the transarticular screws are placed, the posterior capsule of the C1-C2 joints is opened and the cartilage and subchondral bone of the posterior half of the joints are removed with curets. Cancellous bone is then packed into the joints and posterior onlay bone graft is placed over the decorticated arches of C1 and C2.

Direct Polyaxial Screw/Rod Fixation Technique

Direct polyaxial screw fixation of the lateral mass of C1 to the pedicle of C2 has been described by Harms and Melcher and has become the favored method of C1-C2 fixation by many surgeons (**Figure 3**).[52] The polyaxial screws are inserted directly into the lateral mass of C1 and the pedicle of C2, and are connected by longitudinally oriented rods. This fixation has the advantage of not relying on the integrity of the arch of C1 or any structural bone grafts. This method of C1-C2 fixation also allows for a direct reduction of the anterior portion of the C1 ring by pulling the C1 lateral mass screws posteriorly. This can be accomplished even in the setting of a posterior ring of C1 that is rendered incompetent by fracture or laminectomy. This fixation technique is also less dependent upon the position of the patient and the amount of thoracic kyphosis present, because these factors do not typically interfere with the trajectory of the screws. These screws may also be incorporated into longer fixation constructs used for occipitocervical fusions.

The surgical setup and positioning for this direct fixation method are similar to that for placement of transarticular screws. A midline approach is used from the inion down to the spinous process of C4. The upper cervical spine is exposed in a similar fashion as described previously for Magerl screws. The C1-C2 joint is exposed and opened by dissection cephalad to the superior surface of the C2 pars interarticularis. This joint is an important landmark for the accurate placement of the C1 lateral mass screw. The C2 nerve root and its venous plexus are retracted caudally to expose the entry point for the C1 lateral mass screw, which is in the middle of the junction of the C1 posterior arch and the midpoint of the posterior/inferior part of the C1 lateral mass. The entry point (**Figure 4,** *A*) is marked with a small

FIGURE 4

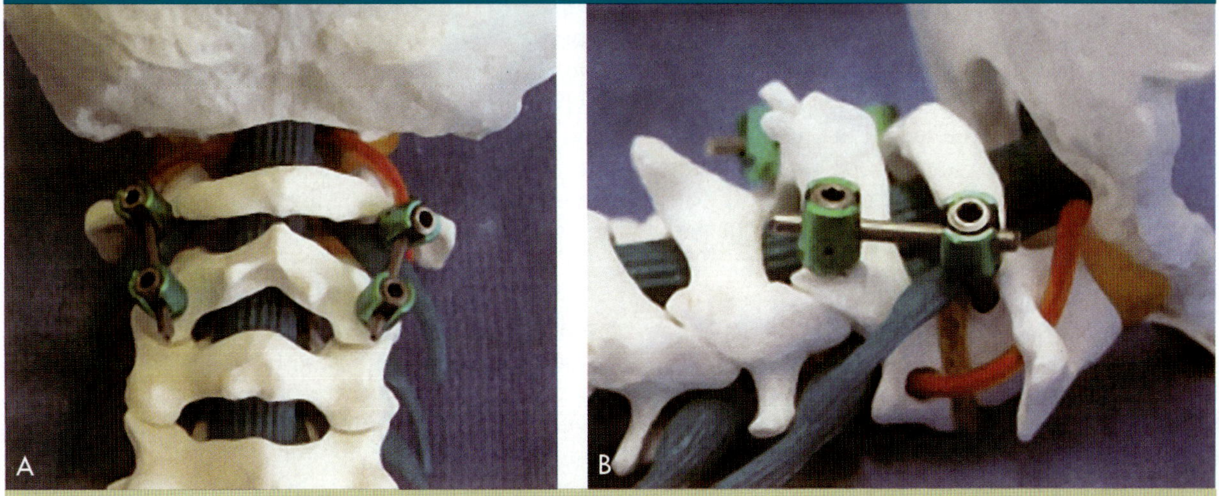

Figure 4 The direct polyaxial screw/rod technique for C1-C2 fixation illustrated on a model of the cervical spine. Note the position of the screws in relation to the C2 nerve root and the vertebral artery. **A,** PA view of the fixation technique. The insertion point of the C1 lateral mass screw can be best appreciated on the lateral view (**B**) at the junction of the posterior ring and lateral mass of C1. (Implants are courtesy of DePuy Spine, Raynham, MA.)

burr to create a pilot hole to prevent slipping of the drill point. The hole is then drilled in a straight or slightly convergent trajectory in the medial/lateral direction and toward the anterior arch of C1 in the cephalad/caudad direction. The drilling is accomplished with guidance from intraoperative landmarks, preoperative fine-cut axial CT images, and lateral fluoroscopic imaging. The hole is then tapped, and a 3.5-mm polyaxial screw is placed through both cortices into the lateral mass of C1. The screw must be of sufficient length to allow the polyaxial portion of the screw to remain dorsal to the bony surface of the posterior arch of C1. The position of the screw is confirmed with biplanar fluoroscopy.

The C2 nerve root and its venous plexus are then retracted cranially and a blunt dissector is used to palpate the medial border of the C2 isthmus. The entry point for the placement of the C2 pedicle screw (**Figure 4,** *A*) is marked with a small burr. This starting point is in the cranial and medial quadrant of the isthmus surface of C2. The drill is directed approximately 20° to 30° medially and approximately 15° cephalad, guided by the superior and medial surface of the C2 isthmus. Once drilled, the integrity of the pilot hole is verified with a blunt probe. The hole is tapped, and a 3.5-mm screw of appropriated length is inserted through both cortices. The screw position is confirmed with biplanar fluoroscopy. Once the screws have been inserted bilaterally, a reduction maneuver may be performed by repositioning the head or by direct manipulation of the C1 and C2 screws. Three-millimeter rods are then placed into the screws and secured with the appropriate locking nuts to maintain alignment. The placement of the screws and rods is illustrated in **Figure 4**. The posterior surface of the C1 ring and the C2 lamina are decorticated and cancellous bone taken from the iliac crest is placed in the prepared fusion bed. An intra-articular fusion may also be performed by removing the cartilage and subchondral bone of the C1-C2 joints as described previously.

Results of Treatment

Results of Magerl's C1-C2 transarticular screw fixation technique have been excellent. Twelve of 12 patients with an acute odontoid fracture obtained a solid arthrodesis.[25] Others have shown lesser rates of union with the Brooks and Gallie techniques.[2,14] McGraw and Rusch,[30] in detailing Gallie's method of posterior C1-C2 fusion, reported 1 nonunion in 15 patients. Fielding et al[2] reported that Gallie fusions resulted in nonunion in 1 of 46 patients. Schatzker et al[53] and others[38] fared worse when treating 15 patients with odontoid fractures operatively with a Gallie-type procedure: 2 of the 15 fusions failed. Brooks and Jenkins[32] reported 13 of 14 successful fusions with their wedge compression technique of C1-C2 sublaminar wiring. Griswold et al[54] improved on this by modifying the Brooks method by using four sublaminar wires and double-twisting them. They believed that the added stability was a major factor in promoting solid fusion in 28 of 29 patients.

The use of posterior interlaminar clamps for C1-C2 fixation was first described in 1982 by Roosen et al[55] and later expounded on by Grob et al.[36] The clinical stability and the ability of this technique to promote union are not yet well established. Furthermore, the technique requires intact posterior arches of C1 and C2 for fixation points, and has another disadvantage of being bulky enough that less surface area in the decorticated bed of C1 and C2 is available on which to place bone graft.

Biomechanical studies have shown that the transarticular screw fixation technique provides significantly higher stiffness than the Gallie or Brooks techniques.[2,14,19,21] The main advantage of the transarticular screw fixation technique is not to make the Gallie fixation unnecessary (since a posterior arthrodesis is always added anyway), but to prevent postoperative translational movements that are responsible for the resubluxation seen with the Gallie and Brooks techniques, and to allow early mobilization without major external support. Actually, it is believed that the subsequent C1-C2 movement following the Brooks- or Gallie-type procedures (but before posterior fusion occurs) is the offending agent in producing nonunions of fusions. Posterior C1-C2 transarticular screw fixation is ideal for strongly stabilizing the articulation, thereby restricting movement and promoting solid fusion. On the other hand, both the Magerl-Gallie method and the direct polyaxial screw/rod construct (with little difference between the two) have been demonstrated to result in stability superior to that of two different wiring-only Gallie techniques.[56]

Results of Atlantoaxial Arthrodesis

Little has been written on the results of C1-C2 fusion specifically for the treatment of transverse ligament injuries, although many reports have been published on the results of atlantoaxial arthrodesis for other indications. Many of these studies combine arthrodesis performed for various conditions ranging from trauma to rheumatoid arthritis, os odontoideum, and congenital atlantoaxial instability. It is likely that the results of these studies can be extrapolated to the treatment of transverse ligament injuries.

Dickman et al[18] reported on the results of treatment of thirty-nine patients with incompetence of the transverse ligament secondary to trauma. They also proposed a classification system for these injuries to help guide treatment decisions (**Figure 1**). Sixteen of their patients had type I injuries (purely ligamentous), while the remaining had type II injuries (fractures that rendered the transverse ligament nonfunctional). Six of the type I injuries were treated with acute surgical intervention with varied techniques. The remaining nine type I injuries were initially managed with a cervical orthosis or halo vest and failed to obtain stability of C1-C2, and subsequently were treated with posterior arthrodesis. All patients with type I injuries were eventually treated surgically, and all went on to a solid arthrodesis. In contrast, all 23 patients with type II injuries were initially treated nonsurgically using a cervical orthosis (7) or halo brace (16). After an average of 13 weeks of treatment, only 26% of these patients had a nonunion with persistent atlantoaxial instability that required surgical treatment. The initial treatment method (cervical orthosis versus halo brace) did not correlate with the development of an unstable nonunion. Based on the results of this study, the authors concluded that disruptions of the substance of the transverse ligament (type I injuries) are incapable of healing and should be treated with early surgery for internal fixation. Surgery for internal fixation of type II injuries should be reserved for patients who develop nonunion with ongoing instability after a reasonable (12-week) trial of halo immobilization.

Biomechanical studies discussed previously have shown that transarticular screw fixation provides significantly higher stiffness when compared to posterior wiring techniques.[36,37,41,42] The main advantage of transarticular screws is not to eliminate the need for posterior wiring and bone grafting (this is usually included in the fixation), but to decrease the postoperative translational motion that is likely to be responsible for recurrent subluxation when posterior wiring is used alone. This motion is also thought to play an important role in the development of nonunion with posterior wiring techniques. The rate of nonunion in most clinical series ranges from 10% to 30%.[2,53,54,57-65] The strength of transarticular screws also affords enough stability to allow early mobilization without the use of rigid postoperative immobilization in the form of a halo.

Subsequent to the description of the technique for transarticular screw placement and the widespread acceptance of the surgical technique, most clinical series have focused on the results of Magerl screw fixation combined with posterior wiring and bone grafting. The clinical and radiographic outcomes of posterior cervical wiring techniques and transarticular screw fixation were reported by Reilly et al.[66] Indications for surgical intervention included odontoid fracture (acute and nonunion), atlantoaxial instability secondary to rheumatoid arthritis, os odontoideum, and tumor. Of those treated with posterior C1-C2 wiring, 71% obtained a solid fusion, compared with 94% of those treated with transarticular screw fixation; this result was statistically significant. The outcome scores of those patients treated with posterior wiring were also significantly worse than those treated with transarticular screws. Complications were also more frequent in the posterior wiring patients, and were frequently related to halo-vest immobilization. The authors concluded that use of posterior C1-C2 transarticular screws, with supplemental C1-C2 wiring, yields a significantly higher fusion and success rate when compared with traditional posterior wiring methods, even when the patients treated with the latter method are immobilized in a halo vest. These higher fusion rates occur without the use of rigid external immobilization, avoid halo-related complications, and yield a significantly decreased reoperation rate.

Dickman and Sonntag[18,33] reported their experiences in treating 121 patients with transarticular screws for atlantoaxial fixation. Atlantoaxial instability was caused by rheumatoid arthritis, C1 or C2 fractures, transverse ligament disruption, os odontoideum, tumor, and infection. Thirteen patients were found to have anomalous vertebral artery anatomy that precluded the insertion of bilateral transarticular screws. These patients were treated with unilateral screw fixation combined with posterior wiring. Of the 226 screws placed, 221 (98%) were positioned satisfactorily while the 5 malpositioned screws did not result in any adverse clinical events. No neurologic complications occurred. After a mean follow-up period of 22 months, 98% of these patients demonstrated a solid arthrodesis. The remaining two patients required occipitocervical fusion to treat the nonunion.

In their original description of the technique for posterior screw/rod fixation, Harms and Melcher[52] also included the results of 37 patients treated with this technique. Indications for atlantoaxial arthrodesis included fracture, os odontoideum, rheumatoid arthritis, rotatory subluxation, osteoarthritis, and congenital malformation. Satisfactory screw placement and reduction were achieved in all patients. No instances of neurologic deterioration or vertebral artery injury were reported. Patients were immobilized in a soft collar postoperatively. At final follow-up, no implant failures were identified and all patients demonstrated evidence of solid arthrodesis on radiographs. This direct screw fixation technique has advantages over transarticular screws, including a lower risk of injury to the vertebral artery because of the specific trajectory of the C2 pedicle screw; individual polyaxial screw placement in C1 and C2 allows for direct manipulation of C1 and C2, therefore simplifying the reduction maneuver and fixation; the integrity of the posterior arch of C1 is not mandatory for stable fixation; and the instrumentation can be incorporated as part of a modular system for occipitocervical fusions. These advantages have been recognized by many spine surgeons and this technique has gained popularity and become the preferred method of C1-C2 fixation for a wide variety of conditions.

References

1. Steel HH: Anatomical and mechanical considerations of the atlanto-axial articulations. *J Bone Joint Surg Am* 1968;50:1481-1482.
2. Fielding JW, Hawkins RJ, Ratzan SA: Spine fusion for atlanto-axial instability. *J Bone Joint Surg Am* 1976;58(3):400-407.
3. Panjabi MM, Dvorák J, Crisco J, Oda T, Grob D: Instability in injury of the alar ligament: A biomechanical model. *Orthopade* 1991;20(2):112-120.
4. Spence KF Jr, Decker S, Sell KW: Bursting atlantal fracture associated with rupture of the transverse ligament. *J Bone Joint Surg Am* 1970;52(3): 543-549.
5. Fielding JW, Cochran GB, Lawsing JF III, Hohl M: Tears of the transverse ligament of the atlas: A clinical and biomechanical study. *J Bone Joint Surg Am* 1974;56(8):1683-1691.
6. Jackson H: The diagnosis of minimal atlanto-axial subluxation. *Br J Radiol* 1950;23(275):672-674.
7. Fielding JW: Normal and selected abnormal motion of the cervical spine from the second cervical vertebra to the seventh cervical vertebra based on cineroentgenography. *J Bone Joint Surg Am* 1964; 46:1779-1781.
8. Weissman BN, Aliabadi P, Weinfeld MS, Thomas WH, Sosman JL: Prognostic features of atlantoaxial subluxation in rheumatoid arthritis patients. *Radiology* 1982;144(4):745-751.
9. Wackenheim A: Occipitalization of the ventral part and vertebralization of the dorsal part of the atlas with insufficiency of the transverse ligament. *Neuroradiology* 1982;24(1):45-47.
10. Bharucha EP, Dastur HM: Craniovertebral anomalies (a report of 40 cases). *Brain* 1964;87: 469-480.
11. McRae DL: Bony abnormalities in the region of the foramen magnum: Correlation of the ana-

tomic and neurologic findings. *Acta Radiol* 1953; 40(2-3):335-354.

12. McRae DL, Barnum AS: Occipitalization of the atlas. *Am J Roentgenol Radium Ther Nucl Med* 1953;70(1):23-46.
13. McRae DL: The significance of abnormalities of the cervical spine. *Am J Roentgenol Rad Ther Nucl Med* 1960;84:3-25.
14. Greenberg AD: Atlanto-axial dislocations. *Brain* 1968;91(4):655-684.
15. Martel W, Tishler JM: Observations on the spine in mongoloidism. *Am J Roentgenol Radium Ther Nucl Med* 1966;97(3):630-638.
16. Dzenitis AJ: Spontaneous atlanto-axial dislocation in a mongoloid child with spinal cord compression: Case report. *J Neurosurg* 1966;25(4): 458-460.
17. Curtis BH, Blank S, Fisher RL: Atlantoxial dislocation in Down's syndrome: Report of two patients requiring surgical correction. *JAMA* 1968;205(6): 464-465.
18. Dickman CA, Greene KA, Sonntag VK: Injuries involving the transverse atlantal ligament: Classification and treatment guidelines based upon experience with 39 injuries. *Neurosurgery* 1996;38(1): 44-50.
19. Dunbar HS, Ray BS: Chronic atlanto-axial dislocations with late neurologic manifestations. *Surg Gynecol Obstet* 1961;113:757-762.
20. Krantz P: Isolated disruption of the transverse ligament of the atlas: An injury easily overlooked at post-mortem examination. *Injury* 1980;12(2): 168-170.
21. Wigren A, Sweden U, Amici F Jr: Traumatic atlanto-axial dislocation without neurological disorder: A case report. *J Bone Joint Surg Am* 1973; 55(3):642-644.
22. Pennecot GF, Leonard P, Peyrot Des Gachons S, Hardy JR, Pouliquen JC: Traumatic ligamentous instability of the cervical spine in children. *J Pediatr Orthop* 1984;4(3):339-345.
23. Fielding JW: Selected observations on the cervical spine in the child. *Curr Pract Orthop Surg* 1973;5: 31-55.
24. Highland TR, Aronson DD: Traumatic rupture of the cervical transverse ligament in a child with a normal odontoid process: A case report. *Spine (Phila Pa 1976)* 1986;11(1):73-75.
25. O'Brien JJ, Butterfield WL, Gossling HR: Jefferson fracture with disruption of the transverse ligament: A case report. *Clin Orthop Relat Res* 1977; 126:135-138.
26. Lipson SJ: Fractures of the atlas associated with fractures of the odontoid process and transverse ligament ruptures. *J Bone Joint Surg Am* 1977; 59(7):940-943.
27. Greene KA, Dickman CA, Marciano FF, Drabier J, Drayer BP, Sonntag VK: Transverse atlantal ligament disruption associated with odontoid fractures. *Spine (Phila Pa 1976)* 1994;19(20): 2307-2314.
28. Dickman CA, Mamourian A, Sonntag VK, Drayer BP: Magnetic resonance imaging of the transverse atlantal ligament for the evaluation of atlantoaxial instability. *J Neurosurg* 1991;75(2):221-227.
29. Simmons E: Alternatives in the surgical stabilization for the upper cervical spine, in Tator CH, ed: *Early Management of Acute Spinal Cord Injury*. New York, NY, Raven, 1982, pp 393-394.
30. McGraw RW, Rusch RM: Atlanto-axial arthrodesis. *J Bone Joint Surg Br* 1973;55(3):482-489.
31. Gallie W: Fractures and dislocations of the cervical spine. *Am J Surg* 1939;46:495-499.
32. Brooks AL, Jenkins EB: Atlanto-axial arthrodesis by the wedge compression method. *J Bone Joint Surg Am* 1978;60(3):279-284.
33. Sonntag VK, Dickman CA: Posterior atlantoaxial wiring techniques, in Dickman CA, Spetzler RF, Sonntag VKH, eds: *Surgery of the Craniovertebral Junction*. New York, NY, Thieme, 1997, pp 783-794.
34. Dickman CA, Crawford NR, Paramore CG: Biomechanical characteristics of C1-2 cable fixations. *J Neurosurg* 1996;85(2):316-322.
35. Crisco JJ III, Panjabi MM, Oda T, Grob D, Dvorak J: Bone graft translation of four upper cervical spine fixation techniques in a cadaveric model. *J Orthop Res* 1991;9(6):835-846.
36. Grob D, Crisco JJ III, Panjabi MM, Wang P, Dvorak J: Biomechanical evaluation of four different posterior atlantoaxial fixation techniques. *Spine (Phila Pa 1976)* 1992;17(5):480-490.
37. Naderi S, Crawford NR, Song GS, Sonntag VK, Dickman CA: Biomechanical comparison of C1-C2 posterior fixations: Cable, graft, and screw combinations. *Spine (Phila Pa 1976)* 1998;23(18): 1946-1956.
38. Magerl F, Seemann PS: Stable posterior fusion of the atlas and axis by transarticular screw fixation, in Kehr P, Weidner A, eds: *Cervical Spine*. New York, NY, Springer-Verlag, 1986, vol 1, pp 322-327.
39. Jeanneret B, Magerl F: Primary posterior fusion C1/2 in odontoid fractures: Indications, technique, and results of transarticular screw fixation. *J Spinal Disord* 1992;5(4):464-475.
40. Grob D, Magerl F: Surgical stabilization of C1 and C2 fractures. *Orthopade* 1987;16(1):46-54.
41. Hajek PD, Lipka J, Hartline P, Saha S, Albright JA: Biomechanical study of C1-C2 posterior arthrodesis techniques. *Spine (Phila Pa 1976)* 1993; 18(2):173-177.

42. Hanson PB, Montesano PX, Sharkey NA, Rauschning W: Anatomic and biomechanical assessment of transarticular screw fixation for atlantoaxial instability. *Spine (Phila Pa 1976)* 1991; 16(10):1141-1145.
43. Hanley EN Jr, Harvell JC Jr: Immediate postoperative stability of the atlantoaxial articulation: A biomechanical study comparing simple midline wiring, and the Gallie and Brooks procedures. *J Spinal Disord* 1992;5(3):306-310.
44. Henriques T, Cunningham BW, Olerud C, et al: Biomechanical comparison of five different atlantoaxial posterior fixation techniques. *Spine (Phila Pa 1976)* 2000;25(22):2877-2883.
45. Kandziora F, Kerschbaumer F, Starker M, Mittlmeier T: Biomechanical assessment of transoral plate fixation for atlantoaxial instability. *Spine (Phila Pa 1976)* 2000;25(12):1555-1561.
46. Wright NM, Lauryssen C, American Association of Neurological Surgeons/Congress of Neurological Surgeons: Vertebral artery injury in C1-2 transarticular screw fixation: Results of a survey of the AANS/CNS section on disorders of the spine and peripheral nerves. *J Neurosurg* 1998;88(4): 634-640.
47. Madawi AA, Casey AT, Solanki GA, Tuite G, Veres R, Crockard HA: Radiological and anatomical evaluation of the atlantoaxial transarticular screw fixation technique. *J Neurosurg* 1997;86(6): 961-968.
48. Farey ID, Nadkarni S, Smith N: Modified Gallie technique versus transarticular screw fixation in C1-C2 fusion. *Clin Orthop Relat Res* 1999;359: 126-135.
49. Coric D, Branch CL Jr, Wilson JA, Robinson JC: Arteriovenous fistula as a complication of C1-2 transarticular screw fixation: Case report and review of the literature. *J Neurosurg* 1996;85(2): 340-343.
50. Campanelli M, Kattner KA, Stroink A, Gupta K, West S: Posterior C1-C2 transarticular screw fixation in the treatment of displaced type II odontoid fractures in the geriatric population—review of seven cases. *Surg Neurol* 1999;51(6):596-601.
51. Abou Madawi A, Solanki G, Casey AT, Crockard HA: Variation of the groove in the axis vertebra for the vertebral artery: Implications for instrumentation. *J Bone Joint Surg Br* 1997;79(5): 820-823.
52. Harms J, Melcher RP: Posterior C1-C2 fusion with polyaxial screw and rod fixation. *Spine (Phila Pa 1976)* 2001;26(22):2467-2471.
53. Schatzker J, Rorabeck CH, Waddell JP: Fractures of the dens (odontoid process): An analysis of thirty-seven cases. *J Bone Joint Surg Br* 1971;53(3): 392-405.
54. Griswold DM, Albright JA, Schiffman E, Johnson R, Southwick W: Atlanto-axial fusion for instability. *J Bone Joint Surg Am* 1978;60(3):285-292.
55. Roosen K, Trauschel A, Grote W: Posterior atlanto-axial fusion: A new compression clamp for laminar osteosynthesis. *Arch Orthop Trauma Surg* 1972;100(1):27-31.
56. Melcher RP, Puttlitz CM, Kleinstueck FS, Lotz JC, Harms J, Bradford DS: Biomechanical testing of posterior atlantoaxial fixation techniques. *Spine (Phila Pa 1976)* 2002;27(22):2435-2440.
57. Anderson LD, D'Alonzo RT: Fractures of the odontoid process of the axis. *J Bone Joint Surg Am* 1974;56(8):1663-1674.
58. Conaty JP, Mongan ES: Cervical fusion in rheumatoid arthritis. *J Bone Joint Surg Am* 1981;63(8): 1218-1227.
59. Dickman CA, Sonntag VK, Papadopoulos SM, Hadley MN: The interspinous method of posterior atlantoaxial arthrodesis. *J Neurosurg* 1991;74(2): 190-198.
60. Ferlic DC, Clayton ML, Leidholt JD, Gamble WE: Surgical treatment of the symptomatic unstable cervical spine in rheumatoid arthritis. *J Bone Joint Surg Am* 1975;57(3):349-354.
61. Fielding JW, Hensinger RN, Hawkins RJ: Os Odontoideum. *J Bone Joint Surg Am* 1980;62(3): 376-383.
62. Glynn MK, Sheehan JM: Fusion of the cervical spine for instability. *Clin Orthop Relat Res* 1983; 179:97-101.
63. Husby J, Sorensen KH: Fracture of the odontoid process of the axis. *Acta Orthop Scand* 1974;45(2): 182-192.
64. Paradis GR, Janes JM: Posttraumatic atlantoaxial instability: The fate of the odontoid process fracture in 46 cases. *J Trauma* 1973;13(4):359-367.
65. Ranawat CS, O'Leary P, Pellicci P, Tsairis P, Marchisello P, Dorr L: Cervical spine fusion in rheumatoid arthritis. *J Bone Joint Surg Am* 1979; 61(7):1003-1010.
66. Reilly TM, Sasso RC, Hall PV: Atlantoaxial stabilization: Clinical comparison of posterior cervical wiring technique with transarticular screw fixation. *J Spinal Disord Tech* 2003;16(3):248-253.

CHAPTER 24

Traumatic Spondylolisthesis of the Axis (Hangman's Fracture)

Kris Radcliff, MD Joseph L. Ferguson, DPT, BS Luciano Miller Reis Rodriques, MD
Jordan Gruskay, BA Alan M. Levine, MD Todd Albert, MD
Alexander R. Vaccaro, MD, PhD

Introduction

Bipedicular or pars interarticularis fractures of the second cervical vertebra have intrigued both anatomists and physicians for well over 1,000 years. The first time that this entity was actually presented in the medical literature was by Rev. Samuel Haughton[1] to describe the fracture-dislocation that occurred with execution by judicial hanging. This particular fracture of the pars interarticularis of the neural arch of C2 has been labeled by many terms—from traumatic spondylolisthesis of the axis,[2-6] to fracture of the axis arch,[7] fracture of the ring of the axis,[8] fracture of the neural arch,[9] and hangman's fracture.[5,10-16] Although there was initially considerable confusion about the mechanisms of these fractures, recent findings have allowed these mechanisms to be more clearly differentiated, leading to the conclusion that the injury resulting from judicial hanging, although similar in bony anatomy to the fracture occurring as a result of motor vehicle accidents, is mechanically a different injury.

As a result of vehicular trauma, a radiographically similar but functionally dissimilar injury to the second cervical vertebra occurs in the same region. The current term, *traumatic spondylolisthesis of the axis*, which is intended to distinguish this injury from a true hangman's fracture, was ascribed to Garber[17] in his 1964 article, but some (eg, Schneider et al[13] in 1965 and Tuite et al[18] as late as 1992) have continued to use the more colorful term "hangman's fracture" to describe the motor vehicle traumatic lesion as opposed to the lesion of judicial injury.

Anatomy and Pathophysiology

The anatomic features of the second cervical vertebra (axis) are distinct from the subaxial vertebrae, the atlas, and the occiput. Most commonly, injuries to the anterior portion of second cervical

Dr. Levine is deceased. At the time this chapter was written Dr. Levine or an immediate family member had received royalties from Elsevier and US Spine; was a member of a speakers' bureau or had made paid presentations on behalf of Accuray; served as a paid consultant to or was an employee of US Spine; and had received research or institutional support from Accuray, Amgen Co., and Medtronic Sofamor Danek. Dr. Albert or an immediate family member serves as a board member, owner, officer, or committee member of American Academy of Orthopaedic Surgeons, the American Orthopaedic Association, the Cervical Spine Research Society, the Council for Value in Spine Care, and the Scoliosis Research Society; has received royalties from DePuy, a Johnson & Johnson company; serves as a paid consultant to or is an employee of DePuy, a Johnson & Johnson company; owns stock or stock options in Bioassets, Biomerix, Breakaway Imaging, Crosstree, Gentis, International Orthopaedic Alliance, Invuity, Paradigm Spine, Pioneer, Reville Consortium, and Vertech; and has received nonincome support (such as equipment or services), commercially derived honoraria, or other non-research-related funding (such as paid travel) from United Healthcare. Dr. Vaccaro or an immediate family member serves as a board member, owner, officer, or committee member of the North American Spine Society, American Spinal Injury Association, and the Cervical Spine Research Society; has received royalties from Aesculap/B.Braun, DePuy, a Johnson & Johnson company, Globus Medical, Medtronic Sofamor Danek, K2M, Stout Medical, Progressive Spinal Technology, and Applied Spinal Intellectual Properties; serves as a paid consultant to or is an employee of K2M; has received research or institutional support from AO North America, DePuy, a Johnson & Johnson company, Medtronic Sofamor Danek, and Stryker; and owns stock or stock options in Globus Medical, Disk Motion Technology, Progressive Spinal Technologies, Advanced Spinal Intellectual Properties, Computational Biodynamics, Stout Medical, Paradigm Spine, K2M, Replication Medica, Spinology, Spine Medica, Orthovita, Vertiflex, Small Bone Technologies, NeuCore, Crosscurrent, Syndicom, In Vivo, Flagship Surgical, Pearl Driver, Location Based Intelligence, and Gamma Spine. None of the following authors or any immediate family member has received anything of value from or owns stock in a commercial company or institution related directly or indirectly to the subject of this chapter: Dr. Radcliff, Mr. Ferguson, Dr. Miller Reis Rodrigues, and Mr. Gruskay.

vertebra are thought to be included in the functional area known as the *upper cervical spine*, whereas injuries to the C2-C3 facet joint have characteristics more similar to injuries of the lower cervical spine.

The structure of the axis is both biomechanically and developmentally unique, distinguishing itself from other vertebrae by the presence of the dens process. The dens process results from a fusion of the axis with the remnant of the vertebral body of the atlas. C2 functions as a transitional region between the upper and the lower portions of the cervical spine due to the position of the two sets of facet joints of the axis. The superior facet joints of C2 lie anterior and lateral to the neural canal in line with the C1-C2 and occipitocervical articulations. The C2 inferior facets lie posterior and lateral to the canal parallel to the facet joints of the lower cervical spine. Therefore, the two sets of C2 joints are functionally and anatomically separated in terms of alignment and motion. The pars interarticularis of C2 experiences significant bending forces due to the spatial separation of load-bearing facets. Because the pars of C2 is a relatively narrow cortical bone with little medullary cavity space, and thus a small cross-sectional area, it is one of the weakest portions of the upper cervical spine. Due to the unique nature of C2, terminology related to the pars interarticularis and pedicles can be confusing in the literature. The pedicles of C2 lie inferior to the superior articular facets and anteromedial to the transverse foramen, while the pars interarticularis is between the superior and inferior articular facets. In addition, the foramen transversarium, through which the vertebral artery passes in the body of C2, is adjacent to the pars.

The C1 and C2 vertebrae are connected by the anterior longitudinal ligament and the strong capsular attachments of the facet joints at the atlantoaxial joint. In addition, C2 is attached directly to the base of the skull and to the ring of C1 by the alar, transverse, and apical ligaments. The joints of the C1-C2 complex are highly congruent, and the joint capsules may be important secondary stabilizers of the craniocervical junction. In particular, the lateral joint height of the C1-C2 joints should not exceed 1.2 mm on a coronal CT scan.[19] This whole complex, including the base of the skull, the atlas, the dens process, and the body of the axis, forms a unique unit referred to as the *upper cervical spine* or the *cervicocranium*.[13] This unique structure, as well as the transitional nature of the vertebra, imparts significant force to the pars interarticularis between the superior and inferior facets of C2 by the entire complex above it. The occipitocervical joint permits only flexion and extension, whereas the atlantoaxial joint allows flexion, extension, rotation, and vertical approximation as well as lateral gliding.[20] Some of these are coupled motions. As a result of the saddle shape of the joint, the atlantoaxial joint's primary motion is rotation. Approximately 50% of the total rotation of the cervical spine occurs at the atlantoaxial joint,[21] with the remainder occurring in the lower cervical spine. Interestingly, the C2-C3 joint exhibits very little motion as compared with that of C1-C2 or even the lower cervical facets. The canal-to-cord ratio is extremely large in the upper cervical spine. The ratio changes at the C2-C3 articulation. At the level of the axis, approximately one-third of the anterior-posterior diameter of the canal is occupied by the dens process, approximately one-third by the cord, and one third is open space.

Several anatomic features of the upper cervical spine, and especially of the C2 vertebral body, seem to predispose this region to injury. First, because the cervicocranium is a mechanically stable complex held together by strong ligamentous attachments, it can bring a significant force to bear on the pars interarticularis or pedicles of C2, which are isolated between the axis of the facets of the upper cervical spine and the facets of the lower cervical spine. The spatial orientation accounts for the position of the fractures that occur in this location. The foramen transversarium is another weak spot in the ring for rotatory injuries and is the location of many atypical hangman's fractures just adjacent to that area. Finally, because of the canal-expanding nature of the fracture and the large canal diameter, fractures through the axis rarely result in neurologic injuries.

Classification and Mechanism of Injury

Several different classification systems have been used for traumatic spondylolisthesis of the axis resulting from trauma to the upper cervical spine. The three types of classification are based on the following: (1) anatomic and/or radiographic characteristics, (2) instability mechanisms, and (3) mechanisms of injury.

Anatomic and radiographic classifications have been proposed based on the work of Francis et al[3] and co-application of the well-established characteristics of White and Panjabi[22] for instability in the lower cervical spine (3.5 mm of translation and 11° of angulation). However, this assessment

FIGURE 1

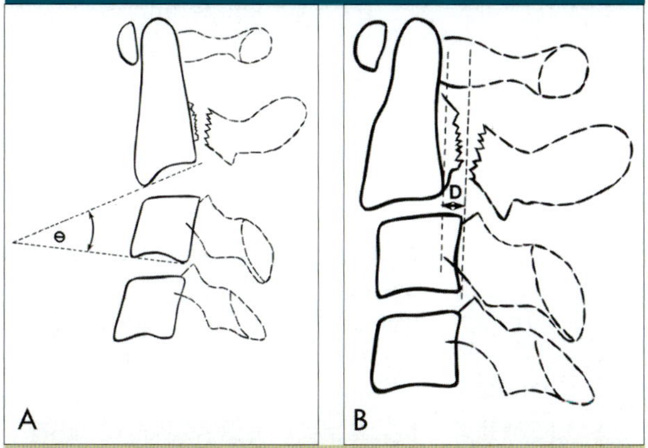

Figure 1 Traumatic spondylolisthesis of the axis is characterized by angulation and translation. The angulation is measured as in **A** and the translation as in **B**. (Reproduced with permission from Levine AM, Edwards CC: Traumatic spondylolisthesis of the axis. *J Bone Joint Surg Am* 1985; 67(2):217-226.)

FIGURE 2

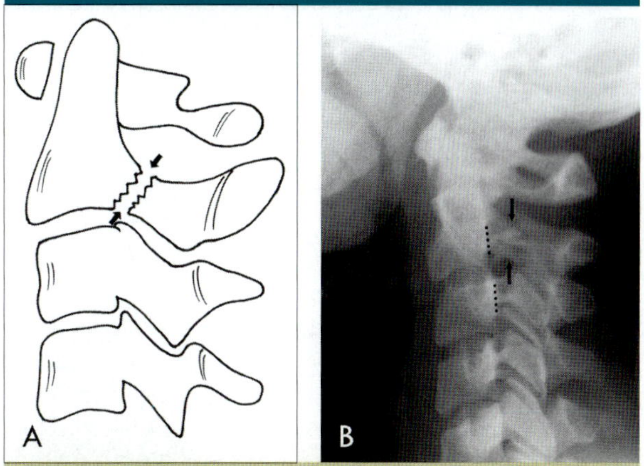

Figure 2 Traumatic spondylolisthesis of the axis can be characterized by the amount of translation and angulation at the fracture site. A type I injury has a fracture through the pedicles of C2 just posterior to the junction of the body and the pedicles and, as noted in the drawing (**A**), the fracture line is either vertical or slightly off vertical (arrows). **B,** It is characterized by minimal translation (≤3 mm) (dotted lines) and essentially no angulation, as shown in the radiograph. (Reproduced from Levine AM: Traumatic spondylolisthesis of the axis [hangman's fracture], in Levine AM, Eismont FJ, Garfin SR, Zigler JE, eds: *Spine Trauma*. Philadelphia, PA, WB Saunders, 1998, pp 278-299.)

does not include neurologic injury or facet status. Additionally, this classification is based on the concept of instability defined as disruption of the anterior elements, which is not relevant to this location and injury subtype.

The most commonly used classification of hangman's fractures is one originally put forth by Effendi et al[8] that was later modified by Levine and Edwards,[4] which allows an understanding of the pathomechanics of the injury and establishes a treatment regimen. The classification is based on defining the amount of deformity between C2 and C3 quantified by angulation and translation. Angulation is measured by angles determined between the inferior end plate of the second cervical vertebra and that of the third cervical vertebra (**Figure 1,** *A*), whereas translation is measured as the distance parallel to the posterior margin of the third cervical vertebra and the posterior margin of the second cervical vertebra at the level of the C2-3 disk space (**Figure 1,** *B*).

Four types of injuries were defined originally,[23] with a fifth type recently included.[24] Type I fractures (fractures through the neural arch at the base of the pedicle) demonstrate less than 3 mm of translation and no angulation at the fracture site. Bilateral fractures occur at the same level in the neural arch at the junction of the body and pedicle in the coronal plane. Type I fractures typically result from a hyperextension and axial load injury,[22] with forces sufficient to fracture the neural arch. Notably, this mechanism does not result in any significant injury to the disk, anterior longitudinal ligament, or posterior longitudinal ligaments. It therefore does not have any angulatory or severe translational instability greater than 3 mm. These fractures are also characterized by absence of deformation of the anterosuperior portion of the C3 body (**Figure 2**). Furthermore, the fracture line is clearly evident on a lateral radiograph. Both fracture lines characteristically lie superimposed and parallel, and a 1- or 2-mm gap is often apparent at the body-pedicle junction.

"Atypical" hangman's fractures are termed type IA traumatic spondylolisthesis of the axis. In contrast to type I fractures, these fracture lines occur at different locations on the C2 arch, usually with one in the vertebral body of C2 with the neural arch spared on that side, and the other on the opposite side, more posterior in the neural arch but generally not at the body-pedicle junction (**Figure 3**). In this injury, the fractures are not visible on lateral films. Because this is a type I injury, there is minimal angulation and translation of the fracture fragments. On radiographic evaluation, there appears to be an elongation of the pars interarticularis and pedicles of C2. The anterior aspect of the C2-C3 articulation appears to be 2 mm to 3 mm anteriorly translated. However, the posterior aspect of the C2-C3 body may appear to

FIGURE 3

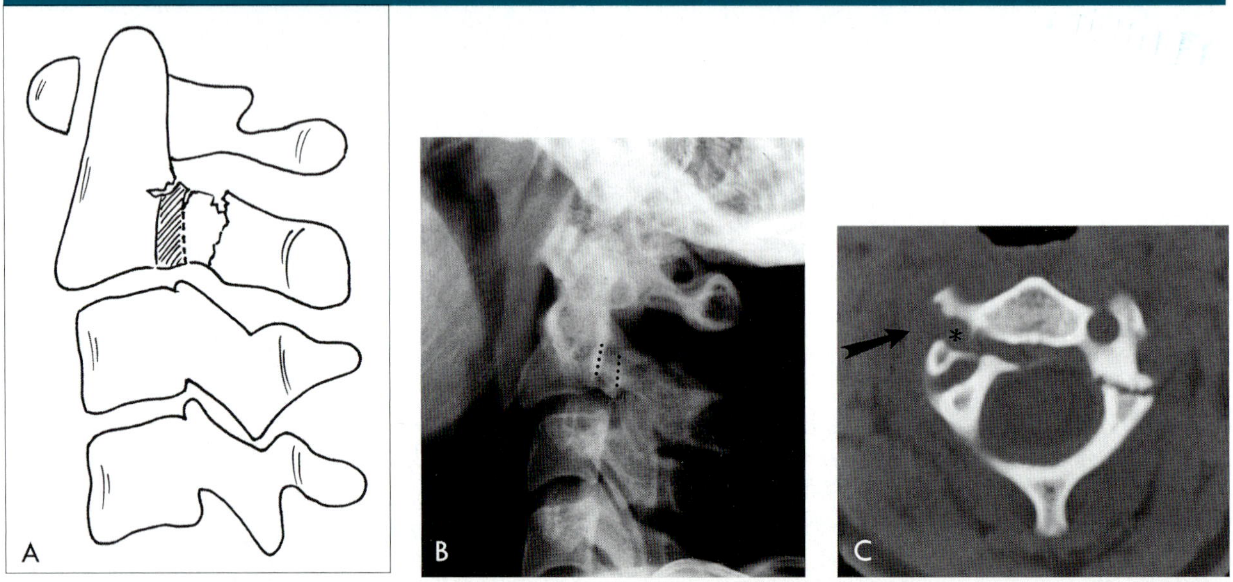

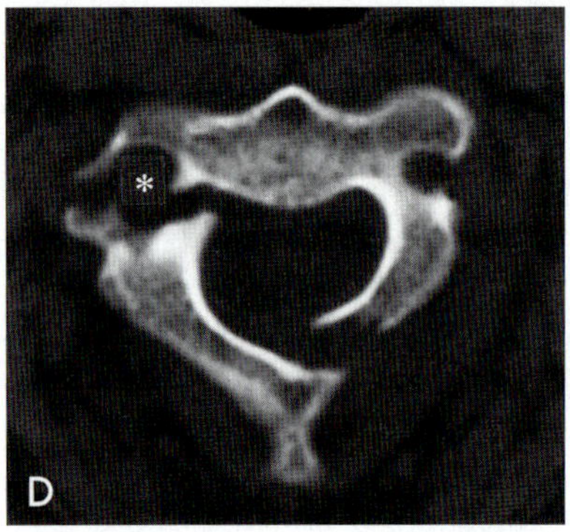

Figure 3 A, The drawing of the atypical or type IA fracture demonstrates the most typical deformity, in which the posterior part of the body appears elongated with minimal angulation and translation. **B,** The lateral radiograph of the cervical spine demonstrates that in this type of fracture, the fracture line is poorly appreciated because of its obliquity. The body of C2 appears to be enlarged but is actually rotated (dotted lines). There is minimal translation. **C,** However, on the CT scan, the oblique nature of the fracture is seen. The fracture line goes through the body on one side and may traverse the foramen for the vertebral artery (asterisk). On the contralateral side it goes more posteriorly through the arch of the axis. It may even pass through the lamina or spinous process (**D**) on the contralateral side. (Reproduced from Levine AM: Traumatic spondylolisthesis of the axis [hangman's fracture], in Levine AM, Eismont FJ, Garfin SR, Zigler JE, eds: *Spine Trauma.* Philadelphia, PA, WB Saunders, 1998, pp 278-299.)

align. In addition, no clear gap or superimposed vertical fracture lines are visible, as they are in a type I injury. In both type I and II injuries, the fracture lines can be clearly defined, especially on a lateral radiograph, without a CT scan. However, in type IA injuries, the fracture lines cannot be identified without a CT scan (**Figure 4**). In a percentage of these patients, the fracture line goes through the foramen transversarium, which may endanger the vertebral artery. The majority of flexion-extension radiographs, which are not recommended in the acute setting, show minimal instability, although in one series, two of the injuries with this radiographic pattern were noted to have more angulation and translation with flexion.[24] The injury mechanism is most probably hyperextension, with an element of lateral bending to yield the asymmetric fracture pattern.

Type II injuries are considered unstable and are subdivided into two separate groups: type II and IIA.[22] Type II injuries are characterized by translation greater than 3 mm and angulation at the fracture site. The degree of translation and angulation seen on the initial radiograph is highly variable and is partially based on the severity of force of injury, the degree of initial displacement, and any reduction maneuvers that have been undertaken. A type II fracture can appear to be a type I fracture on a supine radiograph. As a result of the extension of the neck in that position, the fracture will reduce almost entirely. This is especially true in extremely obese or large-shouldered patients, which results in a relative extension of the neck compared to the head. On careful initial inspection of the screening lateral radiograph, patients almost always demonstrate a compression of the anterosuperior portion of the C3 body (**Figure 5**). Type II injuries (as distinct from the type IIA injuries) are the result of a sequence of forces that commonly occur in vehicular trauma. The initial injurious force is a hyperextension and axial loading force that is sufficient to fracture the neural

FIGURE 4

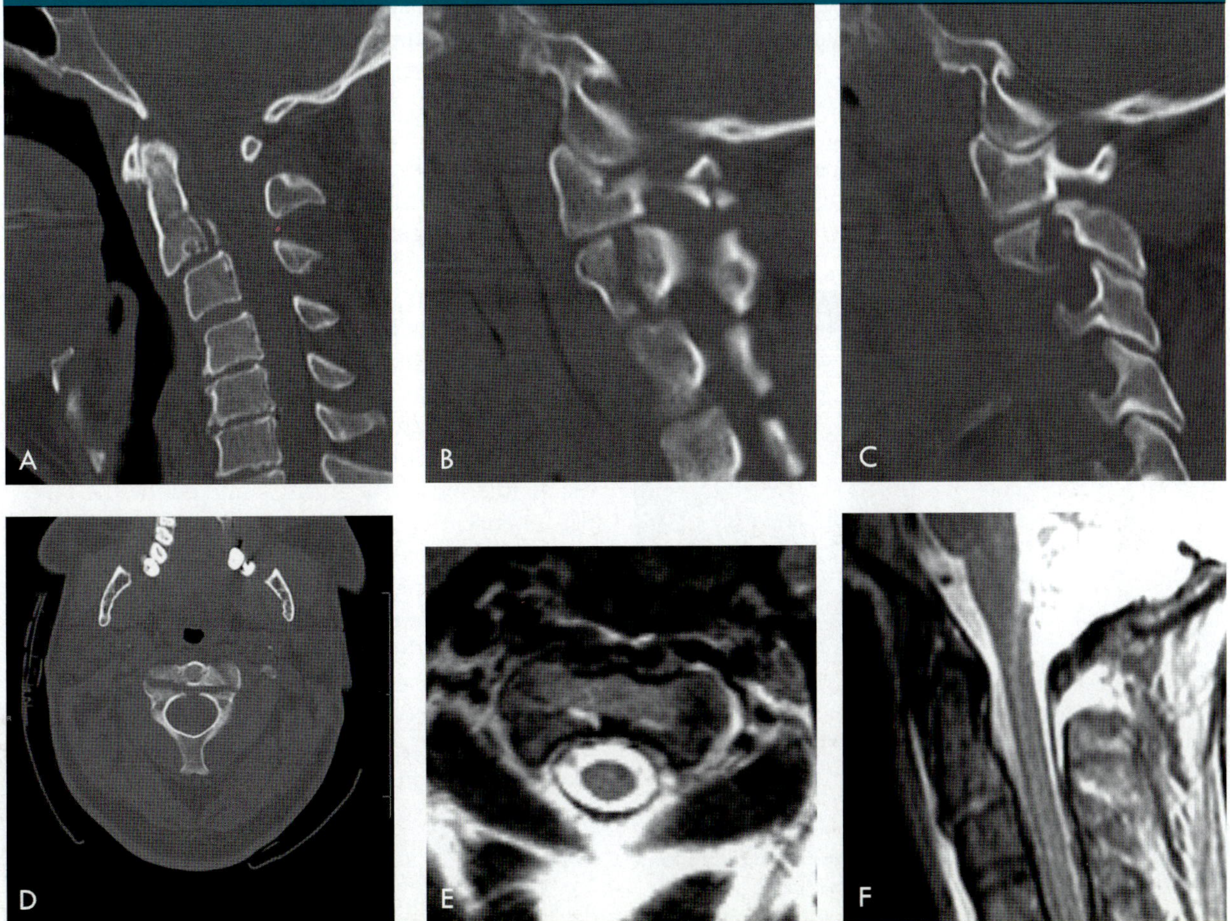

Figure 4 Midsagittal (**A**), parasagittal (**B** and **C**), and axial (**D**) CT images demonstrate an atypical type IA hangman's fracture. The fracture lines are asymmetric with the right fracture line anterior to the left fracture line. Magnetic resonance images in the axial (**E**) and sagittal (**F**) planes demonstrate no spinal cord compression and minimal disk disruption. This patient was neurologically intact and was managed nonsurgically. The fracture lines traverse the right foramen transversarium and therefore a work-up of vertebral artery injury was performed.

arch in a pattern similar to that seen in type I injuries. The fracture lines are usually vertical, fairly close to the body-pedicle junction, and in the coronal plane. A second force causes hyperflexion of the neck after initial disruption of the neural arch. This allows disruption of the C2-C3 disk with compression of the anterosuperior portion of the C3 body by the C2 body. Often, the anterior longitudinal ligament is stripped off the superior 33% to 50% of the front of the C3 body. In the majority of cases, however, the stripping does not disrupt the ligament function, which remains intact. The combined mechanism of hyperextension followed by flexion is frequently a result of the deceleration-acceleration forces in vehicular trauma from a head-on collision. Therefore, unlike a type I fracture, in which the injury is predominantly a bone injury, the instability portion of the type II hangman's fracture is ligamentous, with disruption of the posterior longitudinal ligament and the anulus of the disk. The disruption of the disk occurs in a posterior to anterior direction, with axial compression preserving the anterior longitudinal ligament but resulting in translation and angulation at a fracture site (**Figure 6**). Previously, it was suggested that the mechanism of injury in a type II fracture was that of continued hyperextension after the initial injury. However, the fracture patterns and results of treatment seem to indicate otherwise. Current treatment methods involve the application of longitudinal traction and extension to severely displaced type II injuries. In the majority of patients with type II injuries with 8 mm to 10 mm of displacement, the anterior longitudinal ligament remains intact, allowing application of 30 lb to 40 lb of longitudinal traction to achieve reduction of a deformity without widening the disk space. The majority of the type II injuries are clearly the result of hyperextension followed by flexion, and therefore the deformity, not the fracture, is the result of the flexion component of the injury. As is seen in clinical practice, the deformity is reduced by application of extension and longitudinal traction.

FIGURE 5

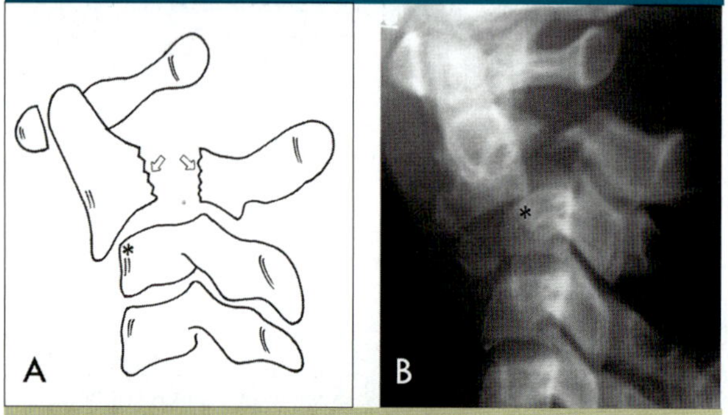

Figure 5 Type II injuries are the result of a hyperextension axial load, which breaks the neural arch, followed by a flexion injury, which results in significant translation. The pattern of the fracture line is similar to that seen with a type I injury. In both the drawing (**A**) and the radiograph (**B**), the fracture line is relatively vertical with wide separation of the fragments (arrows). These are characterized by more than 3 mm of translation and significant angulation as well. They frequently demonstrate a compression of the anterosuperior corner of the body of C3 as a result of the flexion force that caused the anterior translation (asterisk). In this case, avulsion of the anterosuperior corner of the body has occurred. (Reproduced from Levine AM: Traumatic spondylolisthesis of the axis [hangman's fracture], in Levine AM, Eismont FJ, Garfin SR, Zigler JE, eds: *Spine Trauma*. Philadelphia, PA, WB Saunders, 1998, pp 278-299.)

Type IIA injuries are characterized by significant angular deformity and minimal translation in relation to the degree of angular deformity. Angulation in this injury can exceed 15°, whereas translation rarely exceeds 2 mm or 3 mm. Another important differentiating feature on the initial screening radiographs is the position and angle of the fracture line. As previously noted, in type I (**Figure 2**) and II fractures (**Figure 5**), the fracture line is predominantly vertical and adjacent to the body-pedicle junction in the coronal plane. This differentiation is usually made on the basis of radiographic criteria before application of any cervical traction. As described previously, the ratio of angulation to translation, the absence of compression of the anterior portion of the C2 body, and the angulation of the fracture line define the type IIA fracture. Any injury in which 10 lb of traction causes disk-space widening is considered a type IIA fracture. Type IIA fractures are a small percentage (rarely more than 5%) of the larger group of traumatic spondylolistheses. The type IIA fracture line tends to be more oblique, running from anteroinferior to posterosuperior. Interlocking of the fragments may occur, as seen in **Figure 7**, keeping the fracture in an angulated position. Type IIA injuries are most probably the result of a flexion force resulting in failure of the neural arch in tension accompanied by rupture of the posterior aspect of the disk. This must be differentiated from the type II injury for several reasons. First, with the flexion-distraction mechanism of injury, the injury propagates from posterior to anterior along the disk, causing angulation without translation. Application of traction in this injury (because it has a distraction mechanism) will result in an increase in the deformity and widening of the disk

FIGURE 6

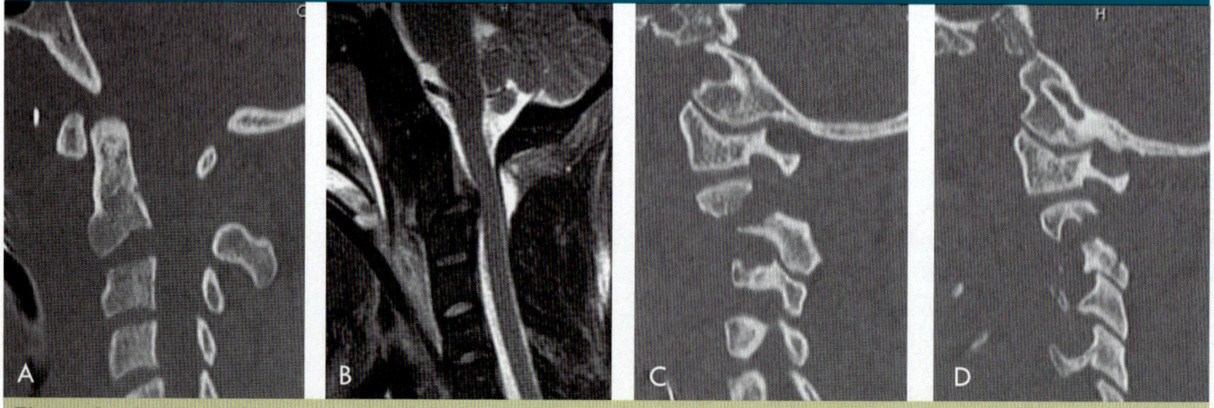

Figure 6 Midsagittal (**A**) and parasagittal (**B** and **C**) CT images demonstrate a displaced type II hangman's fracture. Midsagittal MRI scan (**D**) demonstrates disruption of the posterior anulus and herniation of the intervertebral disk.

FIGURE 7

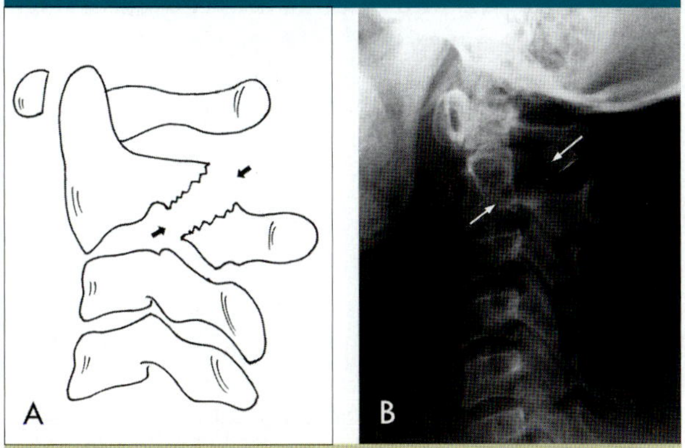

Figure 7 Type IIA traumatic spondylolisthesis differs from type I and II injuries due to the presence of significant angulation at the fracture site. **A** and **B,** Frequently, the fracture lines are more oblique (arrows in **A**) and are not located as close to the junction of the body and the pedicle as in the type I and II injuries. In addition, they are characterized by minimal translation and significant angulation, with widening of the posterior aspect of the disk space. With application of traction, these are the injuries that will demonstrate significant widening of the disk. They represent a flexion-distraction injury, and the deformity will therefore be increased by the addition of further distraction. (Reproduced from Levine AM: Traumatic spondylolisthesis of the axis [hangman's fracture], in Levine AM, Eismont FJ, Garfin SR, Zigler JE, eds: *Spine Trauma*. Philadelphia, PA, WB Saunders, 1998, pp 278-299.)

FIGURE 8

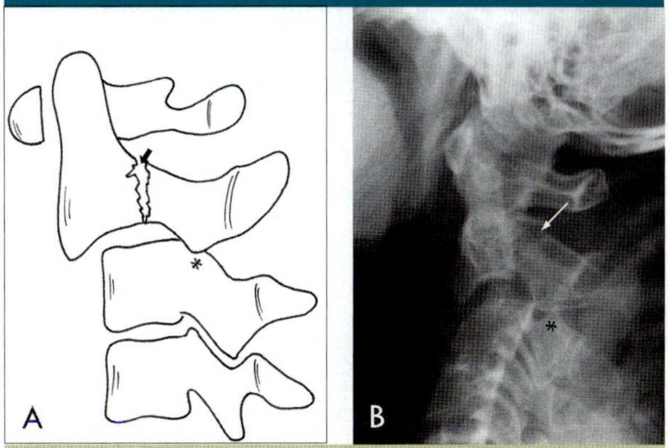

Figure 8 **A** and **B,** Type III traumatic spondylolisthesis of the axis combines fractures of the neural arch with facet injuries at C2-C3. The first type is a bilateral facet dislocation at C2-C3 (asterisk) with a type I hangman's fracture at the base of the body-pedicle junction (arrowhead in **A**). The mechanism most probably is initial flexion-distraction, which causes the dislocation, and then extension, which causes the traumatic spondylolisthesis. Reversing the mechanism would not permit the dislocation to occur, because the inferior facet of C2 would then be detached from the cervicocranium, which serves as the lever for the dislocation. (Reproduced from Levine AM: Traumatic spondylolisthesis of the axis [hangman's fracture], in Levine AM, Eismont FJ, Garfin SR, Zigler JE, eds: *Spine Trauma*. Philadelphia, PA, WB Saunders, 1998, pp 278-299.)

space. In some individuals, as the injury propagates from posterior to anterior by this flexion-distraction mechanism, the anterior longitudinal ligament will be ruptured in distraction. Should that occur, dramatic widening of the disk space can be seen with minimal application of weight. In addition to the previously mentioned characteristic lack of proportionality between angulation and translation, the obliquity of the fracture line in the neural arch and compression of the anterosuperior portion of the C3 vertebral body is rarely seen in type IIA injuries.

The fifth subtype, a type III fracture, combines C2-C3 facet subluxation with fractures of the neural arch. Multiple combinations of these injuries have been reported previously.[4,8,25,26] The most common injury is a bipedicular fracture with a standard bilateral facet dislocation (**Figure 8**). Other combinations occur involving facet fractures or dislocations that include more oblique injuries with unilateral facet fracture-dislocation combined with a contralateral neural arch fracture (**Figure 9**). The critical feature in these injuries is that, as a result of the neural arch fracture, the inferior facets of C2 are free-floating fragments. If bilateral dislocation from C3 occurs, the fracture cannot be reduced by closed methods. The most logical mechanism of this injury is a flexion-distraction mechanism, which produces a bilateral facet dislocation, followed by a hyperextension injury, which causes the type I fracture of the pars. If a fracture of the pars were to occur first, it would then be impossible to dislocate the facet joint at C2-C3 because it would no longer be connected to the cervicocranial segment. The usual methods for reduction of facet dislocations by application of traction are not applicable to this injury pattern. This is because traction applied to the skull by tongs will result in application of traction to the body of C2 but not the C2 inferior facets due to the pars interarticularis fracture.

Finally, bilaminar fractures with facet fracture-dislocations may also result in spondylolisthesis of the axis over C3. Bilaminar fractures of C2 may also result in spondylolisthesis of C2 over C3 and bilateral facet fractures (**Figure 10**). These injuries are similar to other bilateral facet fractures in the cervical spine and are dealt with in the chapter on facet injuries of the cervical spine (chapter 27).

FIGURE 9

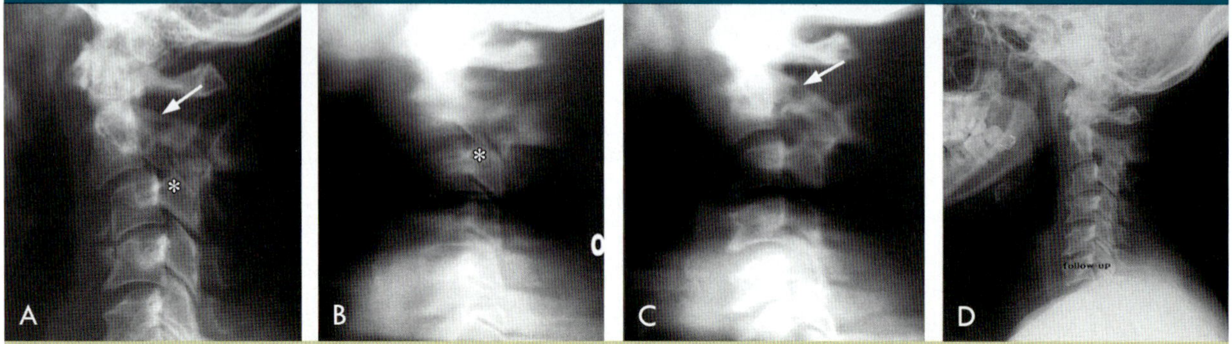

Figure 9 This patient demonstrates one of the variants of the type III injury. **A,** The lateral radiograph shows the fracture through the right side of the pedicle (arrow) and with a dislocation of the left facet joint (asterisk). **B,** Radiograph of the left side demonstrates the facet dislocation (asterisk). **C,** Radiograph of the right side demonstrates the more standard fracture through the neural arch (arrow). **D,** The final lateral view shows the healed stable position. (Reproduced from Levine AM: Traumatic spondylolisthesis of the axis [hangman's fracture], in Levine AM, Eismont FJ, Garfin SR, Zigler JE, eds: *Spine Trauma.* Philadelphia, PA, WB Saunders, 1998, pp 278-299.)

FIGURE 10

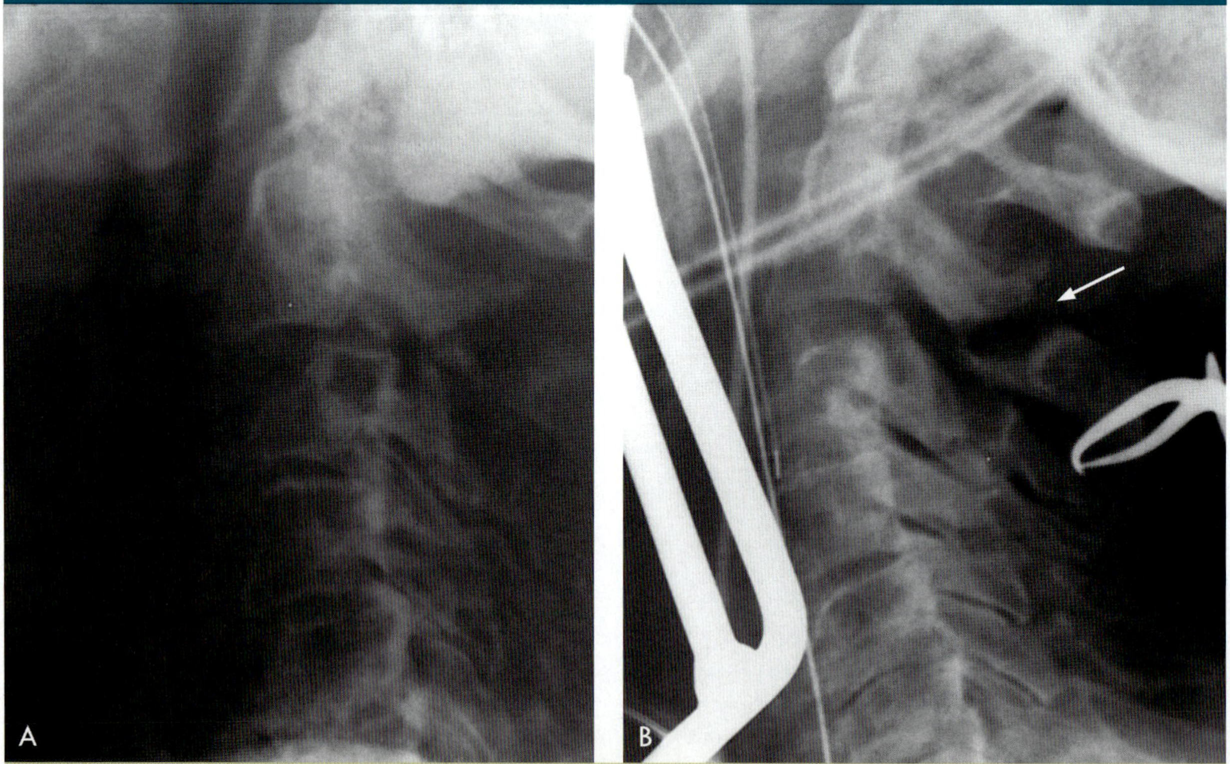

Figure 10 A, This lateral radiograph of an elderly man involved in a motor vehicle accident demonstrates a traumatic spondylolisthesis at C2-C3, which resulted from a bilateral facet fracture with fracture of the lamina at C2-C3. The radiographic picture is similar to that of a traumatic spondylolisthesis with anterior compression to the body of C2 and translation of C2 over C3. **B,** This is easily reduced in traction, and the fracture line was clearly evident (arrow) preoperatively. (Reproduced from Levine AM: Traumatic spondylolisthesis of the axis [hangman's fracture], in Levine AM, Eismont FJ, Garfin SR, Zigler JE, eds: *Spine Trauma.* Philadelphia, PA, WB Saunders, 1998, pp 278-299.)

FIGURE 11

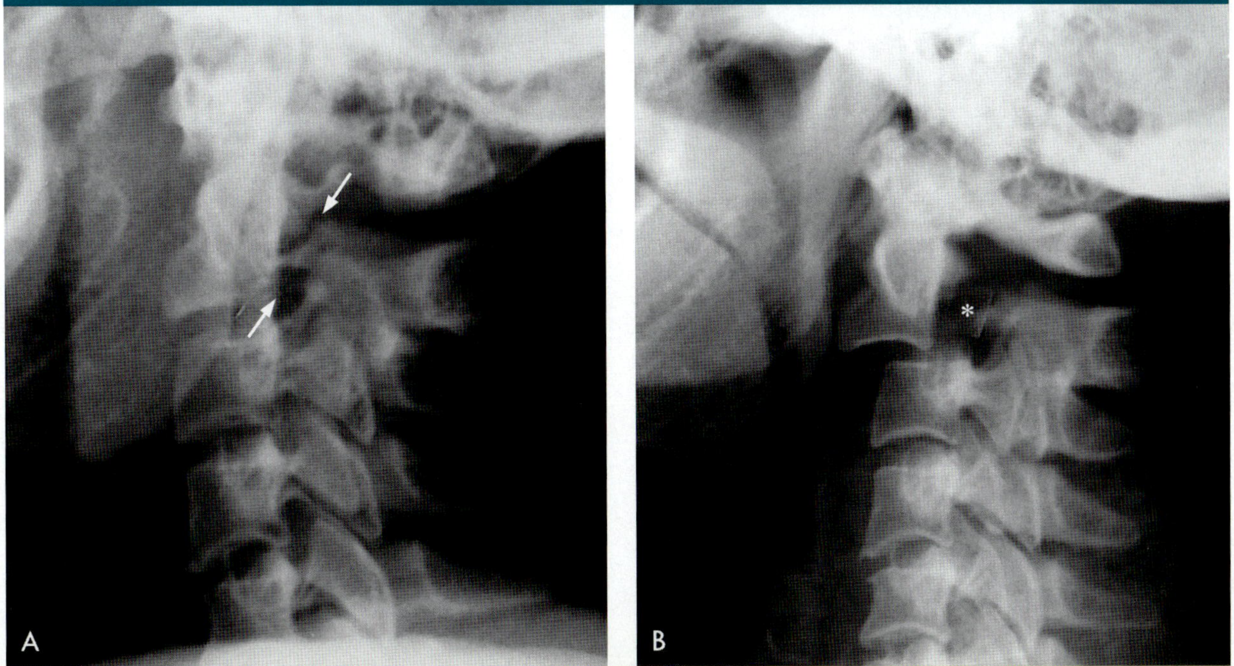

Figure 11 This patient was seen after a motor vehicle accident with what was initially thought to be a type I injury. **A,** The original radiograph was taken in the supine lateral position. Because of the patient's obesity, the neck was in an extended position, and although the fracture line was evident (arrows), the fracture was fully reduced. The patient was discharged in a collar and returned 2 weeks later for follow-up with marked displacement (**B**) and separation of the fracture (asterisk). (Reproduced from Levine AM: Traumatic spondylolisthesis of the axis [hangman's fracture], in Levine AM, Eismont FJ, Garfin SR, Zigler JE, eds: *Spine Trauma*. Philadelphia, PA, WB Saunders, 1998, pp 278-299.)

Radiographic Evaluation

In evaluating the lateral cervical spine radiograph, two factors must be taken into consideration. The first is the position of the patient during radiography, which is most commonly the supine position. Large shoulders may result in relative extension and reduction of the fracture fragments during radiography (**Figure 11**). Conversely, a large occiput relative to the torso may result in relative flexion of the fracture site in a supine patient. This would have the effect of magnifying the apparent fracture displacement. This scenario commonly occurs in pediatric cervical injuries. Type IIA fractures generally are angulated and are reasonably evident on the lateral radiograph, regardless of the patient's position. A true type III injury is also easily identified, because the dislocation is usually seen without difficulty. However, type IA injuries are difficult to diagnose on a plain radiograph. To avoid fracture displacement, dynamic imaging, including flexion-extension radiographs and traction radiographs, is not recommended in the acute setting.

All patients with any type of traumatic spondylolisthesis should have a CT scan of the cervical spine performed to evaluate fracture displacement and evaluate for other intra-axial injuries. The critical feature to observe in the radiologic evaluation of patients with traumatic spondylolisthesis of the axis is the presence of other fractures in both the upper and lower cervical spine (**Figure 12**). In type I fractures, all other hyperextension injuries should be considered, especially in the upper cervical spine. In type II or IIA fractures, both hyperextension and flexion-distraction injuries should be considered. For type IA fractures, lateral bending injuries, such as fracture separations of the articular mass, should be considered. For an atypical hangman's fracture or traumatic spondylolisthesis of the axis, a CT scan is the diagnostic study of choice. A CT scan will demonstrate the location of the breaks within the ring of C2 (**Figure 13**). More importantly, it will reveal whether there is an injury that goes through the vertebral foramen anteriorly. If the fracture pattern is such that it goes through the vertebral foramen, there is a risk of vertebral artery injury, and a digital

FIGURE 12

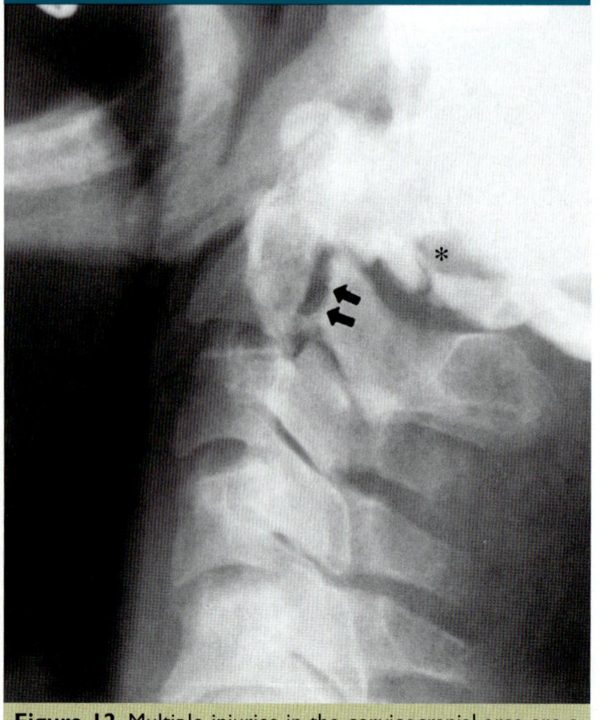

Figure 12 Multiple injuries in the cervicocranial area are a fairly common phenomenon. Usually these injuries have a common mechanism. In this case, both the fracture of the posterior arch of C1 (asterisk) and the type I traumatic spondylolisthesis of the axis (arrows) are the result of a hyperextension–axial load mechanism. Individually, both injuries are stable and require only collar immobilization, and the two injuries together are no more unstable than either one alone. (Reproduced from Levine AM: Traumatic spondylolisthesis of the axis [hangman's fracture], in Levine AM, Eismont FJ, Garfin SR, Zigler JE, eds: *Spine Trauma*. Philadelphia, PA, WB Saunders, 1998, pp 278-299.)

subtraction angiogram or a magnetic resonance angiogram should be done to assess the blood flow in the vertebral artery on that side. This is especially true in the presence of evidence of any neurologic deficit that might be associated with a cerebral infarction based on the vertebral artery injury.

MRI is a useful adjunctive study to evaluate the integrity of the C2-C3 disk in a suspected type II fracture or a type III fracture. MRI is the gold standard to distinguish a type II injury from a type IIA injury. Additionally, because disk herniations are associated with bilateral facet dislocations, if a facet dislocation in a type III hangman's fracture cannot be reduced with the patient awake to signal any change in neurologic status, a preoperative MRI should be used to assess the disk. If no significant disk herniation is seen with a type III injury, the standard surgical treatment can proceed.

Neurologic Injury

In contradistinction to the judicial hanging injury, which results in death by either strangulation or traumatic transection of the cord, traumatic spondylolisthesis of the axis infrequently demonstrates neurologic deficit. Type III injuries are more likely to demonstrate neurologic deficit at the level of injury. Neurologic deficit is infrequently associated with type I and II traumatic spondylolisthesis, but it is more commonly associated with type IA (atypical) and III injuries. Type IA, or atypical hangman's fracture, is believed to be accompanied by a higher incidence of neurologic deficit because the fracture does not symmetrically enlarge the spinal canal.[24] Specifically, a fracture fragment that includes part of the posterior vertebral body wall may retrolisthese into the spinal canal and impinge upon the spinal cord. In addition, with a type IA injury, when the fracture goes through the transverse foramen for the vertebral artery, neurologic deficit may also occur related to vertebral artery disruption. In most type II injuries, the neurologic deficit is usually related to closed head injuries and only infrequently to the level of injury.

Biomechanics of Fixation

There are a variety of fixation options at the C1-C2 level. One study of seven specimens determined that although direct pars interarticularis screw fixation reduces lateral bending, instability is still present in flexion-extension motions. Additionally, posterior C2-C3 fixation was seen to demonstrate increased axial rotational and lateral bending rigidity over anterior plating.[27] Some authors have suggested that C2 pars interarticularis screws may be sufficient in a subset of the population.[28,29] This is in agreement with another study of six cadaver specimens comparing anterior to posterior approaches for type II injuries.[30] The authors of this study found that the posterior approach resulted in increased stiffness over the intact vertebrae in all motions.

Treatment

General Recommendations

The treatment options range from simple cervical immobilization in a collar to halo traction and/or surgery followed by immobilization in an orthosis to anteroposterior fusion. Despite the various classification systems, most clinicians recommend conservative management of hangman's fractures because good results have been reported in multi-

FIGURE 13

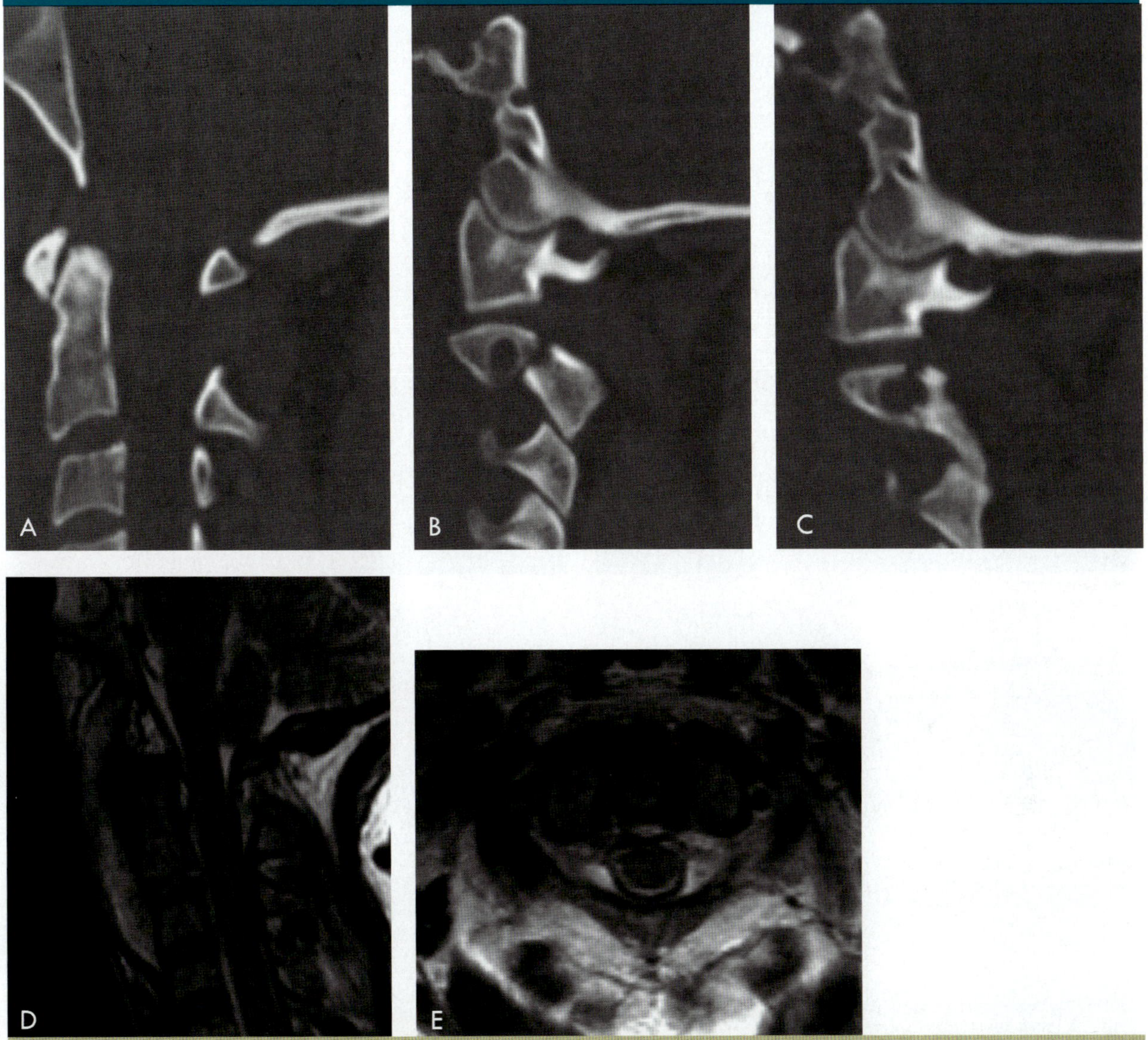

Figure 13 Midsagittal (**A**) and parasagittal (**B** and **C**) CT images display a type I injury with minimal displacement. Midsagittal MRI scans (**D** and **E**) demonstrate possible disruption of the posterior anulus with no intervertebral disk herniation.

ple series.[3,8,31] This entails using external immobilization when a stable reduction can be achieved.

Type I Fractures

Universally, type I fractures are considered to be stable by most experts.[32] The relative benefit of halo immobilization over cervical collar at C2-C3 is controversial.[22,33,34] A cervical orthosis represents the most reasonable immobilization option with minimal risk of complication. Of course, body habitus must be considered. Immobilization in a collar may not be possible in patients who are extremely obese and have a very short neck, and thus halo immobilization should be considered.

In atypical or type IA fractures, an oblique fracture occurs through the body of C2 on one side and the pars or pedicle on the opposite side. The majority of these injuries in patients who are neurologically intact are stable injuries that can be treated with a cervical collar. Union will occur in a slightly displaced position (**Figure 14**), and there will appear to be an elongation of the vertebral body, with anterior translation of approximately 2 mm to 3 mm. Because at least one portion of this fracture is through the cancellous portion of the C2 body, the union rate is extremely high even if reduction is not achieved. Occasionally, a patient will have either a neurologic deficit or a very

FIGURE 14

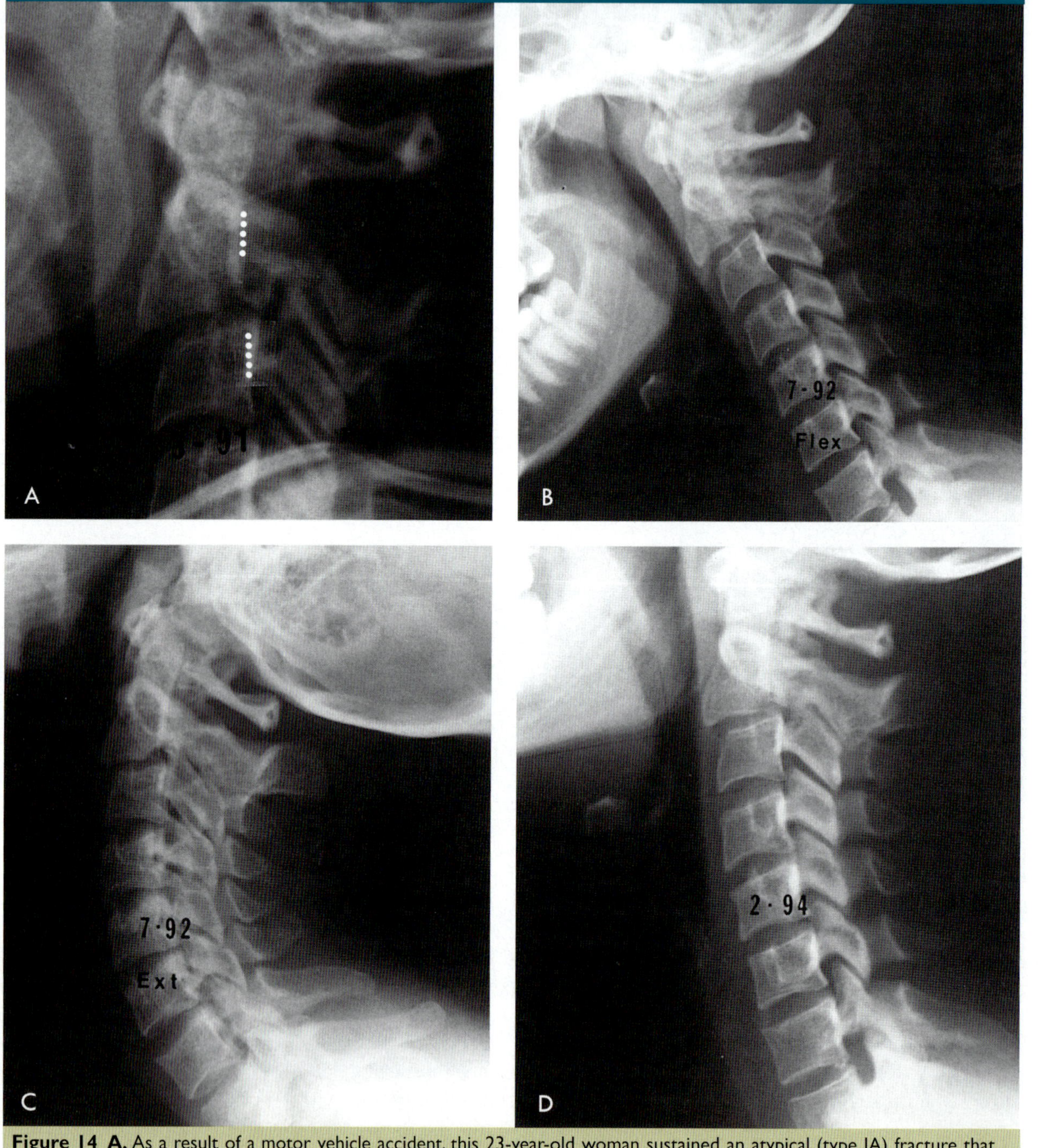

Figure 14 **A,** As a result of a motor vehicle accident, this 23-year-old woman sustained an atypical (type IA) fracture that did not penetrate through the foramen transversarium but did traverse the body of C2 on one side. Slight rotatory translation is evident (dotted lines), but there is essentially no angulation. She was treated in external immobilization for 3 months and then was subjected to extension (**B**) and flexion (**C**) radiographs to test stability. **D,** At 3-year follow-up, the patient was asymptomatic and showed no additional deformity. (Reproduced from Levine AM: Traumatic spondylolisthesis of the axis [hangman's fracture], in Levine AM, Eismont FJ, Garfin SR, Zigler JE, eds: *Spine Trauma*. Philadelphia, PA, WB Saunders, 1998, pp 278-299.)

unstable fracture, in which case traction or even open decompression and fusion may be necessary to achieve reduction of the fracture and the neural canal. Essentially these fractures can be treated as type I even though the mechanism and the fracture pattern differ from a type I fracture.

Type II Fractures

Type II fractures are subdivided into standard type II and type IIA, which are treated differently. The degree of instability varies, but in all cases the thecal sac should not be compressed by this type of fracture, because the neural canal is expanded by the fracture of the neural arch. Although it has been demonstrated that the neural arch fractures as a result of hyperextension and axial load force, the displacement of a type II fracture is a result of the flexion component.

Traction in Type II Fractures

Nonsurgical treatments of this injury have varied dramatically, from simple immobilization to prolonged treatment. Brashear et al[9] and Seljeskog and Chou[14] suggested cervical traction for 6 weeks followed by 2 or 3 months of cervical immobilization in a Minerva cast. Another retrospective study demonstrated a 94.5% union rate at an average 11.5 weeks in 123 patients with hangman's fractures.[3] There was no difference between the results of patients with early immobilization and prolonged halo traction. The effectiveness of early immobilization has been demonstrated in one study of 27 type II and 4 type IIA injuries.[35] All patients received traction to reduce the fracture followed by immediate halo-vest application. Twenty-one of the 27 type II patients and all four of the type IIA patients demonstrated successful union. Those six patients who failed to achieve solid union had an initial angulation of 12° or greater.

Technique for Application of Traction Reduction

The sequence of steps involves application of a halo ring and placement on a RotoRest (KCI, San Antonio, TX) bed with 10 lb of traction, which is increased serially in 5-lb increments until the fracture is reduced. If the height of the interspace appears to be restored and the C2-C3 disk is not increasing pathologically, the weight can be increased to as much as 40 to 45 lb before reduction may be achieved. In addition, placing a roll with a 4-in diameter at approximately the C6 level will allow some extension of the upper cervical spine in a patient with relatively small shoulders, to facilitate completion of the reduction. Both axial distraction and slight extension are required to achieve a reduction of a type II fracture. Once anatomic reduction is achieved, the patient can be left in halo traction for a minimum of 4 weeks until initial healing of the reduced fracture fragments has begun. At the end of 4 weeks, traction can be removed while the patient remains supine on a RotoRest bed for 1 hour. A lateral radiograph should be taken at the end of that 1-hour period. If no redisplacement of the fracture is seen, the patient can then be immobilized in a halo vest. Should there be any change in position with removal of the traction (either angulation or translation), the fracture callus is still too plastic and the patient should then be placed back in traction for an additional week. This whole procedure should be repeated again at the end of 5 weeks from injury or initiation of treatment. If there is still displacement, then the procedure should be repeated at the end of 6 weeks. It is generally not necessary to go beyond 6 weeks in halo traction. Finally, the patient should spend another 6 weeks in a halo vest to complete the treatment program (**Figure 15**). Many adolescents or young adults will have enough fracture callus and a well-opposed fracture that begins to unite by the end of 4 or 5 weeks, which will allow early release from traction. Elderly patients may require the full 6 weeks. For patients who demonstrate increased displacement during the course of nonsurgical treatment, the patient can still be returned to halo traction within the first 2 weeks of injury, and reduction can again be achieved by the use of axial traction and hyperextension. At this point, either the surgical or nonsurgical treatment is undertaken.

Therefore, patients who have moderate degrees of displacement in angulation (less than 5 mm, and less than 10° of angulation), and in whom the displacement can be accepted, can be treated successfully with immediate immobilization in a halo vest. The degree of residual angular deformity or kyphosis between C2 and C3 should be reduced to prevent compensatory deformities and nonunion. Despite the fracture gap, a spontaneous anterior arthrodesis between C2 and C3 occurs in some of these patients. The anterior arthrodesis results from the destruction of the disk and bleeding as the anterior longitudinal ligament is stripped off the body of C3. Nonunion occurs in a small percentage of patients because of the widely displaced fracture fragments. Care must be taken to distinguish type II injuries from type IIA injuries. Type IIA injuries can exhibit either increasing posterior distraction of the disk space or, in the more severe variants, total distraction of the disk space.

Type IIA Injuries

Type IIA fractures must be differentiated from type II fractures, as application of axial traction to a type IIA injury will cause the fracture to displace

FIGURE 15

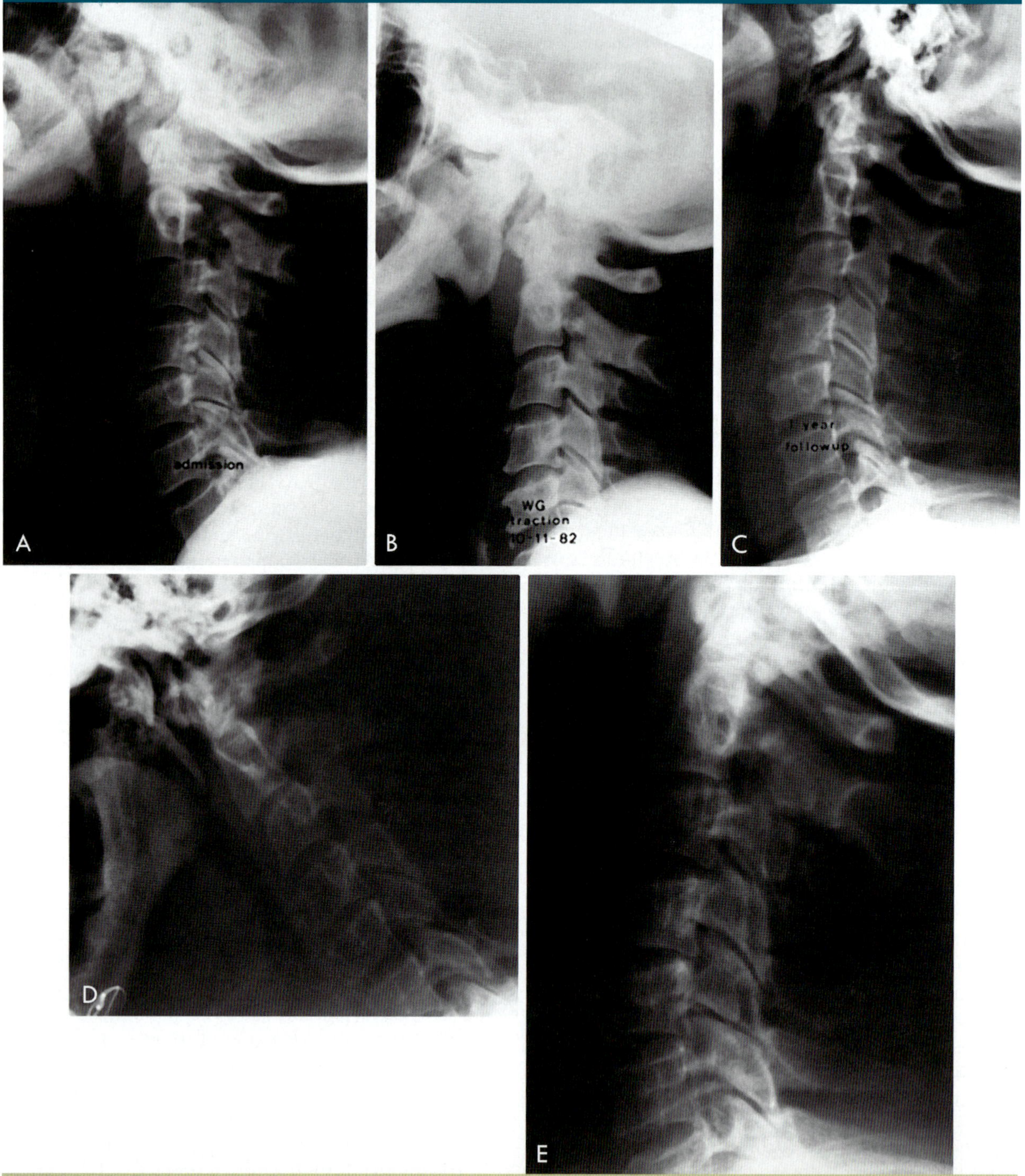

Figure 15 A, This 63-year-old patient with a severely displaced type II traumatic spondylolisthesis of the axis had 12 mm of translation on the initial lateral radiograph. **B,** The patient was placed in halo traction (30 lb) with slight extension of the neck over a roll to achieve anatomic reduction in traction. The patient was maintained in traction for 6 weeks and then immobilized in a halo vest. **C,** On follow-up radiographs at 1 year, the patient demonstrates maintenance of reduction and healing of the traumatic spondylolisthesis of the axis in an anatomic position. **D** and **E,** Flexion-extension radiographs demonstrate the ultimate stability obtained. (Reproduced from Levine AM: Traumatic spondylolisthesis of the axis [hangman's fracture], in Levine AM, Eismont FJ, Garfin SR, Zigler JE, eds: *Spine Trauma*. Philadelphia, PA, WB Saunders, 1998, pp 278-299.)

FIGURE 16

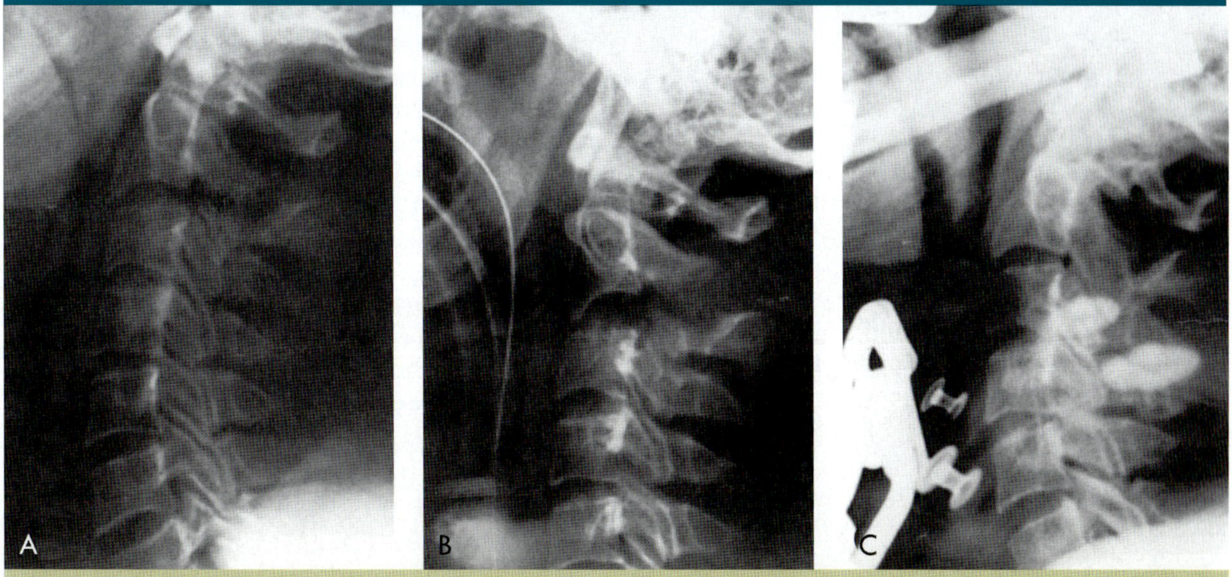

Figure 16 A, This patient had a type IIA traumatic spondylolisthesis that was minimally displaced when seen initially. **B,** Traction of 20 lb was placed on the neck via Gardner-Wells tongs, and the patient had immediate widening of the disk space posteriorly without neurologic deficit. The traction was removed and the patient was placed in a halo vest, and gentle compression was undertaken under radiographic control. **C,** An anatomic reduction was achieved. (Reproduced with permission from Levine AM, Edwards CC: Traumatic spondylolisthesis of the axis. *J Bone Joint Surg Am* 1985;67(2):217-226.)

by widening the disk space. Because the fracture mechanism for type IIA injuries is flexion and distraction, reduction is done by extension and compression. In this group of patients, we recommend nonsurgical treatment that entails immediate application of a halo vest under image intensification to achieve extension and compression (**Figure 16**). The vest generally will need to be tightened after immobilization to achieve slightly more axial compression. The reduction is maintained in that position for 3 months in a halo vest.

For patients in whom there is significant risk from prolonged bed rest, a surgical alternative can be undertaken involving interfragmentary compression and osteosynthesis along the C2 pars interarticularis. The most effective method of achieving stabilization is placement of posterior screws along the pedicles of C2. This method was originally suggested by Judet[36] and described by Roy-Camille et al.[37] The surgeon absolutely must inspect the preoperative CT scan to determine the location of the vertebral artery and the adequacy of the pedicles of C2 to hold a pedicle screw. The patient is placed in a prone position with the head held in a Mayfield head holder. Manipulation of the head in the Mayfield holder before preparation and draping of the sterile field allows optimal alignment. After an image intensifier is positioned to allow visualization of the C2 pedicles in both the AP and lateral projections, a standard midline posterior approach to the C2-C3 facet joints is undertaken. A partial dissection of the C1-C2 interspace is also undertaken, defining the medial side of the pars and pedicles of C2 up to the C1-C2 joint. Subperiosteal dissection along the pars interarticularis of C2 is critical to mobilizing the venous plexus with minimal blood loss. We also prefer a small elevator, such as a Freer, Key elevator, or Penfield 1, over electrocautery for mobilization of the periosteum on C2. The surgeon should have cottonoids and local hemostatic agent immediately available for packing venous bleeding because this technique may be more effective than cautery for control of some bleeding. The C1-C2 joint capsule does not have to be removed, and only the medial side of the C2 pedicle needs to be identified. The surgeon should be able to palpate the medial aspect of the C2 pedicle to direct the trajectory of the screw. The fracture line will be encountered during this portion of the dissection and the reduction is checked under image intensification. The starting point for the entry of the drill or burr is determined both by landmarks and by image intensification. Beginning at a point that is just medial to the facet joints of C2-C3 at its point of connection with the lamina, a high-speed 2-mm burr is used to make a small depression in the bone of theposterior cortex of the C2 pedicle starting point. Using a 2-mm burr or a 3.5-mm drill bit, the posterior fragment of the pedicle of C2 is drilled or burred. This is done under image intensification to verify that the drill is being advanced in the proper anterosuperior direction. This does not have to be monitored by image intensification in the AP plane, as the medial side of the pedicle is directly visualized with the nerve hook held by an assistant. The screw is aimed to parallel this medial cortex of the pedicle (which can be palpated during the burring or drilling process to ensure its integrity) and is angled toward the midline at approximately 15° (**Figure 17,** *A* and *B*). The posterior fragment is overdrilled and the anterior fracture fragment is underdrilled to create interfragmentary compression across the fracture site; this is performed bilaterally. Care must be taken to not displace the fracture when drilling or burring. The hole is then measured with a depth gauge, and a 3.5-mm partially threaded screw is used to lag the posterior fragment to the anterior portion of the body. Generally a 35-mm–long screw that has a 20-mm unthreaded section can be used so that there are no threads across the fracture site (**Figure 17,** *C* and *D*). At this point, the weight is removed from the spine if traction is being used and the final position of fracture alignment is checked (**Figure 17,** *E* through *G*). If the C2-C3 disk is disrupted, then C2-C3 posterior arthrodesis may be considered with lateral mass fixation into C3. This approach should only be undertaken by experienced surgeons particularly familiar with vertebral artery local anatomy because a lateral screw or anterior screw violation will injure the vertebral artery. If a vertebral artery injury is encountered on one side, alternative fixation should be performed contralaterally and the patient should be taken immediately for evaluation and possible embolization.

Another option for stabilization of a displaced type II or Type IIA fracture is the anterior approach. Several authors have suggested an anterior C2-C3 fusion.[38,39] This has several intrinsic liabilities. First, in type II fractures, the only remaining structure to maintain stability is the anterior longitudinal ligament. The nature of the injury means that the posterior arch is incompetent and the disk is disrupted from the posterior aspect of the anulus through to the anterior longitudinal ligament. To achieve an anterior arthrodesis, the anterior longitudinal ligament must be removed to insert the graft, thus decreasing the overall stability of the spine. The use of anterior plate fixation to augment the stability of the construct is routinely performed. Another technical problem is the difficulty in placing the plate and screws in this very proximal location of the upper cervical spine. In particular, the superior laryngeal nerve is endangered by an upper cervical spine approach, which can result in significant risk of dysphagia and aspiration. However, there are at least two recent studies of 28 or more patients (classified as Levine-Edwards type II, IIA, or III) that demonstrate solid fusion of C2-C3 after an anterior fusion with plating.[38,39] Although technically demanding, the anterior approach may be considered a reasonable method for achieving fixation.

Type III Injuries

Patients with type III injuries (ie, traumatic spondylolisthesis of the axis combined with a bilateral facet dislocation at C2-C3) absolutely require surgical intervention. The most common subtype of this injury is the type I bipedicular fracture associated with a standard C2-C3 bilateral facet dislocation. In this situation, the standard posterior approach is used to reduce the facet dislocation and perform a C2-C3 fusion (**Figure 18**). This may be attempted with C2 pedicle screws, or, if surgical fixation in C2 is impossible due to comminution, a C1-C3 fusion.

Results and Complications

Type I Injuries

The treatment of type I injury, or minimally displaced traumatic spondylolisthesis of the axis, is accompanied by few complications and even fewer long-term problems. The union rate of type I fractures, including type IA injuries, since the displacement is minimal, is approximately 98%.[4] Nonunion of a type I fracture is extremely rare (**Figure 19**). Nonunions in this injury can be treated either by osteosynthesis with a pedicle screw across the fracture and compression or by C2-C3 anterior arthrodesis.

Type I Fractures With Associated Injuries

Type I fractures have a high rate of association with other fractures, including the fractures of the posterior arch of C1.[25] The two combined also require collar immobilization for adequate treatment. A less frequently encountered combination is traumatic spondylolisthesis and a posteriorly displaced dens fracture, both resulting from hyperextension–axial load injuries. If the dens fracture is easily reduced or nondisplaced (as it is the more significant injury), it may require collar or halo-vest immobilization, or surgical intervention. Pos-

FIGURE 17

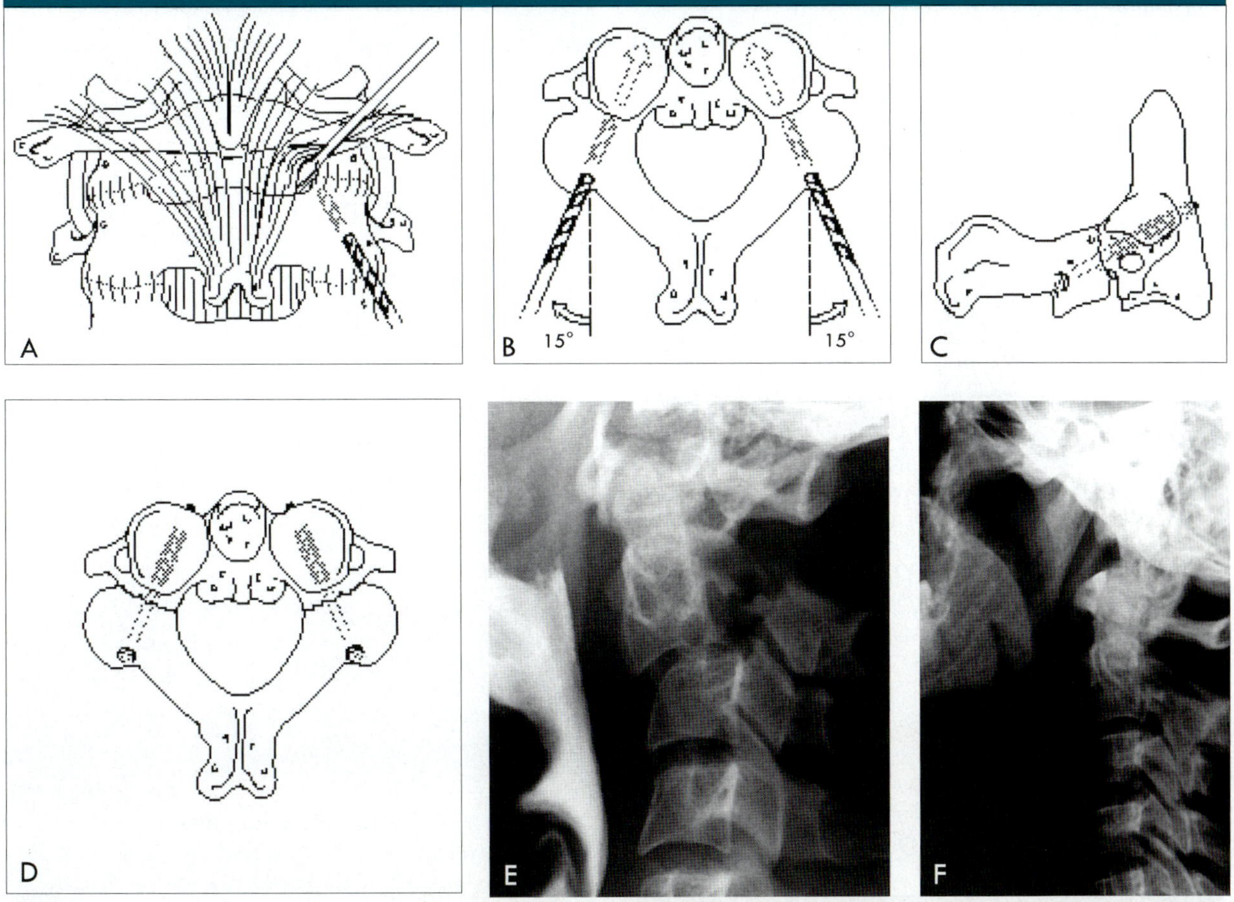

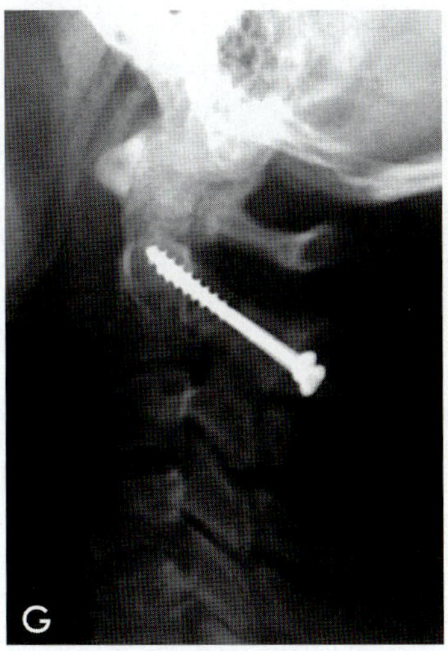

Figure 17 A, Surgical technique for osteosynthesis of a traumatic spondylolisthesis of the axis. The procedure is done with the aid of biplanar image intensification so that the trajectory of the screws can be easily monitored. The initial portion of the dissection requires demonstration of the medial aspect of the pedicle of C2. The facet joint at C1-C2 does not need to be disrupted, but dissection from posterior to anterior toward the facet will usually demonstrate the fracture of the pedicle. Prior to beginning screw insertion, care should be taken that the fracture is as reduced as possible and that a No. 4 Penfield elevator can be placed along the medial border of the pedicle for guidance. **B,** Orientation of the screws along the pedicle in an axial plane. Slight convergence of the screws is desirable. **C,** Orientation across the fracture line from the posterior fracture to the anterior fragment. A partially threaded screw is desirable with usually about 15 mm of thread and 20 mm of shank. The proximal fragment can be overdrilled and lagged to the anterior fragment. **D,** The final axial view. **E,** This patient sustained a displaced type II traumatic spondylolisthesis of the axis as well as other extremity and systemic injuries. Because halo traction and bed rest were not an alternative, the patient was reduced in halo traction (**F**) and then direct screw fixation of the fracture was achieved (**G**). (Reproduced from Levine AM: Traumatic spondylolisthesis of the axis [hangman's fracture], in Levine AM, Eismont FJ, Garfin SR, Zigler JE, eds: *Spine Trauma*. Philadelphia, PA, WB Saunders, 1998, pp 278-299.)

teriorly displaced odontoid fractures treated with traction have been associated with respiratory distress. This should be taken into account when treating this type of injury with cervical flexion, and the issue may be avoided by nasotracheal intubation.[40] The most common long-term problem of type I traumatic spondylolisthesis is the degeneration of the C2-C3 facet joint. Because the mechanism of injury is hyperextension combined with axial loading, the C2-C3 facets are oriented

FIGURE 18

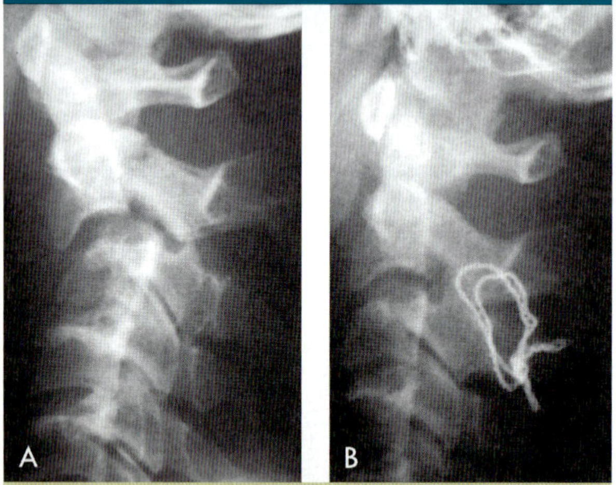

Figure 18 A, This patient sustained a type III traumatic spondylolisthesis of the axis and a dislocation of the C2-C3 facet joints as well as a fracture of the pedicles of C2, which could not be reduced in traction because the facet could not be relocated. **B,** The patient was therefore treated by open reduction and internal fixation of the bilateral facet dislocation followed by external immobilization for healing of the traumatic spondylolisthesis in an anatomic position. (Reproduced from Poss R, Bucholz RW, Frymoyer JW, Gelberman RH, Hensinger RN, Morrey BF, eds: Cervical spine and cord: Trauma, in *Orthopaedic Knowledge Update*, ed 3. Park Ridge, IL, American Academy of Orthopaedic Surgeons, 1990, p 407.)

FIGURE 19

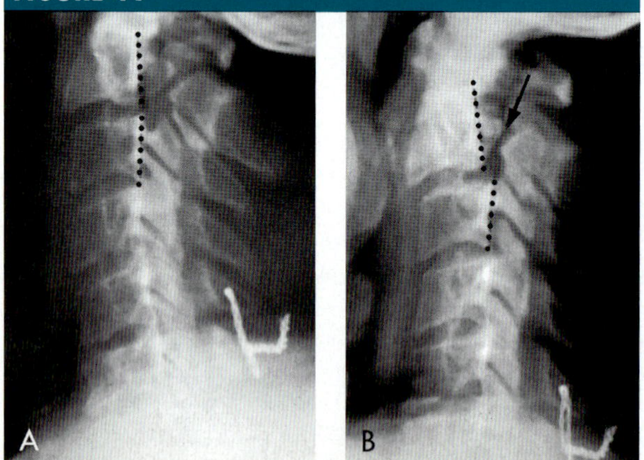

Figure 19 This 41-year-old man sustained a type I traumatic spondylolisthesis of the axis 12 months before these flexion-extension radiographs were taken. **A,** The extension radiograph demonstrates full reduction of the deformity but with a lucent gap in the fracture line after 12 months of orthotic immobilization (dotted line). **B,** The flexion radiograph demonstrates both translation and angulation and widening of the gap in the fracture line (arrow) with sclerotic edges. The patient subsequently underwent arthrodesis for correction of nonunion. (Reproduced with permission from Levine AM, Rhyne AL: Traumatic spondylolisthesis of the axis. *Semin Spine Surg* 1991;3:47-60.)

FIGURE 20

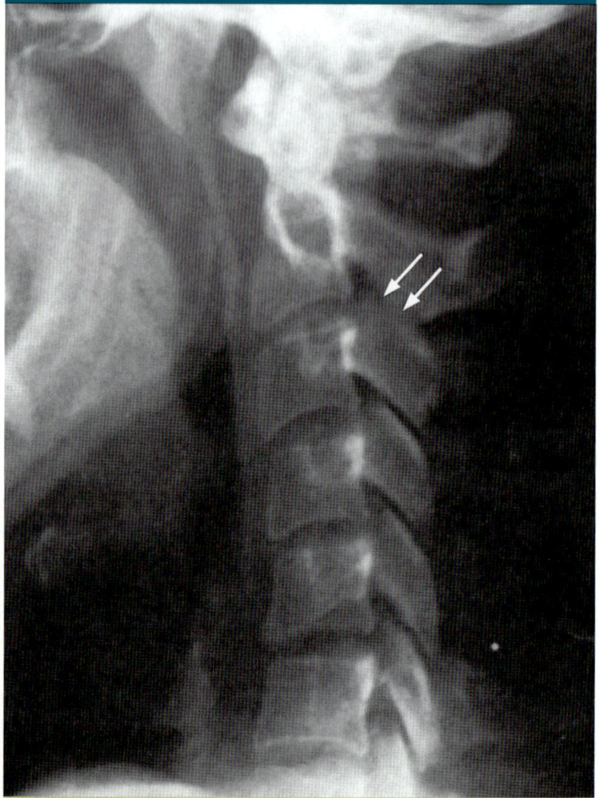

Figure 20 This 27-year-old woman sustained a type I traumatic spondylolisthesis of the axis 3 years before these radiographs were taken. She healed in a completely anatomic position. However, she began to have both weather-related symptoms and intermittent pain, localized specifically to the upper cervical spine and reproduced with pressure over the C2 spinous process. On the flexion-extension radiograph, the patient is noted to have loss of the joint space at C2-C3 (arrows), but she retains minimal motion at that level. (Reproduced with permission from Levine AM, Rhyne AL: Traumatic spondylolisthesis of the axis. *Semin Spine Surg* 1991;3:47-60.)

in such a direction that they will achieve significant loading during that injury. Approximately 10% of patients with this injury will have symptoms and late degenerative changes at that level (**Figure 20**).

Type II Injuries

Type II fractures do not result in C2-C3 degeneration as frequently. The majority of those patients experience spontaneous C2-C3 ankylosis. Approximately 30% of patients with type I injuries who have mobile C2-C3 joints have some degenerative symptoms (**Figure 20**).[41] In the long term, should symptoms become significant enough, they may require a secondary arthrodesis. One series of nine

FIGURE 21

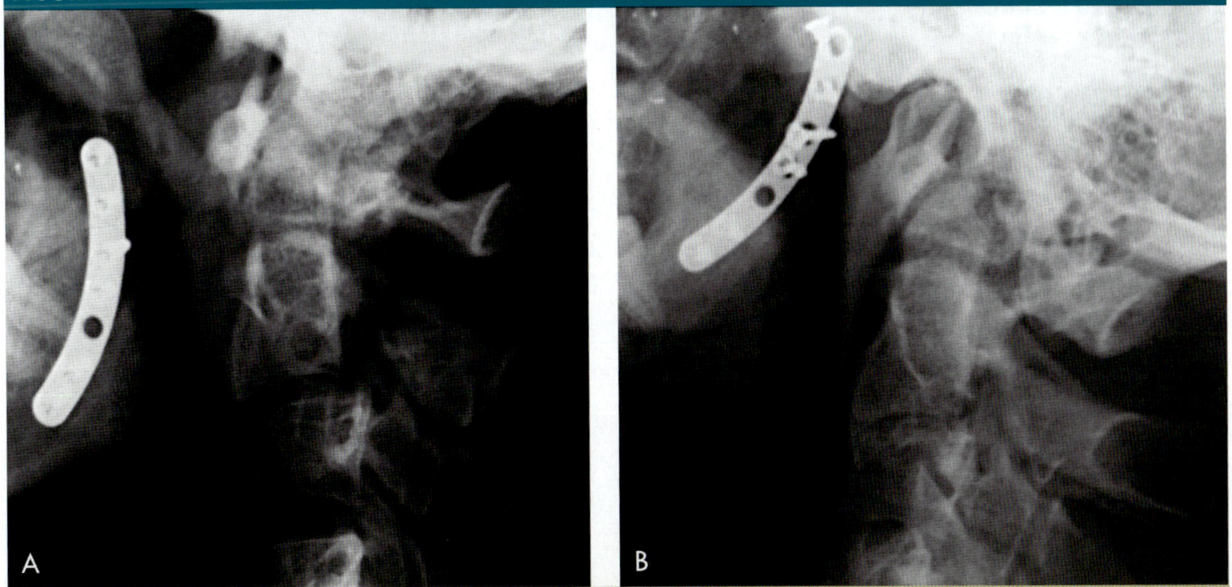

Figure 21 Type II fractures frequently progress to spontaneous ankylosis as a result of the trauma to the disk and the anterior portion of the C3 body. **A,** This patient was involved in a motor vehicle accident and sustained a cervical fracture as well as facial injuries. The amount of displacement was accepted and the patient was placed in a halo vest. **B,** By follow-up 9 months later, a spontaneous anterior C2-C3 arthrodesis had occurred. (Reproduced from Levine AM: Traumatic spondylolisthesis of the axis [hangman's fracture], in Levine AM, Eismont FJ, Garfin SR, Zigler JE, eds: *Spine Trauma*. Philadelphia, PA, WB Saunders, 1998, pp 278-299.)

patients (four with type I, four with type II, and one with type IIA) showed that increased angulation and translation are risk factors for long-term pain after conservative management.[41] These patients were assessed between 21 and 108 months after injury.

Patients with type II traumatic spondylolisthesis of the axis often have head and other injuries in addition to their C2 fracture. Residual translation may predispose patients to risk of nonunion of the pars interarticularis. However, these patients commonly develop anterior ankylosis of the C2-3 disk space (**Figure 21**). The incidence of symptomatic nonunion is relatively low despite the radiographic evidence of no bony continuity across the arch posteriorly. Rarely will a patient have both lack of bony continuity posteriorly and failure to develop ankylosis anteriorly. Although the numbers are very small, the patient with a moderately displaced fracture is somewhat more likely to go on to a symptomatic nonunion than one with a severely displaced fracture with marked destruction of the disk space and anterior portion of the body of C2. Residual angulation may result in a significant kyphotic defect occurring locally at the C2-3 disk space. In the patient with a nonunion and widely displaced fracture fragments, posterior osteosynthesis is not technically possible as it is with the nonunited type I fracture. Nonunions of type II fractures generally require an anterior C2-C3 arthrodesis, which sometimes necessitates osteotomy of the inferior portion of the body of C2 to enter the C2-3 disk space. Dysphagia is common after anterior arthrodesis,[39] although it may abate after 3 years.

Patients with type III injuries constitute a very small group of patients. In all series, they have a high rate of neurologic deficit because of the bilateral facet dislocation.[42] Traditionally, all patients with high levels of quadriplegia have very poor long-term results. In the very small group of patients with either minimal or no neurologic deficit in whom an anatomic reduction can be achieved with arthrodesis, the long-term results are excellent.

Conclusions

Traumatic spondylolisthesis of the axis is a very different injury than the classically defined hangman's fracture that results from judicial hangings. It is often the result of high-speed vehicular trauma and occurs in the younger age groups. The injuries can be classified according to five different types. Treatment of injuries is dictated by displacement. The prognosis for hangman's fractures is generally favorable, with most patients experiencing a full recovery.

References

1. Haughton S: On hanging, considered from a mechanical and physiological point of view. *Philos Mag J* 1866;32(4):23-24.
2. Cornish BL: Traumatic spondylolisthesis of the axis. *J Bone Joint Surg Br* 1968;50(1):31-43.
3. Francis WR, Fielding JW, Hawkins RJ, Pepin J, Hensinger R: Traumatic spondylolisthesis of the axis. *J Bone Joint Surg Br* 1981;63(3):313-318.
4. Levine AM, Edwards CC: The management of traumatic spondylolisthesis of the axis. *J Bone Joint Surg Am* 1985;67(2):217-226.
5. Pepin JW, Hawkins RJ: Traumatic spondylolisthesis of the axis: Hangman's fracture. *Clin Orthop Relat Res* 1981;157:133-138.
6. Sherk HH, Howard T: Clinical and pathologic correlations in traumatic spondylolisthesis of the axis. *Clin Orthop Relat Res* 1983;174:122-126.
7. Marar BC: Fracture of the axis arch: "Hangman's fracture" of the cervical spine. *Clin Orthop Relat Res* 1975;106:155-165.
8. Effendi B, Roy D, Cornish B, Dussault RG, Laurin CA: Fractures of the ring of the axis: A classification based on the analysis of 131 cases. *J Bone Joint Surg Br* 1981;63(3):319-327.
9. Brashear R Jr, Venters GC, Preston ET: Fractures of the neural arch of the axis: A report of twenty-nine cases. *J Bone Joint Surg Am* 1975;57(7):879-887.
10. Bucholz RW: Unstable hangman's fractures. *Clin Orthop Relat Res* 1981;154:119-124.
11. Mollan RA, Watt PC: Hangman's fracture. *Injury* 1982;14(3):265-267.
12. Roda JM, Castro A, Blázquez MG: Hangman's fracture with complete dislocation of C-2 on C-3: Case report. *J Neurosurg* 1984;60(3):633-635.
13. Schneider RC, Livingston KE, Cave AJ, Hamilton G: "Hangman's fracture" of the cervical spine. *J Neurosurg* 1965;22:141-154.
14. Seljeskog EL, Chou SN: Spectrum of the hangman's fracture. *J Neurosurg* 1976;45(1):3-8.
15. Termansen NB: Hangman's fracture. *Acta Orthop Scand* 1974;45(4):529-539.
16. Williams TG: Hangman's fracture. *J Bone Joint Surg Br* 1975;57(1):82-88.
17. Garber JN: Abnormalities of the atlas and axis vertebrae: Congenital and traumatic. *J Bone Joint Surg Am* 1964;46:1782-1791.
18. Tuite GF, Papadopoulos SM, Sonntag VK: Caspar plate fixation for the treatment of complex hangman's fractures. *Neurosurgery* 1992;30(5):761-765.
19. Radcliff KE, Ben-Galim P, Dreiangel N, et al: Comprehensive computed tomography assessment of the upper cervical anatomy: What is normal? *Spine J* 2010;10(3):219-229.
20. Hohl M: Normal motions in the upper portion of the cervical spine. *J Bone Joint Surg Am* 1964;46:1777-1779.
21. Fielding JW: Normal and selected abnormal motion of the cervical spine from the second cervical vertebra to the seventh cervical vertebra based on cineroentgenography. *J Bone Joint Surg Am* 1964;46:1779-1781.
22. White AA, Panjabi MM: *Clinical Biomechanics of the Spine*. Philadelphia, PA, JB Lippincott, 1990, pp 208-215.
23. Levine AM, Rhyne AL: Traumatic spondylolisthesis of the axis. *Semin Spine Surg* 1991;3:47-60.
24. Starr JK, Eismont FJ: Atypical hangman's fractures. *Spine (Phila Pa 1976)* 1993;18(14):1954-1957.
25. Levine AM, Edwards CC: Treatment of injuries in the C1-C2 complex. *Orthop Clin North Am* 1986;17(1):31-44.
26. Dussault RG, Effendi B, Roy D, Cornish B, Laurin CA: Locked facets with fracture of the neural arch of the axis. *Spine (Phila Pa 1976)* 1983;8(4):365-367.
27. Duggal N, Chamberlain RH, Perez-Garza LE, Espinoza-Larios A, Sonntag VK, Crawford NR: Hangman's fracture: A biomechanical comparison of stabilization techniques. *Spine (Phila Pa 1976)* 2007;32(2):182-187.
28. Bristol R, Henn JS, Dickman CA: Pars screw fixation of a hangman's fracture: Technical case report. *Neurosurg* 2005;56(1 Suppl):E204.
29. Dalbayrak S, Yilmaz M, Firidin M, Naderi S: Traumatic spondylolisthesis of the axis treated with direct C2 pars screw. *Turk Neurosurg* 2009;19(2):163-167.
30. Chittiboina P, Wylen E, Ogden A, Mukherjee DP, Vannemreddy P, Nanda A: Traumatic spondylolisthesis of the axis: A biomechanical comparison of clinically relevant anterior and posterior fusion techniques. *J Neurosurg Spine* 2009;11(4):379-387.
31. Greene KA, Dickman CA, Marciano FF, Drabier JB, Hadley MN, Sonntag VK: Acute axis fractures: Analysis of management and outcome in 340 consecutive cases. *Spine (Phila Pa 1976)* 1997;22(16):1842-1852.

32. Isolated fractures of the axis in adults. *Neurosurgery* 2002;50(3 Suppl):S125-S139.

33. Whitehill R, Richman JA, Glaser JA: Failure of immobilization of the cervical spine by the halo vest: A report of five cases. *J Bone Joint Surg Am* 1986;68(3):326-332.

34. Schneider AM, Hipp JA, Nguyen L, Reitman CA: Reduction in head and intervertebral motion provided by 7 contemporary cervical orthoses in 45 individuals. *Spine (Phila Pa 1976)* 2007;32(1): E1-E6.

35. Vaccaro AR, Madigan L, Bauerle WB, Blescia A, Cotler JM: Early halo immobilization of displaced traumatic spondylolisthesis of the axis. *Spine (Phila Pa 1976)* 2002;27(20):2229-2233.

36. Judet R, Roy-Camille R, Saillant G: Fractures du raches cervical. Actualités de Chirurgie Orthopé dique de l'hôpital. *Raymond-Poincaré* 1970;8: 174-195.

37. Roy-Camille R, Saillant G, Bouchet T: Technique du vissage despedicules de C2, in Roy-Camille R, ed: *Cinquiemes Journees d'Orthopedie de la Pitie, Rachis Cervical Superieur*. Paris, France, Masson, 1986, pp 41-43.

38. Xu H, Zhao J, Yuan J, Wang C: Anterior discectomy and fusion with internal fixation for unstable hangman's fracture. *Int Orthop* 2010;34(1): 85-88.

39. Ying Z, Wen Y, Xinwei W, et al: Anterior cervical discectomy and fusion for unstable traumatic spondylolisthesis of the axis. *Spine (Phila Pa 1976)* 2008;33(3):255-258.

40. Harrop JS, Vaccaro A, Przybylski GJ: Acute respiratory compromise associated with flexed cervical traction after C2 fractures. *Spine (Phila Pa 1976)* 2001;26(4):E50-E54.

41. Hadley MN, Browner C, Sonntag VK: Axis fractures: A comprehensive review of management and treatment in 107 cases. *Neurosurgery* 1985; 17(2):281-290.

42. Li XF, Dai LY, Lu H, Chen XD: A systematic review of the management of hangman's fractures. *Eur Spine J* 2006;15(3):257-269.

CHAPTER 25

Subaxial Cervical Spine Burst Fractures

Nancy McLaughlin, MD, PhD, FRCS(C)   Daniel Shedid, MD, Msc, FRCS(C), FABN
Edward C. Benzel, MD

Definition

A burst fracture of the lower cervical spine has been described as an incomplete or complete fragmentation of the vertebral body. Retropulsion of bony fragments of the comminuted vertebral body may result in varying degrees of encroachment upon the spinal canal. Burst fractures are also characterized by the loss of vertebral body height and a widening of the interpedicular distance.[1] Furthermore, one or both adjacent disks may be involved (**Figure 1**).

Pathomechanics

Burst fractures may occur following motor vehicle accidents, falls from a height, contact sports, or diving accidents. They result from severe axial loads, with or without various degrees of flexion,[2] leading to the explosion of the vertebral body. In a study using young male cadaveric cervical spines, Zhu et al[3] demonstrated that instability caused by compressive trauma increased with the level of impact energy. Bony injury, however, occurred only after high-energy trauma (50 J).[3] A biomechanical analysis of compression injuries demonstrated that compressive forces applied to normal spinal segments induced a repeatable sequence of pathologic changes;[4] after bulging of the anulus and end plate and the squeezing of blood out of the vertebral bodies, the end plate cracked, allowing the nucleus pulposus to push into the vertebral body and induce a fracture.[4] Ultimately, it appears that the ultimate compressive strength of the vertebral body depends on the bone mineral content.[5]

Disrupted spinal elements may transiently encroach upon the spinal cord. Such encroachment may, however, decrease following injury. Therefore, postinjury radiographic assessment of spinal canal involvement may not provide an accurate representation of the extent to which the spinal cord was damaged at the time of injury. Carter et al[6] quantified geometric changes in the spinal canal of human cadaveric cervical spine specimens during and after fast axial loading resulting in a burst fracture. They found that immediate postinjury spinal canal midsagittal diameter measurement significantly underestimated the amount of transient canal occlusion occurring during high-rate fractures.[6] Although spinal canal length decreased transiently during impact, it was only partially restored after injury. No correlation was found between transient changes and postinjury values. Chang et al[7] conducted similar biomechanical studies. They found that the midsagittal diameter decreased significantly during impact compared with postinjury measurements, with a small but significant correlation between values.[7] Transient spinal canal occlusion and shortening might induce greater neurologic deficit than that expected from radiologic assessments.[6] This supports the belief that initial mechanical trauma occurring during spinal injury initiates a sequence of closely related events that result in neural injury.[8,9]

Classification

Although classification systems have been proposed to categorize cervical spine injuries, none have gained universal acknowledgment. Cervical injuries are described with regard to injury mechanism,[2,10] pathomorphologic and functional aspects,[11] and radiographic features.[12]

Dr. Shedid or an immediate family member is a member of a speakers' bureau or has made paid presentations on behalf of DePuy, a Johnson & Johnson company; serves as a paid consultant to or is an employee of Baxano; has received research or institutional support from DePuy, a Johnson & Johnson company; and owns stock or stock options in Baxano. Dr. Benzel or an immediate family member has received royalties from AxioMed and DePuy, a Johnson & Johnson company; serves as an unpaid consultant to DePuy, a Johnson & Johnson company; and owns stock or stock options in AxioMed. Neither Dr. McLaughlin nor any immediate family member has received anything of value from or owns stock in a commercial company or institution related directly or indirectly to the subject of this chapter.

FIGURE 1

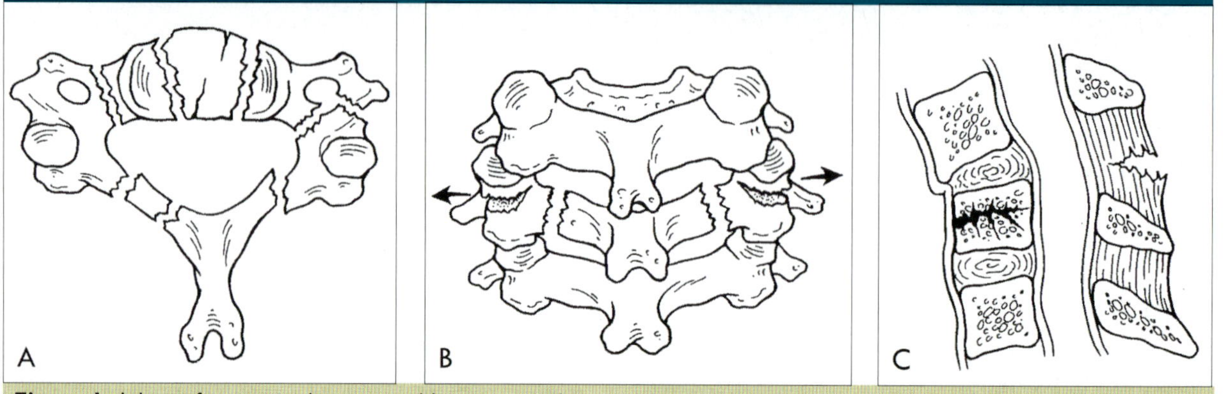

Figure 1 A burst fracture is characterized by an incomplete or complete fragmentation of the vertebral body (**A**), secondary widening of the interpedicular distance (**B**), and a loss of vertebral body height and the involvement of one or both adjacent disks (**C**). (Adapted with permission from Aebi M, Benzel E: Cervical spine burst fractures, in Cervical Spine Research Society, eds: *The Cervical Spine*, ed 3. Philadelphia, PA, Lippincott-Raven Publishers, 1998, pp 465-473.)

TABLE 1

Mechanistic Classification of Closed, Indirect Fracture and Dislocation of the Lower Cervical Spine by Allen et al

Type	Injury Stages
Compression flexion	CF 1-5
Vertical compression	CV 1-3
Distractive flexion	DF 1-4
Compressive extension	CE 1-5
Distractive extension	DE 1-2
Lateral flexion	LF 1-2

(From Allen BL Jr, Ferguson RL, Lehmann TR, O'Brien RP: A mechanistic classification of closed, indirect fractures and dislocations of the lower cervical spine. *Spine (Phila Pa 1976)* 1982;7(1):1-27.)

(Adapted from Aebi M, Benzel E: Cervical spine burst fractures, in Cervical Spine Research Society, eds: *The Cervical Spine*, ed 3. Philadelphia, PA, Lippincott-Raven Publishers, 1998, pp 465-473.)

Allen et al[2] developed a classification scheme based on the mechanism of injury. This scheme divides the cervical spine into two columns: (1) the ventral column, including the posterior longitudinal ligament and structures ventral to it; and (2) the posterior column, including structures dorsal to the posterior longitudinal ligament.[2] Burst fractures correspond to stage 3 vertical compression injury with this system (**Table 1**).

Denis[10] classified fractures of the thoracolumbar spine according to mechanism of injury, radiographic findings, and presence or absence of spine stability. His three-column spine model was introduced for use in the thoracolumbar spine and was then applied to the cervical spine.[10] The middle column is formed by the dorsal wall of the vertebral body, the posterior longitudinal ligament, and dorsal anulus fibrosus. According to this scheme, burst fractures imply failure under compression of both the anterior and middle columns.[10] The recognition of posterior column involvement, however, is important with regard to surgical decision-making.[13]

Magerl et al[11] have established a comprehensive classification system for thoracic and lumbar injuries by taking into consideration the mechanism of injury, pathomorphologic uniformity, and prognostic aspects regarding healing potential. This classification scheme has also been applied to cervical fractures (**Table 2**).

Using preoperative plain radiographs and axial and sagittal CT reconstructed images, McCormack et al[12] developed a grading system based on the amount of damaged vertebral body (extent of comminution), the spread of the fragments in the fracture site (fragment dispersion), and the amount of corrected traumatic kyphosis (**Figure 2**). This load-sharing classification can help estimate the extent of instability of the injured spine and plan surgical intervention.

Vaccaro et al[14] recently defined a new classification system for subaxial cervical trauma. This scheme takes into consideration the injury pattern, severity, treatment consideration, and prognosis. The three main categories identified as independently important to injury classification include injury morphology, discoligamentous complex, and neurologic status[14] (**Table 3**). The injury se-

TABLE 2

Classification of Lower Cervical Spine Injuries by Magerl et al[11]

Type	Description
A	Vertebral body fractures (compressive lesions)
B	Posterior disruptions (distractive lesions)
C	Rotational dislocation combined with type A, B, or both (special lesions)

If no posterior element injury is present, a burst fracture is classified as type A. If posterior element distraction is present, it is classified as type B, whereas if a rotational component is superimposed, it is classified as type C.

(Adapted from Aebi M, Benzel E: Cervical spine burst fractures, in Cervical Spine Research Society, eds: *The Cervical Spine*, ed 3. Philadelphia, PA, Lippincott-Raven Publishers, 1998, pp 465-473.)

verity score resulting from the addition of each weighted score is used to guide treatment options. This subaxial injury classification and severity scale is the first to abandon the mechanism and anatomy characterized by other classification systems in favor of injury morphology and neurologic status.[14]

Diagnosis

Clinical Evaluation

The most important phase in the treatment of the multiply injured patient begins at the scene of the accident. The initial goals of the emergency personnel should be expedient evaluation, extrication, and transport of the patient to the nearest emergency center, without causing or increasing neurologic injury.

At the trauma center, the Advanced Trauma Life Support protocol of resuscitation is implemented.[15] A spine injury must be assumed in all trauma patients until clinically and/or radiologically evaluated. Throughout the initial assessment, spine precautions should be followed. When oxygenation is inadequate and intubation is required, special measures must be taken to protect the uncleared cervical spine. Hypotension must initially be managed with fluids and possibly vasopressors. Although hypovolemia is the most frequent cause of hypotension following trauma, neurogenic shock must be considered, particularly in the presence of bradycardia.

FIGURE 2

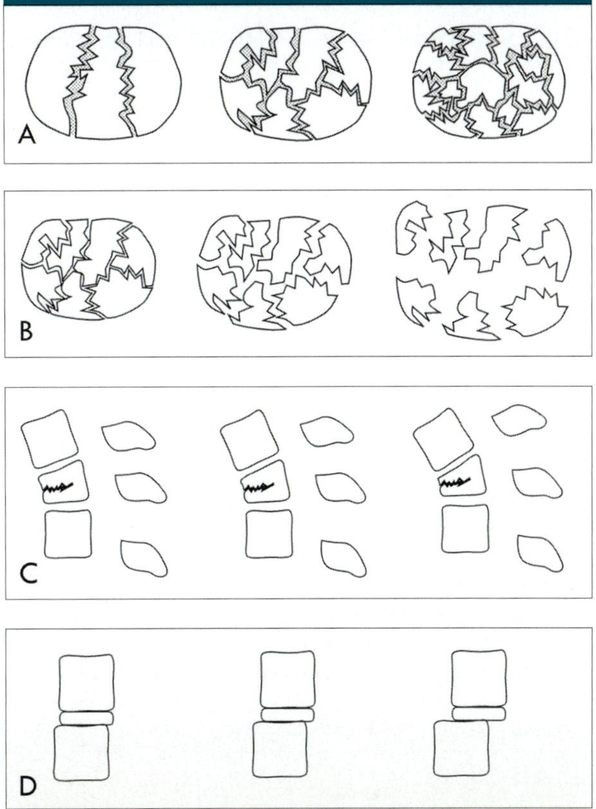

Figure 2 Thoracic and lumbar fracture assessment. **A,** The extent of fracture comminution. **B,** The extent of dispersion of the fragments. **C,** The extent of angular deformation. **D,** The extent of translation (in any plane). These factors are used to determine axial load-bearing capacity (**A**, **B**, and **C**) and the angular and translational deformation resistance ability (**C** and **D**). (Adapted with permission from Benzel E: Trauma, tumor, and infection, in Benzel E, ed: *Biomechanics of Spine Stabilization*. Rolling Meadows, IL, American Association of Neurological Surgeons, 2001, pp 61-82.)

Following stabilization, a thorough physical examination should include inspection and palpation of the head and the entire spine, searching for lacerations, contusions, ecchymoses, swelling, tenderness, gaps, and widened interspinous space. Findings might provide useful information regarding the mechanism of injury that might not have been reported.[16] Any trauma-associated injuries to the head, scapula, pelvis, and long bones should alert the examiner to spinal injury.[17] After the primary assessment is completed, a more detailed neurologic examination must be performed, using validated tools such as the Frankel Neurologic Performance scale[18] or the American Spinal Injury Association (ASIA) classification scheme.[19] Neurologic injury can present as pain, nerve root injury,

TABLE 3

The Sub-axial Injury Classification (SLIC) and Severity Scale

	Points
Morphology	
No abnormality	0
Compression	1
Burst	+1 = 2
Distraction (eg, facet perch, hyperextension)	3
Rotation/translation (eg, facet dislocation, unstable teardrop or advanced staged flexion compression injury	4
Discoligamentous complex (DLC)	
Intact	0
Indeterminate (eg, isolated interspinous widening, MRI signal change only)	1
Disrupted (eg, widening of disk space, facet perch or dislocation)	2
Neurologic status	
Intact	0
Root injury	1
Complete cord injury	2
Incomplete cord injury	3
Continuous cord compression in setting of neuron deficit (neuro modifier)	+1

(Reproduced with permission from Vaccaro AR, Hulbert RJ, Patel AA, et al: The subaxial cervical spine injury classification system: A novel approach to recognize the importance of morphology, neurology, and integrity of the disco-ligamentous complex. *Spine (Phila Pa 1976)* 2007;32(21):2365-2374.)

and partial or complete spinal cord injury. A cord lesion is qualified as incomplete if any residual motor or sensory function more than three segments below the level of injury is preserved.[20] Frequent reevaluation is essential to monitor for subsequent neurologic deterioration or recuperation.

Imaging

All algorithms for cervical spine imaging following trauma should assess the necessity of imaging in addition to determining which, if any, studies to order. Two large studies addressed the question of necessity. The National Emergency X-Radiography Utilization Study (NEXUS) included 34,069 patients with blunt trauma who underwent radiography of the cervical spine.[21,22] NEXUS established five criteria enabling identification of low-risk patients for cervical injury after trauma (**Table 4**).[22] Its sensitivity and specificity were 99.6% and 12.9%, respectively.[22] The Canadian C-Spine rule (CCR) evaluated 8,924 alert and stable trauma patients with plain cervical radiographs.[23] This decision tool is based on three high-risk criteria, five low-risk criteria, and the ability of patients to rotate their necks (**Figure 3**). Its sensitivity and specificity were 100% and 42.5%, respectively.[23] The CCR is believed to be a more accurate tool for the triage of cervical spinal trauma.[24] Therefore, some patients might not need radiographic investigation at all.

Until a few years ago, plain radiography was the initial imaging procedure performed for cervical spine evaluation in trauma patients. A cervical spine series should include a lateral view, AP view, and odontoid view.[25] It is important to visualize the entire cervical spine from the occiput to the superior end plate of the T1 vertebral body. If the cervicothoracic junction is not clearly visualized, an additional swimmer's view or supine oblique views may be necessary.[26] Alignment of the spinolaminar line, bony integrity, cartilage and joint spaces, and soft tissues must be systematically assessed. Three radiographic signs are important in identifying burst fractures:[1] compression of the vertebral body,[2] disruption of the dorsal vertebral body line representing retropulsed bone fragments, and widening of the interpedicular distance.[3] In addition to these signs, subluxation and loss of normal lordosis suggest disruption of the dorsal ligamentous structures and resulting spinal instability.[27] Therefore, what is considered a simple compressive fracture can be unstable, depending on the extent of ligamentous disruption.[28]

TABLE 4

The NEXUS Low-Risk Criteria[a]

Cervical spine radiology is indicated for patients with trauma unless they meet all of the following criteria:
No posterior midline cervical-spine tenderness[b]
No evidence of intoxication[c]
A normal level of alertness[d]
No focal neurologic deficit[e]
No painful distracting injuries[f]

[a]Criteria are from Hoffman et al.[21]

[b]Midline posterior bony cervical spine tenderness is present if the patient reports pain on palpation of the posterior midline neck from the nuchal ridge to the prominence of the first thoracic vertebra, or if the patient evinces pain with direct palpation of any cervical spinous process.

[c]Patients should be considered intoxicated if they have either of the following: a recent history provided by the patient or an observer of intoxication or intoxicating ingestion; or evidence of intoxication on physical examination such as an odor of alcohol, slurred speech, ataxia, dysmetria, or other cerebellar findings, or any behavior consistent with intoxication. Patients may also be considered to be intoxicated if tests of bodily secretions are positive for alcohol or drugs that affect the level of alertness.

[d]An altered level of alertness can include any of the following: a Glasgow Coma Scale score of 14 or less; disorientation to person, place, time, or events; an inability to remember three objects at 5 minutes; a delayed or inappropriate response to external stimuli; or other findings.

[e]A focal neurologic deficit is any focal neurologic finding on motor or sensory examination.

[f]No precise definition of a painful distracting injury is possible. This category includes any condition thought by the clinician to be producing pain sufficient to distract the patient from a second (neck) injury. Such injuries may include, but are not limited to, any long-bone fracture; a visceral injury requiring surgical consultation; a large laceration, degloving injury, or crush injury; large burns; or any other injury causing acute functional impairment. Physicians may also classify any injury as distracting if it is thought to have the potential to impair the patient's ability to appreciate other injuries.

(Adapted with permission from Stiell IG, Clement CM, McKnight RD, et al: The Canadian C-spine rule versus the NEXUS low-risk criteria in patients with trauma. *N Engl J Med* 2003;349(26):2510-2518.)

Flexion-extension radiographs are indicated in patients with normal cervical plain radiographs who report persisting neck pain. Nearly all flexion-extension images, however, reveal no additional abnormalities in patients with blunt trauma.[29] Insko et al[30] evaluated the use of this evaluation strategy in the acute setting and found that 30% were limited by inadequate cervical motion. Acute neck pain and paraspinal muscle spasm may limit the capacity to flex and extend adequately and therefore mask unstable ligamentous injuries.[30] In some cases, flexion-extension radiographs may be useful to exclude delayed instability 2 to 4 weeks after trauma.[31] Literature on fluoroscopic flexion and extension cervical spine evaluations in the obtunded patient is limited. Reports on its safety and its performance as a diagnostic test are divergent.[32,33]

Although plain radiographic evaluation has long been the gold standard, recent data suggest that CT is the best initial imaging procedure for bony cervical spine injury. The reported incidence of missed cervical spine injury in blunt trauma patients evaluated initially with radiographs varies from 0.5 to 61%.[34-37] Occult cervical spinal injuries may result in significant morbidity, with permanent sequelae resulting from delay in diagnosis and treatment in 29% of patients.[35] CT is the preferred initial imaging modality in blunt spinal trauma patients in many centers throughout the world.[38] The sensitivity of CT for detection of spinal fractures ranges from 97% to 100%.[38,39] In addition to being accurate, it reduces patient mobilization and time for spinal evaluation.[40] CT is cost-effective in cases of high or moderate probability of injury.[40] Specific indications for CT and extent of imaging (symptomatic level, not adequately visualized level or complete cervical spine) vary considerably. CT is performed when plain films do not enable optimal visualization of the spine, when unexplained focal pain or neurologic deficit exists with a negative plain film, when soft-tissue swelling is present, or when the plain radiograph is abnormal.[41] Axial CT is limited regarding the

FIGURE 3

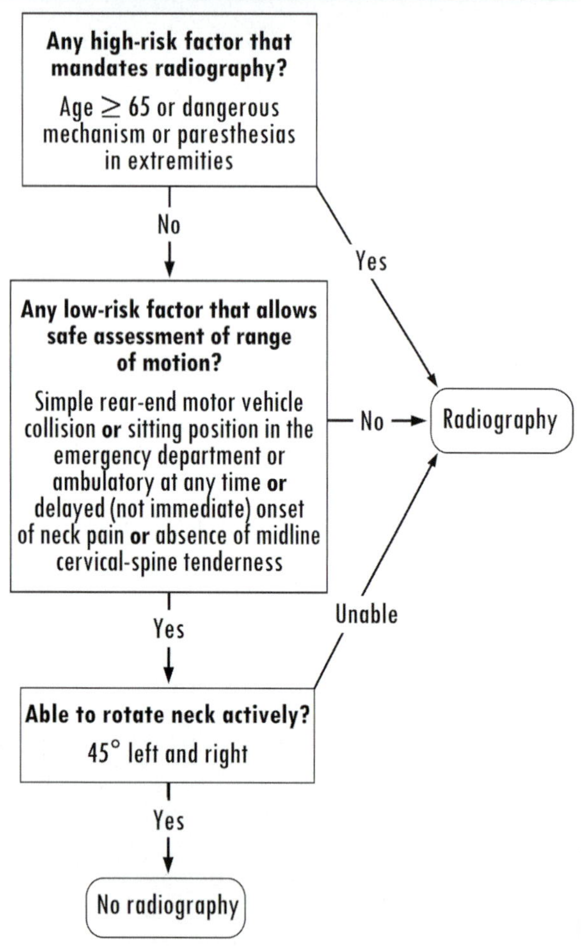

Figure 3 For patients with trauma who are alert (as indicated by a score of 15 on the Glasgow Coma Scale) and in stable condition, and in whom cervical spine injury is a concern, the determination of risk factors guides the use of cervical spine radiography. A dangerous mechanism is considered to be a fall from an elevation ≥ 3 ft or five stairs; an axial load to the head (eg, diving); a motor vehicle collision at high speed (> 100 km/h), or with rollover or ejection; a collision involving a motorized recreational vehicle; or a bicycle collision. A simple rear-end motor vehicle collision excludes being pushed into oncoming traffic, being hit by a bus or large truck, a rollover, and being hit by a high-speed vehicle. (Reproduced with permission from Stiell IG, Clement CM, McKnight RD, et al: The Canadian C-spine rule versus the NEXUS low-risk criteria in patients with trauma. *N Eng J Med* 2003;349(26):2510-2518. © 2006 Massachusetts Medical Society. All rights reserved.)

visualization of subluxations, increases in intervertebral distances, abnormal angulations, and horizontal fractures.[41,42] The advent of helical CT has, however, improved the detection rate of these spinal abnormalities. MRI is the modality of choice in assessing soft-tissue injuries, spinal cord injury, and intervertebral disks and ligaments.[43] It enables differentiation of spinal cord hemorrhage and edema, which can have significant prognostic significance in the final outcome of the motor system.[44] MRI is indicated in the presence of myelopathy, radiculopathy, progressive neurologic deficit, and/or unexpected neurologic deficit not explained by radiographic findings.[41] Moreover, patients with negative cervical plain films and persisting pain after trauma should be evaluated by MRI because of its ability to detect ligamentous injuries that are not evident on plain radiographs or are missed on flexion-extension examinations.[45] Although MRI is sensitive when using it solely to determine ligamentous injury, whether actual spinal instability results from the documented ligamentous injury is debated.[46,47]

Treatment

The initial goal of management of spinal injury is to prevent or minimize the progression of the primary injury. Initial immobilization, cardiopulmonary resuscitation maintaining normotension and normohypoxia, and early reduction and maintenance of spinal alignment are crucial steps. Few pharmaceutical agents have been used for the prevention or treatment of the secondary biochemical injury cascade.

Medical Treatment

Methylprednisolone, the most extensively used medical modality for spinal cord injuries, exerts its effects by decreasing lipid oxidation, stabilizing the cell membranes, enhancing spinal cord blood flow, and decreasing vascular permeability and edema.[48] The routine use of corticosteroids remains controversial because there is insufficient evidence to support treatment standards.[49] Treatment with methylprednisolone is optional in the management of patients with acute cervical spine injury, given that evidence suggesting harmful side effects is more consistent than any suggestion of clinical benefit.[49] Following the National Acute Spinal Cord Injury Study III guidelines, a 24-hour course should be given to patients receiving steroids within the first 3 hours after injury and a 48-hour course if patients received their first dose 3 to 8 hours after injury. In both circumstances, a loading dose of 30 mg/kg should be administered followed by a maintenance dose of 5.4 mg/kg/h for the determined period.[48] Proton pump inhibitors should be used for gastrointestinal ulcer prophylaxis.[50]

Nonsurgical Treatment

The goals of treatment of cervical spinal injury are to provide spinal stability, restore anatomic alignment, preserve and improve neurologic function, and prevent late deformity.[51] After initial radiographic evaluation is completed, patients with significant burst fractures and neural deficits or spinal instability should be placed under craniocervical traction. Closed reduction of dislocations and fractures can be performed with Gardner-Wells tongs in awake and alert patients. Craniocervical traction is initiated by applying 3 lb per rostral level injury.[52] Weight may be added as often as every 10 to 15 minutes if clinical, neurologic, and radiographic monitoring is performed regularly. No upper weight limit has been described in the literature.[52] Any neurologic deterioration or severe pain occurring during reduction warrants a reduction of weight to restore neurologic status and radiographic evaluation using plain films. If vertebral alignment and stability (overdistraction) are not in question, CT and/or MRI should be performed to rule out disk herniation,[53] epidural hematoma,[54] and spinal cord edema.[55] If closed reduction is unsuccessful, external stabilization should be considered before transport to the radiology suite for further assessment or to the operating room for surgical management.[56,57] If closed reduction is successful, traction is continued. In the protocol proposed by Ducker et al,[58] traction was continued for 4 weeks, followed by a halo vest for 8 weeks, and a soft collar for 4 weeks. They observed that less than 10% of pure burst fractures required delayed surgical fusion.[58] The complications associated with bed rest and the cost of care regarding this strategy, however, may be prohibitive. The efficacy of such conservative treatment has been challenged, as discussed below.

Burst fractures in patients who are either neurologically intact or complete and out of spinal shock, without significant dorsal element involvement, may be treated nonsurgically by applying a halo vest or a hard cervicothoracic orthosis for 2 to 3 months. Although the halo vest provides the most rigid external cervical immobilization of all orthoses, it allows considerable segmental motion through a process of paradoxical spinal motion described as "snaking."[59] The residual motion may be clinically significant in patients with very unstable injuries, resulting in neurologic injury, persisting instability, or progressive deformity.[60,61] Fusion was achieved in 85% of patients following immobilization with a halo fixator.[62] Although halo vests allow early patient mobilization and shorten hospital stays, compared with supine cervical traction techniques, complications occur frequently.[61,63,64] Minor complications include pin loosening, pin-site infection, periorbital edema, superficial pressure sores, and cosmetically disfiguring scars. Major complications include dural penetration, osteomyelitis, subdural abscess, cranial nerve palsies, fracture overdistraction, and persistent instability. Flexion-extension lateral radiographs should be obtained when the orthosis is removed to be certain no occult, residual dorsal ligamentous instability is present.

Orthoses failed to maintain reduction of subaxial cervical fracture-dislocation injuries in 7% to 56% of patients.[65] Overall, 30% had recurrent displacement or inadequate alignment during external immobilization and 11% required subsequent surgical treatments.[65] More specifically, 5% of compression fractures of the subaxial cervical spine treated with immobilization for 8 to 12 weeks had persistent instability.[65] Morbidity and mortality associated with external traction/immobilization treatment,[61,63,64] as well as its associated failure rate,[65] underscore the usefulness of internal fixation in the management of cervical spine injuries.

Surgical Indications and Timing

Koivikko et al[66] retrospectively compared traction or halo-vest nonsurgical management with the surgical treatment of 65 cervical burst and flexion teardrop fractures. Patients treated with ventral decompression, bone grafting, and fixation with a Caspar plate were found to have greater neurologic improvement, greater spinal canal diameter, and less kyphotic deformation.[66] Kiwerski[67] studied 273 patients with cervical spine crush fractures, of whom 70 were treated with craniocervical traction and 203 were treated by ventral decompression and fusion. Neurologic improvement was observed in 14% of patients treated nonsurgically and 44% of patients treated surgically.

Many factors should be considered during the decision-making process. Neurologic deficits, extent of spinal canal compromise, the presence of spinal instability, and the potential for deformity of the cervical spine influence management decisions.

Neurologic Involvement

At admission, neurologic assessment may reveal a neurologically normal patient, an incomplete or complete myelopathy, or an isolated radiculopathy. The neurologic response to traction should be noted. Patients with incomplete spinal cord injury

TABLE 5

Quantification of Acute Instability for Subaxial Cervical, Thoracic, and Lumbar Injuries

Condition	Points Assigned[a]
Loss of integrity of anterior (and middle) column[b]	2
Loss of integrity of posterior column(s)[b]	2
Acute resting translational deformity[c]	2
Acute dynamic translation deformity exaggeration[d]	2
Acute dynamic angulation deformity exaggeration[d]	2
Neural element injury[e]	3
Acute disk narrowing at level of suspected pathology	1
Dangerous loading anticipated	1

[a]A score of 5 points or more implies the presence of overt instability. A score of 2 to 4 points implies the presence of limited instability.

[b]By clinical examination, MRI, CT, or radiography. A single point may be allotted if incomplete evidence exists—for example, only MRI evidence of dorsal ligamentous injury (ie, evidence of only interspinous ligament injury on T2-weighted images). Columns are defined as per Denis.[10]

[c]From static resting AP and lateral spine radiographs. Must be the result of an acute clinical process. Tolerance for this criterion is variable with respect to surgeon and clinical circumstances. Guidelines as per White and Panjabi.[72]

[d]From dynamic (flexion-extension) spine radiographs. Recommended only after other mechanisms of instability assessment have been exhausted, and then only by an experienced clinician. Usually indicated only in cervical region. Must be the result of an acute clinical process. Tolerance for this criterion is variable with respect to surgeon's opinion and clinical circumstances. Guidelines as per White and Panjabi.[72]

[e]Three points for cauda equina, 2 points for spinal cord, or 1 point for isolated nerve root neurologic deficit. The presence of neural element injury indicates that a significant spinal deformation occurred at the time of impact, implying that structural integrity may well have been disturbed.

(Adapted from White and Panjabi[72] as modified in Benzel E: Stability and instability of the spine, in Benzel E, ed: *Biomechanics of Spine Stabilization*. Rolling Meadows, IL, American Association of Neurologic Surgeons, 2001 pp 29-43.)

(Adapted from Aebi M, Benzel E: Cervical spine burst fractures, in Cervical Spine Research Society, eds: *The Cervical Spine*, ed 3. Philadelphia, PA, Lippincott-Raven Publishers, 1998, pp 465-473.)

who do not improve following traction, and who are observed to have residual spinal cord compression after traction, should undergo decompression.[68] Patients with complete myelopathy who present with dysfunction of the nerve root distal to the level of fracture after reduction with traction should be considered for surgical decompression to enhance recovery of nerve root function.[69]

Extent of Spinal Canal Compromise

Onset of neurologic injury usually occurs with 30% to 35% of spinal canal encroachment.[70] However, a correlation has been established between neurologic deficit and spinal canal encroachment when canal narrowing is 50% or more.[71] Controversy exists regarding the optimal management of neurologically intact patients presenting with spinal canal narrowing. The retropulsed bony fragment may spontaneously remodel if stability is achieved.

Instability

Clinical instability is defined as "the loss of the ability of the spine, under physiologic loads, to maintain its pattern of displacement so that there is no initial or additional neurologic deficit, no major deformity, and no incapacitating pain."[72] Criteria for the diagnosis of clinical stability have been developed by White and Panjabi (**Table 5**).[72] Holdsworth[73] considered burst fractures to be stable injuries because the dorsal ligaments were intact. However, the flexion component of these injuries is often difficult to assess, rendering burst fractures unstable in the presence of dorsal ligamentous complex disruption.[74] Assessment of burst fracture stability is relevant because unstable injuries are managed differently due to their poorer healing potential. In addition, the presence of distraction or rotational injury of the dorsal osteoligamentous elements may endanger neural integrity and/or cause chronic pain.[11]

Timing of Surgery

Once the decision for surgical intervention has been made, the surgeon must determine when to intervene. If neurologic function is deteriorating, then acute decompression must be performed to treat spinal cord compression. However, in the presence of stable neurologic deficits, there is controversy regarding the timing of surgery.[75] Advocates of early surgery emphasize that early decompression and stabilization decrease ongoing secondary injury to the spinal cord and result in better outcome.[76,77] Early surgery allows early patient mobilization and rehabilitation, decreasing overall morbidity, duration of acute hospitalization, and cost of treatment.[78] The precise time frame to achieve optimal results is, however, unknown. Advocates of delayed surgery stress that the majority of spinal cord damage occurs at the time of injury and that the traumatized spinal cord is extremely vulnerable during the acute phase of injury.[74,79] Marshall et al[79] prospectively examined the frequency of neurologic worsening in 283 patients with acute spinal cord injury. In patients with cervical spine injury, worsening was observed only in patients operated on within 5 days of injury. Other studies concluded similarly that surgery performed within 3 to 5 days have resulted in increased morbidity and mortality.[53,80] However, retrospective studies comparing early versus delayed surgery of complete and incomplete cervical spine injuries have shown no adverse effects of early surgery.[81,82]

If the patient is intact neurologically, there is less debate regarding the timing of surgery, although some might argue that there exists an exaggerated spinal cord vulnerability during the acute period following injury. The urgency of decompression in an intact patient with radiographic evidence of spinal cord compression remains controversial.

Surgical Management

The surgeon must determine the optimal surgical approach in his or her hands. Multiple factors should be considered during this decision-making process.

Ventral Approach

Ventral approaches to the traumatized cervical spine are usually undertaken when there is neurologic compromise secondary to ventral compression, loss of anterior column integrity, and kyphotic deformity. In general, ventral surgery is superior to dorsal surgery.[81,83-85] This approach usually involves minimal blood loss and relatively straightforward access. The ventral approach enables the removal of retropulsed bony fragments under direct vision. Ventral decompression procedures can be performed with or without fusion and with or without instrumentation.

Schulte et al[86] determined the immediate biomechanical stability of the cervical spine without dorsal ligamentous disruption following load deformation. The application of a ventral plate, in addition to a bony strut at the injured cervical level, provided significant reduction in motion in all loading modalities. This construct possessed equal to or greater strength than the intact specimen.[86] Similarly, Grubb et al[87] performed a corpectomy with a release of dorsal ligamentous structures and stabilization with a ventral plate. Instrumented specimens had flexural, lateral bending, and torsional stiffness values that were similar to or greater than those of their paired intact specimens.[87]

Bone mineral density of the specimen used in biomechanical studies is a strong determinant of the degree of stabilization achieved, regardless of the type of plate used.[88] Clinically, the insertion of a bone graft in a well-vascularized bony bed under axial compression with ventral plating optimizes fusion rates.[81] Using a fixation plate, Böhler and Gaudernak[83] consistently achieved solid fusion of the involved region of the cervical spine without recurrence of the deformity. Some studies have not observed an increased bony healing rate associated with ventral plate fixation.[89,90] A review of the relevant published literature demonstrated that the reported nonunion rate with ventral plating is approximately 3%.[91]

If the caudal third of the caudal vertebral body and caudal end plate of the rostral vertebral body are intact, fixation may be limited to the injured segment. In this setting, the caudal screws of a ventral plating system are inserted into the intact lower third of the vertebral body into the subchondral bone (**Figure 4**).

Both unicortical and bicortical screws used with nonlocking ventral plate systems can decrease immediate flexibility of the tested cervical segment.[92] This suggests that unicortical screw fixation can be used for ventral plate fixation with immediate stability comparable to bicortical screw fixation and without the risk of dorsal cortex penetration. In addition, studies have shown that plating with locked fixation screws (fixed moment-arm cantilever beam) provides greater stability than ventral plating with no locking at the screw-plate interface (nonfixed moment-arm cantilever beam).[87,93]

FIGURE 4

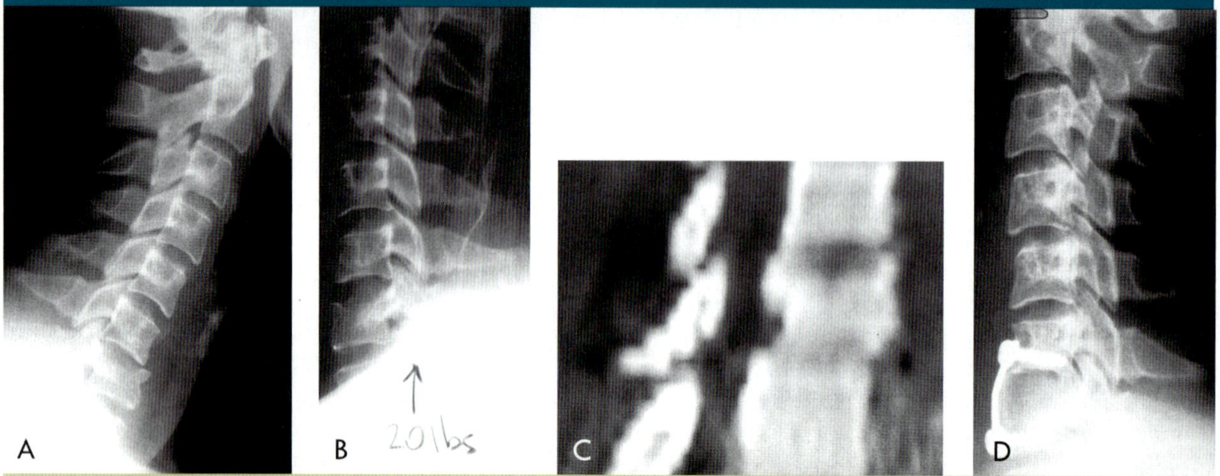

Figure 4 A burst fracture of C7. **A,** Lateral burst with kyphosis deformity. **B,** After axial traction with 20 lb, satisfactory reduction was achieved. **C,** Sagittal CT reconstruction demonstrating the fractured posterior wall of C7. **D,** Following anterior decompression, a monosegmental anterior fusion of C6-C7 using a simple Orozco plate with titanium plasma cover and 3.5-mm screws that did not protrude through the posterior wall was performed. Note that the distal screws are placed in the subchondral bone of the C7 distal end plate. (Adapted from Aebi M, Benzel E: Cervical spine burst fractures, in Cervical Spine Research Society, eds: *The Cervical Spine*, ed 3. Philadelphia, PA, Lippincott-Raven Publishers, 1998, pp 465-473.)

Dorsal Approach

The dorsal approach is indicated for the treatment of dorsal compression of the neural elements and for failure of the posterior column structures, with preservation of the anterior column integrity. Nonetheless, some authors have reported successful stabilization of vertebral body fractures and ventral ligamentous injuries with dorsal constructs.[94,95] Current techniques for posterior cervical spinal stabilization following trauma include wiring techniques, pedicle or lateral mass screws (with or without plates or rods), and laminar clamps.

Dorsal spinal wiring can be applied to spinous processes, facets, and laminae. This technique ensures stability in flexion but not in extension and rotation. Therefore, it is not usually recommended as a stand-alone construct. Neurologic deterioration has been reported following sublaminar wiring, as well as with spinous process wiring in cases where wires were placed too far ventrally.[96]

In cases presenting with dorsal element deficiency requiring dorsal cervical fixation, lateral mass plating with optional C2 and/or C7 pedicle screw placement restores the dorsal tension band and provides effective stabilization.[97] Some authors suggest that halo-vest immobilization is unnecessary and supplemental bone grafting is generally not required for recent trauma patients.[97] Although lateral mass plating systems have been shown to be safe and reliable,[94,98] their use can be problematic in patients with abnormal cervical anatomy and suboptimal bone density.[99] Furthermore, compromised screw placement and implant failure can partially account for the risk of vertebral artery and nerve root injury.[99] Unicortical lateral mass screws provide an equivalent strength with a much lower risk of injury than bicortical screws placed in a similar orientation.[100]

Pedicle screw fixation systems have gained acceptance as an effective and reliable method of spinal stabilization.[101] Cervical pedicle screws have been shown to have significantly higher pull-out strength than lateral mass screws.[102] Given the variations in pedicle anatomy between patients, screw placement may be suboptimal, risking neurovascular complications and fixation failure.[101,103] Imaging techniques that provide an accurate spatial orientation may facilitate pedicle screw placement and help minimize complications.[104,105]

Interlaminar clamps have been shown to be safe and effective as a dorsal stabilization strategy in the lower cervical spine.[106-108] Multilevel fixation with these devices is associated with excessive construct failure and should be avoided.[108] Also, a significant failure rate was found with its use for atlantoaxial arthrodesis.[107,108]

Combined Approach

It has been shown that ventral plating systems are capable of substantially stabilizing the cervical spine in all modes of loading after a burst frac-

FIGURE 5

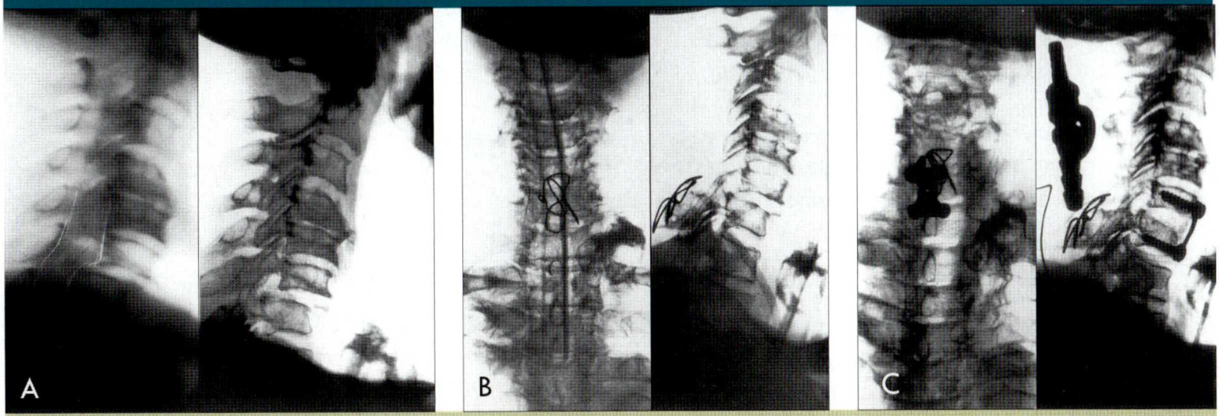

Figure 5 **A,** An 80-year-old man with significant degenerative stiffness in the cervical spine sustained a fracture-dislocation of C6-C7 and incomplete quadriplegia. **B,** Posterior reduction and wire stabilization was inadequate. **C,** Anterior plate fixation was added and provided sufficient stability for rehabilitation without external bracing. The patient became an independent walker. (Adapted from Aebi M, Benzel E: Cervical spine burst fractures, in Cervical Spine Research Society, eds: *The Cervical Spine*, ed 3. Philadelphia, PA, Lippincott-Raven Publishers, 1998, pp 465-473.)

ture.[109,110] Do Koh et al[111] found that ventral plate fixation provides much greater stability in a burst fracture model than in the flexion-distraction injury model. Also, Spivak et al[112] demonstrated that ventral plating alone was able to restore the stability of the cervical spine with dorsal ligamentous injury following corpectomy, but it failed to do so with the addition of bilateral facetectomies.

In the presence of severe dorsal osteoligamentous disruption, although the primary emphasis should be directed ventrally to decompress the spinal cord and establish ventral column integrity, the ventral construct might not be sufficient to ensure stability. In these structures, an additional dorsal stabilization procedure should be considered. By itself, a dorsal stabilization procedure is also likely to result in persistent instability in the presence of a three-column injury (**Figure 5**).[113] There exists evidence suggesting that the combined approach provides significantly better stability than either the ventral or dorsal approach alone.[109,110,112] Indeed, a combined approach or the use of a rigid external immobilization following a ventral approach is often required for three-column injuries.[114-116] In cases of complete myelopathy, the stabilization procedure may be performed in conjunction with foraminotomies, with the goal of improving regional nerve root function.[2,69,71]

A combined single-stage ventral and dorsal decompression, reconstruction, and instrumentation procedure represents a feasible and viable option for the treatment of patients with complex cervical spinal disorders.[117,118] Schultz et al[117] retrospectively studied 72 patients who underwent a combined procedure for complex cervical spine disorders. Their results demonstrated that this technique provides immediate rigid stabilization of the cervical spine, prevents ventral plate failure or strut-graft extrusion, and eliminates the need for halo immobilization postoperatively. In their study population, they observed a higher rate of fusion achieved with this combined approach than with the ventral approach alone.[117] Similarly, McNamara et al[119] performed a single-stage dorsal wiring followed by ventral decompression for the acute surgical management of cervical spine injury in six patients. A halo vest was used for 12 weeks, and then a Philadelphia collar was used for another 4 weeks. Solid fusion was observed in all patients.[119] McAfee et al[115,118] presented two series including patients with cervical spine injuries treated by a single-stage ventral approach, followed by a dorsal approach. Results were satisfactory, with improvement of neurologic deficits and/or reduction of the spinal deformity. Furthermore, because both procedures were performed during one session of general anesthesia, the prevalence of perioperative complications related to the airway was lower than that previously reported in the literature.[118]

Complications

Complications may be a direct result of the cervical spine injury. Frequent evaluations are necessary to detect any clinical deterioration. Ascending paralysis due to ascending central gray-matter necrosis can occur at any time after injury.

Posttraumatic syrinx is documented with MRI.[120] Spinal deformity may be the result of unrecognized instability.[121] In children, paralysis of back muscles caudal to the injury level may result in a scoliotic deformity.

Complications may be related to the management of cervical spine injuries, including complications related to the surgical approach, pseudarthrosis, and instrumentation failure. Ventral approaches carry the risk of injury to the recurrent laryngeal nerve;[122-124] superior laryngeal nerve;[125] cervical sympathetic chain;[124] cranial nerves IX, X, XI, XII;[126-128] spinal cord,[129,130] and carotid[129,131] or vertebral arteries.[132,133] Complications associated with the dorsal approach include injury to the spinal cord,[129,131] nerve roots,[134] and vertebral artery. With both approaches, postoperative epidural hematomas,[135] cerebrospinal fluid leakage,[136] and wound infections[137] rarely occur. Surgery may also induce unrecognized instability. Nonunion or pseudarthrosis (fibrous union) and instrumentation failure are intimately related and may contribute to postoperative spinal deformity. Finally, autologous bone graft harvest is associated with donor-site morbidity.[138]

Systemic complications may also occur during the perioperative period. Gastrointestinal ulcers may occur in up to 40% of patients, usually 10 to 14 days after trauma.[50,139] The administration of methylprednisolone after trauma increases the risk of ulceration. The use of antacids, H2 antagonists, or proton pump inhibitors are important for the prevention and treatment of gastric stress ulcers.[140] Early and adequate caloric replenishment may prevent this complication.[141] Deep venous thrombosis (DVT) is a frequent complication following trauma. The loss of vasomotor tone, immobility, and a hypercoagulation state following trauma all predispose to DVT. The use of low molecular-weight heparins, rotating beds, adjusted-dose heparin, or a combination of modalities is recommended as a prophylactic treatment strategy.[142]

Pulmonary embolism may be minimized by DVT prophylaxis. The paralysis of intercostal muscles and the diaphragm, as well as prolonged immobilization, may lead to hypoventilation, atelectasia, and pneumonia. Intensive respiratory physiotherapy in the awake patient, close monitoring of respiratory parameters, and daily chest radiographs in the intubated patient should be routinely performed.

Skin care is important for immobilized patients.[143] Pressure ulcers should be prevented and aggressively treated if present. Débridement, local wound care, and pressure relief are the mainstays of such treatment. Traction and halo-vest pins must be assessed frequently, as pin loosening and infection are frequently observed.[61,63,64]

Conclusion

Isolated burst fractures of the cervical spine are relatively uncommon. They are caused primarily by axial loading. In the presence of vertebral body collapse, neurologic compromise, or dorsal element injury, surgical intervention should be considered. Ventral decompression and fusion should be undertaken when there is neurologic compromise secondary to ventral compression, loss of anterior column integrity, and kyphotic deformity. The goal of treatment is the attainment of a healing fracture in a stable, well-aligned position, preserving or regaining neurologic function, and preventing late deformity. The dorsal approach is indicated for the treatment of dorsal compression of the neural elements and for failure of the posterior column structures with preservation of the anterior column integrity. A combined ventral and dorsal approach or the use of a rigid external immobilization following a ventral approach may be required for three-column injuries. A thoughtful and orderly evaluation of each case should result in optimal care for patients with cervical spine injuries.

References

1. Daffner RH, Daffner SD: Vertebral injuries: Detection and implications. *Eur J Radiol* 2002;42(2): 100-116.
2. Allen BL Jr, Ferguson RL, Lehmann TR, O'Brien RP: A mechanistic classification of closed, indirect fractures and dislocations of the lower cervical spine. *Spine (Phila Pa 1976)* 1982;7(1):1-27.
3. Zhu Q, Ouyang J, Lu W, et al: Traumatic instabilities of the cervical spine caused by high-speed axial compression in a human model: An in vitro biomechanical study. *Spine (Phila Pa 1976)* 1999; 24(5):440-444.
4. Roaf R: A study of the mechanics of spinal injuries. *J Bone Joint Surg Br* 1960;42:810-823.
5. Hansson T, Roos B, Nachemson A: The bone mineral content and ultimate compressive strength of lumbar vertebrae. *Spine (Phila Pa 1976)* 1980;5(1):46-55.
6. Carter JW, Mirza SK, Tencer AF, Ching RP: Canal geometry changes associated with axial compressive cervical spine fracture. *Spine (Phila Pa 1976)* 2000;25(1):46-54.

7. Chang DG, Tencer AF, Ching RP, Treece B, Senft D, Anderson PA: Geometric changes in the cervical spinal canal during impact. *Spine (Phila Pa 1976)* 1994;19(8):973-980.
8. Ogata T, Nakamura Y, Tsuji K, Okumura H, Kataoka K, Shibata T: Role of aspartate in ischemic spinal cord damage. *J Orthop Res* 1996;14(3): 504-510.
9. Viano DC, King AI, Melvin JW, Weber K: Injury biomechanics research: An essential element in the prevention of trauma. *J Biomech* 1989;22(5): 403-417.
10. Denis F: The three column spine and its significance in the classification of acute thoracolumbar spinal injuries. *Spine (Phila Pa 1976)* 1983;8(8): 817-831.
11. Magerl F, Aebi M, Gertzbein SD, Harms J, Nazarian S: A comprehensive classification of thoracic and lumbar injuries. *Eur Spine J* 1994;3(4): 184-201.
12. McCormack T, Karaikovic E, Gaines RW: The load sharing classification of spine fractures. *Spine (Phila Pa 1976)* 1994;19(15):1741-1744.
13. Wilber RG, Peters JG, Likavec MJ: Surgical techniques in cervical spine surgery, in Errico TJ, Bauer RD, Waugh T, eds: *Spinal Trauma*. Philadelphia, PA, JB Lippincott, 1990.
14. Vaccaro AR, Hulbert RJ, Patel AA, et al: The subaxial cervical spine injury classification system: A novel approach to recognize the importance of morphology, neurology, and integrity of the discoligamentous complex. *Spine (Phila Pa 1976)* 2007; 32(21):2365-2374.
15. American College of Surgeons Committee on Trauma: Initial assessment, in *Advanced Life Support Student Manual*. Chicago, IL, American College of Surgeons, 1997, pp 21-46.
16. Stauffer ES: Management of spine fractures C3 to C7. *Orthop Clin North Am* 1986;17(1):45-53.
17. Saboe LA, Reid DC, Davis LA, Warren SA, Grace MG: Spine trauma and associated injuries. *J Trauma* 1991;31(1):43-48.
18. Frankel HL, Hancock DO, Hyslop G, et al: The value of postural reduction in the initial management of closed injuries of the spine with paraplegia and tetraplegia: I. *Paraplegia* 1969;7(3): 179-192.
19. American Spinal Injury Association: *Standards for Neurologic and Functional Classification of Spinal Cord Injury Revised*. Chicago, IL, American Spinal Injury Association, 1992.
20. Waters RL, Adkins RH, Yakura J, Sie I: Profiles of spinal cord injury and recovery after gunshot injury. *Clin Orthop Relat Res* 1991;267:14-21.
21. Hoffman JR, Wolfson AB, Todd K, Mower WR: Selective cervical spine radiography in blunt trauma: Methodology of the National Emergency X-Radiography Utilization Study (NEXUS). *Ann Emerg Med* 1998;32(4):461-469.
22. Hoffman JR, Mower WR, Wolfson AB, Todd KH, Zucker MI, National Emergency X-Radiography Utilization Study Group: Validity of a set of clinical criteria to rule out injury to the cervical spine in patients with blunt trauma. *N Engl J Med* 2000; 343(2):94-99.
23. Stiell IG, Wells GA, Vandemheen KL, et al: The Canadian C-spine rule for radiography in alert and stable trauma patients. *JAMA* 2001;286(15): 1841-1848.
24. Stiell IG, Clement CM, McKnight RD, et al: The Canadian C-spine rule versus the NEXUS low-risk criteria in patients with trauma. *N Engl J Med* 2003;349(26):2510-2518.
25. MacDonald RL, Schwartz ML, Mirich D, Sharkey PW, Nelson WR: Diagnosis of cervical spine injury in motor vehicle crash victims: How many X-rays are enough? *J Trauma* 1990;30(4):392-397.
26. Jenkins MG, Curran P, Rocke LG: Where do we go after the three standard cervical spine views in the conscious trauma patient? A survey. *Eur J Emerg Med* 1999;6(3):215-217.
27. Webb JK, Broughton RB, McSweeney T, Park WM: Hidden flexion injury of the cervical spine. *J Bone Joint Surg Br* 1976;58(3):322-327.
28. Mazur JM, Stauffer ES: Unrecognized spinal instability associated with seemingly "simple" cervical compression fractures. *Spine (Phila Pa 1976)* 1983; 8(7):687-692.
29. Pollack CV Jr, Hendey GW, Martin DR, Hoffman JR, Mower WR, NEXUS Group: Use of flexion-extension radiographs of the cervical spine in blunt trauma. *Ann Emerg Med* 2001;38(1):8-11.
30. Insko EK, Gracias VH, Gupta R, Goettler CE, Gaieski DF, Dalinka MK: Utility of flexion and extension radiographs of the cervical spine in the acute evaluation of blunt trauma. *J Trauma* 2002; 53(3):426-429.
31. Gebhard JS, Donaldson DH, Brown CW: Soft-tissue injuries of the cervical spine. *Orthop Rev* 1994;Suppl:9-17.
32. Davis JW, Parks SN, Detlefs CL, Williams GG, Williams JL, Smith RW: Clearing the cervical spine in obtunded patients: The use of dynamic fluoroscopy. *J Trauma* 1995;39(3):435-438.
33. Bolinger B, Shartz M, Marion D: Bedside fluoroscopic flexion and extension cervical spine radiographs for clearance of the cervical spine in comatose trauma patients. *J Trauma* 2004;56(1): 132-136.
34. Besman A, Kaban J, Jacobs L, Jacobs LM: False-negative plain cervical spine x-rays in blunt trauma. *Am Surg* 2003;69(11):1010-1014.

35. Davis JW, Phreaner DL, Hoyt DB, Mackersie RC: The etiology of missed cervical spine injuries. *J Trauma* 1993;34(3):342-346.
36. Schenarts PJ, Diaz J, Kaiser C, Carrillo Y, Eddy V, Morris JA Jr: Prospective comparison of admission computed tomographic scan and plain films of the upper cervical spine in trauma patients with altered mental status. *J Trauma* 2001;51(4):663-669.
37. Woodring JH, Lee C: Limitations of cervical radiography in the evaluation of acute cervical trauma. *J Trauma* 1993;34(1):32-39.
38. Griffen MM, Frykberg ER, Kerwin AJ, et al: Radiographic clearance of blunt cervical spine injury: Plain radiograph or computed tomography scan? *J Trauma* 2003;55(2):222-227.
39. Crim JR, Moore K, Brodke D: Clearance of the cervical spine in multitrauma patients: The role of advanced imaging. *Semin Ultrasound CT MR* 2001;22(4):283-305.
40. Blackmore CC, Ramsey SD, Mann FA, Deyo RA: Cervical spine screening with CT in trauma patients: A cost-effectiveness analysis. *Radiology* 1999;212(1):117-125.
41. Van Goethem JW, Maes M, Ozsarlak O, van den Hauwe L, Parizel PM: Imaging in spinal trauma. *Eur Radiol* 2005;15(3):582-590.
42. Woodring JH, Lee C: The role and limitations of computed tomographic scanning in the evaluation of cervical trauma. *J Trauma* 1992;33(5):698-708.
43. Flanders AE, Schaefer DM, Doan HT, Mishkin MM, Gonzalez CF, Northrup BE: Acute cervical spine trauma: Correlation of MR imaging findings with degree of neurologic deficit. *Radiology* 1990;177(1):25-33.
44. Schaefer DM, Flanders AE, Osterholm JL, Northrup BE: Prognostic significance of magnetic resonance imaging in the acute phase of cervical spine injury. *J Neurosurg* 1992;76(2):218-223.
45. Geck MJ, Yoo S, Wang JC: Assessment of cervical ligamentous injury in trauma patients using MRI. *J Spinal Disord* 2001;14(5):371-377.
46. Takhtani D, Melhem ER: MR imaging in cervical spine trauma. *Magn Reson Imaging Clin N Am* 2000;8(3):615-634.
47. Horn EM, Lekovic GP, Feiz-Erfan I, Sonntag VK, Theodore N: Cervical magnetic resonance imaging abnormalities not predictive of cervical spine instability in traumatically injured patients: Invited submission from the Joint Section Meeting on Disorders of the Spine and Peripheral Nerves, March 2004. *J Neurosurg Spine* 2004;1(1):39-42.
48. Bracken MB, Shepard MJ, Holford TR, et al: Administration of methylprednisolone for 24 or 48 hours or tirilazad mesylate for 48 hours in the treatment of acute spinal cord injury: Results of the Third National Acute Spinal Cord Injury Randomized Controlled Trial. National Acute Spinal Cord Injury Study. *JAMA* 1997;277(20):1597-1604.
49. Pharmacological therapy after acute cervical spinal cord injury. *Neurosurgery* 2002;50(3 Suppl):S63-S72.
50. Albert TJ, Levine MJ, Balderston RA, Cotler JM: Gastrointestinal complications in spinal cord injury. *Spine (Phila Pa 1976)* 1991;16(10 Suppl):S522-S525.
51. Aebi M, Mohler J, Zäch GA, Morscher E: Indication, surgical technique, and results of 100 surgically-treated fractures and fracture-dislocations of the cervical spine. *Clin Orthop Relat Res* 1986;203:244-257.
52. Initial closed reduction of cervical spine fracture-dislocation injuries. *Neurosurgery* 2002;50(3 Suppl):S44-S50.
53. Farmer J, Vaccaro A, Albert TJ, Malone S, Balderston RA, Cotler JM: Neurologic deterioration after cervical spinal cord injury. *J Spinal Disord* 1998;11(3):192-196.
54. Key A: Cervical spine dislocations with unilateral facet interlocking. *Paraplegia* 1975;13(3):208-215.
55. Lee AS, MacLean JC, Newton DA: Rapid traction for reduction of cervical spine dislocations. *J Bone Joint Surg Br* 1994;76(3):352-356.
56. Hadley MN, Argires PJ: The acute/emergent management of vertebral column fracture dislocation injuries, in *Neurological Emergencies*. Park Ridge, IL, American Association of Neurological Surgeons, 1994, vol 2, pp 249-262.
57. Kilburn MP, Smith DP, Hadley MN: The initial evaluation and treatment of the patient with spinal trauma, in Batjer HH, Loftus CM, eds: *Textbook of Neurological Surgery: Principles and Practice*. Philadelphia, PA, Lippincott Williams & Wilkins, 2002.
58. Ducker TB, Bellegarrigue R, Salcman M, Walleck C: Timing of operative care in cervical spinal cord injury. *Spine (Phila Pa 1976)* 1984;9(5):525-531.
59. Benzel EC: Spinal orthotics, in Menezes AH, Sonntag VKH, eds: *Principles of Spinal Surgery*. New York, NY, McGraw-Hill, 1996, pp 181-190.
60. Koch RA, Nickel VL: The halo vest: An evaluation of motion and forces across the neck. *Spine (Phila Pa 1976)* 1978;3(2):103-107.
61. Glaser JA, Whitehill R, Stamp WG, Jane JA: Complications associated with the halo-vest: A review of 245 cases. *J Neurosurg* 1986;65(6):762-769.
62. Bucholz RD, Cheung KC: Halo vest versus spinal fusion for cervical injury: Evidence from an outcome study. *J Neurosurg* 1989;70(6):884-892.
63. Baum JA, Hanley EN Jr, Pullekines J: Comparison of halo complications in adults and children. *Spine (Phila Pa 1976)* 1989;14(3):251-252.

64. Hayes VM, Silber JS, Siddiqi FN, Kondrachov D, Lipetz JS, Lonner B: Complications of halo fixation of the cervical spine. *Am J Orthop (Belle Mead NJ)* 2005;34(6):271-276.

65. Treatment of subaxial cervical spinal injuries. *Neurosurgery* 2002;50(3 Suppl):S156-S165.

66. Koivikko MP, Myllynen P, Karjalainen M, Vornanen M, Santavirta S: Conservative and operative treatment in cervical burst fractures. *Arch Orthop Trauma Surg* 2000;120(7-8):448-451.

67. Kiwerski JE: Early anterior decompression and fusion for crush fractures of cervical vertebrae. *Int Orthop* 1993;17(3):166-168.

68. Benzel EC, Larson SJ: Functional recovery after decompressive spine operation for cervical spine fractures. *Neurosurgery* 1987;20(5):742-746.

69. Benzel EC, Larson SJ: Recovery of nerve root function after complete quadriplegia from cervical spine fractures. *Neurosurgery* 1986;19(5):809-812.

70. Ching RP, Watson NA, Carter JW, Tencer AF: The effect of post-injury spinal position on canal occlusion in a cervical spine burst fracture model. *Spine (Phila Pa 1976)* 1997;22(15):1710-1715.

71. Bedbrook GM: Spinal injuries with tetraplegia and paraplegia. *J Bone Joint Surg Br* 1979;61-B(3): 267-284.

72. White AA, Panjabi MM: The problem of clinical instability in the human spine: A systematic approach, in White AA, Panjabi, eds: *Clinical Biomechanics of the Spine*, ed 2. Philadelphia, PA, JB Lippincott, 1990, pp 277-378.

73. Holdsworth F: Fractures, dislocations, and fracture-dislocations of the spine. *J Bone Joint Surg Am* 1970;52(8):1534-1551.

74. Cheshire DJ: The stability of the cervical spine following the conservative treatment of fractures and fracture-dislocations. *Paraplegia* 1969;7(3): 193-203.

75. Vaccaro AR, Daugherty RJ, Sheehan TP, et al: Neurologic outcome of early versus late surgery for cervical spinal cord injury. *Spine (Phila Pa 1976)* 1997;22(22):2609-2613.

76. Papadopoulos SM, Selden NR, Quint DJ, Patel N, Gillespie B, Grube S: Immediate spinal cord decompression for cervical spinal cord injury: Feasibility and outcome. *J Trauma* 2002;52(2): 323-332.

77. Fehlings MG, Perrin RG: The role and timing of early decompression for cervical spinal cord injury: Update with a review of recent clinical evidence. *Injury* 2005;36(Suppl 2):B13-B26.

78. Schlegel J, Bayley J, Yuan H, Fredricksen B: Timing of surgical decompression and fixation of acute spinal fractures. *J Orthop Trauma* 1996; 10(5):323-330.

79. Marshall LF, Knowlton S, Garfin SR, et al: Deterioration following spinal cord injury: A multicenter study. *J Neurosurg* 1987;66(3):400-404.

80. Heiden JS, Weiss MH, Rosenberg AW, Apuzzo ML, Kurze T: Management of cervical spinal cord trauma in Southern California. *J Neurosurg* 1975; 43(6):732-736.

81. Aebi M, Zuber K, Marchesi D: Treatment of cervical spine injuries with anterior plating: Indications, techniques, and results. *Spine (Phila Pa 1976)* 1991;16(3, Suppl)S38-S45.

82. Levi L, Wolf A, Rigamonti D, Ragheb J, Mirvis S, Robinson WL: Anterior decompression in cervical spine trauma: Does the timing of surgery affect the outcome? *Neurosurgery* 1991;29(2):216-222.

83. Böhler J, Gaudernak T: Anterior plate stabilization for fracture-dislocations of the lower cervical spine. *J Trauma* 1980;20(3):203-205.

84. Cabanela ME, Ebersold MJ: Anterior plate stabilization for bursting teardrop fractures of the cervical spine. *Spine (Phila Pa 1976)* 1988;13(8): 888-891.

85. Lambiris E, Zouboulis P, Tyllianakis M, Panagiotopoulos E: Anterior surgery for unstable lower cervical spine injuries. *Clin Orthop Relat Res* 2003;411:61-69.

86. Schulte K, Clark CR, Goel VK: Kinematics of the cervical spine following discectomy and stabilization. *Spine (Phila Pa 1976)* 1989;14(10): 1116-1121.

87. Grubb MR, Currier BL, Shih JS, Bonin V, Grabowski JJ, Chao EY: Biomechanical evaluation of anterior cervical spine stabilization. *Spine (Phila Pa 1976)* 1998;23(8):886-892.

88. Dvorak MF, Pitzen T, Zhu Q, Gordon JD, Fisher CG, Oxland TR: Anterior cervical plate fixation: A biomechanical study to evaluate the effects of plate design, endplate preparation, and bone mineral density. *Spine (Phila Pa 1976)* 2005;30(3): 294-301.

89. Zoëga B, Kärrholm J, Lind B: Plate fixation adds stability to two-level anterior fusion in the cervical spine: A randomized study using radiostereometry. *Eur Spine J* 1998;7(4):302-307.

90. Zdeblick TA, Cooke ME, Wilson D, Kunz DN, McCabe R: Anterior cervical discectomy, fusion, and plating: A comparative animal study. *Spine (Phila Pa 1976)* 1993;18(14):1974-1983.

91. Aebi M, Webb J: The spine, in Muller ME, Allgower M, Schneider R, et al, eds: *Manual of Internal Fixation*, ed 3. Berlin, Germany, Springer, 1991.

92. Lehmann W, Blauth M, Briem D, Schmidt U: Biomechanical analysis of anterior cervical spine plate fixation systems with unicortical and bicortical screw purchase. *Eur Spine J* 2004;13(1):69-75.

93. Spivak JM, Chen D, Kummer FJ: The effect of locking fixation screws on the stability of anterior cervical plating. *Spine (Phila Pa 1976)* 1999;24(4): 334-338.
94. Anderson PA, Henley MB, Grady MS, Montesano PX, Winn HR: Posterior cervical arthrodesis with AO reconstruction plates and bone graft. *Spine (Phila Pa 1976)* 1991;16(3, Suppl)S72-S79.
95. Cooper PR, Cohen A, Rosiello A, Koslow M: Posterior stabilization of cervical spine fractures and subluxations using plates and screws. *Neurosurgery* 1988;23(3):300-306.
96. Lundy DW, Murray HH: Neurological deterioration after posterior wiring of the cervical spine. *J Bone Joint Surg Br* 1997;79(6):948-951.
97. Fehlings MG, Cooper PR, Errico TJ: Posterior plates in the management of cervical instability: Long-term results in 44 patients. *J Neurosurg* 1994;81(3):341-349.
98. Wellman BJ, Follett KA, Traynelis VC: Complications of posterior articular mass plate fixation of the subaxial cervical spine in 43 consecutive patients. *Spine (Phila Pa 1976)* 1998;23(2):193-200.
99. Deen HG, Birch BD, Wharen RE, Reimer R: Lateral mass screw-rod fixation of the cervical spine: A prospective clinical series with 1-year follow-up. *Spine J* 2003;3(6):489-495.
100. Seybold EA, Baker JA, Criscitiello AA, Ordway NR, Park CK, Connolly PJ: Characteristics of unicortical and bicortical lateral mass screws in the cervical spine. *Spine (Phila Pa 1976)* 1999;24(22): 2397-2403.
101. Abumi K, Shono Y, Ito M, Taneichi H, Kotani Y, Kaneda K: Complications of pedicle screw fixation in reconstructive surgery of the cervical spine. *Spine (Phila Pa 1976)* 2000;25(8):962-969.
102. Kowalski JM, Ludwig SC, Hutton WC, Heller JG: Cervical spine pedicle screws: A biomechanical comparison of two insertion techniques. *Spine (Phila Pa 1976)* 2000;25(22):2865-2867.
103. Kast E, Mohr K, Richter HP, Börm W: Complications of transpedicular screw fixation in the cervical spine. *Eur Spine J* 2006;15(3):327-334.
104. Holly LT, Foley KT: Three-dimensional fluoroscopy-guided percutaneous thoracolumbar pedicle screw placement: Technical note. *J Neurosurg* 2003;99(3, Suppl)324-329.
105. Mirza SK, Wiggins GC, Kuntz C IV, et al: Accuracy of thoracic vertebral body screw placement using standard fluoroscopy, fluoroscopic image guidance, and computed tomographic image guidance: A cadaver study. *Spine (Phila Pa 1976)* 2003;28(4):402-413.
106. Maniker AH, Schulder M, Duran HL: Halifax clamps: efficacy and complications in posterior cervical stabilization. *Surg Neurol* 1995;43(2): 140-146.
107. Statham P, O'Sullivan M, Russell T: The Halifax Interlaminar Clamp for posterior cervical fusion: Initial experience in the United Kingdom. *Neurosurgery* 1993;32(3):396-399.
108. Aldrich EF, Weber PB, Crow WN: Halifax interlaminar clamp for posterior cervical fusion: A long-term follow-up review. *J Neurosurg* 1993; 78(5):702-708.
109. Adams MS, Crawford NR, Chamberlain RH, Bse, Sonntag VK, Dickman CA: Biomechanical comparison of anterior cervical plating and combined anterior/lateral mass plating. *Spine J* 2001;1(3): 166-170.
110. Bozkus H, Ames CP, Chamberlain RH, et al: Biomechanical analysis of rigid stabilization techniques for three-column injury in the lower cervical spine. *Spine (Phila Pa 1976)* 2005;30(8): 915-922.
111. Do Koh Y, Lim TH, Won You J, Eck J, An HS: A biomechanical comparison of modern anterior and posterior plate fixation of the cervical spine. *Spine (Phila Pa 1976)* 2001;26(1):15-21.
112. Spivak JM, Bharam S, Chen D, Kummer FJ: Internal fixation of cervical trauma following corpectomy and reconstruction: The effects of posterior element injury. *Bull Hosp Jt Dis* 2000;59(1):47-51.
113. Cybulski GR, Douglas RA, Meyer PR Jr, Rovin RA: Complications in three-column cervical spine injuries requiring anterior-posterior stabilization. *Spine (Phila Pa 1976)* 1992;17(3):253-256.
114. Ulrich C, Wörsdörfer O, Claes L, Magerl F: Comparative study of the stability of anterior and posterior cervical spine fixation procedures. *Arch Orthop Trauma Surg* 1987;106(4):226-231.
115. McAfee PC, Bohlman HH: One-stage anterior cervical decompression and posterior stabilization with circumferential arthrodesis: A study of twenty-four patients who had a traumatic or a neoplastic lesion. *J Bone Joint Surg Am* 1989;71(1): 78-88.
116. Van Peteghem PK, Schweigel JF: The fractured cervical spine rendered unstable by anterior cervical fusion. *J Trauma* 1979;19(2):110-114.
117. Schultz KD Jr, McLaughlin MR, Haid RW Jr, Comey CH, Rodts GE Jr, Alexander J: Single-stage anterior-posterior decompression and stabilization for complex cervical spine disorders. *J Neurosurg* 2000;93(2, Suppl):214-221.
118. McAfee PC, Bohlman HH, Ducker TB, Zeidman SM, Goldstein JA: One-stage anterior cervical decompression and posterior stabilization: A study of one hundred patients with a minimum of two years of follow-up. *J Bone Joint Surg Am* 1995; 77(12):1791-1800.

119. McNamara MJ, Devito DP, Spengler DM: Circumferential fusion for the management of acute cervical spine trauma. *J Spinal Disord* 1991;4(4): 467-471.

120. Hida K, Iwasaki Y, Imamura H, Abe H: Posttraumatic syringomyelia: Its characteristic magnetic resonance imaging findings and surgical management. *Neurosurgery* 1994;35(5):886-891.

121. Vaccaro AR, Silber JS: Post-traumatic spinal deformity. *Spine (Phila Pa 1976)* 2001;26(24, Suppl) S111-S118.

122. Heeneman H: Vocal cord paralysis following approaches to the anterior cervical spine. *Laryngoscope* 1973;83(1):17-21.

123. Tew JM Jr, Mayfield FH: Complications of surgery of the anterior cervical spine. *Clin Neurosurg* 1976;23:424-434.

124. Bertalanffy H, Eggert HR: Complications of anterior cervical discectomy without fusion in 450 consecutive patients. *Acta Neurochir (Wien)* 1989; 99(1-2):41-50.

125. Carrau RL, Cintron FR, Astor F: Transcervical approaches to the prevertebral space. *Arch Otolaryngol Head Neck Surg* 1990;116(9): 1070-1073.

126. Lu J, Ebraheim NA, Nadim Y, Huntoon M: Anterior approach to the cervical spine: Surgical anatomy. *Orthopedics* 2000;23(8):841-845.

127. Fielding JW: Complications of anterior cervical disk removal and fusion. *Clin Orthop Relat Res* 1992;284:10-13.

128. Oh SH, Perin NI, Cooper PR: Quantitative three-dimensional anatomy of the subaxial cervical spine: Implication for anterior spinal surgery. *Neurosurgery* 1996;38(6):1139-1144.

129. Graham JJ: Complications of cervical spine surgery: A five-year report on a survey of the membership of the Cervical Spine Research Society by the Morbidity and Mortality Committee. *Spine (Phila Pa 1976)* 1989;14(10):1046-1050.

130. Flynn TB: Neurologic complications of anterior cervical interbody fusion. *Spine (Phila Pa 1976)* 1982;7(6):536-539.

131. Cloward RB: Complications of anterior cervical disc operation and their treatment. *Surgery* 1971; 69(2):175-182.

132. Golfinos JG, Dickman CA, Zabramski JM, Sonntag VK, Spetzler RF: Repair of vertebral artery injury during anterior cervical decompression. *Spine (Phila Pa 1976)* 1994;19(22): 2552-2556.

133. Smith MD, Emery SE, Dudley A, Murray KJ, Leventhal M: Vertebral artery injury during anterior decompression of the cervical spine: A retrospective review of ten patients. *J Bone Joint Surg Br* 1993;75(3):410-415.

134. Graham AW, Swank ML, Kinard RE, Lowery GL, Dials BE: Posterior cervical arthrodesis and stabilization with a lateral mass plate: Clinical and computed tomographic evaluation of lateral mass screw placement and associated complications. *Spine (Phila Pa 1976)* 1996;21(3):323-329.

135. Scavarda D, Peruzzi P, Bazin A, et al: Postoperative spinal extradural hematomas. 14 cases. *Neurochirurgie* 1997;43(4):220-227.

136. Fountas KN, Kapsalaki EZ, Johnston KW: Cerebrospinal fluid fistula secondary to dural tear in anterior cervical discectomy and fusion: Case report. *Spine (Phila Pa 1976)* 2005;30(10): E277-E280.

137. Shektman A, Granick MS, Solomon MP, Black P, Nair S: Management of infected laminectomy wounds. *Neurosurgery* 1994;35(2):307-309.

138. Silber JS, Anderson DG, Daffner SD, et al: Donor site morbidity after anterior iliac crest bone harvest for single-level anterior cervical discectomy and fusion. *Spine (Phila Pa 1976)* 2003;28(2): 134-139.

139. Bohlman HH: Acute fractures and dislocations of the cervical spine: An analysis of three hundred hospitalized patients and review of the literature. *J Bone Joint Surg Am* 1979;61(8):1119-1142.

140. MacLellan DG, Shulkes A, Hardy KJ: Effect of omeprazole on acute gastric stress ulceration in cervical cord transected rats. *Dig Dis Sci* 1987; 32(4):417-421.

141. Dietz JM, Bertschy M, Gschaedler R, Dollfus P: Reflections on the intensive care of 106 acute cervical spinal cord injury patients in the resuscitation unit of a general traumatology centre. *Paraplegia* 1986;24(6):343-349.

142. Deep venous thrombosis and thromboembolism in patients with cervical spinal cord injuries. *Neurosurgery* 2002;50(3, Suppl):S73-S80.

143. Curry K, Casady L: The relationship between extended periods of immobility and decubitus ulcer formation in the acutely spinal cord-injured individual. *J Neurosci Nurs* 1992;24(4):185-189.

CHAPTER 26
Teardrop Fractures of the Cervical Spine

Yu-Po Lee, MD   Steven R. Garfin, MD

Introduction

Teardrop fractures were first described in 1956 by Kahn and Schneider.[1] They believed that these fractures were created when one vertebral body was crushed by the vertebral body superior to it. This resulted in a fracture in which the anteroinferior corner was separated from the main portion of the vertebral body. To them, this anteroinferior fragment resembled a "drop of water dripping from the vertebral body."[1] They also believed that "acute-flexion" was the mechanism of injury and that displacement of the posterior portion of the vertebral body into the spinal canal was an essential feature of this fracture (**Figure 1**).[1] The authors also noted that patients improved neurologically with decompression and that surgical fixation was frequently necessary to prevent instability and neurologic deterioration.

These views, however, were not shared by everyone. Many authors subsequently published reports disputing the classification and management of teardrop fractures. In 1963, Sir Frank Holdsworth published a paper where he classified teardrop fractures as burst fractures.[2] In 1970, he published another paper in which he classified teardrop fractures as avulsion fractures.[3] Holdsworth believed that these fractures were stable and could be treated nonsurgically. In 1960, Whitley and Forsyth[4] classified these fractures as stable, as did Fielding and Hawkins[5] in the mid-1970s. These authors believed that teardrop fractures were avulsion injuries caused by extension and advocated nonsurgical treatment. To strengthen the argument against surgical intervention for these fractures, many authors pointed to the poor results obtained with surgery for teardrop fractures.[3,6] The results of laminectomy for cervical spine injuries were generally very poor at this

FIGURE 1

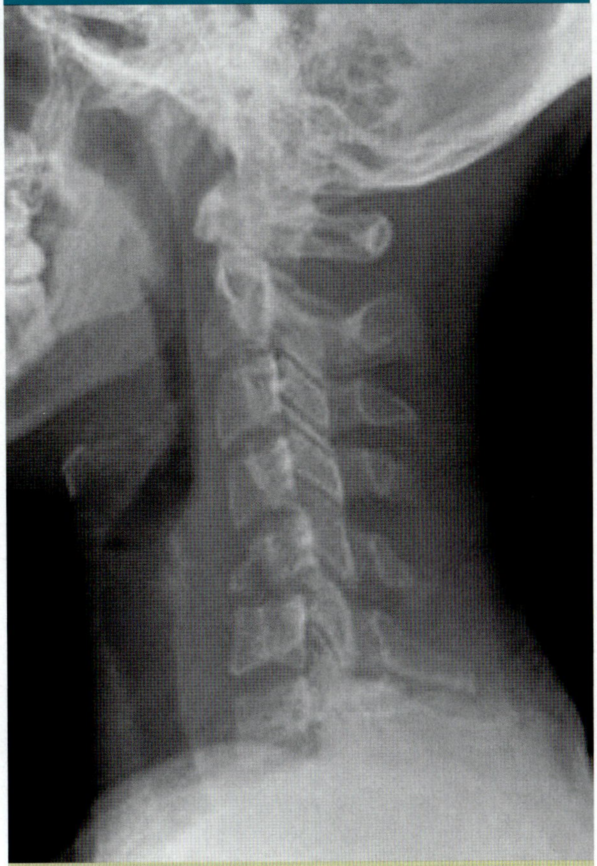

Figure 1 Lateral radiograph of a C5 teardrop fracture. Note the fracture of the anteroinferior corner of the vertebra along with displacement of the remaining vertebral body posteriorly into the spinal canal.

Dr. Lee or an immediate family member is a member of a speakers' bureau or has made paid presentations on behalf of DePuy, a Johnson & Johnson company; and serves as a paid consultant to or is an employee of Nuvasive and Stryker. Dr. Garfin or an immediate family member serves as a board member, owner, officer, or committee member of the Spine Arthroplasty Society; has received royalties from DePuy, a Johnson & Johnson company, and Lippincott; is a member of a speakers' bureau or has made paid presentations on behalf of DePuy, a Johnson & Johnson company; serves as a paid consultant to or is an employee of Applied Spine, Benvenue Medical, Cytonics Corp, DePuy, a Johnson & Johnson company, Disc Dynamics, EBI, Globus Medical, Magnifi Group, Nuvasive, SI Bone, Spinal Kinetics, SpineMark, SpineMedica, and Vertiflex; has received research or institutional support from AO North America, DePuy, a Johnson & Johnson company, EBI, Medtronic, and Synthes; and owns stock or stock options in Cytonics Corp, Orthovita, SI Bone, SpineMark, and SpineMedica.

time, and neurologic worsening was frequently reported after this procedure.[3,6,7] As a result, many surgeons believed that teardrop fractures should be treated nonsurgically. Bedbrook,[8] Cheshire,[9] and Norton[10] all studied nonsurgical treatment of cervical spine injuries and reported good results with a low incidence of late instability after nonsurgical treatment. As a result, surgery for acute teardrop fractures fell out of favor during the 1960s and 1970s.

During the late 1970s and 1980s, however, the belief that acute teardrop fractures were stable was challenged by many authors. In 1979, Bohlman[7] studied 300 patients who had acute cervical spine injuries. Of the 78 patients who were treated nonsurgically, he noted that chronic instability developed in 33 patients (42%). Bohlman emphasized the importance of surgical stabilization for cervical spine injuries, especially if the posterior ligaments were injured. Similar to the earlier studies, Bohlman also observed that patients who had laminectomies tended to have increased rates of mortality and neurologic decline.[3,6,7] He noted, however, that patients who had anterior decompressions and fusions had improved results. As a result, he advocated anterior decompression and fusion and dissuaded the use of laminectomies for teardrop fractures. In 1982, Allen et al[11] published their classification of lower cervical spine injuries. They also believed that teardrop fractures were highly unstable and classified them as compressive flexion stage 5 lesions, which were the most severe injuries in this category. These authors advocated surgical decompression, if necessary, and stabilization for teardrop fractures. Other investigators noted the unstable nature of these fractures and recommended surgical treatment because of the improved results seen with anterior decompression and fusion.[12-24]

Since the original description by Kahn and Schneider, the approach to evaluating and treating teardrop fractures has changed. Part of the problem in evaluating teardrop fractures is that the term "teardrop" is imprecise. This has resulted in some confusion as to what constitutes a teardrop fracture. The characteristic anteroinferior fragment that is associated with teardrop fractures can be seen with other fracture patterns, adding to the confusion in evaluating and treating these fractures. Improved imaging techniques have resulted in a better understanding of the pathoanatomy and complexity of these injuries. Together with improved methods of decompression and stabilization, this understanding has generated a change in opinion as to how teardrop fractures should be managed. This chapter discusses these issues, and outlines the evaluation and management of teardrop fractures.

Mechanism of Injury

Teardrop fractures result from high-energy trauma. Causes of injury typically include motor vehicle accidents, falls from heights, diving injuries, and football injuries.[5,8,9,14,16-19,25-31] As the head strikes a solid object, the energy from the impact is transmitted to the cervical spine. Because the thoracic spine is relatively fixed due to the ribs, the inertial energy from the trunk and extremities is also transmitted to the cervical spine. Thus, the cervical spine is crushed by forces from above and below. A flexion moment is also coupled to this axial load to produce a teardrop fracture.

In the initial description of teardrop fractures by Kahn and Schneider, "acute-flexion" (hyperflexion) was thought to be the primary mechanism of injury for teardrop fractures.[1] Axial loading, to a lesser degree, was also believed to be necessary to produce this fracture pattern. To test this theory, Torg et al[32] evaluated teardrop fractures in 55 football players. Game film was available of eight players and stop-frame analysis was performed on these players. In all cases, the initial point of contact was the crown of the helmet with the neck slightly flexed 20° to 30°. Torg et al believed that this straightened the cervical spine so that the cervical vertebrae were stacked one on top of the other. Because they did not observe excessive flexion in any of the players, they did not believe that hyperflexion was the primary injury mechanism, as originally proposed by Kahn and Schneider. Instead, they determined that the predominant force was axial loading with components of flexion or extension.

Kim et al[26] also believed that teardrop fractures were caused by flexion and axial compression. They felt this caused the anteroinferior margin of the vertebral body to fracture from shear stresses, while the remaining portion of the body displaces posteriorly into the spinal canal. This anterior flexion-compression force is coupled with distractive forces in the posterior elements, resulting in posterior ligamentous injuries. The intervertebral disk is simultaneously disrupted by these forces. A sagittal fracture in the posteriorly displaced fragment is a key component of teardrop fractures and most likely results from compression forces.[32] Torg et al[32] pointed out that Kahn and Schneider did not appreciate this sagittal fracture because they based their observations primarily on lateral radiographs.

It has been observed by some authors that an anteroinferior corner fracture may also result from an extension injury.[4,5,31,33] These fractures are avulsion injuries of the anteroinferior vertebral body and are stable, because there is no associated damage to the posterior elements. Marar and Orth evaluated 45 patients with extension injuries.[33] All of these patients had facial lesions, indicating that extension was the primary mechanism of injury. Of these 45 patients, 24 had the characteristic anteroinferior fragment. Autopsy evaluations in four patients revealed that the anterior longitudinal ligaments were torn in all cases, but the posterior longitudinal ligaments were intact at the level of injury. The capsular ligaments were also intact. The only osseous injury was a spinous process fracture that was found in one case.

When evaluating patients with an anteroinferior corner fracture, it is important to keep in mind that there is a subset of these fractures that may be avulsion fractures caused by an extension moment. Because the posterior elements are not subjected to distractive forces, less injury is typically seen in the posterior elements with these injuries, and they tend to be more stable.[4,26,31] Confusion between these fractures and the more serious teardrop fractures is probably what led Holdsworth and others to classify teardrop fractures as stable injuries. To distinguish these fractures from the more serious teardrop fractures, many authors now refer to these injuries as "extension teardrop fractures." A discussion on how to differentiate the extension fractures from the classic teardrop fractures can be found in the Diagnostic Studies section below.

Classification

One of the difficulties in attempting to classify teardrop fractures is that a triangular anteroinferior fragment can be seen with more than one fracture pattern. As this is also the most recognizable radiographic feature of teardrop fractures, this makes the assessment of these fractures difficult. To complicate matters, the terms "teardrop," "burst," and "compression" have no precise meaning. This in turn has led to some confusion as to what teardrop, burst, and compression fractures truly are. These terms have often been used interchangeably.

In the original description by Kahn and Schneider, the authors referred to teardrop fractures only as "fracture-dislocations."[1] Although they described the triangular anteroinferior fragment, which gave rise to the name "tear-drop," they did not discuss how to classify these fractures, nor did they describe a way to distinguish these fractures from other fractures that may also have an anteroinferior fragment. From the late 1950s to the 1980s, many authors developed classification systems to better characterize cervical spine injuries.[2-5,9,10,34-37] As previously mentioned, Holdsworth[3] classified teardrop fractures as burst fractures in one of his classification systems. Other authors also classified teardrop fractures as burst fractures. The terms "burst fracture" and "teardrop fracture" became synonymous.[2,3,5,9,10,32,34,36]

Although burst fractures and teardrop fractures share some common features, there are distinct differences between these two fracture patterns. In burst fractures, the primary mechanism of injury is generally vertical compression. Allen et al[11] classified these fractures as stage 3 vertical compression injuries. This results in a comminuted fracture where the vertebral body is crushed and the fracture fragments radiate outward in multiple directions, with varying degrees of retropulsion into the spinal canal. This differs from teardrop fractures, in which compression and flexion cause the posterior fragment to shear away from the anteroinferior fragment and displace posteriorly into the spinal canal. The differences in the mechanism of injury account for the variations observed radiographically between these two fractures and also for the higher degree of neurologic injury noted with teardrop fractures. In burst fractures, because the fracture fragments radiate in many directions, the inertial energy from the impact is dissipated along many vectors. With teardrop fractures, the energy is directed posteriorly into the spinal cord. In their evaluation of spinal cord injuries from diving accidents, Aito et al[14] noted that 70% of patients with teardrop fractures had a complete neurologic injury, while only 22% of patients with burst fractures had a complete neurologic deficit. Another important difference between burst and teardrop fractures is the frequency of injury to the posterior osteoligamentous structures. In the classification by Allen et al,[11] the authors noted that burst fractures had posterior osteoligamentous injuries 40% of the time. In teardrop fractures, many authors have observed that the posterior osteoligamentous structures are injured 100% of the time.[26,30-32] Thus, while teardrop and burst fractures may appear similar, there are critical differences that separate the two fracture types. These fractures should not be classified together.

In their classification of cervical fractures and dislocations, Allen et al[11] made note of the fact that the terms "teardrop fracture," "burst fracture," and "wedge fracture" were imprecise. They based their classification system on the mechanism of injury to avoid using these ambiguous terms. They believed that teardrop fractures were caused by compressive flexion. They described five stages of compressive flexion injury.[11] Stage 1 lesions consist of blunting of the anterosuperior vertebral margin of the vertebral body with no evidence of failure of the posterior ligaments. Stage 2 lesions show obliquity of the anterior vertebral body and loss of some height in the anterior body. This results in a beak appearance of the anteroinferior vertebral body. With increased force, the beak is fractured and a stage 3 lesion develops. A stage 4 lesion is similar to a stage 3 lesion, but the posterior fragment is displaced less than 3 mm posteriorly into the spinal canal. Finally, in stage 5 lesions, the posterior fragment is displaced more than 3 mm into the spinal canal and there is also injury to the posterior ligaments. Based on this classification scheme, teardrop fractures should be classified as stage 5 compressive flexion injuries. This fracture pattern has the anteroinferior fragment that is characteristic of teardrop fractures. Additionally, the posterior displacement of the posterior fragment into the spinal canal, which Kahn and Schneider[1] believed was an essential feature of this fracture, is also described. Rupture of the posterior ligaments is a feature of this classification. This is also an important component of teardrop fractures. Furthermore, Allen et al[11] noted a 91% incidence of neurologic injury with stage 5 compressive flexion injuries. Lee et al[31] noted neurologic injury in 87% of the teardrop fractures that they studied. A stage 5 compressive flexion injury is a reasonable classification for teardrop fractures because it accurately describes the fracture pattern and predicts the rate of neurologic injury seen clinically.

Evaluation

Teardrop fractures account for 8% to 15% of all reported cervical spine fractures.[27,28] In a study by Korres et al,[28] the main causes of injury were identified as motor vehicle accidents (63%), falls from heights (21.5%), and diving injuries (13.2%). The mean age of the patients was 35 years (range, 16 to 67 years), and 87% of the patients were male.[28] Other studies have reported similar results.[12,14,16,19,24,26-32,38,39]

These fractures typically occur at C5, but also frequently occur at C4 and C6.[1,16,24,26-32] In a study by Torg et al,[32] teardrop fractures were seen at C5 (74%), C4 (16%), and C6 (10%). Other authors have reported similar results.[26-31] Neurologic injuries are common with teardrop fractures. Kim et al[26] reported that in 45 patients with teardrop fractures, there were 25 complete spinal cord injuries (56%), 14 incomplete injuries (31%), and 6 patients who were intact (13%). In a study by Lee et al,[31] 87% of patients who had teardrop fractures sustained a neurologic injury. In these patients, 67% were quadriplegic or paraplegic, 7% sustained a Brown-Séquard injury, and 13% had a central cord syndrome. Kahn and Schneider[1] noted that anterior cord syndrome was the most common pattern of neurologic injury seen with teardrop fractures. However, it seems that any pattern of neurologic injury is possible, with complete injuries being the most frequent.

It is important to determine the degree of neurologic injury at the time of presentation. It is not only prognostic of neurologic recovery, but it also correlates with the number of complications that the patient is likely to encounter during the course of treatment. Korres et al[28] noted that none of the patients in their study with a complete injury showed any neurologic recovery. Neurologic improvement, however, was noted in six of eight (75%) patients who had an incomplete injury. Koivikko et al[27] reported that the number of complications encountered by patients with teardrop fractures correlated most strongly with the degree of motor impairment and immobility. Of the observed complications, 94% occurred in patients with Frankel grades A through C spinal cord injury. Complications encountered included urologic problems (39%), respiratory difficulties (35%), decubitus ulcers (28%), deep venous thrombosis (9%), and gastrointestinal difficulties (9%).

If the patient remains neurologically stable, the patient should be evaluated for any additional injuries. Teardrop fractures result from high-energy trauma, and patients experience high rates of morbidity and mortality. In the study by Korres et al,[28] 5 of 38 patients (13%) died from pulmonary and gastrointestinal complications. Associated injuries often occur and include head injuries (10%), extremity injuries (25%), pelvic fractures, and injures to the chest and abdomen.[28] The entire spine should also be evaluated for other fractures. Fractures in adjacent vertebrae occur in up to 33% of cases.[26,31] Distant vertebral fractures have been noted in 7% of cases.[26,31]

FIGURE 2

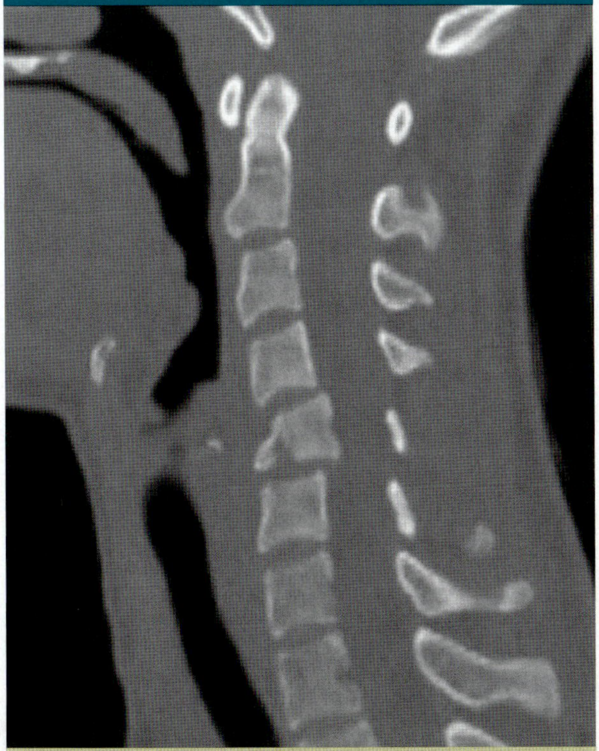

Figure 2 Sagittal CT scan of a C5 teardrop fracture. Note how the anteroinferior corner remains aligned with the inferior vertebra; this feature is also evident in Figure 1.

FIGURE 3

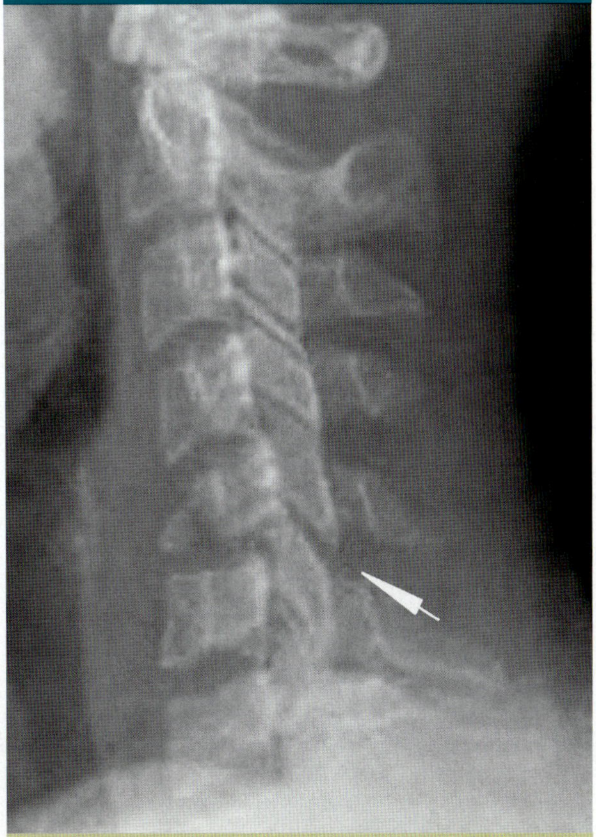

Figure 3 Lateral radiograph of a C5 teardrop fracture. Note the widening of the facet joint and loss of facet-joint parallelism between C5 and C6 (white arrow).

Diagnostic Studies

Imaging studies for evaluation of these patients start with the standard cervical spine trauma series. In most institutions, this includes AP, lateral, and odontoid views of the cervical spine. Cervical spine fractures can be seen on lateral radiographs 75% to 80% of the time.[40] The entire cervical spine and T1 should be visualized. This is especially important in the case of teardrop fractures, as these may occur in the lower cervical spine. If necessary, a swimmer's view may be obtained. If there is difficulty in obtaining a swimmer's view, a CT scan can provide the information. If a fracture of the cervical spine is seen, the entire spine should be imaged to search for any other fractures.

In the original description by Kahn and Schneider,[1] the characteristic features of teardrop fractures included a fracture of the anteroinferior corner of the vertebra along with displacement of the remaining vertebral body posteriorly into the spinal canal (**Figure 1**). The anteroinferior fragment is generally one-third to one-half the size of the vertebral body.[32] This fragment has a quadrilateral appearance in 3% of the cases.[31] Kim et al[26] noted that the anteroinferior fragment was generally aligned with the vertebral body below it, while the posterior portion was displaced posteriorly in all of the cases (100%) (**Figures 1** and **2**). Tonetti et al[41] postulated that this is due to the morphology of the cervical disk. In a histologic analysis of 140 sections, they noted that the ventral anulus was much thicker than the dorsal anulus both in height and in the anterior-posterior dimensions. In addition, the ventral anulus was more robust in comparison to the lateral anulus. They believed that this stronger ventral anulus holds onto the anteroinferior corner of the vertebra, while the rest of the vertebral body is sheared away from it, producing the characteristic teardrop fragment.

In addition to the fracture of the vertebral body, the posterior elements are also injured. Kim et al[26] believed that the posterior displacement of the posterior fragment provided indirect evidence that the posterior ligamentous structures were injured. Other signs that the posterior ligaments may be disrupted include widening of the interlaminar

FIGURE 4

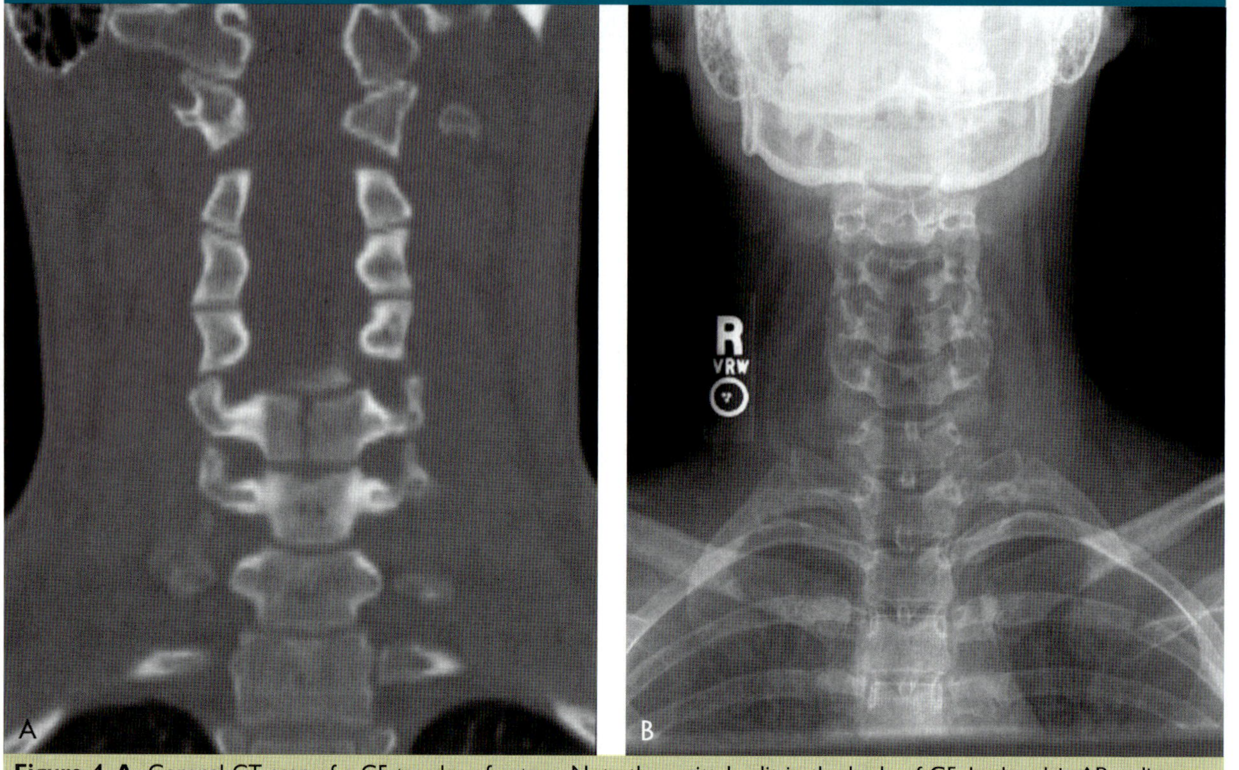

Figure 4 A, Coronal CT scan of a C5 teardrop fracture. Note the sagittal split in the body of C5. In the plain AP radiograph (**B**), it is difficult to visualize the sagittal split.

and interspinous spaces, which indicates injury to the ligamentum flavum and interspinous ligaments, respectively. Also, widening of a facet joint, or loss of facet parallelism, indicates that the facet capsule has been disrupted (**Figure 3**). Kim et al noted widening of the interlaminar and interspinous spaces in 40% of teardrop fractures and facet joint widening in 100% of the cases.[26] Torg et al observed that damage to the posterior ligamentous complex was more severe in patients who were quadriplegic.[32] Other key radiographic features that these authors noted were that the disk space was narrowed in all cases (100%) and kyphotic deformities were seen in 90%.[32]

In addition to plain radiography, CT scans should also be included in the work-up of teardrop fractures. A sagittal split in the posterior fragment will be more easily visualized on CT (**Figure 4**). Kim et al[26] noted a sagittal fracture in the posterior fragment in 39 of 45 cases (87%) in their study. They believed that this sagittal fracture was important clinically, because it was present in 38 of 39 patients (97%) who had a neurologic injury. Conversely, in cases where the sagittal fracture was absent, only one of the six patients (17%) had a neurologic injury.[26] They concluded that the presence of the sagittal split in the posterior fragment was predictive of neurologic injury. Torg et al[32] also noted that patients who had a sagittal split in the posterior fragment tended to have a greater degree of neurologic injury. Of 31 patients who had the sagittal split, 27 (87%) were permanently quadriplegic. When the sagittal split was absent, only one of six patients (17%) had a neurologic injury.[32]

The degree of retropulsion into the spinal canal and spinal canal compromise can be quantified with CT. The correlation between the degree of canal compromise and neurologic recovery, however, remains a topic of debate. Korres et al[28] saw no correlation between the amount of posterior displacement of the posterior fragment and neurologic recovery. Torg et al[32] noted that posterior displacement of the posterior fragment was greater than 2 mm in 40 of 45 patients (88%) who were permanently quadriplegic. In patients who had no permanent neurologic sequelae, the posterior displacement averaged 2 mm (range: 0 to 4 mm).[32]

Fractures in the posterior osseous structures are better visualized with CT. In the study by Kim et al,[26] lamina fractures were present in 38 of 45 cases (84%) (**Figure 5**), and were noted in

FIGURE 5

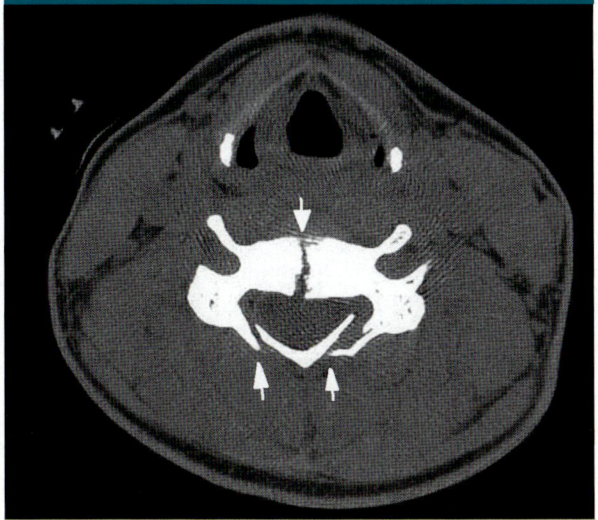

Figure 5 Axial CT scan of a C5 teardrop fracture. Note the sagittal split in the body and the lamina fractures (white arrows).

FIGURE 6

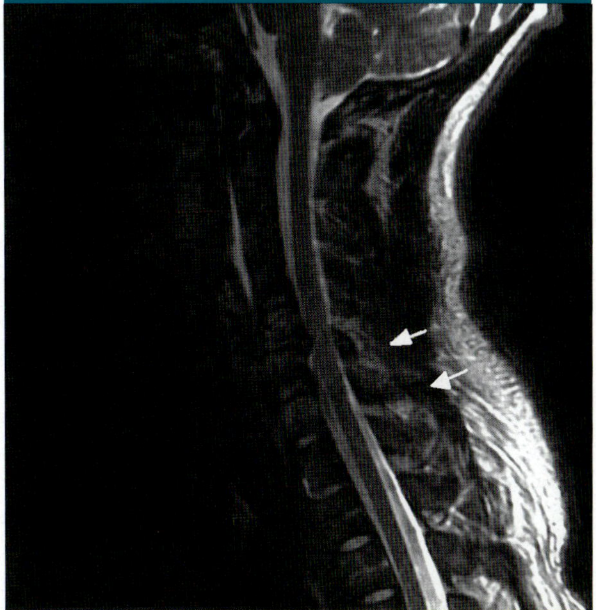

Figure 6 T2-weighted MRI scan of a C5 teardrop fracture. Note hyperintensity in the posterior ligaments (white arrows).

multiple levels in 12 of 38 patients (32%). Although MRI is probably not necessary in most instances, it can be helpful in evaluating for posterior ligamentous injuries when there is no evidence of osseous injuries on radiographs or CT (**Figure 6**).

As previously mentioned, extension teardrop fractures may also have an anteroinferior corner fracture that appears very similar to the classic teardrop fractures. There are some radiographic differences, however, that can be used to differentiate these fractures from one another. In extension teardrop fractures, the characteristic anteroinferior fragment is noted on lateral radiographs. However, posterior displacement of the remaining vertebral body is not typically seen.[26,31] Also, a sagittal fracture in the posterior fragment, which Torg et al[32] and Kim et al[26] believed was a characteristic feature of the classic teardrop fracture, is absent from these fractures as well. Furthermore, the posterior ligamentous structures are generally not injured, and there is no kyphotic deformity of the cervical spine.[26,31,33] These fractures are typically seen at C2, but can occur in the subaxial spine (**Figure 7**).[26,31] In contrast to this, classic teardrop fractures commonly occur at C4-C6.[1,16,24,26-32] It has also been noted that the anteroinferior fragment is smaller in extension teardrop fractures. Lee et al[31] noted that the anteroinferior fragment seen in their extension teardrop fractures never exceeded one-fourth of the vertebral body size.

FIGURE 7

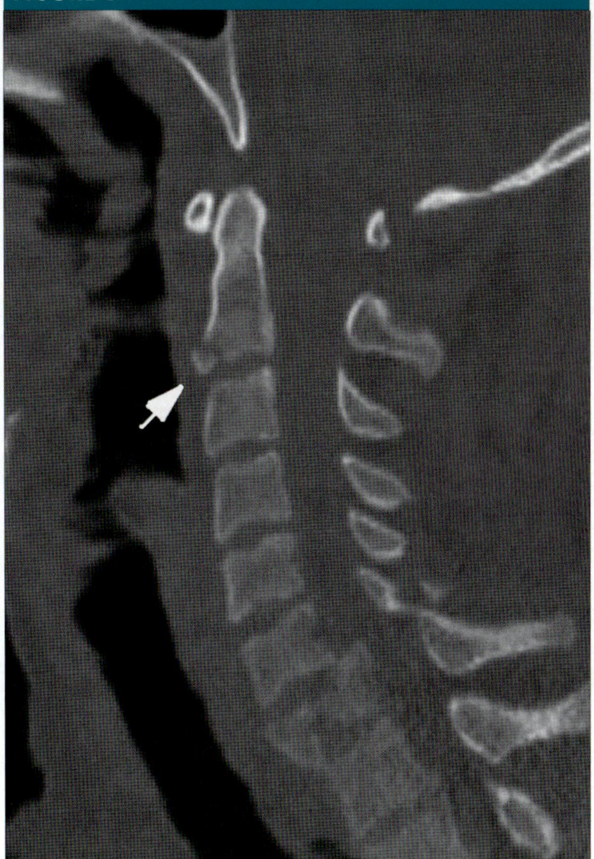

Figure 7 Sagittal CT scan of a C2 extension teardrop fracture (white arrow) and C7 burst fracture.

Nonsurgical Treatment

Nonsurgical treatment may be considered for patients who do not have a neurologic deficit, in whom the fracture is thought to be stable. Teardrop fractures are generally not stable and typically require surgical intervention. The injury through the bone and disk and posterior elements often leads to further anterior settling and kyphosis. Korres et al,[28] however, believed that there was a subset of teardrop fractures that were stable. They noted that in some teardrop fractures, only the anteroinferior corner was fractured. While these patients did have disruption of the posterior ligaments, they did not have posterior displacement of the posterior fragment and a sagittal split was absent from the posterior fragment. Out of the 38 cases they reported, 14 patients had this fracture pattern.[28] They noted neurologic injury in only 13% of these patients. They achieved good or excellent results in 14 out of 15 patients treated nonsurgically.[28] Nonsurgical treatment consisted of 6 weeks in skeletal traction followed by treatment in a Minerva cast or hard cervical collar. They recommended surgical treatment, however, for any other variety of teardrop fracture.

If a patient is unable to undergo surgery, or if surgery must be delayed to stabilize the patient, skeletal traction is recommended. Animal models of spinal cord injury have shown neurologic recovery may be improved with early decompression.[42-44] Clinical studies also support early decompression in patients with spinal cord injuries. In a study by Papadopoulos et al,[45] patients who had spinal cord injuries thought to be due to compression were treated with early decompression in the form of skeletal traction or surgery; 50% of patients treated with immediate decompression showed neurologic improvement, compared with 24% of patients in whom intervention was delayed. Eight of the patients (12%) who had early decompression improved from complete motor quadriplegia to independent ambulation. None of the patients who had delayed treatment showed this amount of recovery.[45] Aebi et al analyzed 100 patients treated surgically for cervical spine injuries. In the patients who showed neurologic recovery, 75% were reduced either by skeletal traction or surgically within 6 hours. The authors concluded that patients recovered better neurologically if they were reduced within 6 hours.[12] However, they also stated that this was not possible in most of their patients due to the time it took to safely extricate the patients, transport them to the hospital, obtain the appropriate imaging studies, and apply the skeletal traction devices or decompress them surgically.[12]

When using skeletal traction, it is important to remember a few key points. Patients with teardrop fractures may have skull fractures as a result of the accident. It is particularly important to check for skull fractures, as application of a skeletal traction device may lead to further injury. Patients with teardrop fractures may have additional injuries in the cervical spine. When examining the radiographs, it is important to check all the levels, in addition to the level of interest, during skeletal traction to make sure that there is no distraction at any other levels. Additionally, if a patient is not going to be treated surgically, or if surgery must be delayed, prophylaxis for deep venous thrombosis should be considered, particularly in immobile patients. However, if an anticoagulant is used, it should be rapidly reversible if surgery is necessary.

Surgical Treatment

As discussed previously, surgical intervention is generally recommended for teardrop fractures. These fractures are often treated surgically because retropulsion of the posterior fragment usually produces neurologic compromise. Surgical decompression relieves the pressure on the spinal cord and improves the chances for neurologic recovery. Furthermore, a sagittal fracture in the posterior fragment compromises the stability of the vertebral column. Additionally, the ligamentous and osseous injuries in the posterior elements, characteristic of teardrop fractures, will most likely result in instability and poor results with nonsurgical treatment. If teardrop fractures were evaluated according to the criteria set by White et al,[46] these fractures would be considered unstable. In teardrop fractures, the anterior and posterior elements are disrupted, the posterior fragment is translated more than 3.5 mm, there is a spinal cord injury, and there is abnormal disk narrowing.

Clinical studies have shown that patients have improved outcomes with surgery. Koivikko et al[27] compared nonsurgical with surgical treatment for both cervical burst and teardrop fractures; 69 patients with unstable cervical burst and teardrop fractures were retrospectively reviewed. In the nonsurgical group, 4 of 18 patients (22%) with either a complete or incompete neurologic injury improved at least one Frankel grade. In the surgical group, 13 of 23 patients (56%) improved at least one Frankel grade. Also, the nonsurgical group had 13° of kyphosis at the injured level compared with the surgical group that had 2° of

FIGURE 8

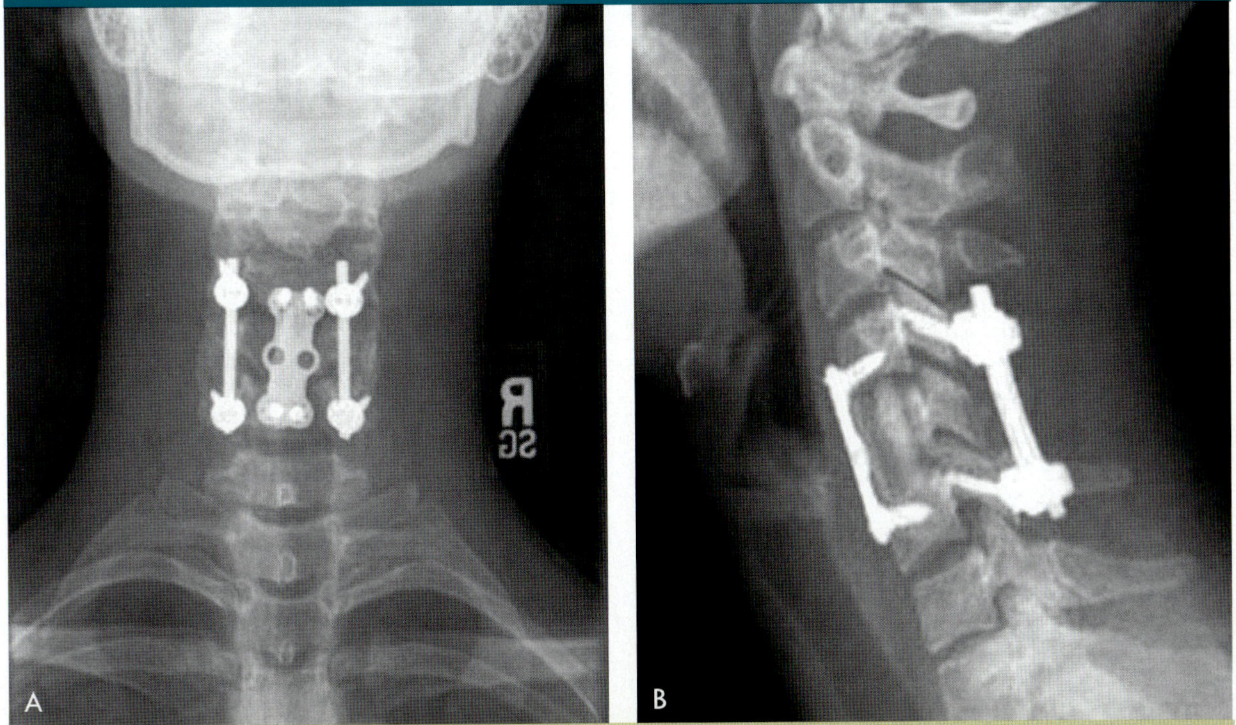

Figure 8 A, Postoperative AP radiograph of a C5 corpectomy and anterior and posterior C4-C6 fusion for a C5 teardrop fracture. **B,** Postoperative lateral radiograph of a C5 corpectomy and anterior and posterior C4-C6 fusion for a C5 teardrop fracture.

lordosis at the end of treatment.[27] In a study by Johnson and Cannon,[38] patients with teardrop fractures were treated with skull traction and converted to a halo vest or Minerva cast after 2 to 6 weeks of traction. Their results demonstrated that none of the patients with complete injuries had any neurologic recovery, while only one of four patients with an incomplete injury showed any significant neurologic improvement. Fisher et al[19] compared the results of patients with teardrop fractures treated with a halo vest versus corpectomy and plating. Of 24 patients in the halo-vest group, two deteriorated neurologically and required surgical intervention, while none in the surgical group deteriorated. At the end of treatment, the nonsurgical group had a kyphosis of 11° compared to 3.5° in the surgical group.[19] Neurologic improvement was not evaluated in this study. Most authors recommend surgery for patients with teardrop fractures as neurologic recovery, and overall alignment, are improved.

Some controversy exists, however, regarding the optimal form of fixation for these fractures. Excellent results have been reported with anterior corpectomy and fusion.[7,13,15-22,27,47,48] The main source of spinal cord compression is attributable to the retropulsed posterior fragment of the vertebral body. By performing a corpectomy, the pressure on the spinal cord is directly relieved. Also, the end plates of the vertebral bodies directly superior and inferior to the fractured vertebra provide a large surface area for fusion. By placing a strut graft and stabilizing it with a plate, the anterior and middle columns are reconstituted, which resists future collapse and kyphosis.

Vertebral body corpectomy and anterior fusion to treat teardrop fractures was initially described by Garger et al[48] in 1969. They reported a case wherein a patient with an incomplete spinal cord injury recovered fully with anterior decompression and fusion with a strut graft obtained from the iliac crest. There have been other reports of good results with anterior decompression and plate fixation. Cabanela and Ebersold[16] reported on eight patients with teardrop fractures who were treated with corpectomy and plate fixation. They also used a halo vest to immobilize their patients after surgery to provide additional support. In five patients who had complete neurologic deficits, all remained complete, but two gained one nerve root level. All three patients who had incomplete neurologic injuries were able to ambulate independently, while one recovered fully. In a study by Aebi et al,[12] 22 patients who had a burst or teardrop fracture were treated with a corpectomy and fusion with a plate. They reported no intraoperative complications, and there were no neurologic deteriorations. In the patients with complete neurologic injuries, there were no improvements. However, the patients with incomplete lesions improved one Frankel grade "on average." The authors did not specify how much neurologic improvement occurred individually.

Posterior decompression and fusion has also been reported as a means of treating teardrop fractures.[9,10,39,49-51] In the original description by Kahn and Schneider,[1] decompressive laminectomy and sectioning of the dentate ligament was recommended for patients with neurologic injury. Unfortunately, the results of laminectomy alone were very poor and often resulted in neurologic and radiographic decline.[9,10,39,49-51] This led many authors to recommend posterior fusion as an adjunct to posterior decompression.[9,10,39,49-51] However, the results of posterior decompression and fusion for teardrop fractures have not been as good as the results achieved with anterior decompression and fusion. In his series of 300 patients, Bohlman[7] noted improved neurologic recovery in patients who had anterior decompression and fusions compared with those who had posterior decompression and fusions. He believed that any protruding bone or disk material could be removed anteriorly, providing better direct decompression than that afforded indirectly with laminectomy. In a report by Cybulski et al,[18] 21 patients who failed posterior wiring and bone grafting for cervical trauma (including 7 teardrop fractures) were reported. These authors also determined that anterior decompression and fusion with plating was a superior method of treatment.

For a one-level decompression, a single-level corpectomy and anterior plating is generally sufficient. If two levels are involved, anterior corpectomies and anterior plating with supplemental posterior stabilization should be considered (**Figure 8**). Studies have shown that the strut graft is subjected to greater cantilever forces when a multilevel corpectomy is performed.[52-55] Also, since the posterior elements are disrupted in these cases as well, a stronger construct may be necessary. Performing an anterior corpectomy and plating, augmented with posterior spinal fusion when a multilevel corpectomy is performed, generally provides the necessary rigidity to allow the cervical spine to fuse and to prevent kyphosis.

References

1. Kahn EA, Schneider RC: Chronic neurological sequelae of acute trauma to the spine and spinal cord: I. The significance of the acute-flexion or tear-drop fracture-dislocation of the cervical spine. *J Bone Joint Surg Am* 1956;38-A(5): 985-997.
2. Holdsworth F: Fractures, dislocations, and fracture-dislocations of the spine. *J Bone Joint Surg Br* 1963;45(1):6-20.
3. Holdsworth F: Fractures, dislocations, and fracture-dislocations of the spine. *J Bone Joint Surg Am* 1970;52(8):1534-1551.
4. Whitley JE, Forsyth HF: The classification of cervical spine injuries. *Am J Roentgenol Radium Ther Nucl Med* 1960;83:633-644.
5. Fielding JW, Hawkins RJ: Roentgenographic diagnosis of the injured neck. *Instr Course Lect* 1976; 25:149-170.
6. Wharton GW: Routine laminectomy for spinal injury criticized. *JAMA* 1970;211:913-917.
7. Bohlman HH: Acute fractures and dislocations of the cervical spine: An analysis of three hundred hospitalized patients and review of the literature. *J Bone Joint Surg Am* 1979;61(8):1119-1142.
8. Bedbrook GM: Pathological principles in the management of spinal cord trauma. *Paraplegia* 1966; 4(1):43-56.
9. Cheshire DJ: The stability of the cervical spine following the conservative treatment of fractures and fracture-dislocations. *Paraplegia* 1969;7(3): 193-203.
10. Norton WL: Fractures and dislocations of the cervical spine. *J Bone Joint Surg Am* 1962;44: 115-139.
11. Allen BL Jr, Ferguson RL, Lehmann TR, O'Brien RP: A mechanistic classification of closed, indirect fractures and dislocations of the lower cervical spine. *Spine (Phila Pa 1976)* 1982;7(1):1-27.
12. Aebi M, Mohler J, Zäch GA, Morscher E: Indication, surgical technique, and results of 100 surgically-treated fractures and fracture-dislocations of the cervical spine. *Clin Orthop Relat Res* 1986;203:244-257.
13. Aebi M, Zuber K, Marchesi D: Treatment of cervical spine injuries with anterior plating: Indications, techniques, and results. *Spine (Phila Pa 1976)* 1991;16(3, Suppl):S38-S45.
14. Aito S, D'Andrea M, Werhagen L: Spinal cord injuries due to diving accidents. *Spinal Cord* 2005; 43(2):109-116.
15. Bell GD, Bailey SI: Section II: General orthopaedics. Anterior cervical fusion for trauma. *Clin Orthop Relat Res* 1977;128:155-158.

16. Cabanela ME, Ebersold MJ: Anterior plate stabilization for bursting teardrop fractures of the cervical spine. *Spine (Phila Pa 1976)* 1988;13(8):888-891.

17. Capen DA, Garland DE, Waters RL: Surgical stabilization of the cervical spine: A comparative analysis of anterior and posterior spine fusions. *Clin Orthop Relat Res* 1985;196:229-237.

18. Cybulski GR, Douglas RA, Meyer PR Jr, Rovin RA: Complications in three-column cervical spine injuries requiring anterior-posterior stabilization. *Spine (Phila Pa 1976)* 1992;17(3):253-256.

19. Fisher CG, Dvorak MF, Leith J, Wing PC: Comparison of outcomes for unstable lower cervical flexion teardrop fractures managed with halo thoracic vest versus anterior corpectomy and plating. *Spine (Phila Pa 1976)* 2002;27(2):160-166.

20. Garvey TA, Eismont FJ, Roberti LJ: Anterior decompression, structural bone grafting, and Caspar plate stabilization for unstable cervical spine fractures and/or dislocations. *Spine (Phila Pa 1976)* 1992;17(10 Suppl):S431-S435.

21. Gassman J, Seligson D: The anterior cervical plate. *Spine (Phila Pa 1976)* 1983;8(7):700-707.

22. Goffin J, van Loon J, Van Calenbergh F, Plets C: Long-term results after anterior cervical fusion and osteosynthetic stabilization for fractures and/or dislocations of the cervical spine. *J Spinal Disord* 1995;8(6):500-508.

23. McAfee PC, Bohlman HH: One-stage anterior cervical decompression and posterior stabilization with circumferential arthrodesis: A study of twenty-four patients who had a traumatic or a neoplastic lesion. *J Bone Joint Surg Am* 1989;71(1):78-88.

24. Toh E, Nomura T, Watanabe M, Mochida J: Surgical treatment for injuries of the middle and lower cervical spine. *Int Orthop* 2006;30(1):54-58.

25. Fuentes JM, Bloncourt J, Vlahovitch B, Castan P: Tear drop fractures: Contribution to the study of the mechanism of osteo-disco-ligamentous lesions. *Neurochirurgie* 1983;29(2):129-134.

26. Kim KS, Chen HH, Russell EJ, Rogers LF: Flexion teardrop fracture of the cervical spine: Radiographic characteristics. *AJR Am J Roentgenol* 1989;152(2):319-326.

27. Koivikko MP, Myllynen P, Karjalainen M, Vornanen M, Santavirta S: Conservative and operative treatment in cervical burst fractures. *Arch Orthop Trauma Surg* 2000;120(7-8):448-451.

28. Korres DS, Stamos K, Andreakos A, Spyridonos S, Kavadias K: The anterior inferior angle fracture of a lower cervical vertebra. *Eur Spine J* 1994;3(4):202-205.

29. Korres DS, Zoubos AB, Kavadias K, Babis GC, Balalis K: The "tear drop" (or avulsed) fracture of the anterior inferior angle of the axis. *Eur Spine J* 1994;3(3):151-154.

30. Lee C, Kim KS, Rogers LF: Sagittal fracture of the cervical vertebral body. *AJR Am J Roentgenol* 1982;139(1):55-60.

31. Lee C, Kim KS, Rogers LF: Triangular cervical vertebral body fractures: Diagnostic significance. *AJR Am J Roentgenol* 1982;138(6):1123-1132.

32. Torg JS, Pavlov H, O'Neill MJ, Nichols CE Jr, Sennett B: The axial load teardrop fracture: A biomechanical, clinical and roentgenographic analysis. *Am J Sports Med* 1991;19(4):355-364.

33. Marar BC, Orth MC: The pattern of neurological damage as an aid to the diagnosis of the mechanism in cervical-spine injuries. *J Bone Joint Surg Am* 1974;56(8):1648-1654.

34. Harris JH Jr, Edeiken-Monroe B, Kopaniky DR: A practical classification of acute cervical spine injuries. *Orthop Clin North Am* 1986;17(1):15-30.

35. Rogers WA: Fractures and dislocations of the cervical spine; an end-result study. *J Bone Joint Surg Am* 1957;39(2):341-376.

36. Stauffer ES: Subaxial injuries. *Clin Orthop Relat Res* 1989;239:30-39.

37. Stauffer ES, Kelly EG: Fracture-dislocations of the cervical spine: Instability and recurrent deformity following treatment by anterior interbody fusion. *J Bone Joint Surg Am* 1977;59(1):45-48.

38. Johnson JL, Cannon D: Nonoperative treatment of the acute tear-drop fracture of the cervical spine. *Clin Orthop Relat Res* 1982;168:108-112.

39. Signoret F, Jacquot FP, Feron JM: Reducing the cervical flexion tear-drop fracture with a posterior approach and plating technique: An original method. *Eur Spine J* 1999;8(2):110-116.

40. Blahd WH Jr, Iserson KV, Bjelland JC: Efficacy of the posttraumatic cross table lateral view of the cervical spine. *J Emerg Med* 1985;2(4):243-249.

41. Tonetti J, Potton L, Riboud R, Peoc'h M, Passagia JG, Chirossel JP: Morphological cervical disc analysis applied to traumatic and degenerative lesions. *Surg Radiol Anat* 2005;27(3):192-200.

42. Delamarter RB, Sherman JE, Carr JB: 1991 Volvo Award in experimental studies: Cauda equina syndrome: neurologic recovery following immediate, early, or late decompression. *Spine (Phila Pa 1976)* 1991;16(9):1022-1029.

43. Dolan EJ, Tator CH, Endrenyi L: The value of decompression for acute experimental spinal cord compression injury. *J Neurosurg* 1980;53(6):749-755.

44. Guha A, Tator CH, Endrenyi L, Piper I: Decompression of the spinal cord improves recovery after acute experimental spinal cord compression injury. *Paraplegia* 1987;25(4):324-339.

45. Papadopoulos SM, Selden NR, Quint DJ, Patel N, Gillespie B, Grube S: Immediate spinal cord decompression for cervical spinal cord injury: Feasibility and outcome. *J Trauma* 2002;52(2): 323-332.

46. White AA III, Johnson RM, Panjabi MM, Southwick WO: Biomechanical analysis of clinical stability in the cervical spine. *Clin Orthop Relat Res* 1975;109:85-96.

47. Bohlman HH, Anderson PA: Anterior decompression and arthrodesis of the cervical spine: Long-term motor improvement. Part I—Improvement in incomplete traumatic quadriparesis. *J Bone Joint Surg Am* 1992;74(5):671-682.

48. Garger WN, Fisher RG, Halfmann HW: Vertebrectomy and fusion for "tear drop fracture" of the cervical spine: Case report. *J Trauma* 1969;9(10): 887-893.

49. Murphy MJ, Daniaux H, Southwick WO: Posterior cervical fusion with rigid internal fixation. *Orthop Clin North Am* 1986;17(1):55-65.

50. Nazarian SM, Louis RP: Posterior internal fixation with screw plates in traumatic lesions of the cervical spine. *Spine (Phila Pa 1976)* 1991;16 (3, Suppl):S64-S71.

51. Stauffer ES: Management of spine fractures C3 to C7. *Orthop Clin North Am* 1986;17(1):45-53.

52. Sasso RC, Ruggiero RA Jr, Reilly TM, Hall PV: Early reconstruction failures after multilevel cervical corpectomy. *Spine (Phila Pa 1976)* 2003;28(2): 140-142.

53. Singh K, Vaccaro AR, Kim J, Lorenz EP, Lim TH, An HS: Biomechanical comparison of cervical spine reconstructive techniques after a multilevel corpectomy of the cervical spine. *Spine (Phila Pa 1976)* 2003;28(20):2352-2358.

54. Singh K, Vaccaro AR, Kim J, Lorenz EP, Lim TH, An HS: Enhancement of stability following anterior cervical corpectomy: A biomechanical study. *Spine (Phila Pa 1976)* 2004;29(8):845-849.

55. Vaccaro AR, Daugherty RJ, Sheehan TP, et al: Neurologic outcome of early versus late surgery for cervical spinal cord injury. *Spine (Phila Pa 1976)* 1997;22(22):2609-2613.

CHAPTER 27
Cervical Facet Fractures and Dislocations

Kris Radcliff, MD Marcos Andre Sonagli, MD Lawrence Delasotta, MD, MPH
Nina Singh, MD Elizabeth Morrison, MD Alan M. Levine, MD
Alexander R. Vaccaro, MD, PhD

Introduction

Injuries involving the posterior articular pillar or facets of the vertebral elements can occur anywhere in the spine. The cervical spine is the most common location of facet fractures or dislocations. Injuries at C5-C6 are the most common among all types of facet injuries, followed in frequency by injuries at C4-C5, C6-C7, C3-C4, C2-C3, and C7-T1.[1,2] The advent of CT with three-dimensional reconstruction and MRI has significantly improved the recognition and treatment of these injuries.

Anatomy and Biomechanics

The facet joints are the only true synovial joints in the spine. The joint itself is an arthrodial joint with a synovial membrane and fibrous capsule. Articular capsules within the facet joint are significant stabilizers of the cervical spine. The articular surface extends approximately 1 sq cm. The facet joint forms the posterior border of the neuroforamen with the anteromedial border of the foramen formed by the joint of Luschka (uncovertebral joint). Understanding the posterior topographic anatomy of the lateral mass is critical to appropriate placement of screws and instrumentation (**Figure 1**). The posterior aspect of the lateral mass is convex, and there is a natural concavity at the junction that separates the hillock from lamina and spinous process.[3] The true dimensions of the dome-shaped posterior aspect of the facet joint measure slightly less than 1 cm in mediolateral and inferosuperior dimensions.

Together, the superior and inferior facet joints comprise the lateral mass.[4] The vertebral artery lies directly anterior to the midpoint of the lateral mass from C3 through C5 and medial edge of the facet joint at C6.[5] The exiting nerve root lies directly beneath the caudal half of the inferior facet. The pedicle lies directly anterior to the midpoint of the superior facet. The facet joint capsule is an important stabilizer of the posterior ligamentous complex (PLC) of the spine.[6,7]

The facet joints of the upper cervical spine (levels cephalad to C2-C3) are located in close proximity to the anterior portion of the vertebral ring, and exhibit a different anatomic configuration than the joints of the lower cervical spine. Injuries to the C2-C3 facet joint are grouped with lower cervical spine joint injuries. In addition, cervical facet joints have an elliptical configuration conforming to the articular surfaces and are oriented slightly medially or laterally, depending on the individual vertebra. In the upper segments, the

---

Dr. Levine is deceased. At the time this chapter was written, Dr. Levine or an immediate family member had received royalties from Elsevier and US Spine; was a member of a speakers' bureau or had made paid presentations on behalf of Accuray; served as a paid consultant to or was an employee of US Spine; and had received research or institutional support from Accuray, Amgen, and Medtronic Sofamor Danek. Dr. Vaccaro or an immediate family member serves as a board member, owner, officer, or committee member of the North American Spine Society, American Spinal Injury Association, and the Cervical Spine Research Society; has received royalties from Aesculap/B. Braun, DePuy, a Johnson & Johnson company, Globus Medical, Medtronic Sofamor Danek, K2M, Stout Medical, Progressive Spinal Technology, and Applied Spinal Intellectual Properties; serves as a paid consultant to or is an employee of K2M; has received research or institutional support from AO North America, DePuy, a Johnson & Johnson company, Medtronic Sofamor Danek, and Stryker; and owns stock or stock options in Globus Medical, Disc Motion Technologies, Progressive Spinal Technologies, Advanced Spinal Intellectual Properties, Computational Biodynamics, Stout Medical, Paradigm Spine, K2M, Replication Medical, Spineology, SpineMedica, Orthovita, Vertiflex, Small Bone Technologies, NeuCore, Crosscurrent, Syndicom, In Vivo, Flagship Surgical, Pearl Diver, Location Based Intelligence Inc., and Gamma Spine. None of the following authors or any immediate family member has received anything of value from or owns stock in a commercial company or institution related directly or indirectly to the subject of this chapter: Dr. Radcliff, Dr. Sonagli, Dr. Delasotta, Dr. Singh, and Dr. Morrison.

FIGURE 1

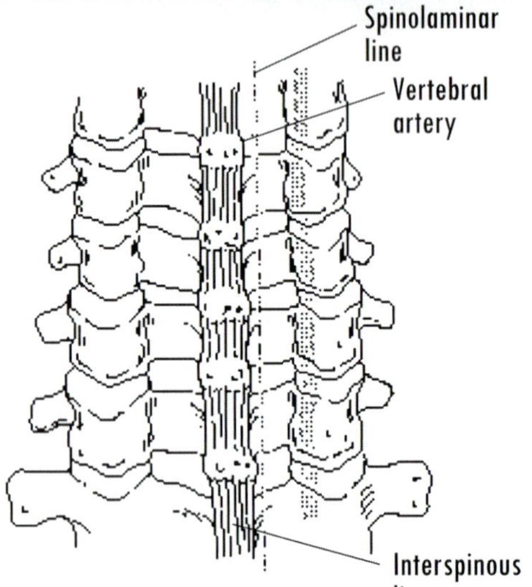

Figure 1 This illustration shows the topographic anatomy of the posterior aspect of the cervical spine. Proper positioning of wire constructs requires penetration of the posterior elements at the level of the spinolaminar line rather than in the spinous process. Proper screw placement uses the anatomy of the facet joint to avoid medial placement of the screw and penetration of the vertebral artery, which courses anterior to the medial half of the facet. The posterior aspect of the facet forms a little hillock, as described by Raymond Roy-Camille, with the valley on its medial side formed by the posterior aspect of the lamina. (Reproduced from Levine AM: Facet fractures and dislocations, in Levine AM, Eismont FJ, Garfin SF, Zigler JE, eds: *Spine Trauma*. Philadelphia, PA, WB Saunders, 1998, pp 331-366.)

facet joints are canted slightly medial, whereas in the lower segments they are angled slightly lateral as the transition is made into the thoracic spine.[2,5] As described by Lysell,[4] a coupled motion occurs with axial rotation and lateral bending. This is a result of the shape of the facet joints. In the upper cervical spine, 2° of rotation occur for every 3° of lateral bending, whereas in the lower cervical spine, only 1° of rotation occurs for every 7.5° of lateral bending. It is possible that the increased compliance to rotation with lateral bending may account for the fact that fewer unilateral facet fractures and dislocations occur in the upper cervical spine than in the lower.

Classification of Facet Injuries

Facet fractures were classified by Allen et al,[8] a scheme later modified by Harris et al.[9] This method of classification attributed a mechanism of injury to radiographic appearance and injury severity. Within the Allen classification, facet dislocations are classified as "distractive flexion" injuries[8] and subclassified into four stages. Subclassifications include: stage 1, facet subluxation; stage 2, unilateral facet dislocation; stage 3, bilateral facet dislocation with approximately 50% vertebral displacement; and stage 4, unstable or floating spine.

The Sub-axial Injury Classification (SLIC) and Severity Scale was developed by Vaccaro et al[10] to address previous classification deficiencies. This system accounts for injury severity and injury patterns to provide the clinician with treatment option recommendations and injury prognoses.[10] Six clinical categories were defined to include spinal level, injury morphology, bony injury description, discoligamentous complex (DLC) injury, neurologic status, and confounders (ie, ankylosing spondylitis, diffuse idiopathic skeletal hyperostosis, stenosis, prior surgery). Focus is placed upon injury morphology, DLC injury, and neurologic status. A severity scale is applied within each category (**Table 1**). When more than one vertebral level is injured, each individual level is scored independently. SLIC scores between 1 and 3 are normally treated with nonsurgical management. A score ≥ 5 indicates surgical treatment, while a score of 4 suggests either nonsurgical or surgical treatment.

Clinical Presentation

Facet joint injuries usually result from high-energy trauma, particularly motor vehicle accidents. Patients typically report unilateral or bilateral axial neck pain. Patients may have paresthesia, palsy, or weakness at the level of the exiting nerve root.[11,12] Patients may also have incomplete or complete spinal cord injury syndrome.[13,14]

Diagnostic Imaging

All patients with suspected cervical spine trauma should be evaluated with standard radiographs that include AP, lateral, and open-mouth odontoid views.[15,16] The entire cervical spine from occiput to C7 should be easily visualized.[17,18] Radiographic technique or patient body habitus, however, may limit visualization of the cervicothoracic junction and it is important to note that a fracture of C7 or dislocation at the C7-T1 junction occurs in 17% of all cervical injuries.[2]

Dynamic (flexion-extension) radiographs provide information regarding abnormal motion within the spine segments. White et al[19] studied 17 vertebral motion segments under physiologic flexion and extension loads. They reported spinal

TABLE 1

Subaxial Injury Classification (SLIC) and Severity Scale

Category	Subcategory	Points
Morphology	No abnormality	0
	Compression	1
	Burst	2
	Distraction (eg, facet patch, hyperextension)	3
	Rotation/translation (eg, facet dislocation, unstable teardrop, or advanced-stage flexion compression injury)	4
Discoligamentous complex (DLC)	Intact	0
	Indeterminate (eg, isolated interspinous widening, MRI signal change only)	1
	Disrupted (eg, widening of disk space, facet patch, or dislocation)	2
Neurologic status	Intact	0
	Root injury	1
	Complete cord injury	2
	Incomplete cord injury	3
	Continuous cord compression in setting of neuro deficit (neuro modifier)	+1

(Adapted with permission from Vaccaro AR, Hulbert RJ, Patel AA, et al: The subaxial cervical spine injury classification system: A novel approach to recognize the importance of morphology, neurology, and integrity of the disco-ligamentous complex. *Spine (Phila Pa 1976)* 2007;32(21):2365-2374.)

instability as angulation greater than 11° compared to adjacent levels of more than 3.5 mm of anterior displacement on flexion-extension radiographs.[19] Several authors have reported the use of acute flexion-extension radiographs to evaluate overall stability.[6] However, in the period immediately after injury, flexion-extension radiographs may be insufficient to exclude even extensive damage to the posterior structures of the cervical spine for several reasons, including paraspinal muscle spasm. Additionally, if critical instability is present, forced flexion and extension may potentially compromise neurologic function. Other biomechanical studies have questioned the sensitivity of flexion-extension radiographs.[7] They found that after sectioning all the posterior ligaments, destroying both facet joints, and then sectioning the posterior longitudinal ligament, only 69% of the cadavers showed increased intervertebral motion according to the criteria of White et al.[19] This study suggests that flexion and extension radiographs exhibit poor sensitivity for detection of posterior cervical spine injury.[7]

CT is a common screening tool for bony injuries after high speed trauma. Axial CT images and sagittal reconstructions aid in the visualization of posterior structures. CT reconstructions also visualize small or minimally displaced fractures of the lamina and facets that can be missed on plain radiographs.[20] A CT scan should be performed on all patients with facet fractures.[21]

MRI is highly sensitive for soft-tissue injuries, including the spinal cord and nerve roots, intervertebral disks, and posterior ligaments. However, MRI may have reduced specificity for soft-tissue injuries compared to actual anatomic findings.[22]

Specific Injury Pathomechanics

Facet Dislocations/Ligamentous Injuries

The spectrum of facet dislocations includes facet subluxations, "perched" facets, and even bilateral facet dislocations.[23] Distractive injuries result from damage to the posterior soft-tissue structures of the cervical spine, including the facet capsules.[24] Because these are flexion-distraction injuries, they

FIGURE 2

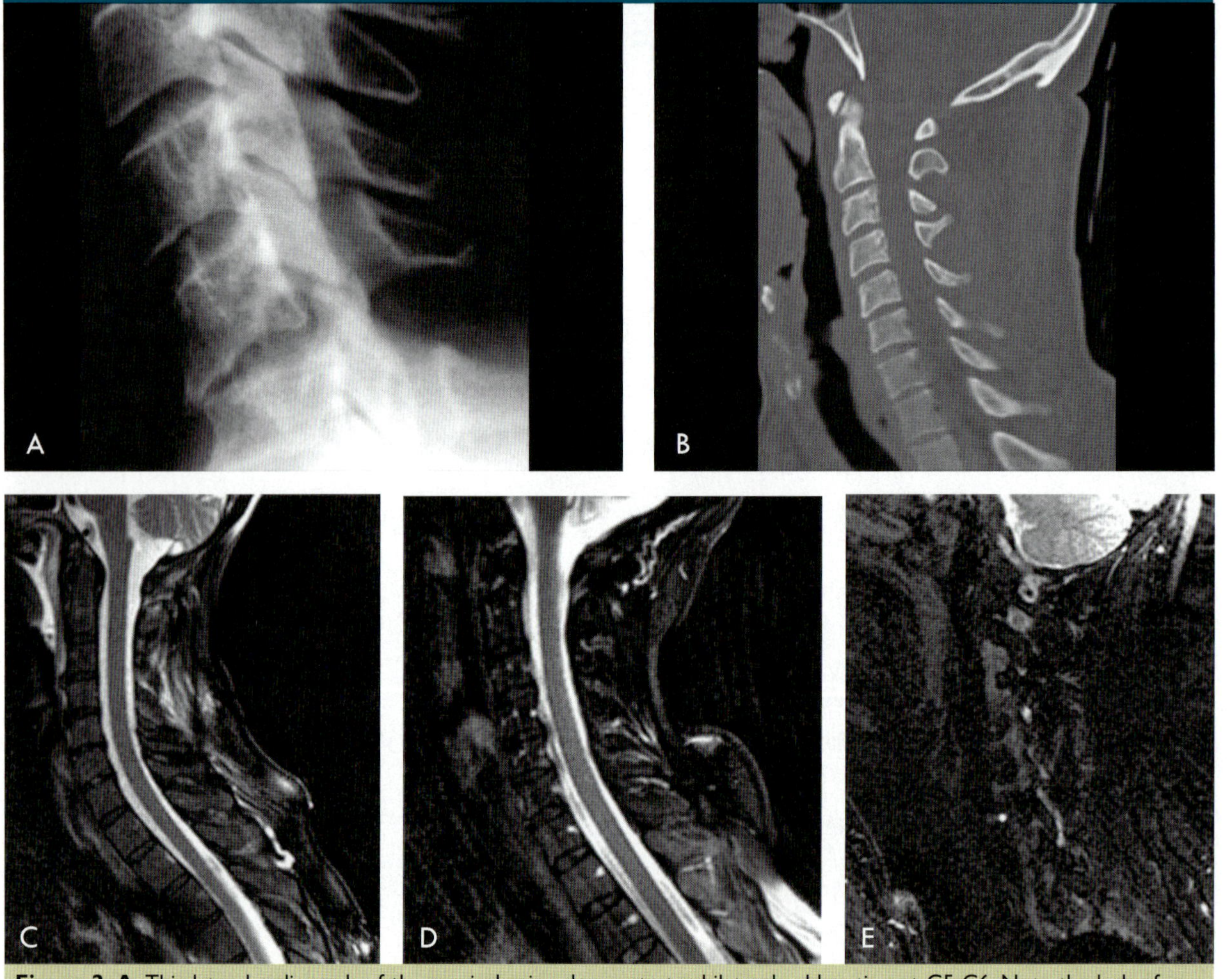

Figure 2 **A,** This lateral radiograph of the cervical spine demonstrates bilateral subluxation at C5-C6. Note the lack of rotation but the significant angulation and widening of the interval between the spinous processes posteriorly. **B,** A midsagittal CT scan may demonstrate no pathologic widening in isolated PLC injury. **C,** Midsagittal MRI of the same patient demonstrates isolated supraspinous ligament injury. **D,** Note the extensive posterior soft-tissue swelling, which correlates with underlying PLC injury. **E,** The clinician should carefully inspect the facet joint capsules on the parasagittal MRI view for signs of capsular injury, as seen on this parasagittal short-tau inversion recovery (STIR) image. (Panel A is reproduced from Levine AM: Facet fractures and dislocations, in Levine AM, Eismont FJ, Garfin SF, Zigler JE, eds: *Spine Trauma*. Philadelphia, PA, WB Saunders, 1998, pp 331-366.)

form a spectrum from minor tearing, or "sprains," of supraspinous, interspinous, and facet capsules, to complete disruption (with disruption of the disk) in the more severe variations of the injury.[25] Integrity of the facet capsule is thought to differentiate minor strain/sprain injuries from significant disruptive injuries.[26] In the most minor degrees of injury, the posterior ligaments are disrupted, but there is no translation or vertebral body rotation. **Figure 2** illustrates the spectrum of PLC injury from likely ligamentous sprain to isolated PLC injury. **Figure 2** also illustrates significant damage to the PLC and intervertebral disk which presents only as isolated PLC injury.

Facet subluxation (**Figure 2,** *E*) is considered to be a flexion-distraction injury that represents a sprain of the posterior cervical ligamentous elements. Thus, there is a partial disruption of the interspinous and supraspinous ligaments and partial disruption of the facet capsules.[27] Facet subluxation is defined by a widening of the joint and interspinous distance on a flexion radiographic view (similar to PLC injury in **Figure 2,** *D*). The inferior articular processes are subluxated superiorly and anteriorly with reference to the superior articular processes. This usually results in slight kyphosis (< 10° on a lateral radiograph).[8] On an extension view, facet subluxation may reduce com-

FIGURE 3

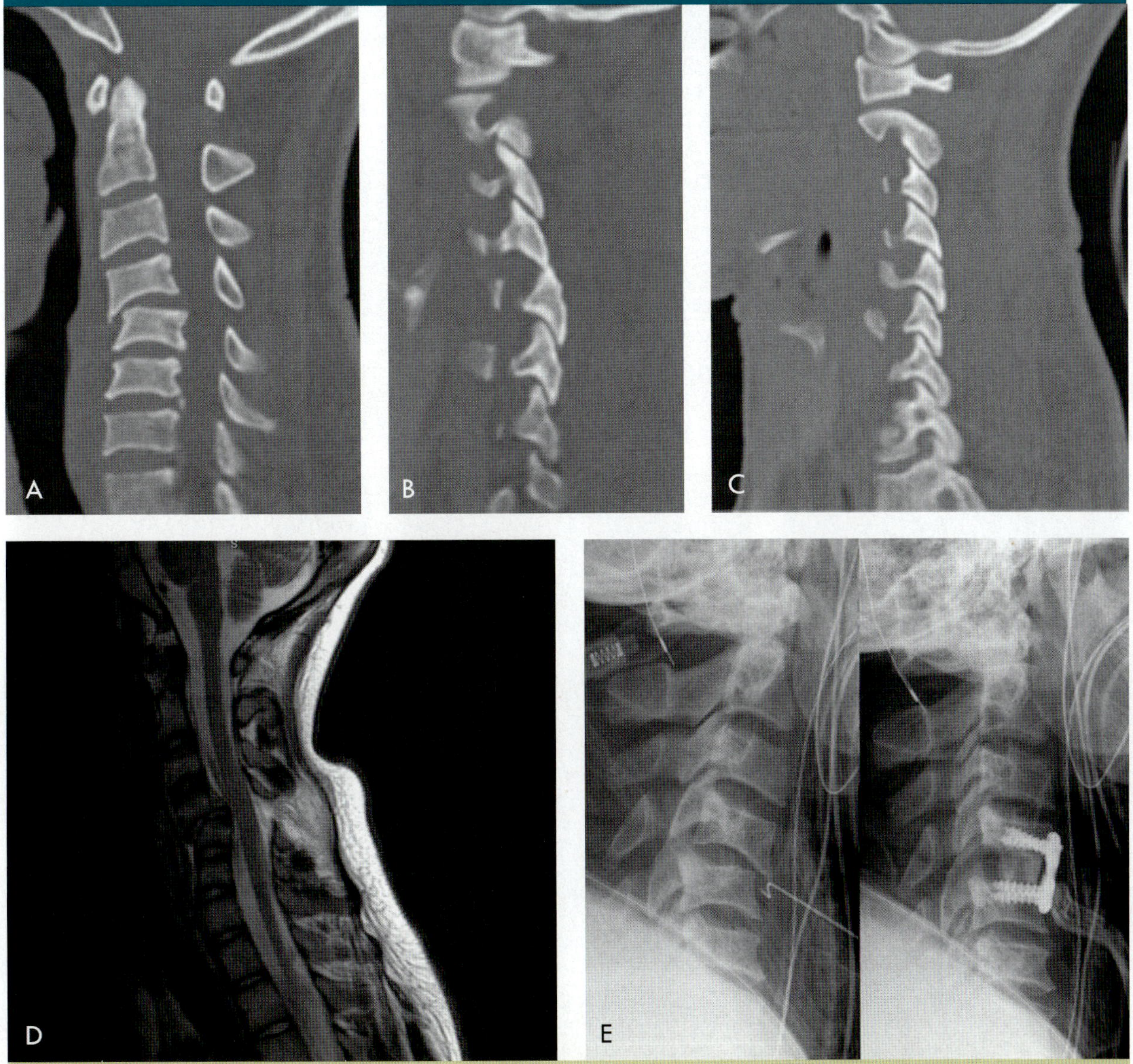

Figure 3 Perched facets. **A,** This midsagittal CT reconstruction demonstrates anterolisthesis and significant kyphosis at C4-C5. **B,** The parasagittal CT view through the midpoint of the lateral masses demonstrates a perched C4-C5 facet. **C,** The contralateral facets are subluxed. **D,** Midsagittal MRI scan demonstrates significant disk herniation posterior to the C4 vertebral body. **E,** Open reduction through an anterior approach and diskectomy was performed followed by stabilization in this man with a complete spinal cord injury.

pletely into normal alignment and may therefore be missed.[28]

Perched facets are the next most severe flexion-distraction injury mechanism (**Figure 3**). In this injury, the inferior articular process slides both superior and anterior to the tip of the superior articular process.[29] The result is significant kyphosis of the affected level, which often exceeds the kyphosis of a true bilateral facet dislocation. Some translation is noted on the lateral radiograph, but it is generally less than that noted with a bilateral facet dislocation. In addition, on the lateral radiograph, marked spreading of the distance between the adjacent spinous processes is noted. This "perching" can usually be delineated on a lateral spine radiograph. The AP radiograph does not depict any rotation, but it can show an increase in distance between the adjacent spinous processes.[30] MRI may be indicated to rule out a large intervertebral disk herniation as an etiology of a neurologic deficit.[31] MRI may show partial disruption of the posterior anulus of the involved disk.[32] The

FIGURE 4

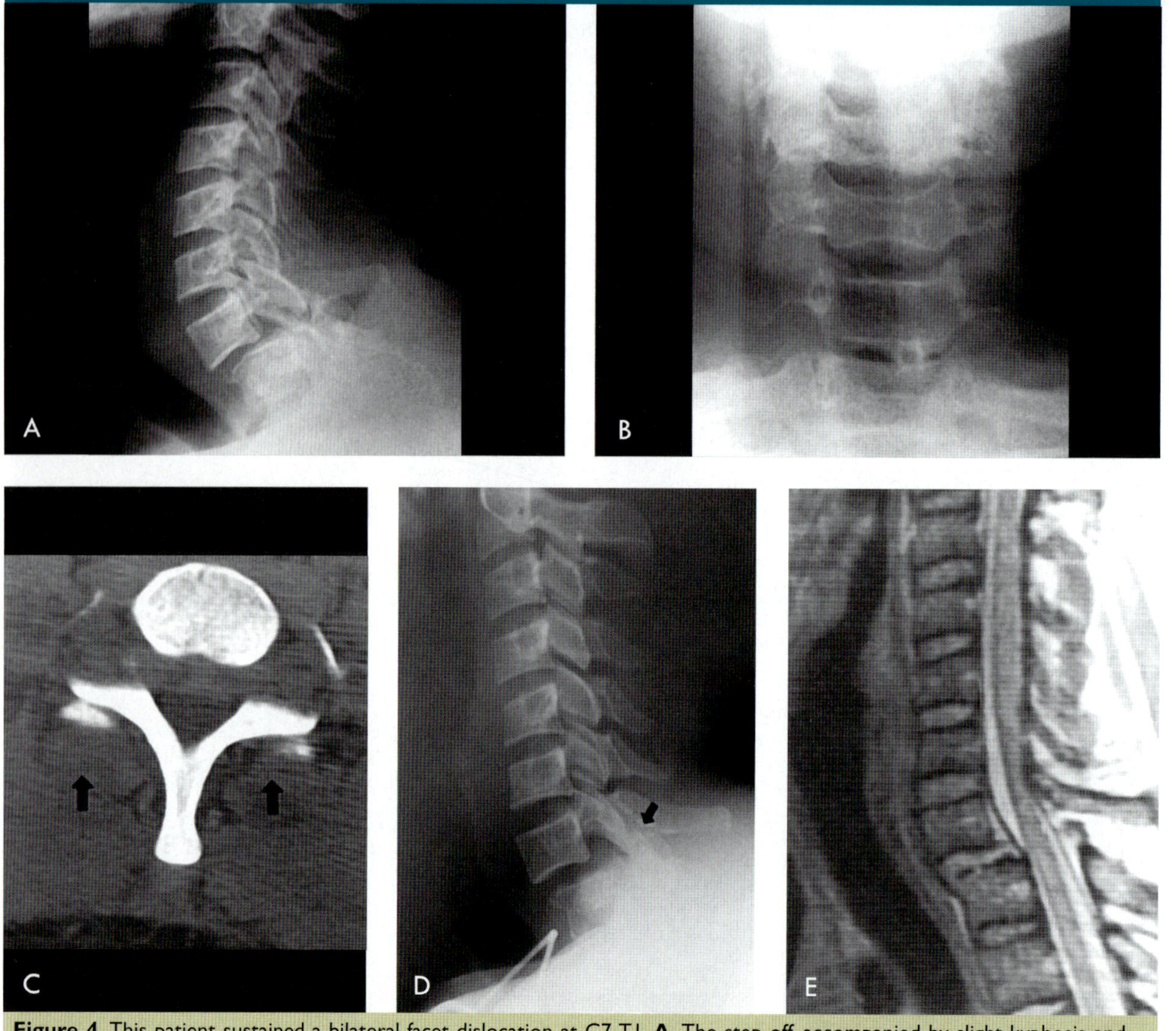

Figure 4 This patient sustained a bilateral facet dislocation at C7-T1. **A,** The step-off, accompanied by slight kyphosis and narrowing of the disk space, is evident on the lateral radiograph. **B,** The AP radiograph demonstrates widening of the interspinous distance but no rotational abnormality. **C,** After the patient was placed in traction, a CT scan was obtained, which showed the dislocated facets (arrows) on the axial view. **D,** Because of the patient's size and the distal position of the dislocation in the cervical spine, the dislocation could not be reduced using traction. The arrow indicates the perched facet complex. **E,** MRI was done because the facet dislocation would have to be reduced with the patient under anesthesia. No disk herniation was observed, but stripping of the posterior longitudinal ligament was evident. (Reproduced from Levine AM: Facet fractures and dislocations, in Levine AM, Eismont FJ, Garfin SF, Zigler JE, eds: *Spine Trauma*. Philadelphia, PA, WB Saunders, 1998, pp 331-366.)

injury essentially involves complete disruption of the intraspinous and supraspinous ligaments as well as facet capsules. The injury is also associated with rupture of the ligamentum flavum, and partial disruption of the posterior anulus.[33] The degree of disruption of the adjacent soft tissues is generally comparable to that of a bilateral facet dislocation. As with bilateral facet subluxation, perched bilateral SLIC Score of 5, consistent with surgical intervention.[10]

Facet dislocation is the most severe stage of flexion-distraction injury, resulting in a failure of the PLC and disk[8] in more than 82% of cases.[34] The injury results in distraction and translation of the inferior facets so that they come to rest anterior to the superior facets of the lower level and lock in that position (**Figure 4**). The result is less angulation than is noted with a bilateral perched facet (approximately 10°), but considerably more translation of the superior segment over the inferior segment (approximately 50% or 5 mm to 6 mm).[2] Unilateral injuries are considered to result in approximately 25% spondylolisthesis. Both the inferior and superior articular processes remain intact. A small chip fracture may occasionally be evident (usually comprising less than 25% of the height of either the superior or inferior facet).[35] The injury is reasonably distinct on a lateral cervical spine radiograph. On the lateral radiograph (**Figure 4,** *A*) an overlap is often seen corresponding to the amount of translation and angulation. The AP radiograph (**Figure 4,** *B*) does not show findings significantly different from those of a bilateral perched facet, although the widening of the interspinous distances may not be as significant as with a bilateral perched facet. The injury can be further defined by several radiologic techniques, including oblique or pillar views (**Figure 5**), which demonstrate the dislocation on both sides and may be useful in helping to differentiate a unilateral facet dislocation from a bilateral facet dislocation. In addition, a CT scan, although parallel to the plane of injury, demonstrates the juxtaposition of the superior and inferior articular processes. This will appear as an "empty" facet sign on axial cuts, which is pathognomonic of the injury (**Figure 4,** *C*).[20] MRI will clearly define the disruption of the disk at the involved segment and may be helpful in differentiating an extruded fragment in patients who are either neurologically intact or compromised (**Figure 4,** *E*).[36] This severe translational deformity is often accompanied by complete disruption of the interspinous and supraspinous ligaments, facet capsules, ligamentum flavum, and possibly a significant portion of the disk.[2] This is a flexion instability injury with a minimum SLIC score of 6 (morphology = 4; DLC = 2), consistent with surgical intervention.[10] The degree of spinal cord compression is exacerbated in patients with preexisting spinal stenosis. In a cadaveric study, the degree of canal occlusion following a bilateral facet dislocation was found to be 88% in those with stenotic canals and 35% in those with normal canal diameters.[37]

Unilateral facet injuries are a result of rotational and distraction injuries. As is the case with their bilateral counterparts, unilateral subluxation, perched facet, and dislocation represent a progression of injury. The mechanism for unilateral facet injuries is a flexion-rotation and distraction force.[8,38] This rotational element is most easily seen on a lateral cervical radiograph, and the severity of the rotational abnormality increases proportionately to the amount of disruption and translation of the facet. Thus, a unilateral subluxation will have less rotational abnormality than a unilateral dislocation.[39] On a lateral radiograph, this is noted as a difference in the appearance of the vertebral bodies proximal and distal to the injury level (**Figure 6**). On one section of the spine, the two lateral edges of the posterior aspect of the vertebral body will be superimposed, appearing as a single line. The other section of the spine will demonstrate a rotational abnormality where the two posterior edges of the cervical body do not overlap, thus appearing as two separate edges. In addition, the apparent translation of the vertebral body is actually the rotational abnormality. This results in an apparent foreshortening of one segment of the spine with reference to the other. Thus, on a lateral radiograph, one vertebral body of the injured level appears longer than its counterpart, either above or below it. Lastly, malrotation of the spinous processes at the level of the injury will also be apparent on AP radiographs. A unilateral dislocation will have characteristically less translation than that noted in a bilateral facet dislocation (3 mm versus 4 mm to 6 mm, or 25% versus 50% translation). As with bilateral dislocations, unilat-

FIGURE 5

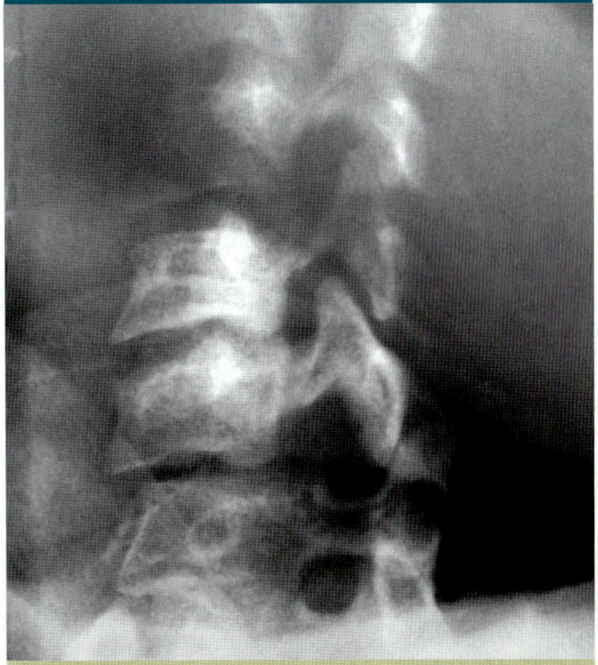

Figure 5 Oblique radiograph reveals a bilateral facet dislocation at C6-C7. Note that the intact inferior facet at C6 as well as the intact superior facet at C7 have been juxtaposed. (Reproduced from Levine AM: Facet fractures and dislocations, in Levine AM, Eismont FJ, Garfin SF, Zigler JE, eds: *Spine Trauma*. Philadelphia, PA, WB Saunders, 1998, pp 331-366.)

FIGURE 6

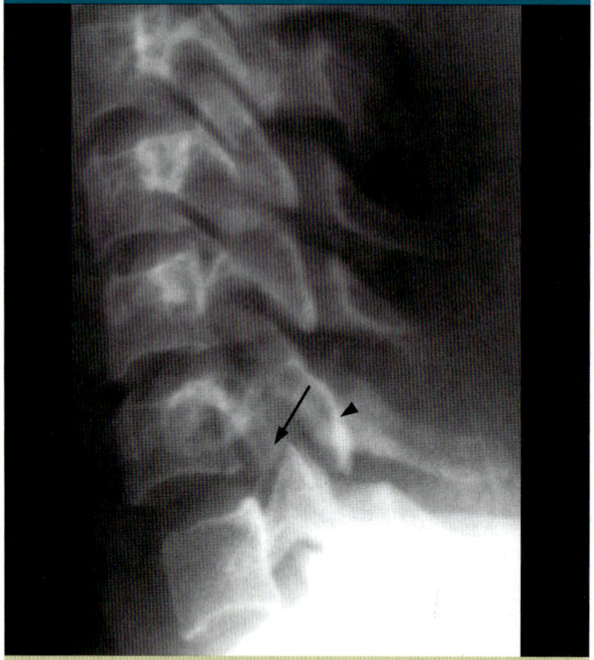

Figure 6 This lateral radiograph of the cervical spine shows a unilateral facet dislocation in a 19-year-old woman at the C6-C7 level. Note the rotational deformity indicated by the apparent widening of the anteroposterior width of the C6 body with reference to the C7 body. In addition, the two facets at C6-C7 are well visualized, and the normal inferior facet of C6 (arrowhead) can be differentiated from the dislocated inferior C6 facet (arrow). (Reproduced from Levine AM: Facet fractures and dislocations, in Levine AM, Eismont FJ, Garfin SF, Zigler JE, eds: *Spine Trauma*. Philadelphia, PA, WB Saunders, 1998, pp 331-366.)

FIGURE 7

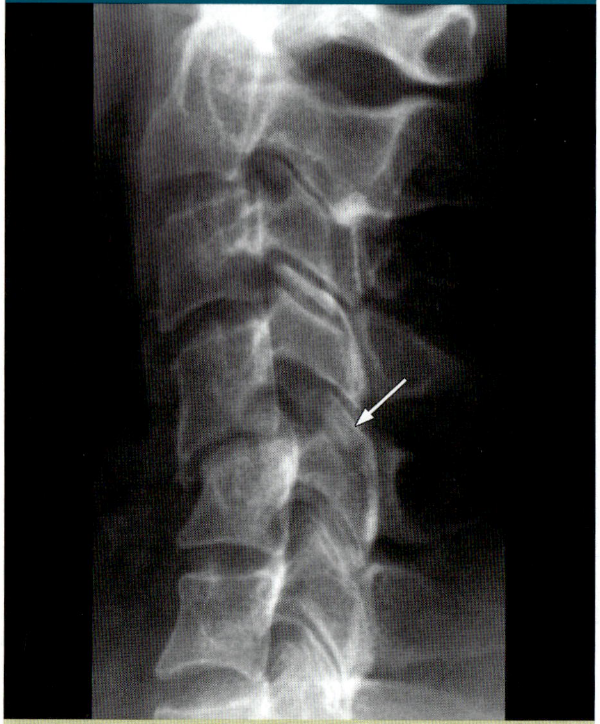

Figure 7 This radiograph of a bilateral facet fracture at C4-C5 in a 40-year-old woman shows displacement and angulation similar to that shown in Figure 5. In addition, there is an absence of rotational deformity, demonstrated either by foreshortening of the affected bodies or by evidence of the biconcave nature of the posterior aspect of the body. The bilateral fractures of the superior facet of C5 are suggested (arrow) on the lateral radiograph, but are best demonstrated on lateral CT or by CT reconstructions. (Reproduced from Levine AM: Facet fractures and dislocations, in Levine AM, Eismont FJ, Garfin SF, Zigler JE, eds: *Spine Trauma*. Philadelphia, PA, WB Saunders, 1998, pp 331-366.)

eral dislocations will show an "empty" facet sign on axial CT scan. MRI may be used to assess the injured disk.[40,41] Significant ligamentous disruption is necessary to achieve the dislocation. If the facet is not removed in the reduction process, the resultant instability is a coupled flexion-rotation.[42,43] Understanding the nature of the disruption is important to comprehend the necessity for a reduction maneuver, as opposed to simple traction, to achieve reduction.[44] Because the flexion and the rotation are a coupled motion, pure restriction of flexion in the case of intact facets after a dislocation results in spinal stability.[45]

Facet Fractures

Facet fractures result from a combination of flexion and a translation or shearing injury (**Figure 7**). Depending on the degree of initial flexion, the location of the fracture may differ. Superior (**Figure 8**) and inferior facet fractures are similar clinically and biomechanically.[46] In the absence of distractive forces to disengage the facet capsules,[47] facet fractures (**Figure 9**) may occur due to a combination of flexion and shear forces. The shear vector results in fracture due to facet impingement and subsequent fracture. Facet injuries associated with vertebral body fracture result from flexion-compression forces, in which the axis of rotation is within the spinal canal.[38] Thus the anterior vertebral body experiences compressive forces, while posterior elements undergo tensile forces. Finally, unilateral facet injuries commonly occur due to rotatory forces.[48] Facet fractures can result in vertebral artery injury (**Figure 9**, *C* through *E*). Angiography (either CT or MRI) may be indicated preoperatively to document the status of the vertebral arteries when planning instrumentation or decompression. Superior facet fractures may be more likely to result in injury to the exiting nerve root because the root is directly adjacent to the fracture.[2,49] If the shearing injury is severe, the posterior longitudinal ligament and the disk may be disrupted, and in the most severe form of injury, total disruption of the disk occurs with marked instability.[50] The degree of translation is related to the severity of injury. These injuries also may be vertically unstable if significant shear has been imparted to the spine, so they may provide classic examples of the positive stretch test by the criteria of White et al.[19] Regardless of the type of fracture (inferior versus superior facet), the intraspinous and supraspinous ligaments are attenuated but are generally not completely disrupted. This may be accompanied by a bilaminar fracture or spinous process fracture. The facet capsule is disrupted, because the injury usually occurs at either the superior or inferior limits of the capsule, with the facet complex instability occurring through the bony margin of the superior or inferior facet. The ligamentum flavum may be disrupted. The anulus is generally not as severely disrupted as in dislocations, because there is no little or no flexion component to the injury. Slight disk injury may occur, but generally without disruption of the anulus. As opposed to dislocations, the neurologic injury with facet fractures is most prominently related to translation of the two vertebral segments and not the extrusion of disk material. Unlike those used in bilateral facet dislocations, constructs to stabilize this fracture must be able to impart a resistance to translation, rather than purely to flexion. The final variant of bilateral facet injuries is a unilateral fracture combined with a contralateral dislocation (**Figures 9** and **10**). This is the rarest of the bilateral facet injuries. It includes both flexion and rotational components and results in complex instability. The exact mechanism of injury is difficult to establish.

Unilateral facet fractures (**Figures 11** and **12**) result from a rotational, flexion, and shear vector applied to the spine. As with unilateral ligamentous injuries, unilateral fractures may be missed on initial screening because the fracture may be fully reduced in the supine position and apparent translation, even in an erect posture, may be minimal.

The final type of fracture is the separation of the articular mass.[44,51,52] The characteristic pattern (**Figure 13**) is a fracture through the pedicle and a longitudinal fracture through the lamina, parallel to the articular process on the same side. It occurs very infrequently as a bilateral injury and is most common as a unilateral injury. This injury, as opposed to the previous two types of facet fractures, is most probably an extension-rotation injury resulting in a fracture of the pedicle and a vertical fracture of the lamina. Associated with this are injuries to the facet capsules, both above and below the fractures. One of the two (usually the lower) is significantly more unstable. The entire lateral mass is a free-floating fragment and thus the rotational instability cannot be stabilized over a single level. Lateral radiographs are similar to those seen in other unilateral facet injuries with rotation across the fracture segment noted by a difference in orientation of the vertebral bodies. As well, there is elongation and evident foreshortening of the two adjacent vertebral bodies. The degrees of translation and angulation are similar to those seen with other unilateral facet fractures.[44] The AP radiograph will likewise show horizontalization of the lateral mass and may reveal the laminar fracture as well. The injury is best seen on CT scan, which demonstrates the characteristic pattern of the fracture through the pedicle, or through the foramen for the vertebral artery, with a second fracture line through the lamina that frees and separates the entire lateral mass (**Figure 13,** *B*).[53]

FIGURE 8

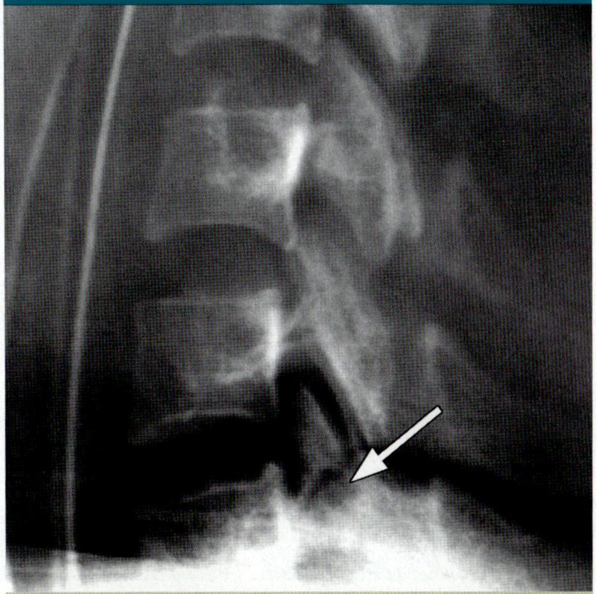

Figure 8 A fracture of the superior facet of C7 is clearly visualized on this lateral radiograph (arrow). No associated deformity is seen because it was reduced with 20 lb of traction. (Reproduced from Levine AM: Facet fractures and dislocations, in Levine AM, Eismont FJ, Garfin SF, Zigler JE, eds: *Spine Trauma.* Philadelphia, PA, WB Saunders, 1998, pp 331-366.)

FIGURE 9

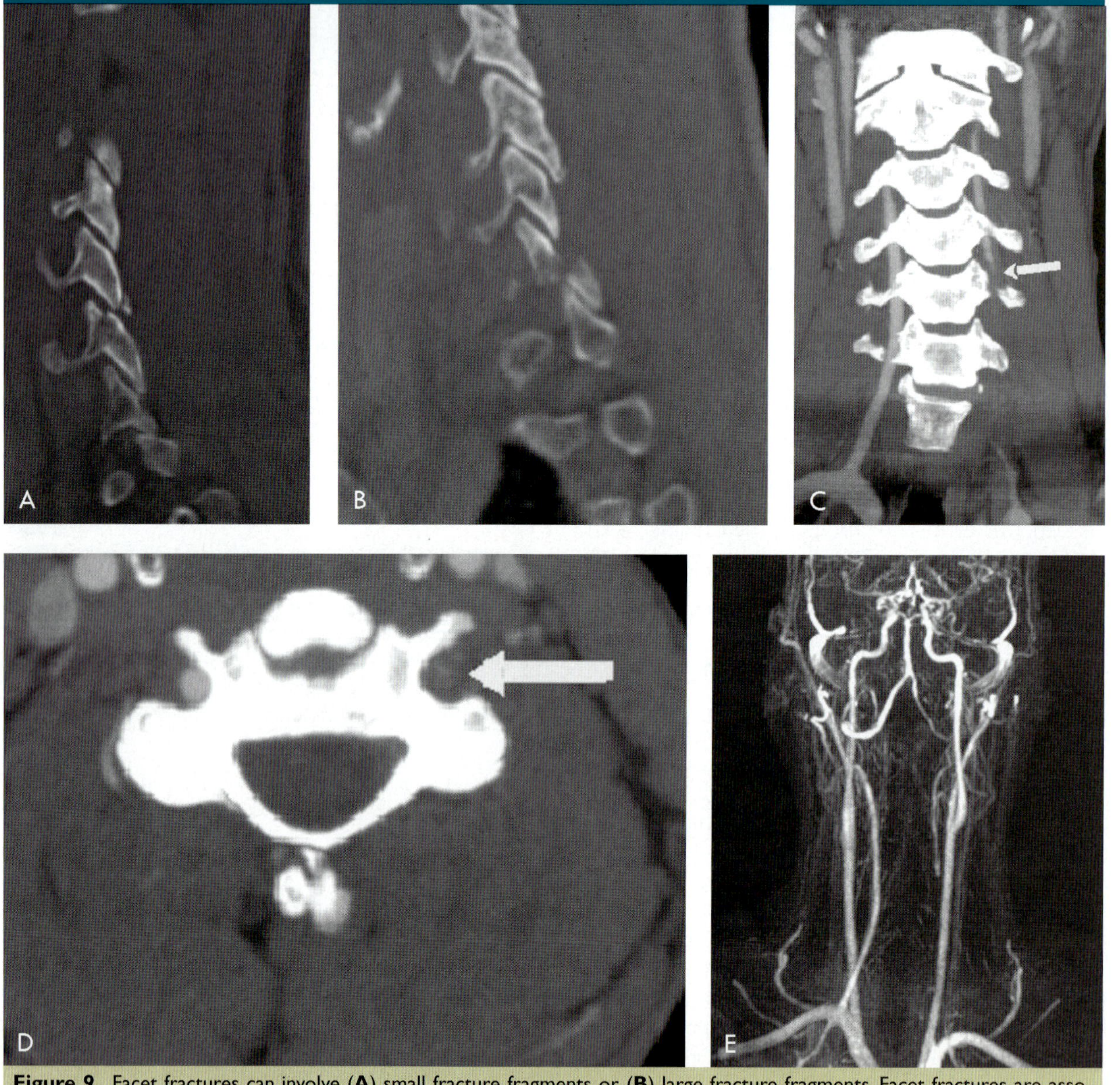

Figure 9 Facet fractures can involve (**A**) small fracture fragments or (**B**) large fracture fragments. Facet fractures are associated with a high rate of vertebral artery injuries. This angiogram demonstrates a left vertebral artery injury (arrow) on coronal (**C**) and axial CT (**D**). Three-dimensional reconstruction (**E**) shows the absence of a left vertebral artery.

Any of these injuries can occur in multiple combinations. Double-level unilateral facet fractures, double-level fracture-separations of the articular mass, or alternate-level injuries can occur. In terms of instability, each of these injuries needs to be considered as a separate entity. If the total injury pattern is difficult to classify, then each individual injury can be considered as a separate unit and treated individually.

Initial Treatment and Timing of MRI

Patients should undergo medical stabilization according to the Advanced Trauma Life Support protocol as described in chapter 2 on patient transport and stabilization. Once the patient is in a monitored setting and is hemodynamically stable, then the spinal injury may be treated. Neurologic

FIGURE 10

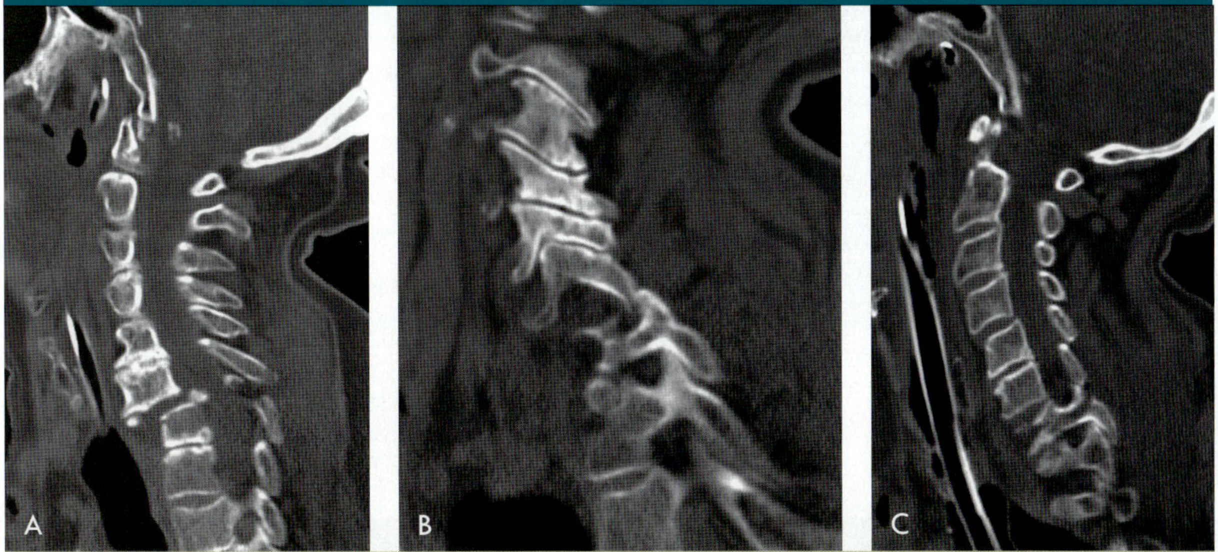

Figure 10 Combined facet fracture/dislocation. **A,** Midsagittal CT scan shows extensive spondylosis and acute anterolisthesis of C6-C7. **B,** Parasagittal CT scan reveals dislocation of the left C6 facet. **C,** Parasagittal CT scan shows displaced fracture of the right C7 pedicle with displacement.

examination should be performed by an experienced observer and assessed as intact, complete spinal cord injury, or incomplete spinal cord injury, with or without a nerve root injury. Patients should be placed on spinal precautions and immobilized without excessive manipulation. Pharmacologic management, including administration of steroids at NASCIS (National Acute Spinal Cord Injury Study)–recommended dosing, may be considered, although the use of steroids is controversial.[2,54]

Significant controversy exists over the timing and indications of MRI in cervical facet dislocations.[22,55] MRI provides valuable information about the status of the intervertebral disk to distinguish annular disruption from true herniation. Theoretically, a closed reduction maneuver may displace a herniated intervertebral disk fragment into the spinal cord.[56] The clinical implication of this is often benign because no cases of a permanent neurologic deficit in an awake, alert, and cooperative patient following closed skeletal reduction of a cervical dislocation have been reported. MRI assists clinical decision making to plan cervical dislocation reduction.

Initial management of patients with perched or dislocated facets is triaged according to neurologic status, not severity of dislocation.[2,57,58] Furthermore, it is critical to assess the patient's mental status and cooperativeness. A cooperative patient can accurately report his or her function and follow commands during a neurologic examination.

FIGURE 11

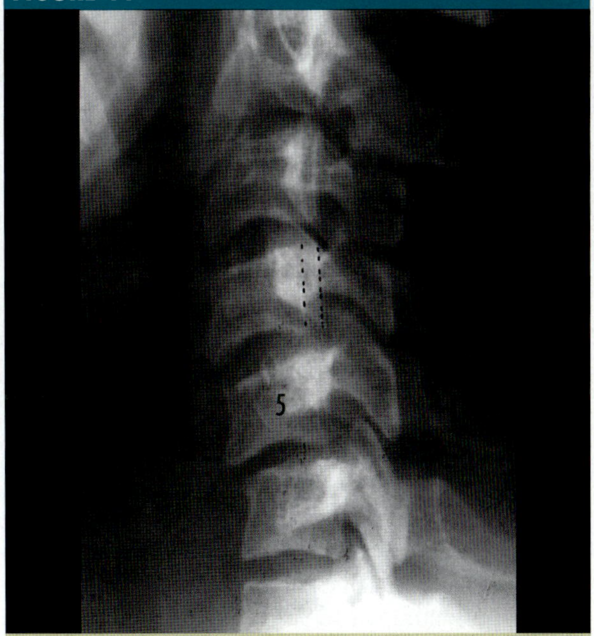

Figure 11 This 19-year-old man was injured in a vehicle accident. Lateral radiograph shows the unilateral facet fracture, which is a fracture separation of the articular mass of C5, and a rotational deformity at both C5-C6 and C4-C5. This is evident from the apparent elongation of the diameter of C5 with reference to C6 and also by the clear appearance of the two posterior edges of the concave vertebral body at C4. (Reproduced from Levine AM: Facet fractures and dislocations, in Levine AM, Eismont FJ, Garfin SF, Zigler JE, eds: *Spine Trauma*. Philadelphia, PA, WB Saunders, 1998, pp 331-366.)

FIGURE 12

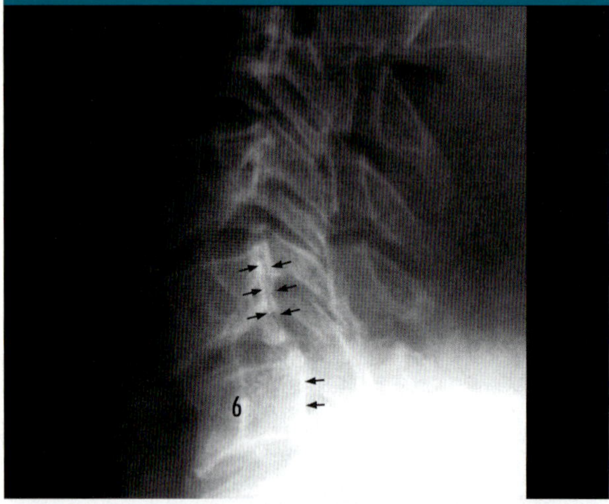

Figure 12 This radiograph demonstrates the more subtle findings of a unilateral facet fracture or dislocation with rotational abnormality. The injury in this patient occurred at the C5-C6 level, demonstrating minimal apparent anterior translation; however, the rotational abnormality is evident. There is a single, posterior line of the vertebral body of C6 (two arrows), but both posterolateral edges of the body of C5 are evident because of the difference in rotation between the two levels (six arrows). Also, there is a difference in the apparent anteroposterior width of C5 versus C6 (C6 appearing to be slightly longer). (Reproduced from Levine AM: Facet fractures and dislocations, in Levine AM, Eismont FJ, Garfin SF, Zigler JE, eds: *Spine Trauma*. Philadelphia, PA, WB Saunders, 1998, pp 331-366.)

FIGURE 13

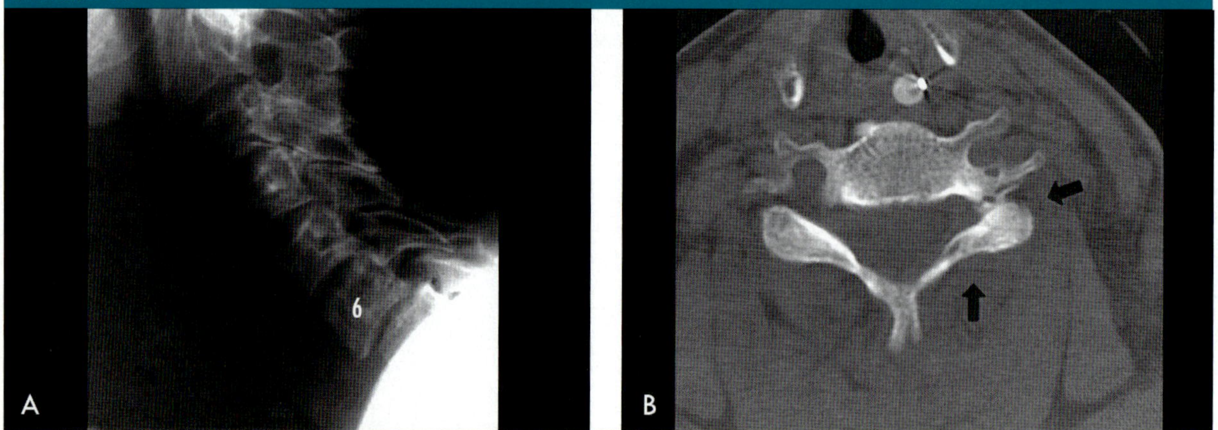

Figure 13 This elderly woman sustained an extension and lateral bending injury in a motor vehicle accident and reported neck pain and radiculopathy. **A,** The lateral radiograph showed a 4-mm step-off with the patient in an erect position. **B,** The two fracture lines in this injury are a vertical fracture in the lamina along the facet-laminar junction and a second fracture through the pedicle (arrows). Stabilization of this injury requires three-level plating. Because the fracture of the C6 lateral mass destabilizes both the C5-C6 and the C6-C7 joints on the affected side, the construct must involve C5 through C7. (Reproduced from Levine AM: Facet fractures and dislocations, in Levine AM, Eismont FJ, Garfin SF, Zigler JE, eds: *Spine Trauma*. Philadelphia, PA, WB Saunders, 1998, pp 331-366.)

Therefore, a cooperative patient can report neurologic changes associated with reduction of a spinal dislocation before irreversible damage is rendered to the spine. Multiple case reports document the successful identification and reversal of neurologic deficits in awake, cooperative patients.[59,60] Uncooperative patients with facet injuries who are neurologically intact should undergo MRI before any treatment to evaluate the integrity of the intervertebral disk. Conversely, patients with complete spinal cord injury may benefit from early closed reduction before MRI to reduce tension on the spinal cord as rapidly as possible.[34]

Definitive Treatment

Closed Reduction

The goal of treatment of facet fractures and dislocations is restoration of the anatomic alignment of the spine, alleviating impingement on the spinal cord and nerve roots, and achieving long-term stability. The reduction of a facet dislocation facilitates restoration of anatomic alignment and decreases neurologic compression (**Figure 14**).

Prior to reduction, the surgeon should (1) confirm the diagnosis of facet injury, (2) understand the biomechanical forces that caused the facet dis-

FIGURE 14

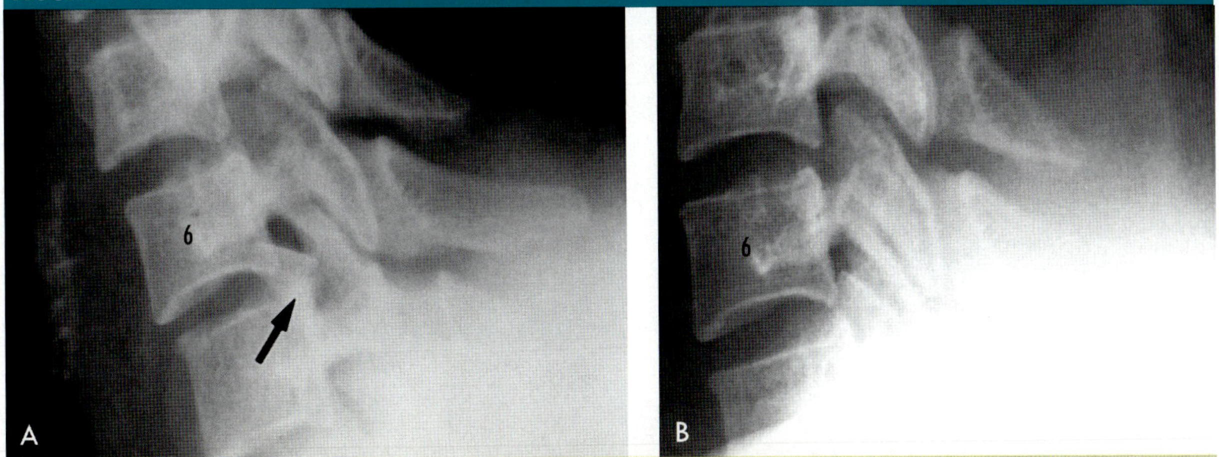

Figure 14 These lateral cervical spine radiographs demonstrate the ease of reduction of a unilateral facet fracture. **A,** The unreduced position with the fracture fragment (arrow) is evident on this view. **B,** With 20 lb of traction applied through Gardner-Wells tongs, the rotational and translational deformities were completely reduced for this C6-C7 fracture. If this had been a unilateral facet dislocation, pure traction with 20 lb would not have changed the deformity. (Reproduced from Levine AM: Facet fractures and dislocations, in Levine AM, Eismont FJ, Garfin SF, Zigler JE, eds: *Spine Trauma.* Philadelphia, PA, WB Saunders, 1998, pp 331-366.)

location (flexion-distraction, rotation, hyperflexion), (3) understand the patient's neurologic state, and (4) plan subsequent decompression and stabilization.[61] Reduction should be performed only in a setting in which an operating room is immediately available in the event of neurologic decompensation. Reduction should be performed by an experienced surgeon, because gentle manipulation including flexion or rotational maneuvers may be necessary to disengage and then re-engage the facet fragments (**Figure 15**).

Closed reduction may be beneficial in spinal cord injury because facet dislocations may result in tensile forces that lead to ischemic spinal cord events, as well as potential spinal cord impingement at the posterosuperior aspect of the caudal vertebral body.[62] Vaccaro and Nachwalter[34] reported 11 consecutive patients with cervical spine dislocations who met the clinical criteria for an awake closed traction reduction. Disk herniations were identified in 2 of 11 patients before reduction. Awake closed traction reduction was successful in 9 of the 11 patients. Of the nine patients with a successful closed reduction, two had disk herniations before reduction, and five had disk herniations after reduction. No patient had neurologic worsening after attempted awake closed traction reduction. However, there are reports of patients with transient neurologic deficits after closed reduction maneuvers. Caution should especially be exercised in the setting of ossification of the posterior longitudinal ligament or preexisting cervical stenosis.[56]

Animal studies have shown that the extent of neurologic injury after spinal cord compression is related to both the rate of injury and the duration of compression. Basic animal research has demonstrated that a relatively brief window of 1 to 3 hours is available, after which injury to the spinal cord caused by mechanical compression may become irreversible. However, these are findings observed in a laboratory environment.[52,63] Although some spine surgeons advocate early reduction for indirect decompression of facet dislocations, the ideal timing of decompression remains unknown.[64] Aebi et al[65] reviewed 100 cervical injuries and found that 25% of the patients who underwent reduction within 6 hours of injury had greater neurologic recovery. Another study found that prompt reduction within 4 hours facilitates recovery even in neurologically compromised patients.[66]

Treatment of Specific Injuries

Facet Subluxations

A bilateral facet subluxation injury actually poses a significant diagnostic and therapeutic dilemma for clinicians, particularly in an emergency situation, because patients with facet subluxation injuries have the potential for progression of their cervical deformity. According to the SLIC classification,

FIGURE 15

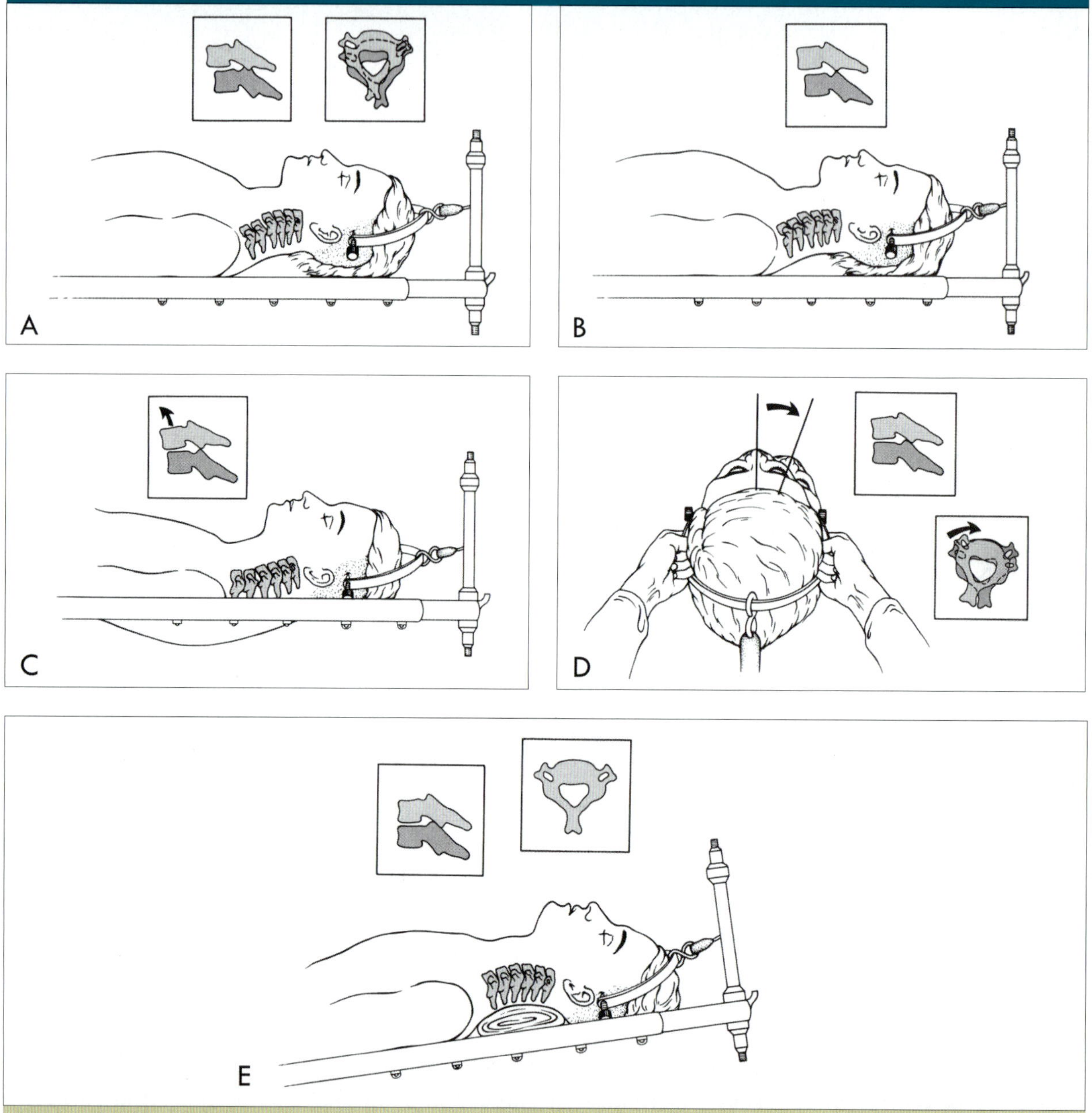

Figure 15 A, Initial position of a unilateral facet dislocation in both the sagittal and axial planes. **B,** Traction allows some distraction but not reduction. **C,** Flexion of the neck increases the distraction but the dislocation remains. **D,** Lateral tilt away from the side of dislocation unlocks the dislocation. **E,** Extension and return of the neck to the neutral position completes the reduction. (Reproduced with permission from Bucholz RW: Lower cervical spine injuries, in Browner BD, Jupiter JB, Levine AM, Trafton PG, eds: *Skeletal Trauma: Fractures, Dislocations, Ligamentous Injuries*. Philadelphia, PA, WB Saunders, 1992, vol 1, p 638.)

bilateral facet subluxations are given a minimum score of 3 (morphology = 3), which may increase depending upon extent of DLC injury and neurologic status.[10] Careful documentation of DLC injury and neurologic injury are necessary to appropriately triage and treat these patients. Controversy exists about what connotes pathologic subluxation and/or normal range of motion.

Therefore, MRI may be useful in these patients to document DLC integrity. Ideally, neurologically intact patients with isolated bilateral facet subluxations and no obvious ligamentous injury on MRI should be managed in a halo vest (pinless or pin design) or hard collar to maintain alignment.[67,68] The patient should undergo supervised flexion-extension exercises 6 weeks after injury to assess for any evidence of instability. Consideration may be given to early surgical intervention in noncompliant patients.

Treatment of Perched or Dislocated Facets

According to the SLIC classification, distractive facet injuries have a morphology score of 3. Translational or rotational injuries may reflect a more severe underlying injury and increase the morphology subscore to 4 points.[10] Patients will typically have a DLC injury subscore of at least 2, which, combined with the morphology score, suggests surgical intervention.[10] Single-level anterior cervical diskectomy and fusion or a single-level posterior cervical fusion using lateral mass screws are acceptable alternatives.[69] Choice of surgical intervention is dictated by the presence and location of neurologic compression.

Patients with unilateral facet injuries may be treated with anterior cervical diskectomy and fusion, posterior cervical fusion, or nonsurgical management with an orthosis.[70,71] Although generally neurologically intact, unilateral facet injuries are serious injuries that generally result in significant pain and disability compared to the general population.[72] Nonsurgically treated patients report worse outcomes than those treated surgically.[72,73] The presence of comorbidities, associated injuries, and advanced age adversely impact clinical outcomes.[72]

Patients with facet dislocation may be treated with an anterior or posterior surgical approach. Reduction may be performed posteriorly with a partial facetectomy followed by reduction and stabilization. Care should be taken to ensure that there is no significant disk herniation within the spinal canal before reduction to minimize the risk of spinal cord compression and quadriparesis.[74,75] Reduction and stabilization may also be performed via an anterior cervical approach using Caspar pins as joysticks in the vertebral bodies (**Figures 16** and **17**). Another consideration is the use of Gardner-Wells tongs, a vertebral body spreader, or lamina spreader to distract and then effect reduction. A subtle fracture of the inferior end plate of the cephalad vertebra following a facet injury has been associated with failure of anterior cervical diskectomy and plating.[76] **Figure 18** illustrates a case of a facet dislocation in which the patient also had an end-plate fracture of C7. Anterior cervical diskectomy was followed by posterior cervical instrumentation and fusion to reduce the risk of subsidence due to the end-plate fracture. A recent prospective, consecutive case series identified a 13% radiographic failure rate associated with isolated anterior cervical diskectomy and fusion.[76] Posterior approaches may also be performed using lateral mass screws (**Figures 17; 18,** *F*; and **19**) or, in rare cases, pedicular fixation (**Figures 18,** *F* and **20**). Of the fixation techniques, the non-FDA (US Food and Drug Administration)–approved use of lateral mass screws has increased significantly because the rigidity of the construct. Cervical pedicle screws (**Figure 20**) afford the most rigid fixation in flexion, extension, rotation, and lateral bending forces. However, there is significant risk of vertebral artery injury in placement of cervical pedicle screws between C2 and C6. Cervical pedicle screws may therefore be most appropriate for subacute or chronic dislocations requiring rigid fixation, such as in **Figure 20**. We will place pedicle screws at C7 or T1 if necessary for stabilization if the vertebral artery is not at risk.

Facet Fractures

Facet fractures with translation or rotation often reflect a potentially unstable clinical situation and are given a subscore of 4 points according to the SLIC system.[10] DLC integrity may also be compromised, resulting in significant instability that may require surgical intervention. The surgical approach is usually a single-level anterior cervical diskectomy and fusion or a single- or two-level posterior cervical fusion.[77,78] The surgical approach is dictated by associated pathology.[79,80] Unilateral facet fractures in which the fragment height is greater than 40% of the contralateral lateral mass or has an absolute height greater than 1 cm are at increased risk for failure of nonsurgical treatment.[81]

Floating Lateral Mass

Cervical floating lateral mass injuries are considered uniformly unstable. Several retrospective reviews have shown that nonsurgical treatment is usually unsuccessful, and early single-level anterior arthrodesis has a favorable outcome. If a posterior approach is chosen, a two-level fusion incorporating the level above and below the injury is necessary.[82,83]

Flexion Compression Injuries

Flexion compression injuries are translation/rotation injuries that often result in teardrop fractures of the spine. These injuries are discussed in chapter 26.

FIGURE 16

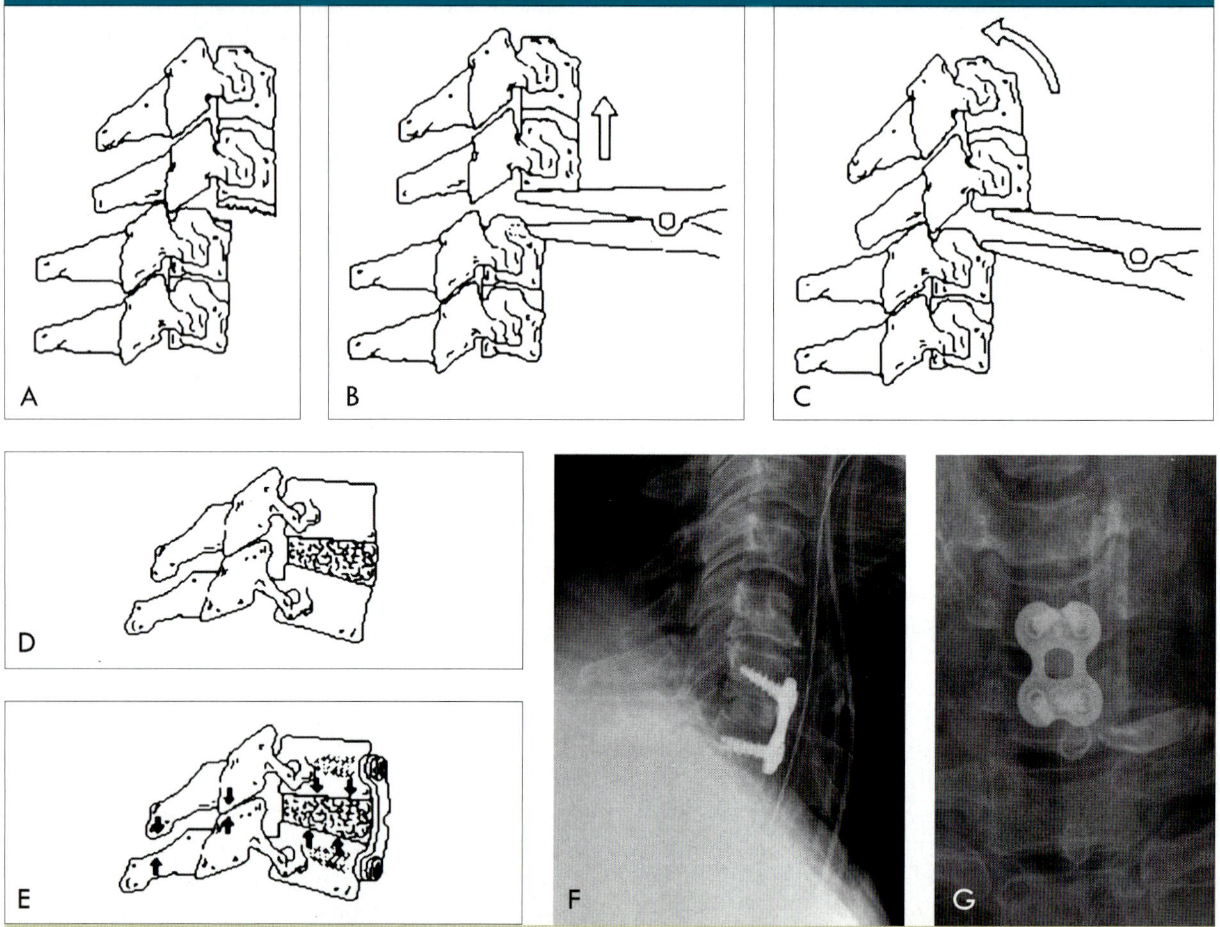

Figure 16 Technique of anterior reduction of bilateral facet dislocation with a large disk extrusion. **A,** Complete diskectomy is done initially to remove the extruded fragment from the canal. **B,** Either a laminar spreader or a Caspar distractor is placed deep within the disk space and symmetric distraction is applied to disengage the facets. Axial traction is also applied. Once the facets are disengaged, the superior body is pushed posteriorly while the distraction is released to achieve the reduction. **C,** The ability to achieve a reduction can be blocked by inserting the distractor into the anterior portion of the disk space, resulting in asymmetric distraction. **D,** The tricortical graft is created in a routine fashion, with the exception that it is slightly tapered. **E,** The plate is then contoured slightly so that the graft is compressed and the posterior elements are not fixed in distraction, but rather aid in the load sharing with the anterior graft and hardware. **F,** This patient sustained a bilateral facet dislocation and underwent an anterior cervical diskectomy, reduction with lamina spreader, and interbody graft placement with plate (**G**). (Panels A through E are reproduced from Levine AM: Facet fractures and dislocations, in Levine AM, Eismont FJ, Garfin SF, Zigler JE, eds: *Spine Trauma.* Philadelphia, PA, WB Saunders, 1998, pp 331-366.)

Complications

Missed Diagnoses

The most catastrophic complication is failure to diagnose an unstable facet injury. Facet subluxations are most likely to be misdiagnosed because initial radiographs may appear normal, particularly if the cervical spine is extended in a cervical collar. **Figure 2,** *C* through *E* demonstrates PLC injury that may be missed unless there is a high degree of suspicion.[16] Unilateral facet injuries are also commonly misdiagnosed. In addition, the step-offs are subtle. Thus, the rotational abnormality may not be seen by the examining physician. Because the neurologic consequences can be alarming, a high degree of suspicion must be maintained when evaluating for a potential cervical spine injury.[84]

Neurologic Injury

Neurologic injury may occur because of several factors. Size of the neural canal (which is a developmental factor), degree of translation experienced at the time of injury (which is a reflection of the type and severity of force applied to the spine), and presence or absence of a disk herniation are

FIGURE 17

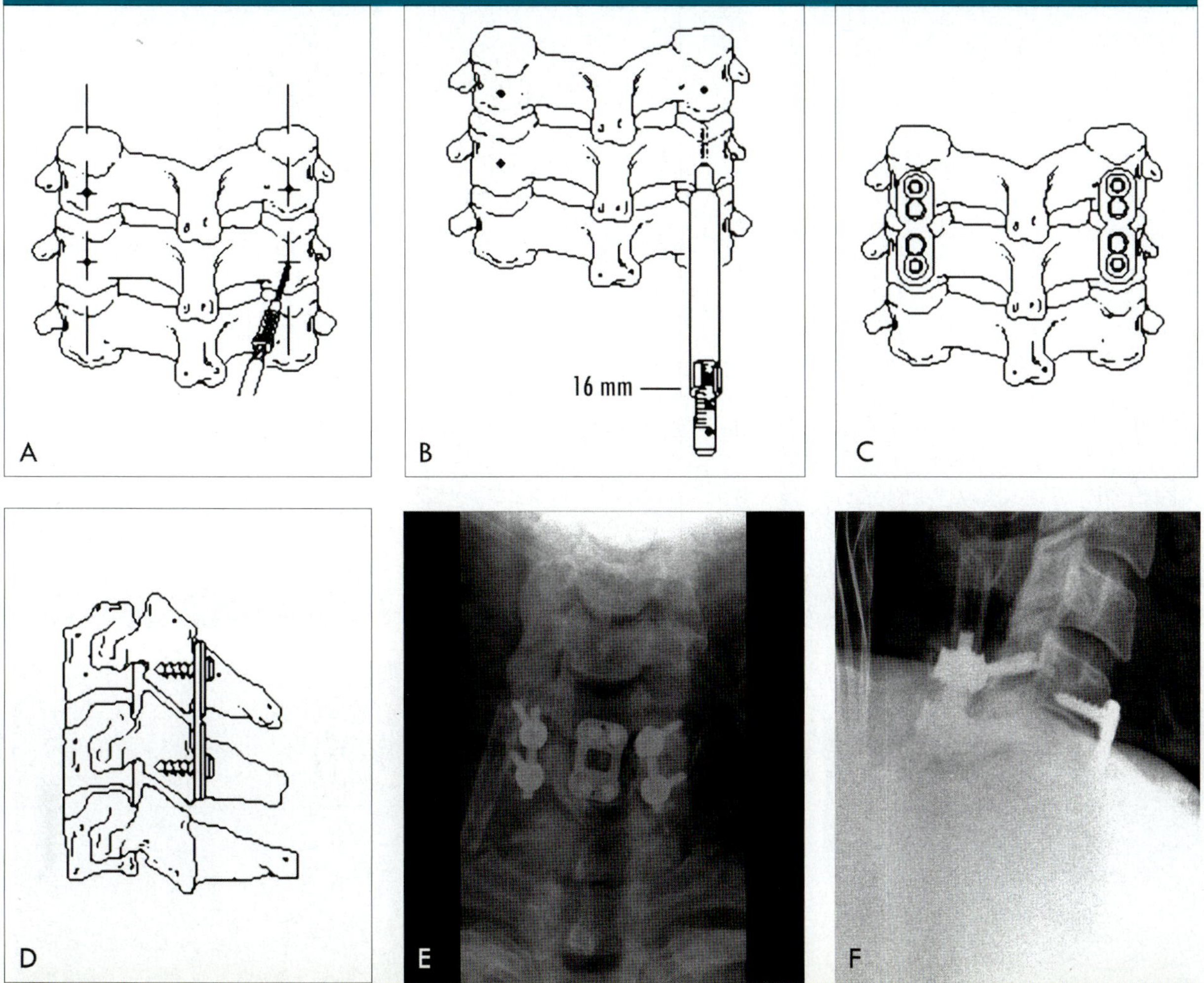

Figure 17 Lateral mass plating technique. After exposure of the posterior aspect of the spine, careful delineation of the anatomy of the lateral mass is necessary. **A,** Once the entire lateral mass is exposed at both levels, a burr with a 2-mm tip is used to make a small depression at the center of the lateral mass, to keep the drill from "walking" out of position when drilling is begun. The trajectory of the drill that can be used with a drill stop is 10° lateral and perpendicular to the lateral mass in a cephalocaudad direction. In fact, about 10° of superior angulation with reference to the posterior aspect of the lateral mass achieves the best position. **B,** After bicortical penetration with the drill, the hole is measured with a depth gauge and tapped. A plate is selected with the proper hole spacing (generally about 13 mm in the average person). **C,** When the two-hole plate is placed over them, the previously drilled holes should lie at the extremes of the holes in the plate, so that application of the plate creates slight compression and lordosis. **D,** Proper screw position avoids both the nerve root and the unfused facet joints. **E** and **F,** Example of an anterior cervical diskectomy followed by posterior cervical stabilization with lateral mass screws due to the presence of an end-plate fracture anteriorly. (Panels A through D are reproduced from Levine AM: Facet fractures and dislocations, in Levine AM, Eismont FJ, Garfin SF, Zigler JE, eds: *Spine Trauma*. Philadelphia, PA, WB Saunders, 1998, pp 331-366.)

most typical. Almost 50% of patients with high degrees of translation but intact neural arches, such as occurs in bilateral facet dislocations and fractures, experience either complete or incomplete quadriplegia.[31,56] These may be associated with disk injuries, which will further aggravate the degree of translation. The patient with a congenitally large neural canal is less likely to sustain neurologic injury, even with the acute reduction in effective canal diameter experienced with bilateral facet dislocation. Facet fractures, especially those of the superior facet, cause narrowing of the neural foramen and root injuries at that level. Patients with unilateral facet fractures and dislocations without significant disk disruption may demonstrate unilateral root injuries. A more severe unilateral injury with an associated disk disruption may not only result in a root injury but might also

FIGURE 18

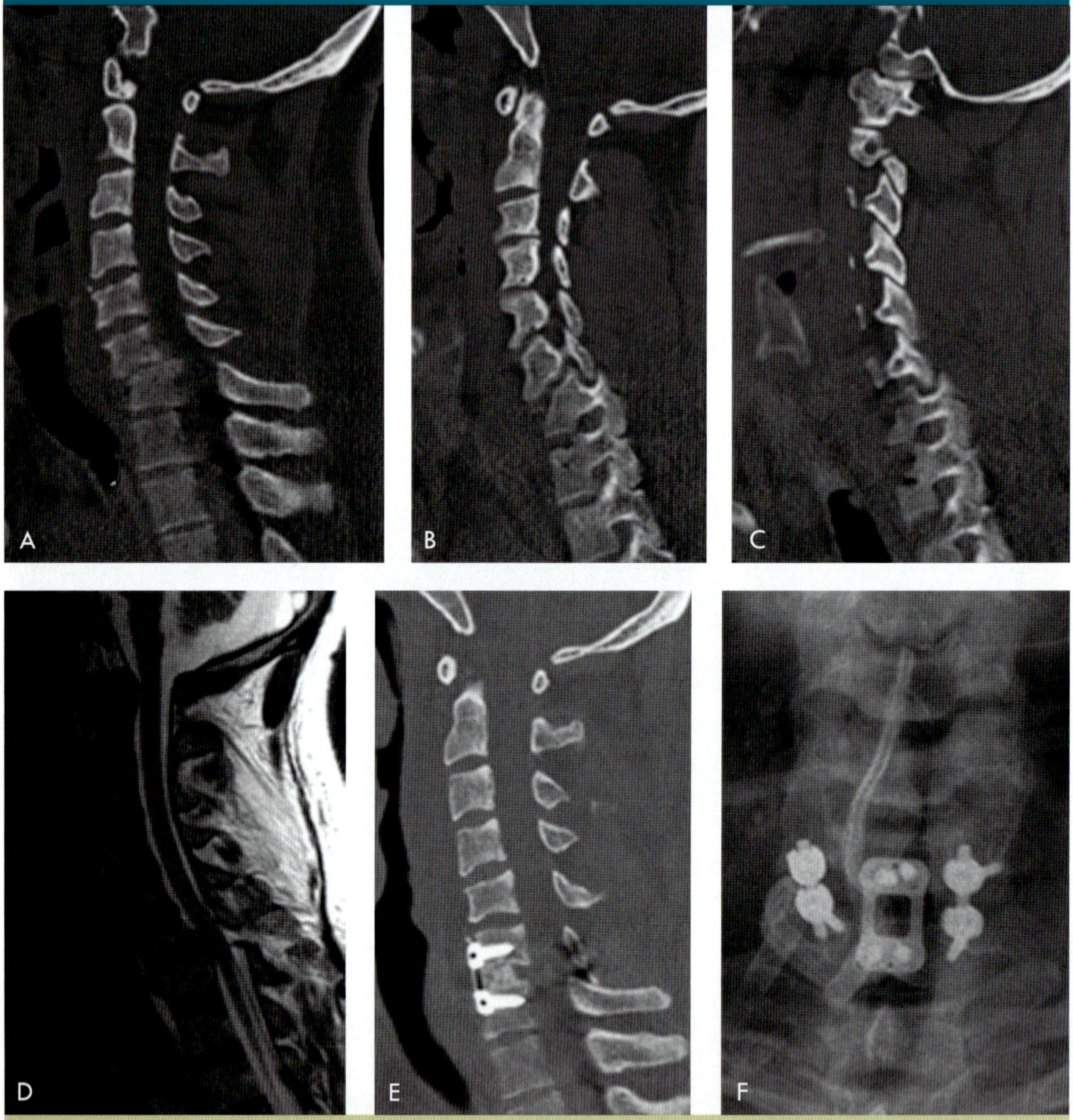

Figure 18 **A,** Midsagittal CT scan demonstrates acute anterolisthesis of C6-C7 and a C7 superior endplate fracture. **B,** Parasagittal CT scan shows dislocation of the left C6 facet. **C,** Parasagittal CT scan demonstrates displacement of the right C6 facet. **D,** Midsagittal MRI scan shows a large disk herniation posterior to the C6 vertebral body and extensive PLC destruction. **E** and **F,** The patient underwent anterior cervical diskectomy followed by posterior instrumentation with lateral mass screws at C6 and pedicle screws at C7 due to the C7 end-plate fracture.

result in an asymmetric cord injury, such as Brown-Séquard hemiplegia. Incomplete or complete quadriplegia are typical in more dense injuries. Roy-Camille and Mazel[3] found that 24% of patients with unilateral facet dislocation had cord symptoms that ranged from incomplete to complete lesions—68% had radicular symptoms; a total of 92% had some neurologic injury. Patients with bilateral facet fractures and dislocations experience acute narrowing of the neural canal with essentially intact neural arches. This creates significant encroachment on the dural sac, and in patients with congenitally smaller canals, the rate of cord injury rises dramatically even in the ab-

FIGURE 19

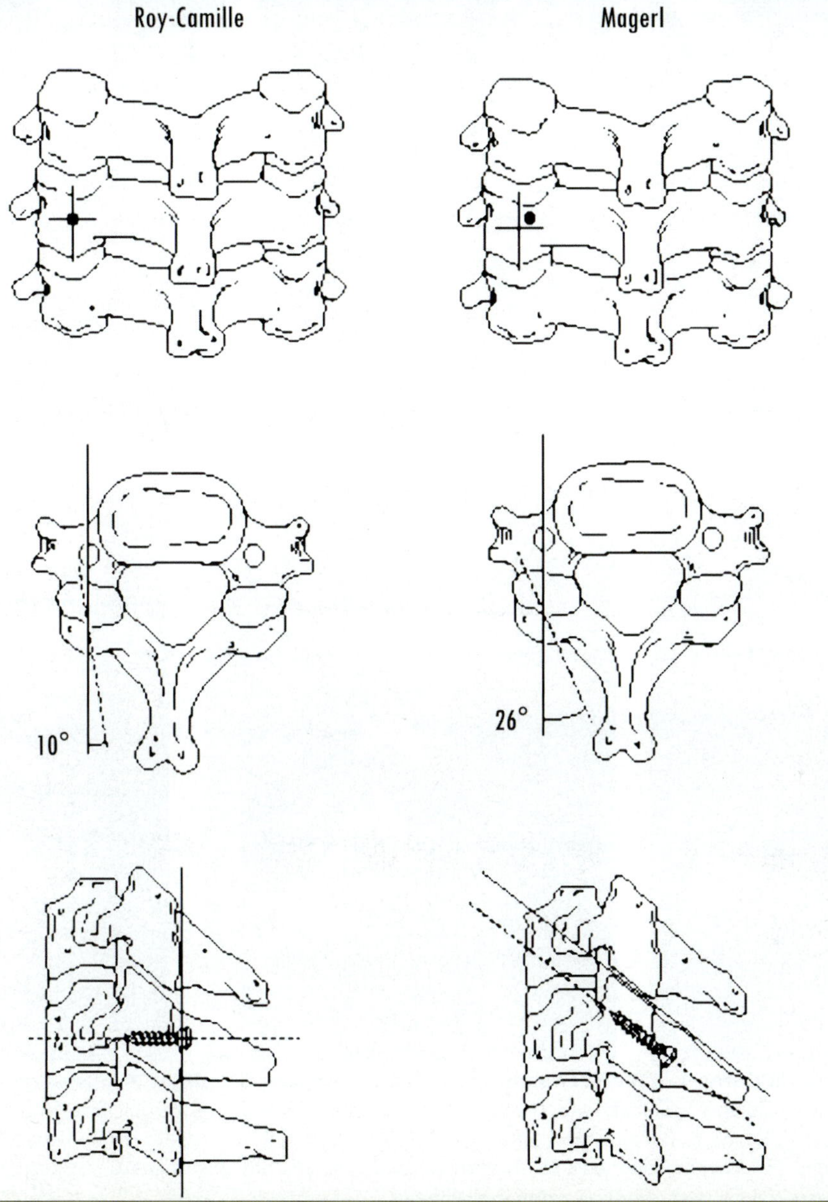

Figure 19 These drawings demonstrate the difference in the trajectory of the screw placement between the original Roy-Camille technique of screw insertion and the modification by Magerl.[77] (Reproduced from Levine AM: Facet fractures and dislocations, in Levine AM, Eismont FJ, Garfin SF, Zigler JE, eds: *Spine Trauma*. Philadelphia, PA, WB Saunders, 1998, pp 331-366.)

sence of disk herniation. Of patients with bilateral dislocations, a higher rate of cord symptoms (41%) and a lower rate of radicular symptoms (32%) are noted.

Neurologic deterioration may occur and has been reported in as many as 6% of patients with spinal cord injury.[31] Improper or inadequate immobilization, hypotension, epidural hematoma, and vertebral artery injury are possible culprits. Immediate reversal of the cause is crucial.

Halo Immobilization and Surgery

Halo immobilization lacks the ability to resist rotation in the midcervical spine.[73] Pin loosening, infection, pressure sores, intracranial pin intrusion, and nerve injury are other possible complications associated with halos.[68] Surgical complications include vascular and neurologic injury, dural tears, infection, esophageal injuries, and hardware failure.[67,85]

FIGURE 20

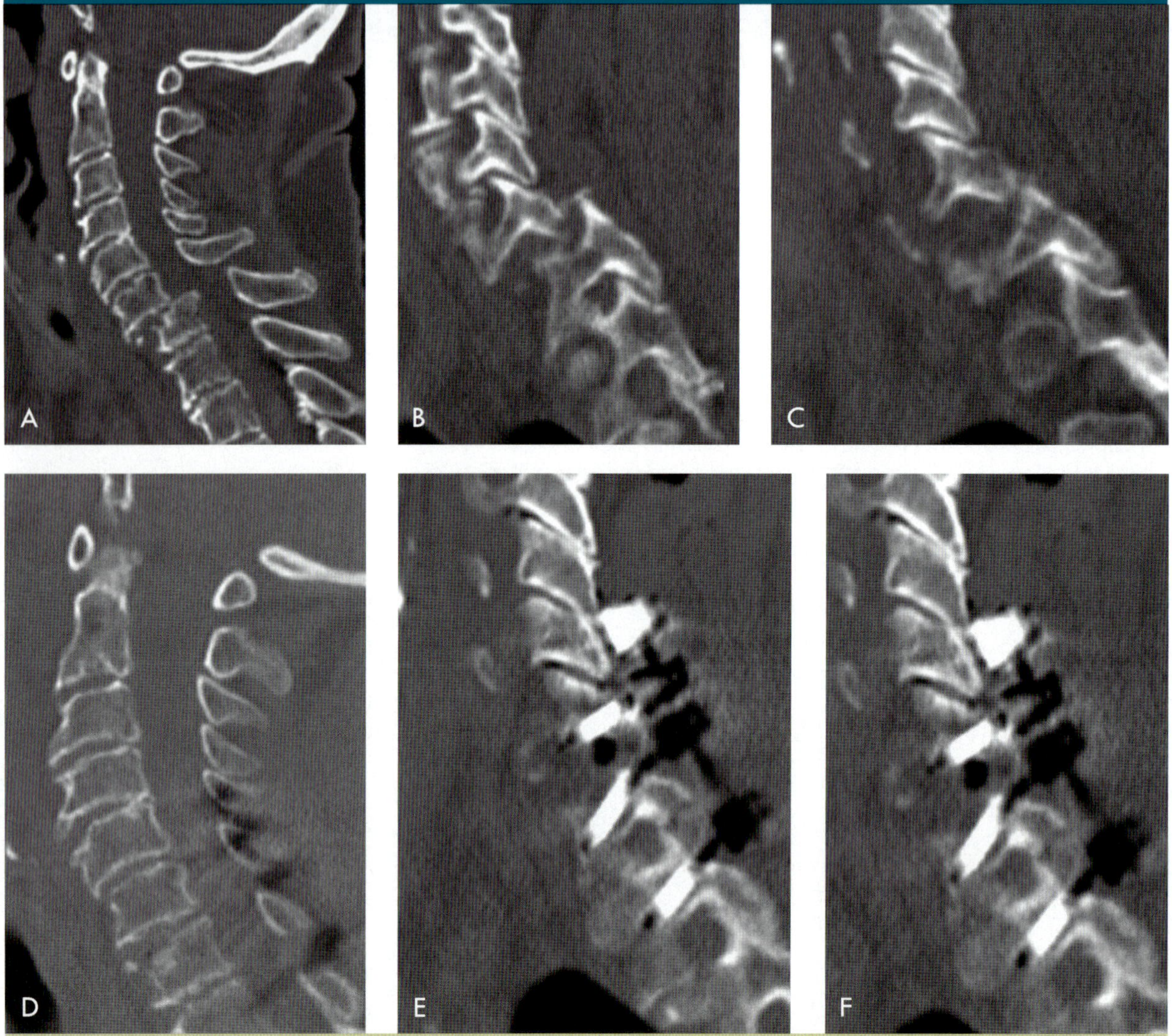

Figure 20 Cervical pedicle screws. This patient presented with a chronic facet dislocation. **A,** Midsagittal CT scan demonstrates anterolisthesis of C6 on C7. Left (**B**) and right (**C**) parasagittal CT views show chronic facet anterolisthesis and extreme foraminal stenosis. **D** and **E,** Postoperative left and right parasagittal CT scans demonstrate partial facectomy of the superior facet and inferior facet and transpedicular fixation at C6, C7, and T1 along with lateral mass fixation at C5. **F,** Postreduction midsagittal CT scan displays anatomic alignment.

Vertebral Artery Injury

Vertebral artery injury (VAI) may present a spectrum of signs and symptoms ranging from no symptoms to stroke and death. Neurologic sequelae may develop from vertebral artery obstruction, thrombus formation with subsequent embolization, obstruction of blood flow into the posterior inferior cerebellar arteries, and anterior spinal artery compromise.[86] Vertebral arteries are at risk for injury with blunt cervical spine trauma and may be present in up to 11% of patients.[87,88] Furthermore, 70% of all traumatic VAIs will have an associated cervical spine fracture.[89] VAIs can be described as intimal tears, dissections, pseudoaneurysms, occlusions, and transections. Intimal tears are just that, allowing the torn intima to intermittently swing into the vessel lumen. An arterial dissection allows blood to collect in the vessel wall, creating a false lumen that can then obstruct the lumen and result in thrombus formation at the dissection site. A pseudoaneurysm may form within an extravascular hematoma, while a severe vessel injury can result in complete occlusion. The most severe form of VAI is a transaction, which often leads to death.

Three types of cervical fractures have been identified as placing patients at significant risk for developing VAI: transverse foramen fractures, subluxations, and C1-C3 fractures. A patient developed bilateral facet fractures, illustrated in **Figure 9,** *A* and *B*, and developed subsequent severe VAI (**Figure 9,** *C* through *E*). Some surgeons will even limit screening to patients with neurologic deficits that are most likely vascular in nature. The gold standard for screening has been cerebral angiography. Less invasive modalities are available, including duplex scanning, magnetic resonance angiography, and CT angiography, but unfortunately the sensitivity of these studies is less optimal. Biffl et al[89] recommend low-dose systemic heparin therapy with a partial thromboplastin time goal of 40 to 50 seconds. Oral anticoagulation therapy then follows for 3 to 6 months or until angiography results have returned to normal. Patients who are unable to receive heparin are treated with antiplatelet therapy instead. This algorithm was supported by a retrospective study of 38 patients with VAI by Biffl et al[88] in 2000. Outcomes for patients treated with systemic heparin were compared to the outcomes of patients who had not received heparin therapy. The result was a threefold higher risk for posterior circulation stroke and a tenfold greater risk of poor neurologic outcome in the group that did not receive heparin therapy. Many centers following surgical stabilization of associated spinal injuries recommend oral antiplatelet therapy for 3 months following VAI identification.

Treatments of symptomatic VAI include anticoagulation, blood pressure control, thrombolytic therapy, and endovascular and surgical procedures.

Conclusion

Injuries to the facets in the cervical spine encompass a very broad spectrum of injuries—bilateral and unilateral fractures and dislocations, in a variety of patterns. These represent less of a spectrum of injury than a group of injuries to a specific anatomic structure. The effective treatment requires a precise understanding of the pathologic characteristics, the mechanism of injury, and the resultant instabilities. The final result depends on a critical appreciation of which treatment modalities can effectively control the resultant instability in each particular injury pattern.

References

1. Vaccaro A, Anderson P: Cervical spine trauma, in Vaccaro A, ed: *Cervical Spine Trauma*. Philadelphia, PA, Wolters Kluwer Pharma Solutions, 2010, pp 383-399.
2. Kwon BK, Vaccaro AR, Grauer JN, Fisher CG, Dvorak MF: Subaxial cervical spine trauma. *J Am Acad Orthop Surg* 2006;14(2):78-89.
3. Roy-Camille R, Mazel G: Les fractures-separation du massif articulaire, in *Sixiemes Journees D'Orthopedie de la Pitie*. 1988, pp 104-107.
4. Lysell E: Motion in the cervical spine: An experimental study on autopsy specimens. *Acta Orthop Scand* 1969;Suppl 123:1+.
5. Marco R, An HS: Spinal anatomy and approaches, in Garfin SR, Fardon DF, eds: *Orthopaedic Knowledge Update: Spine*, ed 2. Rosemont, IL, American Academy of Orthopaedic Surgeons, 2002, pp 7-14.
6. Subramanian N, Reitman CA, Nguyen L, Hipp JA: Radiographic assessment and quantitative motion analysis of the cervical spine after serial sectioning of the anterior ligamentous structures. *Spine (Phila Pa 1976)* 2007;32(5):518-526.
7. Brown T, Reitman CA, Nguyen L, Hipp JA: Intervertebral motion after incremental damage to the posterior structures of the cervical spine. *Spine (Phila Pa 1976)* 2005;30(17):E503-E508.
8. Allen BL Jr, Ferguson RL, Lehmann TR, O'Brien RP: A mechanistic classification of closed, indirect fractures and dislocations of the lower cervical spine. *Spine (Phila Pa 1976)* 1982;7(1):1-27.
9. Harris JH Jr, Edeiken-Monroe B, Kopaniky DR: A practical classification of acute cervical spine injuries. *Orthop Clin North Am* 1986;17(1):15-30.
10. Vaccaro AR, Hulbert RJ, Patel AA, et al: The subaxial cervical spine injury classification system: A novel approach to recognize the importance of morphology, neurology, and integrity of the disco-ligamentous complex. *Spine (Phila Pa 1976)* 2007;32(21):2365-2374.
11. Jacobs B: Cervical fractures and dislocations (C3-7). *Clin Orthop Relat Res* 1975;109:18-32.
12. Horlyck E, Rahbek M: Cervical spine injuries. *Acta Orthop Scand* 1974;45(6):845-853.
13. Bohlman HH: Acute fractures and dislocations of the cervical spine: An analysis of three hundred hospitalized patients and review of the literature. *J Bone Joint Surg Am* 1979;61(8):1119-1142.
14. Rogers WA: Fractures and dislocations of the cervical spine: An end-result study. *J Bone Joint Surg Am* 1957;39(2):341-376.
15. Patel AA, Dailey A, Brodke DS, et al: Subaxial cervical spine trauma classification: The Subaxial Injury Classification system and case examples. *Neurosurg Focus* 2008;25(5):E8.

16. Harris JH, Edeiken-Monroe B: *The Radiology of Acute Cervical Spine Trauma*. Baltimore, MD, Williams & Wilkins, 1987.
17. Scher AT: The value of the anteroposterior radiograph in 'hidden' fractures and dislocations of the lower cervical spine: A case report. *S Afr Med J* 1979;55(6):221-224.
18. Babcock JL: Cervical spine injuries: Diagnosis and classification. *Arch Surg* 1976;111(6):646-651.
19. White AA III, Johnson RM, Panjabi MM, Southwick WO: Biomechanical analysis of clinical stability in the cervical spine. *Clin Orthop Relat Res* 1975;109:85-96.
20. Shanmuganathan K, Mirvis SE, Levine AM: Rotational injury of cervical facets: CT analysis of fracture patterns with implications for management and neurologic outcome. *AJR Am J Roentgenol* 1994;163(5):1165-1169.
21. Webb JK, Broughton RB, McSweeney T, Park WM: Hidden flexion injury of the cervical spine. *J Bone Joint Surg Br* 1976;58(3):322-327.
22. Vaccaro AR, Madigan L, Schweitzer ME, Flanders AE, Hilibrand AS, Albert TJ: Magnetic resonance imaging analysis of soft tissue disruption after flexion-distraction injuries of the subaxial cervical spine. *Spine (Phila Pa 1976)* 2001;26(17):1866-1872.
23. Durbin FC: Fracture-dislocations of the cervical spine. *J Bone Joint Surg Br* 1957;39-B(1):23-38.
24. Woodring JH, Goldstein SJ: Fractures of the articular processes of the cervical spine. *AJR Am J Roentgenol* 1982;139(2):341-344.
25. Miller LS, Cotler HB, De Lucia FA, Cotler JM, Hume EL: Biomechanical analysis of cervical distraction. *Spine (Phila Pa 1976)* 1987;12(9):831-837.
26. Onan OA, Heggeness MH, Hipp JA: A motion analysis of the cervical facet joint. *Spine (Phila Pa 1976)* 1998;23(4):430-439.
27. Braakman M, Braakman R: Hyperflexion sprain of the cervical spine: Follow-up of 45 cases. *Acta Orthop Scand* 1987;58(4):388-393.
28. Brav EA, Miller JA, Bouzard WC: Traumatic dislocation of the cervical spine: Army experience and results. *J Trauma* 1963;3:569-582.
29. Ellis VH: Injuries of the cervical vertebrae: President's address. *Proc R Soc Med* 1946;40(1):19-26.
30. Shapiro SA: Management of unilateral locked facet of the cervical spine. *Neurosurgery* 1993;33(5):832-837.
31. Robertson PA, Ryan MD: Neurological deterioration after reduction of cervical subluxation: Mechanical compression by disc tissue. *J Bone Joint Surg Br* 1992;74(2):224-227.
32. Doran SE, Papadopoulos SM, Ducker TB, Lillehei KO: Magnetic resonance imaging documentation of coexistent traumatic locked facets of the cervical spine and disc herniation. *J Neurosurg* 1993;79(3):341-345.
33. Vaccaro AR, Falatyn SP, Flanders AE, Balderston RA, Northrup BE, Cotler JM: Magnetic resonance evaluation of the intervertebral disc, spinal ligaments, and spinal cord before and after closed traction reduction of cervical spine dislocations. *Spine (Phila Pa 1976)* 1999;24(12):1210-1217.
34. Vaccaro AR, Nachwalter RS: Is magnetic resonance imaging indicated before reduction of a unilateral cervical facet dislocation? *Spine (Phila Pa 1976)* 2002;27(1):117-118.
35. Holdsworth F: Fractures, dislocations, and fracture-dislocations of the spine. *J Bone Joint Surg Am* 1970;52(8):1534-1551.
36. Eismont FJ, Arena MJ, Green BA: Extrusion of an intervertebral disc associated with traumatic subluxation or dislocation of cervical facets: Case report. *J Bone Joint Surg Am* 1991;73(10):1555-1560.
37. Ivancic PC, Pearson AM, Tominaga Y, Simpson AK, Yue JJ, Panjabi MM: Mechanism of cervical spinal cord injury during bilateral facet dislocation. *Spine (Phila Pa 1976)* 2007;32(22):2467-2473.
38. Braakman R, Vinken PJ: Unilateral facet interlocking in the lower cervical spine. *J Bone Joint Surg Br* 1967;49(2):249-257.
39. Rorabeck CH, Rock MG, Hawkins RJ, Bourne RB: Unilateral facet dislocation of the cervical spine: An analysis of the results of treatment in 26 patients. *Spine (Phila Pa 1976)* 1987;12(1):23-27.
40. Rizzolo SJ, Piazza MR, Cotler JM, Balderston RA, Schaefer D, Flanders A: Intervertebral disc injury complicating cervical spine trauma. *Spine (Phila Pa 1976)* 1991;16(6, Suppl)S187-S189.
41. Berrington NR, van Staden JF, Willers JG, van der Westhuizen J: Cervical intervertebral disc prolapse associated with traumatic facet dislocations. *Surg Neurol* 1993;40(5):395-399.
42. de Oliveira JC: Anterior reduction of interlocking facets in the lower cervical spine. *Spine (Phila Pa 1976)* 1979;4(3):195-202.
43. Hadley MN, Fitzpatrick BC, Sonntag VK, Browner CM: Facet fracture-dislocation injuries of the cervical spine. *Neurosurgery* 1992;30(5):661-666.
44. Duggal N, Chamberlain RH, Park SC, Sonntag VK, Dickman CA, Crawford NR: Unilateral cervical facet dislocation: Biomechanics of fixation. *Spine (Phila Pa 1976)* 2005;30(7):E164-E168.
45. Crutchfield WG: Skeletal traction in treatment of injuries to the cervical spine. *J Am Med Assoc* 1954;155(1):29-32.
46. Scher AT: Articular pillar fractures of the cervical spine: Diagnosis on the anteroposterior radiograph. *S Afr Med J* 1981;60(25):968-969.

47. Braakman R, Vinken PJ: Old luxations of the lower cervical spine. *J Bone Joint Surg Br* 1968; 50(1):52-60.

48. Beyer CA, Cabanela ME, Berquist TH: Unilateral facet dislocations and fracture-dislocations of the cervical spine. *J Bone Joint Surg Br* 1991;73(6): 977-981.

49. Rizzolo SJ, Vaccaro AR, Cotler JM: Cervical spine trauma. *Spine (Phila Pa 1976)* 1994;19(20): 2288-2298.

50. Sim E: Vertical facet splitting: A special variant of rotary dislocations of the cervical spine. *J Neurosurg* 1995;82(2):239-243.

51. Levine AM, Mazel C, Roy-Camille R: Management of fracture separations of the articular mass using posterior cervical plating. *Spine (Phila Pa 1976)* 1992;17(10, Suppl):S447-S454.

52. Tarlov IM: Spinal cord compression studies: III. Time limits for recovery after gradual compression in dogs. *AMA Arch Neurol Psychiatry* 1954; 71(5):588-597.

53. Jeanneret B, Gebhard JS, Magerl F: Transpedicular screw fixation of articular mass fracture-separation: Results of an anatomical study and operative technique. *J Spinal Disord* 1994;7(3):222-229.

54. Ito Y, Sugimoto Y, Tomioka M, Kai N, Tanaka M: Does high dose methylprednisolone sodium succinate really improve neurological status in patient with acute cervical cord injury? A prospective study about neurological recovery and early complications. *Spine (Phila Pa 1976)* 2009;34(20): 2121-2124.

55. Grauer JN, Vaccaro AR, Lee JY, et al: The timing and influence of MRI on the management of patients with cervical facet dislocations remains highly variable: A survey of members of the Spine Trauma Study Group. *J Spinal Disord Tech* 2009; 22(2):96-99.

56. Wimberley DW, Vaccaro AR, Goyal N, et al: Acute quadriplegia following closed traction reduction of a cervical facet dislocation in the setting of ossification of the posterior longitudinal ligament: Case report. *Spine (Phila Pa 1976)* 2005; 30(15):E433-E438.

57. Star AM, Jones AA, Cotler JM, Balderston RA, Sinha R: Immediate closed reduction of cervical spine dislocations using traction. *Spine (Phila Pa 1976)* 1990;15(10):1068-1072.

58. Lee AS, MacLean JC, Newton DA: Rapid traction for reduction of cervical spine dislocations. *J Bone Joint Surg Br* 1994;76(3):352-356.

59. Mahale YJ, Silver JR, Henderson NJ: Neurological complications of the reduction of cervical spine dislocations. *J Bone Joint Surg Br* 1993;75(3): 403-409.

60. Fried LC: Cervical spinal cord injury during skeletal traction. *JAMA* 1974;229(2):181-183.

61. Initial closed reduction of cervical spine fracture-dislocation injuries. *Neurosurgery* 2002; 50(3, Suppl)S44-S50.

62. Rihn JA, Fisher C, Harrop J, Morrison W, Yang N, Vaccaro AR: Assessment of the posterior ligamentous complex following acute cervical spine trauma. *J Bone Joint Surg Am* 2010;92(3):583-589.

63. Carlson GD, Minato Y, Okada A, et al: Early time-dependent decompression for spinal cord injury: Vascular mechanisms of recovery. *J Neurotrauma* 1997;14(12):951-962.

64. Fehlings MG, Sekhon LH, Tator C: The role and timing of decompression in acute spinal cord injury: What do we know? What should we do? *Spine (Phila Pa 1976)* 2001;26(24, Suppl): S101-S110.

65. Aebi M, Zuber K, Marchesi D: Treatment of cervical spine injuries with anterior plating: Indications, techniques, and results. *Spine (Phila Pa 1976)* 1991;16(3, Suppl)S38-S45.

66. Wolf A, Levi L, Mirvis S, et al: Operative management of bilateral facet dislocation. *J Neurosurg* 1991;75(6):883-890.

67. Bucholz RD, Cheung KC: Halo vest versus spinal fusion for cervical injury: Evidence from an outcome study. *J Neurosurg* 1989;70(6):884-892.

68. Perry J: The halo in spinal abnormalities: Practical factors and avoidance of complications. *Orthop Clin North Am* 1972;3(1):69-80.

69. Forsyth HF, Alexander E Jr, Davis C Jr, Underdal R: The advantages of early spine fusion in the treatment of fracture-dislocation of the cervical spine. *J Bone Joint Surg Am* 1959;41-A(1):17-36.

70. Nassr A, Lee JY, Dvorak MF, et al: Variations in surgical treatment of cervical facet dislocations. *Spine (Phila Pa 1976)* 2008;33(7):E188-E193.

71. Toh E, Nomura T, Watanabe M, Mochida J: Surgical treatment for injuries of the middle and lower cervical spine. *Int Orthop* 2006;30(1):54-58.

72. Dvorak MF, Fisher CG, Aarabi B, et al: Clinical outcomes of 90 isolated unilateral facet fractures, subluxations, and dislocations treated surgically and nonoperatively. *Spine (Phila Pa 1976)* 2007; 32(26):3007-3013.

73. Anderson PA, Budorick TE, Easton KB, Henley MB, Salciccioli GG: Failure of halo vest to prevent in vivo motion in patients with injured cervical spines. *Spine (Phila Pa 1976)* 1991;16(10, Suppl): S501-S505.

74. Mahale YJ, Silver JR: Progressive paralysis after bilateral facet dislocation of the cervical spine. *J Bone Joint Surg Br* 1992;74(2):219-223.

75. Marshall LF, Knowlton S, Garfin SR, et al: Deterioration following spinal cord injury: A multicenter study. *J Neurosurg* 1987;66(3):400-404.

76. Johnson MG, Fisher CG, Boyd M, Pitzen T,

Oxland TR, Dvorak MF: The radiographic failure of single segment anterior cervical plate fixation in traumatic cervical flexion distraction injuries. *Spine (Phila Pa 1976)* 2004;29(24):2815-2820.

77. Heller JG, Carlson GD, Abitbol JJ, Garfin SR: Anatomic comparison of the Roy-Camille and Magerl techniques for screw placement in the lower cervical spine. *Spine (Phila Pa 1976)* 1991; 16(10, Suppl):S552-S557.

78. Dvorak MF, Fisher CG, Fehlings MG, et al: The surgical approach to subaxial cervical spine injuries: An evidence-based algorithm based on the SLIC classification system. *Spine (Phila Pa 1976)* 2007;32(23):2620-2629.

79. Paxinos O, Ghanayem AJ, Zindrick MR, et al: Anterior cervical discectomy and fusion with a locked plate and wedged graft effectively stabilizes flexion-distraction stage-3 injury in the lower cervical spine: A biomechanical study. *Spine (Phila Pa 1976)* 2009;34(1):E9-E15.

80. Kim SM, Lim TJ, Paterno J, Park J, Kim DH: A biomechanical comparison of three surgical approaches in bilateral subaxial cervical facet dislocation. *J Neurosurg Spine* 2004;1(1):108-115.

81. Spector LR, Kim DH, Affonso J, Albert TJ, Hilibrand AS, Vaccaro AR: Use of computed tomography to predict failure of nonoperative treatment of unilateral facet fractures of the cervical spine. *Spine (Phila Pa 1976)* 2006;31(24): 2827-2835.

82. Do Koh Y, Lim TH, Won You J, Eck J, An HS: A biomechanical comparison of modern anterior and posterior plate fixation of the cervical spine. *Spine (Phila Pa 1976)* 2001;26(1):15-21.

83. Lifeso RM, Colucci MA: Anterior fusion for rotationally unstable cervical spine fractures. *Spine (Phila Pa 1976)* 2000;25(16):2028-2034.

84. Harrop JS, Sharan AD, Vaccaro AR, Przybylski GJ: The cause of neurologic deterioration after acute cervical spinal cord injury. *Spine (Phila Pa 1976)* 2001;26(4):340-346.

85. Heller JG, Silcox DH III, Sutterlin CE III: Complications of posterior cervical plating. *Spine (Phila Pa 1976)* 1995;20(22):2442-2448.

86. Fassett DR, Dailey AT, Vaccaro AR: Vertebral artery injuries associated with cervical spine injuries: A review of the literature. *J Spinal Disord Tech* 2008;21(4):252-258.

87. Stauffer ES: Management of spine fractures C3 to C7. *Orthop Clin North Am* 1986;17(1):45-53.

88. Biffl WL, Moore EE, Elliott JP, et al: The devastating potential of blunt vertebral arterial injuries. *Ann Surg* 2000;231(5):672-681.

89. Biffl WL, Ray CE Jr, Moore EE, et al: Treatment-related outcomes from blunt cerebrovascular injuries: Importance of routine follow-up arteriography. *Ann Surg* 2002;235(5):699-707.

CHAPTER 28
Hyperextension Injuries of the Cervical Spine

Robert P. Norton, MD Gregory S. McDowell, MD Frank P. Cammisa, Jr, MD, FACS
Frank J. Eismont, MD

Key Points

- There is a spectrum of injuries involving both the osseous and soft-tissue structures of the cervical spine when it is subjected to supraphysiologic hyperextension forces, with the severity and mode of failure dependent on variations in head position, forces applied, and age-dependent anatomic characteristics of the individual.
- A thorough and timely assessment, including a full history, physical examination, complete radiographic evaluation, and CT and MRI when indicated, should be performed on persons who have neck pain or neurologic symptoms following a hyperextension injury.
- Hyperextension teardrop fractures are characterized by a small teardrop fragment from the anteroinferior end plate of the vertebral body, commonly occurring at C2, best appreciated on lateral radiographs. The majority are best managed conservatively. These are distinctly different than the "teardrop fractures" associated with flexion-axial loading injuries, which are very often unstable, frequently associated with paralysis, and often require surgical treatment.
- A hyperextension injury may rarely result in isolated anterior longitudinal ligament or disk disruption without vertebrae involvement.
- Patients with ankylosing spondylitis, congenital cervical stenosis, or spondylotic stenosis have an increased risk of spinal cord injury when subjected to a hyperextension force as compared to patients with normal cervical spine anatomy who have similar injuries.
- SCIWORA is an acronym used to describe an acute spinal cord injury resulting in some degree of paralysis without evidence of vertebral fracture on radiography or CT imaging. This syndrome predominantly occurs in children.
- Whiplash represents a constellation of injuries to the soft tissues of the cervical spine following an acceleration-deceleration motion, with the facet joints and intervertebral disks most likely responsible for chronic pain. Early active treatment strategies with education and reassurance are most effective.
- Hyperextension fracture-dislocations are characterized with failure of the anterior column in tension and the posterior column via facet dislocation or fracture. Radiographic evaluation is often misleading due to partial reduction with the patient lying supine in a neutral position. MRI is useful to confirm diagnosis and aid in management.

Introduction

Hyperextension injuries of the cervical spine have long been regarded as less significant contributors to the overall incidence of spine lesions acquired traumatically, and yet this mechanism clearly has been demonstrated to play a role in a variety of pathologic entities. These include: atlantooccipital dislocations; fractures of the posterior arch of C1; dens fractures; hangman's fractures; extension teardrop injuries; anterior longitudinal ligament (ALL) or disk disruptions; central cord syndromes in spondylotic, stenotic, or ankylosed spines; spinal cord injury without radiographic abnormality (SCIWORA); whiplash; and complex high-velocity fracture-dislocations.

Dr. McDowell or an immediate family member has received research or institutional support from Stryker; and owns stock or stock options in Johnson & Johnson and Merck. Dr. Cammissa or an immediate family member has received royalties from Nuvasive, HydroCision, K2M, and Orthovita; serves as a paid consultant to or is an employee of Centinal Spine, Disc Motion Technologies, HydroCision, K2M, Orthovita, Paradigm Spine, and Vertebral Technologies; and owns stock or stock options in Alphatech Spine, Disc Motion Technologies, HealthpointCapital, HydroCision, K2M, Mazor Robotics, NuVasive, Paradigm Spine, Orthovita, Royer, Scient'x USA, Spinal Kinetics, and Vertebral Technologies. Dr. Eismont or an immediate family member serves as a paid consultant to or is an employee of Alphatech Spine; and owns stock or stock options in Alphatech Spine. Neither Dr. Norton nor any immediate family member has received anything of value from or owns stock in a commercial company or institution related directly or indirectly to the subject of this chapter.

For the purpose of this chapter, we address only the lesions of the subaxial spine because the others have been discussed elsewhere in this book. We attempt to better clarify the common biomechanics, while emphasizing the varied etiology, presentation, evaluation, and treatment of these injuries.

Etiology, Epidemiology, and Pathomechanics of Hyperextension Injuries

When the cervical spine is subjected to supraphysiologic hyperextension moments, either secondary to a direct blow to the forehead or through acceleration mechanisms such as seen in whiplash, it may fail subtly or quite dramatically. In part, the mode of failure can be attributed to variations in head position and the forces applied. A spectrum of injuries involves both the osseous and soft-tissue structures of the cervical spine; the severity of injury depends on the integrity of the spinal cord and the mechanical stability of the spine.[1] The mode of failure will also be affected to a great extent by the age-dependent anatomic characteristics of the individual. The pediatric spine will fail differently from the middle-aged or elderly spine, or the spine affected by advanced spondylosis, stenosis, or ankylosing conditions. In children younger than 10 years of age, flexion and extension are centered around C2-C3; however, after 10 years of age, they move caudally to C4-C5 and C5-C6.[2] The pediatric atlantooccipital joint allows 25° of extension, whereas the adult atlantooccipital joint permits only 15°of extension.[2] Further cervical extension comes from the vertebral segments below, with an overall greater degree of motion throughout the cervical spine in children compared to adults. With regard to the elderly, the cervical spine may fail with low loading rates in addition to injuries seen with high loading rates typically seen in younger patients.[3] Additionally, the elderly may be more vulnerable to axial loading due to reduced bone mineral content.[4] As the cervical spine stiffens in the elderly as a result of degenerative changes, the range of motion likewise decreases with age.[5] Injury subsequently is most likely to occur at or adjacent to the stiff portion of the cervical spine. Although hyperextension injuries are often seen in the upper cervical spine of the general population, the elderly are more prone to this type of injury in the mid and lower cervical spine.[6]

No single classification scheme for cervical injury explains the diversity seen in radiographic and clinical findings. Whitehill's[7] review of classification schemes relating to subaxial fractures in the adult discusses taking each individual case through a so-called injury analysis that combines the mechanistic elements of six injury categories affecting Holdsworth's two-column spine and the biomechanical force vectors involved.[8] For the purposes of this chapter, we have adopted a scheme that relies on commonly used descriptive terms for hyperextension injuries.

The function of the spine is to transmit physiologic loads, to allow for controlled active and constrained passive motion, and to protect the neural elements. The lordotic subaxial spine enables flexibility, postural balance, and shock absorption, with both disk and facet joints sharing in carrying compressive load.[9] This anatomy, however, can be the site of stress concentration in traumatic hyperextension, given the high stiffness and large moment of inertia attributed to the thoracic spine below and the head above.

From a biomechanical standpoint of examining hyperextension trauma to the cervical spine, injury occurs to the cervical spine and associated soft tissues when physiologic ranges of extension and lateral tilting are exceeded by a particular loading force.[1] Cadaveric models have demonstrated that high compressive loading rates lower the threshold for injury,[10] in addition to independent factors such as patient age and alignment of the cervical spine at time of impact.[11,12] These hyperextension injuries are a result of either direct contact, such as from an impact to the face or forehead seen most often in unrestrained motor vehicle accidents,[13] elderly patients falling from a height,[3] and athletic injuries in the young, or from a noncontact incident such as whiplash.[14] In patients who do sustain a spinal cord injury following a hyperextension motion, a central cord syndrome most commonly occurs.

Which loads and patterns of loading in hyperextension are excessive, and when is motion abnormally large either in translation or angulation such that it might permit injury to the cord or cervical nerve roots? White et al[15] were the first to look at this from a sound biomechanical perspective. They subscribed to a practical definition of stability. Instability is defined as the loss of the spine's ability under physiologic loads to maintain normal relationships to avoid neural injury. This can be expanded to include avoidance of deficit progression, incapacitating deformity, or intractable pain. Ultimately, their cadaveric testing model, in which they sectioned constraining soft tissues from anterior to posterior and subjected spines to hyperextension loads, allowed for the definition of more objective radiographic criteria for impending instability. Their results demonstrated remarkably small increments of change in angular and translational displacement until the posterior longitudinal ligament (PLL) was sectioned, at which time catastrophic failure ensued without warning. No motion segments that exhibited less than 2.7 mm of linear translation or 10.7° of angular displacement were observed to fail. These values subsequently served as guidelines for the development of their instability diagnostic checklist[15] (**Table 1**). The checklist should serve as a guide for the experienced interpreter. However, problems can arise in its use, as noted by Whitehill.[7] Recently, more detailed anatomic scoring methods have been proposed based on modern three-dimensional imaging modalities.[16]

Shono et al[17] were able to demonstrate that predictable anterior avulsion fractures, and ALL and disk disruptions, as well as posterior element fractures in compression, are seen with hyperextension in immature calf spines. This conclusion was supported by the work of White et al in elderly cadaveric spines.[15] These investigators' experimental findings corroborate several good postmortem pathologic studies that elucidate the variety of typical hyperextension injuries seen[18-20] (**Figure 1**).

These injuries are not uncommon. Kiwerski[21] described a series of 1,687 patients with cervical spine injury treated in Poland over 23 years. Twenty-six percent of these patients had a hyperextension mechanism. The average age of the patients with an extension injury was 53 years. Twenty-five percent had complete spinal cord lesions, 61% had incomplete lesions, and 13% were without neurologic deficit. Lesions were more commonly seen from C5 to T1 (n = 177), but the 120 hyperextension lesions from C1 to C3 represented 68% of all injuries at these levels. Interestingly, other authors have noted that C5-C6 is a common site for hyperextension injury, a fact attributed to its high underlying mobility.[22] The outcome with extension injuries as a whole was better than that with flexion or axial load injuries, with 61% demonstrating improvement neurologically. Mortality, however, was high (21%), a fact that may be attributed to the advanced age of the patients as a whole.

Meyer[23] wrote of the experience at Northwestern University's Spine Injury Center over 27 years

TABLE 1

Guidelines for the Evaluation of Clinical Stability of the Adult Cervical Spine

Any one of the following three conditions are indicative of instability or potential instability:
1. All the anterior or all the posterior elements are destroyed.
2. There is > 3.5 mm of anterolisthesis and retrolisthesis on resting lateral or flexion-extension radiographs.
3. There is > 11° of angular deformity as compared to either adjacent motion segment on resting lateral or flexion-extension radiographs.

(Adapted with permission from White AA III, Johnson RM, Panjabi MM, Southwick WO: Biomechanical analysis of clinical stability in the cervical spine. *Clin Orthop Relat Res* 1975;109:85-96.)

FIGURE 1

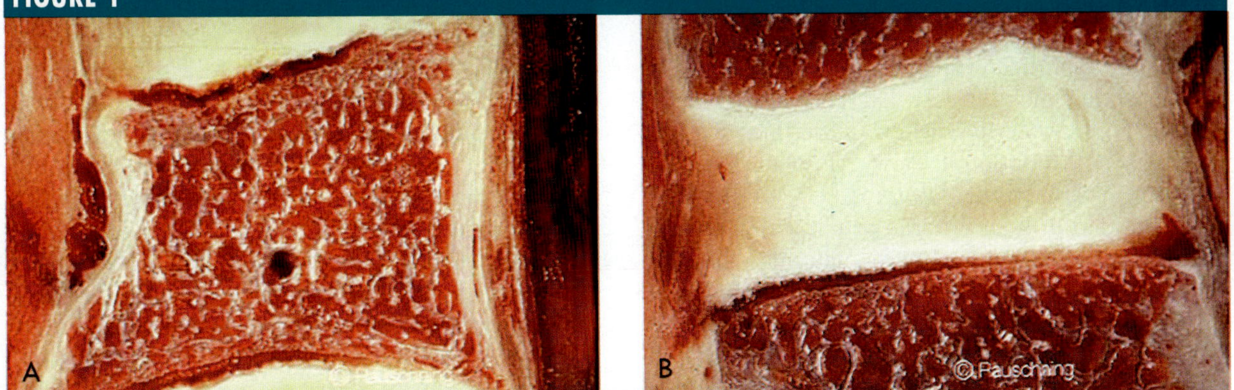

Figure 1 These cryosections of the spine represent the types of cervical spine injuries that are seen in fatalities and associated with hyperextension injuries of the cervical spine: **A,** a C5 superior end-plate avulsion; **B,** a C6-C7 disk avulsed from the C7 superior end plate. (Courtesy of Dr. Wolfgang Rauschning, Uppsala University, Uppsala, Sweden.)

with 1,626 patients who sustained cervical spine fractures. Of these, 532 (33%) were due to hyperextension, second only to the frequency of flexion injuries. Twenty-six percent of the patients had complete spinal cord lesions, 35% had incomplete lesions, and 39% had no neurologic deficit. Bohlman's[24] series of 300 hospitalized patients over 22 years included a number with presumed hyperextension injury, although a complete definition of mechanism is limited by the author's description of the lesions. Similarly, Holdsworth's[8] series includes descriptions of classic hyperextension injuries. Burke[25] and Forsyth,[18] among others, have published specifically on hyperextension injuries, further elaborating their diverse characteristics and unique subtypes. We will discuss each subtype in more detail, but first it will be useful to elaborate on the clinical and radiographic evaluation of these patients.

Clinical and Radiographic Assessment

The clinical and radiographic assessment of persons who have neck pain or neurologic symptoms following hyperextension injury should be thorough. It begins with a careful history. A review of the patient's past medical history, including any history of previous trauma, is important. If the patient has acute symptoms, it may be appropriate for a full trauma evaluation to be performed with careful attention being paid to cervical immobilization throughout. The physical examination must include a detailed neurologic and skeletal examination. It is imperative that the clinician search for occult signs of closed head injury, orbital or facial fractures, cranial nerve injuries, and injury to soft-tissue structures of the neck, including the musculature, larynx, esophagus, and great vessels, all of which have been noted to be injured with hyperextension.

The radiographic evaluation must include a full trauma series, including AP, lateral, oblique, and lateral swimmer's views (when needed), as well as an open-mouth odontoid view. The plain film criteria for instability were described by White et al[15] and included in their criteria for clinical instability. The finding of a prevertebral hematoma is highly suggestive of a cervical spine injury and this can certainly include those with a hyperextension injury. A retropharyngeal space measuring greater than 5.0 mm as measured in front of C3 or a retrotracheal distance greater than 15 mm to 18 mm as measured in front of C6 is abnormal. Penning[26] described large increases (up to 12.3 mm) above the upper limit of normal in prevertebral soft-tissue measurements following hyperextension injury. Changes were most readily seen from C1 to C4 in the retropharyngeal space, regardless of injury location. Furthermore, he defined the upper limits of normal for prevertebral space measurement in 50 uninjured patients. Longitudinal follow-up of these hematomas revealed rapid decreases in size over 1 week and near normalcy typically within 2 to 3 weeks. Thus, the prevertebral hematoma should be considered a significant red flag for acute or subacute hyperextension injuries. In a study by Edeiken-Monroe et al,[27] the combination of diffuse prevertebral soft-tissue widening and normal cervical vertebrae alignment was the only radiographic finding in 30% of the patients who sustained a hyperextension dislocation injury. Scher[28] has described additional plain-film radiographic findings that are highly suggestive of hyperextension injury. These include small triangular avulsion fractures from the anteroinferior edge of a vertebral body (**Figure 2**), disk-space widening, fractures of the posterior elements without obvious anterior column bony abnormalities (**Figure 3**), and retrolisthesis of a cranial-on-caudal vertebral body.[28]

If the radiographs of patients with neck pain are cleared of obvious fracture, subluxation, and angulation (ie, gross instability) by a qualified radiologist or knowledgeable physician, flexion-extension radiographs should not be obtained. Wang et al[29] reported finding only one positive study in 290 patients in an emergency department setting. These patients should be immobilized in a rigid cervical collar and reevaluated with new radiographs in 7 to 10 days when muscular splinting may have resolved, allowing for recognition of occult instabilities. If the plain radiographs remain normal, lateral flexion-extension radiographs are obtained. If these are also normal, the collar may be discontinued.

CT and MRI both have roles to assist the clinician in recognizing occult injury to soft-tissue or bony elements of the cervical spine. CT has gained widespread acceptance as the primary imaging modality due to its high sensitivity and specificity with regard to picking up fractures missed or incompletely visualized on conventional radiography[1] (**Figure 4**). Furthermore, CT can be performed in a very short period of time. However, a potential disadvantage of CT as an initial radiographic assessment is that facet joint gapping, intervertebral distraction, and subtle malalignment may be difficult to assess on axial imaging alone without coronal or midsagittal reconstruction. CT

FIGURE 2

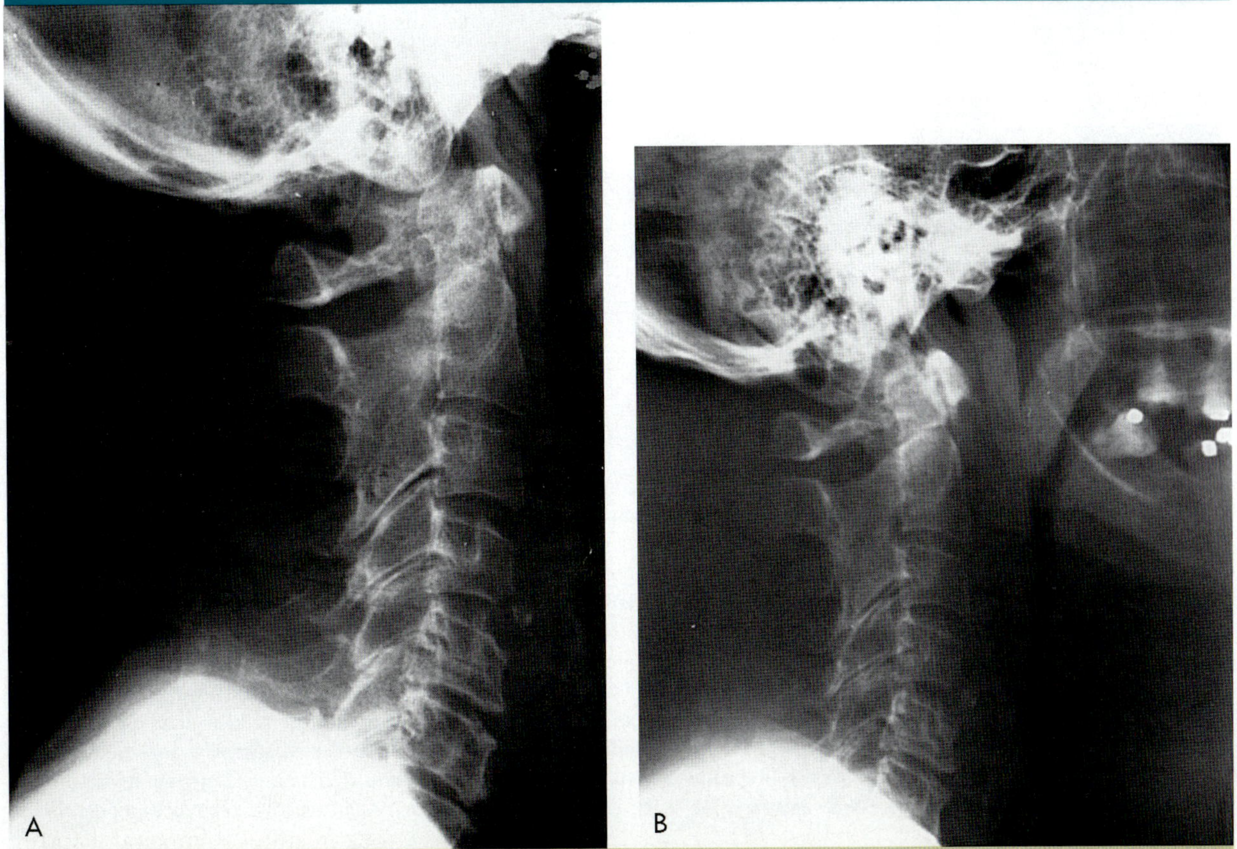

Figure 2 This patient was seen in the emergency department following a motor vehicle accident. She had significant facial lacerations and ecchymosis and reported some mild neck pain. No tenderness to palpation was noted posteriorly. **A,** The lateral cervical spine radiograph shows diffuse spondylosis consistent with her age, and the anterior aspect of the C4 vertebral body gives an excellent demonstration of a "teardrop fracture" of the anteroinferior portion of the vertebral body. This is consistent with a significant hyperextension injury. There is some slight rotation of the anterior fragment and one can also see that there is no sclerosis at the site of fracture, indicating that this is a new injury. The soft tissue swelling measures 8 mm in front of C3. Anything more than 5 mm is abnormal and consistent with a new injury. **B,** This radiograph taken 1 day later shows an increase in the soft-tissue swelling to 16 mm. The patient was neurologically normal and flexion-extension views did not show evidence of instability, so she was immobilized for 6 weeks in a rigid collar. (Reproduced from McDowell GS, Cammisa FP, Eismont FJ: Hyperextension injuries of the cervical spine, in Levine AM, Eismont FJ, Garfin SR, Zigler JE, eds: *Spine Trauma*. Philadelphia, PA, WB Saunders, 1998, pp 367-386.)

angiography with intravenous contrast is another imaging modality gaining acceptance for the evaluation of the vertebral arteries. MRI has emerged as a tool that is invaluable in diagnosing hyperextension injuries of the cervical spine and will clearly show epidural hematomas, spinal cord edema, ligamentous disruptions, and disk herniations. Data reported by Benzel et al[30] as well as by Davis et al[31] show that MRI is able to detect a high percentage of trauma patients with significant occult disk, ligament, or soft-tissue abnormalities. In their report of 130 patients who had normal radiographs following trauma, 50 had recognizable injuries of soft tissue, bone, or disk on MRI scans. Goldberg et al[32] have also shown that MRI is particularly helpful in recognizing and aiding in treatment decisions for patients with hyperextension injury. They noted that MRI enabled the clinician to correctly recognize occult injuries of the longitudinal ligaments (**Figure 5**), disks, and posterior elements (whether bony, capsular, or ligamentous), as well as contusion injuries of the cord, stenosis of the spinal canal, and associated soft-tissue injuries of the anterior neck. The study by Schaefer et al[33] of 57 patients with cervical spine injuries revealed that MRI may not always detect cord injury, but when it does, it is often able to distinguish between intramedullary hematoma (group I), edema involving more than one motion segment (group II), and edema involving one motion

FIGURE 3

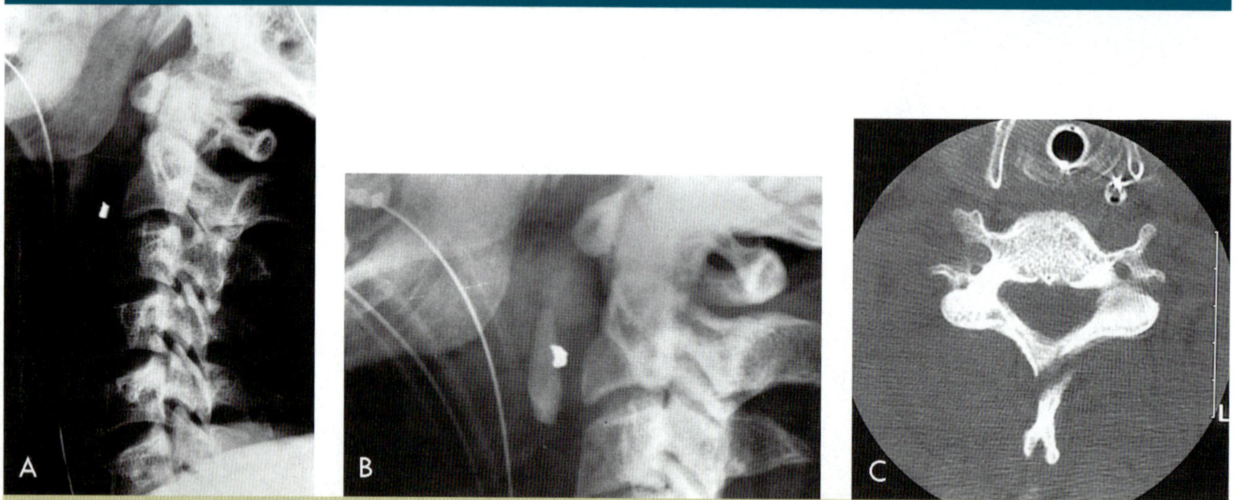

Figure 3 This patient was brought to the emergency department following a motor vehicle accident in which he sustained significant trauma to the face. He had multiple comminuted fractures of the mandible and had significant respiratory distress that required intubation. He was neurologically normal, but he did have neck pain with palpation in the lower cervical spine. **A,** This lateral cervical spine radiograph shows normal alignment of the spine but there is inadequate visualization of the lower cervical spine. The patient was immobilized awaiting further evaluation. What appears to be a foreign body is seen in the retropharyngeal area anterior to the C2-C3 disk. **B,** A cone-down radiograph reveals that this foreign body was actually a tooth that had broken loose at the time of the mandibular fractures. Care was taken to remove this before extubation. **C,** This CT scan clearly shows a fracture of the spinous process of C6. This is consistent with the facial injuries and a cervical spine hyperextension injury. Once extubated, flexion-extension radiographs revealed no significant instability and the patient was immobilized in a rigid collar for 6 weeks. (Reproduced from McDowell GS, Cammisa FP, Eismont FJ: Hyperextension injuries of the cervical spine, in Levine AM, Eismont FJ, Garfin SR, Zigler JE, eds: *Spine Trauma*. Philadelphia, PA, WB Saunders, 1998, pp 367-386.)

segment (group III). These diagnoses will often aid the clinician in prognosticating final motor outcome. The median percentage motor recovery for the three groups was, respectively, 9%, 41%, and 72% at a mean follow-up of 8 months.

Interventional techniques such as diagnostic and therapeutic facet and nerve root blocks as well as cervical diskography may help to better evaluate patients with subtle clinical presentations or ongoing pain in the face of a "normal" workup. The risks of cervical diskography and studies describing its lower predictive value make its widespread usefulness controversial.[34] As discussed by McLain,[35] however, the zygapophyseal joint is a structure noted to be innervated with mechanoreceptors and, as Barnsley et al[36] have pointed out, zygapophyseal joint pain may well be the most common basis for chronic pain following injuries such as whiplash (54% prevalence). They described its diagnosis with double-blind controlled diagnostic blocks of medial branches of the cervical dorsal rami that supply the target joint. The patients' response to some of these interventional techniques, coupled with sound clinical judgment, may help aid the clinician in predicting their potential response to cervical arthrodesis. The use of a diagnostic external fixator was described for the same purpose, but never progressed to any practical applications.[37]

Prompt recognition and the maintenance of a high index of suspicion for occult lesions will aid in the appropriate diagnosis and treatment of acute cervical hyperextension injuries. The patient who exhibits subacute or chronic symptoms that persist in the face of an initially negative screening examination should be fully evaluated to ensure that a treatable lesion does not exist.

Hyperextension Teardrop Fractures

Reports of hyperextension teardrop fractures of the cervical spine are few in the literature,[18,27,38-40] whereas several series report larger numbers of patients with flexion teardrop fractures.[41-43] The differences between these two entities with regard to mechanism, radiographic and clinical findings, and treatment and outcome, are substantial. Failure to recognize the difference between these two injuries could result in inappropriate treatment.

The flexion teardrop fracture was first described by Schneider and Kahn in 1956.[42] Later series of

FIGURE 4

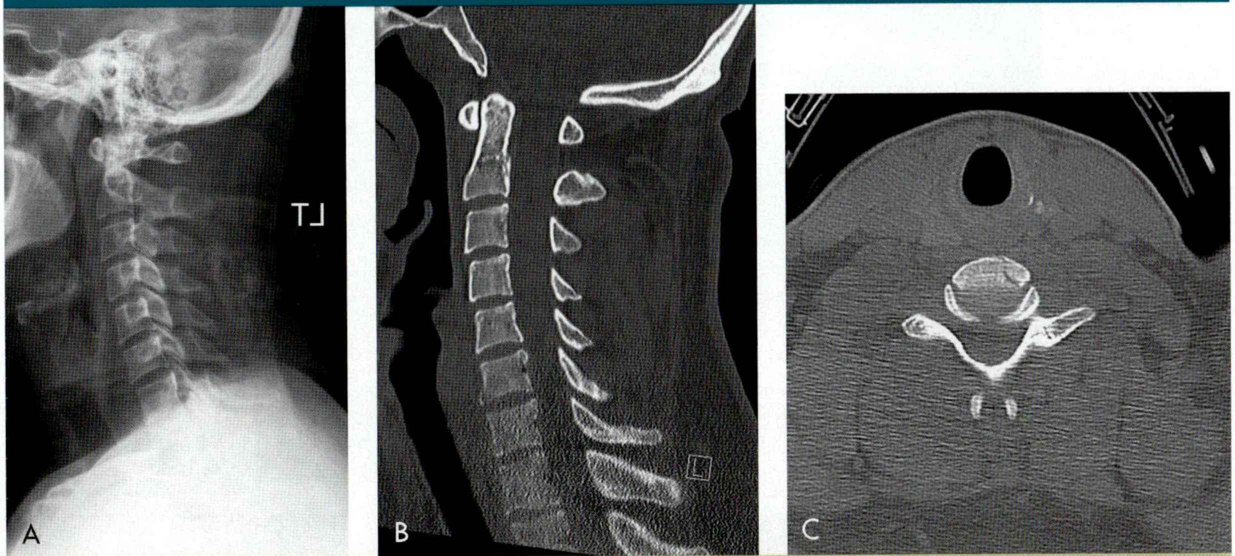

Figure 4 This patient was involved in a motor vehicle accident and sustained lacerations to his forehead. He was neurologically normal. **A,** This lateral radiograph shows no gross abnormality. The soft-tissue swelling in front of C3 is slightly increased at 6 mm. There is a slight indication of opening at the C6-C7 level, with slightly increased distance between the spinous processes of C6 and C7 compared to other levels. **B,** This midsagittal CT scan reconstruction shows a small avulsion fracture of the anterior inferior aspect of the C6 vertebral body. **C,** This CT scan through the inferior end plate of C6 shows that there is a small avulsion fracture of the anterior inferior end plate of C6 consistent with a hyperextension injury. This patient was immobilized in a rigid collar for 3 weeks, and at that time he had no neck pain and a flexion-extension radiograph showed no evidence of instability. His collar was then discontinued.

larger numbers of patients described its occurrence in football players sustaining axial loads on their helmets with their necks slightly flexed (n = 45) and in patients involved in diving and vehicular accidents or falls (n = 55).[41,43] The characteristic radiographic features of the flexion–axial load injury are an anteroinferior avulsion fracture and a sagittal midbody fracture, usually occurring at the C4 through C6 level in association with posterior laminar fractures[41,43] (**Figure 6**). The triangular fragment remains aligned with the anterior margin of the spine.[40] Significant neurologic injury and quadriplegia are common, occurring in 45 of 55 patients in the series of Torg et al[43] and 39 of 45 patients in the series of Kim et al.[41] Prognosis for neurologic recovery is grim. Definitive management of these injuries will often require anterior decompression with circumferential fusion to attain decompression and stability.

In contradistinction to this, the extension teardrop fracture constituted a larger percentage of patients (13 of 20) with hyperextension injury as reported by Edeiken-Monroe et al[27] and similarly reported by Levine and Lutz.[40] The characteristic radiographic feature is a small teardrop fragment, which is avulsed via its attachments to Sharpey's fibers of the anulus from the anteroinferior end plate of the vertebral body (**Figure 2**) and is usually malrotated 35° from its resting position.[40] Lateral radiographs enable the appreciation of the triangular configuration of the avulsed fragment, with its vertical dimension equal to or greater than its transverse dimension.[1] CT helps to better characterize the fracture and evaluate for additional bony injuries (**Figure 4**). Commonly occurring at C2, and sometimes associated with a vacuum disk or disk-space widening,[27] the soft-tissue component of the injury can be defined on MRI.[44] In addition, MRI will identify spinal cord edema and contusion. In younger patients, the avulsion most commonly follows a greater degree of traumatic force, most often seen in the lower cervical spine, and is often associated with extensive soft-tissue swelling and spinal cord injury.[1] However, in the weak spine, a smaller degree of traumatic force is required to produce this avulsion with associated minimal or no soft-tissue swelling and no neurologic deficit.[1] Posterior element fractures may occur, but the midsagittal body fracture that is commonly seen in the flexion–axial load injury is absent. Neurologic injury was reported as rare by Levine and Lutz,[40] although central cord syndromes were not uncommonly noted by Edeiken-Monroe et al.[27] Lee et al[45] found neurologic deficits

FIGURE 5

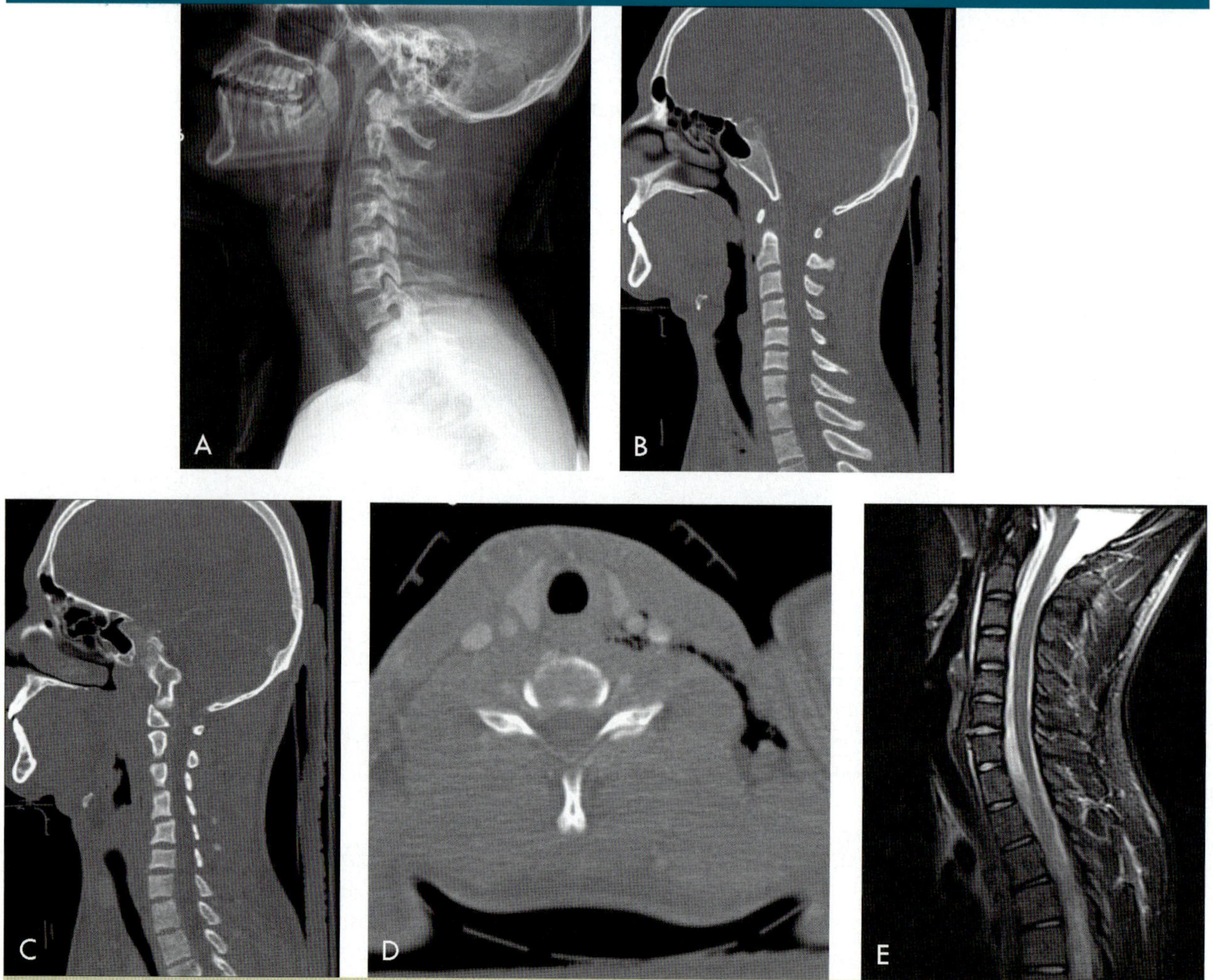

Figure 5 This patient was ejected from a motor vehicle resulting in a pneumothorax and was resuscitated following placement of chest tubes. The subcutaneous air can be seen in the cervical spine radiograph (**A**). The alignment of the spine appears normal. The patient was neurologically normal. **B,** Reconstructed sagittal CT scan slightly off midline shows a very small avulsion fracture from the anterior inferior aspect of the C6 vertebral body. This is barely visible. **C,** Midsagittal CT scan shows no abnormality other than the subcutaneous air. **D,** This axial CT scan visualizes the small anterior avulsion fracture from the anterior inferior aspect of C6. **E,** This MRI scan demonstrates complete destruction of the ALL and a widening of the disk space anteriorly at C6-7. This is certainly consistent with the patient's significant facial trauma. This patient was immobilized in a rigid cervical collar and later evaluated for instability.

to be similar to those found in hyperextension dislocation, with central cord syndrome seen in up to 80% of patients. Dynamic radiographic evidence of instability was rare, with only 4 of 24 patients demonstrating it in the series of Levine and Lutz.[40] The majority of these patients are best managed conservatively in an external cervical orthosis, and most go on to stability uneventfully without surgical arthrodesis. In the series reported by Levine and Lutz,[40] 21 of 24 patients achieved bony union and 2 of the remaining 3 patients achieved stable fibrous union at a mean follow-up of 2.5 years.

Anterior Longitudinal Ligament and Disk Disruptions

Cases reported in the literature describe hyperextension injuries of the cervical spine resulting in varying degrees of paralysis without evidence of vertebral fracture or dislocation.[19,46-50] The exact mechanism of this lesion is not clearly defined and has been the subject of debate for many years.[6,18,46,47,51-57] Just as hyperextension injuries may involve failure of bone anteriorly, the ALL itself and disk may fail in tension, producing a primarily soft-tissue injury. The radiographic pre-

FIGURE 6

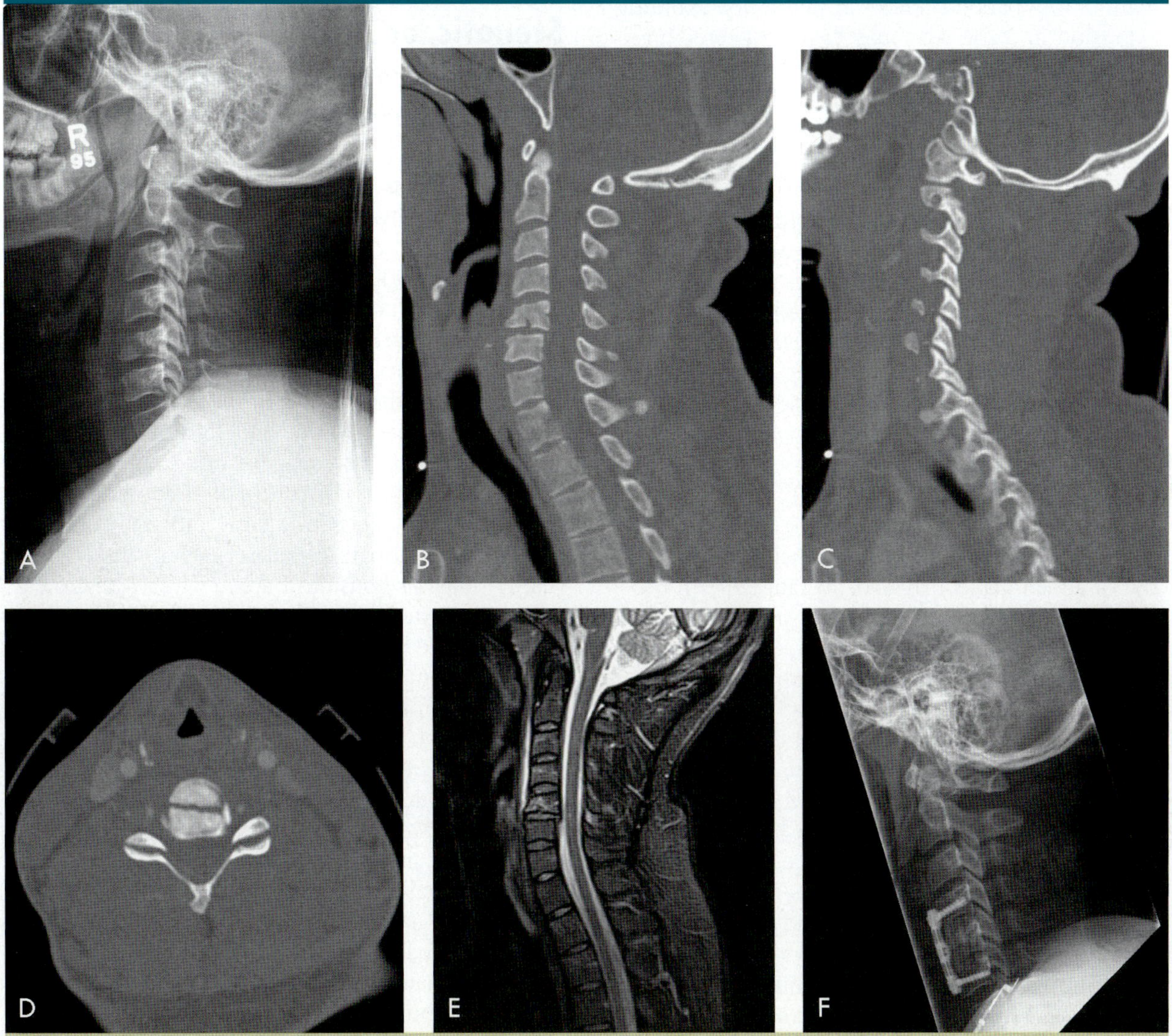

Figure 6 This patient was involved in a motorcycle accident and sustained a C5 fracture. **A,** This lateral radiograph shows fracture lines consistent with a flexion–axial loading injury with retropulsion of the inferior aspect of the C5 vertebral body and some comminution of the anterior aspect of the C5 vertebral body. Some widening of the C5-C6 facet joints can be seen. The patient also has the expected increased soft-tissue swelling noted at the C3 level. **B,** This midsagittal reconstructed CT image shows the retrolisthesis of C5 into the spinal canal and the typical anterior fracture that is most obvious at the inferior aspect of the C5 vertebral body. **C,** Parasagittal reconstructed CT scan showing the widening of the C5-C6 facet joint. **D,** This axial CT image through the inferior aspect of the C5 vertebral body shows the coronal fracture through the C5 vertebral body and also the widening of the facet joints posteriorly, especially on the left side. **E,** Midsagittal T2-weighted fat-saturated MRI scan shows increased signal intensity between the spinous processes of C5 and C6 consistent with ligamentous disruption. **F,** Because this patient was neurologically normal but was thought to be unstable at this level, he was treated with an anterior cervical partial corpectomy and reconstruction with fibula allograft and titanium plates with screws. He was immobilized for 8 weeks in a rigid cervical collar.

sentation may vary from subtle to dramatic. Taylor and Blackwood[58] described the interesting case of a 31-year-old Scottish miner who in 1948 had fallen downstairs on his face and was rendered completely quadriplegic. Their discussion reveals the frustrations associated with negative plain radiographic and myelographic assessment of this patient, whose stormy course was complicated by ascending paralysis and eventual death. Their anatomic dissection showed an ALL and disk disruption with associated intramedullary hemorrhage and edema of the cord. The deformity reduced unrecognizably in flexion. The authors advise maintaining patients' necks in neutrality, avoiding extension in those who may have suspected hyperextension-induced insufficiencies of the ALL and disk.

Hayes et al[59] likewise described a 68-year-old male who sustained a severe cervical hyperextension injury while body surfing but had no evidence of vertebral fracture or subluxation. On post mortem examination, the patient was found to have sustained severe disk injuries at C3-C4, C4-C5, and C5-C6, with associated rupture of the ALL at each of these levels and focal cord hemorrhage at these three corresponding levels. The authors argued that the cord contusion was likely a result of transient disk retropulsion or a pincer-like process resulting from a transient vertebral retrolisthesis.

Loading rates of ligaments have been implicated as determining sites of failure, whether at the bony site of attachment or in midsubstance.[60,61] In the final analysis, the weakest link in the chain will fail first, a property determined undoubtedly by the tissue characteristics of the individual. In cadaveric preparations, if the ALL is severed and a hyperextension moment is placed on the spine, the intervertebral disk will rupture, allowing for retrolisthesis of the body above. Marar[19] showed that subtle retrolisthesis may be a helpful clue to recognizing hyperextension-induced disk injury in the spine.

If conventional radiography and CT imaging are negative in a patient who has sustained myelopathic findings on clinical examination, MRI is warranted (**Figure 5**). Studies have indicated a correlation exists between abnormal MRI findings and the severity of neurologic injury,[57] therefore making MRI a possible diagnostic as well as prognostic modality.

Gupta et al[51] identified 15 patients at their institution who sustained a neurologic deficit following a hyperextension injury to the cervical spine without radiographic evidence of fracture. Upon MRI examination, six patients had a traumatic intervertebral disk herniation causing the paralysis.[51]

The definitive management of patients with ALL or disk disruptions has not been clarified, yet it remains logical that this condition represents a significant instability. The nonsurgical approach would be mandating 2 or 3 months of rigid immobilization followed by flexion-extension radiographs to determine stability. The other option would be to perform an anterior cervical diskectomy and fusion supplemented with plate and screws.

Hyperextension in Spondylotic, Stenotic, or Ankylosed Spines

Hyperextension Injuries in Patients With Ankylosing Spondylitis

The evaluation and treatment of hyperextension injuries to the cervical spine in patients with ankylosing spondylitis (AS) poses significant challenges to the clinician. Algorithms in management that are ordinarily applied to patients with cervical injury require modification. Clinical suspicion must remain particularly high for occult injury, and the acute and definitive management must be modified in consideration of the patient's underlying abnormalities of bone and soft tissue. The propensity for associated vascular and neural injury and preexisting abnormalities of alignment further compound the decision-making process. Patients with diffuse idiopathic skeletal hyperostosis (DISH) may also sustain fractures in association with hyperextension injuries. Although more rarely reported in the literature than AS, extension is a more common mechanism than flexion in creating complex skeletal and severe neurologic injury in such patients. Twelve of 14 fractures reported by Mirkovic et al[62] in patients with DISH occurred at either C5-C6 or C6-C7, and the authors described good results with surgical reduction, fusion, and instrumentation.

AS, originally described by Marie and Strümpell in 1897 and 1898, is an inflammatory seronegative spondyloarthropathy that may begin with general inflammation and a radiographic picture of osteopenia, but progress to painless ossification of the spine. More commonly seen in males, its incidence in the general population is roughly 2 in 1,000. The disease is characterized by bilateral sacroiliitis and the formation of stiff joints by the consolidation of the articular surfaces.[63] Spine flexibility and chest expansion are reduced. This is typically seen in a patient with an elevated erythrocyte sedimentation rate (ESR) who is rheumatoid factor—and antinuclear antibody–negative but human leukocyte antigen–positive—such as seen in patients with respiratory failure and pneumonia.

Seventy-five percent of patients with AS in whom the duration of disease is 16 years or more[65] develop cervical ankylosis. Ossification of the ligaments results in syndesmophyte formation and generates the appearance of a "bamboo spine" on plain radiographs. This ankylosis creates a cylinder of bone about the spinal cord that is rigid, brittle, and osteoporotic. When stressed, therefore, a tremendous lever arm exists for fracture initiation. It is not surprising that these patients present in their fifth and sixth decades, commonly after falls or vehicular accidents, with unstable spine fractures ranging from the occult to the catastrophic[66-70] (**Figure 7**). Occasionally, the patient will present after trivial or no injury at all with a presumed stress fracture. Compared to the general population, patients with AS have a fourfold risk of sustaining a spinal fracture, and hyperextension is a more common mechanism than hyperflexion-induced fractures in these patients.[71] Other hyperextension injuries, such as odontoid fractures, may be prone to occur in patients with AS and cervical flexion deformities and have been reported.[72] Bohlman's[24] series of 300 cervical injuries described 8 patients with AS, 7 of whom had neurologic deficits. Four of these had significant epidural hematomas, a complication not seen in the 292 other patients. Murray and Persellin[69] reviewed the literature on fractures in AS in 1981 and added 8 additional patients from their own experience to present a total of 83 patients, 77 of whom were male. Their review suggests that hyperextension is clearly the most common mechanism of injury.

Fractures can occur at any region of the spine in patients with AS with only minimal trauma, and may occur at multiple sites. Furthermore, previous spine fractures treated with spinal instrumentation may decrease the risk of refracture at that level; however, there may be an increased risk of fracture occurring adjacent to the instrumentation due to the instrument-induced formation of a rigid moment arm.[64] The most common site of fracture in patients with AS is the cervical spine or at the cervicothoracic junction (75%).[73] The most common type is a transverse fracture through the calcified intervertebral disk (70%), most often C5-C6 or C6-C7, although the fracture can also occur through the body, commonly its cranial portion.[69,74] In addition, fractures are highly unstable due to the ossification of the ligamentous structures that "break" during the initial injury,[64] the fractures extend across the anterior and posterior columns,[71,75,76] and the fractures tend to be displaced. Epidural hematomas may accompany cervical fractures in AS;[71,75] therefore, in cases of neurologic deterioration with an established spinal cord injury, or a free interval between the trauma and the onset of neurologic signs, epidural hematoma must be ruled out.[24,75]

The patient may have an unsuspected injury and neck pain alone or a painful flexion deformity. Pain should not be attributed to arthritis, even

FIGURE 7

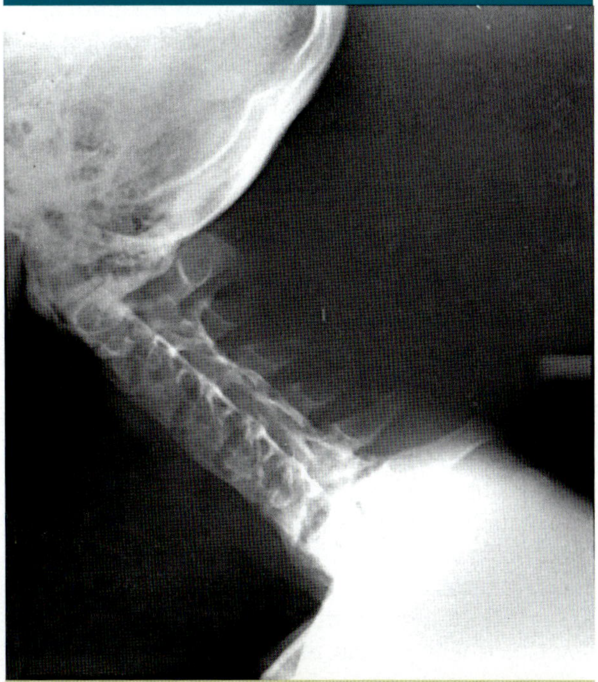

Figure 7 This middle-aged man had AS but had a functional alignment of his spine. He had not had any significant spine pain for several years. He was in a motor vehicle accident, however, several months before this radiograph was taken. The lateral view shows that the patient has a very straight cervical spine. Also, between C6 and C7, there is a lucent line through the disk space and through the facet joints that cannot be seen at any other level. This was a fracture that had not been recognized at the time of the accident and one can see that some kyphosis and subluxation is beginning to develop at this level. This patient later developed a chin-on-chest deformity that required cervical osteotomy to improve his daily function. (Reproduced from McDowell GS, Cammisa FP, Eismont FJ: Hyperextension injuries of the cervical spine, in Levine AM, Eismont FJ, Garfin SR, Zigler JE, eds: *Spine Trauma*. Philadelphia, PA, WB Saunders, 1998, pp 367-386.)

after trivial injury. Simmons[77] cautioned that it is those with neck pain and no deformity who may have an acute or subacute fracture, a condition that, left untreated, may well progress to a chin-on-chest deformity.

Significant morbidity and mortality are the rule with these fractures. Ultimately, one-third of these patients die as the result of the injury, while 22% to 45% persist with significant paralysis, initially present in greater than one-half.[69,78] Murray and Persellin[69] observed a trend that death has been more common in the group treated surgically (45%) than in the group treated nonsurgically (29%), but this was a retrospective review of the literature in which the treatment groups were not matched for injury severity.

The early management of the patient requires having a high index of suspicion for the injury. Rescue squad personnel must be attentive to the need to place a patient's head in the "normal" resting position for immobilization. This requires communication with the patient and his or her family and modification of protocols regarding field collar immobilization. The physician should continue to observe these precautions and should avoid the use of traction in extension or even neutral positioning. Excessive traction will frequently overdistract or malalign the spine.[79] It is often best to immediately apply a halo vest in the patient's normal preinjury posture. This allows the patient to be further assessed and safely mobilized while the physician decides whether surgical treatment would be beneficial.

The radiographic evaluation may be complicated by distortion of normal anatomy and lack of displacement on plain radiographs. The inherent abnormalities of deformity, fusion, and osteopenia associated with AS can mask injuries on plain radiographs. Therefore, a high index of suspicion must be maintained. Plain films should alert the physician to the diagnosis of AS and may demonstrate the fracture. Most authors suggest using reformatted CT to generate orthogonal images (coronal and sagittal) to avoid missing transverse (axial plane) vertebral fractures and to better evaluate the cervicothoracic junction.[80-82] MRI should be obtained if there is any neurologic abnormality, especially considering the propensity for epidural hematoma formation. Dynamic radiographs are not necessary and may be hazardous. Throughout the evaluation, extreme caution with positioning and careful supervision of the procedures must be observed.

There are no established treatment guidelines for cervical fractures in AS.[71] Proponents of both conservative[78,83-85] and surgical management[86-88] exist. Many authors support conservative treatment, and argue that higher rates of morbidity and mortality are associated with surgery,[71] especially respiratory complications.[75] Nonsurgical therapy includes prolonged bed rest, either in traction or in a cervical collar, or use of a halo vest for early mobilization.[76] One must remember that a patient with AS has lungs that are less compliant with restricted intercostal motion and may be further restricted by the halo vest. Rarely, with halo-vest immobilization, a fracture may become redisplaced, with resultant failed union and neurologic deterioration. Rowed[89] found that 4 of 21 patients immobilized in a halo vest had a recurrent dislocation. In addition, pin-site infections, skin breakdown, and pneumonia further complicate halo use. Halo-vest immobilization alone, however, has allowed most patients to heal solidly without incident. It will often take 4 months of halo-vest immobilization to achieve adequate fracture healing.

At present, the indications for surgery include the patient in whom reduction has failed (**Figure 8**), who has significant canal compromise with neurologic impairment, or who has ascending paralysis due to epidural hematoma.[77,90] They also include those patients unable or unwilling to tolerate halo-vest immobilization. These patients all require instrumented fusion and may require neural decompression. Current surgical procedures include posterior instrumentation and fusion, combined anterior and posterior instrumentation and fusion, and, rarely, a pure anterior approach.[71] Appropriate aftercare may still require the use of a halo vest if the bone quality is poor. Few believe the fracture should be used as an occasion to correct a chin-on-chest deformity if this deformity was present before the injury.[82]

In summary, significant hyperextension injuries to the cervical spine in patients with AS are easily missed unless one maintains a high level of suspicion. Cautious evaluation and immobilization are indicated, each of which should be performed with respect to the patient's preinjury cervical alignment. Routine in-line traction may be harmful by creating a hyperextension bending moment or overdistracting the spine. The possibility of an epidural hematoma must be considered in patients with neurologic deficits because this group of patients is predisposed to this complication.

Hyperextension Injuries in Patients With Congenital Cervical Stenosis

Hyperextension injuries in young persons with congenital cervical stenosis have an increased risk for spinal cord injuries as compared to similar injuries in patients with normal cervical canal size. An increasing body of literature concerning younger patients with sports-related injuries supports this contention. Sports-related spinal cord injuries, however, likely constitute a small (2%) proportion of all patients seen with spinal cord injury.[91] Additionally, athletic injuries are thought to be more commonly seen with hyperflexion or axial loading. Patients with neurapraxia, however, may have a higher incidence of hyperextension injuries.[92] Because of the personal impact of these occasionally devastating injuries on the young person and the medicolegal implications relating to physician permission for return to sports after a

FIGURE 8

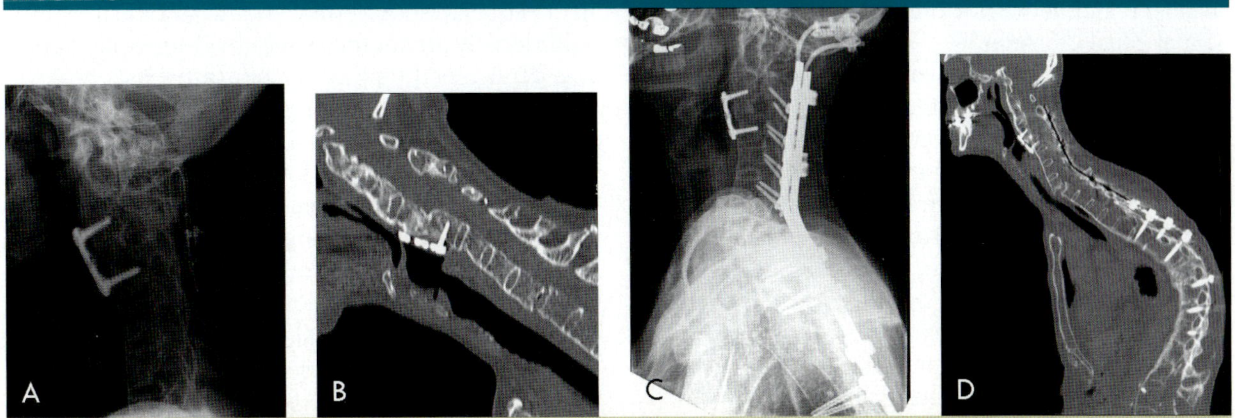

Figure 8 This patient has AS that was diagnosed when he was a teenager. He was involved with a minor fall in the past and sustained a C3-C4 fracture that was treated surgically. The patient is now 1 year after a new minor fall and is having persistent pain at the base of his neck. **A,** This standing lateral radiograph of the cervical spine shows that the patient already is tipping forward and is unable to look straight ahead. **B,** This reconstructed CT scan shows a new fracture at the C7-T1 level and an air vacuum sign in the C7-T1 disk. His spine is otherwise fused above and below this level. **C,** Because of the long-term pain and failure of previous treatment with halo vests and rigid cervical collars, he underwent surgical correction with a posterior laminectomy followed by a correction of his deformity by 38°. The instrumentation extends from occiput to L2. This postoperative standing lateral radiograph shows that the patient is able to see straight ahead. **D,** At this time, the patient is 3 weeks following his correction and is able to have a forward gaze. This sagittal reconstructed CT scan shows that the anterior fracture site is not yet healed, but is expected to heal in time. Supplementation with an anterior bone graft with plate and screws is sometimes necessary.

transient neurologic injury, further attention will be devoted to this clinical entity.

Hinck et al[93] originally described the picture of congenital cervical stenosis in children in 1962. More recently, Torg et al[92] described transient quadriplegia in football players with congenital stenosis. This study complements a growing body of literature on congenital stenotic patients sustaining hyperextension injuries in football, rugby, body surfing, and other sports.[91,94-99] Additional published reviews emphasize that patients with postsurgical, posttraumatic, and congenitally fused vertebrae are also at risk of spinal cord injury with hyperextension.[92,100] This likely is a result of hypermobility or secondary degenerative arthrosis developing above or below a fused motion segment.[100]

Torg et al[92] described the typical case of a young male athlete sustaining a hyperextension cervical injury with an acute transient neurapraxia of the cervical cord. Generally, the neurapraxia consists of burning dysesthesias and motor weakness, lasting 10 to 15 minutes but occasionally as long as 2 days. The athlete commonly has had no prodromal symptoms or history of previous injury.[92] This picture of transient quadriplegia or the milder form of central cord dysfunction known as "burning hands" syndrome[101] must be distinguished on the field from the athlete who exhibits symptoms of unilateral upper extremity neurologic dysfunction known as the "burner" or "prolonged burner," which represents a traction or direct blow injury to the brachial plexus or cervical nerve root(s).[102]

Commonly, plain radiographs are normal after transient quadriplegia. However, Torg et al[92] described 32 patients with neurapraxia in their study, 17 of whom were noted to have normal radiographs, but who otherwise met criteria for congenital spinal stenosis. Seventeen of 32 patients were also thought to have hyperextension as the mechanism for their injuries. The plain radiographic criteria for stenosis, as described by Pavlov, is when the ratio of sagittal spinal canal diameter divided by the vertebral body is less than 0.80, as compared to a normal of 0.98 in controls.[92] This technique avoids errors in measurements of sagittal spinal canal diameters referable to variations in target distances of radiographic equipment. It is the diameter of the spinal canal between the third and sixth vertebra that is most important to evaluate. Traditionally, clinicians have thought of congenital stenosis when AP sagittal diameters measure less than 14 mm on standard radiographs as measured from the midposterior aspect of the body to the spinolaminar line. The normal diameter is 17 to 18 mm as measured at a target distance of 6 feet. CT scanning is also easily available and allows for direct measurement of spinal canal diameter.[103]

The incidence of transient quadriplegia as reported by Torg et al[104] was 1.3 in 10,000 in a 1984 survey of 503 National Collegiate Athletic Association football programs. This contrasts with 6.0 in 10,000 for four-extremity paresthesias.[92] Speer and Bassett[102] reported an incidence of 5 to 10 per 100 for prolonged "burners" and a 4-year career incidence of up to 50% for burners in varsity collegiate football players.

Taylor[47] demonstrated in cadavers with myelography that infoldings of the ligamentum flavum occur with hyperextension resulting in 30% narrowing of the thecal canal outline. Breig et al[105] demonstrated that the spinal cord actually thickens as tension is released on it with shortening as might be seen in hyperextension injuries. This further reduces the potential free space constituting a safe zone for impingement.[105] Penning[90] described a "pincer effect," which in hyperextension squeezes the spinal cord between the posteroinferior portion of the vertebral body and the subjacent posterior elements. Additionally, hyperextension causes the PLL and the ligamentum flavum to actually thicken secondary to stress relaxation.[92] All of these aforementioned events result in cord compression and ultimately cause transient disruption of axonal cell membrane permeability.[106] These pathomechanical factors help explain why, in persons with congenitally stenotic canals, neurologic injury might occur with greater frequency.

What should the clinician do after recognizing this injury pattern? Clearly, in the field, a patient presenting with neurapraxia must be carefully stabilized and removed promptly from the playing field for a complete neurologic and musculoskeletal examination including radiographs and in some instances MRI. Clinical evaluation alone may be insufficient even for patients presenting solely with pain. The need for a cervical CT scan will vary, but is strongly advocated by some as an excellent way of evaluating congenital stenosis.[96] A Torg ratio of less than 0.8 is highly sensitive of significant cervical spine stenosis, but has poor predictive value.[107] Therefore, some authors recommend the use of MRI to determine the size of the spinal cord and functional reserve of the spinal canal.[108]

Torg et al[109] found a strong and inverse relationship between the risk of recurrent transient neurapraxia and the Torg ratio in adult athletes who returned to their sport. However, the data of Torg et al[92] do not indicate that these persons are predisposed to more severe injuries with permanent sequelae should they choose to return.[91,98] Additionally, in another study by Torg et al,[110] it was determined that no relationship exists between a congenitally narrowed cervical canal and irreversible injury to the spinal cord. On the contrary, other studies have found a significantly narrower cervical spinal canal in patients who sustained permanent neurologic deficit from spine trauma compared with patients who sustained no neurologic deficit.[111,112] Nevertheless, some believe the presence of congenital stenosis alone should potentially preclude participation in contact sports.[96] Athletes with congenital stenosis who have experienced transient quadriparesis should be advised that there is a 56% chance of recurrence of the transient quadriparesis if they continue participation in contact sports and high-risk activities.[110]

Unfortunately, the relationship between cervical stenosis and sports-related neurapraxia has not been examined as extensively in children as in adults.[113] Boockvar et al[113] set out to do just this when they measured the sagittal canal diameter and Torg ratio in 13 children who had a sports-related cervical neurapraxia. They found that, contrary to adult athletes, pediatric athletes with cervical neurapraxia do not demonstrate congenital cervical canal stenosis as defined by the Torg ratio or sagittal diameter. The authors concluded that the occurrence of cervical neurapraxia in pediatric athletes can more likely be attributed to the greater mobility of the pediatric spine rather than congenital cervical spinal stenosis.

In the case of progressive neurologic deterioration after a hyperextension injury in a patient with cervical spinal stenosis, urgent decompression may be warranted. In patients with mild cervical stenosis or in elderly debilitated patients with severe stenosis who would not be considered surgical candidates, conservative treatment such as immobilization in a cervical collar and physical therapy may be used.[114]

The role of the clinician should be expanded to assist in prevention through protective equipment modification, training, and rule changes. The addition of shoulder and neck rolls, modifications in face masks, and changes in the posterior trim lines of helmets are examples of sensible equipment modifications. These biomechanical principles were studied by Carter and Frankel[115] in their evaluation of hyperextension injuries in football players using free body diagrams of helmeted cervical spines. Training programs emphasizing neck strengthening serve as additional prevention. Rule

FIGURE 9

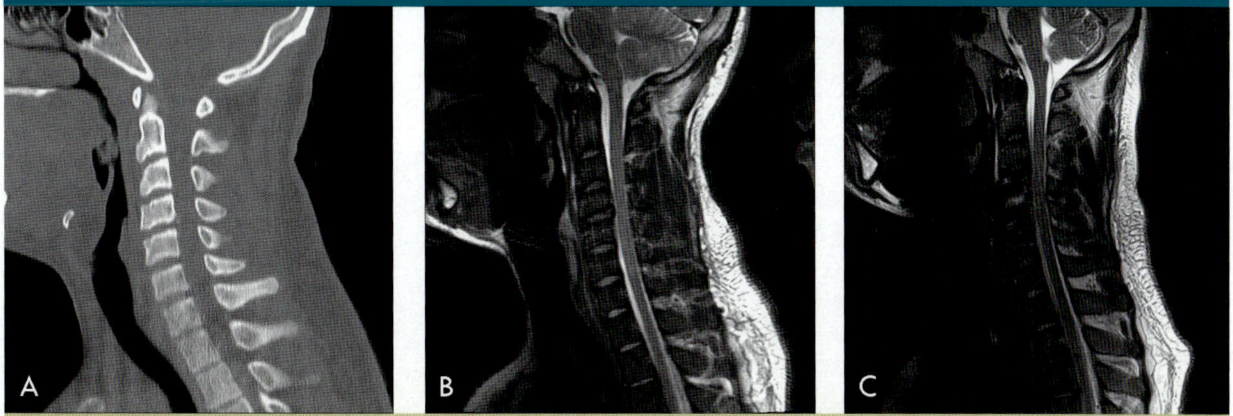

Figure 9 This 18-year-old collegiate football player had persistent recurrent pain radiating into his left shoulder with persistent significant weakness after practice with contact. He was refractory to conservative measures. **A,** Midsagittal reconstructed CT scan showing the vertebral body diameter and spinal canal diameter. The Torg ratio at C4 is 0.58 and the Torg ratio at C5 is 0.61. **B,** The patient has a bulging or small extruded disk at C4-C5. It can be seen that it is central, but it also extended more to his symptomatic left side. **C,** Two months following an anterior diskectomy and fusion at C4-C5, the spinal canal is still diffusely small from the inferior portion of C3 through the midportion of C5. Although patients can usually return to football following a single-level anterior fusion, if the spinal canal is still severely narrowed, better judgment might restrict a patient to less violent sport activities.

changes regarding spearing (1976) and existing rules regarding face-masking address risky tackling techniques. At present, the clinician's role must be to recognize, treat, and appropriately advise the player with congenital stenosis and previous hyperextension injury who participates in high-risk activities (**Figure 9**).

Hyperextension Injuries in Patients With Spondylotic Stenosis

Like patients with congenital stenosis, those with cervical spondylosis and stenosis have significant risk of neurologic injury with hyperextension. In middle-aged and elderly patients, minor hyperextension injuries may result in serious damage to the spinal cord[116] (**Figure 10**). Disk degeneration and associated protrusion, facet hypertrophy, hypertrophic and infolded ligamentum flavum, and posterior end-plate osteophyte formation all result in significant reduction in the space available for the spinal cord. Soft tissues that are likely to fail under hyperextension loading include the ALL, the disk, and the PLL.

A common presentation is that of an elderly person who has struck his or her forehead, either in a fall or vehicular accident, and who demonstrates the findings of a central cord syndrome (**Figure 11**). Misdiagnosis is frequent in this group of patients.[24] There are multiple reasons for this, including (1) the subtleties of abnormal physical findings in mild central cord lesions, (2) inadequate radiographs, (3) radiographs that appear strikingly normal except for spondylosis, (4) failure to recognize subtle radiographic findings suggestive of significant hyperextension injury, and (5) impaired patient-physician communication secondary to advanced age or closed head injury. Prevertebral swelling and/or hematomas may occur and may be massive. Both Smith et al[117] and Howcroft and Jenkins[118] presented case reports of elderly patients with near-fatal asphyxia after sustaining this lesion before evacuation of the hematomas and tracheostomy.

Another associated soft-tissue lesion reported in the anterior neck includes esophageal perforation with the potential for life-threatening mediastinitis, a complication reported by several authors.[119,120] Additionally, retropharyngeal abscess with airway obstruction and tetraplegia has been described in the elderly with hyperextension.[121] Traumatic dissection of the extracranial internal carotid artery when hyperextension is combined with lateral bending was described by Stringer and Kelly[122] in six patients.

It is generally recognized that a congenitally narrow cervical canal is a risk factor in the development of myelopathy in patients with cervical spondylosis.[123-125] Yue et al[126] set out to directly compare the Torg ratio between patients with myelopathy secondary to cervical spondylosis and the nonspondylotic, nonmyelopathic population. They

FIGURE 10

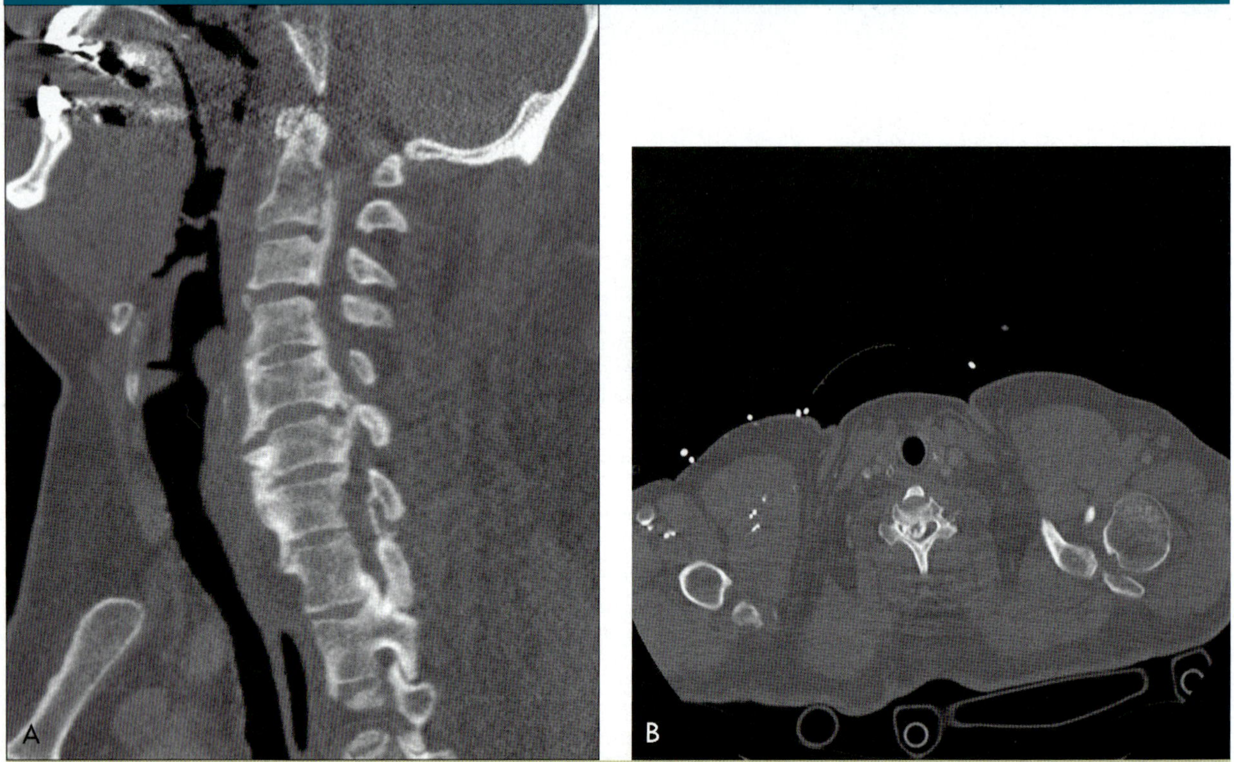

Figure 10 This elderly gentleman was transported to a trauma center after falling 36 hours previously. Although this was only a minor low-energy fall, he had hyperextension of the cervical spine resulting in complete quadriplegia. There is no function in any muscle C5 or lower. Because the patient had a pacemaker, an MRI scan could not be obtained. **A,** This reconstructed sagittal CT scan shows that he has a combination of DISH and ossification of the PLL. The only level that appears not be fused is his C3-C4 level, which would be consistent with his level of paralysis. **B,** This axial CT image shows that his osteophyte at the C6 level actually has fractures. The severe extent of the spinal canal narrowing is apparent. This patient had actually been completely asymptomatic before his fall. This patient remained a high-level complete quadriplegic.

determined that the Torg ratio is significantly lower in patients with cervical spondylotic myelopathy compared with the normal population, irrespective of sex and age, and that the Torg ratio could possibly be used as an index for predicting future development of cervical spondylotic myelopathy.

MRI is particularly important in the evaluation of these patients. MRI may help differentiate traumatic from degenerative changes (spinal cord edema, hematoma, or prevertebral hematoma) because radiographic findings seen in spondylosis and acute trauma overlap.[4] However, differentiating acute traumatic cord edema from preexisting myelomalacia in cervical spondylosis may prove more difficult.[4]

The care of the elderly spinal cord–injured patient will usually require a team approach and a period of rehabilitation. Most patients with central cord lesions will walk and regain bowel and bladder control, but upper extremity deficits are likely to persist. The need for decompression or stabilization, or both, must be individualized (**Figure 12**). In general, if the neurologic improvement is rapid, then nonsurgical care is continued. If the improvement is slow or static at an unacceptable level and the stenosis is severe, then surgical decompression would be electively performed.

Spinal Cord Injury Without Radiographic Abnormality (SCIWORA)

SCIWORA is an acronym used to describe an acute spinal cord injury resulting in some degree of sensory or motor deficit without evidence of vertebral fracture or malalignment on plain radiographs and CT scans.[51,57,127-132] The first to report it was Burke;[133] however, Pang and Wilberger[129] were the first to coin and define the acronym. SCIWORA is a syndrome that can occur in all

FIGURE 11

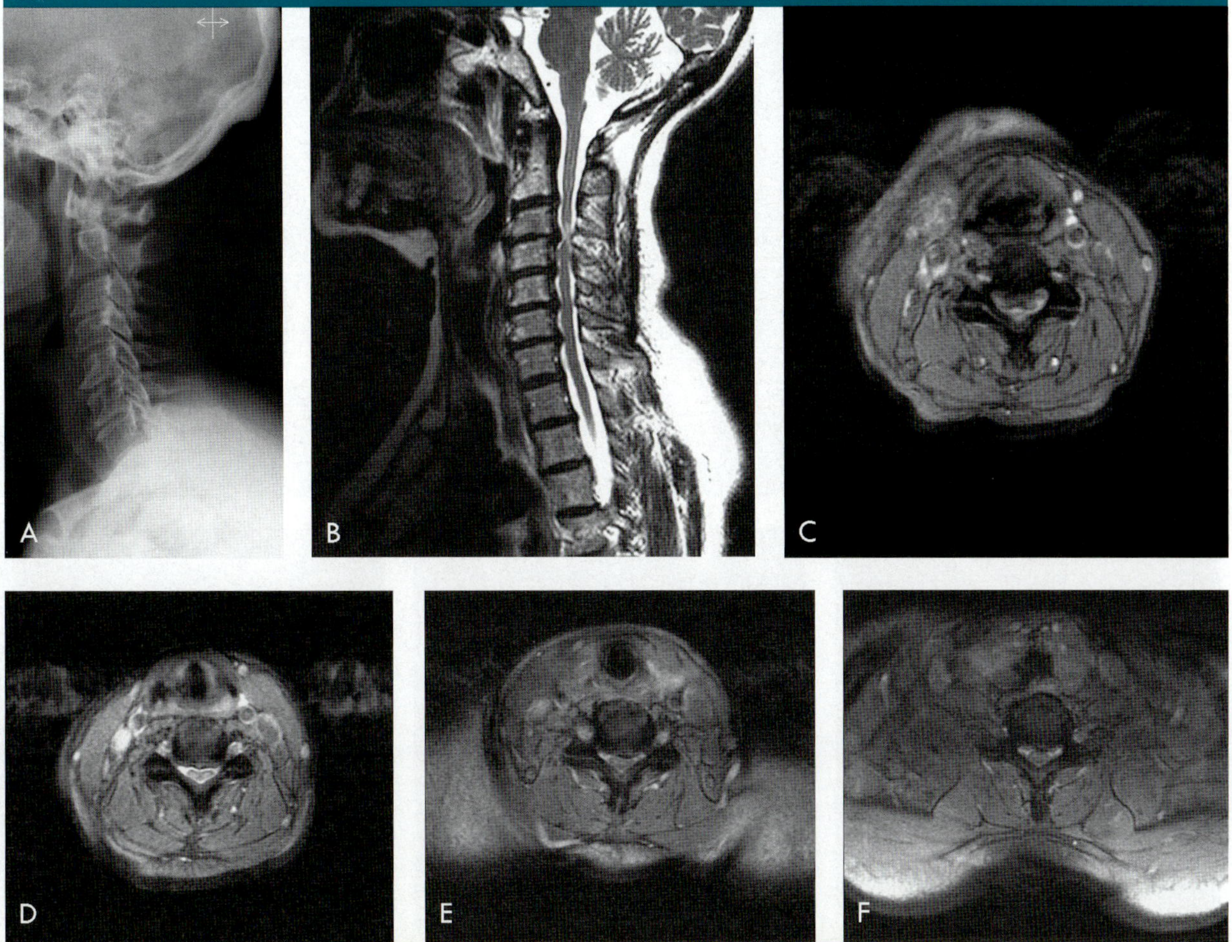

Figure 11 This 65-year-old woman had a minor hyperextension injury as a result of a fall at home. Following the fall, significant myelopathy with gross ataxia developed. **A,** This lateral radiograph shows moderate spondylosis but normal alignment of the spine. Neck pain has never been a significant problem for her. **B,** Midsagittal MRI scan shows diffuse stenosis from the superior portion of C3 down through the superior portion of C7. She has obvious myelomalacia at the C3-C4 level. **C,** Transverse T2-weighted MRI scan at the C3-C4 level. **D,** Transverse T2-weighted MRI scan at the C4-C5 level. **E,** Transverse T2-weighted MRI scan at the C5-C6 level. **F,** Transverse T2-weighted MRI scan at the C6-C7 level.

ages, but is predominantly found in the pediatric population.[53,134-136]This traditional definition does not include the use of MRI.

Four mechanisms of injury, including hyperextension, flexion, distraction, and spinal cord ischemia, have all been implicated in SCIWORA.[136,137] During hyperextension, the interlaminar ligaments bulge forward into the spinal canal while the cord concomitantly thickens as it shortens, both of which critically reduced the canal space.[138] In addition, rupture of the ALL, shearing of the intervertebral disk from end plates, and retrodisplacement of the upper vertebra can occur.[138] Various degrees of spinal cord injury can occur, ranging from complete cord transaction to incomplete paralysis with expected improvement.[138]

Launay et al,[127] who performed a meta-analysis on all reported cases of SCIWORA, found 392 published cases in the literature with 90% of the cases occurring in children. Of reported spinal cord injury cases in children, the incidence of SCIWORA is 34.8%.[138] Of the pediatric cases reported by Launay et al, motor vehicle accident was the most common cause, followed by fall from a height, sports-related injury, birth trauma, and child abuse, in descending order. The specific mechanisms included flexion, distraction, extension, and crush. As expected, MRI demonstrated both extraneural injuries such as disk herniations, ligament disruptions, and hematomas, as well as intrinsic neural injuries with edema, hemorrhage, etc. Follow-up MRI was found to be necessary

FIGURE 11 *(CONTINUED)*

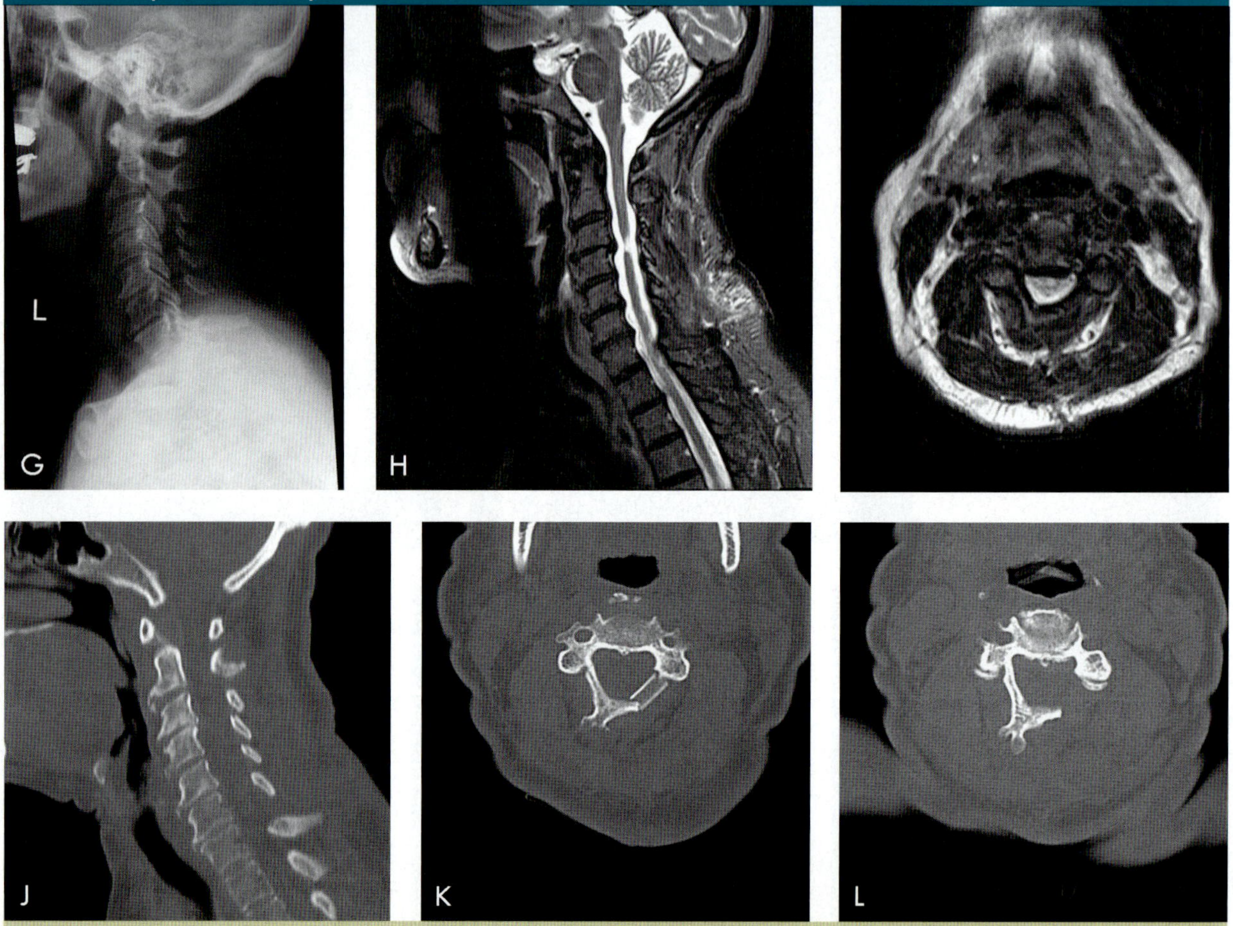

Figure 11 *(continued)* **G,** This lateral radiograph was taken 8 weeks after C3 to C6 posterior cervical laminaplasty. **H,** Midsagittal MRI scan showing that the spine has been completely decompressed from C3 to C7; the area of myelomalacia can still be seen. There is more than adequate room for the spinal cord at all levels. **I,** Transverse T2-weighted MRI scan at the C3-C4 level postoperatively shows that there is more than adequate room around the spinal cord at this level, which had previously been the tightest. The myelomalacia can still be seen. **J,** Midsagittal CT scan shows a marked opening of the spinal canal over these levels. The C7 lamina was left in place and only the superior portion of the C7 lamina was removed. **K,** At 8 weeks, this axial image shows the hinge side of the laminaplasty is completely healed at C3. The allograft bone used for reconstruction can be seen. **L,** This axial CT scan at the C4 level shows the hinge side is completely healed at this level. No bone graft was placed at this level.

because in some instances, injury did not appear immediately. External immobilization for 12 weeks was recommended by the authors to help prevent recurrence of these injuries. Although 44% of the patients did not recover, 39% of the patients had a complete recovery. Other authors have published similar series regarding these patients.[129,139,140]

By definition, these cases of SCIWORA should not include patients with radiographic abnormalities, but it should be kept in mind that 10% to 12% of initial pediatric spine trauma radiographs are misinterpreted as normal.[141,142]

Several important characteristics of the immature spine may account for the normal radiographic appearance in the face of high-energy injuries that have rendered the patient neurologically impaired. The first of these is the greater tissue compliance or elasticity seen in ligaments and joint capsules of children, which may allow for transient subluxations without gross mechanical failure. This laxity was described by Cattell and Filtzer[143] in their article on pseudosubluxation in children based on a review of 160 normal subjects. Second, the planes of the cervical facets in children are more horizontal and thus possess greater mobility and less stability.[129] Third, the intervertebral disk and anulus in children are high in water content and subsequently exceptionally

FIGURE 12

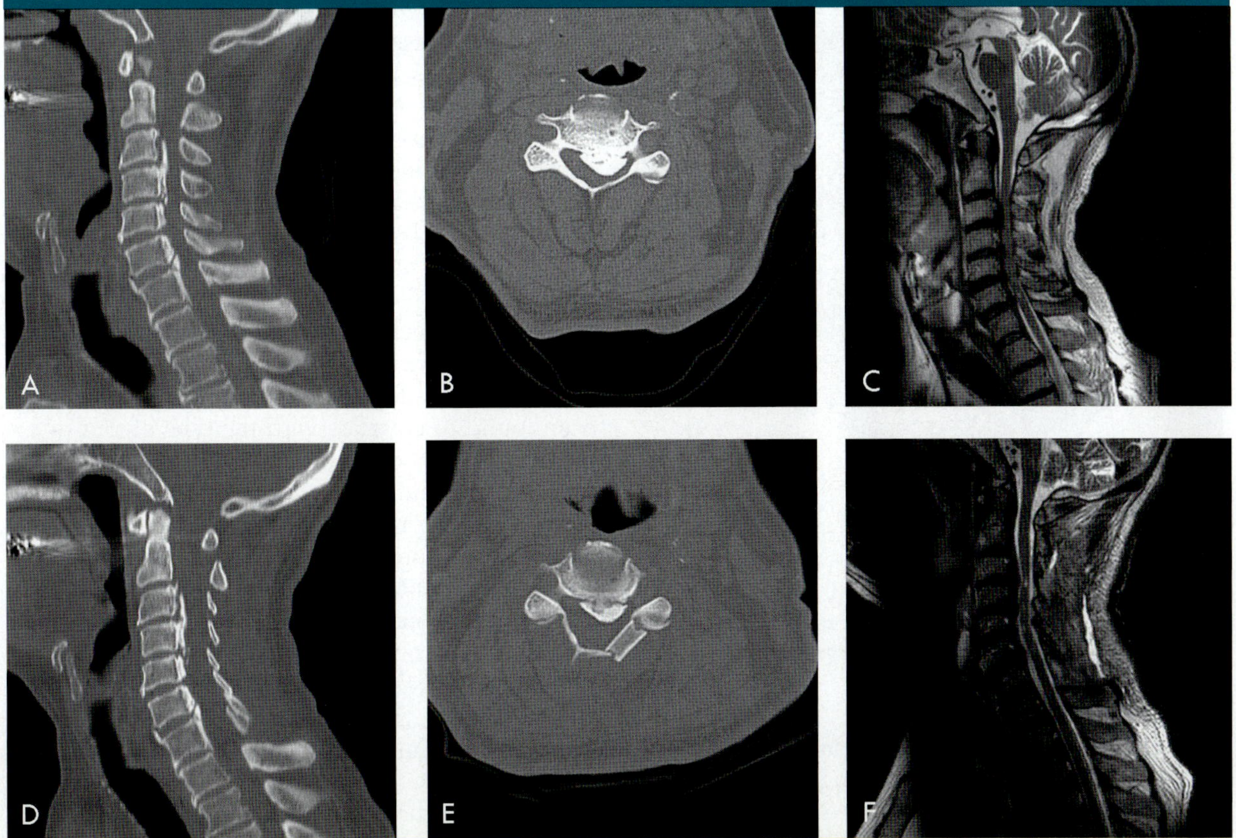

Figure 12 This patient noted some lack of coordination following a minor motor vehicle accident. **A,** Midsagittal CT reconstruction shows that the patient has ossification of the PLL. **B,** Transverse image at C3 shows the severe extent of the spinal canal compromise. **C,** Midsagittal MRI scan shows severe spinal cord compression from the top of C3 to the superior portion of C7. Several areas of myelomalacia can be seen within the spinal cord. **D,** The patient was treated with a laminaplasty from C3 through C7. This midsagittal image shows that the spinal canal has been significantly expanded. **E,** Axial CT image shows how the spinal canal has been significantly expanded at this level and the hinge side of the laminaplasty is healed at 8 weeks. The allograft is not yet healed. **F,** Midsagittal postoperative MRI scan shows that there is adequate room around the spinal cord at all levels. Multiple areas of myelomalacia are still seen. At this time, the patient had significant improvement of the myelopathy.

expandable longitudinally.[138,144] Fourth, the vertebral bodies are wedged anteriorly.[145-147] Fifth, the uncinate process of the adult vertebrae is yet to develop in children under 10 years of age.[148,149] Sixth, the large head of a child compared to the relatively small nuchal musculature predisposes the spine to gross displacement when subjected to external forces.[150] Finally, and most important, as demonstrated by Aufdermaur[151] in his elegant pathologic study of 12 children, catastrophic failure in the immature spine nearly always occurs through the cartilaginous end plate (**Figure 13**). The end plate or physis is the weak link in the child and fractures through it are commonly missed unless they are complete and seen on stress radiographs.

In patients with SCIWORA, however, even stress radiographs of the neck may be normal. This in part may be related to patient compliance or protective splinting, but may also be due to incomplete mechanical failure. It may also suggest that complete physeal failure contributes to only a portion of these clinical presentations. Pang and Wilberger,[129] in their comprehensive treatise on this subject, described 24 patients with SCIWORA seen over 20 years at the Children's Hospital of Pittsburgh. Eighteen of the patients had voluntary flexion-extension films done acutely and none revealed an abnormality. All 24 eventually received dynamic films and only 1 patient had radiographic instability. With MRI, it may be possible in the future to detect most of these injuries of the

FIGURE 13

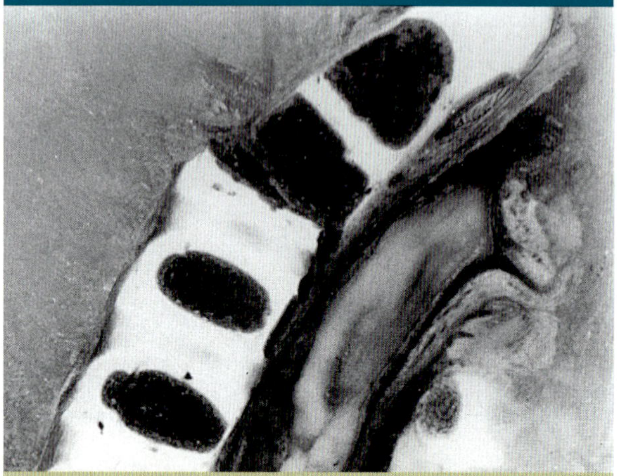

Figure 13 This cryomicrotome section was made through the cervical spine of a young child who had presented with a high-level complete quadriplegia. This is a hyperextension-type injury and the disruption is through the end plate at the bottom of the vertebral body. This is often the anatomic appearance of those cases presenting with SCIWORA. (Courtesy of Dr. Jose Becerra, Miami, FL.)

cartilaginous end plate and determine the role that they might have played in allowing for neurologic compromise.

In the series by Pang and Wilberger,[129] hyperextension alone was the presumed mechanism of injury in 10 of 24 patients. Seven of the 10 patients were more than 8 years old. The majority of the lesions involved the lower cervical cord (C5 through C8 root level), while the five cases of upper cord injury were in the minority and only seen in children under 8 years of age. The younger children with upper cord injuries seemed to have an increased likelihood of serious injury in general. Corroborating physical signs such as chin lacerations, mandibular fractures, facial injuries, and frontal skull injuries were commonly seen to support a hyperextension injury. Overall, 58% sustained a complete or serious cord injury and the final outcome did not seem to be affected significantly by age or treatment.[129]

Management of these patients begins with neutral cervical immobilization in the field and the hospital until screening radiographs can be performed. To accomplish this, the small child and infant may require a roll to be placed under his or her shoulders to compensate for the disproportionately large size of the head. Associated basic life and trauma resuscitations take priority over all further work-up. Avoidance of hypotension may be critical to maintaining adequate spinal cord perfusion pressures. Some authors recommend the administration of a 24-hour course of high-dose corticosteroids within 8 hours after the injury.[127,152] The potential risks and benefits of this must be measured and it is no longer considered mandatory.

Complete cervical spine radiographs and CT should be obtained immediately. When a neurologic deficit is diagnosed in the face of normal plain radiographs or CT, MRI should be performed, which may be the only way of demonstrating neural (edema and hemorrhage) and extraneural (ligamentous injuries, disk protrusions, and compressive extradural hematomas) injuries.[127,128,153] In addition, MRI abnormalities have been found to correlate with the type of neurologic injury.[51,127,154,155] Finally, follow-up MRI has been recommended because of the possibility that SCIWORA may recur,[135,156,157] following inadequate treatment and premature spine mobilization. Recurrent SCIWORA has been reported to result in more severe deficits than the initial presentation.[153,156] Dynamic radiographs are recommended by some clinicians to assess potential spine instability; however, this study may cause additional injury in the acute setting.

Definitive management of the spine may require no more than the use of a secure rigid collar.[135,157,158] Most authors recommend immobilization with bracing for 12 weeks;[128,136] however, Bosch et al[159] recently performed a retrospective review of all the cases of SCIWORA at Children's Hospital of Pittsburgh between 1965 and 1999 and determined that a case-by-case evaluation is required for the treatment of SCIWORA and that bracing may not be uniformly indicated. Those patients with demonstrable instability will be best treated with cervical arthrodesis. Follow-up dynamic radiographs are mandatory in all patients. Evolving neurologic deficits were reported in one-half of Pang and Wilberger's patients, which mandates emergency reevaluation.[129] Consideration should be given to decompression and fusion if a structural lesion is found. Laminectomy alone in the pediatric spine renders the patient prone to the eventual development of kyphosis and, in general, is contraindicated. If the progression of neurologic deficit is related to evolving edema, hemorrhage, or watershed infarction in the absence of neural compression,[129] then the management of these patients may be primarily medical and supportive.

The neurologic status at admission of children with SCIWORA has been found to be the only predictor of long-term outcome.[138] Poor prognosis has been associated with an initial severe neural injury; however, good recovery has been associated with initial mild to moderate neural injury.[127,153,156] In addition, MRI findings of complete cord disruption or major cord hemorrhage (greater than 50% cross-sectional area of the cord shows evidence of hemorrhage) correlate with a poor outcome.[128] Minor hemorrhage (less than 50% cross-sectional area of the cord shows evidence of hemorrhage) or edema only without hemorrhage correlate with a moderate to good recovery.[135,146,160,161] Patients without any evidence of MRI abnormality who do have documented clinical SCIWORA have an excellent prognosis for complete recovery.[53,155]

Whiplash (Acceleration-Deceleration Injury to the Cervical Spine)

Whiplash injuries, or acceleration-deceleration injuries of the neck, have been commonly referred to as cervical sprains. Although some whiplash injuries may indeed represent minor ligamentous injuries of the ALL experienced under tension, the syndrome likely represents a constellation of injuries rarely dramatically evident at initial or follow-up examination. The foundations of the syndrome appear to be an injury of both the anterior and posterior column soft-tissue structures. There is as well a plethora of potential associated injuries of the head and neck. The approach to patients with whiplash must be to methodically search for underlying pathologic changes that can cause persistent symptoms.

Most people involved in a motor vehicle collision do not develop neck pain; however, studies have shown that between 15% and 40% of people with whiplash injuries develop chronic neck pain and 5% to 10% of these people will have constant, severe pain with permanent partial or total disability.[162-171] Giannoudis et al[172] set out to retrospectively investigate the incidence of whiplash in patients sustaining high-energy trauma. They found the incidence of whiplash to be low following high-energy polytrauma compared to the high incidence reported following low-energy trauma, and that no dose-response relationship appears to exist between the magnitude of trauma severity and the incidence of whiplash injury.

A large body of literature has been written on this topic. For the purposes of this chapter, we discuss first the experimental studies relating to the mode of injury and then the clinical presentation, evaluation, treatment options, and outcome.

Basic experimentation as it relates to whiplash has centered on defining the biomechanical forces seen in acceleration injuries and the resultant diverse injury patterns. During a rear-end collision, the torso displaces forward and upward. The head lags behind the torso, resulting in a forced extension of the lower cervical spinal levels and a resultant S-shaped curve. The head is then accelerated forward along with the torso to force the neck into flexion.[169]

It is thought that potential injury to facet joints, disks, and ligaments during the whiplash event are due to an abnormal amount of motion occurring within and between individual motion segments of the cervical spine, with greater changes in velocity correlating directly with greater injury to the passenger.[162] However, other research suggests that acceleration of the struck vehicle rather than the change in velocity may better correlate with injury during a whiplash event.[173-175]

In 1955, Severy et al[176] reported on the photometric and biomechanical evaluation of controlled low-speed rear-end collisions using human subjects and models. The seats in the vehicles tested were without headrests and the subjects were unrestrained. The magnitudes of head acceleration were far greater than that of vehicle acceleration. At 10 mph, 11g was seen by the driver and 122° of neck extension was noted with subsequent rebound flexion.[176] Out of this work grew an interest in automobile seat and restraint design changes that have attempted to lower the incidence of neck injury in vehicular accidents. The use of headrests, however, has not uniformly been shown statistically to reduce the incidence of whiplash,[177] which may be in part due to driver/passenger positioning at the time of the crash. Most would agree, however, that properly positioned headrests are of benefit.

The collision severity clearly influences peak translational and angular accelerations. Williams and McKenzie[178] reported that for a 12g impact, head horizontal acceleration climbs to greater than 50g for a period of approximately 40 msec. Higher impacts (20g) clearly exceed the tensile strength of the cervical spine's soft tissue and bony structures.[178]

Macnab[179] reviewed his clinical experience and discussed experimental work relating to monkeys sustaining various degrees of hyperextension injury. The pathologic findings included injuries to the sternocleidomastoid, longus colli, esophagus, ALL, and vertebral disk with retropharyngeal hematomas, findings that might help explain many of the clinical reports of the whiplash patient. The author did not address possible compression injuries of the posterior column or associated head injuries.[179] Posterior capsular and cartilaginous injuries are common, however, and these experimental changes were reviewed by La Rocca.[180] Recent work by Barnsley et al[36] suggests that the facet joint may be the first site of "contact" in hyperextension and that the zygapophyseal joints are likely to be one of the most important sources of segmental pain generation in whiplash. Additionally, Hohl[181] has shown that the zygapophyseal joints as well as the intervertebral disks develop an incidence (39%) of degenerative changes within the first decade after whiplash that is six times higher than normal.

A variety of hemodynamic, behavioral, and biochemical disturbances have been reported to occur in rats after whiplash injury, specifically disturbances in postural regulation of blood flow and variations in brain neurotransmitter levels. Associated learning impairment and overaggressive behaviors were also observed.[182] Additionally, subcortical electroencephalographic changes have been seen in monkeys following whiplash.[183]

Yoganandan et al[14] set out to replicate soft-tissue injuries in cadaveric models and found that the application of a whiplash acceleration may induce soft-tissue and ligamentous injury. Furthermore, they found that subtle yet clinically relevant injuries may be missed with CT and radiography imaging techniques. Ito et al[184] recently performed a biomechanical investigation to determine the soft-tissue injury threshold during a whiplash simulation. They found the injury threshold peak acceleration of their whole cervical spine with muscle force replication model was 5g, evidenced by a 39.8% increased C5-C6 extension neutral zone. Furthermore, greater accelerations resulted in spread of injury to involve C4-C5 to C7-T1.

Clinical series reporting manifestations of whiplash describe several features that are summarized by La Rocca.[180] The principal symptoms are neck pain and stiffness, reported in 97% to 100% and 78% to 95% of patients, respectively. Forty percent to 72% reported significant headaches, often occipital. Studies have demonstrated sources for chronic cervicogenic headache to include the atlanto-occipital joint, upper cervical disk herniations, injury to the facet joints, or discogenic pain from C2-C3 and C3-C4.[162,185-187] At least one-third of patients had shoulder or arm pain.[181,188,189] Without evidence of neural compression on imaging and no objective neurologic deficits, arm pain may be better termed referred pain rather than radiculopathy and may be referred to the arm from a discogenic source[162,190,191] or, less commonly, from a facet joint.[162,192,193] Arm pain may also be due to shoulder pathology, which may be primary in nature or secondarily referred from the neck.[192,194,195] Many patients (40% to 60%) described having symptoms of psychological distress including irritability, insomnia, and anxiety. Some reported dysphagia, visual blurring, tinnitus, and vertigo, the first perhaps related to retropharyngeal hematoma or occult esophageal injury and the latter three to vertebral artery spasm.[196] The literature contains reports of esophageal injury,[119,121,197] sternocleidomastoid rupture,[198] temporomandibular joint arthritis,[199,200] vestibular injury,[201] thoracic outlet syndrome,[202] and cerebral or ocular injury[203,204] in association with whiplash, which may be responsible for generating further occult symptoms. Although many people who sustain a whiplash injury develop acute neck pain, between 60% and 85% will recover completely.[162,163,165,167,170,171]

Physical findings may reveal decreased range of motion and point tenderness while objective neurologic signs are rarely found. Radiographs are typically normal. However, 20 of 146 radiographs in Hohl's[181] series revealed a "sharp reversal of lordosis," which may have been indicative of occult disk, capsular, or ligamentous injuries. Interestingly, 60% of these patients went on to develop significant degenerative changes at the same level of the mild kyphosis, which was seen to be commonly C4-C5 or C5-C6.[181] Dynamic radiographs, although important to obtain, rarely add information in whiplash. MRI and invasive diagnostic procedures, such as diskography and diagnostic facet blocks, may help to better localize the site of symptomatic injury (**Figure 14**).

Although a clinical history and physical examination do not identify any one structural cause for chronic neck pain from a whiplash event, it is important to identify or exclude more serious injuries and establish the whiplash associated disorder grade.[205-208] Evidence suggests that the facet joints and intervertebral disks are the most common source of chronic neck pain due to injury following a whiplash event.[163,168,205,206,209-221] Acute injury secondary to muscle and ligaments may likewise occur; however, there is no evidence to support chronic neck pain from whiplash to be the result of a chronically strained muscle or sprained ligament.[174]

Cervical facet joints, which are innervated by the medial branches of the cervical dorsal rami, can be diagnosed as a source of pain after being anesthetized.[209] Likewise, diskography may be used to identify pathologic disks in the cervical spine.[190,191,222] In general, imaging is not helpful for the diagnosis of whiplash.

Multiple prognostic factors have been identified; however, it is a high initial intensity of pain that has been reported as the strongest predictor of poor outcome.[162,170,171,223] A study by Côté et al[170] found female sex, older age, radicular symptoms, multiple areas of pain, and being unprepared for impact to all portend a worse prognosis. Interestingly, Côté et al[224] observed in another study that intensive health care early after whiplash is associated with slower recovery. Williamson et al[225] performed a systematic literature review and found that self-efficacy and posttraumatic distress may be associated with the development of late whiplash syndrome. However, in another systematic review, Scholten-Peeters et al[171] found that female sex, older age, high acute psychological response, rear-end collision, angular deformity of the neck, and compensation were not associated with a poor prognosis.

Treatment of whiplash can be challenging and frustrating for the patient and physician alike. The overlay of secondary gain seen with unsettled litigation can further complicate an already clouded clinical presentation. Claims of personal injury are filed in a high percentage of cases.[180] Interestingly, however, Macnab[179] reported that 45% of patients continued to have some symptoms 2 years or more after settlement. He described these symptoms as "nuisance-like" rather than "significantly disabling." Hohl[181] also stated that only 38% of patients were asymptomatic at 5-year follow-up if settlement was achieved more than 18 months after injury. Pearce[189] maintained that despite this, 79% of his 100 patients returned to work by 1 month and 94% by 1 year.

Multiple studies have demonstrated that early, active treatment strategies including physical therapy, analgesics, education and reassurance, and quick return to preinjury activity are most effective for whiplash patients.[162,163,205,226-242] Furthermore, rest and immobilization with a soft cervical collar are in general not helpful and are contraindicated.[162,163,168,226,243,244] Two prospective trials done in Europe have helped to better our understanding of treatment. The blinded study of age- and sex-matched patients by Mealy et al[245] revealed that the subgroup treated with early mobilization and a supervised physical therapy program of stretching, heat, and ice improved pain scores and mobility above that of rest and soft collar use alone. However, the work of Pennie and Agambar[9] work contradicts that of Mealy et al.[245] They advocated the use of a molded rigid collar in slight flexion for best pain relief.

FIGURE 14

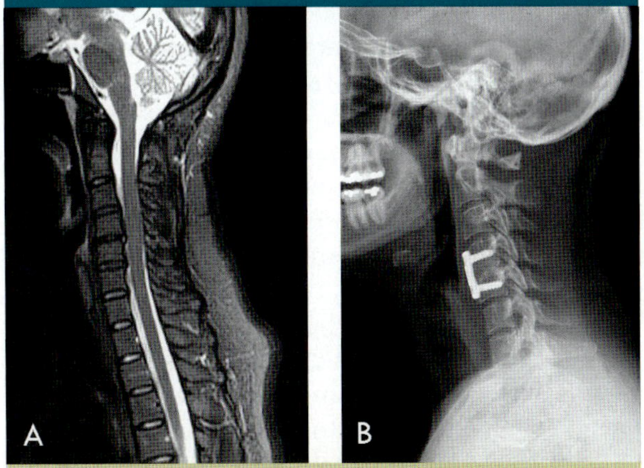

Figure 14 This young woman was involved in a cervical hyperextension followed by flexion injury of her cervical spine several years previously. She had persistent neck pain and pain radiating toward her shoulder and she also had significant facial pain. **A,** This T2-weighted midsagittal MRI scan shows that there is a tear of the posterior anulus at the C4-C5 level. C4-selective nerve root injections were found to give the patient significant improvement of her pain. Based on this, it was assumed that the abnormality at this level was responsible for her symptoms. **B,** She was treated with a single-level anterior diskectomy and fusion, taking care to remove the posterior anulus and the PLL at that level. The patient had some improvement of her pain, but it has persisted to some degree at 6 months following the surgery despite having a solid fusion. This demonstrates the difficulty of correctly diagnosing the source of pain and the difficulty of successfully treating it following cervical whiplash injuries.

Along with analgesics and physical therapy for the treatment of chronic neck pain associated with whiplash, recent work suggests that therapeutic and diagnostic facet injections may be of some distinct benefit to patients, as discussed previously. Intra-articular corticosteroid or local anesthetic injections have been found to produce short-term relief of facet joint pain. Peloso et al[246] performed a retrospective review of the literature and found intramuscular injections of lidocaine for chronic mechanical neck disorders and intravenous injection of methylprednisone for acute whiplash to be effective short-term treatments. Evidence now supports the use of radiofrequency neurotomy for the treatment of chronic neck pain in patients with proven facet joint involvement following anesthetic blocks of the medial branches of the corresponding dorsal rami.[162,168,247,248] Pain relief lasts approximately 8 to 12 months and can be repeated indefinitely[162] There is no evidence supporting the use of trigger-point injections or cervical epidural corticosteroid injections for neck pain relief, and there is no consensus regarding the efficacy of spinal manipulation therapy,[162] despite the fact that it remains a popular treatment modality used by patients.[249,250]

Surgery may be considered in the patient with severe chronic neck pain with significant impairment who has failed nonsurgical intervention. The role of selective cervical arthrodesis in patients with substantial segmental dysfunction has not yet been clearly established, but may be appropriate for those with significant disability beyond 1 to 2 years and supporting studies that suggest segmental instability or arthrosis. Diskography may be useful in identifying painful cervical disks. Anterior cervical diskectomy and fusion would theoretically relieve pain by eliminating motion if the involved facet joint and disk were proven to be the source of the pain. It is hoped that MRI and perhaps invasive techniques will help to guide the clinician in the future. Prevention remains the mainstay of effective treatment at this time.

Overall prognosis of patients having whiplash is highly variable, ranging from complete recovery to persistent disability. This variability could be a reflection of cultural expectations of different societies, variable case identification of studies, or outcome assessments of studies.[168]

Complex High-Energy Hyperextension Fracture-Dislocations

Dislocation of the cervical spine is a rare manifestation of hyperextension injury. Some authors have grouped significant failures of the anterior column in tension without associated subluxations together with this lesion. Hyperextension fracture-dislocations present characteristically with failure of the anterior column in tension and the posterior column via facet dislocation or posterior element fracture.[27,38,44] The latter is a dramatic presentation ultimately representing three-column instability, the likes of which are not seen in other hyperextension injuries. In reality, combined mechanisms with initial hyperflexion in rapid deceleration injuries may be responsible for allowing facet dislocation to occur before the patient's head strikes an object, imparting hyperextension.

Several case reports have been published describing patients who have sustained high-energy hyperextension injuries in motor vehicle accidents presenting with head and facial injuries, posterior ring fractures of C1 (two of four patients), and subaxial fracture-dislocations.[251-253] Varying degrees of frank dislocation were present, from less than 25% subluxation and perched facets in one report[253] to 100% displacement in another.[251] Interestingly, neurologic injury was not noted in all patients as posterior element fractures at the site of dislocation can contribute to indirect decompression of the spinal cord.[251]

Clinically, there are often signs of blunt facial trauma and acute central cord syndrome following a severe hyperextension force to the cervical spine, which can result in momentary posterior dislocation of the involved vertebrae. The ALL, anulus, intervertebral disk, PLL, ligamentum flavum, and paraspinal muscles can all be disrupted.[1] In approximately two-thirds of the cases, an avulsion fracture off the anteroinferior end plate of the involved vertebra occurs.[44]

Radiographic evaluation is often misleading due to the absence of gross dislocation of vertebrae on lateral radiographs, which immediately realign after removal of the impacting force. In some cases, jumped or locked facets can occur. However, the presence of normally aligned vertebrae with diffuse prevertebral soft-tissue swelling should raise suspicion.

Harris and Yeakley[44] performed MRI of the cervical spines of eight patients with hyperextension-dislocation and signs of cervical myelopathy. None of the patients showed radiographic evidence of other cervical spine injuries. All the cases demonstrated ligamentous injury to occur at the same level as the MRI evidence of damage within the spinal cord. Some showed widening of the disk space, posterior bulging or herniation of the nucleus pulposus, and some showed disruption of the ligamentum flavum. In addition, all cases demonstrated diffuse prevertebral soft-tissue hemorrhage. The authors recommend obtaining MRI to confirm the diagnosis and aid in management of suspected hyperextension-dislocation of the cervical spine.

Definitive management consists of a careful reduction and stabilization of the spine. Early resolution of myelopathy associated with transient acute central cord syndrome and resorption of the prevertebral soft-tissue swelling have the potential to mislead clinicians into a false impression that the injury is healed or at least of minor significance.[44] However, it should be recognized that the cervical spine will continue to be unstable. Given the extreme disruption of all three columns, circumferential surgical arthrodesis with instrumentation is usually indicated, although a more conservative instrumented one-column approach has been advocated by some authors.[251,252] The small numbers of patients with this specific lesion reported may not allow for a meaningful prediction of outcome.

Summary

We have discussed the etiology, pathomechanics, evaluation, and treatment of a wide variety of clinical entities presenting after hyperextension injuries. The wide variation in clinical presentation is presumed to be a function of differences in load magnitudes, vectors, and points of application. More important, the presentation also appears to be age- and tissue-dependent. Concomitant spinal cord injuries are seen in those with underlying spondylosis, stenosis, and ankylosis, as well as in children with normal-appearing spines. Whiplash remains a challenging condition.

References

1. Rao SK, Wasyliw C, Nunez DB Jr: Spectrum of imaging findings in hyperextension injuries of the neck. *Radiographics* 2005;25(5):1239-1254.
2. Jagannathan J, Dumont AS, Prevedello DM, Shaffrey CI, Jane JA Jr: Cervical spine injuries in pediatric athletes: Mechanisms and management. *Neurosurg Focus* 2006;21(4):E6.
3. Pintar FA, Yoganandan N, Voo L: Effect of age and loading rate on human cervical spine injury threshold. *Spine (Phila Pa 1976)* 1998;23(18): 1957-1962.
4. Ehara S, Shimamura T: Cervical spine injury in the elderly: Imaging features. *Skeletal Radiol* 2001; 30(1):1-7.
5. Kuhlman KA: Cervical range of motion in the elderly. *Arch Phys Med Rehabil* 1993;74(10): 1071-1079.
6. Regenbogen VS, Rogers LF, Atlas SW, Kim KS: Cervical spinal cord injuries in patients with cervical spondylosis. *AJR Am J Roentgenol* 1986; 146(2):277-284.
7. Whitehill R: Fractures of the lower cervical spine: Subaxial fractures in the adult. *Semin Spine Surg* 1991;3:71-86.
8. Holdsworth F: Fractures, dislocations, and fracture-dislocations of the spine. *J Bone Joint Surg Am* 1970;52(8):1534-1551.
9. Pennie BH, Agambar LJ: Whiplash injuries: A trial of early management. *J Bone Joint Surg Br* 1990; 72(2):277-279.
10. Yoganandan N, Sances A Jr, Pintar F, et al: Injury biomechanics of the human cervical column. *Spine (Phila Pa 1976)* 1990;15(10):1031-1039.
11. Nuscholtz GS, Huelke DE, Lux P, et al: Cervical spine injury mechanisms. *Proceedings of the 27th Stapp Car Crash Conference*. Warrendale, PA, Society of Automotive Engineers, 1983, pp 179-197.
12. Maiman DJ, Yoganandan N: Biomechanics of cervical spine trauma. *Clin Neurosurg* 1991;37: 543-570.
13. Hart RA, Mayberry JC, Herzberg AM: Acute cervical spinal cord injury secondary to air bag deployment without proper use of lap or shoulder harnesses. *J Spinal Disord* 2000;13(1):36-38.
14. Yoganandan N, Cusick JF, Pintar FA, Rao RD: Whiplash injury determination with conventional spine imaging and cryomicrotomy. *Spine (Phila Pa 1976)* 2001;26(22):2443-2448.
15. White AA III, Johnson RM, Panjabi MM, Southwick WO: Biomechanical analysis of clinical stability in the cervical spine. *Clin Orthop Relat Res* 1975;109:85-96.
16. Mirza S, Chapman J, Anderson P, et al: Assessment of instability in the lower cervical spine: Application of the White and Panjabi criteria and anatomic scoring to cervical spine injuries. Presented at the *20th Annual Meeting of the Cervical Spine Research Society*. Palm Beach, FL, Dec 5-7, 1996, Poster No. 20.
17. Shono Y, McAfee PC, Cunningham BW: Mechanisms of compression injuries in the cervical spine: Non-destructive and destructive investigative methods. Research award paper. Presented at the *20th Annual Meeting of the Cervical Spine Research Society*. Palm Desert, CA, Dec 3-5, 1992.
18. Forsyth HF: Extension injuries of the cervical spine. *J Bone Joint Surg Am* 1964;46:1792-1797.
19. Marar BC: Hyperextension injuries of the cervical spine: The pathogenesis of damage to the spinal cord. *J Bone Joint Surg Am* 1974;56(8):1655-1662.
20. Kinoshita H, Hirakawa H: Pathological studies and pathological principles on the management of extension injuries of the cervical spine. *Paraplegia* 1989;27(3):172-181.
21. Kiwerski J: The influence of the mechanism of cervical spine injury on the degree of the spinal cord lesion. *Paraplegia* 1991;29(8):531-536.
22. Colachis SC Jr, Strohm BR: Radiographic studies of cervical spine motion in normal subjects: Flexion and hyperextension. *Arch Phys Med Rehabil* 1965;46(11):753-760.
23. Meyer P Jr: Cervical spine fractures: Changing management concepts, in Bridwell KJ, Dewald RL, eds: *The Textbook of Spinal Surgery*. Philadelphia, PA, JB Lippincott, 1991, p 1004.
24. Bohlman HH: Acute fractures and dislocations of the cervical spine: An analysis of three hundred hospitalized patients and review of the literature. *J Bone Joint Surg Am* 1979;61(8):1119-1142.

25. Burke DC: Hyperextension injuries of the spine. *J Bone Joint Surg Br* 1971;53(1):3-12.
26. Penning L: Prevertebral hematoma in cervical spine injury: Incidence and etiologic significance. *AJR Am J Roentgenol* 1981;136(3):553-561.
27. Edeiken-Monroe B, Wagner LK, Harris JH Jr: Hyperextension dislocation of the cervical spine. *AJR Am J Roentgenol* 1986;146(4):803-808.
28. Scher AT: Hyperextension trauma in the elderly: An easily overlooked spinal injury. *J Trauma* 1983; 23(12):1066-1068.
29. Wang JC, Hatch JD, Delamarter RB, et al: Emergent cervical flexion and extension radiographs in acutely injured patients. Presented at the *24th Annual Meeting of the Cervical Spine Research Society*. Palm Beach, FL, Dec 5-7, 1996, Abstract No. 23.
30. Benzel EC, Hart BL, Ball PA, et al: The definition of soft tissue injury associated with acute cervical spine trauma by MRI. Presented at the *20th Annual Meeting of the Cervical Spine Research Society*. Palm Desert, CA, Dec 3-5, 1992, Abstract No. 6.
31. Davis SJ, Teresi LM, Bradley WG Jr, Ziemba MA, Bloze AE: Cervical spine hyperextension injuries: MR findings. *Radiology* 1991;180(1):245-251.
32. Goldberg AL, Rothfus WE, Deeb ZL, Frankel DG, Wilberger JE Jr, Daffner RH: Hyperextension injuries of the cervical spine: Magnetic resonance findings. *Skeletal Radiol* 1989;18(4):283-288.
33. Schaefer DM, Flanders AE, Osterholm JL, Northrup BE: Prognostic significance of magnetic resonance imaging in the acute phase of cervical spine injury. *J Neurosurg* 1992;76(2):218-223.
34. Darden BV II, Connor PM: Cervical discography: Complications and clinical efficacy. Presented at the *20th Annual Meeting of the Cervical Spine Research Society*. Palm Desert, CA, Dec 3-5, 1992, Abstract No. 25.
35. McLain RF: Innervation of human cervical facets. Presented at the *20th Annual Meeting of the Cervical Spine Research Society*. Palm Desert, CA, Dec 3-5, 1992, Abstract No. 13.
36. Barnsley N, Bogduk N, Lord S, et al: Cervical zygapophysial joint pain in whiplash: A double-blind, controlled prevalence study. Presented at the *20th Annual Meeting of the Cervical Spine Research Society*. Palm Desert, CA, Dec 3-5, 1992, Abstract No. 8.
37. Panjabi MM, Lydon C, Vasavada DG, et al: Biomechanical evaluation of diagnostic external fixation. Presented at the *20th Annual Meeting of the Cervical Spine Research Society*. Palm Desert, CA, Dec 3-5, 1992, Abstract No. 19.
38. Gehweiler JA Jr, Clark WM, Schaaf RE, Powers B, Miller MD: Cervical spine trauma: The common combined conditions. *Radiology* 1979;130(1): 77-86.
39. Levine AM, Fischgrund J, Edwards CC: Fractures of the C1–2 complex: Concurrent spinal injuries. Presented at the *20th Annual Meeting of the Cervical Spine Research Society*. Palm Desert, CA, Dec 3-5, 1992, Abstract No. 50.
40. Levine AM, Lutz B: Extension teardrop injuries of the cervical spine. Presented at the *20th Annual Meeting of the Cervical Spine Research Society*. Palm Desert, CA, Dec 3-5, 1992, Abstract No. 49.
41. Kim KS, Chen HH, Russell EJ, Rogers LF: Flexion teardrop fracture of the cervical spine: Radiographic characteristics. *AJR Am J Roentgenol* 1989; 152(2):319-326.
42. Kahn EA, Schneider RC: Chronic neurological sequelae of acute trauma to the spine and spinal cord: I. The significance of the acute-flexion or tear-drop fracture-dislocation of the cervical spine. *J Bone Joint Surg Am* 1956;38-A(5): 985-997.
43. Torg JS, Pavlov H, O'Neill MJ, Nichols CE Jr, Sennett B: The axial load teardrop fracture: A biomechanical, clinical and roentgenographic analysis. *Am J Sports Med* 1991;19(4):355-364.
44. Harris JH, Yeakley JW: Hyperextension-dislocation of the cervical spine: Ligament injuries demonstrated by magnetic resonance imaging. *J Bone Joint Surg Br* 1992;74(4):567-570.
45. Lee JS, Harris JH Jr, Mueller CF: The significance of prevertebral soft tissue swelling in extension teardrop fracture of the cervical spine. *Emerg Radiol* 1997;4(3):132-139.
46. Barnes R: Paraplegia in cervical spine injuries. *J Bone Joint Surg Br* 1948;30B(2):234-244.
47. Taylor AR: The mechanism of injury to the spinal cord in the neck without damage to vertebral column. *J Bone Joint Surg Br* 1951;33-B(4):543-547.
48. McMillan BS, Silver JR: Extension injuries of the cervical spine resulting in tetraplegia. *Injury* 1987; 18(4):224-233.
49. Martin D, Schoenen J, Lenelle J, Reznik M, Moonen G: MRI-pathological correlations in acute traumatic central cord syndrome: Case report. *Neuroradiology* 1992;34(4):262-266.
50. Kinoshita H: Pathology of cervical intervertebral disc injuries. *Paraplegia* 1993;31(9):553-559.
51. Gupta SK, Rajeev K, Khosla VK, et al: Spinal cord injury without radiographic abnormality in adults. *Spinal Cord* 1999;37(10):726-729.
52. Hayashi K, Yone K, Ito H, Yanase M, Sakou T: MRI findings in patients with a cervical spinal cord injury who do not show radiographic evidence of a fracture or dislocation. *Paraplegia* 1995;33(4):212-215.

53. Kothari P, Freeman B, Grevitt M, Kerslake R: Injury to the spinal cord without radiological abnormality (SCIWORA) in adults. *J Bone Joint Surg Br* 2000;82(7):1034-1037.

54. Saruhashi Y, Hukuda S, Katsuura A, Asajima S, Omura K: Clinical outcomes of cervical spinal cord injuries without radiographic evidence of trauma. *Spinal Cord* 1998;36(8):567-573.

55. Chen TY, Lee ST, Lui TN, et al: Efficacy of surgical treatment in traumatic central cord syndrome. *Surg Neurol* 1997;48(5):435-441.

56. Schneider RC, Cherry G, Pantek H: The syndrome of acute central cervical spinal cord injury; with special reference to the mechanisms involved in hyperextension injuries of cervical spine. *J Neurosurg* 1954;11(6):546-577.

57. Tewari MK, Gifti DS, Singh P, et al: Diagnosis and prognostication of adult spinal cord injury without radiographic abnormality using magnetic resonance imaging: Analysis of 40 patients. *Surg Neurol* 2005;63(3):204-209.

58. Taylor AR, Blackwood W: Paraplegia in hyperextension cervical injuries with normal radiographic appearances. *J Bone Joint Surg Br* 1948;30B(2):245-248.

59. Hayes KC, Askes HK, Kakulas BA: Retropulsion of intervertebral discs associated with traumatic hyperextension of the cervical spine and absence of vertebral fracture: An uncommon mechanism of spinal cord injury. *Spinal Cord* 2002;40(10):544-547.

60. Matyas JR: *The Structure and Function of Tendon and Ligament Insertions into Bone*. Thesis. Ithaca, NY, Cornell University, 1985.

61. Shea M, Wittenberg RH, Edwards WT, White AA III, Hayes WC: In vitro hyperextension injuries in the human cadaveric cervical spine. *J Orthop Res* 1992;10(6):911-916.

62. Mirkovic S, Jain P, Meyer PR, et al: Cervical fractures in DISH: Surgical and clinical evaluation. Presented at the *24th Annual Meeting of the Cervical Spine Research Society*. Palm Beach, FL, Dec 5-7, 1996, Poster No. 20.

63. Ball GV: Ankylosing spondylitis, in McCarty D, ed: *Arthritis and Allied Conditions*, ed 11. Philadelphia, PA, Lea & Febiger, 1989, pp 934-941.

64. Samartzis D, Anderson DG, Shen FH: Multiple and simultaneous spine fractures in ankylosing spondylitis: Case report. *Spine (Phila Pa 1976)* 2005;30(23):E711-E715.

65. Wilkinson M, Bywaters EG: Clinical features and course of ankylosing spondylitis; as seen in a follow-up of 222 hospital referred cases. *Ann Rheum Dis* 1958;17(2):209-228.

66. Foo D, Bignami A, Rossier AB: Two spinal cord lesions in a patient with ankylosing spondylitis and cervical spine injury. *Neurology* 1983;33(2):245-249.

67. Grisolia A, Bell RL, Peltier LF: Fractures and dislocations of the spine complicating ankylosing spondylitis: A report of six cases. *J Bone Joint Surg Am* 1967;49(2):339-344.

68. Ho EK, Chan FL, Leong JC: Postsurgical recurrent stress fracture in the spine affected by ankylosing spondylitis. *Clin Orthop Relat Res* 1989;247:87-89.

69. Murray GC, Persellin RH: Cervical fracture complicating ankylosing spondylitis: A report of eight cases and review of the literature. *Am J Med* 1981;70(5):1033-1041.

70. Osgood C, Martin LG, Ackerman E: Fracture-dislocation of the cervical spine with ankylosing spondylitis: Report of two cases. *J Neurosurg* 1973;39(6):764-769.

71. Payer M: Surgical management of cervical fractures in ankylosing spondylitis using a combined posterior-anterior approach. *J Clin Neurosci* 2006;13(1):73-77.

72. Kaplan SL, Tun CG, Sarkarati M: Odontoid fracture complicating ankylosing spondylitis: A case report and review of the literature. *Spine (Phila Pa 1976)* 1990;15(6):607-610.

73. Hunter T, Dubo H: Spinal fractures complicating ankylosing spondylitis. *Ann Intern Med* 1978;88(4):546-549.

74. Harding JR, McCall IW, Park WM, Jones BF: Fracture of the cervical spine in ankylosing spondylitis. *Br J Radiol* 1985;58(685):3-7.

75. Ticó N, Ramon S, Garcia-Ortun F, et al: Traumatic spinal cord injury complicating ankylosing spondylitis. *Spinal Cord* 1998;36(5):349-352.

76. Taggard DA, Traynelis VC: Management of cervical spinal fractures in ankylosing spondylitis with posterior fixation. *Spine (Phila Pa 1976)* 2000;25(16):2035-2039.

77. Simmons EH: The surgical correction of flexion deformity of the cervical spine in ankylosing spondylitis, in Sherk HH, Dunn EJ, Eismont FJ, et al, eds: *The Cervical Spine*, ed 2. Philadelphia, PA, JB Lippincott, 1989, pp 573-598.

78. Weinstein PR, Karpman RR, Gall EP, Pitt M: Spinal cord injury, spinal fracture, and spinal stenosis in ankylosing spondylitis. *J Neurosurg* 1982;57(5):609-616.

79. Podolsky SM, Hoffman JR, Pietrafesa CA: Neurologic complications following immobilization of cervical spine fracture in a patient with ankylosing spondylitis. *Ann Emerg Med* 1983;12(9):578-580.

80. Fishman EK, Magid D, Morgan RH: Cervical fracture in ankylosing spondylitis: Value of multidimensional imaging. *Clin Imaging* 1992;16(1):31-33.

81. Fitt G, Hennessy O, Thomas D: Case report 709: Transverse fracture with epidural and small paravertebral hematomata, in a patient with ankylosing spondylitis. *Skeletal Radiol* 1992;21(1):61-63.
82. Hershman EB, Bercik RJ, Allen SC, Fielding JW: Correction of chin-on-chest deformity in ankylosing spondylitis through a fracture site: A case report. *Clin Orthop Relat Res* 1985;201:201-204.
83. Apple DF Jr, Anson C: Spinal cord injury occurring in patients with ankylosing spondylitis: A multicenter study. *Orthopedics* 1995;18(10):1005-1011.
84. Graham B, Van Peteghem PK: Fractures of the spine in ankylosing spondylitis: Diagnosis, treatment, and complications. *Spine (Phila Pa 1976)* 1989;14(8):803-807.
85. Hunter T, Dubo HI: Spinal fractures complicating ankylosing spondylitis: A long-term followup study. *Arthritis Rheum* 1983;26(6):751-759.
86. Böhler J, Gaudernak T: Anterior plate stabilization for fracture-dislocations of the lower cervical spine. *J Trauma* 1980;20(3):203-205.
87. Detwiler KN, Loftus CM, Godersky JC, Menezes AH: Management of cervical spine injuries in patients with ankylosing spondylitis. *J Neurosurg* 1990;72(2):210-215.
88. Fox MW, Onofrio BM, Kilgore JE: Neurological complications of ankylosing spondylitis. *J Neurosurg* 1993;78(6):871-878.
89. Rowed DW: Management of cervical spinal cord injury in ankylosing spondylitis: The intervertebral disc as a cause of cord compression. *J Neurosurg* 1992;77(2):241-246.
90. Penning L: Some aspects of plain radiography of the cervical spine in chronic myelopathy. *Neurology* 1962;12:513-519.
91. Bailes JE, Hadley MN, Quigley MR, Sonntag VK, Cerullo LJ: Management of athletic injuries of the cervical spine and spinal cord. *Neurosurgery* 1991;29(4):491-497.
92. Torg JS, Pavlov H, Genuario SE, et al: Neurapraxia of the cervical spinal cord with transient quadriplegia. *J Bone Joint Surg Am* 1986;68(9):1354-1370.
93. Hinck VC, Hopkins CE, Savara BS: Sagittal diameter of the cervical spinal canal in children. *Radiology* 1962;79:97-108.
94. Cheng CL, Wolf AL, Mirvis S, Robinson WL: Bodysurfing accidents resulting in cervical spinal injuries. *Spine (Phila Pa 1976)* 1992;17(3):257-260.
95. Epstein JA, Carras R, Hyman RA, Costa S: Cervical myelopathy caused by developmental stenosis of the spinal canal. *J Neurosurg* 1979;51(3):362-367.
96. Ladd AL, Scranton PE: Congenital cervical stenosis presenting as transient quadriplegia in athletes: Report of two cases. *J Bone Joint Surg Am* 1986;68(9):1371-1374.
97. Ohwada T, Tachibana S, Wada K, et al: Cervical myelopathy due to developmental stenosis of the spinal canal. *Orthop Trans* 1978;2:32.
98. Scher AT: Diversity of radiological features in hyperextension injury of the cervical spine. *S Afr Med J* 1980;58(1):27-30.
99. Starshak RJ, Kass GA, Samaraweera RN: Developmental stenosis of the cervical spine in children. *Pediatr Radiol* 1987;17(4):291-295.
100. Scher AT: Cervical spine fusion and the effects of injury. *S Afr Med J* 1979;56(13):525-527.
101. Maroon JC: 'Burning hands' in football spinal cord injuries. *JAMA* 1977;238(19):2049-2051.
102. Speer KP, Bassett FH III: The prolonged burner syndrome. *Am J Sports Med* 1990;18(6):591-594.
103. Stanley JH, Schabel SI, Frey GD, Hungerford GD: Quantitative analysis of the cervical spinal canal by computed tomography. *Neuroradiology* 1986;28(2):139-143.
104. Torg JS, Vegso JJ, Sennett B, Das M: The National Football Head and Neck Injury Registry: 14-year report on cervical quadriplegia, 1971 through 1984. *JAMA* 1985;254(24):3439-3443.
105. Breig A, Turnbull I, Hassler O: Effects of mechanical stresses on the spinal cord in cervical spondylosis: A study on fresh cadaver material. *J Neurosurg* 1966;25(1):45-56.
106. Torg JS, Thibault LE, Sennett B, Pavlov H: The Nicolas Andry Award: The pathomechanics and pathophysiology of cervical spinal cord injury. *Clin Orthop Relat Res* 1995;321:259-269.
107. Andrews FJ: Transient cervical neurapraxia associated with cervical spine stenosis. *Emerg Med J* 2002;19(2):172-173.
108. Herzog RJ, Wiens JJ, Dillingham MF, Sontag MJ: Normal cervical spine morphometry and cervical spinal stenosis in asymptomatic professional football players: Plain film radiography, multiplanar computed tomography, and magnetic resonance imaging. *Spine (Phila Pa 1976)* 1991;16(6, Suppl):S178-S186.
109. Torg JS, Corcoran TA, Thibault LE, et al: Cervical cord neurapraxia: Classification, pathomechanics, morbidity, and management guidelines. *J Neurosurg* 1997;87(6):843-850.
110. Torg JS, Naranja RJ Jr, Pavlov H, Galinat BJ, Warren R, Stine RA: The relationship of developmental narrowing of the cervical spinal canal to reversible and irreversible injury of the cervical spinal cord in football players. *J Bone Joint Surg Am* 1996;78(9):1308-1314.

111. Eismont FJ, Clifford S, Goldberg M, Green B: Cervical sagittal spinal canal size in spine injury. *Spine (Phila Pa 1976)* 1984;9(7):663-666.

112. Matsuura P, Waters RL, Adkins RH, Rothman S, Gurbani N, Sie I: Comparison of computerized tomography parameters of the cervical spine in normal control subjects and spinal cord-injured patients. *J Bone Joint Surg Am* 1989;71(2): 183-188.

113. Boockvar JA, Durham SR, Sun PP: Cervical spinal stenosis and sports-related cervical cord neurapraxia in children. *Spine (Phila Pa 1976)* 2001;26(24):2709-2713.

114. Epstein NE: Laminectomy for cervical myelopathy. *Spinal Cord* 2003;41(6):317-327.

115. Carter DR, Frankel VH: Biomechanics of hyperextension injuries to the cervical spine in football. *Am J Sports Med* 1980;8(5):302-309.

116. Scher AT: Serious cervical spine injury in the older rugby player: An indication for routine radiological examination. *S Afr Med J* 1983;64(4): 138-140.

117. Smith JP, Morrissey P, Hemmick RS, Haas AF, Bodai BI: Retropharyngeal hematomas. *J Trauma* 1988;28(4):553-554.

118. Howcroft AJ, Jenkins DH: Potentially fatal asphyxia following a minor injury of the cervical spine. *J Bone Joint Surg Br* 1977;59(1):93-94.

119. Agha FP, Raji MR: Oesophageal perforation with fracture dislocation of cervical spine due to hyperextension injury. *Br J Radiol* 1982;55(653): 369-372.

120. Latimer EA III, Clevenger FW, Osler TM: Tear of the cervical esophagus following hyperextension from manual traction: Case report. *J Trauma* 1991;31(10):1448-1449.

121. Robinson MH, Young JD, Burge PD: Retropharyngeal abscess, airway obstruction, and tetraplegia after hyperextension injury of the cervical spine: Case report. *J Trauma* 1992;32(1):107-109.

122. Stringer WL, Kelly DL Jr: Traumatic dissection of the extracranial internal carotid artery. *Neurosurgery* 1980;6(2):123-130.

123. Edwards WC, LaRocca H: The developmental segmental sagittal diameter of the cervical spinal canal in patients with cervical spondylosis. *Spine (Phila Pa 1976)* 1983;8(1):20-27.

124. Hayashi H, Okada K, Hamada M, Tada K, Ueno R: Etiologic factors of myelopathy: A radiographic evaluation of the aging changes in the cervical spine. *Clin Orthop Relat Res* 1987;214:200-209.

125. Murone I: The importance of the sagittal diameters of the cervical spinal canal in relation to spondylosis and myelopathy. *J Bone Joint Surg Br* 1974;56(1):30-36.

126. Yue WM, Tan SB, Tan MH, Koh DC, Tan CT: The Torg-Pavlov ratio in cervical spondylotic myelopathy: A comparative study between patients with cervical spondylotic myelopathy and a nonspondylotic, nonmyelopathic population. *Spine (Phila Pa 1976)* 2001;26(16):1760-1764.

127. Launay F, Leet AI, Sponseller PD: Pediatric spinal cord injury without radiographic abnormality: A meta-analysis. *Clin Orthop Relat Res* 2005;433: 166-170.

128. Grabb PA, Pang D: Magnetic resonance imaging in the evaluation of spinal cord injury without radiographic abnormality in children. *Neurosurgery* 1994;35(3):406-414.

129. Pang D, Wilberger JE Jr: Spinal cord injury without radiographic abnormalities in children. *J Neurosurg* 1982;57(1):114-129.

130. Dare AO, Dias MS, Li V: Magnetic resonance imaging correlation in pediatric spinal cord injury without radiographic abnormality. *J Neurosurg* 2002;97(1, Suppl):33-39.

131. Grabb PA, Albright AL: Spinal cord injury without radiographic abnormality in children, in Wilkins RH, Rengachari SS, eds: *Neurosurgery*, ed 2. New York, NY, McGraw Hill Publications, 1996, pp 2667-2670.

132. Pang D, Sahrarkar K, Sun PP: Pediatric spinal cord and vertebral column injuries, in Youman JR, ed: *Neurological Surgery*, ed 4. Philadelphia, PA, WB Saunders, 1996, pp 1991-2037.

133. Burke DC: Traumatic spinal paralysis in children. *Paraplegia* 1974;11(4):268-276.

134. Kokoska ER, Keller MS, Rallo MC, Weber TR: Characteristics of pediatric cervical spine injuries. *J Pediatr Surg* 2001;36(1):100-105.

135. Kriss VM, Kriss TC: SCIWORA (spinal cord injury without radiographic abnormality) in infants and children. *Clin Pediatr (Phila)* 1996;35(3): 119-124.

136. Pang D, Pollack IF: Spinal cord injury without radiographic abnormality in children—the SCIWORA syndrome. *J Trauma* 1989;29(5): 654-664.

137. Pollack IF, Pang D: Spinal cord injury without radiographic abnormality (SCIWORA), in Pang D, ed: *Disorders of the Pediatric Spine*. New York, NY, Raven Press, 1995, pp 509-516.

138. Pang D: Spinal cord injury without radiographic abnormality in children, 2 decades later. *Neurosurgery* 2004;55(6):1325-1343.

139. Hill SA, Miller CA, Kosnik EJ, Hunt WE: Pediatric neck injuries: A clinical study. *J Neurosurg* 1984;60(4):700-706.

140. Ruge JR, Sinson GP, McLone DG, Cerullo LJ: Pediatric spinal injury: The very young. *J Neurosurg* 1988;68(1):25-30.

141. Orenstein JB, Klein BL, Ochsenschlager DW: Delayed diagnosis of pediatric cervical spine injury. *Pediatrics* 1992;89(6 Pt 2):1185-1188.

142. Dietrich AM, Ginn-Pease ME, Bartkowski HM, King DR: Pediatric cervical spine fractures: Predominantly subtle presentation. *J Pediatr Surg* 1991;26(8):995-1000.

143. Cattell HS, Filtzer DL: Pseudosubluxation and other normal variations in the cervical spine in children: A study of one hundred and sixty children. *J Bone Joint Surg Am* 1965;47(7):1295-1309.

144. Henrys P, Lyne ED, Lifton C, Salciccioli G: Clinical review of cervical spine injuries in children. *Clin Orthop Relat Res* 1977;129:172-176.

145. Bailey DK: The normal cervical spine in infants and children. *Radiology* 1952;59(5):712-719.

146. Fesmire FM, Luten RC: The pediatric cervical spine: Developmental anatomy and clinical aspects. *J Emerg Med* 1989;7(2):133-142.

147. Sullivan CR, Bruwer AJ, Harris LE: Hypermobility of the cervical spine in children; a pitfall in the diagnosis of cervical dislocation. *Am J Surg* 1958; 95(4):636-640.

148. Braakman R, Penning L: *Injuries of the Cervical Spine*. Amsterdam, The Netherlands, Excerpta Medica, 1971.

149. Toendury G: The cervical spine, its development and changes during life. *Acta Orthop Belg* 1959; 25:602-626.

150. Pang D, Wilberger JE Jr: Traumatic atlanto-occipital dislocation with survival: Case report and review. *Neurosurgery* 1980;7(5):503-508.

151. Aufdermaur M: Spinal injuries in juveniles: Necropsy findings in twelve cases. *J Bone Joint Surg Br* 1974;56B(3):513-519.

152. Bracken MB, Shepard MJ, Collins WF, et al: A randomized, controlled trial of methylprednisolone or naloxone in the treatment of acute spinal-cord injury: Results of the Second National Acute Spinal Cord Injury Study. *N Engl J Med* 1990; 322(20):1405-1411.

153. Yamaguchi S, Hida K, Akino M, Yano S, Saito H, Iwasaki Y: A case of pediatric thoracic SCIWORA following minor trauma. *Childs Nerv Syst* 2002; 18(5):241-243.

154. Graber MA, Kathol M: Cervical spine radiographs in the trauma patient. *Am Fam Physician* 1999; 59(2):331-342.

155. Kulkarni MV, McArdle CB, Kopanicky D, et al: Acute spinal cord injury: MR imaging at 1.5 T. *Radiology* 1987;164(3):837-843.

156. Marinier M, Rodts MF, Connolly M: Spinal cord injury without radiographic abnormality (SCIWORA). *Orthop Nurs* 1997;16(5):57-65.

157. Osenbach RK, Menezes AH: Spinal cord injury without radiographic abnormality in children. *Pediatr Neurosci* 1989;15(4):168-175.

158. Lang SM, Bernardo LM: SCIWORA syndrome: Nursing assessment. *Dimens Crit Care Nurs* 1993; 12(5):247-254.

159. Bosch PP, Vogt MT, Ward WT: Pediatric spinal cord injury without radiographic abnormality (SCIWORA): The absence of occult instability and lack of indication for bracing. *Spine (Phila Pa 1976)* 2002;27(24):2788-2800.

160. Dickman CA, Zabramski JM, Hadley MN, Rekate HL, Sonntag VK: Pediatric spinal cord injury without radiographic abnormalities: Report of 26 cases and review of the literature. *J Spinal Disord* 1991;4(3):296-305.

161. Turgut M, Akpinar G, Akalan N, Ozcan OE: Spinal injuries in the pediatric age group: A review of 82 cases of spinal cord and vertebral column injuries. *Eur Spine J* 1996;5(3):148-152.

162. Schofferman J, Bogduk N, Slosar P: Chronic whiplash and whiplash-associated disorders: An evidence-based approach. *J Am Acad Orthop Surg* 2007;15(10):596-606.

163. Spitzer WO, Skovron ML, Salmi LR, et al: Scientific monograph of the Quebec Task Force on Whiplash-Associated Disorders: Redefining "whiplash" and its management. *Spine (Phila Pa 1976)* 1995;20(8, Suppl)1S-73S.

164. Bogduk N, Yoganandan N: Biomechanics of the cervical spine: Part 3. Minor injuries. *Clin Biomech (Bristol, Avon)* 2001;16(4):267-275.

165. Radanov BP, Sturzenegger M, Di Stefano G: Long-term outcome after whiplash injury: A 2-year follow-up considering features of injury mechanism and somatic, radiologic, and psychosocial findings. *Medicine (Baltimore)* 1995;74(5): 281-297.

166. Gozzard C, Bannister G, Langkamer G, Khan S, Gargan M, Foy C: Factors affecting employment after whiplash injury. *J Bone Joint Surg Br* 2001; 83(4):506-509.

167. Berglund A, Alfredsson L, Cassidy JD, Jensen I, Nygren A: The association between exposure to a rear-end collision and future neck or shoulder pain: A cohort study. *J Clin Epidemiol* 2000; 53(11):1089-1094.

168. Rodriquez AA, Barr KP, Burns SP: Whiplash: Pathophysiology, diagnosis, treatment, and prognosis. *Muscle Nerve* 2004;29(6):768-781.

169. Barnsley L, Bogduk N: Medial branch blocks are specific for the diagnosis of cervical zygoapophyseal joint pain. *Reg Anesth* 1993;18(6):343-350.

170. Côté P, Cassidy JD, Carroll L, Frank JW, Bombardier C: A systematic review of the prognosis of acute whiplash and a new conceptual framework

to synthesize the literature. *Spine (Phila Pa 1976)* 2001;26(19):E445-E458.

171. Scholten-Peeters GG, Verhagen AP, Bekkering GE, et al: Prognostic factors of whiplash-associated disorders: A systematic review of prospective cohort studies. *Pain* 2003;104(1-2):303-322.

172. Giannoudis PV, Mehta SS, Tsiridis E: Incidence and outcome of whiplash injury after multiple trauma. *Spine (Phila Pa 1976)* 2007;32(7): 776-781.

173. Krafft M, Kullgren A, Tingvall C, Boström O, Fredriksson R: How crash severity in rear impacts influences short- and long-term consequences to the neck. *Accid Anal Prev* 2000;32(2):187-195.

174. Centeno CJ, Freeman M, Elkins WL: A review of the literature refuting the concept of minor impact soft tissue injury. *Pain Res Manag* 2005;10(2): 71-74.

175. Brault JR, Wheeler JB, Siegmund GP, Brault EJ: Clinical response of human subjects to rear-end automobile collisions. *Arch Phys Med Rehabil* 1998;79(1):72-80.

176. Severy DM, Mathewson JH, Bechtol CO: Controlled automobile rearend collisions, an investigation of related engineering and medical phenomena. *Can Serv Med J* 1955;11(10):727-759.

177. Olney DB, Marsden AK: The effect of head restraints and seat belts on the incidence of neck injury in car accidents. *Injury* 1986;17(6): 365-367.

178. Williams JF, McKenzie JA: The effect of collision severity on the motion of the head and neck during "whiplash." *J Biomech* 1975;8(3-4):257-259.

179. Macnab I: Acceleration injuries of the cervical spine. *J Bone Joint Surg Am* 1964;46:1797-1799.

180. La Rocca H: Cervical sprain syndrome-diagnosis, treatment, and long-term outcome, in Frymoyer JW, ed: *The Adult Spine: Principles and Practice*. New York, NY, Raven Press, 1991, pp 31-41.

181. Hohl M: Soft-tissue injuries of the neck in automobile accidents: Factors influencing prognosis. *J Bone Joint Surg Am* 1974;56(8):1675-1682.

182. Boismare F, Boquet J, Moore N, Chretien P, Saligaut C, Daoust M: Hemodynamic, behavioral and biochemical disturbances induced by an experimental cranio-cervical injury (whiplash) in rats. *J Auton Nerv Syst* 1985;13(2):137-147.

183. Liu YK, Chandran KB, Heath RG, Unterharnscheidt F: Subcortical EEG changes in rhesus monkeys following experimental hyperextension-hyperflexion (whiplash). *Spine (Phila Pa 1976)* 1984;9(4):329-338.

184. Ito S, Ivancic PC, Panjabi MM, Cunningham BW: Soft tissue injury threshold during simulated whiplash: A biomechanical investigation. *Spine (Phila Pa 1976)* 2004;29(9):979-987.

185. Schofferman J, Garges K, Goldthwaite N, Koestler M, Libby E: Upper cervical anterior diskectomy and fusion improves discogenic cervical headaches. *Spine (Phila Pa 1976)* 2002;27(20): 2240-2244.

186. Lord SM, Barnsley L, Wallis BJ, Bogduk N: Third occipital nerve headache: A prevalence study. *J Neurol Neurosurg Psychiatry* 1994;57(10): 1187-1190.

187. Chen TY: The clinical presentation of uppermost cervical disc protrusion *Spine (Phila Pa 1976)* 2000;25(4):438-442.

188. Maimaris C, Barnes MR, Allen MJ: 'Whiplash injuries' of the neck: A retrospective study. *Injury* 1988;19(6):393-396.

189. Pearce JM: Whiplash injury: A reappraisal. *J Neurol Neurosurg Psychiatry* 1989;52(12): 1329-1331.

190. Slipman CW, Plastaras C, Patel R, et al: Provocative cervical discography symptom mapping. *Spine J* 2005;5(4):381-388.

191. Schellhas KP, Garvey TA, Johnson BA, Rothbart PJ, Pollei SR: Cervical diskography: Analysis of provoked responses at C2-C3, C3-C4, and C4-C5. *AJNR Am J Neuroradiol* 2000;21(2): 269-275.

192. Dwyer A, Aprill C, Bogduk N: Cervical zygapophyseal joint pain patterns: I. A study in normal volunteers. *Spine (Phila Pa 1976)* 1990;15(6): 453-457.

193. Cooper G, Bailey B, Bogduk N: Cervical zygapophysial joint pain maps. *Pain Med* 2007;8(4): 344-353.

194. Gorski JM, Schwartz LH: Shoulder impingement presenting as neck pain. *J Bone Joint Surg Am* 2003;85-A(4):635-638.

195. Chauhan SK, Peckham T, Turner R: Impingement syndrome associated with whiplash injury. *J Bone Joint Surg Br* 2003;85(3):408-410.

196. Janecki CJ Jr, Lipke JM: Whiplash syndrome. *Am Fam Physician* 1978;17(4):144-151.

197. Stringer WL, Kelly DL Jr, Johnston FR, Holliday RH: Hyperextension injury of the cervical spine with esophageal perforation: Case report. *J Neurosurg* 1980;53(4):541-543.

198. Schuyler-Hacker H, Green R, Wingate L, Sklar J: Acute torticollis secondary to rupture of the sternocleidomastoid. *Arch Phys Med Rehabil* 1989; 70(12):851-853.

199. Heise AP, Laskin DM, Gervin AS: Incidence of temporomandibular joint symptoms following whiplash injury. *J Oral Maxillofac Surg* 1992; 50(8):825-828.

200. Weinberg S, Lapointe H: Cervical extension-flexion injury (whiplash) and internal

derangement of the temporomandibular joint. *J Oral Maxillofac Surg* 1987;45(8):653-656.

201. Chester JB Jr: Whiplash, postural control, and the inner ear. *Spine (Phila Pa 1976)* 1991;16(7): 716-720.
202. Capistrant TD: Thoracic outlet syndrome in whiplash injury. *Ann Surg* 1977;185(2):175-178.
203. Kelley JS, Hoover RE, George T: Whiplash maculopathy. *Arch Ophthalmol* 1978;96(5):834-835.
204. Kischka U, Ettlin T, Heim S, Schmid G: Cerebral symptoms following whiplash injury. *Eur Neurol* 1991;31(3):136-140.
205. McClune T, Burton AK, Waddell G: Whiplash associated disorders: A review of the literature to guide patient information and advice. *Emerg Med J* 2002;19(6):499-506.
206. Bogduk N: The neck. *Baillieres Clin Rheumatol* 1999;13(2):261-285.
207. Kasch H, Bach FW, Jensen TS: Handicap after acute whiplash injury: A 1-year prospective study of risk factors. *Neurology* 2001;56(12):1637-1643.
208. Kasch H, Stengaard-Pedersen K, Arendt-Nielsen L, Staehelin Jensen T: Pain thresholds and tenderness in neck and head following acute whiplash injury: A prospective study. *Cephalalgia* 2001; 21(3):189-197.
209. Lord SM, Barnsley L, Wallis BJ, Bogduk N: Chronic cervical zygapophysial joint pain after whiplash: A placebo-controlled prevalence study. *Spine (Phila Pa 1976)* 1996;21(15):1737-1745.
210. Barnsley L, Lord SM, Wallis BJ, Bogduk N: The prevalence of chronic cervical zygapophysial joint pain after whiplash. *Spine (Phila Pa 1976)* 1995; 20(1):20-26.
211. Bogduk N, Aprill C: On the nature of neck pain, discography and cervical zygapophysial joint blocks. *Pain* 1993;54(2):213-217.
212. Barnsley L, Lord S, Bogduk N: Whiplash injury. *Pain* 1994;58(3):283-307.
213. Cusick JF, Pintar FA, Yoganandan N: Whiplash syndrome: Kinematic factors influencing pain patterns. *Spine (Phila Pa 1976)* 2001;26(11): 1252-1258.
214. Davis CG: Injury threshold: Whiplash-associated disorders. *J Manipulative Physiol Ther* 2000;23(6): 420-427.
215. Grauer JN, Panjabi MM, Cholewicki J, Nibu K, Dvorak J: Whiplash produces an S-shaped curvature of the neck with hyperextension at lower levels. *Spine (Phila Pa 1976)* 1997;22(21): 2489-2494.
216. Jónsson H Jr, Cesarini K, Sahlstedt B, Rauschning W: Findings and outcome in whiplash-type neck distortions. *Spine (Phila Pa 1976)* 1994;19(24): 2733-2743.
217. Kullgren A, Krafft M, Nygren A, Tingvall C: Neck injuries in frontal impacts: Influence of crash pulse characteristics on injury risk. *Accid Anal Prev* 2000;32(2):197-205.
218. Panjabi MM, Cholewicki J, Nibu K, Grauer JN, Babat LB, Dvorak J: Mechanism of whiplash injury. *Clin Biomech (Bristol, Avon)* 1998;13(4-5): 239-249.
219. Kaneoka K, Ono K, Inami S, Hayashi K: Motion analysis of cervical vertebrae during whiplash loading. *Spine (Phila Pa 1976)* 1999;24(8): 763-770.
220. Siegmund GP, Myers BS, Davis MB, Bohnet HF, Winkelstein BA: Mechanical evidence of cervical facet capsule injury during whiplash: A cadaveric study using combined shear, compression, and extension loading. *Spine (Phila Pa 1976)* 2001; 26(19):2095-2101.
221. Thunberg J, Hellström F, Sjölander P, Bergenheim M, Wenngren B, Johansson H: Influences on the fusimotor-muscle spindle system from chemosensitive nerve endings in cervical facet joints in the cat: Possible implications for whiplash induced disorders. *Pain* 2001;91(1-2):15-22.
222. Grubb SA, Kelly CK: Cervical discography: Clinical implications from 12 years of experience. *Spine (Phila Pa 1976)* 2000;25(11):1382-1389.
223. Hendriks EJ, Scholten-Peeters GG, van der Windt DA, Neeleman-van der Steen CW, Oostendorp RA, Verhagen AP: Prognostic factors for poor recovery in acute whiplash patients. *Pain* 2005; 114(3):408-416.
224. Côté P, Hogg-Johnson S, Cassidy JD, Carroll L, Frank JW, Bombardier C: Early aggressive care and delayed recovery from whiplash: Isolated finding or reproducible result? *Arthritis Rheum* 2007;57(5):861-868.
225. Williamson E, Williams M, Gates S, Lamb SE: A systematic literature review of psychological factors and the development of late whiplash syndrome. *Pain* 2008;135(1-2):20-30.
226. Allen M, Barron S, Broudo M, et al: *British Columbia Whiplash Initiative–A Comprehensive Syllabus*. Vancouver, BC, Physical Medicine Research Foundation, 1997.
227. Peeters GG, Verhagen AP, de Bie RA, Oostendorp RA: The efficacy of conservative treatment in patients with whiplash injury: A systematic review of clinical trials. *Spine (Phila Pa 1976)* 2001;26(4): E64-E73.
228. Rosenfeld M, Gunnarsson R, Borenstein P: Early intervention in whiplash-associated disorders: A comparison of two treatment protocols. *Spine (Phila Pa 1976)* 2000;25(14):1782-1787.
229. Söderlund A, Olerud C, Lindberg P: Acute whiplash-associated disorders (WAD): The effects of early mobilization and prognostic factors in

long-term symptomatology. *Clin Rehabil* 2000; 14(5):457-467.

230. Eck JC, Hodges SD, Humphreys SC: Whiplash: A review of a commonly misunderstood injury. *Am J Med* 2001;110(8):651-656.

231. Sterner Y, Löfgren M, Nyberg V, Karlsson AK, Bergström M, Gerdle B: Early interdisciplinary rehabilitation programme for whiplash associated disorders. *Disabil Rehabil* 2001;23(10):422-429.

232. Goodman R, Frew LJ: Effectiveness of progressive strength resistance training for whiplash: A pilot study. *Physiother Can* 2000;52:211-214.

233. Borchgrevink GE, Kaasa A, McDonagh D, Stiles TC, Haraldseth O, Lereim I: Acute treatment of whiplash neck sprain injuries: A randomized trial of treatment during the first 14 days after a car accident. *Spine (Phila Pa 1976)* 1998;23(1):25-31.

234. Berg HE, Berggren G, Tesch PA: Dynamic neck strength training effect on pain and function. *Arch Phys Med Rehabil* 1994;75(6):661-665.

235. Highland TR, Dreisinger TE, Vie LL, Russell GS: Changes in isometric strength and range of motion of the isolated cervical spine after eight weeks of clinical rehabilitation. *Spine (Phila Pa 1976)* 1992;17(6, Suppl):S77-S82.

236. Jordan A, Bendix T, Nielsen H, Hansen FR, Høst D, Winkel A: Intensive training, physiotherapy, or manipulation for patients with chronic neck pain: A prospective, single-blinded, randomized clinical trial. *Spine (Phila Pa 1976)* 1998;23(3):311-319.

237. Levoska S, Keinänen-Kiukaanniemi S: Active or passive physiotherapy for occupational cervicobrachial disorders? A comparison of two treatment methods with a 1-year follow-up. *Arch Phys Med Rehabil* 1993;74(4):425-430.

238. Randløv A, Ostergaard M, Manniche C, et al: Intensive dynamic training for females with chronic neck/shoulder pain: A randomized controlled trial. *Clin Rehabil* 1998;12(3):200-210.

239. Viljanen M, Malmivaara A, Uitti J, Rinne M, Palmroos P, Laippala P: Effectiveness of dynamic muscle training, relaxation training, or ordinary activity for chronic neck pain: Randomised controlled trial. *BMJ* 2003;327(7413):475.

240. Kay TM, Gross A, Goldsmith C, et al: Exercises for mechanical neck disorders. *Cochrane Database Syst Rev* 2005;3(3):CD004250.

241. Chiu TT, Lam TH, Hedley AJ: A randomized controlled trial on the efficacy of exercise for patients with chronic neck pain. *Spine (Phila Pa 1976)* 2005;30(1):E1-E7.

242. Ylinen J, Takala EP, Nykänen M, et al: Active neck muscle training in the treatment of chronic neck pain in women: A randomized controlled trial. *JAMA* 2003;289(19):2509-2516.

243. Gennis P, Miller L, Gallagher EJ, Giglio J, Carter W, Nathanson N: The effect of soft cervical collars on persistent neck pain in patients with whiplash injury. *Acad Emerg Med* 1996;3(6): 568-573.

244. Gross AR, Aker PD, Goldsmith CH, Peloso P: Physical medicine modalities for mechanical neck disorders. *Cochrane Database Syst Rev* 2000;(2): CD000961.

245. Mealy K, Brennan H, Fenelon GC: Early mobilization of acute whiplash injuries. *Br Med J (Clin Res Ed)* 1986;292(6521):656-657.

246. Peloso PM, Gross AR, Haines TA, Trinh K, Goldsmith CH, Aker P: Medicinal and injection therapies for mechanical neck disorders: A Cochrane systematic review. *J Rheumatol* 2006;33(5): 957-967.

247. Lord SM, Barnsley L, Wallis BJ, McDonald GJ, Bogduk N: Percutaneous radio-frequency neurotomy for chronic cervical zygapophyseal-joint pain. *N Engl J Med* 1996;335(23):1721-1726.

248. McDonald GJ, Lord SM, Bogduk N: Long-term follow-up of patients treated with cervical radiofrequency neurotomy for chronic neck pain. *Neurosurgery* 1999;45(1):61-68.

249. Gross AR, Hoving JL, Haines TA, et al: A Cochrane review of manipulation and mobilization for mechanical neck disorders. *Spine (Phila Pa 1976)* 2004;29(14):1541-1548.

250. Hoving JL, Koes BW, de Vet HC, et al: Manual therapy, physical therapy, or continued care by a general practitioner for patients with neck pain: A randomized, controlled trial. *Ann Intern Med* 2002;136(10):713-722.

251. Baker RP, Grubb RL Jr: Complete fracture-dislocation of cervical spine without permanent neurological sequelae: Case report. *J Neurosurg* 1983;58(5):760-762.

252. Pitman MI, Pitman CA, Greenberg IM: Complete dislocation of the cervical spine without neurological deficit: A case report. *J Bone Joint Surg Am* 1977;59(1):134-135.

253. Scher AT: Dislocation of the cervical spine—a rare manifestation of hyperextension injury: A report of 2 cases. *S Afr Med J* 1979;55(24):998-999.

CHAPTER 29
Compression Fractures of the Thoracic and Lumbar Spine

Michael Linn, MD Choll W. Kim, MD, PhD Mark Valente, DO

Key Points

- Most thoracic and lumbar compression fractures without posterior osseoligamentous injury are stable and can be treated nonsurgically.
- Surgical treatment is reserved for pain and disability due to kyphosis that results in sagittal imbalance.
- Late pain due to vertebral compression fractures often occurs in the low back as a result of compensatory hyperlordosis of the lumbar spine.
- Surgical treatment is most common for painful osteoporotic compression fractures and pathologic fractures due to malignancy.
- Posterior vertebral resection osteotomies are useful for treatment of symptomatic focal kyphosis in patients who cannot tolerate anterior exposures.
- Minimally invasive treatment options, such as percutaneous cement augmentation and thoracoscopic surgery, are available to hasten recovery in older, frail patients.

Introduction

Compression wedge fractures account for the vast majority of osseous injuries of the thoracolumbar spine. In their study of 2,404 blunt trauma patients, Holmes et al[1] found that the thoracolumbar junction is the most commonly injured area in the thoracic and lumbar spine. Compression fractures were the most common injury in the thoracic spine (52%) and were second only to transverse process fractures (37% versus 31%) in the lumbar spine. The injury mechanism involves a combination of forward flexion and axial compressive loading, producing a characteristic wedge-shaped vertebral deformity.

Prior to the use of axial CT imaging of the spine, all fractures resulting from spinal compression had been grouped similarly. Little emphasis was placed on the presence or absence of retropulsed bony fragments within the vertebral canal.[2-5] With improved spinal imaging modalities, newer classification systems have been developed for spinal trauma.[4-8] Pure compression fractures are now frequently defined as isolated failure of the anterior column in compression. Flexion forces compress the anterior column of the spine while creating tensile forces in the ligaments of the posterior column. The middle column is often intact and thus the neurologic elements are spared injury.[9] This chapter focuses on vertebral compression fractures without posterior column injury in terms of their etiology, biomechanical principles, treatment, and prognosis.

Etiology

Violent trauma is the most common cause of compression fractures in young and middle-aged people. Motor vehicle accidents and vertical plunges represent the largest sources, followed by sports and recreational activities.[9-24] A high incidence of compression fractures (up to 30%) is seen in airplane pilots after use of an ejection seat.[25-27] In the elderly, osteoporosis is the most common cause of simple wedge compression fractures of the spine.[28-32] Patients with osteoporotic bone may suffer from injury with only minor trauma and even with bending forward or lifting.

Although the thoracolumbar junction is the most frequently affected area in spinal compression injuries, certain injury mechanisms have a predilection for specific spinal levels. For example, falling onto the buttocks, as occurs in parachute landings, most commonly results in L1 vertebral body fractures.[33-35] Flexion-compression injuries from aircraft ejections most commonly involve the

Dr. Kim or an immediate family member serves as a board member, owner, officer, or committee member of Society for Minimally-Invasive Spine Surgery; has received royalties from Hydrocision; is a member of a speakers' bureau or has made paid presentations on behalf of Globus Medical, Synthes, and Spineview; serves as a paid consultant to or is an employee of Globus Medical, Synthes, and Spineview; and owns stock or stock options in Globus Medical. Dr. Valente or an immediate family member serves as a paid consultant to or is an employee of Surgical Salient Technologies. Neither Dr. Linn nor any immediate family member has received anything of value from or owns stock in a commercial company or institution related directly or indirectly to the subject of this chapter.

FIGURE 1

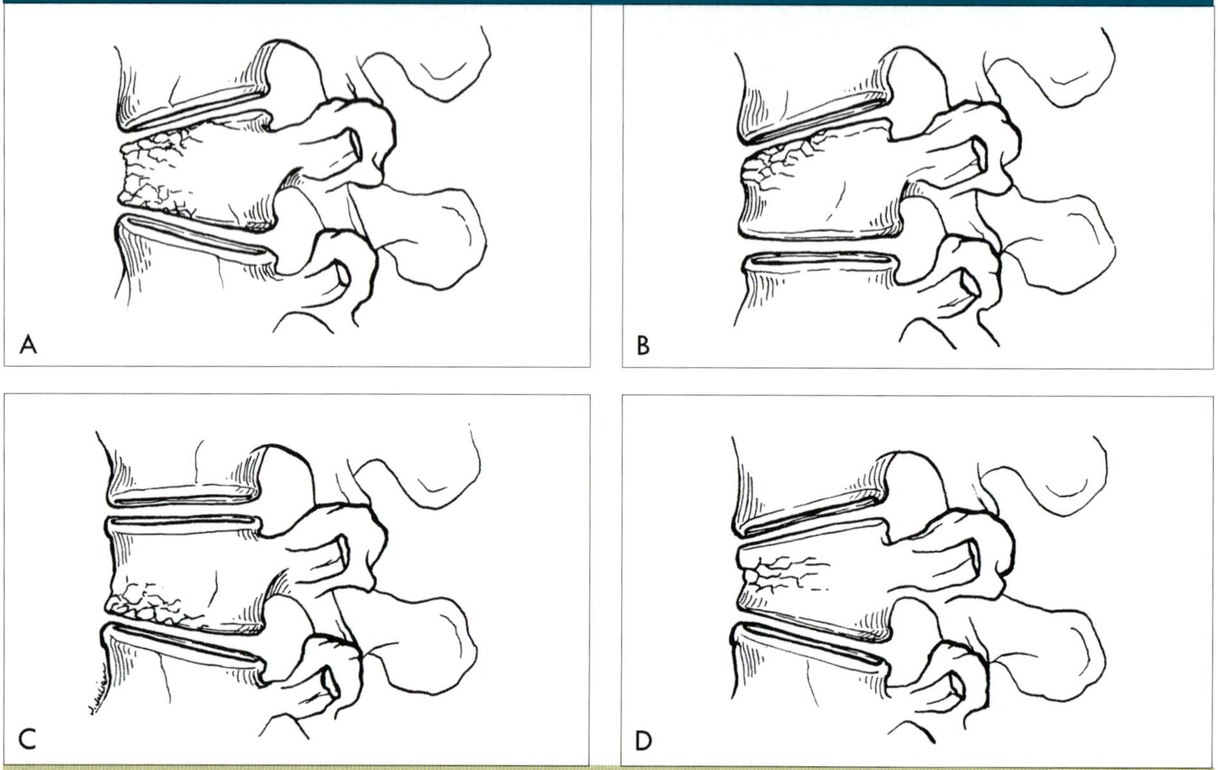

Figure 1 Four subtypes of wedge compression fractures as described by Denis.[7] **Type A** involves a fracture of the superior and inferior end plates. **Type B,** the most common type, involves failure of the superior vertebral end plate with compression of a portion of the superior one-half of the anterior vertebral body. **Type C** is an isolated failure of the inferior end plate with involvement of the inferior half of the vertebral body. **Type D** results in failure of the central aspect of the anterior body with relative preservation of the superior and inferior end plates. (Reproduced from Cohen MS, Blair B, Garfin SR: Thoracolumbar compression fractures, in Levine AM, Eismont FJ, Garfin SR, Zigler JE, eds: *Spine Trauma.* Philadelphia, PA, WB Saunders, 1998, pp 388-401.)

midthoracic spinal levels.[25,26] Osteoporotic compression fractures occur most frequently at two sites: the mid-thoracic region (T6-T8) and the thoracolumbar junction (T12-L1).[36]

Classification

Four subtypes of anterior wedge compression fractures have been identified by Denis (**Figure 1**).[7] The most common, type B, results in failure of the superior end plate with osseous compression of the cancellous bone of the proximal half of the vertebral body. The compression is usually symmetric bilaterally. Less common patterns of injury involve failure of both end plates (type A), isolated failure of the inferior end plate (type C), and failure of the anterior vertebral body (type D). The lateral wedge compression fracture is a relatively uncommon injury. It accounts for between 8% and 14% of all wedge compression injuries and is most frequently seen in the midlumbar region of the spine.[7,37,38] The fracture is believed to be due to the same mechanism as that for anterior compression fractures, except for asymmetric collapse of the vertebral body in the sagittal plane (**Figure 2**).

Biomechanics

The mechanism of injury in all wedge compression fractures involves an axially directed central compressive force in combination with an eccentric compressive force. The latter force falls anterior to the axis of rotation (center of the nucleus pulposus) and results in a "flexion" bending moment (**Figure 3,** *A*). If the forces are great enough to overcome the intrinsic mechanical strength of the vertebral body, an anterior wedge deformity results. The forces lead to progressive vertebral body compression until the energy becomes dissipated and the intrinsic bone strength is equal

FIGURE 2

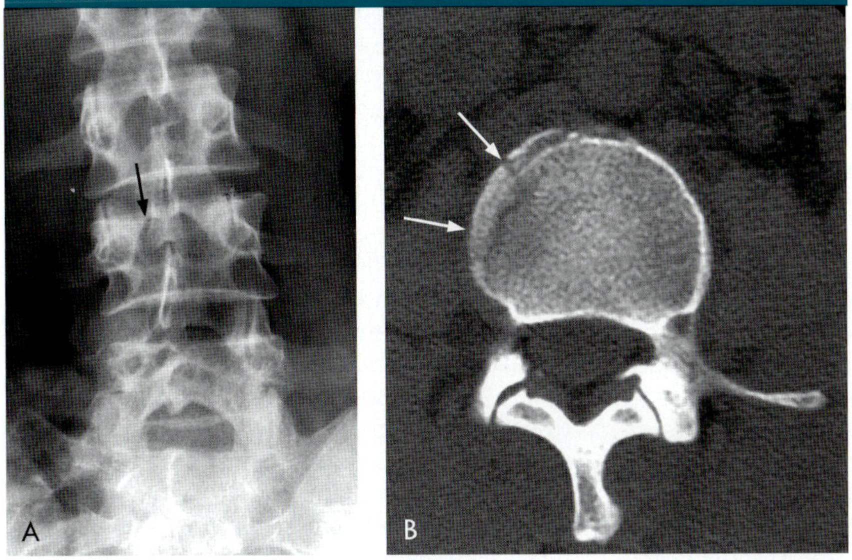

Figure 2 AP radiograph (**A**) and CT scan (**B**) of a lateral wedge compression fracture of L4. The AP film shows asymmetric collapse of the vertebral body (arrow). The CT scan through L4 in the axial plane reveals the asymmetric fracture of the vertebral body (arrows). (Reproduced from Cohen MS, Blair B, Garfin SR: Thoracolumbar compression fractures, in Levine AM, Eismont FJ, Garfin SR, Zigler JE, eds: *Spine Trauma*. Philadelphia, PA, WB Saunders, 1998, pp 388-401.)

FIGURE 3

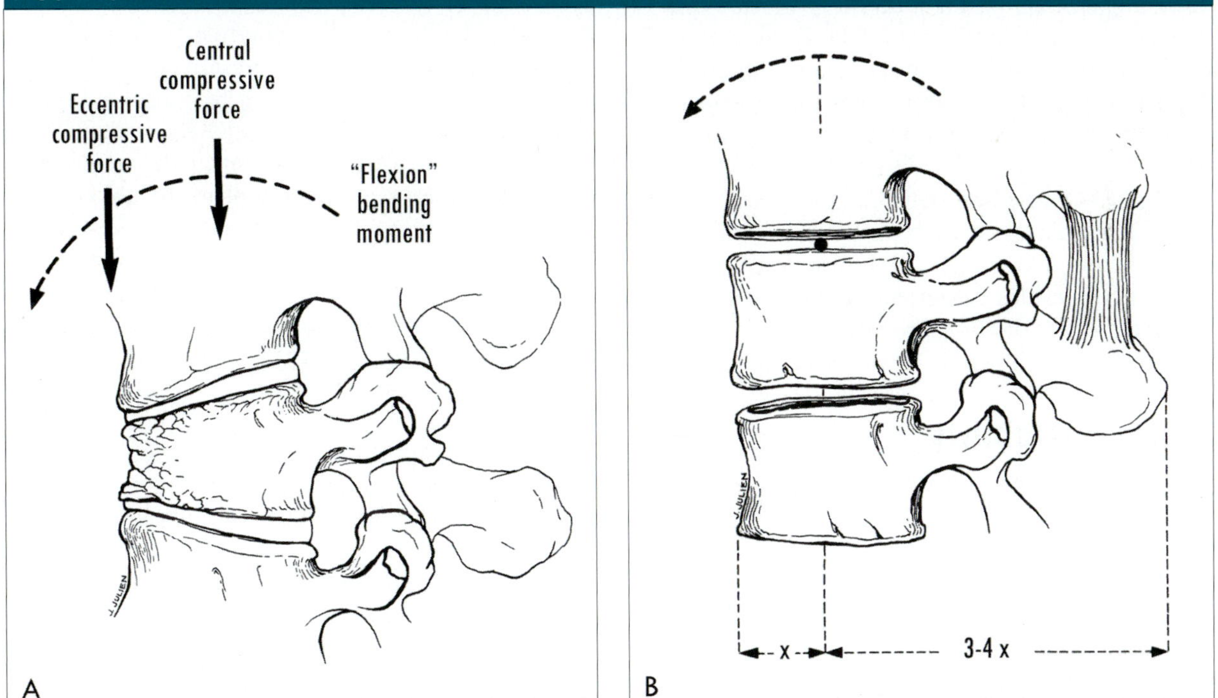

Figure 3 A, Mechanism of anterior wedge compression fractures of the thoracolumbar spine. An axial centrally directed force works in combination with an eccentric compressive force anteriorly. The latter induces a flexion bending moment. If the forces are great enough to overcome the intrinsic strength of the vertebral body, an anterior wedge compression fracture results. **B,** When a flexion force is placed on the spine, a fulcrum exists in the middle column (black dot). The ligaments of the posterior column can resist nearly 400 lb of tensile force before failure. As the distance to the fulcrum is asymmetric (× versus 3-4 ×), a greater load is placed on the anterior elements causing a fracture before the failure of the posterior elements. (Reproduced from Cohen MS, Blair B, Garfin SR: Thoracolumbar compression fractures, in Levine AM, Eismont FJ, Garfin SR, Zigler JE, eds: *Spine Trauma*. Philadelphia, PA, WB Saunders, 1998, pp 388-401.)

to or greater than the remaining compressive forces.

The pathologic sequence of vertebral body failure was described by Roaf.[39,40] With pure flexion-compression forces, failure occurs first in the vertebral body end plate. This is because the intact disk has only limited compressibility and transmits the load to the contiguous bone. Further compression leads to fracture of the vertebral cortical shell. This is followed by compression of the subcortical cancellous vertebral bone.

In pure flexion-compression injuries, the middle column remains intact and acts as a hinge. The posterior ligaments resist tensile forces, and their failure has been shown to be anatomically impossible before anterior column compression in pure flexion-compression injuries.[41] With the middle column acting as a fulcrum, the spine acts as a simple lever system. As the distance from the posterior elements to the fulcrum is greater than the distance from the anterior elements to the fulcrum, any distracting force on the posterior ligaments creates a compressive force on the vertebral body with three to four times greater magnitude (**Figure 3,** *B*). The breaking point for the posterior ligaments is nearly 400 lb, which generates a force of 1,200 lb to 1,600 lb on the anterior column, greatly exceeding their fracture point.[41] With the relative greater strength of the posterior ligaments, failure is only seen in injuries involving other forces besides flexion alone. Rotational forces can easily disrupt any of the spinal ligaments.[39]

Clinical Instability

Mechanical stability reflects the ability of the spine under physiologic loading to limit subsequent deformation and neurologic compromise.[42-44] Mild wedge compression fractures are generally considered stable injuries. Panjabi et al[45] have emphasized that biomechanically, the middle column is the primary determinant of stability. As compression fractures have, by definition, intact middle columns, they are inherently stable. In more severe wedge compression fractures, stability depends on two factors: the ability of the anteriorly compressed vertebra (anterior column) to withstand further compressive loading, and the ability of the interspinous and other posterior ligaments (posterior column) to resist tensile forces. As early as 1949, Nicoll[37] recognized that wedge compression fractures could be unstable if rupture of the posterior ligaments occurred. Failure of these ligaments allows the spine to bend around the hinge of the middle column and further compress the anterior vertebral body. Ching et al[46] assessed the residual stability of thoracolumbar spine fractures as a function of the type of injury. They found increased instability in the sagittal plane in flexion-distraction injuries of 126% compared with only 40% in pure compression fractures. Similarly, flexion-distraction injuries showed an increased torsional instability of 62% compared with the torsional instability for compression fractures, which increased only 3%.

The ability of compressed vertebrae to withstand loading has been studied in vitro. Plaue[47] studied cadaveric specimens and found that compressed vertebral bodies were able to withstand greater than 60% of their original load-bearing capacity. At 50% compression, the vertebral body maintains nearly 100% of its original load-bearing ability.[47] It is believed that stability is maintained from impaction of the cancellous vertebral bone. Keaveny et al[48] have also shown that after compression fracture, elasticity of the vertebral body decreases, while overall strength remains unchanged. Some wedge compression fractures may continue to collapse as a result of continued mechanical loads.[2,3,37,49,50] The greater the wedging and kyphotic deformity, the greater the moment arm. The greater the moment arm, the greater the tendency toward further progression.[32,42] A vicious circle can thus ensue.

Another consideration in vertebral body integrity following compression injury involves the occasional occurrence of posttraumatic osteonecrosis (Kümmell's disease).[37,42,51-57] In this condition, increased radiodensity of the vertebral body is seen on the radiograph in association with collapse days to years after the injury. Pathologic specimens suggest that vascular insult at the time of injury leads to subsequent bone death.[55,58-60] Although some think the likelihood of posttraumatic osteonecrosis increases with severity of injury,[37,42] some cases occur with only minor anterior vertebral wedging.[53,54] This emphasizes the need for close clinical and radiographic follow-up of all spinal compression injuries to identify the small group of patients who may develop neurologic injury due to progressive focal kyphosis.[55]

The other major determining factor in the stability of compression injuries is the integrity of the posterior osseoligamentous complex (posterior column). As described previously, anterior vertebral collapse places tensile forces on the posterior ligaments approximately one-fourth to one-third as great as the anterior compressive forces. A widened interspinous process distance in simple compression fractures is often thought to represent posterior column tension failure.[61-63] Neumann et al,[64] using a cadaver model, found that instability exists if a relative increase in interspinous process distance of greater than 33 mm is seen on AP radiographs. However, the posterior spinous ligaments are not taut in neutral position, and flexion of the normal spine leads to a physiologic increase in the interspinous process distance. In turn, compression fractures are routinely associated with an increased interspinous process distance geometrically proportional to the deformity of the anterior wedged vertebra.[7,8]

White and Panjabi[42] state that wedging of greater than 50% of the vertebral body is suggestive of posterior ligamentous disruption and instability. This value is cited frequently in the literature and is generally accepted as the cut-off for wedge compression fracture stability.[4,15,44,65-70] However, this figure is based on "biomechanical theory" as representing greater likelihood of posterior ligamentous failure. It is not known exactly how much separation of the posterior elements can reliably be correlated with structural failure of the posterior ligaments. Interestingly, Roaf[39] was unable to cause complete rupture of the posterior ligaments with flexion-compression injuries in cadaveric spines. He found that additional rotatory forces are necessary to produce posterior ligamentous rupture. The integrity of the posterior spinous ligaments may depend on the magnitude, direction, and rate of the applied forces, as well as the patient's age and location of the fracture. Flexion radiographs may be helpful in determining the status of the posterior spinal column soft tissues. MRI has made it possible to identify injuries to the posterior ligamentous structures as noted by increased signal intensity between spinous processes on T2-weighted images.[71] At this time, it can only be concluded that the probability of mechanical instability in wedge compression fractures is increased by several interrelated factors: (1) severity of vertebral wedging and comminution, (2) the presence of posttraumatic osteonecrosis, and (3) injury of the posterior osseoligamentous complex.[42,72]

Diagnosis

The diagnosis of wedge compression fractures depends on a careful review of the AP and lateral radiographs, as well as CT imaging. The AP view shows loss of vertebral height, which is usually symmetric. The lateral view reveals wedging of the vertebral body with loss of the anterior body height. The posterior vertebral body height is characteristically unchanged. The plain films must be scrutinized for subtle abnormalities to rule out more severe injuries. For example, if the AP and/or lateral radiographs reveal widening of the interpedicular distance of the fractured vertebral body, a more serious burst fracture has occurred (involvement of the middle column). Similarly, any disruption of the posterior vertebral body cortex on the lateral film denotes a burst injury as opposed to a pure compression injury. Disruption of this line, by definition, implies middle column involvement.[73] Further evaluation with high-resolution CT scanning is the imaging modality of choice to fully identify the fracture pattern (**Figure 4**).

The severity of compression fractures may be defined by the percentage of anterior vertebral body collapse and corresponding kyphotic deformity. The percentage collapse may be calculated by measuring the remaining anterior vertebral body height, divided by the average height of the anterior vertebral bodies above and below the level of injury, as measured on the lateral radiograph.[42] Alternatively, it can be calculated by dividing the remaining anterior vertebral body height by the posterior vertebral body height of the involved vertebra. The angular deformity is measured by the Cobb angle between the first intact end plate on either side of the injured segment.[74]

Thoracic Compression Fractures (T2-T10)

The upper thoracic spine, because of the rib cage, has unique mechanical characteristics and must be discussed separately. The rib cage stiffens the motion segments at each level in the thoracic spine, resisting bending and axial rotation forces. In vitro studies have shown that the load-bearing capacity of the isolated spine can support two to three times greater compressive loads before instability occurs with the addition of the rib cage. Furthermore, the rib cage increases the bending stiffness of the spine in flexion by 27%.[74] Considerable force is necessary to produce a compression injury of the thoracic spine. These fractures are associated with a high degree of concomitant injuries to the chest, head, and cervical spine.[2,15,65,69,75] Several reports show dislocations of the manubriosternal joint in high thoracic compression fractures due to the large forces accompanying these injuries.[42,76]

Another important difference between the thoracic spine and the lumbar spine is the presence of the spinal cord. In this region, the spinal canal is narrowed, with less free space between the cord

FIGURE 4

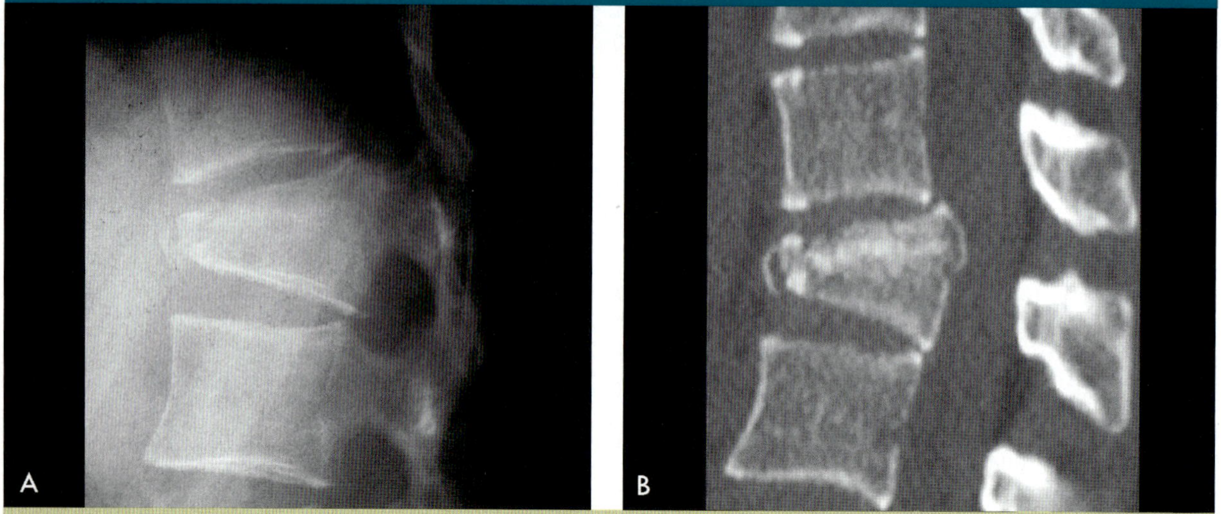

Figure 4 Treatment of focal kyphosis with severe anterior height loss. Lateral radiograph (**A**) and midsagittal CT reconstruction (**B**) of T12 compression fracture shows 24° focal kyphosis and 73% anterior height loss. This 32-year-old female sustained a fall onto the buttocks while taking a jump on an inner-tube snow jump. No posterior tenderness was noted and imaging studies showed no interspinous splaying or changes in facet-joint morphology. After nonsurgical treatment with a custom-molded thoracolumbosacral orthosis for 12 weeks, no further kyphosis was seen. At 4-year follow-up, the patient maintained full preinjury activities with only intermittent mild back pain.

FIGURE 5

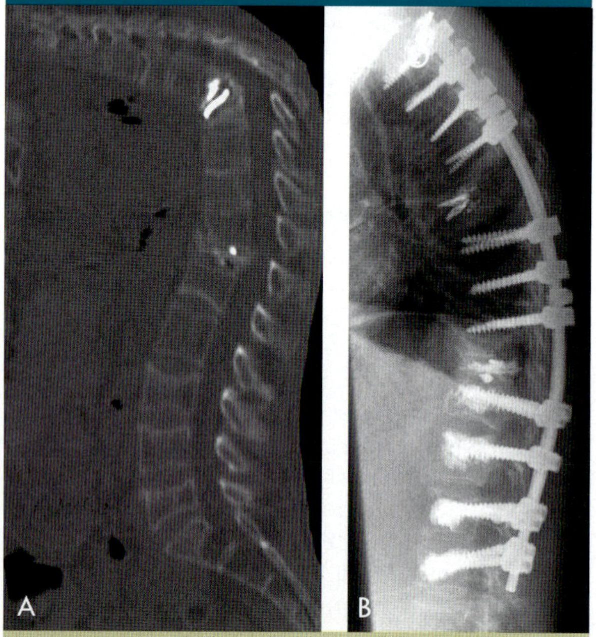

Figure 5 Multiple wedge compression fractures in a 34-year-old patient with osteogenesis imperfecta. **A,** Sagittal reconstruction CT showing compression fractures of T6, T7, T8, and T12 causing severe sagittal imbalance and 102° thoracic kyphosis. **B,** Standing lateral radiograph 12 months after surgical treatment with T6, T7, and T8 posterior shortening pedicle subtraction osteotomies, correction was maintained to 26° of thoracic kyphosis. Instrumented fusion from T2-L4 includes cement augmentation of T2, T3, L1, L2, L3, and L4 pedicle screws.

and the osseous ring. The central thoracic spine also has a relatively sparse blood supply.[43,69] Because of this, spinal cord injury may occur with a lower percentage of compression or degree of kyphosis than in the lumbar spine. Kyphosis may be especially severe in multiple thoracic wedge compression fractures (**Figure 5**). These are the primary exception to the rule that pure flexion-compression injuries do not cause acute neurologic loss.[5,44,65]

Thoracolumbar Compression Fractures (T11-L5)

The great majority of compression fractures occur at the thoracolumbar junction (T11-L2), where there is a fulcrum of motion between the relatively stiff thoracic spine and the mobile lumbar spine.[2,5,9,10,15,31,37,38,70,77-80] This region accounts for 54% to 70% of wedge compression fractures in reported series.[7,9,38,70,79,80] This is also the most common region for multiple wedge compression injuries, with a lesser peak in the midthoracic region.[79]

The lower lumbar spine (L3-L5) constitutes only a minority of wedge compression injuries. Biomechanical evidence suggests that the lower lumbar vertebrae are mechanically stronger than the upper lumbar vertebrae.[17] Well-developed paraspinal musculature likely improves mechanical support of this region, while a lordotic posture resists anterior compression forces.

Treatment

Nearly all thoracic and lumbar compression fractures without posterior element injuries are considered stable. Fractures between T2 and T10 are believed to be stable injuries because of the rib cage functioning as a stabilizing outrigger.[2,3] However, much higher forces are necessary to cause compression injuries in this area compared with the thoracolumbar junction. The classic management of stable thoracolumbar compression fractures consists of postural reduction and immobilization in a well-fitting orthosis for 6 to 12 weeks. Patients likely benefit from active mobilization. Because progression of deformity occurs early in the treatment process, frequent imaging is recommended. Progression of kyphosis is most frequent in early healing, with progression greater than 10° resulting in significantly more pain.[81] At our institution, we obtain weekly radiographs for 2 to 3 weeks, and then continue them monthly until pain is resolved or the pain level remains stable.

Historically, compression fractures greater than 50% of the original height of the vertebral body in physiologically young patients were believed to be unstable, with the potential for further progression and collapse.[4,15,42,65-70] However, it is likely that these patients also had unrecognized posterior ligamentous disruption and not pure compression injury alone. Severely kyphotic compression fractures with instability and no posterior ligamentous injury are uncommon; thus, no long-term clinical studies of sufficient sample size exist. Today, most spine surgeons do not use anterior height loss or degree of kyphosis alone in the decision for surgical treatment. The integrity of the posterior elements is of higher importance. This is reflected in contemporary classification schemes that place higher significance on the status of the posterior elements in the determination of spinal instability.[82,83] Recent findings now suggest that in the absence of posterior ligamentous injury and neurologic compromise, even burst fractures with 50% height loss are best treated nonsurgically.[84]

Surgical Treatment

Surgical treatment of thoracic and lumbar compression fractures is indicated for persistent pain, neural compression, and/or deformity causing sagittal imbalance. Less severe injuries may also be treated surgically in certain clinical scenarios (**Figure 6**). For example, surgery may be beneficial for the polytrauma patient in whom brace wear and compliance with precautions are difficult. Surgical fixation allows earlier mobilization and rehabilitation, which reduces multiple medical risks such as pneumonia, deep venous thrombosis, decubitus ulcers, and depression caused by prolonged bed rest and loss of independence.

More often, surgical treatment is employed well after the initial injury. Late surgical reconstruction addresses chronic pain due to residual kyphosis. In the past, treatment of compression fractures with laminectomy and consequent removal of the posterior osseoligamentous complex is thought to increase the risk of progressive kyphosis.[3,12,42,65,85-88] A kyphotic deformity causes an increase in the eccentric distribution of force throughout the spine, overstretching the posterior muscle fibers beyond their optimal sarcomere overlap. This places the muscle fibers at a physiologic disadvantage.[89] As a kyphotic deformity increases, the moment arm further increases the demand on the muscles to maintain an erect posture.[32,90] The combination of suboptimal muscle fiber overlap and the increased moment arm caused by a forward-leaning posture can lead to pain and early fatigue.[91] Increased kyphosis also increases the need for compensatory hyperlordosis of the cervical and/or lumbar spine to maintain an erect posture.[11,31,44,68] At higher degrees of hyperlordosis, pain may result due to compression of the facet joints (**Figure 7**).

Day and Kokan[92] studied 220 patients and found half to have residual symptoms, 25% disabling. The severity of compression correlated with a negative outcome, with lumbar fractures causing more pain than thoracic fractures. Soreff[93] reviewed 147 compression injuries and found that objective radiographic abnormalities correlated with symptoms and disability. Härkönen et al[75,94,95] reviewed 242 Finnish patients with thoracic and lumbar fractures and found approximately 75% of patients reporting late occasional or continuous pain. Kyphotic deformity again correlated with poor clinical results. In addition, they found age greater than 40 years to predispose toward pain and disability. Gertzbein[72] performed a prospective multicenter study on thoracic and lumbar spine fractures, including a subset of 104 compression fractures. He found a positive relationship between the presence of a kyphotic deformity at 1 year postinjury and pain. In particular, an increased incidence of moderate to severe pain was noted in kyphotic deformities of greater than 30°. When pain is present, low back pain is more common than pain at the site of injury.[37,38] Thus, late pain

FIGURE 6

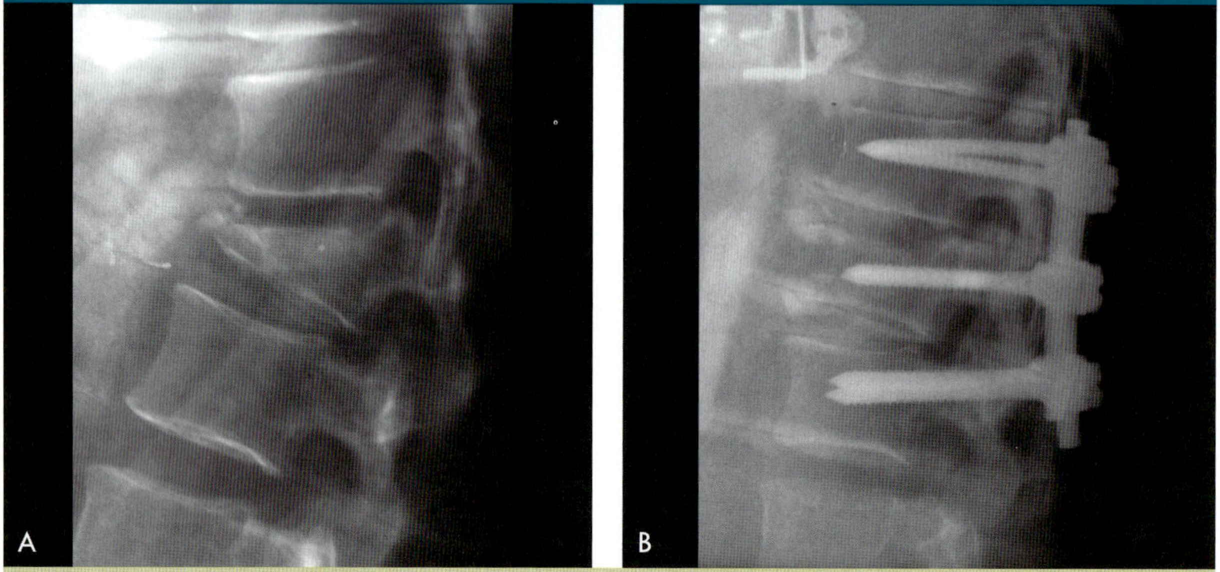

Figure 6 Short-segment posterior fixation of focal kyphosis with severe anterior height loss. **A,** Lateral radiograph of T12 compression fracture shows 23° focal kyphosis and 78% anterior height loss. Surgical treatment with pedicle screws at the level of the fracture provides segmental fixation and a three-point bending moment that allows substantial reduction of kyphosis. **B,** Improvement to 8° of lordosis is shown in a 6-month postoperative lateral radiograph.

FIGURE 7

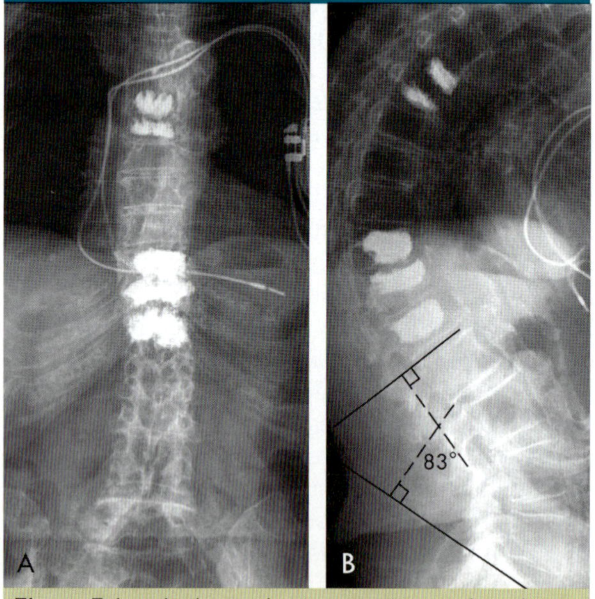

Figure 7 Low back pain due to compensatory hyperlordosis of the lumbar spine in a 78-year-old female reporting persistent low back pain after previous T6, T7, T11, T12, and L1 kyphoplasties. T6 and T7 procedures were approximately 8 months before the T11-L1 procedures. Each procedure provided significant improvement in upper back and midback pain. Low back pain is likely due to compensatory hyperlordosis of the lumbar spine causing impingement of facet joints and spinous processes. **A,** Standing AP radiograph shows neutral coronal alignment. **B,** Standing lateral radiograph shows lordosis angle of 83° (marked with black lines).

attributable to compression fractures is likely due more to sagittal imbalance than the degree of focal kyphosis at the injury site.[96,97] This may explain why several early studies were not able to correlate the degree of compression with clinical outcomes, as sagittal imbalance was not well appreciated at that time.[37,38]

Special Situations/Populations

Multiple Wedge Compression Fractures

The treatment of multiple, adjacent wedge compression fractures is poorly defined. As previously mentioned, the severe kyphosis resulting from these injuries may cause neurologic compromise.[5,44,65] This may occur in the patient with preexisting stenosis, which may be exacerbated by the spinal cord being draped over a kyphotic edge. In cases without neurologic involvement, several reports show multiple wedge compression injuries leading to progressive deformity and spinal instability.[65,79] At present, no clear guidelines exist for these injuries. For example, should two adjacent wedge compression injuries, 30% each, be considered a stable injury, or is this equivalent to one 60% vertebral body compression fracture? Theoretically, the probability of posterior ligamentous failure is not additive, as the tensile forces are spread over two adjacent intervertebral segments. However, the magnitude of the acute kyphosis resulting from multiple anterior wedge fractures is indeed additive and must be considered. The greater the angular deformity, the greater the chance for additional angulation due to the increased moment arm related to the deformity and the greater degree of sagittal imbalance.

Pediatric Compression Fractures

Several differences make spinal compression fractures in children different from those in adults. Vertebral bodies in children are well mineralized, and the spinal column in children is more elastic. This makes fractures of the spine in children uncommon. The disks are healthy and have a high turgor pressure. This allows the transmission of force to multiple spinal levels. Finally, the vertebral body epiphyses are open. This allows for a remodeling of the compressed vertebra, and an infrequent occurrence of late kyphotic deformities.

Several reports on thoracolumbar compression fractures in children between the age of 2 and 15 years exist and document the differences between this age group and adults.[13,21,98,99] Multiple-level compression injuries are the rule, constituting between 66% and 90% of reported series. It should be noted that some authors have remarked on the relative difficulty in interpretation of radiographic studies, particularly CT scans, in pediatric patients with compression fractures, making the diagnosis at times difficult.[9] The average patient has two to four affected vertebrae, with 11 compressed vertebrae being the highest number reported.[98] The primary location of fractures in this age group is the thoracic spine, especially midthoracic. At follow-up, some restoration of vertebral height is seen in almost all patients. Recovery of vertebral height is proportional to the severity of the compression and the age of the patient. Restoration is generally complete before 10 years of age. A slight, clinically insignificant scoliosis (less than 10°) is common and is believed to be secondary to uneven compression of the epiphysis. Progression of deformity is uncommon, as are posttraumatic degenerative changes.

Follow-up studies indicate that, even in children, several patients report long-term back pain after compression fractures, up to a mean of 16 years after injury.[13] Back pain affects from 38% to 67% of patients and is generally mild and intermittent without functional disability.[13,21,99] Treatment of these fractures is generally symptomatic in the younger age groups. Short-term bed rest is followed by early mobilization with or without extension supports. By approximately 10 years of age, the thoracolumbar spine approaches the adult spine in biomechanical properties, and by the teenage years, the indications for surgical treatment are similar to those for adults.[23]

Osteoporotic Compression Fractures

Osteoporosis is a common problem throughout the world, affecting an estimated 75 million people in the United States, Europe, and Japan.[36] As the average life expectancy increases, osteoporosis and osteoporotic fractures increase in number as well. The rate of osteoporotic fractures increases with age, with a prevalence of 20% in 50-year-old women increasing to 64.5% in women older than 90 years of age.[100-103] In one population-based study, 74% to 90.8% of women with fractures had either moderate trauma or no trauma at all.[104] Compression loading to the spine is increased in normal daily events such as coughing, laughing, or running. With healthy bone, this is of little consequence as the disk distributes the load throughout the vertebral body and the normal bone can more adequately handle the increased load. With osteoporosis and aging, the disks cannot distribute loads effectively, the core musculature weakens, and, most importantly, the bone itself is much weaker. As the load-bearing capacity of the spine decreases with age, minor events, such as simple bending or lifting, can lead to atraumatic vertebral compression fractures.[105-108] Osteoporotic vertebral fractures occur most frequently in older women, but there is also an increasing number of young patients with osteoporotic compression fractures, frequently related to immunosuppressive and high-dose steroid therapy.[109-111] Another population at risk for osteoporotic compression fractures is patients with ankylosing spondylitis, in whom multiple compression fractures in the thoracic and lumbar spine can lead to kyphosis over multiple levels and severe sagittal imbalance.[112]

Osteoporotic vertebral fractures are most common in the midthoracic region and at the thoracolumbar junction. These two regions are subjected to the greatest compressive stresses due to the thoracic kyphosis and the motion between the rigid thorax and the mobile lumbar spine. Three types of osteoporotic vertebral fractures occur: wedge, biconcave, and crush. Wedge fractures are the most common, and make up 51% of all osteoporotic vertebral fractures. In wedge fractures, the posterior wall is relatively undamaged while the anterior vertebral body is compressed. Biconcave or "cod-fish" fractures are the next most frequent, making up 17%. Biconcave fractures only have compression in the central portion of the vertebral

FIGURE 8

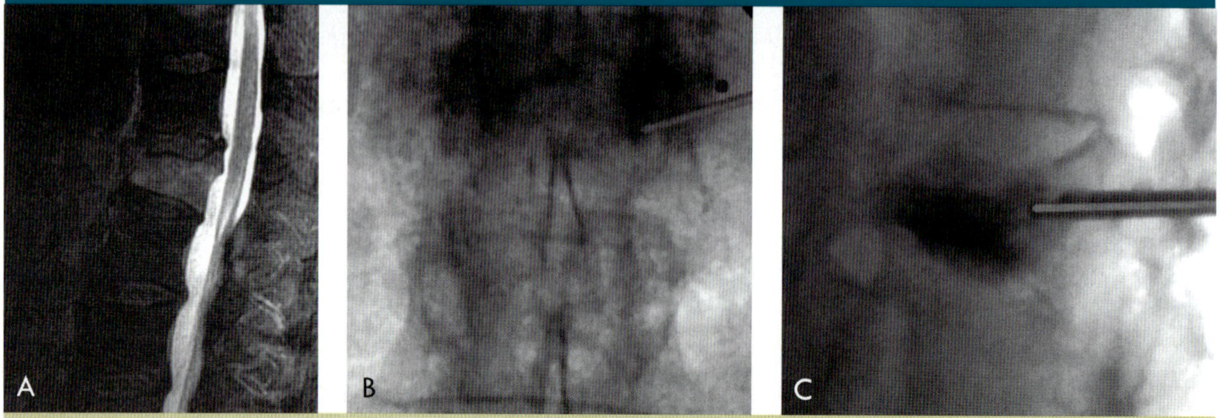

Figure 8 Osteoporotic compression fractures treated with kyphoplasty. A 78-year-old man with T12 osteoporotic compression fractures reporting severe pain for 3 months. **A,** MRI shows compression and height loss. Image-guided virtual fluoroscopy is used during cannula insertion in the anteroposterior (**B**) and lateral (**C**) planes. Image-guided virtual fluoroscopy is used to place the transpedicular cannula. Live, lateral C-arm imaging is used during cement injection (**C**).

body, with preservation of height of the anterior and posterior end plates. Crush fractures are the third most common injury, comprising 13% of all fractures. Crush injuries are simply the compression of the entire vertebral body. A combination of these patterns exist in 4% of osteoporotic fractures.[100]

The diagnosis of osteoporotic compression fractures is based chiefly on radiographic and MRI studies. On plain radiographs, the extent of osteoporosis can be seen as a decrease in both number and size of trabeculae in the cancellous vertebral body. It requires up to 30% loss of bone mineral, however, before changes become obvious on plain radiographs. Therefore, other, more sensitive methods are required to determine those at risk. Currently, dual-energy x-ray absorptiometry (DEXA) remains the modality of choice for determining bone mineral density. Furthermore, the definition of these fractures has been debated, making diagnosis even more unclear.[100,113,114] Over 700,000 clinically symptomatic osteoporotic vertebral fractures occur every year in the United States.[115] It is estimated that clinically diagnosed fractures account for approximately one-third of all osteoporotic vertebral fractures.[100]

These fractures are no longer treated with orthoses, as most elderly patients cannot tolerate bracing. Early mobilization and avoidance of prolonged bed rest is important. The risk of progressive collapse and neurologic injury warrants close clinical and radiographic follow-up. Surgical treatment of osteoporotic compression fractures has evolved considerably in the last several years. New techniques such as kyphoplasty and the development of minimally invasive surgery of the spine have made surgery a much more appealing option (**Figure 8**).

Despite these advances, the surgical treatment of osteoporotic vertebral fractures is still complicated by the inherent poor bone stock of the osteoporotic spine. Hooks have been known to cause further fractures in the lamina or pull out entirely, as their force is localized on one small area of osteoporotic bone. Sublaminar wires may simply slide through the bone like a cheese slicer. The large cortical purchase of pedicle screws allows for the most rigid fixation but they may also pull out.[116] Cement-augmented pedicle screws significantly improve pull-out strength and may decrease the incidence of clinical failures (**Figure 5**).[117-119] In patients that cannot tolerate an anterior approach (such as lung disease, previous abdominal surgery), an alternative technique is to perform a posterior shortening resection osteotomy (**Figure 9**).

Both vertebroplasty and kyphoplasty involve augmenting the osteoporotic vertebra with polymethylmethacrylate cement. Pain is diminished through the stabilization of microfractures, the prevention of further fracture, and possibly the cauterization of nociceptive nerves.[120,121] Vertebroplasty successfully decreases pain in 80% of patients, but cement leakage may occur in 40% of patients with a 6% moderate complication rate.[122] However, vertebroplasty cannot reduce the fracture, reduce kyphotic deformity, or restore the vertebral height. Kyphoplasty uses a balloon tamp to reduce the fracture and restore the vertebral height. The balloon creates a cavity in the vertebral body that allows for low-pressure injection of cement, unlike the higher-pressure injection needed in vertebroplasty. The cavity expansion creates a sclerotic rim of bone that further serves to decrease the leakage of cement. Eighty percent to 90% of patients describe pain relief, and moderate height restoration occurs in 70% of cases.[123]

Recently, the use of vertebroplasty has been questioned in the treatment of compression fractures. In 2009, Kallmes et al[124] published a randomized trial of vertebroplasty in the treatment of osteoporotic fractures in 131 patients compared to sham surgery alone. They did not show a statistically significant benefit for vertebroplasty, but did show a trend with less pain at 1 month than the control arm.

A meta-analysis published by Bouza et al[125] in 2006 compared kyphoplasty and vertebroplasty in the treatment of vertebral compression fractures. Kyphoplasty showed a significant improvement over medical therapy for pain intensity, mobility, vertebral collapse, kyphotic deformity, development of new vertebral fractures, and decreased hospital stay. It also significantly reduced the degree of kyphotic deformity and had a significantly lower leakage rate than vertebroplasty, but had no other significant differences.[125]

Another randomized controlled trial compared kyphoplasty to nonsurgical care in a study of 300 patients followed up to 1 month posttreatment.[126] The investigators found that kyphoplasty significantly decreased pain and there was no increased risk of adverse events in the surgical group.[126]

FIGURE 9

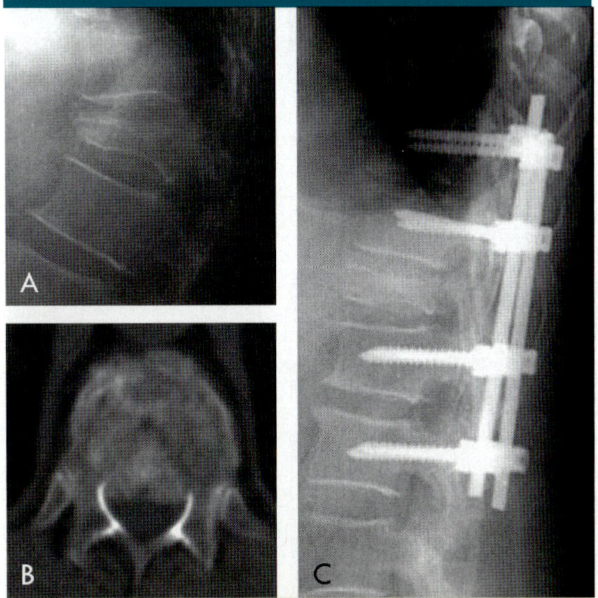

Figure 9 Osteoporotic compression fractures treated with posterior vertebral subtraction osteotomy. A 73-year-old man with a T12 osteoporotic compression fracture reported worsening pain, urinary retention, and gait disturbance for 4 weeks. **A,** Lateral radiograph shows compression and height loss of T12. **B,** Axial CT image shows disruption and retropulsion of the posterior wall. **C,** Lateral standing radiograph shows a posterior approach with T12 pedicle subtraction osteotomy used for decompression, kyphosis correction, and stabilization.

Pathologic Compression Fractures

Compression fractures accompany a variety of systemic disorders involving bone. In the child, spinal compression fractures are associated with lymphoma, eosinophilic granuloma, Gaucher's disease, the mucopolysaccharidoses, osteogenesis imperfecta, and idiopathic juvenile osteoporosis.[10] In older patients, common causes of pathologic fracture include metastatic disease and infection. Many fractures due to malignancy can be treated symptomatically. Bracing is recommended only if there is a decrease in pain and improvement in quality of life. In our experience, most tumor patients do not tolerate brace wear.

The goal of treatment of spinal metastatic disease is palliative, not curative. All treatment should be directed toward improving the patient's quality of life by decreasing pain and minimizing neurologic deficit. Traditionally, radiation therapy has been the treatment of choice, along with chemotherapy, for nonsurgical management. Katagiri et al[127] found that, using nonsurgical treatment alone, 67% of patients obtained pain relief, 64% showed functional improvement, and 66% had stable or improved neurologic function following treatment. The use of radiation for bone metastases has been proven to be successful for palliative care.[128] Bisphosphonates can also be added to a treatment regimen to decrease the tumor-driven osteoclastic enhancement, thereby decreasing the lytic activity of the tumor on the surrounding bone and decreasing pain.[129,130]

More recently, surgical treatment with modern techniques of decompression and spinal reconstruction is effective for pain relief and neurologic recovery. A randomized, prospective clinical trial showed that surgical decompression and stabilization is superior to radiation therapy alone in cases where there is neurologic deficit.[131] Improvements were also found in tiredness, nausea, anxiety, drowsiness, appetite, and well-being.[132] The type of surgery performed is dependent on the individ-

FIGURE 10

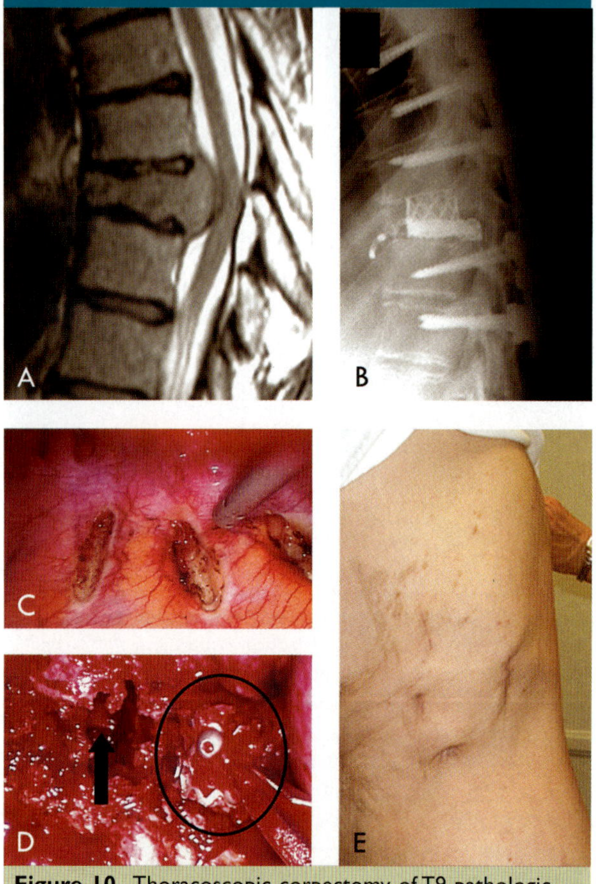

Figure 10 Thoracoscopic corpectomy of T9 pathologic fracture in a 64-year-old woman with multiple myeloma. **A,** Sagittal T2-weighted MRI scan; **B,** Postoperative lateral radiograph; **C,** Intraoperative photograph through endoscope with rib heads marked with electrocautery; **D,** Decompression site (arrow) before cage insertion (circle); and **E,** Postoperative clinical photograph showing the four small incisions 4 weeks after surgery.

ual patient, the extent of the disease, and the properties of the tumor.[133] En bloc spondylectomy, intralesional excision, or cord decompression with spinal stabilization are all options for treatment.[133] Minimally invasive spine surgery has been shown to decrease the pain, blood loss, respiratory difficulty, and prolonged hospitalization for degenerative spinal conditions.[134] Such goals are even more important in tumor patients who are frail and have a limited life expectancy (**Figure 10**).[135]

References

1. Holmes JF, Miller PQ, Panacek EA, Lin S, Horne NS, Mower WR: Epidemiology of thoracolumbar spine injury in blunt trauma. *Acad Emerg Med* 2001;8(9):866-872.
2. Bohlman HH: Treatment of fractures and dislocations of the thoracic and lumbar spine. *J Bone Joint Surg Am* 1985;67(1):165-169.
3. Rothman RH, Simeone FA, eds: *The Spine*, ed 2. Philadelphia, PA, Saunders, 1982, vol 2.
4. Ferguson RL, Allen BL Jr: A mechanistic classification of thoracolumbar spine fractures. *Clin Orthop Relat Res* 1984;189:77-88.
5. McAfee PC, Yuan HA, Fredrickson BE, Lubicky JP: The value of computed tomography in thoracolumbar fractures: An analysis of one hundred consecutive cases and a new classification. *J Bone Joint Surg Am* 1983;65(4):461-473.
6. Bucholz RW, Gill K: Classification of injuries to the thoracolumbar spine. *Orthop Clin North Am* 1986;17(1):67-73.
7. Denis F: The three column spine and its significance in the classification of acute thoracolumbar spinal injuries. *Spine (Phila Pa 1976)* 1983;8(8): 817-831.
8. Denis F: Spinal instability as defined by the three-column spine concept in acute spinal trauma. *Clin Orthop Relat Res* 1984;189:65-76.
9. Glass RB, Sivit CJ, Sturm PF, Bulas DI, Eichelberger MR: Lumbar spine injury in a pediatric population: Difficulties with computed tomographic diagnosis. *J Trauma* 1994;37(5): 815-819.
10. Dickson JH, Harrington PR, Erwin WD: Results of reduction and stabilization of the severely fractured thoracic and lumbar spine. *J Bone Joint Surg Am* 1978;60(6):799-805.
11. Edwards CC, Levine AM: Early rod-sleeve stabilization of the injured thoracic and lumbar spine. *Orthop Clin North Am* 1986;17(1):121-145.
12. Flesch JR, Leider LL, Erickson DL, Chou SN, Bradford DS: Harrington instrumentation and spine fusion for unstable fractures and fracture-dislocations of the thoracic and lumbar spine. *J Bone Joint Surg Am* 1977;59(2):143-153.
13. Horal J, Nachemson A, Scheller S: Clinical and radiological long term follow-up of ventebral fractures in children. *Acta Orthop Scand* 1972;43(6): 491-503.
14. Kilcoyne RF, Mack LA, King HA, Ratcliffe SS, Loop JW: Thoracolumbar spine injuries associated with vertical plunges: Reappraisal with computed tomography. *Radiology* 1983;146(1): 137-140.
15. Meyer PR Jr: Posterior stabilization of thoracic, lumbar, and sacral injuries. *Instr Course Lect* 1986; 35:401-419.
16. Osebold WR, Weinstein SL, Sprague BL: Thoracolumbar spine fractures: Results of treatment. *Spine (Phila Pa 1976)* 1981;6(1):13-34.

17. Perey O: Fracture of the vertebral end-plate in the lumbar spine; an experimental biochemical investigation. *Acta Orthop Scand Suppl* 1957;25:1-101.
18. Odom JA, Brown CW, Messner DG: Tubing injuries. *J Bone Joint Surg Am* 1976;58A:733.
19. Marcus NA, Sweetser ER, Benson RW: Hot-air ballooning injuries. *Am J Sports Med* 1981;9(5): 318-321.
20. Keene JS: Thoracolumbar fractures in winter sports. *Clin Orthop Relat Res* 1987;216:39-49.
21. Hubbard DD: Injuries of the spine in children and adolescents. *Clin Orthop Relat Res* 1974;100: 56-65.
22. Herkowitz HN, Samberg LC: Vertebral column injuries associated with tobogganing. *J Trauma* 1978;18(12):806-810.
23. Rockwood CA, Wilkins KE, King RE, eds: *Fractures in Children*. Philadelphia, PA, Lippincott, 1984.
24. Alexander MJ: Biomechanical aspects of lumbar spine injuries in athletes: A review. *Can J Appl Sport Sci* 1985;10(1):1-20.
25. Hirsch C, Nachemsson A: Clinical observations on the spines of ejected pilots. *Ind Med Surg* 1963;32:28-29.
26. Lyons TJ, Ficke AJ: Cases from the aerospace medicine residents' teaching file: Case #17. An aviator with multiple compression fractures of the spine secondary to high speed ejection. *Aviat Space Environ Med* 1987;58(4):379-381.
27. Visuri T, Aho J: Injuries associated with the use of ejection seats in Finnish pilots. *Aviat Space Environ Med* 1992;63(8):727-730.
28. Boukhris R, Becker KL: The inter-relationship between vertebral fractures and osteoporosis. *Clin Orthop Relat Res* 1973;90:209-216.
29. De Smet AA, Robinson RG, Johnson BE, Lukert BP: Spinal compression fractures in osteoporotic women: Patterns and relationship to hyperkyphosis. *Radiology* 1988;166(2):497-500.
30. Härmä M, Heliövaara M, Aromaa A, Knekt P: Thoracic spine compression fractures in Finland. *Clin Orthop Relat Res* 1986;205:188-194.
31. Howorth MB: Fracture of the spine. *Am J Surg* 1956;92(4):573-593.
32. White AA III, Panjabi MM, Thomas CL: The clinical biomechanics of kyphotic deformities. *Clin Orthop Relat Res* 1977;128:8-17.
33. Ciccone R, Richman RM: The mechanism of injury and the distribution of 3000 fractures and dislocations caused by parachute jumping. *J Bone Joint Surg Am* 1948;30(1):77-97.
34. Grech P: Falls from coconut trees. *East Afr Med J* 1964;41:63-68.
35. Petras AF, Hoffman EP: Roentgenographic skeletal injury patterns in parachute jumping. *Am J Sports Med* 1983;11(5):325-328.
36. Haczynski J, Jakimiuk A: Vertebral fractures: A hidden problem of osteoporosis. *Med Sci Monit* 2001;7(5):1108-1117.
37. Nicoll EA: Fractures of the dorso-lumbar vertebral column. *J Bone Joint Surg Br* 1949;31B:367-394.
38. Westerborn A, Olsson O: Mechanics, treatment and prognosis of fractures of the dorso-lumbar spine. *Acta Chir Scand* 1951;102(1):59-83.
39. Roaf R: A study of the mechanics of spinal injuries. *J Bone Joint Surg Br* 1960;42:810-823.
40. Roaf R: Biomechanics of injuries of the spinal column, in Vinken PJ, Bruyn GW, eds: *Handbook of Clinical Neurology*. New York, NY, American Elsevier, 1975, pp 123-140.
41. Brown T, Hansen RJ, Yorra AJ: Some mechanical tests on the lumbosacral spine with particular reference to the intervertebral discs; a preliminary report. *J Bone Joint Surg Am* 1957;39(5): 1135-1164.
42. White AA, Panjabi MM, eds: *Clinical Biomechanics of the Spine*. Philadelphia, PA, Lippincott, 1978.
43. White AA III, Panjabi MM, Posner I, Edwards WT, Hayes WC: Spinal stability: Evaluation and treatment. *Instr Course Lect* 1981;30:457-483.
44. Whitesides TE Jr: Traumatic kyphosis of the thoracolumbar spine. *Clin Orthop Relat Res* 1977;128: 78-92.
45. Panjabi MM, Oxland TR, Kifune M, Arand M, Wen L, Chen A: Validity of the three-column theory of thoracolumbar fractures: A biomechanic investigation. *Spine (Phila Pa 1976)* 1995;20(10): 1122-1127.
46. Ching RP, Tencer AF, Anderson PA, Daly CH: Comparison of residual stability in thoracolumbar spine fractures using neutral zone measurements. *J Orthop Res* 1995;13(4):533-541.
47. Plaue R: Mechanics of vertebral compression fracture (static pressure studies in dead vertebrae). *Zentralbl Chir* 1973;98(21):761-770.
48. Keaveny TM, Wachtel EF, Guo XE, Hayes WC: Mechanical behavior of damaged trabecular bone. *J Biomech* 1994;27(11):1309-1318.
49. Baab OD, Howorth MB: Fractures on the dorsal and lumbar vertebrae. *J Am Med Assoc* 1951; 146(2):97-100.
50. Rockwood CA, Green DP, eds: *Fractures in Adults*, ed 2. Philadelphia, PA, Lippincott, 1984, vol 2.
51. Bedbrook GM: Stability of spinal fractures and fracture dislocations. *Paraplegia* 1971;9(1):23-32.
52. Benedek TG, Nicholas JJ: Delayed traumatic vertebral body compression fracture; part II: Pathologic features. *Semin Arthritis Rheum* 1981;10(4): 271-277.

5: Thoracolumbar Injuries

53. Benedek TG, Nicholas JJ, Reece GJ: Kummell's disease: A rare cause of post-traumatic back pain. *Arthritis Rheum* 1980;23:653.
54. Brower AC, Downey EF Jr: Kümmell disease: Report of a case with serial radiographs. *Radiology* 1981;141(2):363-364.
55. Kaneda K, Asano S, Hashimoto T, Satoh S, Fujiya M: The treatment of osteoporotic-posttraumatic vertebral collapse using the Kaneda device and a bioactive ceramic vertebral prosthesis. *Spine (Phila Pa 1976)* 1992;17(8, Suppl):S295-S303.
56. Nicholas JJ, Benedek TG, Reece GJ: Delayed traumatic vertebral body compression fracture; part I: Clinical features. *Semin Arthritis Rheum* 1981;10(4):264-270.
57. Resnick D, Niwayama G, eds: *Diagnosis of Bone and Joint Disorders*, ed 2. Philadelphia, PA, Saunders, 1988, vols 2-6.
58. Schinz HW, Baensch FE, eds: *Roentgen Diagnostics*. New York, NY, Grune & Stratton, 1964, vol 2.
59. Schmorl G, Junghanns H, eds: *The Human Spine in Health and Disease; Anatomicopathologic Studies*. New York, NY, Grune & Stratton, 1959.
60. Leidholt JD, Young JJ, Hahn HR, Jackson RE, Gamble WE, Miles JS: Evaluation of late spinal deformities with fracture-dislocations of the dorsal and lumbar spine in paraplegics. *Paraplegia* 1969;7(1):16-28.
61. Gehweiler JA Jr, Daffner RH, Osborne RL Jr: Relevant signs of stable and unstable thoracolumbar vertebral column trauma. *Skeletal Radiol* 1981;7(3):179-183.
62. Holdsworth F: Fractures, dislocations, and fracture-dislocations of the spine. *J Bone Joint Surg Am* 1970;52(8):1534-1551.
63. Holdsworth FW, Hardy A: Early treatment of paraplegia from fractures of the thoraco-lumbar spine. *J Bone Joint Surg Br* 1953;35-B(4):540-550.
64. Neumann P, Nordwall A, Osvalder AL: Traumatic instability of the lumbar spine: A dynamic in vitro study of flexion-distraction injury. *Spine (Phila Pa 1976)* 1995;20(10):1111-1121.
65. Bradford DS, Akbarnia BA, Winter RB, Seljeskog EL: Surgical stabilization of fracture and fracture dislocations of the thoracic spine. *Spine (Phila Pa 1976)* 1977;2(3):185-196.
66. Esses SI: The placement and treatment of thoracolumbar spine fractures: An algorithmic approach. *Orthop Rev* 1988;17(6):571-584.
67. Jacobs RR, Asher MA, Snider RK: Thoracolumbar spinal injuries: A comparative study of recumbent and operative treatment in 100 patients. *Spine (Phila Pa 1976)* 1980;5(5):463-477.
68. Jacobs RR, Casey MP: Surgical management of thoracolumbar spinal injuries: General principles and controversial considerations. *Clin Orthop Relat Res* 1984;189:22-35.
69. King AG: Spinal column trauma. *Instr Course Lect* 1986;35:40-51.
70. Weitzman G: Treatment of stable thoracolumbar spine compression fractures by early ambulation. *Clin Orthop Relat Res* 1971;76:116-122.
71. Brightman RP, Miller CA, Rea GL, Chakeres DW, Hunt WE: Magnetic resonance imaging of trauma to the thoracic and lumbar spine: The importance of the posterior longitudinal ligament. *Spine (Phila Pa 1976)* 1992;17(5):541-550.
72. Gertzbein SD: Scoliosis Research Society: Multicenter spine fracture study. *Spine (Phila Pa 1976)* 1992;17(5):528-540.
73. Daffner RH, Deeb ZL, Rothfus WE: The posterior vertebral body line: Importance in the detection of burst fractures. *AJR Am J Roentgenol* 1987;148(1):93-96.
74. Andriacchi T, Schultz A, Belytschko T, Galante J: A model for studies of mechanical interactions between the human spine and rib cage. *J Biomech* 1974;7(6):497-507.
75. Härkönen M, Kataja M, Lepistö P, Paakkala T, Pätiälä H, Rokkanen P: Fractures of the thoracic spine: Clinical and radiological results in 98 patients. *Arch Orthop Trauma Surg* 1979;94(3):179-184.
76. Scher AT: Associated sternal and spinal fractures: Case reports. *S Afr Med J* 1983;64(3):98-100.
77. Kelly RP, Whitesides TE Jr: Treatment of lumbodorsal fracture-dislocations. *Ann Surg* 1968;167(5):705-717.
78. Riggins RS, Kraus JF: The risk of neurologic damage with fractures of the vertebrae. *J Trauma* 1977;17(2):126-133.
79. Sutherland CJ, Miller F, Wang GJ: Early progressive kyphosis following compression fractures: Two case reports from a series of "stable" thoracolumbar compression fractures. *Clin Orthop Relat Res* 1983;173:216-220.
80. Young MH: Long-term consequences of stable fractures of the thoracic and lumbar vertebral bodies. *J Bone Joint Surg Br* 1973;55(2):295-300.
81. McLain RF, Sparling E, Benson DR: Early failure of short-segment pedicle instrumentation for thoracolumbar fractures: A preliminary report. *J Bone Joint Surg Am* 1993;75(2):162-167.
82. Magerl F, Aebi M, Gertzbein SD, Harms J, Nazarian S: A comprehensive classification of thoracic and lumbar injuries. *Eur Spine J* 1994;3(4):184-201.
83. Vaccaro AR, Lehman RA Jr, Hurlbert RJ, et al: A new classification of thoracolumbar injuries: The importance of injury morphology, the integrity of the posterior ligamentous complex, and neuro-

logic status. *Spine (Phila Pa 1976)* 2005;30(20): 2325-2333.

84. Wood K, Buttermann G, Mehbod A, et al: Operative compared with nonoperative treatment of a thoracolumbar burst fracture without neurological deficit: A prospective, randomized study. *J Bone Joint Surg Am* 2003;85-A(5):773-781.
85. Whitesides TE, Shah S Ghazanfar A: On the management of unstable fractures of the thoracolumbar spine: Rationale for use of anterior decompression and fusion and posterior stabilization. *Spine (Phila Pa 1976)* 1976;1(2):99-107.
86. Roberts JB, Curtiss PH Jr: Stability of the thoracic and lumbar spine in traumatic paraplegia following fracture or fracture-dislocation. *J Bone Joint Surg Am* 1970;52(6):1115-1130.
87. Morgan TH, Wharton GW, Austin GN: The results of laminectomy in patients with incomplete spinal cord injuries. *Paraplegia* 1971;9(1):14-23.
88. Lonstein JE: Post-laminectomy kyphosis. *Clin Orthop Relat Res* 1977;128:93-100.
89. Morgan DL, Proske U: Popping sarcomere hypothesis explains stretch-induced muscle damage. *Clin Exp Pharmacol Physiol* 2004;31(8):541-545.
90. Böhler L, Böhler J, eds: *The Treatment of Factures*, ed 5. New York, NY, Grune & Stratton, 1956, vol 3.
91. Orchowski J, Polly DW Jr, Klemme WR, Oda I, Cunningham B: The effect of kyphosis on the mechanical strength of a long-segment posterior construct using a synthetic model. *Spine (Phila Pa 1976)* 2000;25(13):1644-1648.
92. Day B, Kokan P: Compression fractures of the thoracic and lumbar spine from compensable injuries. *Clin Orthop Relat Res* 1977;124:173-176.
93. Soreff J: *Assessment of Late Results of Traumatic Compression Fractures of the Thoracolumbar Vertebral Bodies*. Karolinska Hospital, Stockholm, Sweden, 1977.
94. Härkönen M, Kataja M, Keski-Nisula L, Paakkala T, Pätiälä H, Rokkanen P: Fractures of the lumbar spine: Clinical and radiological results in 94 patients. *Arch Orthop Trauma Surg* 1979;94(1): 43-48.
95. Härkönen M, Kataja M, Keski-Nisula L, Paakkala T, Pätiälä H, Rokkanen P: Injuries of the thoracolumbar junction: Clinical and radiological results in 149 patients. *Arch Orthop Trauma Surg* 1979;94(1):35-41.
96. Been HD, Poolman RW, Ubags LH: Clinical outcome and radiographic results after surgical treatment of post-traumatic thoracolumbar kyphosis following simple type A fractures. *Eur Spine J* 2004;13(2):101-107.
97. Heary RF, Bono CM: Pedicle subtraction osteotomy in the treatment of chronic, posttraumatic kyphotic deformity. *J Neurosurg Spine* 2006;5(1): 1-8.
98. Hegenbarth R, Ebel KD: Roentgen findings in fractures of the vertebral column in childhood examination of 35 patients and its results. *Pediatr Radiol* 1976;5(1):34-39.
99. Hubbard DD: Fractures of the dorsal and lumbar spine. *Orthop Clin North Am* 1976;7(3):605-614.
100. Cooper C, O'Neill T, Silman A, European Vertebral Osteoporosis Study Group: The epidemiology of vertebral fractures. *Bone* 1993;14(Suppl 1): S89-S97.
101. Melton LJ III, Kan SH, Frye MA, Wahner HW, O'Fallon WM, Riggs BL: Epidemiology of vertebral fractures in women. *Am J Epidemiol* 1989; 129(5):1000-1011.
102. Melton LJ III, Lane AW, Cooper C, Eastell R, O'Fallon WM, Riggs BL: Prevalence and incidence of vertebral deformities. *Osteoporos Int* 1993;3(3): 113-119.
103. O'Neill TW, Felsenberg D, Varlow J, Cooper C, Kanis JA, Silman AJ: The prevalence of vertebral deformity in european men and women: The European Vertebral Osteoporosis Study. *J Bone Miner Res* 1996;11(7):1010-1018.
104. Cooper C, Atkinson EJ, O'Fallon WM, Melton LJ III: Incidence of clinically diagnosed vertebral fractures: A population-based study in Rochester, Minnesota, 1985-1989. *J Bone Miner Res* 1992; 7(2):221-227.
105. Buchanan JR, Myers CA, Greer RB III: A comparison of the risk of vertebral fracture in menopausal osteopenia and other metabolic disturbances. *J Bone Joint Surg Am* 1988;70(5):704-711.
106. Buchanan JR, Myers CA, Greer RB: Determinants of atraumatic vertebral fracture rates in menopausal women: Biologic v mechanical factors. *Metabolism* 1988;37(4):400-404.
107. Ekin JA, Sinaki M: Vertebral compression fractures sustained during golfing: Report of three cases. *Mayo Clin Proc* 1993;68(6):566-570.
108. Gershon-Cohen J, Rechtman AM, Schraer H, Blumberg N: Asymptomatic fractures in osteoporotic spines of the aged. *J Am Med Assoc* 1953; 153(7):625-627.
109. Katz IA, Epstein S: Posttransplantation bone disease. *J Bone Miner Res* 1992;7(2):123-126.
110. Rich GM, Mudge GH, Laffel GL, LeBoff MS: Cyclosporine A and prednisone-associated osteoporosis in heart transplant recipients. *J Heart Lung Transplant* 1992;11(5):950-958.
111. Van Cleemput J, Daenen W, Nijs J, Geusens P, Dequeker J, Vanhaecke J: Timing and quantification of bone loss in cardiac transplant recipients. *Transpl Int* 1995;8(3):196-200.

112. Ralston SH, Urquhart GD, Brzeski M, Sturrock RD: Prevalence of vertebral compression fractures due to osteoporosis in ankylosing spondylitis. *BMJ* 1990;300(6724):563-565.

113. Lauritzen JB: Hip fractures: Incidence, risk factors, energy absorption, and prevention. *Bone* 1996;18(1, Suppl)65S-75S.

114. Marshall D, Johnell O, Wedel H: Meta-analysis of how well measures of bone mineral density predict occurrence of osteoporotic fractures. *BMJ* 1996;312(7041):1254-1259.

115. Riggs BL: Overview of osteoporosis. *West J Med* 1991;154(1):63-77.

116. Blam OG, Cotler JM: Fractures in the stiff and osteoporotic spine, in Browner BD, Jupiter JB, Levine AM, Trafton PG, eds: *Skeletal Trauma: Basic Science, Management, and Reconstruction*. Philadelphia, PA, Saunders, 2003, pp 1004-1006.

117. Cook SD, Salkeld SL, Stanley T, Faciane A, Miller SD: Biomechanical study of pedicle screw fixation in severely osteoporotic bone. *Spine J* 2004;4(4): 402-408.

118. Wuisman PI, Van Dijk M, Staal H, Van Royen BJ: Augmentation of (pedicle) screws with calcium apatite cement in patients with severe progressive osteoporotic spinal deformities: An innovative technique. *Eur Spine J* 2000;9(6):528-533.

119. Mobbs RJ, Szkandera B, Blum P: Posterior femoral cutaneous nerve entrapment neuropathy: Operative exposure and technique. *Br J Neurosurg* 2002; 16(3):309-311.

120. Wilson DR, Myers ER, Mathis JM, et al: Effect of augmentation on the mechanics of vertebral wedge fractures. *Spine (Phila Pa 1976)* 2000;25(2): 158-165.

121. Garfin SR, Yuan HA, Reiley MA: New technologies in spine: Kyphoplasty and vertebroplasty for the treatment of painful osteoporotic compression fractures. *Spine (Phila Pa 1976)* 2001;26(14): 1511-1515.

122. Cornell CN, Lane JM, Poynton AR: Orthopedic management of vertebral and long bone fractures in patients with osteoporosis. *Clin Geriatr Med* 2003;19(2):433-455.

123. Lieberman IH, Dudeney S, Reinhardt MK, Bell G: Initial outcome and efficacy of "kyphoplasty" in the treatment of painful osteoporotic vertebral compression fractures. *Spine (Phila Pa 1976)* 2001; 26(14):1631-1638.

124. Kallmes DF, Comstock BA, Heagerty PJ, et al: A randomized trial of vertebroplasty for osteoporotic spinal fractures. *N Engl J Med* 2009;361(6): 569-579.

125. Bouza C, López T, Magro A, Navalpotro L, Amate JM: Efficacy and safety of balloon kyphoplasty in the treatment of vertebral compression fractures: A systematic review. *Eur Spine J* 2006;15(7): 1050-1067.

126. Wardlaw D, Cummings SR, Van Meirhaeghe J, et al: Efficacy and safety of balloon kyphoplasty compared with non-surgical care for vertebral compression fracture (FREE): A randomised controlled trial. *Lancet* 2009;373(9668):1016-1024.

127. Katagiri H, Takahashi M, Inagaki J, et al: Clinical results of nonsurgical treatment for spinal metastases. *Int J Radiat Oncol Biol Phys* 1998;42(5): 1127-1132.

128. Fine PG: Palliative radiation therapy in end-of-life care: Evidence-based utilization. *Am J Hosp Palliat Care* 2002;19(3):166-170.

129. Berenson JR, Lipton A: Bisphosphonates in the treatment of malignant bone disease. *Annu Rev Med* 1999;50:237-248.

130. Falkmer U, Järhult J, Wersäll P, Cavallin-Ståhl E: A systematic overview of radiation therapy effects in skeletal metastases. *Acta Oncol* 2003;42(5-6): 620-633.

131. Patchell RA, Tibbs PA, Regine WF, et al: Direct decompressive surgical resection in the treatment of spinal cord compression caused by metastatic cancer: A randomised trial. *Lancet* 2005; 366(9486):643-648.

132. Wai EK, Finkelstein JA, Tangente RP, et al: Quality of life in surgical treatment of metastatic spine disease. *Spine (Phila Pa 1976)* 2003;28(5): 508-512.

133. Tomita K, Kawahara N, Kobayashi T, Yoshida A, Murakami H, Akamaru T: Surgical strategy for spinal metastases. *Spine (Phila Pa 1976)* 2001; 26(3):298-306.

134. Schwender JD, Holly LT, Rouben DP, Foley KT: Minimally invasive transforaminal lumbar interbody fusion (TLIF): Technical feasibility and initial results. *J Spinal Disord Tech* 2005;18(Suppl): S1-S6.

135. Amini A, Beisse R, Schmidt MH: Thoracoscopic spine surgery for decompression and stabilization of the anterolateral thoracolumbar spine. *Neurosurg Focus* 2005;19(6):E4.

CHAPTER 30
Flexion-Distraction Injuries of the Thoracic and Lumbar Spine

Frank J. Eismont, MD   Esteban Cuartas, MD

Key Points

- Combined multiple series in the literature indicate there is a 45% chance of a patient with a thoracic or lumbar flexion-distraction spine injury to have an intra-abdominal injury that requires surgery.
- Up to 85% of patients with a flexion-distraction injury of the thoracic or lumbar spine have an associated anterior vertebral compression fracture or burst fracture.
- A patient with a flexion-distraction injury of the thoracic or lumbar spine who has a deformity equal to 17% to 20% of kyphosis will most likely require surgical treatment.
- Surgery, when indicated, is usually two or three vertebral levels and is always posterior surgery with screws and rods or hooks and rods to restore the spinal alignment and the posterior column tension band.
- Beware of using a posterior compression instrumentation system when there is a concomitant herniated disk or burst fracture; this can produce paralysis.

Introduction

Flexion-distraction injuries of the thoracic and lumbar spine were first described by G.Q. Chance in 1948.[1] He did not mention a mechanism of injury in his three cases, but he included an example and a drawing showing the typical posterior distraction and the commonly seen anterior vertebral body wedging. He also noted that hyperextension should achieve an excellent reduction and that bone-to-bone opposition should allow healing and provide an excellent clinical prognosis. Although there have since been significant additions to these concepts concerning mechanism of injury, further classification of the pathology, and alternative treatment options, Chance's astute clinical observations have generally remained true.

In a mechanistic sense, the term flexion-distraction injury refers to a failure in tension of the posterior and middle columns during an acute spinal flexion.[2] In practice, however, the term also encompasses those injuries accompanied by an anterior compression or burst component. The crucial point is to identify the distractive disruption of the posterior elements, because this will dictate appropriate assessment and treatment.

The purpose of this chapter is to facilitate prompt recognition and appropriate treatment of patients with flexion-distraction injuries of the thoracic and lumbar spine. Thoracic and lumbar spine facet dislocations are discussed in the following chapter.

Seat Belts

Although any accident providing significant forward flexion combined with distraction can produce thoracic or lumbar flexion-distraction injury, it is most commonly the result of a motor vehicle accident (MVA) with the victim wearing a lap seat belt.

The question of whether seat belt use predisposes to any particular injury was first raised in 1962 by Garrett and Braunstein[3] in their article entitled "The Seat Belt Syndrome." They believed that the use of a lap seat belt made injuries to the lumbar spine "somewhat more frequent." This has subsequently been further developed and discussed in many articles.[4-15]

Anderson et al[4] studied the association of various spine injuries with types of restraints used and occupant position in the vehicle. They reviewed 303 patients admitted to a level I trauma center with spine or abdominal injuries as a result of MVAs over a 5-year period from 1984 to 1988. Thirteen (81%) of the 16 patients with lumbar flexion-distraction injuries were restrained, compared to 8 (14%) of 59 patients with cervical spine injuries. Also, none of the 59 cervical injuries or 71 thoracic injuries were using lap belts

Dr. Eismont or an immediate family member has received royalties from Alphatec Spine; serves as a paid consultant to or is an employee of Alphatech Spine; and owns stock or stock options in Alphatech Spine. Neither Dr. Cuartas nor any immediate family member has received anything of value from or owns stock in a commercial company or institution related directly or indirectly to the subject of this chapter.

alone, but 10 (62%) with lumbar flexion-distraction injuries were using lap belts without a shoulder harness. In this series, 26.8% of all those injured in MVAs used some type of restraint, with 13.9% using lap and shoulder restraints and 8.3% using lap belts.

Furthermore, although only 12.9% of all victims in their study were known to be rear-seat passengers, 67% of those with lumbar flexion-distraction injuries were rear-seat passengers. This association is not surprising considering that most vehicles with lap-only seat restraints have these in the rear seat.

In this same review by Anderson et al,[4] 32% of patients with small bowel injuries and 29% of patients with colon injuries were wearing lap belts alone, compared with 10% of patients with liver injuries, 3% of those with spleen injuries, and 8% of patients with pancreas injuries. Those using lap belts alone were ten times more likely to have a small bowel injury compared to those passengers using no restraints, and those using lap-shoulder harnesses were 4.4 times more likely to have small bowel injuries compared with those using no restraints.

Because the mechanisms of hollow viscus injury and of lumbar spine flexion-distraction injuries are similar in those using lap seat belts, we would expect many patients to have injuries to both of these areas. In fact, in this same review, 10 of the 16 patients with lumbar flexion-distraction injuries had hollow viscus injuries. Nine had small bowel injuries and seven had colon injuries requiring surgery.

School-aged children are at higher risk for seat-belt syndrome, particularly its more severe forms. Several reports document the higher incidence of abdominal injuries as well as neurologic injury.[16-21]

There are many possible reasons why this flexion-distraction injury of the spine has occurred so often in young children. One is that they may be limited to riding in the back seat, which more commonly has only lap seat belts. Another is that biomechanically, the center of gravity is higher in a child than in an adult.[22] With the pelvis fixed to the vehicle with a lap seat belt, the flexion-distraction forces may be increased relative to the strength of the bone and ligaments.[14] There is also concern that in children, for various anatomic reasons, the seat belts tend to be worn too high to grab the pelvis, as they do in adults, and instead compress only the mid-abdomen and flexible lumbar spine. Finally, due to discomfort, some children may elect to wear shoulder/lap belts as lap belts only.

Multiple case reports document this increased severity in young children. In one case report,[17] three children in a head-on collision were restrained passengers. They were all 9 to 12 years of age, and all sustained blunt abdominal injuries along with thoracolumbar flexion-distraction injuries resulting in paraplegia. Another case report documents a complete spinal cord and cauda equina avulsion in a 14-year-old boy who was wearing a lap belt.[23] A series of 27 pediatric Chance fractures that presented to the British Columbia Children's Hospital between 1984 and 2001 revealed a 30% incidence of neurologic injury.[24]

The American Academy of Pediatrics recommends using booster seats in this age group to elevate the children and permit the restraints to fit more snugly.[25] However, these are not foolproof; in one case report, an improperly fastened booster displaced during deceleration and subjected a child to fatal neck injuries.[26]

These statistics should warn us that any patient brought to the hospital for evaluation of injuries sustained in an MVA and especially in those patients with a seat belt contusion of the abdomen or a history of being a rear-seat occupant or a history of lap seat belt use should be thoroughly evaluated for both lumbar spine flexion-distraction injuries and for hollow viscus injuries.

Although we have emphasized these injuries and their association with seat belts, it should be positively mentioned that seat restraints have reduced fatalities 40% to 50%.[3,27-29] Also, considering nonfatal crash victims, restrained occupants generally have less severe injuries than those not restrained.[30,31] In a study at the Maryland Institute for Emergency Medical Services Systems, unrestrained occupants had a mean injury severity score of 22.9 compared with those restrained occupants with a mean injury severity score of 10.8, which is a significant difference ($P < .0005$).[30] They also found that the medical cost was significantly reduced in those restrained victims ($P < .025$). In a review of 1,019 spine fracture patients conducted through the Scoliosis Research Society, Gertzbein[6] found that there was a highly significant relationship between wearing a seat belt and neurologic status. Those wearing a belt were much less likely to have a complete paralysis ($P = 0.007$).

According to data from the US Department of Transportation,[32,33] shoulder seat-belt usage has steadily increased from 58% in 1994, to 67% in 1999, 73% in 2001, and 80% in 2004. For 2004, on a national level, front-seat restraint use in pas-

TABLE 1

Correlation of Injuries With the Type of Restraint Used in Head-on MVAs

	Two-Point or Lap Belt	Three-Point	Airbag + Three-Point	Totals
Flexion-distraction injury of the spine	13 of 16 (81%)	11 of 15 (73%)	2 of 6 (33%)	26 of 37 (70%)
Intra-abdominal injury requiring laparotomy	8 of 16 (50%)	4 of 15 (26.7%)	0 of 6	12 of 37 (32%)
Spinal cord or cauda equina injury	3 of 16 (19%)	0 of 15	0 of 6	3 of 37 (8%)
Burst component	5 of 16 (31%)	11 of 15 (73%)	5 of 6 (83%)	21 of 37 (54%)

(Adapted from Ball ST, Vaccarro AR, Albert TJ, Cotler JM: Injuries of the thoracolumbar spine associated with restraint use in head-on motor vehicle accidents. *J Spinal Disord* 2000;13(4):297-304.)

senger cars was associated with a 45% lower mortality after a motor vehicle crash. Also, ejection from vehicles was associated with 74% mortality. Restraint use was associated with a 1% ejection rate compared to 29% for unrestrained passengers.

Since 1990, rear-seat restraints have included lap-shoulder restraints. The increased use of airbags has also likely reduced the incidence of these flexion-distraction injuries, although specific data are not available. The Department of Transportation estimates that at a national level, airbag use decreases mortality by 14% when used alone.[32]

Ball et al[34] studied thoracolumbar injuries and their association with restraint use. They reviewed 221 patients treated for thoracolumbar fractures at a level I trauma center from 1988 to 1998. Out of this group, only 37 patients had well-documented restraint use (**Table 1**). There was an apparent lower incidence of flexion-distraction injuries with three-point restraints and airbags, when compared to lap belts. Interestingly, they noted a higher incidence of burst fractures in the patients with three-point restraints (80%) than in those with lap belts (28.6%). Also of note is the high overall incidence of a flexion-distraction component to the injuries (70%). The authors suggest that a three-point restraint brings the instantaneous axis of rotation closer to and even posterior to the middle column, thereby causing a compressive force to the anterior and middle columns. At the same time, it appears to decrease the distractive forces posteriorly, as evidenced by a lower incidence of neurologic injury.

Biomechanics of Injury

Flexion-distraction injuries should involve a forward flexion with the axis of rotation in the middle column of the spine or slightly anterior to it. This would explain the posterior column separations commonly seen, as well as axial load injuries such as wedge compression fractures or burst fractures, which are seen in up to 70% of these injuries. What is not immediately evident is how these injury patterns are caused by a lap belt, which sits far anterior to the spine.

Research presented by Begeman and Prasad[35] in 1973 helps to explain these associated anterior vertebral body wedge compression and burst fractures. They found that with rapid deceleration using lap belts and using lap-shoulder restraints, the initial loading of the spine was actually an axial load (**Figure 1**). This peaked rapidly, and slowly decreased throughout the deceleration. There was also a second peak in the axial loading at the termination of the deceleration injury when the torso was thrown back into the seat. Begeman and Prasad also found that greater axial loads were seen in the upright spine supported by a combined lap and shoulder harness. The magnitude of the initial axial loading was proportional to the deceleration gravity force g. Hence, there is more likely to be an associated anterior vertebral wedge compression fracture when the initial deceleration g-force is the greatest. Conversely, injury is likely to be limited to the posterior flexion-distraction

FIGURE 1

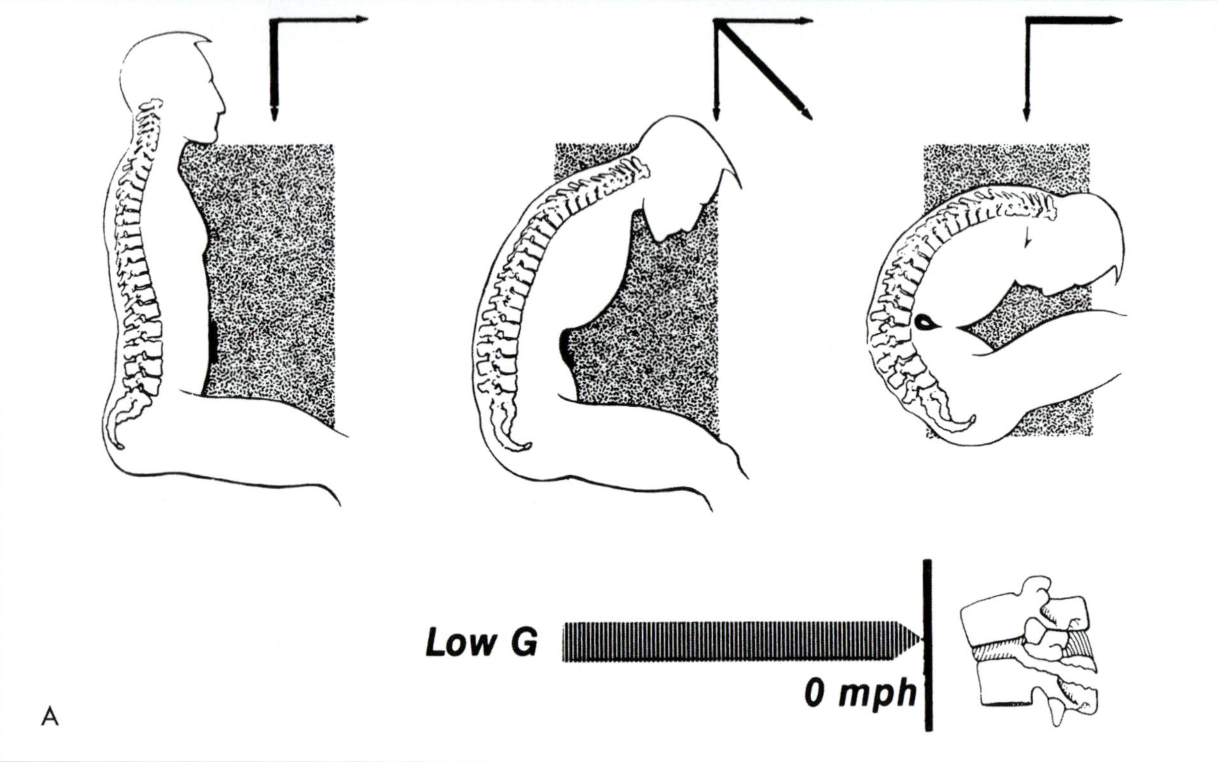

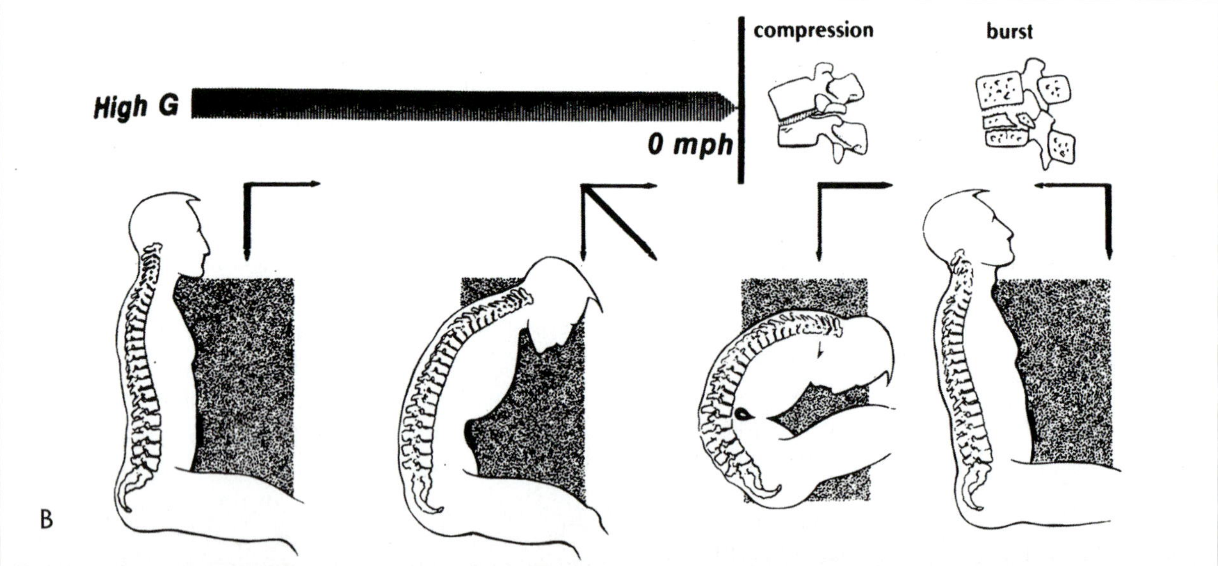

Figure 1 A, This shows a flexion-distraction injury occurring with low *g* forces. The axial component of the force is relatively small, and hence no wedge compression fracture or burst fracture occurs. A typical distraction injury of the posterior elements of the spine occurs. **B,** In sudden deceleration injuries with high *g* forces, there is an initial significant axial load force that can result in either a wedge compression fracture or burst fracture anteriorly. As the injury progresses, the standard posterior distraction injury occurs. At the termination of the motion the body is thrown back into the sitting position and further injury to the vertebral body may occur at this time. (Reproduced with permission from Gertzbein SD, Court-Brown CM: Flexion-distraction injuries of the lumbar spine: Mechanisms of injury and classification. *Clin Orthop Relat Res* 1988; 227:52-60.)

component when the initial deceleration g-force is smaller.

Hoshikawa et al[36] reproduced these injuries by combining a flexed posture of the spine and a compressive load. A compressive force applied to a flexed spine can be divided into an anterior axial compressive force and a posterior distractive force. The angle of flexion of the spine at the time of the compressive force determines the motion axis of fracture (MAF), which is the point of transition from anterior compression to posterior distraction. The MAF is more anterior for larger flexion angles and more posterior for smaller angles. For a larger flexion angle, a smaller compressive force is required to cause the posterior elements to fail in tension and the anterior elements in compression. This model, as opposed to those using a combination of bending moments and distractive forces, can bring the MAF from the anterior to the middle column, thus recreating the common clinical situation of a burst component. According to this model, to effectively recreate a flexion-distraction injury with a burst component, the spine must be compressed while flexed. In MVAs, this combination of vectors is given by the fact that the spine is initially inclined posteriorly and the deceleration force applies compression.

Other basic research concerning flexion-distraction injuries of the lumbar spine has been performed using isolated two-vertebrae segments in mechanical testing.[11,37] The first point of substantial structural injury occurred between a mean flexion angulation of 16°[11] and 20°.[23] In another model, Nagel et al[38] demonstrated a flexion-extension range of motion increase at L1-L2 from 8.4° (neutral zone) to 17.3° after disruption of supraspinous and interspinous ligaments, ligamentum flavum, facet joints, posterior longitudinal ligament, and anulus. Neumann et al[39] demonstrated a "potential instability" with focal kyphosis of 12° to 19°, as well as "total instability" with flexion greater than 22°. Neumann et al studied criteria for instability by using a dynamic loading model of flexion-distraction injuries (without burst or compression components). They found that there was impending instability with less than 12° of flexion or greater than 20-mm increase in interspinous distance, and total instability less than 19° or greater than 33-mm increase in interspinous distance.[39] It is unclear how these numbers translate to the clinical situation, where there is often a compression or burst component as well as a partial reduction of the deformity before radiographic studies. However, these are surprisingly close to the angulations cited in clinical reviews beyond which nonsurgical treatment failed (ie, 20° by Glassman et al[7] in 1992 and 17° by LeGay et al[10] in 1990).

Clinical Assessment

As noted in the discussion concerning seat belts, the clinician should be wary of spine flexion-distraction injury in any patient with a history of involvement in an MVA, especially with documented use of a seat belt. The suspicion should be raised further if the victim is a child, a back-seat occupant, and if only a lap restraint was used. Both the spine and abdominal injuries may be subtle and are at risk for delayed diagnosis.

The diagnosis of spine injuries can be delayed in polytrauma patients for several reasons. Stanislas et al[40] noted a 3.6% occurrence of delayed diagnosis in a review of 110 spine injuries. In their series, delayed diagnosis was associated with Glasgow Coma Scale less than 11, high-velocity trauma, head injury, and distracting pelvic or lower extremity injuries.[40]

Patients with flexion-distraction injuries in particular seem to be at risk for delayed diagnosis. A recent review of more than 300 patients treated at a level I trauma center for acetabular fractures found a 13% rate of coincident spine injuries.[41] Of note, three spine injuries had an 8.6-day delay in diagnosis, two of them being flexion-distraction injuries. One of these patients was initially neurologically intact at presentation, and subsequently developed a T7-T8 dislocation with complete paraplegia on the eighth hospital day.

Delay in diagnosis of abdominal injuries in children with seat-belt syndrome has also been commonly described. Initial radiographic and CT examination is often falsely negative. Some of the patients have presented late (at 4 to 6 weeks after their accident)[14] with intestinal obstruction due to narrowed ischemic bowel or obstructing hernias through the mesentery or even hernias through the posterior abdominal fascia.[42] One case report describes an enterocolic fistula diagnosed 4 months after an L3-L4 Chance fracture in a 9-year-old boy. This child presented with late-onset and persistent abdominal symptoms including vomiting and diarrhea.[16]

For these reasons, some authors advocate exploratory laparotomy or laparoscopy in all children with a lumbar spine injury and abdominal wall contusion—the "seat-belt sign" (**Figure 2**).[18] Indeed, the incidence of an associated abdominal injury requiring surgery (**Figure 3**) is 45% according to a combined review of 10 series of patients

FIGURE 2

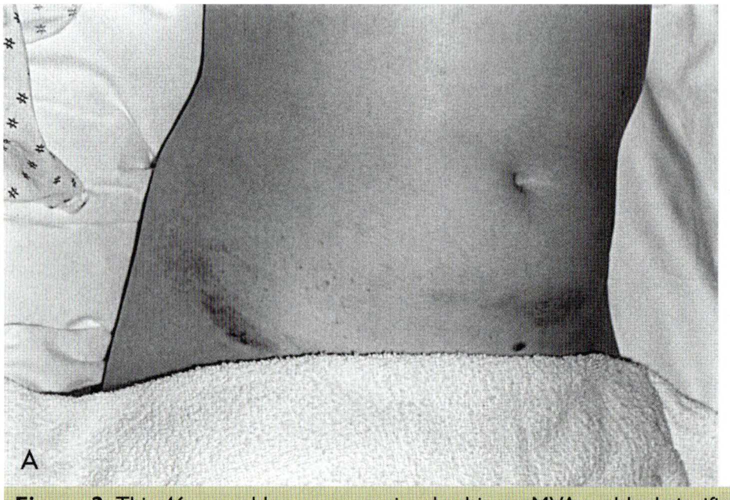

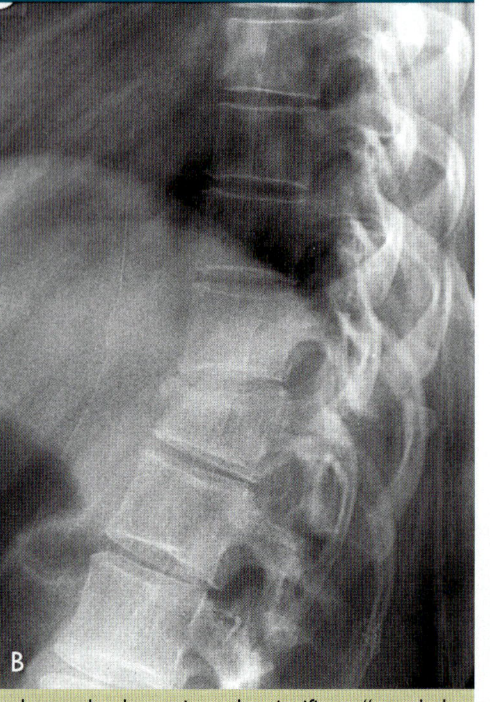

Figure 2 This 46-year-old woman was involved in an MVA and had significant thoracolumbar pain and a significant "seat-belt sign." **A,** This photograph of the patient's lower abdomen shows the typical ecchymoses consistent with a seat-belt injury. This should alert the clinician to possible hollow viscus injury and to flexion-distraction injuries of the spine. This patient did not have an associated intra-abdominal injury. **B,** This lateral radiograph of the thoracolumbar junction reveals a flexion-distraction injury of T11. This could easily be mistaken for a benign compression fracture of T11. (Reproduced from Eismont FJ: Flexion-distraction injuries of the thoracic and lumbar spine, in Levine AM, Eismont FJ, Garfin SR, Zigler JE, eds: *Spine Trauma*. Philadelphia, PA, WB Saunders, 1998, pp 402-414.)

(**Table 2**).[2,4,5,7,8,10,12-14,43] The spectrum of abdominal injuries includes both hollow and solid viscus injuries, as well as vascular disruptions (aortic and mesenteric) and abdominal wall herniations.[20,28,44]

Physical examination should always be comprehensive for accident victims, but special attention should be given to palpation of the spine for tenderness and for any gaping space between adjacent posterior elements.

The abdomen should also be inspected for any seat-belt sign (ie, any ecchymoses or contusion of the abdomen) (**Figure 2**). One series of 61 children with seat-belt ecchymoses showed a 64% incidence of significant abdominal injury, 23% incidence of hollow viscus injury, and 21% incidence of lumbar spine injury.[45]

Neurologically, the majority of patients with lumbar flexion-distraction injuries remain normal. In his series of 19 patients, Denis[2] reported that none had paralysis secondary to their seat belt-type injury. Other series, however, have had up to 30% of patients with paralysis.[14] In the sum of the 10 series of patients (**Table 2**), the chance of paralysis is 13%. Although it is extremely uncommon, patients may also develop a progressive paraparesis secondary to an associated epidural hematoma at the site of a flexion-distraction injury of the lumbar spine. In most cases, in patients with no neurologic deficit, immobilization in the supine position on a rotating treatment frame or rigid bed will tend to reduce and stabilize the injury until definitive treatment with bracing or surgery can be performed.

There are also several case reports in the literature of unusual presentations. These include one in an adult snowboarder,[46] two caused by a squatting exercise machine,[47] and two in pregnant women after MVAs.[48] These cases serve to remind the surgeon to maintain a high level of vigilance.

Radiographic Assessment

Plain radiographs will usually be adequate to demonstrate most flexion-distraction injuries of the lumbar spine. However, CT scans have been shown to be more sensitive than plain radiographs

FIGURE 3

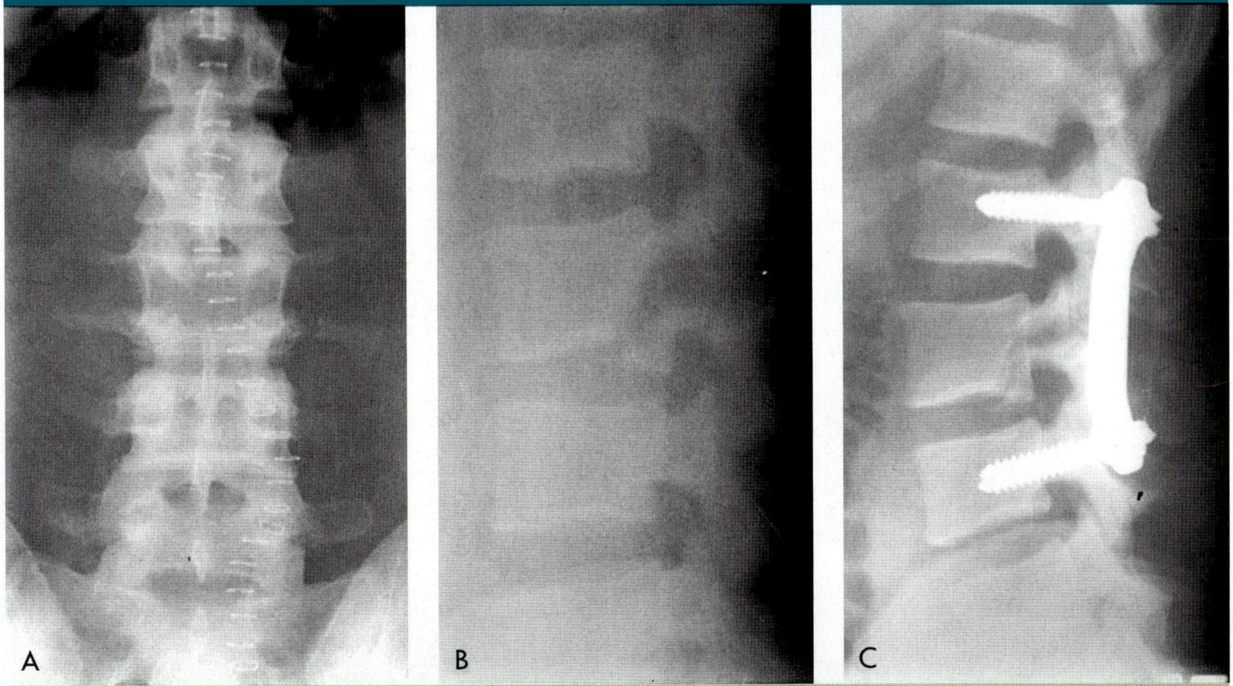

Figure 3 This young man was involved in an MVA and was using a lap seat belt at the time of the injury. He had sustained a rupture of his colon, which was diagnosed and treated acutely. He was immobilized on a rigid oscillating bed before and after the abdominal surgery until it was certain that his bowel repair was satisfactory. **A,** AP radiograph shows anterior abdominal skin clips overlying the lumbar spine. It can be seen quite clearly that the L3 transverse processes, as well as the pedicles, are split. **B,** Lateral film shows that the injury line goes through the inferior end plate of L3 and into the L3-4 disk space. **C,** Postoperative lateral view shows that the fracture has been well reduced. Considering the pattern of the injury, it was not possible to use a shorter construct. This patient was fully mobilized following the spine surgery that facilitated his recovery. (Reproduced from Eismont FJ: Flexion-distraction injuries of the thoracic and lumbar spine, in Levine AM, Eismont FJ, Garfin SR, Zigler JE, eds: *Spine Trauma*. Philadelphia, PA, WB Saunders, 1998, pp 402-414.)

TABLE 2

Patients Requiring Abdominal Surgery and Patients With Paralysis Following Flexion-Distraction Injury

Series	Patients Requiring Abdominal Surgery	Patients With Paralysis
Anderson et al[4]	10/16	—
Dehner[5]	3/7	0/7
Denis[2]	—	0/19
Gertzbein and Court-Brown[43]	9/19	5/19
Glassman et al[7]	5/12	0/12
Gumley et al[8]	8/20	2/20
LeGay et al[10]	7/18	2/18
Newman et al[12]	4/9	2/9
Reid et al[13]	3/7	1/7
Rumball and Jarvis[14]	4/10	3/10
Totals	53/118 = 45%	16/121 = 13%

(Reproduced from Eismont FJ: Flexion-distraction injuries of the thoracic and lumbar spine, in Levine AM, Eismont FJ, Garfin SR, Zigler JE, eds: *Spine Trauma*. Philadelphia, PA, WB Saunders, 1998, pp 402-414.)

FIGURE 4

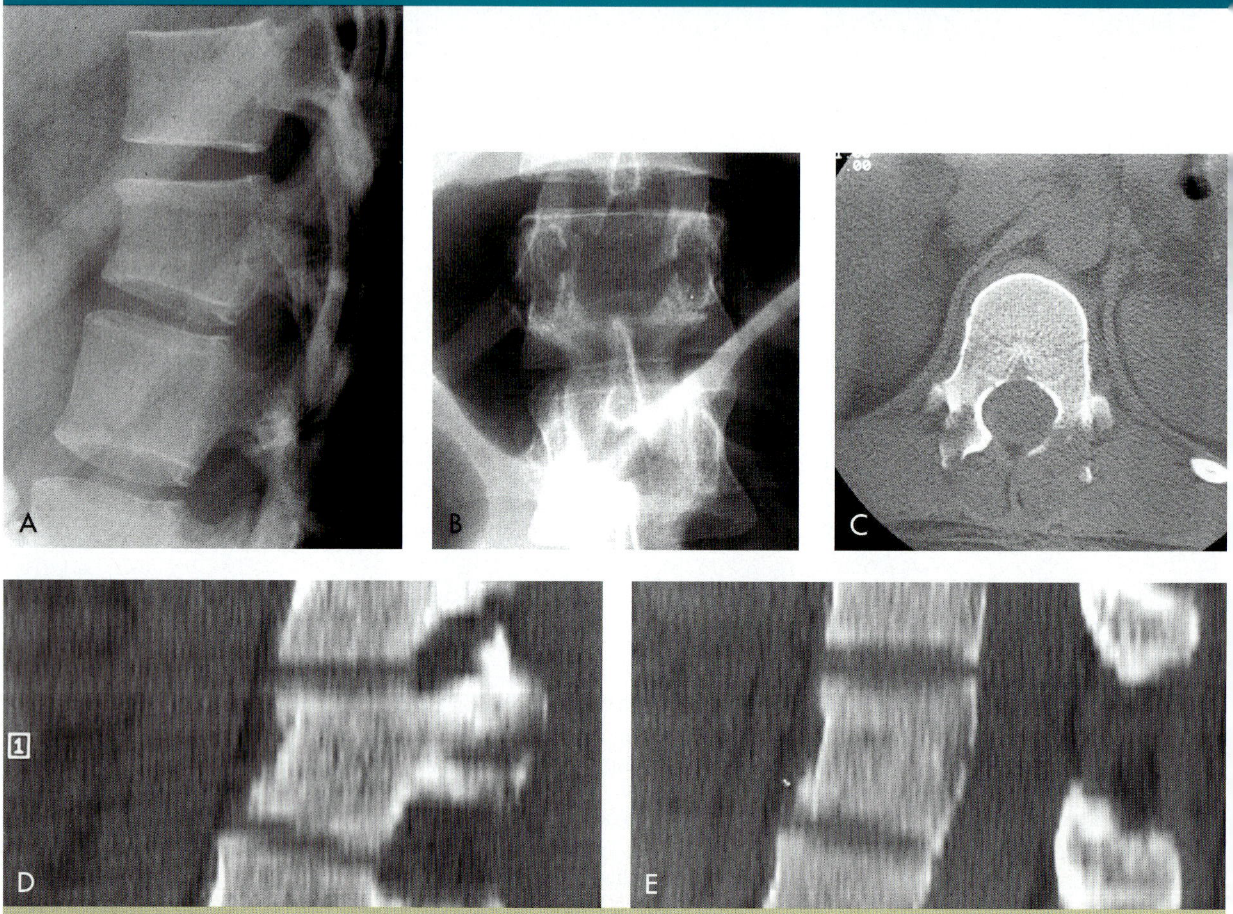

Figure 4 An excellent radiographic example of the flexion-distraction injury as originally described by Chance. **A,** The cone-down lateral radiograph shows the T12 vertebra is slightly compressed anteriorly as with a wedge compression fracture and is distracted posteriorly with the fracture line proceeding through the pedicles. **B,** This cone-down AP film shows that the fracture line divides the pedicles of T12 bilaterally. It can also be appreciated that there is significant spread between the spinous process of T11 and the spinous process of T12. **C,** A typical-appearing CT section through the level of injury. The fracture lines are not clearly defined because the cut is exactly parallel to the line of injury. **D,** With reconstruction, it can be seen that the fracture line proceeds directly through the pedicle. **E,** This midsagittal CT reconstruction shows that the fracture line goes into the posterior aspect of the vertebral body. This also very clearly shows the spread of the T11 and T12 spinous processes posteriorly. (Reproduced from Eismont FJ: Flexion-distraction injuries of the thoracic and lumbar spine, in Levine AM, Eismont FJ, Garfin SR, Zigler JE, eds: *Spine Trauma*. Philadelphia, PA, WB Saunders, 1998, pp 402-414.)

in detecting spinal injuries. Sheridan et al[49] reviewed 78 patients with thoracolumbar spine injuries and found this to be true for both thoracic (97% versus 62%) and lumbar (95% versus 86%) fractures. These authors suggest that in high-energy trauma patients, CT scans may actually be reasonable screening examinations from both economic and practical points of view. CT scans are also useful screening modalities in patients who are otherwise obtunded or intubated.

The bony anatomy of the injury is best demonstrated by CT scan. It is essential to obtain thin cuts and good sagittal and coronal reconstructions (**Figure 4**). Standard transverse cuts with the CT scanner will tend to minimize or may even miss the injury if the cuts are too wide, especially because the plane of injury is horizontal and parallel to the CT cuts. The CT scan is especially helpful in those victims with anterior vertebral body axial-load injuries (up to 85% of cases) to be certain that there is no burst fracture present (up to 15% of cases). This is especially important information if surgery is planned, as it will dictate whether or not compression forces can be used to help achieve reduction.

It is important to document the degree of angulation, any splaying of the spinous processes, the integrity of the posterior elements, and the con-

TABLE 3

MRI Findings: MRI Features Associated With Flexion-Distraction Spinal Trauma

Type of Injury	Percentage of Patients	No. of Patients
Bony Findings		
Pedicle disruption	96	23/24
Bilateral pedicle disruption	71	17/24
Sandwich sign	50	12/24
Facet disruption	71	17/24
Laminar fracture	21	5/24
Vertebral body disruption	100	24/24
Contiguous injury	83	20/24
Noncontiguous injury	33	8/24
Soft-Tissue Findings		
Subcutaneous fat disruption	100	24/24
Epidural hematoma	88	21/24
Paravertebral hematoma	83	20/24
Disk disruption	54	13/24
Psoas muscle edema	29	7/24
Cord disruption	33	8/24

(Adapted from Groves CJ, Cassar-Pullicino VN, Tins BJ, Tyrrell PN, McCall IW: Chance-type flexion-distraction injuries in the thoracolumbar spine: MR imaging characteristics. *Radiology* 2005;236(2): 601-608.)

comitant presence of a burst or compression component. The naked facet sign—where one facet either inferior or superior can be seen in an axial cut without its corresponding facet—has been proposed as an indicator of instability, especially in the lumbar spine.[50-53]

For any patient with a neurologic deficit or any patient scheduled for surgery, it is also important to obtain an MRI scan or a myelogram followed by a CT scan if for some reason the MRI is contraindicated. This is necessary because these patients may also have disk abnormalities or unsuspected spinal stenosis which might alter the treatment plan.[15]

MRI can be especially helpful in discerning the full extent of the osseoligamentous injury. Groves et al[54] reviewed the MRI findings in 24 patients with flexion-distraction injuries (**Table 3**). T1-weighted images were better for visualizing the vertebral body and posterior neural arch fractures, whereas pedicular and soft-tissue injuries were best seen on T2-weighted images. They describe a "sandwich sign" in the fractured pedicles (**Figure 5**). This consists of a linear layer of low signal intensity (hemorrhage), framed by two layers of high signal intensity (edema), and is seen only on T2-weighted and short-tau inversion recovery images. The sandwich sign was present in 50% of their patients. It is noteworthy that they found a 33% rate of noncontiguous spine injuries, as well as a 56% rate of "empty facet sign."

Adams et al[55] found that MRI can be valuable as a screening examination in critically injured patients with unresolved tenderness at multiple levels, neurologic complaints such as radiculopathy or myelopathy, or decreased levels of consciousness. They found that a screening MRI confirmed previous CT diagnoses in 83 of 97 patients (86%), reclassified injuries as degenerative changes in 12 of 97 (13%), and uncovered 2 previously undiagnosed distraction-type ligamentous injuries. In both of these cases, treatment was modified, and one of these was a Chance fracture that underwent surgical stabilization.

Although not commonly employed, ultrasound has been shown to be of some potential use in evaluating the posterior ligament complex in patients in whom MRI is contraindicated (eg, patients with pacemakers or ferromagnetic valves).[56]

These injuries are best classified according to Gertzbein and Court-Brown[43] (**Figure 6**), as their system addresses both the flexion-distraction component as well as any vertebral body axial-load injuries that may be present. It is a modification of the classification systems of Gumley et al[8] and Denis.[2] Type I is used to categorize the posterior fracture, which symmetrically splits the spinous process, laminae, pedicles, and transverse processes. Type II denotes that the fracture is similar to type I but the fracture line enters at the base of the spinous process. Type III denotes that the fracture posteriorly is asymmetric, involving more of the posterior elements on one side than the other. Gertzbein and Court-Brown[43] found that 10% of their injuries were type I, 65% were type II, and 25% were type III.

The injury involving the disk or vertebral body is categorized as A when the injury exits through the disk, as B when the injury is limited to the body, and as C when the bony injury proceeds through an end plate and into the disk. C-1 denotes an injury through the superior end plate and C-2 denotes an injury through the inferior end plate. Gertzbein and Court-Brown found that 5% of their injuries were type A, 20% were type B, 25% were type C-1, and 50% were type C-2.

Finally, the state of the vertebral body is assessed. A typical wedge compression fracture is classified type D; if there is an associated vertebral burst fracture, it is classified type E; and if the vertebral body is intact, it is classified as type F. They found that 70% of their injuries were type D, 15% were type E, and 15% were type F.

Treatment

The initial assessment has been discussed already; emphasis is placed on recognition of the spine injury and adequate evaluation of intra-abdominal injury, which is seen in 45% of these patients. The abdominal evaluation may include a peritoneal lavage, minilaparotomy, or both.

Associated bowel disruption obviously takes priority over surgical treatment of the spine injury. If the bowel surgery involves the colon, spine surgery should be postponed until it is certain that there will be no bouts of septicemia. If the surgery involves the duodenum or jejunum, however, and the general surgeons are pleased with the adequacy of repair, then spine surgery could be performed at any time.

The spine can be initially treated with bed rest on a rigid turning frame. This allows adequate stabilization of the spine injury, and lying supine on a rigid surface may even achieve some degree of injury reduction. At this point, decisions are made concerning surgical or nonsurgical treatment. Surgery is usually recommended under the following circumstances:

(1) A progressive neural deficit with proven neural compression.

(2) A static neural deficit that occurred at the time of injury with seat-belt flexion-distraction injury is usually due to tensile disruption of the neural elements and is not often associated with residual neural compression. Surgery is most helpful in these patients to stabilize the spine to facilitate mobilization and rehabilitation (**Figure 7**).

(3) In the multiple trauma patient, to allow rapid mobilization that may be needed to help with pulmonary function and skin care.

(4) Flexion-distraction injuries in which the original deformity is 17° or more. This recommendation is based on reviews of flexion-distraction injuries that found poor results with nonsurgical treatment if the original deformity was greater than 17° (Le Gay et al[10]) or 20° (Glassman et al[7]).

(5) Injuries with primarily soft-tissue involvement. These injuries, such as the type IIA (Gertzbein and Court-Brown classification[43]), will generally heal poorly and will do best with surgical treatment.

For those patients who are neurologically intact and have an isolated flexion-distraction injury, the decision between surgical and nonsurgical treatment is a relatively easy one. In that uniform group of patients (isolated injury in a neurologically intact patient), the decision concerning the type of treatment is based on the presumed outcome for spinal stability and the ability to obtain a reduction.

The first issue centers on understanding the nature of the injury. Looking at all classifications of injury, three common generic injury types exist. The first comprises purely bony injuries with a

FIGURE 5

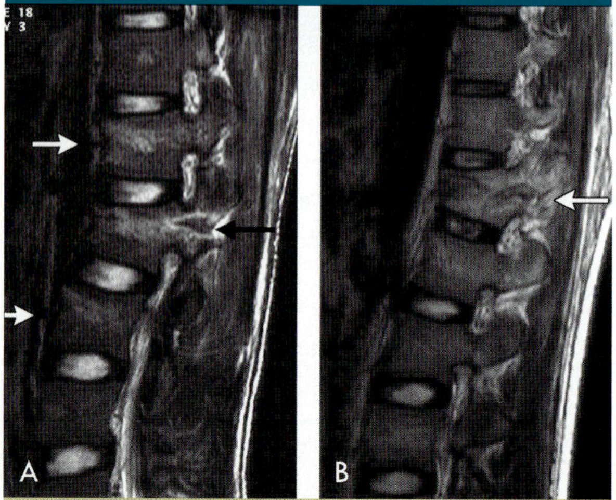

Figure 5 MRI features of the sandwich sign. **A,** Sagittal short-tau inversion recovery MRI scan shows the sandwich sign (black arrow)—an area of low-signal–intensity hemorrhage within the pedicular fracture, encased by a rim of edema. Note the linear areas of edema in the two adjacent injured vertebral bodies (white arrows). **B,** Sagittal T2-weighted turbo spin-echo image shows a horizontal fracture in the pedicle of T12, with linear adjacent zones of high and low signal intensity that produce a sandwich sign (arrow). The fracture extends into the vertebra and is associated with an anterosuperior wedge-shaped fracture of the vertebral body. (Reproduced with permission from Groves CJ, Cassar-Pullicino VN, Tins BJ, Tyrrell PN, McCall IW: Chance-type flexion-distraction injuries in the thoracolumbar spine: MR imaging characteristics. *Radiology* 2005; 236(2):601-608.)

FIGURE 6

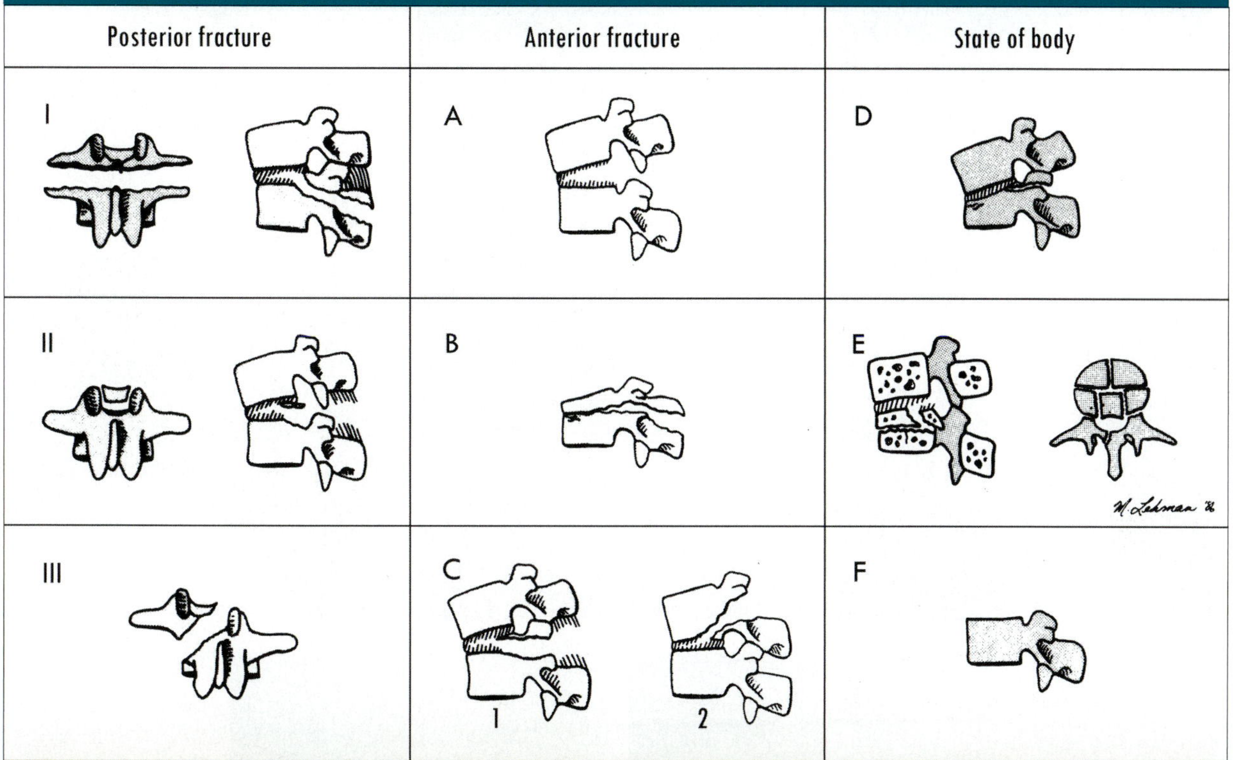

Figure 6 This illustrations depict a useful classification system for discussing flexion-distraction injuries of the spine. A posterior fracture is characterized as I, where the fracture proceeds through the superior aspect of the spinous process through the pedicle and transverse processes; II, where the fracture line enters at the base of the spinous process; or III, where the fracture lines enter obliquely involving more of the posterior elements on one side than the other. The anterior fracture is either categorized as A, which shows the plane of injury going through the disk space only; B, which shows the plane of injury is a fracture line through the vertebral body proceeding from posterior to anterior; C-1, which breaks through the superior end plate of the vertebral body and into the disk space; or C-2, which proceeds through the inferior end plate of the vertebral body and into the disk space. The state of the vertebral body is categorized as D, which represents a simple anterior wedge compression fracture; E, which denotes a burst fracture component; or F, which denotes an intact vertebral body. (Reproduced with permission from Gertzbein SD, Court-Brown CM: Flexion-distraction injuries of the lumbar spine: Mechanisms of injury and classification. *Clin Orthop Relat Res* 1988;227:52-60.)

fracture line through the spinous process, lamina, pedicle, and body. If these heal in a relatively anatomic position, no potential instability can exist. The second group of injuries are combined osseoligamentous injuries, with either posterior element disruption through the ligamentous complex together with a body fracture or posterior element fracture through the bony portion with an anterior disk disruption. The former most commonly results in ligamentous instability even if an anatomic reduction can be obtained. The latter can have a variable outcome. The third type is the purely ligamentous disruption (facet dislocations), which always result in instability and most often cannot be anatomically reduced.

Thus, for the purely bony injuries, the sole element in decision making is the ability to obtain and maintain a satisfactory reduction. The only indication for surgery in this patient group with a purely bony injury is the inability to obtain a satisfactory reduction of the kyphosis. This most often can be achieved with the use of a well-fitted hyperextension brace. This could be achieved with either a Jewett hyperextension brace or a custom-made thoracolumbosacral orthosis (TLSO) molded in hyperextension. Reduction, if obtained, is usually maintained. For the combined osseoligamentous injuries, the outcome with reference to stability can be mixed. Thus for those in whom a satisfactory reduction of deformity can be achieved nonsurgically, two potential options exist. The first is to treat the patient nonsurgically for 3 months and, if instability is present on flexion-extension radiographs at that time, then surgical stabilization

FIGURE 7

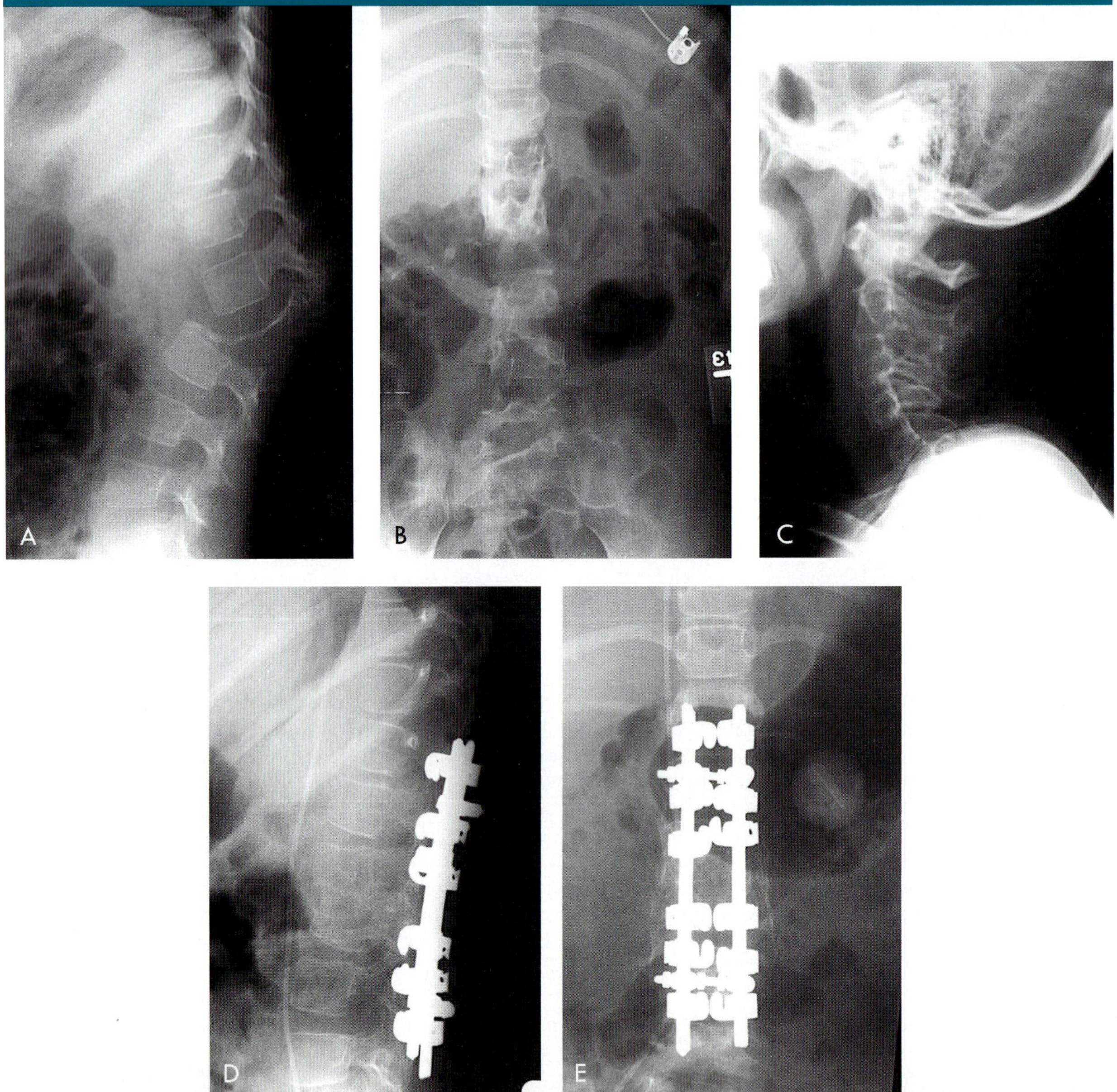

Figure 7 This 6-year-old girl was involved in an MVA and presented to the hospital with a high-level quadriplegia as well as an obvious thoracolumbar spine injury. **A,** Because of a severe respiratory problem and a persistently febrile course, stabilization of her spine could not be performed. This lateral radiograph was taken approximately 5 weeks after injury. There is complete disruption of L2 on L3. **B,** This AP view shows good alignment in the sagittal plane, but significant widening of the posterior elements between L2 and L3 can be clearly seen. **C,** The alignment of the cervical spine always remained normal and no obvious fracture could be seen. This is a good example of SCIWORA (spinal cord injury without radiographic abnormality). **D,** This lateral radiograph was taken approximately 1 year after the original injury and approximately 10 months after the spine reconstruction, which was done through a posterior approach with resection of the lamina of L2 and a posterolateral diskectomy and excision of the early callus to allow reduction. **E,** AP radiograph taken at the same time shows satisfactory healing of the fusion laterally. This construct is considerably longer than what is usually required to stabilize a flexion-distraction injury and was necessitated by the severity of the injury and the deformity. Small, low-profile hooks and rods were used because of her small pedicles at 6 years of age and to minimize hardware prominence.

can be undertaken. The second option is to undertake surgical stabilization initially, based on the presumption that complete posterior ligamentous disruption at a high-stress area like the thoracolumbar or lumbar spine will predictably result in instability and symptoms requiring surgery. Initial treatment, especially if the construct can be kept relatively short, may shorten the overall clinical course. Obviously, if satisfactory reduction of alignment cannot be achieved in these osseoligamentous injuries, then surgical reduction and stabilization will yield a better result.

The final group of purely ligamentous injuries, bilateral facet dislocations, are closely related to a similar entity in the cervical spine. However, in the thoracolumbar spine, it was recognized very early that these are frequently irreducible and have very poor clinical outcomes when treated nonsurgically. Thus, irrespective of the clinical and neurologic status of the patient, these need to be treated surgically. As a result of the distinct nature of this injury, its surgical management is covered in detail in the following chapter.

Once the decision has been made to treat this injury with surgery, the exact details of surgery must be planned based on the injury pattern. Because these injuries all involve predominantly posterior disruption, a posterior approach is always indicated. In trying to correct this type of problem via anterior spine surgery, the spine is further destabilized and the mechanical advantage for correction of the deformity is lost. Spinal instrumentation should always be used and adequate autogenous bone grafting should also be performed. The instrumentation ensures immediate correction of the deformity and the bone grafting ensures the permanency of the correction.

Laminectomy is not necessary unless there are circumstances such as a dural tear that needs to be repaired or a symptomatic epidural hematoma that needs to be evacuated. Performing a laminectomy will usually add to the number of spinal levels that need to be instrumented and fused. Treatment of this type of injury with a laminectomy alone is never indicated. It is recommended to perform a small laminotomy before reduction to remove the disrupted ligamentum flavum, which is often infolded into the spinal canal, and to evacuate the hematoma. Additionally, the surgeon should undercut the adjacent lamina to ensure no neural compression.[57] The reduction can then be more safely achieved.

Patient positioning for surgery is best accomplished on a frame that provides maximal extension forces to facilitate reduction. A four-poster frame is our preference because it allows the abdomen to be completely free while allowing reduction of the spinal deformity. The initial localizing radiograph will usually show that the majority of the deformity has already been corrected.

During surgical exposure, extra care is taken to protect the dura and neural elements, which may be quite exposed due to the posterior distraction injury. Also, in those patients with complete paraplegia following a flexion-distraction injury of the spine, it is not uncommon to see the dura and neural elements completely severed from the initial injury; the surgeon should be prepared to perform dural repairs or subarachnoid shunts at the time of the surgery.[58]

From the preoperative studies, it should be determined if there is an associated burst fracture (up to 15% of cases) or disk disruption (at least 5% of cases). The presence of either of these will necessitate removal of the bone or disk fragments from the spinal canal and fixation with a neutralization type of instrumentation. The decompression can be accomplished through a standard laminotomy if the injury is at the level of the cauda equina, or can be done through a transpedicular posterolateral decompression if the injury is at the level of the spinal cord or conus medullaris. Instrumentation of the spine under these circumstances is best accomplished with the use of pedicle screws at two or three vertebral levels and rods to provide neutralization and correct the initial kyphosis. In the lumbar spine, this type of short construct will provide the best results with the least risk. In the thoracic or thoracolumbar spine, longer systems that provide distraction and three-point bending will also give satisfactory results (**Figure 8**). If the approach described above is not taken, the bone or disk fragments may further intrude into the spinal canal with resultant neurologic deterioration.

Now that the most dangerous possibilities have been considered, we will discuss treatment of the more common flexion-distraction injury with no significant bone or disk fragments intruding into the spinal canal. The surgery should involve as short a segment as possible that will allow reconstruction of the posterior column.[15,43] This will most commonly involve two and occasionally three levels (ie, one and occasionally two motion segments). It is important to minimize the number of levels fused (**Figure 9**) because most of these injuries occur in the midlumbar spine, where preservation of mobile levels is essential to reduce degenerative changes and low back pain at adjacent levels in the future.[59,60] In most of these cases,

FIGURE 8

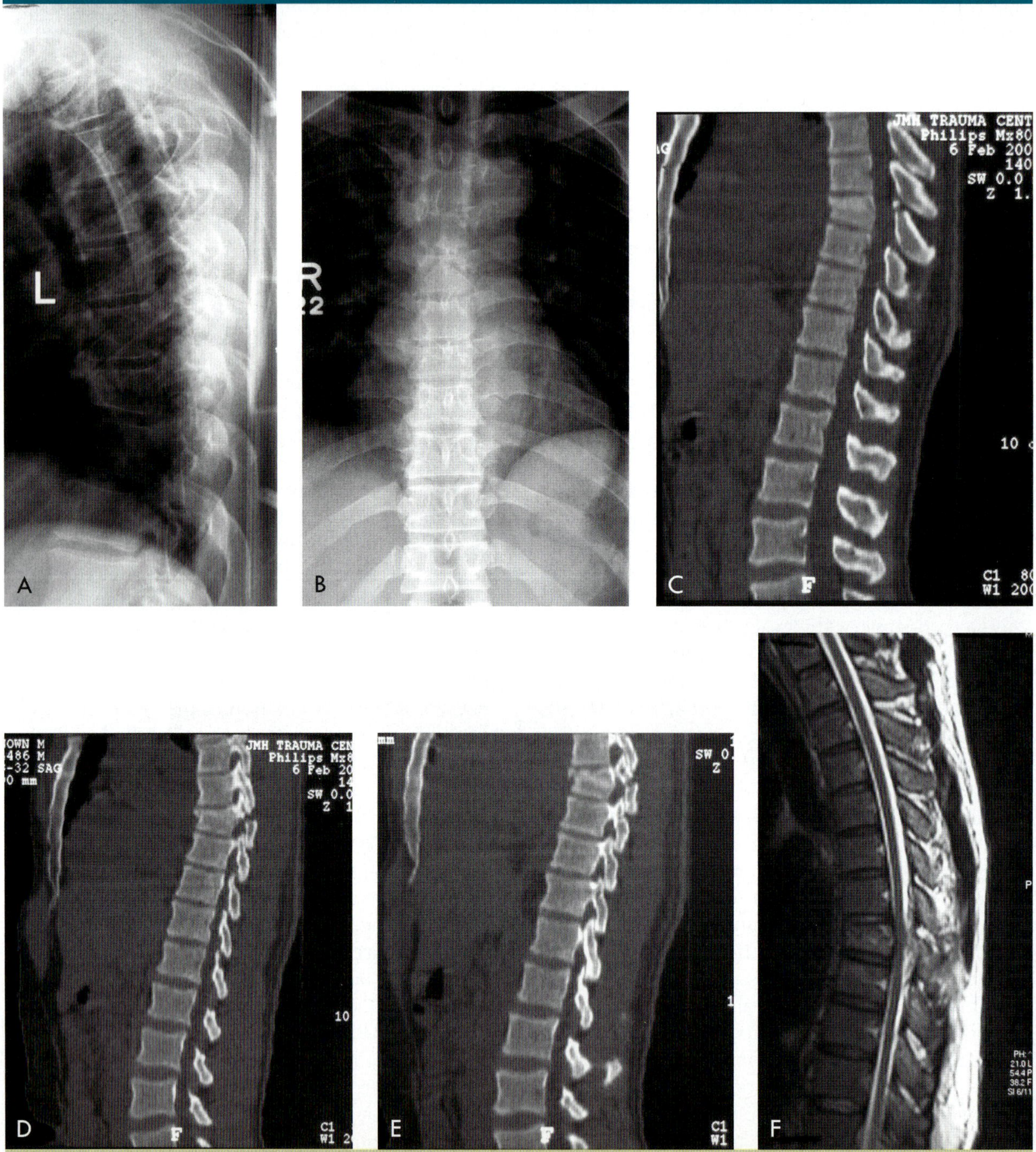

Figure 8 A 46-year-old man sustained this flexion-distraction injury of the T8 level of the spine. **A,** This lateral radiograph shows what could be misinterpreted as a minor compression fracture of the T8 vertebra. **B,** AP radiograph illustrates again what appears to be a minor compression fracture of the T8 vertebra. **C,** This midsagittal reconstructive CT scan shows that the T8 vertebral body fracture is actually a minor burst fracture. It also shows that there is a fracture through the superior portion of the T8 lamina, which is consistent with the flexion-distraction injury. **D,** Right-sided sagittal image indicates that the T8 pars is fractured. **E,** Left-sided reconstructive sagittal CT scan shows that the left pars interarticularis is also fractured. **F,** T2-weighted MRI shows posterior impingement on the spinal cord on this midsagittal image; this is most likely a combination of blood and infolded ligamentum flavum.

FIGURE 8 *(CONTINUED)*

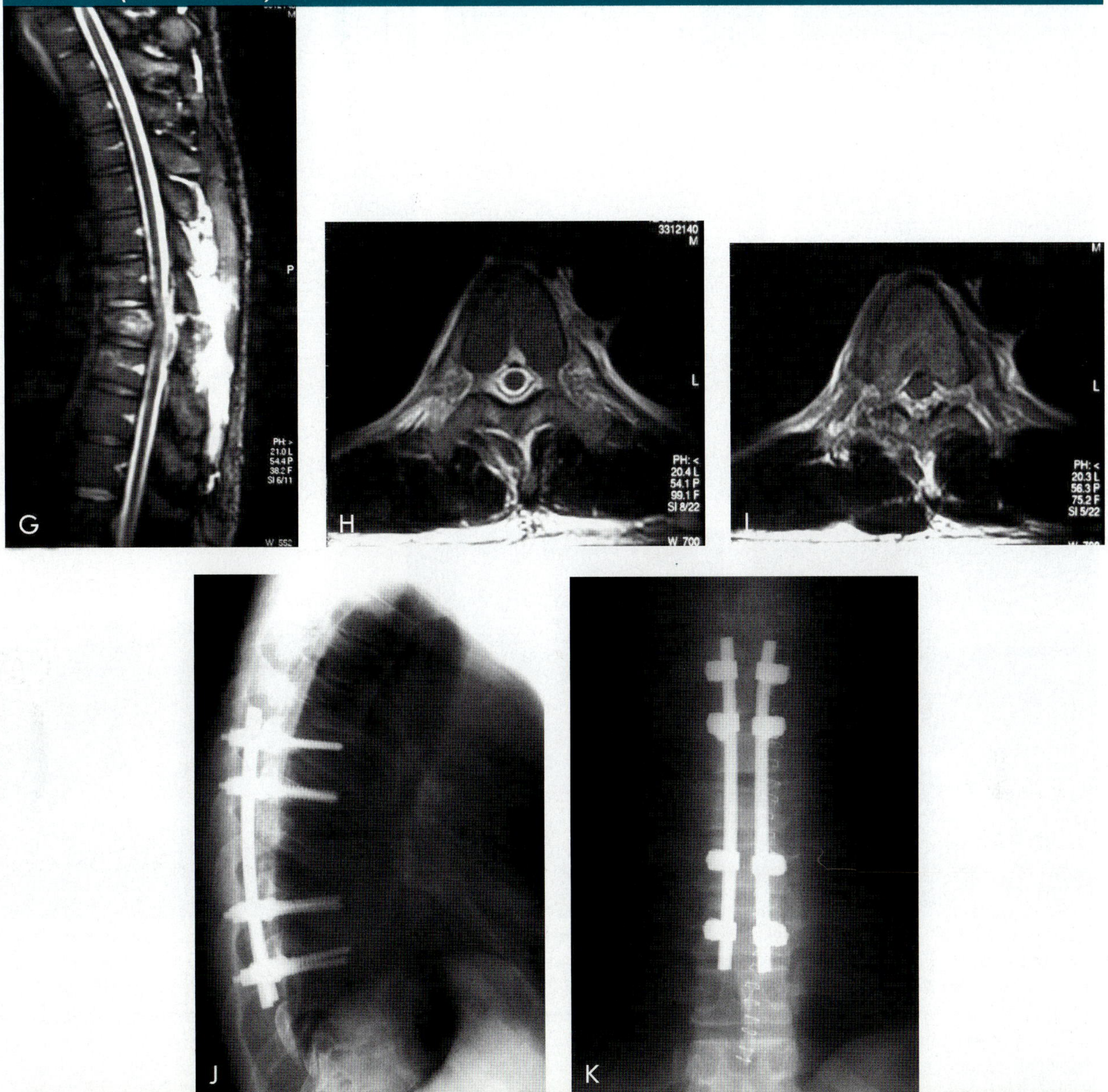

Figure 8 (*continued*) **G,** Midsagittal short-tau inversion recovery MRI sequence shows all of the posterior ligament and soft-tissue injuries. The soft-tissue disruption posteriorly is the white area. **H,** This transverse T2-weighted image is just below the level of injury and shows a normal spinal cord with adequate white cerebrospinal fluid around the spinal cord. **I,** Transverse T2-weighted image at the level of injury demonstrates infolded ligamentum posteriorly, which is significantly compressing the dural sac. There is no cerebrospinal fluid around the spinal cord at this level. **J,** This patient was treated with posterior laminotomy to remove the buckled ligamentum flavum and local posterior hematoma. He was not considered a reliable patient for follow-up and hence his spine was stabilized over a total of five levels instead of the usual three levels. This lateral radiograph shows good alignment of the spine. **K,** Postoperative AP radiograph again illustrates a normal alignment of the spine. This patient was myelopathic preoperatively with marked hyperreflexia, which resolved postoperatively.

compression instrumentation using pedicle screws and rods will achieve a satisfactory reduction. Pedicle screws offer the advantage of not protruding into the spinal canal and can avoid the production of additional "steel stenosis" due to laminar hooks. Hooks and rods can be used in patients with small pedicles provided that there is adequate room in the spinal canal (**Figure 7**).

FIGURE 9

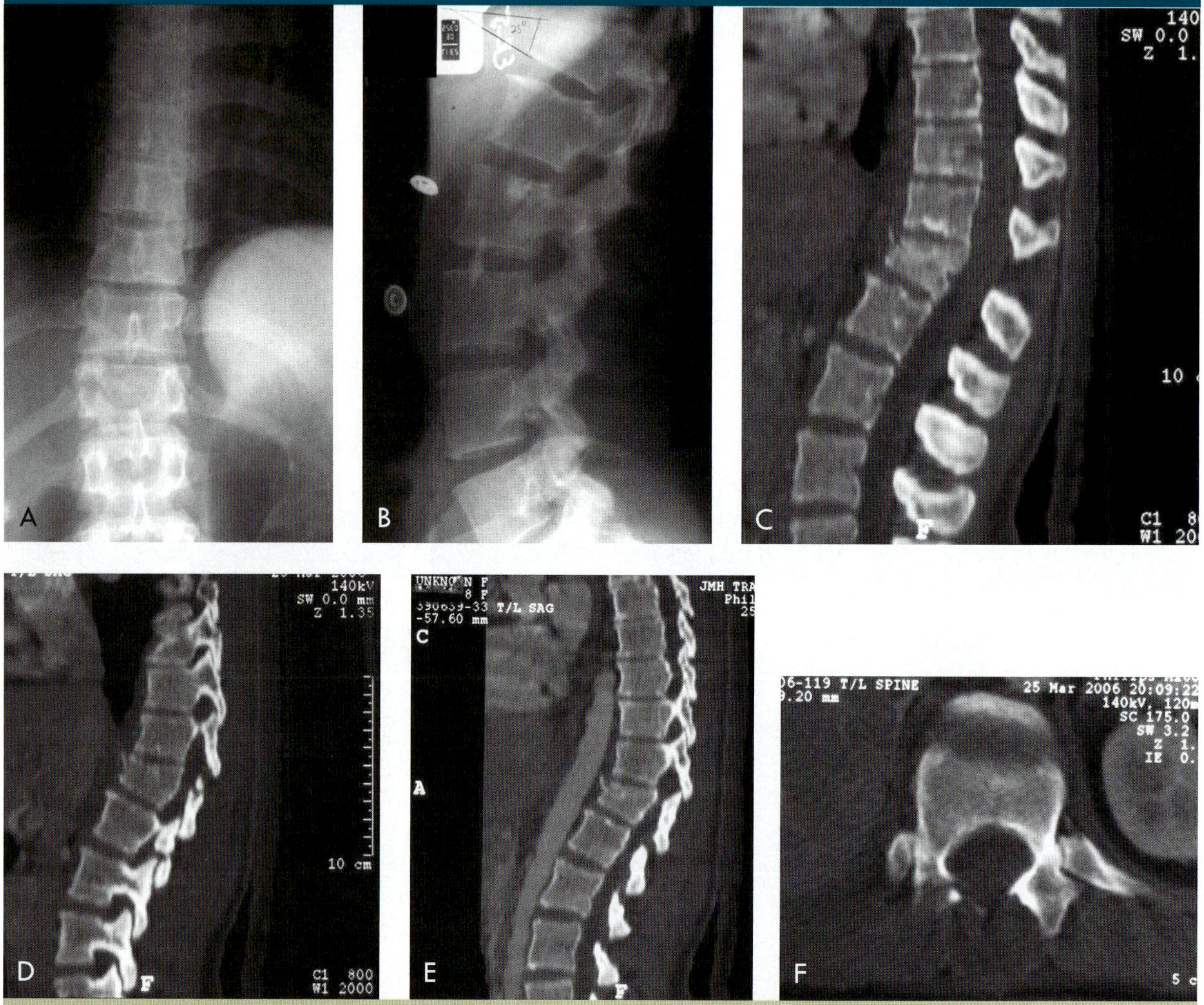

Figure 9 This 27-year-old woman was involved in a motor vehicle accident and sustained a significant flexion-distraction injury of the spine. She was neurologically normal. **A,** AP radiograph shows separation at the T11-T12 interspace. The right T12 pedicle has a transverse fracture. **B,** This lateral radiograph of her lumbar spine just misses her T12 fracture. **C,** Midsagittal reconstructive CT image shows a compression of T12 combined with a slight burst component. The posterior spread of the spinous processes is easily seen. Her kyphosis at this level measured 25°. **D,** This right-side midsagittal image shows that there has been disruption through the T11-T12 facet joint with significant separation present. **E,** Left-side sagittal image shows significant subluxation of the left-sided facet at T11-T12. **F,** Transverse image of T12 shows the "empty facet" sign.

Finkelstein et al,[57] as well as others, advocate for single-level fixation in flexion-distraction injuries without burst components. In a review of 21 injuries that underwent single level fixation, Finkelstein et al had no problems related to the number of levels fixed. After anatomic reductions, they placed hook/pedicle screw–rod constructs in neutral position. Their results indicate that reduction and restoration of the disrupted posterior tension band are adequate.

The posterolateral elements that are spanned by the instrumentation are decorticated with a burr and copious amounts of autologous bone graft are placed over these levels.

Even though these constructs are quite stable, patients are usually fitted with a TLSO, which they wear when out of bed. Once mobilized in their orthosis/brace, patients are encouraged to be as active as possible. The brace is worn for 3 months and flexion-extension radiographs are then taken without the brace. If no motion is seen at the levels where instrumentation and fusion were performed, the brace is discontinued and the patient is gradually allowed to resume

FIGURE 9 *(CONTINUED)*

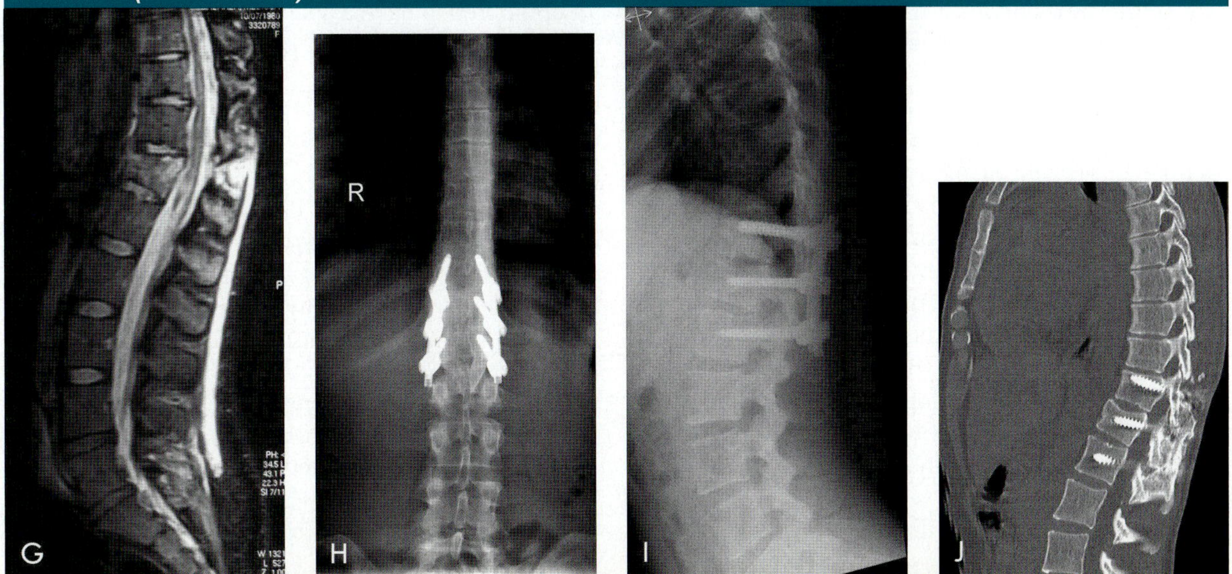

Figure 9 *(continued)* **G,** Midsagittal MRI scan indicates there is some infolded ligamentum flavum that is protruding into the spinal canal from the posterior elements. It also shows the disruption of the interspinous ligament between T12 and L1. **H,** At slightly more than 1 year after injury, this AP radiograph demonstrates normal alignment of the spine and normal position of the screws and rods. **I,** Lateral radiograph shows that her kyphosis has been markedly reduced and at this time her spinal sagittal alignment is normal. **J,** Sagittal image through the fusion shows a solid fusion from T11-L1. With the severe amount of angulation that was present and the severe amount of disruption, and considering that there was a component of the burst fracture, it was necessary to perform a fusion over these three vertebral levels to ensure adequate reduction and maintenance of reduction. The patient at this time has some local back pain but obviously no problems with spinal instability.

all preinjury activities by 6 months after the injury.

In those patients with flexion-distraction injuries with no paralysis, minimal deformity, and primarily bone injury, nonsurgical treatment may be the best option. If this course is taken, a custom-made TLSO is fitted with the patient lying prone and slightly hyperextended. The fitting is usually done within the first day. Once it is ready, the patient is taught how to roll into the two-piece brace and apply it and tighten it while still lying down. The patient is then taught how to get out of bed safely and ambulate under the direct supervision of a physical therapist. The patient is allowed out of the brace when in bed but instructed to always use it when out of bed. When in bed, the patient is encouraged to lie prone and hyperextend the injury.

After being out of bed and ambulating for 12 to 24 hours, a new standing radiograph is obtained. If there is no loss of position as indicated by an increase in angulation or displacement, then the patient is discharged from the hospital and scheduled for regular follow-up as an outpatient at short initial intervals and longer final intervals. If there is a deterioration in spinal alignment, the patient is readmitted for surgical treatment of the spine injury.

Results

The literature is sparse concerning the clinical results of patients who have been treated for flexion-distraction injuries of the thoracic and lumbar spine. The Scoliosis Research Society's prospective review, including all types of thoracic and lumbar spine fractures, has established some general principles that apply to treating these injuries.[6]

A positive relationship was found between the amount of kyphotic deformity present at 1 year after injury and the amount of pain that was present at 1 year for all fracture patients, including those treated surgically as well as nonsurgically ($P < 0.02$). A kyphosis greater than 30° was also associated with an increased incidence of more intense back pain, but no statistical significance could be determined because the numbers of patients allowed to keep this degree of deformity was very small.

Three publications dealing specifically with flexion-distraction injuries of the thoracic and lumbar spine address the patient's pain at follow-up. In the series of Glassman et al,[7] 10 of 12 (83%) had no significant pain at follow-up. Of the two patients with pain, one had been treated surgically and one had been treated conservatively. In the series of LeGay et al,[10] 13 (76%) of 17 patients had no pain or mild pain at follow-up and the majority of patients had been treated nonsurgically (ie, only 3 [18%] of those with follow-up had been treated surgically). In the series of surgically treated patients described by Triantafyllou and Gertzbein,[15] 16 patients had been treated with one-level fusions and 14 (87%) had no pain or mild pain at the time of follow-up. The results from each of these reviews show that the majority of patients with these spine fractures do relatively well with regard to pain.

The only articles specifically addressing function at follow-up were those by LeGay et al[10] and Finkelstein et al.[57] In the series reported by LeGay et al,[10] 11 of 17 (65%) of the patients reported they were able to participate in all normal activities and 4 (24%) reported that they had to slightly alter their activities because of their injuries. The remaining two patients had a major change in their activities, but both had sustained multiple injuries, which probably contributed to their limitations. In the series described by Finkelstein et al,[57] at an average follow-up of 29 months, 88% of patients reported minimal disability on the Oswestry score.

The results concerning paralysis are very vague. We know that approximately 13% of patients with these flexion-distraction injuries have some degree of paralysis, but each series of patients is so small that no comments can be made regarding the outcome of the paralysis and its relationship to the type of treatment given.

Summary

Flexion-distraction injuries of the thoracic and lumbar spine are often seen in young rear-seat passengers using lap seat-belt restraints alone. A surprising 45% of these patients have significant bowel injuries that may be occult. Spinal surgery is indicated for those patients with initial kyphotic deformities of greater than 17° to 20°, especially when associated with ligamentous and disk injuries and with pars interarticularis fractures. Short surgical constructs using compression or neutralization are extremely effective in treating these injuries. Special care should be taken with those patients with associated burst fracture or disk disruption to avoid neurologic deterioration. Fortunately, the vast majority of patients with this type of spine injury have a successful final outcome regarding pain, function, and stability.

References

1. Chance GQ: Note on a type of flexion fracture of the spine. *Br J Radiol* 1948;21(249):452-453.
2. Denis F: Spinal instability as defined by the three-column spine concept in acute spinal trauma. *Clin Orthop Relat Res* 1984;189:65-76.
3. Garrett JW, Braunstein PW: The seat belt syndrome. *J Trauma* 1962;2:220-238.
4. Anderson PA, Rivara FP, Maier RV, Drake C: The epidemiology of seatbelt-associated injuries. *J Trauma* 1991;31(1):60-67.
5. Dehner JR: Seatbelt injuries of the spine and abdomen. *Am J Roentgenol Radium Ther Nucl Med* 1971;111(4):833-843.
6. Gertzbein SD, Scoliosis Research Society: Scoliosis Research Society: Multicenter spine fracture study. *Spine (Phila Pa 1976)* 1992;17(5):528-540.
7. Glassman SD, Johnson JR, Holt RT: Seatbelt injuries in children. *J Trauma* 1992;33(6):882-886.
8. Gumley G, Taylor TK, Ryan MD: Distraction fractures of the lumbar spine. *J Bone Joint Surg Br* 1982;64(5):520-525.
9. Howland WJ, Curry JL, Buffington CB: Fulcrum fractures of the lumbar spine: Transverse fracture induced by an improperly placed seat belt. *JAMA* 1965;193:240-241.
10. LeGay DA, Petrie DP, Alexander DI: Flexion-distraction injuries of the lumbar spine and associated abdominal trauma. *J Trauma* 1990;30(4):436-444.
11. Neumann P, Osvalder AL, Nordwall A, Lövsund P, Hansson T: The mechanism of initial flexion-distraction injury in the lumbar spine. *Spine (Phila Pa 1976)* 1992;17(9):1083-1090.
12. Newman KD, Bowman LM, Eichelberger MR, et al: The lap belt complex: Intestinal and lumbar spine injury in children. *J Trauma* 1990;30(9):1133-1140.
13. Reid AB, Letts RM, Black GB: Pediatric Chance fractures: Association with intra-abdominal injuries and seatbelt use. *J Trauma* 1990;30(4):384-391.
14. Rumball K, Jarvis J: Seat-belt injuries of the spine in young children. *J Bone Joint Surg Br* 1992;74(4):571-574.
15. Triantafyllou SJ, Gertzbein SD: Flexion distraction injuries of the thoracolumbar spine: A review. *Orthopedics* 1992;15(3):357-364.

16. Letts M, Davidson D, Fleuriau-Chateau P, Chou S: Seat belt fracture with late development of an enterocolic fistula in a child: A case report. *Spine (Phila Pa 1976)* 1999;24(11):1151-1155.

17. Santschi M, Echavé V, Laflamme S, McFadden N, Cyr C: Seat-belt injuries in children involved in motor vehicle crashes. *Can J Surg* 2005;48(5): 373-376.

18. Beaunoyer M, St-Vil D, Lallier M, Blanchard H: Abdominal injuries associated with thoraco-lumbar fractures after motor vehicle collision. *J Pediatr Surg* 2001;36(5):760-762.

19. Fakhry SM, Watts DD, Luchette FA, EAST Multi-Institutional Hollow Viscus Injury Research Group: Current diagnostic approaches lack sensitivity in the diagnosis of perforated blunt small bowel injury: Analysis from 275,557 trauma admissions from the EAST multi-institutional HVI trial. *J Trauma* 2003;54(2):295-306.

20. Muñiz AE, Haynes JH: Delayed abdominal aortic rupture in a child with a seat-belt sign and review of the literature. *J Trauma* 2004;56(1):194-197.

21. Tyroch AH, McGuire EL, McLean SF, et al: The association between Chance fractures and intra-abdominal injuries revisited: A multicenter review. *Am Surg* 2005;71(5):434-438.

22. Palmer CE: The center of gravity of the human body during growth: I. An improved apparatus for determining the center of gravity. *Am J Phys Antropol* 1928;11(3):423-455.

23. Tubbs RS, Golden B, Doyle S, Grabb PA, Oakes WJ: Lap-belt injury with complete avulsion of the spinal cord and cauda equina. *Clin Anat* 2006; 19(7):665-668.

24. Reilly M, Torrång A, Klint A: Re-use of case-control data for analysis of new outcome variables. *Stat Med* 2005;24(24):4009-4019.

25. Committee on Injury and Poison Prevention, American Academy of Pediatrics: Selecting and using the most appropriate car safety seats for growing children: Guidelines for counseling parents. *Pediatrics* 2002;109(3):550-553.

26. Byard RW, Noblett H: Child booster seats and lethal seat belt injury. *J Paediatr Child Health* 2004;40(11):639-641.

27. Evans L: The effectiveness of safety belts in preventing fatalities. *Accid Anal Prev* 1986;18(3): 229-241.

28. Rutledge R, Thomason M, Oller D, et al: The spectrum of abdominal injuries associated with the use of seat belts. *J Trauma* 1991;31(6): 820-826.

29. Sullivan P: Number of traffic deaths plummets, experts say MDs can help trend continue. *CMAJ* 1991;145(3):249.

30. Kaplan BH, Cowley RA: Seatbelt effectiveness and cost of noncompliance among drivers admitted to a trauma center. *Am J Emerg Med* 1991;9(1):4-10.

31. Reath DB, Kirby J, Lynch M, Maull KI: Injury and cost comparison of restrained and unrestrained motor vehicle crash victims. *J Trauma* 1989;29(8): 1173-1177.

32. National Highway Traffic Safety Administration: *Occupant Protection Facts*. Washington, DC, Department of Transportation, 2004.

33. Williams AF, Wells JK, Lund AK: Seat belt use in cars with airbags. *Am J Public Health* 1990;80(12): 1514-1516.

34. Ball ST, Vaccaro AR, Albert TJ, Cotler JM: Injuries of the thoracolumbar spine associated with restraint use in head-on motor vehicle accidents. *J Spinal Disord* 2000;13(4):297-304.

35. Begeman PC, Prasad P: Spinal loads resulting from -G acceleration. *Proceedings of the 17th Stapp Car Crash Conference*. New York, NY, Society of Automotive Engineers, 1973.

36. Hoshikawa T, Tanaka Y, Kokubun S, Lu WW, Luk KD, Leong JC: Flexion-distraction injuries in the thoracolumbar spine: An in vitro study of the relation between flexion angle and the motion axis of fracture. *J Spinal Disord Tech* 2002;15(2): 139-143.

37. Osvalder AL, Neumann P, Lövsund P, Nordwall A: A method for studying the biomechanical load response of the (in vitro) lumbar spine under dynamic flexion-shear loads. *J Biomech* 1993;26(10): 1227-1236.

38. Nagel DA, Koogle TA, Piziali RL, Perkash I: Stability of the upper lumbar spine following progressive disruptions and the application of individual internal and external fixation devices. *J Bone Joint Surg Am* 1981;63(1):62-70.

39. Neumann P, Nordwall A, Osvalder AL: Traumatic instability of the lumbar spine: A dynamic in vitro study of flexion-distraction injury. *Spine (Phila Pa 1976)* 1995;20(10):1111-1121.

40. Stanislas MJ, Latham JM, Porter KM, Alpar EK, Stirling AJ: A high risk group for thoracolumbar fractures. *Injury* 1998;29(1):15-18.

41. Archdeacon MT, Anderson R, Harris AM, Wilber JH: Concomitant fractures of the acetabulum and spine: A retrospective review of over 300 patients. *J Trauma* 2006;60(3):609-612.

42. Wang SF, Tiu CM, Chou YH, Chang T: Obstructive intestinal herniation due to improper use of a seat belt: A case report. *Pediatr Radiol* 1993;23(3): 200-201.

43. Gertzbein SD, Court-Brown CM: Flexion-distraction injuries of the lumbar spine: Mechanisms of injury and classification. *Clin Orthop Relat Res* 1988;227:52-60.

44. Prince JS, LoSasso BE, Senac MO Jr: Unusual seat-belt injuries in children. *J Trauma* 2004; 56(2):420-427.
45. Sivit CJ, Taylor GA, Newman KD, et al: Safety-belt injuries in children with lap-belt ecchymosis: CT findings in 61 patients. *AJR Am J Roentgenol* 1991;157(1):111-114.
46. Okamoto K, Doita M, Yoshikawa M, Manabe M, Sha N, Yoshiya S: Lumbar Chance fracture in an adult snowboarder: Unusual mechanism of a Chance fracture. *Spine (Phila Pa 1976)* 2005;30(2): E56-E59.
47. Gallo RA, Reitman RD, Altman DT, Altman GT, Jones CB, Chapman JR: Flexion-distraction injury of the thoracolumbar spine during squat exercise with the Smith machine. *Am J Sports Med* 2004; 32(8):1962-1967.
48. Tanchev P, Dikov D, Novkov H: Thoracolumbar distraction fractures in advanced pregnancy: A contribution of two case reports. *Eur Spine J* 2000;9(2):167-170.
49. Sheridan R, Peralta R, Rhea J, Ptak T, Novelline R: Reformatted visceral protocol helical computed tomographic scanning allows conventional radiographs of the thoracic and lumbar spine to be eliminated in the evaluation of blunt trauma patients. *J Trauma* 2003;55(4):665-669.
50. Harris MB, Chang DS, Shilt JS, Villarraga ML, Thomas KA, Stelly MV: Modeling of the naked facet sign in the lumbar spine. *J Spinal Disord Tech* 2002;15(6):495-501.
51. Harris MB, Stelly MV, Villarraga ML, Schroeder AC, Thomas KA: Modeling of the naked facet sign in the thoracolumbar spine. *J Spinal Disord* 2001; 14(3):252-258.
52. Lingawi SS: The naked facet sign. *Radiology* 2001; 219(2):366-367.
53. O'Callaghan JP, Ullrich CG, Yuan HA, Kieffer SA: CT of facet distraction in flexion injuries of the thoracolumbar spine: The "naked" facet. *AJR Am J Roentgenol* 1980;134(3):563-568.
54. Groves CJ, Cassar-Pullicino VN, Tins BJ, Tyrrell PN, McCall IW: Chance-type flexion-distraction injuries in the thoracolumbar spine: MR imaging characteristics. *Radiology* 2005;236(2):601-608.
55. Adams JM, Cockburn MI, Difazio LT, Garcia FA, Siegel BK, Bilaniuk JW: Spinal clearance in the difficult trauma patient: A role for screening MRI of the spine. *Am Surg* 2006;72(1):101-105.
56. Moon SH, Park MS, Suk KS, et al: Feasibility of ultrasound examination in posterior ligament complex injury of thoracolumbar spine fracture. *Spine (Phila Pa 1976)* 2002;27(19):2154-2158.
57. Finkelstein JA, Wai EK, Jackson SS, Ahn H, Brighton-Knight M: Single-level fixation of flexion distraction injuries. *J Spinal Disord Tech* 2003; 16(3):236-242.
58. Kitchel SH, Eismont FJ, Green BA: Closed subarachnoid drainage for management of cerebrospinal fluid leakage after an operation on the spine. *J Bone Joint Surg Am* 1989;71(7):984-987.
59. Cochran T, Nachemson A: Long-term anatomic and functional changes in patients with adolescent idiopathic scoliosis treated with the Milwaukee brace. *Spine (Phila Pa 1976)* 1985;10(2): 127-133.
60. Cochran T, Irstam L, Nachemson A: Long-term anatomic and functional changes in patients with adolescent idiopathic scoliosis treated by Harrington rod fusion. *Spine (Phila Pa 1976)* 1983; 8(6):576-584.

CHAPTER 31

Facet Fractures and Dislocations of the Thoracolumbar Spine

Mara Karamitopoulos, MD Kris Radcliff, MD Alana J. Arnold, BS Alan M. Levine, MD
Alexander R. Vaccaro, MD, PhD

Introduction

Flexion-distraction mechanisms produce a wide variety of injuries in the thoracolumbar spine. Prognostically, it is most effective to consider flexion-distraction injuries in the thoracolumbar spine as being divided into three major categories. The first category includes the pure bony flexion-distraction injuries, which are characterized by a fracture line propagating from posterior to anterior through the spinous process and lamina, into the pedicles, and into the vertebral body (Chance fracture). The second major category has both a bony and ligamentous injury component. One injury variant occurs through the interspinous ligament and facet capsules in the posterior column, followed by bony injury occurring at the base of the pedicle into the vertebral body. A related injury is the converse—the fracture line occurring through the posterior bony elements and then proceeding anteriorly into the disk space. In children, this may appear as a variant in which the cartilaginous end plate separates from the vertebral body instead of the usual discal injury. The third category involves a purely ligamentous injury. Again, the line of injury emanates from posterior through the interspinous ligament into the facet capsule and then across, from a posteroanterior direction into the joint, hinging off the anterior longitudinal ligament. Although this injury greatly resembles bilateral facet dislocations in the cervical spine, the analogous characteristics of cervical and thoracolumbar injuries have not been discussed frequently. The similarities between bilateral facet dislocations in the cervical spine and those in the thoracolumbar spine make analysis of components of diagnosis, treatment, and prognosis more reasonable. This chapter discusses the pure ligamentous variant of the flexion-distraction injury, drawing on similarities to other flexion-distraction injuries in other areas of the spine. The differences between this injury and other flexion-distraction injuries of the thoracolumbar spine are emphasized as well.

Dr. Levine is deceased. At the time this chapter was written, Dr. Levine or an immediate family member had received royalties from Elsevier and US Spine; was a member of a speakers' bureau or had made paid presentations on behalf of Accuray; served as a paid consultant to or was an employee of US Spine; and had received research or institutional support from Accuray, Amgen, and Medtronic Sofamor Danek. Dr. Vaccaro or an immediate family member serves as a board member, owner, officer, or committee member of the North American Spine Society, American Spinal Injury Association, and the Cervical Spine Research Society; has received royalties from Aesculap/B. Braun, DePuy, a Johnson & Johnson company, Globus Medical, Medtronic Sofamor Danek, K2M, Stout Medical, Progressive Spinal Technologies, and Applied Spinal Intellectual Properties; serves as a paid consultant to or is an employee of K2M; has received research or institutional support from AO North America, DePuy, a Johnson & Johnson company, Medtronic Sofamor Danek, and Stryker; and owns stock or stock options in Globus Medical, Disk Motion Technology, Progressive Spinal Technologies, Advanced Spinal Intellectual Properties, Computational Biodynamics, Stout Medical, Paradigm Spine, K2M, Replication Medical, Spinology, Spine Medica, Orthovita, Vertiflex, Small Bone Technologies, NeuCore, Crosscurrent, Syndicom, In Vivo, Flagship Surgical, Pearl Diver, Location Based Intelligence, and Gamma Spine. None of the following authors or any immediate family member has received anything of value from or owns stock in a commercial company or institution related directly or indirectly to the subject of this chapter: Dr. Karamitopoulos, Dr. Radcliff, and Ms. Arnold.

Anatomy

The distribution of these injuries in the thoracic, lumbar, and lumbosacral spine strongly suggests that the variation in the anatomy of the facet complex plays a large role in the genesis of this injury. The majority of these injuries occur at the thoracolumbar junction, with 40% in one series[1] occurring at the T12-L1 interspace and 60% at the thoracolumbar junction. Other authors, including Lewis and McKibbin,[2] showed that 51% of all facet dislocations occurring outside of the cervical spine occurred at the thoracolumbar junction. The possibility of a bilateral facet dislocation occurring in the thoracic region of the spine is more remote,[3] owing to both the orientation of the facet joints and the supporting structures of the ribs. The orientation of the facet joints in the thoracic spine is essentially coronal, with slight orientation toward the anterior portion of the spine. The predominant reason for the rare occurrence of facet injuries at this level is the large amount of energy required to disrupt the rib cage. Thus, rather than the orientation of the facet joints, the junctional nature of the T12-L1 interspace is the chief reason for the high occurrence of injuries at that location. There is a reasonably rigid segment above, in the thoracic spine, with a transitional-level facet joint occurring at T12-L1. The orientation of the facet joints at the thoracolumbar junction has not converted to the sagittal plane, as seen in the lower lumbar spine, thus making a flexion moment more likely to cause dissociation of the superior and inferior facets. With progression more caudally in the spine, the facet joints are oriented almost purely in a sagittal plane, with slight convergence of approximately 10° to 15° toward the midline. The junctional nature of the T12-L1 facet and, to a lesser extent, the L1-L2 facet as a transition between the coronal plane of the thoracic joints and the parasagittal plane of the lumbar joints adds to the overall junctional nature of this level. Thus, the combination of the facet orientation, and the fact that a significant lever arm occurs above the level that is most often disrupted, provides the rationale for the frequent involvement of this level.

Another site of peak occurrence of facet injuries is located at the L5-S1 joint in the spine. As we shall see, the mechanism of injury is often very different from that occurring at the thoracolumbar junction; again, however, this represents a transitional zone. The sacrum forms a rigid kyphotic segment that is connected to the more flexible portion of the lumbar spine. In this area, the anatomic configuration of the facet joint contributes less to the occurrence of injury than does the transitional nature of the L5-S1 articulation.

Mechanism of Injury

The predominant mechanism of injury for the majority of bilateral facet dislocations occurring in the thoracic and the lumbar spine is flexion and distraction. Holdsworth and Hardy[4] originally thought that this injury was the result of severe flexion alone, resulting in failure of the posterior elements. As in the cervical spine, to cause anterior translation of the more superior segment over the inferior segment, it is necessary to distract the posterior ligamentous tissues so that the facet joints can clear one another as flexion occurs. Kelly and Whitesides[5] recognized this bilateral facet dislocation as a rare flexion-distraction injury. It is important to differentiate facet dislocations from fracture-dislocations in the thoracolumbar spine. Facet dislocations represent a continuum of injuries, ranging from a pure ligamentous bilateral facet dislocation with little or no body disruption, to a dislocation with anterior column comminution, to a dislocation associated with a burst fracture of the inferior level, and, finally, to a fracture-dislocation as the result of shear injury. If a relatively pure mechanism of flexion and distraction occurs, the injury will be reflected predominantly in ligamentous disruption. That is, as the distraction portion of the injury occurs, the interspinous ligament, facet capsules, and ligamentum flavum are disrupted and fail in tension. The inferior facet at the injury segment is distracted to a point at which it clears the tip of the superior facet, and as flexion occurs, disruption of the posterior longitudinal ligament and disk takes place in a posterior-to-anterior direction. The anterior longitudinal ligament is generally spared, because the center of rotation for this injury is approximately located at this juncture. In pure distraction injuries, all ligamentous connections are disrupted.[6] The anterior longitudinal ligament may, depending on the degree of flexion, be stripped off of the superior portion of the more caudal body in the injury segment. What is more important is that if the flexion is greater, the probability exists that the anteroinferior portion of the upper vertebral body will be jammed into the superoanterior portion of the inferior body, thus causing some fracturing of the anterior portion of the inferior body. This is a limited vertebral column injury with no significance to the ultimate degree of stability. In this injury mechanism, there is no comminution of the posterior vertebral body and its cortex. The posterior vertebral wall is spared and remains intact, as it has been cleared by the initial distraction portion of the mechanism. Thus, depending on the degree of flexion imparted during the injury, the anterior column injury may simply consist of disk disruption up to but not including the anterior longitudinal ligament; or it may result in stripping of the anterior longitudinal ligament from the anterior portion of the body, with the ligament remaining intact; or, finally, a triangular fracture may occur off of the anterior portion of the inferior body, which generally remains in continuity with the intact anterior longitudinal ligament. If after the dislocation occurs, an axial loading force is imparted to the injured segment, a burst fracture may be associated with the facet dislocation. Treatment of this combined injury needs to take into account both the facet dislocation and the disruption of the vertebral body or the burst fracture component. Occasionally a unilateral facet dislocation can occur as a result of both flexion-distraction and rotation forces.[7]

Facet dislocations must be carefully differentiated from a fracture-dislocation of the thoracolumbar spine. In that type of injury, there is little or no distraction imparted to the posterior elements. Thus, as the translational deformity occurs by application of a shear force, the posterior elements (facets) are fractured, with the remainder of the injury line proceeding either through the disk or the vertebral body. There are many variants of this fracture-dislocation, which may include partial distraction of the posterior elements with either complete or incomplete fracture of one or both of the facets. This may also include a shear-type mechanism combined with axial compression, which causes a burst-type injury to accompany the shear component. In this case, comminution of the entire vertebral body occurs, involving not only the anterior but also the posterior vertebral columns. A third variant of this shear injury is one in which a rotational moment is imparted. In this case, one facet is generally fractured and the other may be dislocated or may even remain intact, with obliteration of the canal due to a shearing rotational force. It is important to differentiate the flexion-distraction (bilateral facet dislocation) injury from the shear injuries, as the degree of instability is much more significant in the latter. Recognition of the difference between these two injuries may make a critical difference in operative planning.

True bilateral facet dislocations at the lumbosacral junction are very rare and directly related to mechanism of injury. At the lumbosacral junction, the majority of injuries tend to be associated with major pelvic trauma. Thus, the cause of the injury is frequently either a fall from a height, where the direction of impact of the patient's pelvis and sacrum determines the force applied, or ejection from a motorcycle or motor vehicle. This is significantly different from the previously mentioned mechanisms for flexion-distraction–type injuries. Thus, as demonstrated in a variety of case reports and other published material, many of these patients have associated sacral fractures or other disruptions about the pelvis. Examination of imaging studies is also critical in these patients, as up to 10% of lumbosacral dislocations can be initially missed because of the high incidence of associated life-threatening injuries.[8]

Facet dislocations at the thoracolumbar spine, as is the case with other flexion-distraction injuries, are the result of similar types of trauma resulting in the spectrum of spinal injury. In one large series of bilateral facet dislocations,[1] the most common cause (approximately 47%) of flexion-distraction injuries was motor vehicle accidents. Falls and direct trauma accounted for fewer cases of flexion-distraction injury. Any mechanism that pins the pelvis in a fixed location (eg, a seatbelt), or a free fall with resultant motion of the chest cage after the lumbosacral spine and pelvis are pinned at a fixed angle, can result in this type of flexion and distraction mechanism to the spine. The use of lap belts alone, as opposed to seatbelts and shoulder harnesses, has been implicated as a cause of flexion-distraction injuries.

Patient Evaluation

The initial evaluation of patients with possible facet injuries in the thoracolumbar spine is similar to that described for other types of major trauma. The critical steps, as outlined in previous chapters, begin with a comprehensive evaluation of the patient in an organized and sequential manner. The injury severity score[9] in a large series of these injuries[1] was 33 for thoracic injuries and 25 for lumbar injuries. Approximately half of all patients with this injury will have some other serious trauma as a result of the force of the impact, reflecting the high degree of force necessary to create this particular injury pattern. There is a known association between intra-abdominal trauma and flexion-distraction injuries in the thoracolumbar spine. Approximately 50% of all of the injuries that result from motor vehicle accidents with the use of lap belts include some degree of intra-abdominal injury,[10,11] and the hallmarks of abdominal trauma in spinal injury patients have been well described.[12,13] The only unique distinguishing feature on initial evaluation is the kyphosis that may be associated with facet dislocations in the thoracolumbar spine. This is a more fixed kyphosis than is present with burst fractures, as a result of the locking of the facets. It has significant implications both for diagnosis and for treatment. It is critical to palpate the entire length of the spine in a potentially injured patient. Most patients present in the supine position and will need to be rolled gently into a semilateral position for the examiner to be able to palpate any deformity along the thoracolumbar spine. It has been shown

FIGURE 1

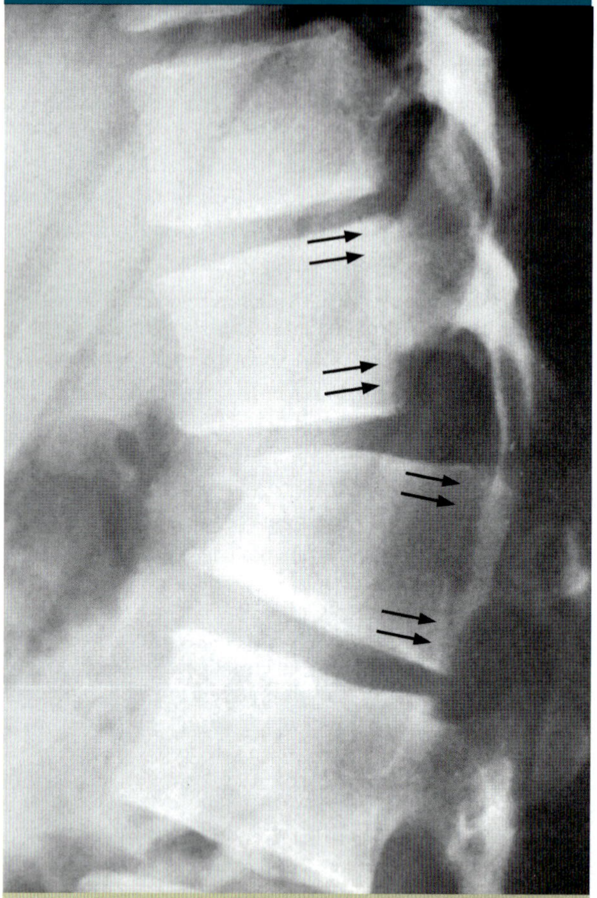

Figure 1 Lateral pretreatment radiograph of this T12-L1 bilateral facet dislocation demonstrates significant translation out of proportion to the degree of body comminution. In addition, the posterior walls of both the superior and inferior vertebral bodies are intact (arrows). (Reproduced with permission from Levine AM, Bosse M, Edwards CC: Bilateral facet dislocation in the thoracolumbar spine. *Spine (Phila Pa 1976)* 1988;13(6):630-640.)

that patients with dislocations have a significant kyphotic deformity.[1] This is much more obvious than bilateral facet dislocations in the cervical spine, especially when it occurs in the area from T11 to L4.

Evaluation of the patient's neurologic status by thorough physical examination is critical and can have implications for treatment. These are devastating injuries, and the incidence of complete and irrevocable paraplegia is higher in thoracolumbar facet-dislocations than in any other single type of spinal injury. Depending on the series, approximately 90% of the patients with bilateral facet dislocations occurring in the thoracic spine (above T10) will have complete paraplegia,[1,3,14,15] but only 60% of the patients with bilateral facet dislocations below T10 will have complete paraplegia at the time of presentation.[1] The percentage of patients with significant spinal cord injury is much higher for bilateral facet dislocations in the thoracic and lumbar spine than for any other type of spinal fracture. Even teardrop fractures and bilateral facet dislocations in the cervical spine do not demonstrate a neural injury incidence of 80%, and burst fractures of the thoracolumbar spine do not exceed a 40% neural injury rate. Thus, if a patient with a thoracolumbar dislocation is placed in the supine position, the extension of the thoracolumbar spine at the level of the relatively fixed kyphotic deformity causes further narrowing of the canal. It is possible to demonstrate that a patient with an incomplete spinal injury from a bilateral facet dislocation who is placed in the lateral position with the knees flexed will regain some function that was lost when the same patient was placed in the supine position. Therefore, patients with incomplete injury who have a demonstrated facet dislocation should be placed in the lateral position with the spine slightly flexed, should their concomitant injuries make such positioning feasible. This minimizes the intrusion of the superior facets into the canal and may preserve some function.

Radiologic Evaluation

The radiographic evaluation of these patients is another critical step in formulating accurate diagnosis and treatment. Once the patient has been carefully examined for neurologic status as well as deformity, appropriate imaging studies are performed. The gold standard is for the patient to undergo a thin-slice multidetector CT of the entire spinal axis. In facilities without routine CT imaging in the emergency department, plain radiographs are performed. Standard plain radiographic work-up in a polytrauma patient includes at least a lateral cervical spine radiograph, AP and lateral views of the thoracic spine, AP and lateral views of the lumbar spine, a chest radiograph, and AP view of the pelvis. If an injury at the thoracolumbar junction is suspected, additional spot radiographs are taken with the beam centered on this junction to optimally define the injury. Facet dislocations in the thoracolumbar spine have a very distinctive radiologic appearance that is frequently evident on the plain radiographs.

Several features can be gleaned from the lateral radiographs. The integrity of the posterior walls of the two vertebrae that make up the injury segment should be carefully inspected (**Figure 1**). In distinction to fracture-dislocations, the height and concave contour of the posterior wall at both levels remains totally intact. There is also significant translation of the superior level over the inferior level. The range of translation is from approximately 10% to 60% (mean, 40%) based on the width of the intact body. The integrity of the posterior wall is easier to evaluate in the lumbar spine than it is in the thoracic region, and CT reconstructions can clarify that differentiation. As mentioned previously, the anterior portion of the vertebral body may in fact be slightly compressed. This does not change the nature of the injury. It is simply a manifestation of the angle of flexion of the superior body at the time of impact, and the anterior column can vary from having no bony injury, to slight compression (approximately 20%), to a small fragmentary avulsion off the anterosuperior corner that remains attached to the anterior longitudinal ligament (**Figure 2**). Facet dislocation in the thoracic spine can be more difficult to appreciate on a lateral radiograph than a similar injury in the lumbar spine. In only approximately 33% of dislocations that occur in the thoracic spine are facet dislocations clearly demonstrated on the lateral radiograph; whereas in the thoracolumbar junction and the lumbar spine, approximately 75% are clearly demonstrated.

Interpretation of the AP radiograph is also important to help distinguish between a facet dislocation and a fracture-dislocation (shear injury). The majority of shear injuries demonstrate bidirectional displacement. If this is a straight bilateral facet dislocation, the AP film will show relatively satisfactory alignment of the upper and lower portions of the injury segment. In contrast, shear injuries usually demonstrate lateral translation on the AP view. Lateral translation cannot easily occur if the inferior facet of the level above is intact and is wedged firmly within the spinal canal. An increased space between the spinous processes is easily identified on the AP radograph due to distraction of the posterior vertebral body. In addition, facet dislocations in both the thoracic and lumbar spine can be differentiated from burst fractures by the unchanged interpedicular distance. The neural canal ring is not disrupted in this flexion-distraction injury. Hence, the interpedicular distance should remain constant.

Preoperative evaluation with a CT scan is routine for these patients. Sagittal reconstructions constitute one of the most effective means to demonstrate the degree of canal compromise (**Figure 3,** *A*). Furthermore, parasagittal CT views are excellent for identification of specific facet pathology, such as dislocation (**Figure 3,** *B* and *C*). As demonstrated by Gellad et al,[14] the midsagittal reconstruction can be very effective in determining prognosis. Based on a true measurement of the residual midsagittal diameter, they found that patients who were neurologically intact or who had incomplete lesions at the time of presentation had a residual midsagittal diameter ranging from 8 mm to 15 mm (mean, 11.2 mm). The patients who were neurologically complete at the time of presentation had a midsagittal diameter ranging from 5 mm to 8.5 mm (mean, 6.6 mm). The canal diameter is larger and the space required for the neural elements is smaller in the lumbar spine; in the thoracic spine, the converse is true.

FIGURE 2

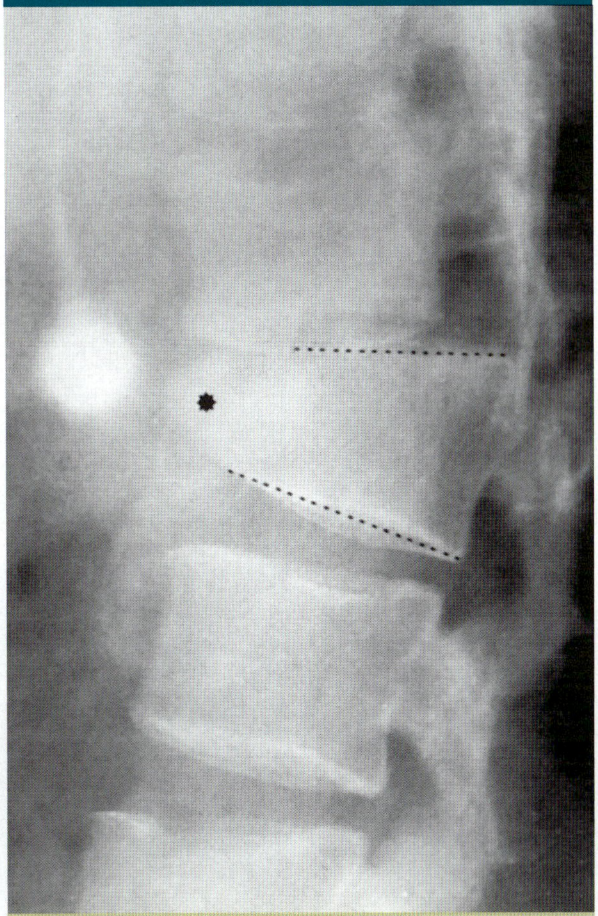

Figure 2 Lateral radiograph demonstrates anterior compression of the lower vertebral segment (dotted lines). In addition, a small fragment from the anterosuperior portion of the body (asterisk) frequently is fractured off as the anterior longitudinal ligament is stripped from the body. (Reproduced with permission from Levine AM, Bosse M, Edwards CC: Bilateral facet dislocation in the thoracolumbar spine. *Spine (Phila Pa 1976)* 1988;13(6):630-640.)

FIGURE 3

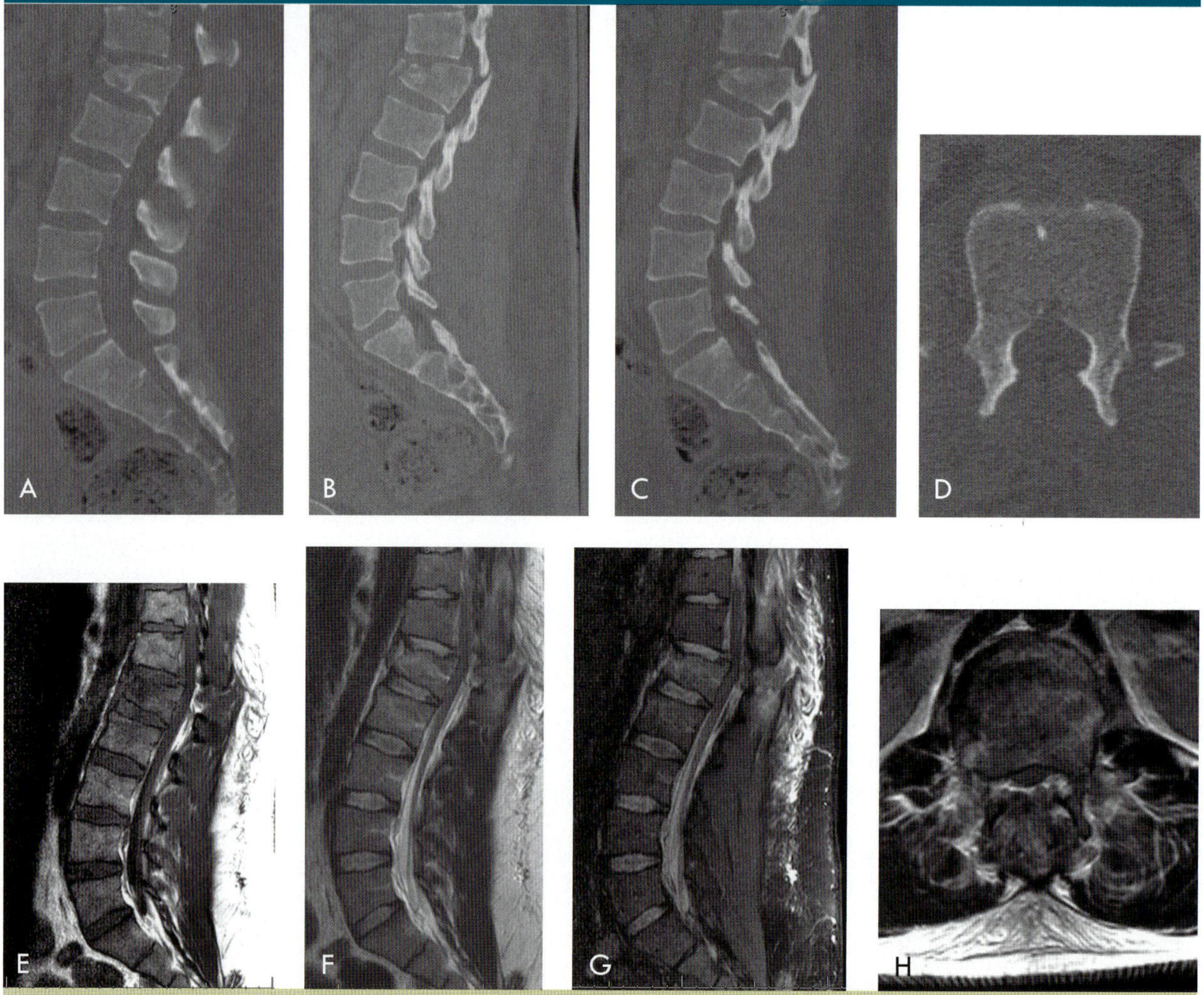

Figure 3 **A,** Midsagittal CT scan demonstrates anterolisthesis of T12 on L1. **B** and **C,** Parasagittal CT scans show anterior dislocation of inferior facet of T12 over the superior facet of L1. **D,** Axial CT section through the pedicles of L1 display empty facets of L1. Midsagittal T1 (**E**), T2 (**F**), and short-tau inversion recovery (STIR) (**G**) MRI scans show extensive posterior ligamentous complex injury. **H,** Axial MRI scan demonstrates contusion of the conus medullaris and epidural hematoma.

Generally, 3-mm axial CT sections are used. The "empty" facet sign as described by O'Callaghan et al[16] and Denis[17] is present in the large majority of patients (**Figure 3,** *D*). Other features noted on the axial sections of the CT scan are marked compromise in the canal diameter and residual area on static analysis.[14,18-22] Canal compromise can result from intervertebral disk herniation or from the posterior-superior corner of the caudal vertebral body. **Figure 3,** *H* illustrates severe conus medullaris compression from anterolisthesis. The CT scan can be used to critically evaluate all of the spinal elements and to better understand the nature of the instability.[9]

MRI may also serve as an important adjunct imaging modality in these patients, especially when the magnitude of injury to the posterior ligamentous complex (PLC), intervertebral disks, and spinal cord are not adequately appreciated on radiographs and CT. Recent classification schemes for thoracolumbar injury have extensively discussed the importance of the PLC in overall stability and as a determinant of treatment.[23-25] As MRI becomes more readily available, the efficacy of this modality in determining the integrity of the PLC has been the subject of much investigation. T1-weighted MRI is excellent for resolution of anatomic structures (**Figure 3,** *E*) but is not sensitive for identification of acute injury. Most authors consider the T2-weighted fat-suppressed images to provide the most accurate assessment of PLC integrity (**Figure 3,** *F*).[26-28] The most sensitive modality is considered to be the short-tau inversion recovery (STIR) sequence (**Figure 3,** *G*) because only fluid has a bright signal intensity on STIR. Recent literature has also provided varying data in terms of the true sensitivity and specificity of MRI for this purpose.[24,29-32] In a retrospective study by Haba et al[30] comparing intraoperative findings with preoperative MRI, the sensitivity and specificity of MRI in identifying injury to the supraspinous and interspinous ligaments was 90.5% and 94.3%, respectively. By contrast, another recent study found the specificity of MRI for PLC injury diagnosis to be much lower (53% to 65%).[24] These results suggest that MRI alone is not sufficient for diagnosis of posterior ligamentous injury. However, when used in conjunction with a thorough clinical examination and appropriate radiography, MRI may prove a useful tool to ascertain the extent of posterior ligamentous injury. MRI is also useful for identification of suspected disk herniation. On the axial MRI scan (**Figure 3,** *H*), the conus medullaris is impinged upon the posterior superior corner of L1 although there is no intervertebral disk herniation that is compressing the thecal sac.

Treatment

As mentioned previously, purely ligamentous flexion-distraction injuries of the thoracolumbar spine are unstable and potentially devastating injuries. These injuries do not allow for predictable healing, as might be expected from an injury with a bony component (ie, Chance fracture) (**Figure 4,** *A* through *C*). The various elements of **Figure 4** illustrate a patient with a combined bone and soft-tissue flexion-distraction injury. The patient experienced a horizontal fracture (**Figure 4,** *B*) and dislocation (**Figure 4,** *C*) through facets, which resulted in significant anterolisthesis of T11 on T12. Hence, surgical reduction in a timely manner is imperative to stabilize these injuries and to preserve function, especially in those with incomplete neurologic deficits (**Figure 4,** *E* and *F*). Postural reduction is ineffective in bilateral facet dislocations,[33] and may, in fact, account for the 13% failure rate originally reported by Frankel et al.[34] Nonsurgical reduction of these injuries is often impossible because of the degree of disruption of ligamentous structures. The disruption of the interspinous ligament facet capsules, ligamentum flavum, and disk is very similar to that which occurs in bilateral facet dislocations in the cervical spine. However, it is impossible to apply equivalent amounts of axial traction to disengage the facets and allow postural reduction. Even if nonsurgical reduction was achievable, the risks of significant kyphotic deformity and redislocation are high. Disruption of the PLC and the anulus leads to chronic instability in the majority of cases (**Figure 4,** *E*).[22,35] Thus, the consensus among most authors is that the treatment goals for bilateral facet dislocations are reduction of the deformity, adequate decompression of the dural contents, and stabilization, with resultant fusion of the spine. The posterior approach allows exposure of the spinal injury and correction of the deformity,[20,22,36-44] using pedicle screw fixation to rigidly stabilize the spinal segments (**Figure 4,** *G* and *H*). Recognition of the severity and the significance of the disk disruption at the injury segment between the two dislocated levels is a central concept in the management of thoracolumbar bilateral facet dislocations. As mentioned before, MRI scans should be evaluated to ascertain the status of the disk. Both anterior[45] and posterior interbody[46,47] approaches to decompression have been described to deal with the extruded disk, and the surgeon's experience and personal preference should guide this decision.[47]

Posterior Approach to Flexion-Distraction Injuries

The initial consideration in surgical treatment of facet dislocations in the thoracolumbar spine is positioning. Hyperextension positioning for both thoracic and lumbar injuries is counterproductive, because postural reduction does not occur. Generally, reduction can be aided by placement of the patient in the prone position with the table flexed to accommodate the resting position of the spine. This causes relaxation of the posterior elements and makes reduction of the dislocated facets easier. This positioning can be done either on a spinal frame that allows the position to be changed from flexion to extension during the procedure (Wilson frame) or on longitudinal rolls, with the table flexed at the outset. We prefer a Jackson frame, which allows the abdomen and pelvis to remain free while the chest and iliac crest are supported. This is particularly important in flexion-distraction injuries given the association with hollow viscus abdominal injuries. A midline approach is used. The defect between the spinous processes at the level of injury is almost always palpable. On incision of the skin, the massive disruption of the soft tissues is usually evident. In the thoracic spine, this may take the form of a subcutaneous dissection over the posterior aspect of the chest

FIGURE 4

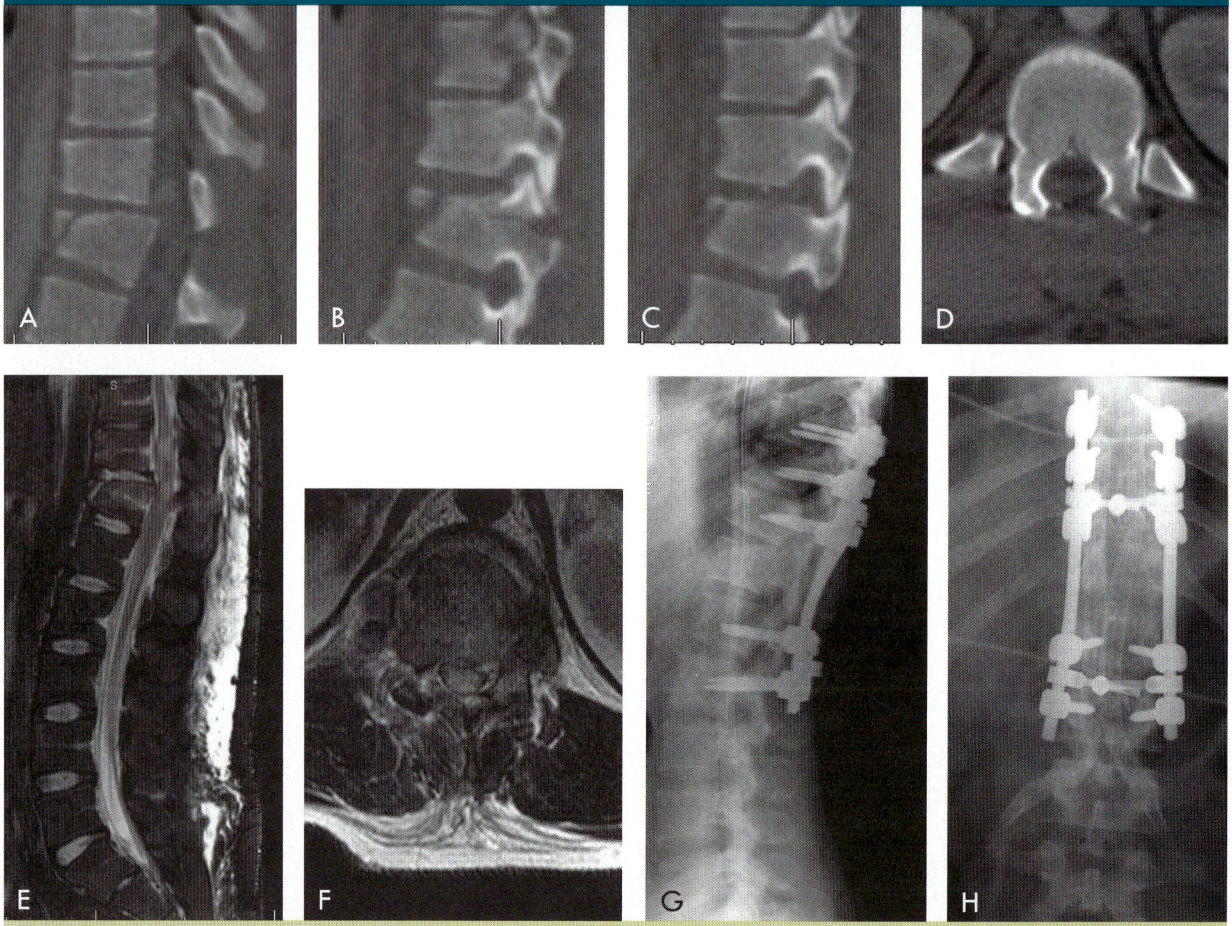

Figure 4 **A,** Midsagittal CT scan demonstrates anterior flexion teardrop fracture. Parasagittal CT scans demonstrate fracture (**B**) and dislocation (**C**) through the facets resulting in anterolisthesis of T11 on T12. **D,** Axial CT scan displays "empty facet" on the left and fracture of the right facet. **E,** Midsagittal MRI scan demonstrates significant injury to the PLC at the fracture/dislocation level. **F,** The significant edema and injury to the conus medullaris is visible on this axial MRI scan. **G** and **H,** The patient underwent posterior reduction, decompression, and stabilization.

wall on both sides, with a large hematoma. The surgeon should identify soft-tissue degloving injuries preoperatively and consider plastic surgery consultation as needed. The defect may, however, simply be evident in either the thoracic or the lumbar spine as one that is visible and palpable immediately after incision of the skin. Careful dissection is necessary along intact spinous processes at least one segment distal or proximal to the injury segment. Dissection at the level of the injury should be avoided until more proximal and distal segments are exposed. Subperiosteal dissection of the proximal and distal segments will then place the intermediate soft tissues on stretch, and they can be gradually and gently stripped from their attachments on the spinous processes of the two involved vertebrae. Care must be taken in the midline, however, to avoid dissection, as there are frequently no structures superficial to the dural sac. Furthermore, it is not uncommon to identify a traumatic dural tear that will need to be repaired at the time of the surgery. If the soft tissues are significantly disrupted and devascularized, they can be débrided at the time of exposure. Once exposure is completed down to the level of injury, care is taken to expose the facet joints. The cartilage of the superior facet will be evident in the wound dorsal to the bony elements of the inferior facet. The disrupted ligamentum flavum and interspinous ligament can be very carefully débrided from the injured interspace to allow visualization of the spinal canal elements. In the thoracic spine, it is not unusual to encounter complete disruption of the dural tube in patients with complete injuries.[48] When looking into the disrupted segment, no structures may be visible except the posterior wall of the vertebral bodies. If the dural sac is intact, the disrupted soft tissues are removed sufficiently to evaluate it. Before achieving reduction of the dislocation, it is reasonable to denude the cartilage from the exposed superior facets. Resecting the superior facets is not recommended, as this will result in increased instability and more difficulty in attaining adequate fixation.

Reduction of the Dislocation

Once the level is thoroughly débrided of soft tissues and the anatomy is fully visualized, a laminar spreader can be placed at the base of the two spinous processes of the involved levels (**Figure 5**). Generally, neither towel clips nor any other bone-holding clamps allow sufficient gradual pressure to achieve this reduction, and a large amount of distractive force is necessary to disengage the facets at almost any level from T2 down to L5. The laminar spreader is gently distracted, one click at a time, until the tip of the inferior facet just reaches the level of the tip of the dislocated superior facet. The amount of force required to achieve this distraction can be minimized by placing the patient in slight flexion. This will recreate, to some degree, the direction of the injury, but not enough to cause any damage to the dural contents. Once the sufficient amount of distraction has been achieved to disengage the facets, it is recommended that the towel clips, or other bone-holding forceps, be placed on the spinous processes on either side of the injury, and while the surgeon gently rotates the laminar spreader to cause the inferior segment to translate anteriorly, the assistant, with the bone-holding clamps, pushes forward on the inferior segment, and pulls gently back on the superior segment until the facet tips are in proper alignment. At that point, the laminar spreader tension is gently reduced, allowing the facets to seat in normal alignment. It will generally not be possible to effect a complete and symmetric reduction at this point. However, once the facets are in proper orientation to each other, the table can be gently brought to either a neutral position or to a position of very slight extension.

Stabilization

The consideration of methods of stabilization can be based both on the biomechanical constraints of the injury and on personal preference. Therefore, the decision about the type of instrumentation needs to be based on a combination of parameters.

FIGURE 5

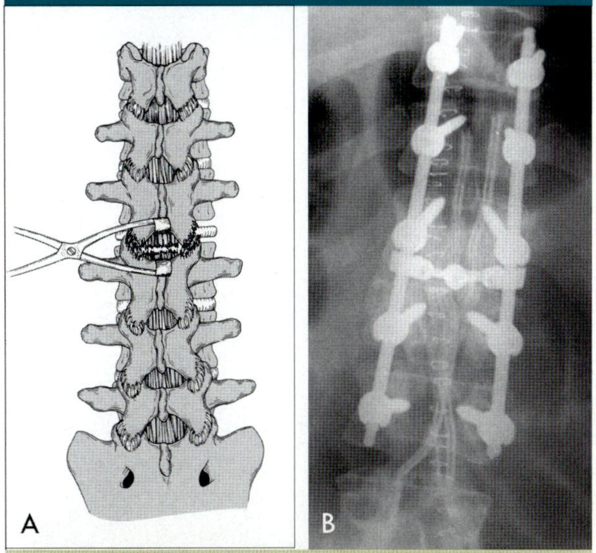

Figure 5 It should be possible to accomplish reduction of bilateral facet dislocation in the lumbar spine in a controlled fashion with preservation of the facets to allow reestablishment of stability. Dissection of the soft tissues is accomplished, and the facet dislocations are identified. Ruptured ligamentum flavum is removed, as are the disrupted facet capsules. Cartilage is removed for the superior facet of the lower level under direct vision. **A,** A laminar spreader is then placed between the two spinous processes and is gently manipulated until the facets are distracted. When the tips of the facets are disengaged, the laminar spreader is tipped, pushing the inferior facet anteriorly and pulling the superior facets posteriorly. The distraction on the laminar spreader is then released, allowing the facets to engage in a normal position. An interspinous wire is placed across the involved level and tightened to complete the reduction and reestablish stability. A short rod-sleeve construct can then be applied. **B,** After reduction, short-segment posterior instrumentation is adequate to maintain alignment in the absence of severe vertebral body comminution. The slight distraction applied by the rod-sleeve construct does not cause redislocation, as the primary force is lordotic, which counteracts the flexion moment of the original injury. (Panel **A** is reproduced with permission from Levine AM: Lumbar and sacral spinal trauma, in Browner BD, Jupiter JB, Levine AM, et al, eds: *Skeletal Trauma: Fractures, Dislocations, Ligamentous Injuries.* Philadelphia, PA, WB Saunders, 1992, vol 1, p 844.)

Typically, we prefer short-segment posterior instrumentation for flexion-distraction injuries that do not involve significant vertebral body comminution. Transpedicular fixation affords three-column stability. Due to the facet injury, we will place a cross link and local bone graft augmented with autogenous iliac crest bone graft to facilitate fusion (**Figure 6**). Depending on the degree of bony comminution and the fracture, surgeons may

FIGURE 6

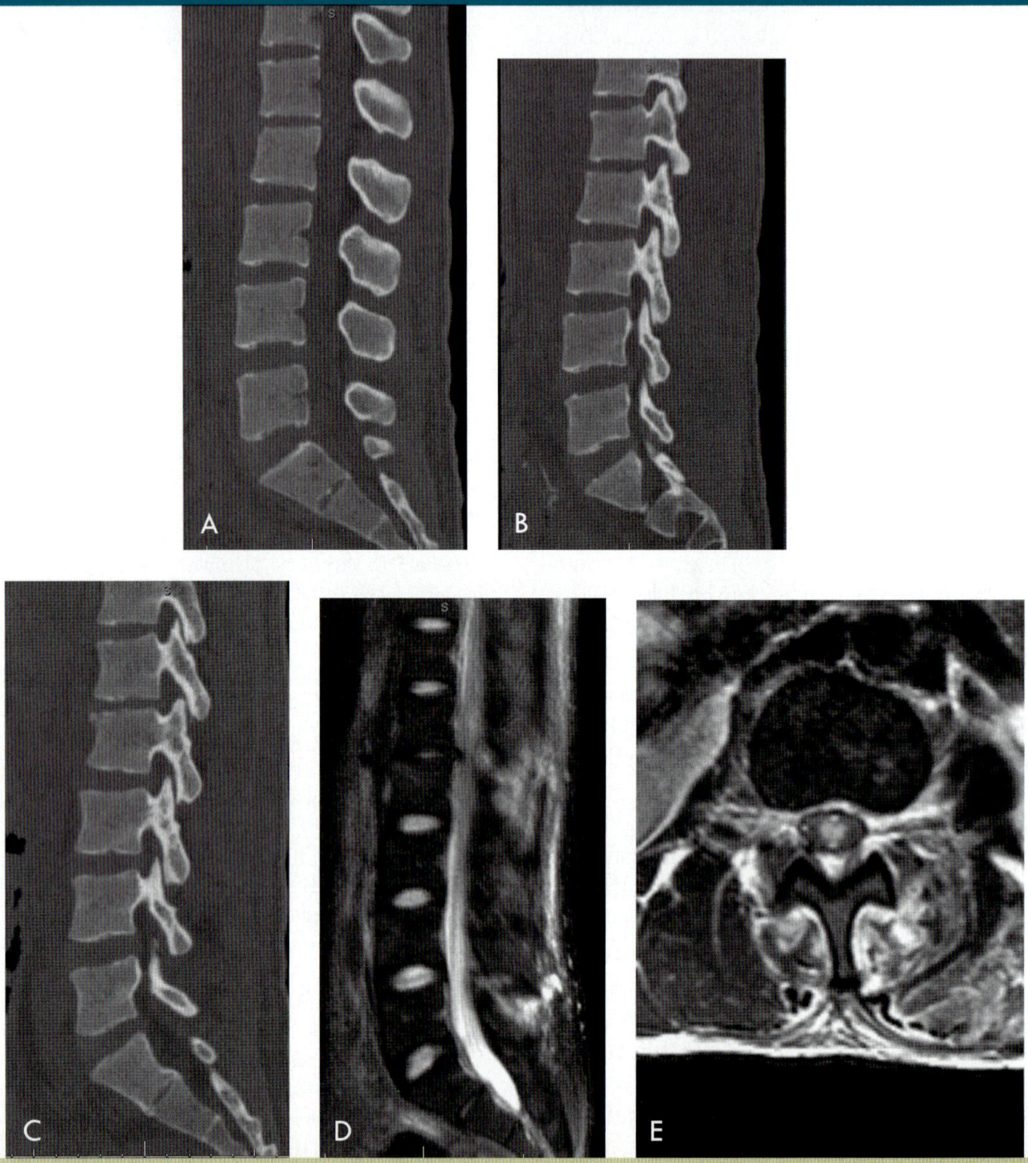

Figure 6 **A,** Midsagittal CT scan was read by radiologist as "anatomic alignment" after a restrained front-end motor vehicle collision with a seatbelt injury. The L12 interspace appears to have regional kyphosis and a small posterior avulsion. **B** and **C,** Parasagittal CT scans demonstrate no significant bony malignment. **D,** Midsagittal T2-weighted MRI scan demonstrates destruction of the PLC at the involved level and a posterior disk herniation. Also note the significant signal change in the conus medullaris at this level. **E,** Axial MRI scan demonstrates significant T2 signal uptake in the conus medullaris at the involved level.

also consider instrumentation one level cephalad and one level caudal to the injury level (**Figure 7**).

Results

Because there is little comminution of the posterior walls, anatomic restoration of the canal area is generally adequate. Neurologic recovery, however, has not been conclusively correlated with the adequacy of canal restoration and is quite unpredictable in most patients with this injury. The injuries described in this chapter are extremely high-energy injuries with an inordinately high rate of neurologic deficit. Thus, because of the rigidity of the neural ring and of the structures in the thoracic spine, and because of the inordinate amount of force required to cause disruption of the thoracic spine (which is protected by the rib cage), the majority of patients are complete paraplegics

FIGURE 6 *(CONTINUED)*

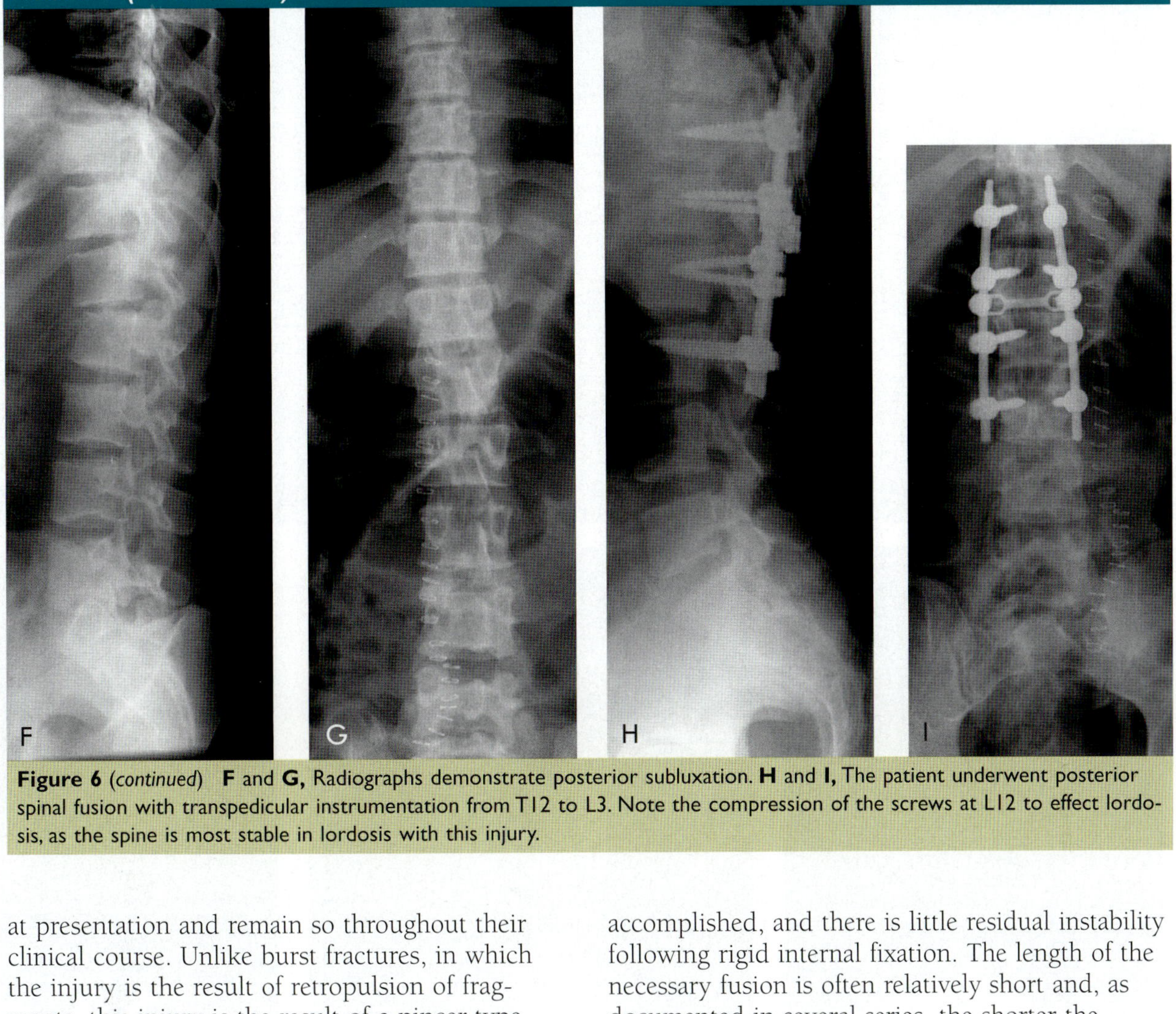

Figure 6 *(continued)* **F** and **G,** Radiographs demonstrate posterior subluxation. **H** and **I,** The patient underwent posterior spinal fusion with transpedicular instrumentation from T12 to L3. Note the compression of the screws at L12 to effect lordosis, as the spine is most stable in lordosis with this injury.

at presentation and remain so throughout their clinical course. Unlike burst fractures, in which the injury is the result of retropulsion of fragments, this injury is the result of a pincer-type movement, with the intact neural arches essentially pinching off the dural sac, either flattening it completely or (in several patients with thoracic injuries) completely transecting the cord and dural sac. Patients who present with incomplete neurologic deficit as a result of lesions below T10 have an optimum chance for substantial neurologic recovery.[1] No matter how severe the initial neurologic injury at presentation, if any function is present, and if the surgery is done in an emergent fashion, excellent recovery has been documented in several series. Radiographically, the results with these patients are most satisfying. Because little comminution and little intrinsic bony instability remain once the reduction has been achieved, anatomic restoration and maintenance of reduction is highly probable. Loss of correction is infrequent if adequate fixation techniques are used. There is little tendency for development of kyphosis or loss of height once relocation of the facets has been accomplished, and there is little residual instability following rigid internal fixation. The length of the necessary fusion is often relatively short and, as documented in several series, the shorter the length of instrumentation for fractures, the greater the likelihood for fusion to occur across the segments.

Complications

Failure to recognize the pure distraction injury[39] with complete ligamentous disruption can result in an unstable construct. The most devastating complication is neural compression from retropulsion of disk material. A proper understanding of the pathophysiology of this injury and appropriate preoperative work-up should obviate the occurrence of that problem. Additionally, the stability of the reconstruction may be compromised if the operating surgeon decides to resect the facets in an attempt to make reduction easier. With proper technique, it is possible to achieve relocation without excessive application of force in any direction. Should the injury become more destabilized

FIGURE 7

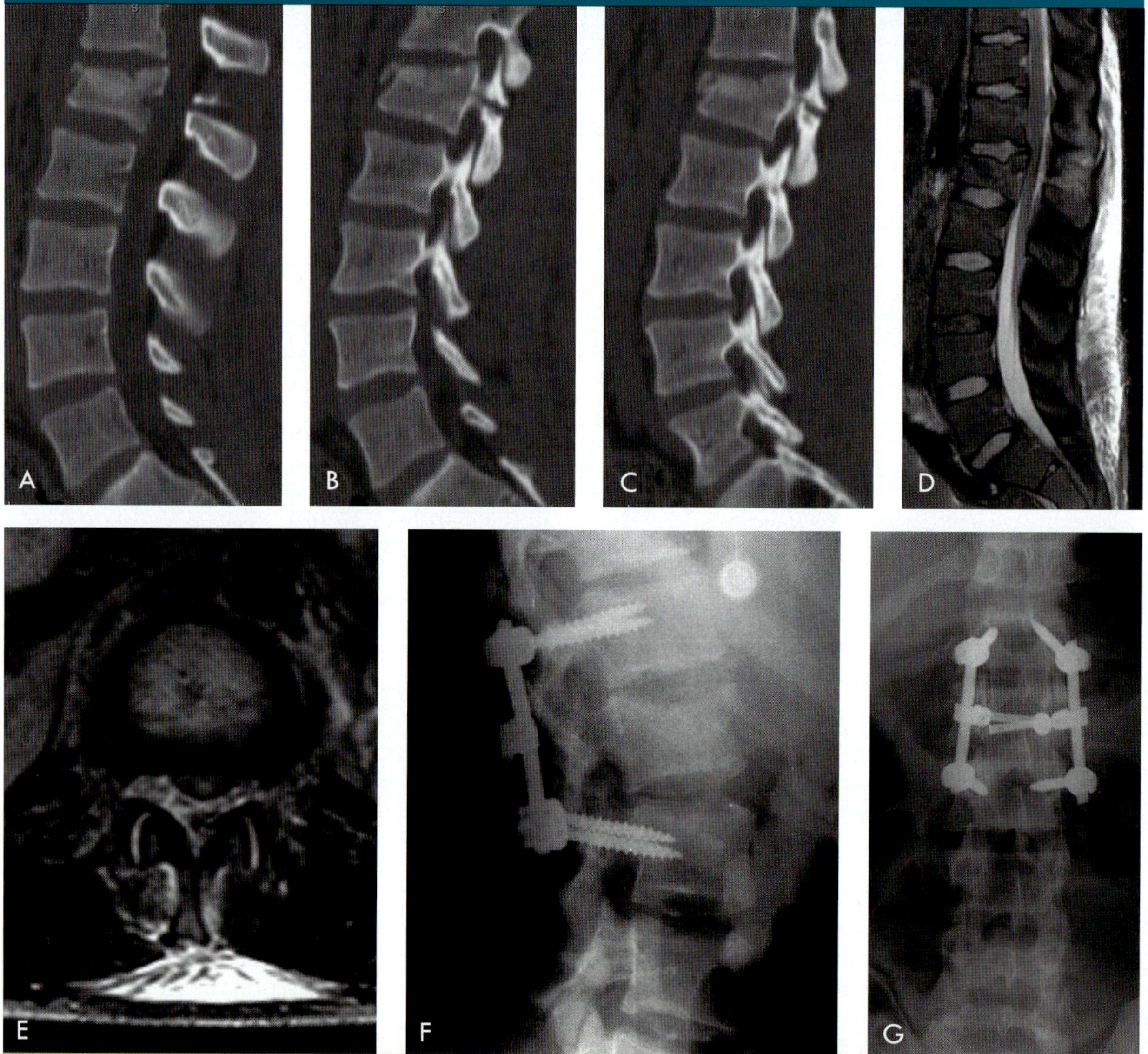

Figure 7 **A,** Midsagittal CT scan demonstrates mild anterolisthesis of T12 on L1. **B** and **C,** Bilateral superior facet fractures are present that traverse through the L1 pedicles. **D,** The PLC has been disrupted. **E,** Contusion in the conus medullaris and epidural hematoma is evident on this axial MRI scan. **F** and **G,** Monosegmental reduction and instrumentation from T12 to L2 to facilitate restoration of alignment and early patient mobilization.

by resection of necessary components, then loss of position and nonunion will be more common postoperative problems.

References

1. Levine AM, Bosse M, Edwards CC: Bilateral facet dislocations in the thoracolumbar spine. *Spine (Phila Pa 1976)* 1988;13(6):630-640.
2. Lewis J, McKibbin B: The treatment of unstable fracture-dislocations of the thoraco-lumbar spine accompanied by paraplegia. *J Bone Joint Surg Br* 1974;56-B(4):603-612.
3. Sharafuddin MJ, Hitchon PW, el-Khoury GY, Dyste GN: Locked facets in the thoracic spine: Report of three cases and a review. *J Spinal Disord* 1990;3(3):255-258.
4. Holdsworth FW, Hardy A: Early treatment of paraplegia from fractures of the thoraco-lumbar spine. *J Bone Joint Surg Br* 1953;35-B(4):540-550.
5. Kelly RP, Whitesides TE Jr: Treatment of lumbodorsal fracture-dislocations. *Ann Surg* 1968; 167(5):705-717.
6. Carl A, Hash L: Distraction injury of the thoracic spine: Report of two cases. *J Bone Joint Surg Am* 1994;76(4):605-607.

7. Lucas MJ, Berg EE: Unilateral thoracic facet dislocation. *Clin Orthop Relat Res* 1997;335:162-165.
8. Shen FH, Crowl A, Shuler TE, Feldenzer JA, Leivy SW: Delayed recognition of lumbosacral fracture dislocations in the multitrauma patient: The triad of transverse process fractures, unilateral renal contusion and lumbosacral fracture dislocation. *J Trauma* 2004;56(3):700-705.
9. Baker SP, O'Neill B, Haddon W Jr, Long WB: The injury severity score: A method for describing patients with multiple injuries and evaluating emergency care. *J Trauma* 1974;14(3):187-196.
10. Anderson PA, Henley MB, Rivara FP, Maier RV: Flexion distraction and Chance injuries to the thoracolumbar spine. *J Orthop Trauma* 1991;5(2): 153-160.
11. Triantafyllou SJ, Gertzbein SD: Flexion distraction injuries of the thoracolumbar spine: A review. *Orthopedics* 1992;15(3):357-364.
12. Crawford CH III, Puno RM, Campbell MJ, Carreon LY: Surgical management of severely displaced pediatric seat-belt fracture-dislocations of the lumbar spine associated with occlusion of the abdominal aorta and avulsion of the cauda equina: A report of two cases. *Spine (Phila Pa 1976)* 2008;33(10):E325-E328.
13. Soderstrom CA, McArdle DQ, Ducker TB, Militello PR: The diagnosis of intra-abdominal injury in patients with cervical cord trauma. *J Trauma* 1983;23(12):1061-1065.
14. Gellad FE, Levine AM, Joslyn JN, Edwards CC, Bosse M: Pure thoracolumbar facet dislocation: Clinical features and CT appearance. *Radiology* 1986;161(2):505-508.
15. Kinoshita H: Pathology of spinal cord injuries due to fracture-dislocations of the thoracic and lumbar spine. *Paraplegia* 1996;34(1):1-7.
16. O'Callaghan JP, Ullrich CG, Yuan HA, Kieffer SA: CT of facet distraction in flexion injuries of the thoracolumbar spine: The "naked" facet. *AJR Am J Roentgenol* 1980;134(3):563-568.
17. Denis F: The three column spine and its significance in the classification of acute thoracolumbar spinal injuries. *Spine (Phila Pa 1976)* 1983;8(8): 817-831.
18. Gehweiler JA Jr, Daffner RH, Osborne RL Jr: Relevant signs of stable and unstable thoracolumbar vertebral column trauma. *Skeletal Radiol* 1981; 7(3):179-183.
19. Manaster BJ, Osborn AG: CT patterns of facet fracture dislocations in the thoracolumbar region. *AJR Am J Roentgenol* 1987;148(2):335-340.
20. Durward QJ, Schweigel JF, Harrison P: Management of fractures of the thoracolumbar and lumbar spite. *Neurosurgery* 1981;8(5):555-561.
21. Ullrich C, Yuan HA: Computed tomography with sagittal-coronal reconstruction images in thoracolumbar spinal fracture. *Orthop Rev* 1979;8: 59-63.
22. Whitesides TE Jr: Traumatic kyphosis of the thoracolumbar spine. *Clin Orthop Relat Res* 1977;128: 78-92.
23. Vaccaro AR, Lehman RA Jr, Hurlbert RJ, et al: A new classification of thoracolumbar injuries: The importance of injury morphology, the integrity of the posterior ligamentous complex, and neurologic status. *Spine (Phila Pa 1976)* 2005;30(20): 2325-2333.
24. Vaccaro AR, Rihn JA, Saravanja D, et al: Injury of the posterior ligamentous complex of the thoracolumbar spine: A prospective evaluation of the diagnostic accuracy of magnetic resonance imaging. *Spine (Phila Pa 1976)* 2009;34(23): E841-E847.
25. Vaccaro AR, Lim MR, Hurlbert RJ, et al: Surgical decision making for unstable thoracolumbar spine injuries: Results of a consensus panel review by the Spine Trauma Study Group. *J Spinal Disord Tech* 2006;19(1):1-10.
26. Emery SE, Pathria MN, Wilber RG, Masaryk T, Bohlman HH: Magnetic resonance imaging of posttraumatic spinal ligament injury. *J Spinal Disord* 1989;2(4):229-233.
27. Lee HM, Kim HS, Kim DJ, Suk KS, Park JO, Kim NH: Reliability of magnetic resonance imaging in detecting posterior ligament complex injury in thoracolumbar spinal fractures. *Spine (Phila Pa 1976)* 2000;25(16):2079-2084.
28. Schweitzer KM, Vaccaro AR, Harrop JS, et al: Interrater reliability of identifying indicators of posterior ligamentous complex disruption when plain films are indeterminate in thoracolumbar injuries. *J Orthop Sci* 2007;12(5):437-442.
29. Dai LY, Ding WG, Wang XY, Jiang LS, Jiang SD, Xu HZ: Assessment of ligamentous injury in patients with thoracolumbar burst fractures using MRI. *J Trauma* 2009;66(6):1610-1615.
30. Haba H, Taneichi H, Kotani Y, et al: Diagnostic accuracy of magnetic resonance imaging for detecting posterior ligamentous complex injury associated with thoracic and lumbar fractures. *J Neurosurg* 2003;99(1, Suppl):20-26.
31. Oner FC, van Gils AP, Dhert WJ, Verbout AJ: MRI findings of thoracolumbar spine fractures: A categorisation based on MRI examinations of 100 fractures. *Skeletal Radiol* 1999;28(8):433-443.
32. Terk MR, Hume-Neal M, Fraipont M, Ahmadi J, Colletti PM: Injury of the posterior ligament complex in patients with acute spinal trauma: Evaluation by MR imaging. *AJR Am J Roentgenol* 1997; 168(6):1481-1486.

33. Davies WE, Morris JH, Hill V: An analysis of conservative (non-surgical) management of thoracolumbar fractures and fracture-dislocations with neural damage. *J Bone Joint Surg Am* 1980;62(8): 1324-1328.
34. Frankel HL, Hancock DO, Hyslop G, et al: The value of postural reduction in the initial management of closed injuries of the spine with paraplegia and tetraplegia: I. *Paraplegia* 1969;7(3): 179-192.
35. Holdsworth F: Fractures, dislocations, and fracture-dislocations of the spine. *J Bone Joint Surg Am* 1963;52(8):1534-1551.
36. Bedbrook GM: Treatment of thoracolumbar dislocation and fractures with paraplegia. *Clin Orthop Relat Res* 1975;112:27-43.
37. Bohlman HH: Treatment of fractures and dislocations of the thoracic and lumbar spine. *J Bone Joint Surg Am* 1985;67(1):165-169.
38. Ferguson RL, Allen BL Jr: A mechanistic classification of thoracolumbar spine fractures. *Clin Orthop Relat Res* 1984;189:77-88.
39. Levine AM, Edwards CC: Complications in the treatment of acute spinal injury. *Orthop Clin North Am* 1986;17(1):183-203.
40. McAfee PC, Bohlman HH, Yuan HA: Anterior decompression of traumatic thoracolumbar fractures with incomplete neurological deficit using a retroperitoneal approach. *J Bone Joint Surg Am* 1985; 67(1):89-104.
41. McAfee PC, Yuan HA, Frederickson BE, Lubicky JP: The value of computed tomography in thoracolumbar fractures: An analysis of one hundred consecutive cases and a new classification. *J Bone Joint Surg Am* 1983;65(4):461-473.
42. Rothman RH, Simeone FA, eds: *The Spine*. Philadelphia, PA, WB Saunders, 1982.
43. Stauffer ES, Neil JL: Biomechanical analysis of structural stability of internal fixation in fractures of the thoracolumbar spine. *Clin Orthop Relat Res* 1975;112:159-164.
44. White AA III, Panjabi MM, Posner I, Edwards WT, Hayes WC: Spinal stability: Evaluation and treatment. *Instr Course Lect* 1981;30:457-483.
45. Tsirikos AI, Saifuddin A, Noordeen MH, Tucker SK: Traumatic lumbosacral dislocation: Report of two cases. *Spine (Phila Pa 1976)* 2004;29(8): E164-E168.
46. Deniz FE, Zileli M, Cağli S, Kanyilmaz H: Traumatic L4-L5 spondylolisthesis: Case report. *Eur Spine J* 2008;17(Suppl 2):S232-S235.
47. Song KJ, Lee KB: Bilateral facet dislocation on L4-L5 without neurologic deficit. *J Spinal Disord Tech* 2005;18(5):462-464.
48. Silvestro C, Francaviglia N, Bragazzi R, Piatelli G, Viale GL: On the predictive value of radiological signs for the presence of dural lacerations related to fractures of the lower thoracic or lumbar spine. *J Spinal Disord* 1991;4(1):49-53.

CHAPTER 32
Thoracolumbar Burst Fractures

Juan M. Raposo, MD Christopher M. Bono, MD Bradford L. Currier, MD

Key Points

- Burst fractures result from high-energy axial loading on the spine.
- They occur primarily at the thoracolumbar junction from T11 to L2.
- Burst fractures may be stable or unstable injuries.
- A key determinant of fracture stability is the integrity of the posterior ligamentous complex.
- Stable injuries may be treated nonsurgically while unstable injuries should be treated with internal fixation to prevent progressive deformity and/or loss of neurologic function.

Introduction

Burst fractures are injuries caused by an axial load and are typically associated with high-energy mechanisms such as falls from a height, motor vehicle accidents, or high-speed recreational activities. The radiographic hallmarks of burst fractures include loss of posterior body height, fragment retropulsion, canal compromise, interpedicular widening, and kyphosis. These fractures may occur at any level in the spine, although they are most frequently observed near the junction of the thoracic and lumbar spine (T11-L2).[1-10] This propensity for the thoracolumbar junction results from the anatomic and biomechanical factors related to the transition between the rigid, kyphotic thoracic cage and the more mobile, lordotic lumbar vertebrae.

In 1963, Holdsworth[11] was the first to coin the term "burst" fracture in describing fractures resulting from extreme flexion. Contemporary biomechanical studies have demonstrated that the primary mechanism of injury is actually axial compression.[12,13] In practice, however, pure axial compression injuries are rarely seen in isolation, and secondary forces acting in flexion, extension, or rotation are frequently observed in conjunction.

Many classification systems proposed over the years have sought to define clinically unstable fracture patterns in an attempt to guide therapeutic decisions. To date, no universally accepted classification system or treatment algorithm exists. Numerous studies have reported satisfactory results in stable burst fractures treated nonsurgically.[11,14-16] Meanwhile, it is generally accepted that clearly unstable burst fractures should be treated with internal fixation; however, the optimal surgical approach remains a topic of ongoing debate.[3,17-26]

The purpose of this chapter is to discuss the pertinent anatomic, clinical, and radiographic properties of burst fractures as a prelude to a comprehensive overview of the current treatment guidelines in practice for these enigmatic fractures.

Thoracolumbar Anatomy

Despite regional morphological variations, thoracic and lumbar vertebrae share several analogous structures (**Figure 1**). The burst fracture pattern primarily involves the vertebral body. Thus, an intimate understanding of this structure, as well as its differences in the thoracic and lumbar spine, is important.

Vertebral Body

Thoracic vertebral bodies are roughly heart-shaped in axial cross section. Subtle wedging of the vertebral bodies collectively produces about 20° to 40° of physiologic thoracic kyphosis.[27,28] The intervertebral disks and adjacent end plates are relatively parallel and contribute little to normal thoracic kyphosis. This is distinct from the lumbar spine, in which physiologic lumbar lordosis, ranging from 40° to 60°, is produced primarily by sagittal asymmetry of the intervertebral disks, with larger anterior versus posterior heights, interposed

Dr. Bono or an immediate family member serves as a board member, owner, officer, or committee member of American Academy of Orthopaedic Surgeons and the North American Spine Society; and has received nonincome support (such as equipment or services), commercially derived honoraria, or other non-research-related funding (such as paid travel) from Barricaid. Dr. Currier or an immediate family member serves as a board member, owner, officer, or committee member of the Cervical Spine Society, the North American Spine Society, the Lumbar Spine Research Society, and the Council for Value in Spine Surgery; and has received royalties from DePuy, a Johnson & Johnson company, and Stryker. Neither Dr. Raposo nor any immediate family member has received anything of value from or owns stock in a commercial company or institution related directly or indirectly to the subject of this chapter.

FIGURE 1

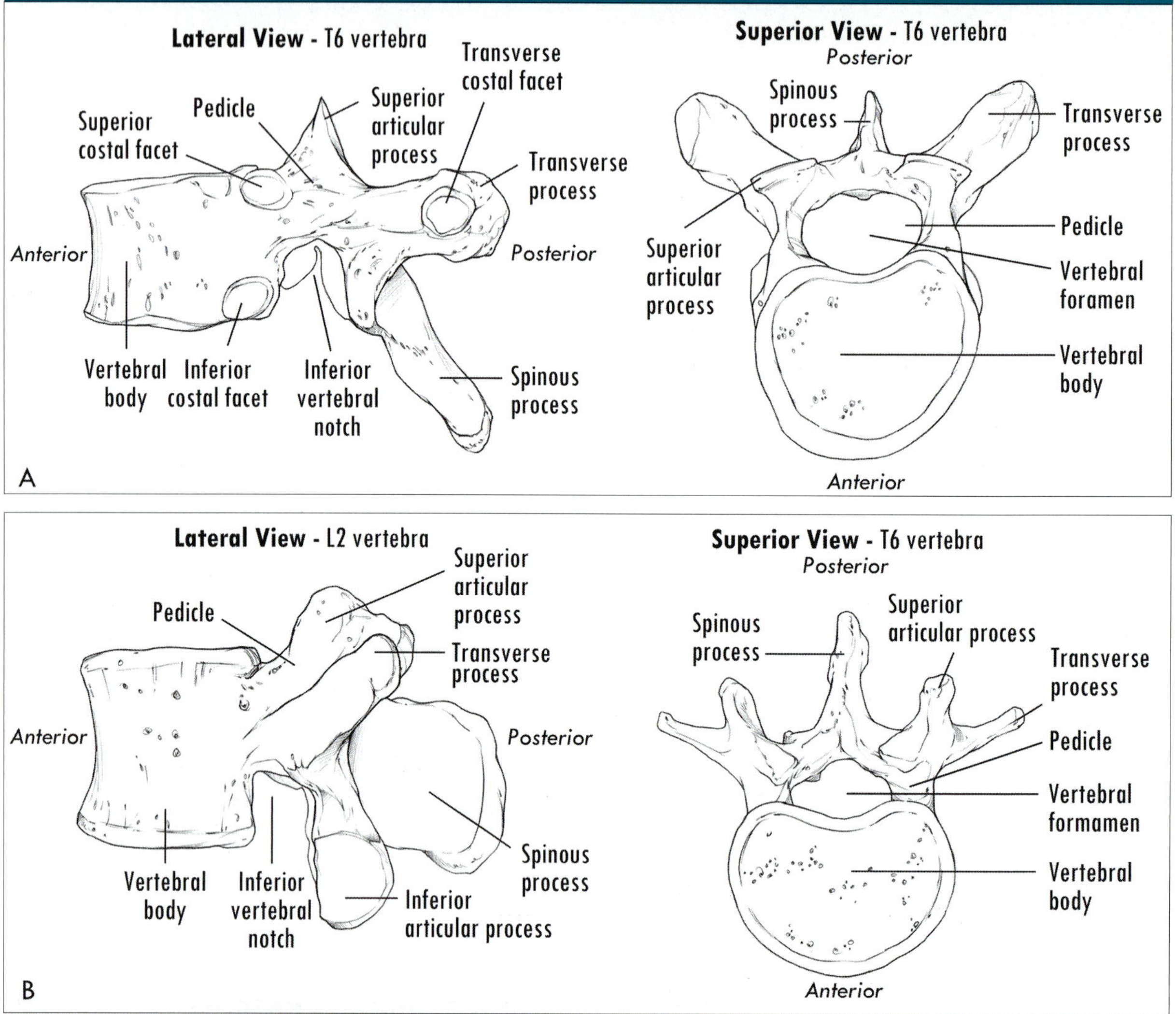

Figure 1 Anatomic and morphologic characteristics of representative thoracic and lumbar vertebra: **A,** representative thoracic vertebra; **B,** representative lumbar vertebra.

between nonwedged vertebral bodies.[27,29] Vertebral body dimensions are relatively small in the upper thoracic spine. They progressively increase in size from cranial to caudad to mechanically sustain increasing proportions of body weight.[30,31]

Sagittal Alignment

The transition between thoracic kyphosis and lumbar lordosis occurs between the T11 and L2 levels. This is conventionally referred to as the thoracolumbar junction. As such, it is normally straight in both the sagittal and coronal planes.[30] Any degree of measured kyphosis after burst fracture can therefore be considered abnormal unless there was a preexisting deformity. This is in contrast to the middle and upper thoracic (T2-T10) and lower lumbar spine (L3-S1), where measured (or absolute) kyphosis must be considered to be superimposed on preexisting physiologic kyphosis or lordosis, respectively. For example, an absolute measurement of 30° of kyphosis between T5 and T7 after a T6 burst fracture may only represent 20° of kyphotic deformity if one assumes that the normal preinjury kyphosis was 10°. In contrast, 10° of absolute measured kyphosis between L3 and L5 after an L4 burst fracture probably represents 20° to 30° of relative kyphosis. Unfortunately, there is a wide range of what can be considered normal thoracic and lumbar sagittal alignment. This makes kyphosis measurements difficult in regions other than the thoracolumbar junction.

FIGURE 2

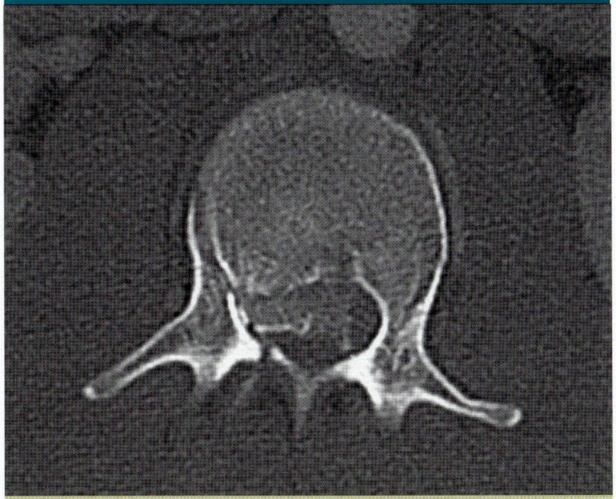

Figure 2 Axial CT image of an L2 burst fracture with significant retropulsion. Despite severe narrowing of the spinal canal, this patient had a normal neurologic examination except for decreased pin-prick sensation in the anterior right thigh. This resolved postoperatively following anterior decompression and L1 through L3 fusion.

FIGURE 3

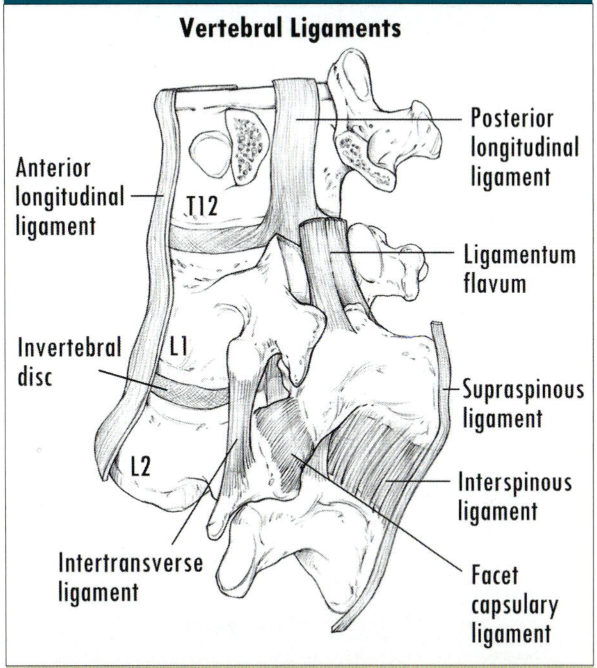

Figure 3 The posterior ligamentous complex (PLC), consisting of the interspinous ligament, supraspinous ligament, ligamentum flavum, and facet capsules.

Spinal Canal

The spinal canal is smaller in the thoracic spine than the lumbar spine.[32] Among other factors, such as the nature of its neural contents, these dimensional constraints make the spinal cord much more susceptible to small amounts of thoracic canal compromise than the conus medullaris or cauda equina at the thoracolumbar junction or lumbar spine. This helps explain why upper and middle thoracic burst fractures with minimal posterior vertebral body fragment retropulsion can be associated with severe, often complete, spinal cord injuries, while thoracolumbar burst fractures with comparatively impressive amounts of canal compromise can be present in neurologically intact patients (**Figure 2**).

Interaction With the Ribs

The thoracic spine gains additional stability by its interaction with the rib cage.[33] This occurs at two specific locations.[33] A single rib head articulates with hemifacets along the posterolateral aspect of the thoracic vertebral bodies, effectively bridging the disk spaces with the costovertebral joint. As the rib curves posterolaterally, it articulates with the anterior aspect of the transverse process and is stabilized by costotransverse ligaments. These articulations make the thoracic spine more stable, but less mobile, than the lumbar spine. This may also help explain the greater likelihood of neurologic deficit with thoracic burst fractures, as a greater amount of energy would be necessary to cause an injury here than in the lumbar spine.

Posterior Ligamentous Complex

The posterior ligamentous complex (PLC) is a term that refers to several important stabilizing ligaments. These include the interspinous ligaments, supraspinous ligaments, ligamentum flavum, and facet capsules (**Figure 3**). Combined, these structures act as a posterior tension band that limits the amount of flexion that can be safely tolerated by the neural elements. The PLC can be disrupted with burst fractures in which a flexion moment is imparted in addition to axial compressive load.

Clinical and Radiographic Evaluation

The initial evaluation of a patient with a suspected thoracolumbar injury should begin with a primary survey to carefully assess airway, breathing, and circulation. Appropriate resuscitative measures should be undertaken and strict spinal precautions observed. As part of a routine work-up for the multiply injured trauma patient, a lateral cervical spine, AP chest, and pelvic radiograph should always be performed. Thoracolumbar injuries are

FIGURE 4

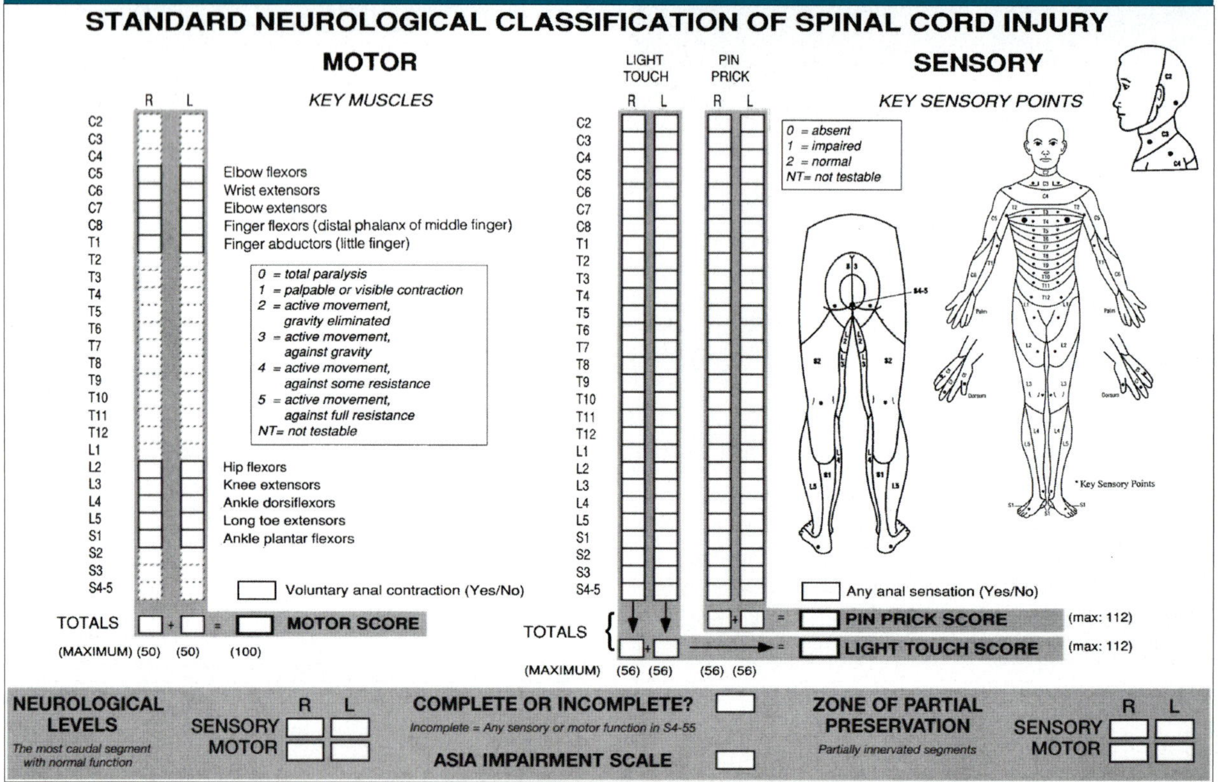
STANDARD NEUROLOGICAL CLASSIFICATION OF SPINAL CORD INJURY

MOTOR

KEY MUSCLES

R L

C2 C3 C4 C5 C6 C7 C8 T1 T2 T3 T4 T5 T6 T7 T8 T9 T10 T11 T12 L1 L2 L3 L4 L5 S1 S2 S3 S4-5

Elbow flexors
Wrist extensors
Elbow extensors
Finger flexors (distal phalanx of middle finger)
Finger abductors (little finger)

0 = total paralysis
1 = palpable or visible contraction
2 = active movement, gravity eliminated
3 = active movement, against gravity
4 = active movement, against some resistance
5 = active movement, against full resistance
NT= not testable

Hip flexors
Knee extensors
Ankle dorsiflexors
Long toe extensors
Ankle plantar flexors

Voluntary anal contraction (Yes/No)

TOTALS + = MOTOR SCORE

(MAXIMUM) (50) (50) (100)

LIGHT TOUCH

PIN PRICK

R L R L

SENSORY

KEY SENSORY POINTS

0 = absent
1 = impaired
2 = normal
NT= not testable

* Key Sensory Points

Any anal sensation (Yes/No)

TOTALS

PIN PRICK SCORE (max: 112)

LIGHT TOUCH SCORE (max: 112)

(MAXIMUM) (56) (56) (56) (56)

NEUROLOGICAL LEVELS
The most caudal segment with normal function

R L
SENSORY
MOTOR

COMPLETE OR INCOMPLETE?
Incomplete = Any sensory or motor function in S4-S5

ASIA IMPAIRMENT SCALE

ZONE OF PARTIAL PRESERVATION
Partially innervated segments

R L
SENSORY
MOTOR

Figure 4 ASIA scoring system.

often the result of high-energy mechanisms, and concomitant injuries in the abdomen, thorax, and urologic systems are frequently seen. A careful assessment of the patient's neurologic status is of paramount importance. Fractures presenting with a neurologic deficit are indicative of an unstable injury.

The incidence of neurologic deficit in the setting of a burst fracture has been reported to range between 32 and 47 percent.[34,35] The American Spinal Injury Association (ASIA) has developed a useful five-tiered scoring system for neurologic function following trauma (**Figure 4**). It requires careful muscle and sensory grading at each myotomal and dermatomal level. The degrees of neurologic involvement range from A (complete spinal injury) to E (no neurologic deficits), with varying degrees of incomplete neurologic injury in between. Patients with incomplete lesions, characterized by intact perianal sensation (ie, sacral root sparing), have been demonstrated to have a significantly better prognosis for neurologic recovery than patients with complete injuries.[36] This distinction should be made after spinal shock has resolved.[37,38]

Spinal fractures are often first recognized by CT of the chest or abdomen. If a single thoracic or thoracolumbar injury is detected, complete radiographs of the entire spine should be obtained, as the rate of concomitant, noncontiguous spinal injury can be as high as 11%.[39] At times, dedicated CT scans or MRI may be required to better characterize the injury pattern and determine the most appropriate choice of treatment.

Plain Radiographs

Lateral View

Lateral films can be used to assess sagittal alignment. This is usually neutral at the thoracolumbar junction. Kyphosis can be measured using the Cobb method or the posterior vertebral body tangent method. In the thoracolumbar spine, the Cobb method has been demonstrated to be more reliable.[40] It involves measuring the angle between the superior end plate of the nearest uninjured cranial vertebra and the inferior end plate of the nearest uninjured caudal vertebra (**Figure 5**). The percentage of height loss of the injured vertebral body is a useful calculation that can be made using a lateral radiograph. It is based on comparing

FIGURE 5

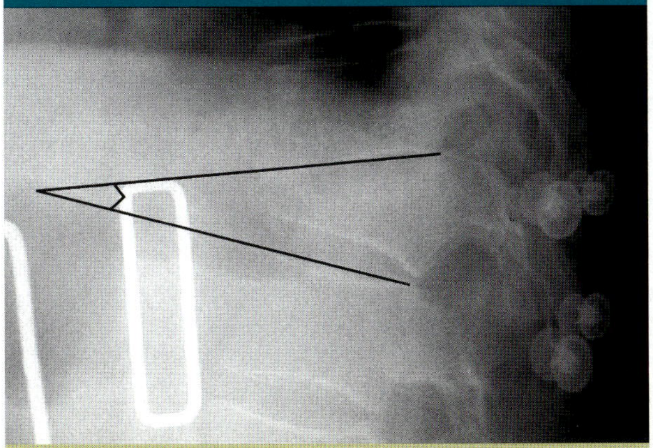

Figure 5 Lateral radiograph measuring fracture kyphosis by the Cobb method.

FIGURE 7

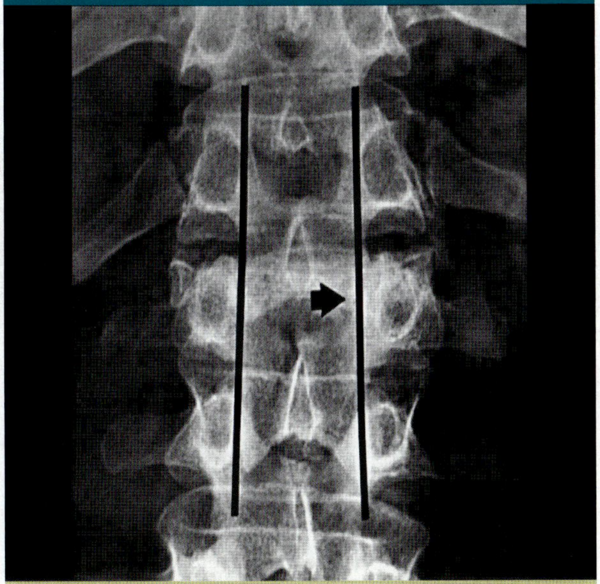

Figure 7 AP radiograph demonstrating interpedicular widening at L1 (arrow). The height of the vertebral body is also decreased. (Reproduced from Scheffer MM, Currier BL: Thoracolumbar burst fractures, in Levine AM, Eismont FJ, Garfin SR, Zigler JE, eds: *Spine Trauma*. Philadelphia, PA, WB Saunders, 1998, pp 428-451.)

values of the injured segment to those of adjacent cranial and caudal uninjured vertebrae. Anterior and posterior vertebral body height should be measured separately to more accurately detect compression of one or both regions. Although by itself not a sufficient criterion, loss of greater than 50% of vertebral body height is suggestive of PLC disruption.[41] Posterior vertebral body fragment retropulsion can usually be appreciated on the lateral radiograph (**Figure 6**).

FIGURE 6

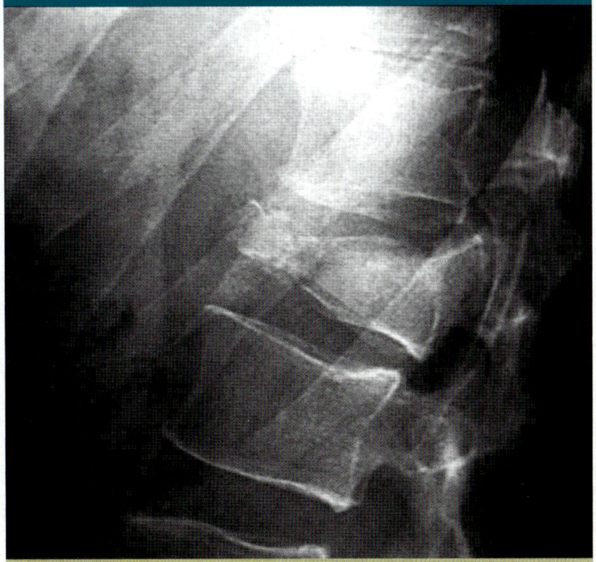

Figure 6 Lateral radiograph demonstrating kyphotic deformity and retropulsion of a posterior vertebral body fragment into the canal. (Reproduced from Scheffer MM, Currier BL: Thoracolumbar burst fractures, in Levine AM, Eismont FJ, Garfin SR, Zigler JE, eds: *Spine Trauma*. Philadelphia, PA, WB Saunders, 1998, pp 428-451.)

Anteroposterior View

Coronal alignment of the spine can be assessed using the AP radiograph. Mild degrees of coronal angulation are frequently associated with thoracolumbar burst fractures. The relative distance between the spinous processes should be assessed systematically. Widening between the spinous processes can suggest PLC disruption. In addition, longitudinal malalignment of the spinous processes can be an indication of rotation (which may suggest the injury is indeed a fracture-dislocation rather than a burst fracture). Rotation can also be judged by the relationship of the pedicles to the spinous process at the same level. Normally, interpedicular width should successively increase from cranial to caudal. Abnormal interpedicular widening is a frequent finding with burst fractures (**Figure 7**); it is the radiographic representation of lateral splaying of the posterolateral vertebral body fragments.

Computer Tomography

CT is more sensitive than plain radiographs in detecting burst fractures.[42,43] Many fractures that appear to be simple compression fractures on plain radiographs demonstrate posterior vertebral body involvement on CT. Helical CT has revolutionized the ability to rapidly obtain a high-quality scan and may soon replace plain radiographs as an initial screening tool.[42]

Thin-cut (1-mm to 1.5-mm) slices should be obtained through the level of injury, as well as normal adjacent levels. The dimensional effects of retropulsed bone fragments on the spinal canal are readily appreciated.[44] Posterior column injuries, such as facet dislocations, facet fractures, and pedicle fractures, are also clearly visualized. Lamina fractures that occur concomitantly with a burst fracture are often associated with posterior dural tears and nerve root entrapment (**Figure 8**).[45,46] This can influence treatment decision making.

Subtle translational deformities (as may occur with fracture-dislocations) or flexion-distraction (Chance-type or seatbelt) injuries, can be missed using only axial CT images. This can lead to misdiagnosis as a burst fracture if the posterior vertebral body is involved. At times, a missing or incompletely visualized superior facet from the subjacent vertebrae, or so-called "empty" facet sign, may be present (**Figure 9,** *A* through *C*). Axial CT images must be considered in concert with plain radiographs or sagittal and coronal reconstructed CT images (**Figure 9,** *D*).

FIGURE 8

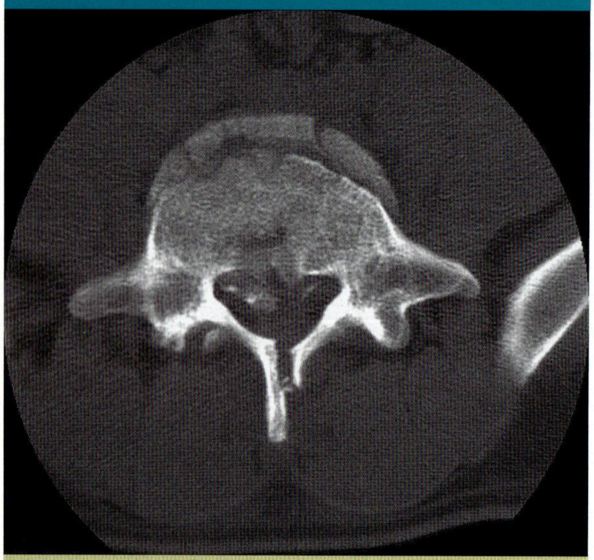

Figure 8 Axial CT of an L5 burst fracture with an associated sagittal split of the lamina.

CT Assessment of the Spinal Canal

Different methods of quantifying canal compromise have been detailed. To our knowledge, the superiority or reproducibility of one versus another has not been clearly demonstrated. In addition, no single method is able to reliably predict neurologic involvement.

Midsagittal canal diameter is among the simpler measurements. It is the distance between the posterior aspect of the displaced wall fragment and the anterior aspect of the lamina. To calculate the percentage of canal compromise, this value can be compared to the sagittal diameters of adjacent uninjured levels above and below the fracture.

Several authors have stated that this method can underestimate the amount of neural compression, purporting that cross-sectional area measurements are more representative.[44,47,48] Unfortunately, area measurements are difficult and cumbersome to perform, even with the advanced imaging software that is currently available. Perhaps more important than quantifying the exact magnitude of canal compromise, axial CT images can be used for preoperative planning.

Magnetic Resonance Imaging

MRI is superior to CT in evaluating the neural elements, the intervertebral disks, and the spinal

FIGURE 9

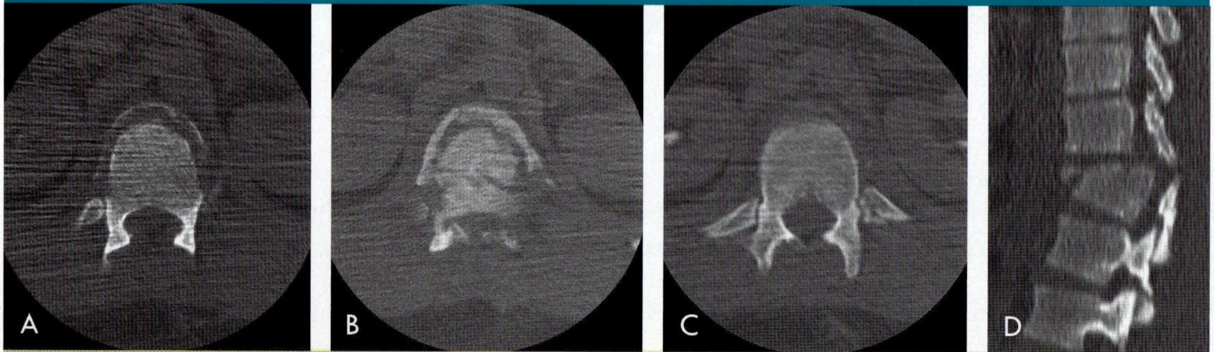

Figure 9 **A-C,** Contiguous (cranial to caudal) axial CT images of a T12 burst fracture demonstrating "empty" facet sign suggestive of a fracture-dislocation. **D,** Sagittally reconstructed CT image showing fracture-dislocation at the T12-L1 facet.

FIGURE 10

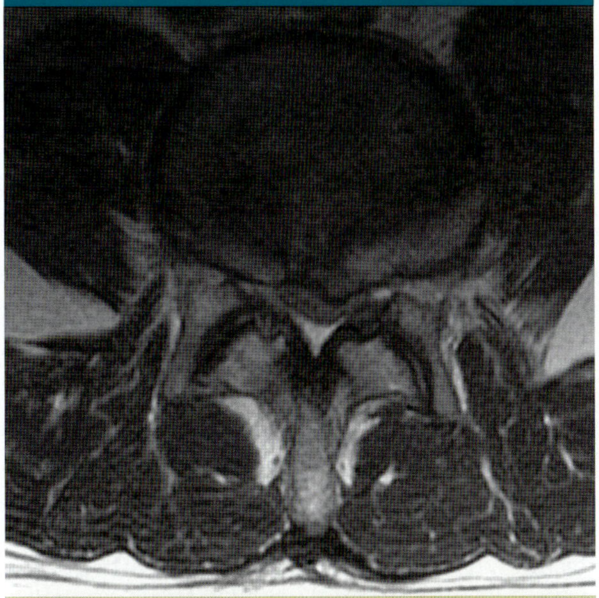

Figure 10 T2 axial MRI scan showing compression of the cauda equina.

FIGURE 11

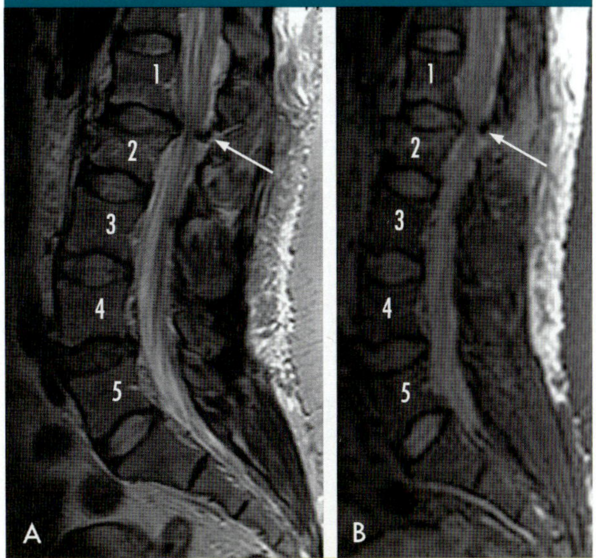

Figure 11 A, Sagittal T2 MRI scan demonstrates disruption of the ligamentum flavum posteriorly at the level of L1-L2 disk (white arrow). **B,** Sagittal STIR fast-spin echo image demonstrates increased soft-tissue edema at the level of L1-L2 interspinous space and evidence of posterior ligamentous injury.

ligaments. Spinal cord or cauda equina compression is clearly visualized using MRI (**Figure 10**). Edema within the spinal cord can be appreciated and may be associated with a poorer prognosis for neurologic recovery.[49-53] Spinal cord transection, although rare after burst fractures, can be detected using MRI. Nerve root entrapment within a lamina fracture can also be seen on axial images.

With increasing availability, MRI assessment of the spinal ligaments is becoming more commonplace. It can be used to assess the integrity of the posterior longitudinal ligament (PLL), the ligamentum flavum, and the interspinous and supraspinous ligaments. The integrity of the PLL, although not of mechanical significance, can affect the ability to indirectly reduce retropulsed bony fragments. Brightman et al[54] found that an intact PLL, as visualized by MRI, was associated with better canal clearance through posterior distraction instrumentation than if the PLL was disrupted.

With a growing trend toward nonsurgical treatment of burst fractures, MRI has become a popular method of assessing the PLC.[55] T2-weighted images are more useful than T1-weighted images. They show greater contrast between the ligaments, such as the ligamentum flavum, and the neighboring cerebrospinal fluid. Tissue edema is detectable as increased signal on T2-weighted images. Short tau inversion recovery (STIR) images may be the most sensitive in detecting edema within the soft tissues; however, this is at the expense of image clarity.

MRI findings within the PLC may vary. Mild increased signal between spinous processes on T2-weighted images might be indicative of a benign ligament sprain that is not mechanically unstable. Bright and expansive signal extending from the tip of the spinous process to the interlaminar interval is indicative of gross PLC disruption and the potential for mechanical instability (**Figure 11**). Varying gradations of less pronounced signal enhancement are more difficult to interpret, because their relationship to physical continuity of the ligaments is not clear. Oner et al[56] have developed a grading system to help differentiate these varying degrees of ligamentous injury. Although the prognostic significance of such a grading system remains to be demonstrated, in one study, PLC disruption was predictive of recurrence of kyphosis in surgically treated patients at final follow-up.[56]

Classification Systems and Fracture Stability

Over the past 50 years, numerous classification systems for thoracolumbar injuries have been devised with the dual purpose of describing

FIGURE 12

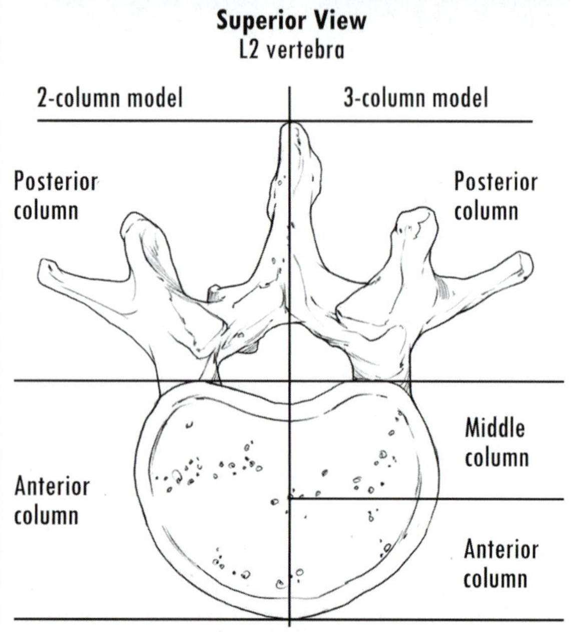

Figure 12 Schematic diagram comparing two-column and three-column models of the spine.

commonly seen fractures and establishing treatment guidelines based on these identifiable patterns of injury. Many of these schemes have been based on anatomic or mechanistic patterns of injury, while the treatment guidelines proposed have been loosely based on the ill-defined concept of stability. Burst fractures, which are among the most common injuries seen in this region of the spine, have had an especially tumultuous heritage for being ambiguously defined and poorly understood.

Historical Perspective

In 1949, Nicoll[57] divided fractures of the spine into stable and unstable fracture patterns based on the risk of progressive deformity and described a basic treatment algorithm for each pattern of injury. Holdsworth[11,58] later expanded on this stability-based classification model, dividing fractures into six categories based on their mechanism of injury. Under his classification scheme, burst fractures, along with wedge fractures and extension injuries, were considered stable injuries. Kelly and Whitesides[59] identified unstable burst fractures as "the most common cause of neural injury in the thoracolumbar region." Whitesides[60] was the first to effectively define the two-column concept by comparing the spine to a construction crane, with compression-resisting vertebral bodies and intervertebral disks corresponding to the boom, and tension-resisting posterior elements represented as guy ropes. Currently, the two most widely used classification systems in use are the Denis[35,61] classification system, which is based on the three column theory of spinal stability, and the AO classification system of Magerl et al,[34] based on the two-column model of the spine (**Figure 12**).

The Three-Column Model

In 1983, Denis[35] introduced the concept of the middle column, arguing that isolated posterior ligamentous injury is not sufficient to create instability. In his description of 412 thoracolumbar injuries, Denis emphasized the importance of an intact middle column in conferring structural stability to the injured spine. Major spine fractures were divided into four categories: (1) compression fractures, (2) burst fractures, (3) seatbelt injuries, and (4) fracture-dislocations.[35] Under this model, burst fractures result from a failure of the anterior and middle columns under axial load and are considered to be inherently unstable.

McAfee et al[43] used CT to analyze the mechanism of failure of the middle column in keeping with the three-column model. Unlike Denis, they differentiated between stable and unstable burst fractures, placing the emphasis on the integrity of the posterior elements, instead of the middle column.[43]

The Two-Column Model

In 1994, Magerl et al[34] proposed a comprehensive alphanumeric classification system for thoracolumbar injuries based on a retrospective review of over 1,400 fractures that adhered to the two-column concept as originally described by Whitesides.[60] Fractures were divided, based on pathomorphologic characteristics, into three main types: A (compression), B (distraction), and C (rotation). Burst fractures were classified as compression injuries and further subdivided into nine subgroups. The overall frequency of neurologic injury observed in type A3 burst fractures was 32% and was found to vary by subgroup.

Fracture Stability

At the root of the debate regarding the appropriate treatment of thoracolumbar burst fractures lies the question: What constitutes an unstable burst fracture?

White and Panjabi[62] defined unstable fractures as those that are likely to progress to symptomatic posttraumatic deformity and/or neurologic loss if

TABLE 1

TLICS Scoring System

Injury Characteristics	Points
Injury morphology	
Compression	1
Flexion burst	2
Translation-rotational injury	3
Distraction injury	4
	1 to 4
PLC integrity	
Intact	0
Indeterminate	2
Injured	3
	0 to 3
Neurologic involvement	
Intact	0
Nerve root	2
Cord, conus medullaris	
Complete	2
Incomplete	3
Cauda equina	3
	0 to 3
Total severity score	**1 to 10**

(Reproduced from Vaccaro AR, Lehman RA Jr, Hurlbert RJ, et al: A new classification of thoracolumbar injuries: The importance of injury morphology, the integrity of the posterior ligamentous complex, and neurologic status. *Spine (Phila Pa 1976)* 2005;30(20): 2325-2333.)

left untreated. Degrees of instability resulting from thoracolumbar burst fractures can be viewed conceptually as a continuum, ranging from a superior end-plate fracture of the vertebral body with little posterior involvement, minimal fracture kyphosis, and no neurologic deficits to fracture with significant loss of vertebral height, obvious kyphotic deformity, and progressive neurologic loss.

At present, PLC integrity is considered to be the most important determinant of mechanical stability of a fracture.[11,14,16,58,63] Varying methods to determine or, more accurately, infer PLC integrity have been proposed over the years. Point tenderness with palpation over the interspinous process region has been purported to be a useful clinical finding. The magnitude of segmental kyphosis felt to be indicative of instability has ranged from 20° to 35°.[43,63] Some use standing films to judge if

TABLE 2

Proposed Treatment Algorithm Based on TLICS Score

TLICS Score	Treatment
≤ 3	Nonsurgical
4	Surgical or nonsurgical
≥ 5	Surgical

(Reproduced from Vaccaro AR, Lehman RA Jr, Hurlbert RJ, et al: A new classification of thoracolumbar injuries: The importance of injury morphology, the integrity of the posterior ligamentous complex, and neurologic status. *Spine (Phila Pa 1976)* 2005;30(20): 2325-2333.)

kyphosis increases with upright posture, although exact numerical criteria have not been described. MRI has been touted as the most direct noninvasive method of ligamentous inspection, though validating studies are lacking.[56]

Thoracolumbar Injury Classification and Severity Score

The Thoracolumbar Injury Classification and Severity Score (TLICS) proposed by Vacccaro et al[64] combines features of a classification scheme and treatment algorithm. Injury morphology, PLC integrity, and neurologic status are the three critical factors assigned points based on severity (**Table 1**). Injuries graded with a composite score of 5 points or greater are considered surgical cases (**Table 2**). The TLICS has demonstrated good interobserver and intraobserver reliability.[65] The overall simplicity of this scoring system makes it a potentially useful clinical adjunct in the classification and treatment of thoracolumbar injuries.

Nonoperative Management

Most stable thoracolumbar burst fractures can be treated nonsurgically if the patient has no neurologic deficit.[14,63,66-69] This presumes a minimum definition of a mechanically stable injury as having an intact PLC. The clinical challenge is predicting, based on injury characteristics, which fractures are stable or unstable (ie, if the PLC is functionally intact). Clear-cut criteria do not exist.[41] This is partially a result of inconsistent, and at times ambiguous, descriptions of injuries reported in outcomes literature.

Various forms of nonsurgical management can be used.[14,63,66-71] Progressive mobilization and observation without an external support device might be used for some injuries.[63] This rests on the belief that if the injury is inherently stable, then external immobilization offers little to prevent subsequent deformity. External orthoses can be used for more substantial fractures. Hyperextension devices, such as a Jewett brace, can counteract sagittal flexion forces; however, they offer minimal resistance to rotation or lateral flexion. Custom-fit clamshell devices, such as a thoracolumbar sacral orthosis (TLSO), provide multiplanar support, which may be more appropriate for burst fractures.

Several studies have evaluated the ability of external orthoses to immobilize the thoracic and thoracolumbar spine.[72-74] Most braces have demonstrated increased motion across the lumbosacral junction.[73,74] One study compared a corset, a rigid brace, and a plaster jacket with and without a thigh cuff, reporting that the plaster jackets provided the best immobilization of the L1-L3 segments.[74]

Patients with mechanically unstable fractures who may be too sick to undergo surgery might be treated nonsurgically by extended bed rest and continued spinal precautions.[70,71,75] Some complications of prolonged recumbency, such as decubitus ulcers and diminished pulmonary function, can be mitigated with the use of a RotaRest™ bed (Kinetic Concepts, Inc [KCI], San Antonio, Texas);[70] this is a specially designed bed that continuously rotates from side to side. Trapdoors in the bed allow the posterior skin to be inspected without moving the patient. Chemical thromboprophylaxis should be considered in such patients. Generally, this should be started within 72 hours, particularly in patients with spinal cord injury (SCI).

Authors' Suggested Treatment Guidelines

An intact PLC should be considered a prerequisite for nonsurgical care. Some authors feel that more than 50% canal compromise is an indication for surgical decompression and/or stabilization. However, there are little data to support this practice routinely in a neurologically intact patient with an intact PLC. Kyphosis more than 25° to 30° and/or anterior height loss of greater than 50% is highly suggestive of posterior ligament injury. We use MRI to confirm the integrity of the PLC in equivocal cases. However, there is literature reporting nonsurgical care for some patients with neurologic deficits.[76,77] We believe that nonsurgical management should be reserved for cases in which the patient is medically unfit to undergo surgery.

We prefer to treat stable burst fractures using a custom-made form-fitting TLSO. The patient is maintained in a flat position until the brace is applied. Prior to ambulation, standing radiographs in the brace are obtained. The kyphotic angle and height loss should be measured and compared with initial values. If kyphosis or height loss increases, the integrity of the posterior ligaments should be more closely evaluated. Patients are followed closely with standing radiographs at weekly intervals until the stability of the fracture and compliance of the patient can be ensured. Typically, the brace is worn at all times for 3 months. In more stable injuries, patients may be allowed to sleep without the brace after 3 to 6 weeks. Bracing the patient in a hyperextended position to decrease deformity is thought to be important by some. However, a more realistic goal is for the fracture to heal with minimal additional height loss or kyphosis. Patients should be advised to avoid lifting more than 5 to 10 lb, twisting, and bending. They are instructed to call if they develop progressive pain, deformity, or any neurologic symptoms.

Published Outcomes

Nonsurgical Management in Neurologically Intact Patients

Weinstein et al[15] documented results of nonsurgical treatment of stable thoracolumbar burst fractures in 42 patients without neurologic deficit followed for 11 to 55 years. Average kyphosis in flexion was 26° and in extension, 17°. However, the degree of kyphosis did not correlate with degree of pain or function at final follow-up. No case of neurologic deterioration was reported. Low pain scores were documented, with no patient using narcotics for pain control. Eighty-eight percent of patients returned to work in their preinjury occupation.

Shen and Shen[63] retrospectively reviewed the outcomes of nonsurgical treatment of 38 patients with thoracolumbar burst fractures without neurologic deficit. Excluded were those injuries with posterior arch fractures, dislocation, or kyphosis more than 35°, presumably because these injury features strongly suggested PLC disruption. All patients were permitted early ambulation, while only nine patients were treated in a brace. Average kyphosis increased from 20° to 24° over an average follow-up period of 4 years. Thirty-two patients had no or mild pain, four had moderate pain, and two patients had severe pain; both eventually underwent surgery more than 1 year after injury. Most importantly, there was no correlation between kyphosis or canal compromise and clinical outcome. Seventy-six percent of patients returned to their preinjury occupation. Complications included transient hematuria and urinary retention in three and six patients, respectively.

Aligizakis et al[78] followed 60 consecutive neurologically intact patients with thoracolumbar burst fractures treated with an orthosis for an average of 42 months. Initial and final kyphosis averaged 6° and 8°, respectively. Ninety-one percent had a satisfactory functional outcome and 83% reported slight or no pain and returned to preinjury activity level. Three patients developed a urinary tract infection successfully treated with antibiotics.

Another group reported the results of twenty-four neurologically intact patients with burst fractures.[67] Treatment consisted of a TLSO, Jewett hyperextension brace, or a hyperextension cast and early ambulation. No patient developed a neurologic deficit. A statistically insignificant increase in kyphosis was observed.

Clinical Comparisons of Nonsurgical Versus Surgical Treatment

The outcomes of surgical and nonsurgical management of thoracolumbar burst fractures have been compared in several studies.[14,16,79] In a classic report, Willén et al[79] compared the results of surgical versus nonsurgical management of unstable thoracolumbar fractures in a group of neurologically intact patients. Longer hospital stays (80 days versus 30 days) and greater duration of immobilization (67 days versus 18 days) were documented in the nonsurgical group. While kyphosis at final follow-up was greater in the nonsurgical group, the degree of deformity did not affect functional outcomes. No patient had neurologic deterioration. There was no difference in pain scores or rates of return to work between the two groups.

In a more recent study, Shen et al[14] prospectively compared outcomes of patients treated with posterior surgery or nonsurgical management for thoracolumbar burst fractures without neurologic deficit. Patients with posterior arch fractures and facet dislocations were excluded. Nonsurgical treatment included hyperextension brace and early ambulation in 47 patients; surgical treatment included short-segment pedicle screw fixation in 33 patients. Outcome scores were better in the surgical group at 3 months; however, at 6 months and 2 years, the scores were not statistically significantly different. Kyphosis correction and pain scores were also initially better in the surgical group, but again, this benefit was not demonstrable at final follow-up.

Wood et al[16] published the results of a well-designed prospective randomized controlled study comparing surgical and nonsurgical treatment of stable thoracolumbar burst fractures in patients without neurologic deficit. Patients with suspected or confirmed posterior ligamentous disruption were excluded. Nonsurgical care included a brace or cast followed by early mobilization; surgical treatment was either anterior or posterior surgery. There were no statistically significant differences in kyphosis, functional outcome, or pain scores between the two groups. Importantly, surgically treated patients tended to have higher pain scores and more complications.

From these data, the main benefit of surgical treatment of unstable fractures in neurologically intact patients appears to be earlier mobilization. Although the reported risk for secondary neurologic compromise is low, this potential remains a concern for most practitioners. For so-called stable fractures with intact posterior ligaments in neurologically intact patients, the data strongly suggest that nonsurgical management, consisting of bracing and early mobilization, is an effective treatment method. What are lacking from these studies, however, are clear recommendations of how to determine or define the integrity of the PLC.

Nonsurgical Management of Patients With Neurologic Deficit

Dendrinos et al[77] found that no patient with a thoracolumbar burst fracture associated with a complete injury (Frankel grade A) demonstrated neurologic recovery, regardless of whether surgical or nonsurgical treatment was employed. Others have also found comparable recovery rates in patients with incomplete neural deficits treated with or without surgery. Burke and Murray,[76] in a review of the results in 89 patients, documented neurologic recovery in 35% and 38% of nonsurgically and surgically treated patients, respectively.

Neurologic Outcomes and Canal Compromise

Although it seems counterintuitive, the degree of neurologic deficit does not appear to be predictable based on the amount of canal stenosis. The degree of deficit is probably more influenced by the instantaneous canal compromise that occurs at the time of impact, which may be substantially more than what is detectable on initial imaging.[80]

Wessberg et al[81] studied canal remodeling in 115 patients treated with posterior distraction instrumentation (2 levels above and below injured vertebrae) by measuring the midsagittal diameter and the cross-sectional area of the spinal canal. Immediately following surgery, the mean canal clearance ranged from 49% to 72% of normal. At final follow-up, the mean canal measurements were 87% of normal, indicating that the retropulsed bony fragments continue to resorb over time. Canals with greater amounts of initial compromise demonstrated greater amounts of clearance. Canal clearance was not significantly different between patients operated on early (less than 3 days) or late (more than 3 days). Dai[82] retrospectively reviewed the CT scans and plain radiographs of 83 patients with thoracolumbar burst fractures treated surgically or nonsurgically. At 12-month follow-up, the spinal canal underwent substantial remodeling, regardless of the type of treatment.

In another review, Kim et al[83] found the average amount of canal compromise was greater in patients with neural deficit (mean of 52%) versus those who are neurologically intact (mean of 35%). However, the average amount of canal clearance was not different for those who demonstrated neural recovery (20%) versus those who did not (23%). A more important predictor of neurologic deficit was the presence of posterior ligamentous disruption (61% versus 25% for patients with and without deficit, respectively). Unfortunately, the study did not specify the method by which the integrity of the PLC was determined.

In an analysis of various radiological canal measurements in patients with burst fractures and neural deficit, Vaccaro et al[84] found the only measurement that correlated with neural status was the sagittal-to-transverse ratio. The absolute cross-sectional area, sagittal canal diameter, and transverse diameter by themselves were not correlative. Another group found that 25%, 50%, and 75% canal compromise corresponded to a 0.29, 0.51, and 0.71 predictive value for the presence (but not severity) of a neural deficit, respectively.[85] In a similar study, 45% canal compromise and posterior column injury was predictive of the presence of neurologic injury at the L1 level.[47] Again, the severity of deficit could not be correlated. By measuring the cross-sectional area of the canal, one study found that 1.0 cm^2 was the critical level below which all patients had some degree of neurologic deficit, while patients with 1.0 to 1.25 cm^2 of canal area had no or incomplete neural injuries.[86]

It appears that patients are more likely to have a neurologic deficit if they have canal compromise, but if they are neurologically intact, the amount of canal compromise is not predictive of outcome.

Surgical Management

Surgical treatment includes stabilization and fusion with or without decompression. The goals of surgery are to restore/maintain spinal alignment and stability until solid bony fusion is achieved. In cases of neurologic deficit and canal compromise, decompression is targeted at maximizing the space available for the neural elements with the hope that this will maximize neurologic recovery. Both anterior and posterior procedures can be used to achieve these goals.

Overview of Surgical Options

There is considerable controversy regarding the indications and optimal method of surgical treatment of thoracolumbar burst fractures. For stabilization, some advocate posterior surgery while others believe that anterior or combined anterior and posterior surgery is preferred.[3,19,20,23,34,87-92] In patients with neurologic deficit (in particular those with incomplete deficits), most surgeons would agree that a decompressive maneuver is warranted. Indirect reduction of displaced vertebral body fragments can be achieved through distraction and realignment with posterior instrumentation. Data suggest that this is more effective if the PLL is intact and if surgery is performed less than 2 to 4 days from injury.[93] It appears that direct fragment removal through an anterior approach offers the best anatomic decompression, although the neurologic benefits have not been conclusively established.[22,91] Direct fragment removal and interbody reconstruction can also be performed through an all-posterior-lateral approach. Several anterior and posterior instrumentation systems are available for stabilization.

Suggested Surgical Indications

A progressive neurologic deficit is an indication for urgent decompression. Progressive kyphotic deformity is a result of mechanical instability, which warrants surgical stabilization. Injury characteristics that are highly suggestive of PLC disruption are (1) progressive kyphotic deformity, (2) kyphosis greater than 25° to 30°, (3) vertebral body height loss greater than 50%, and (4) MRI evidence of PLC disruption. Patients with neurologic deficit associated with canal compromise are typically decompressed.

Posterior Stabilization Techniques

Pedicle Screws

The role of posterior surgery for burst fractures is primarily for realignment and stabilization. This can be accomplished using a variety of constructs; pedicle screw fixation is among the more popular methods.[4,17-19,94,95] At a minimum, the level above and below the fracture should be included in the fusion (ie, short-segment instrumentation). Some prefer inclusion of two levels above and below the fracture. Short-segment instrumentation can lead to high rates (as high as 50%) of pedicle screw breakage or failure.[17,96] This is thought to be the result of continued cyclic loading amplified by anterior column deficiency. In our experience, a short screw inserted into the pedicle of the injured vertebra appears to decrease the rate of instrumentation failure, much in the same way that Edwards sleeves provided a third point to resist bending moments. Transpedicular intracorporeal bone grafting was introduced in an attempt to reconstitute the vertebral body height. However, this has not diminished the rate of instrumentation failure with short-segment pedicle screw stabilization.[18,97]

The load-sharing classification system proposed by McCormack et al[98] addresses the need for supplementary anterior fusion in the setting of anterior column deficiency. Point totals are given to quantify the degree of vertebral body comminution, fracture apposition, and deformity. In a subsequent study by Parker et al,[92] 39 patients with mild to moderate (load-sharing score up to more than 6) anterior column deficiency were successfully treated with posterior short-segment instrumentation alone. There were no implant failures and the average loss of correction at last follow-up was 4°. Importantly, all patients were braced postoperatively for a period of 4 to 6 months. In cases of significant anterior column deficiency, we do not recommend short-segment instrumentation as a stand-alone procedure.

Hooks and Wires

Prior to development of pedicle screws, hook-based constructs were a common method of fracture stabilization. Although a useful option, this technique has lost its popularity as it requires inclusion of at least two to three segments above and below the injury. Sublaminar wire constructs are an unpopular means of stabilization of unstable burst fractures.

Posterior Decompression Techniques

Indirect Decompression

Indirect reduction, a concept that relies on longitudinal distraction along the fractured segment, works through ligamentotaxis of the displaced posterior vertebral fragments. With distraction, an intact PLL and/or posterior anulus are thought to pull the fragments back into place. One group[10] used this technique in 22 junctional (T11 to L2) burst fractures, reporting an average 28% improvement in canal compromise. Although patients with an incomplete neurologic injury improved an average of 1.8 Frankel grades, the rate of neurologic recovery or injury could not be predicted based on the amount of canal clearance. A cadaveric study found a relationship between measured vertebral height loss/kyphosis and spinal canal compromise with simulated burst fractures.[99] Interestingly, extension of the motion segment (a commonly performed maneuver to reduce burst fractures) did not affect canal clearance.

Indirect reduction has not been uniformly endorsed. Disruption of the PLL appears to compromise its effectiveness.[55] One group documented an average improvement in canal compromise of only 19% (57% preoperatively versus 38% postoperatively) after posterior distractive instrumentation in 30 patients.[23] Independent of canal clearance, incomplete (Frankel grades B through D) injuries improved one or more grades. Although the authors felt that disruption of the PLL was a contributing factor to the modest effects on canal clearance, they did not perform MRI to assess the PLL. From these findings, they inferred that more than 50% canal compromise might be indicative of PLL disruption, and that decompression should be performed through an anterior approach in these cases.

A greater delay from injury to operation is thought to compromise the efficacy of indirect canal clearance. One surgeon found that surgery performed within 1 week led to an average of 33% improvement of canal compromise.[100] Surgery done 1 week or 2 weeks after injury resulted in 24% and 0% improvement, respectively. As with other reports, all incomplete injuries improved by one or more Frankel grades regardless of canal clearance. Others[93] have found modestly better canal clearance in patients stabilized within 4 days (56% to 38% canal compromise) compared with those fixed more than 4 days after injury (52% to 44%, $P = 0.05$).

Direct Decompression Through a Posterior Approach

Several posterior methods of decompressing the spinal canal have been advocated. Simple decompressive laminectomy has fallen out of favor because it causes further posterior destabilization and can lead to progressive kyphotic deformity, particularly if adequate fixation is not achieved.

FIGURE 13

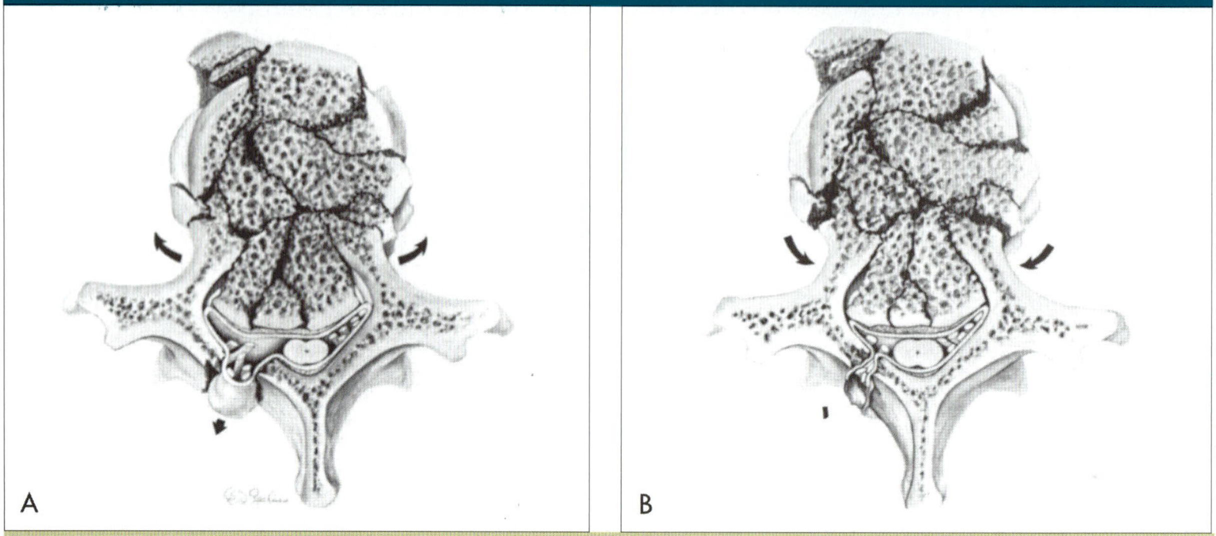

Figure 13 Proposed mechanism of injury for lamina fracture associated with entrapped neural elements. **A,** During axial loading, the pedicles are spread laterally, the lamina fractures, and the posterior vertebral body is retropulsed into the canal, resulting in protrusion of the dura and nerve rootlets into the laminar fracture defect. **B,** With dissipation of the axial load, the dura and nerve rootlets may become entrapped in the laminar fracture gap as the posterior elements recoil. (Reproduced with permission from Cammisa FP Jr, Eismont FJ, Green BA: Dural laceration occurring with burst fractures and associated laminar fractures. *J Bone Joint Surg Am* 1989;71(7):1044-1052.)

Furthermore, direct removal of retropulsed vertebral body fragments via a standard laminectomy can necessitate undue manipulation of the spinal cord.

Alternative methods of anterior canal decompression through an all-posterior approach have been developed. Silvestro et al[101] used a posterolateral approach to reduce the displaced vertebral body fragments to clear the spinal canal in 31 patients. Their technique includes removal of the facet joint and/or pedicle to gain access to the posterior vertebral body lateral to the spinal cord or cauda equina. Supplementation with a pedicle screw construct was used. They reported statistically significant decreases in canal compromise as measured by CT, with neurologic improvement in 96% of cases.

Some authors have recommended the use of intraoperative ultrasound to assess canal patency after distraction with reduction.[102,103] In a prospective study by Eismont et al,[102] intraoperative ultrasonography demonstrated persistent cord or root compression in 12 of 16 burst fractures after Harrington rod distraction instrumentation. Patients with incomplete reduction of the canal underwent posterolateral decompression. Eight of the 12 fractures were evaluated postoperatively with CT and all 8 showed normal or near-normal canal patency.

Concomitant Lamina Fracture

The combination of a burst fracture with a concomitant lamina fracture can be associated with a dural tear and entrapped nerve roots (**Figure 13**). This was first recognized and reported by Cammisa et al.[45] They demonstrated a high rate of dural lacerations with this injury pattern and subsequently recommended posterior laminectomy for exploration and dural repair before any planned anterior procedure.

Anterior Decompression

Anterior decompression is the most direct method of clearing the spinal canal after a burst fracture. The majority of the injured vertebral body along with the adjacent intervertebral disks can be removed. Retropulsed fragments are carefully removed to relieve pressure on the spinal cord or cauda equina. The highest rates of neurologic recovery have been reported after anterior decompressive surgery for burst fractures in patients with incomplete neural injuries. One report documented a median of two Frankel grades in patients undergoing anterior decompression within 48 hours.[104]

Timing of Decompression

It has been suggested that the time elapsed from injury to surgical decompression can influence the rate of neurologic recovery. Most of the studies on timing of surgical decompression have primarily included patients with cervical SCI. In addition, previous studies have been limited by inconsistent definitions of early and late treatment.

Vaccaro et al,[105] in a prospective, randomized controlled trial comparing early (less than 72 hours) with late (more than 5 days) decompression of patients with cervical SCI, reported no difference in terms of functional or neurologic improvement. One major limitation of this study was that 20 of the 62 patients enrolled were lost to follow-up. In their systematic review of the literature, Fehlings and Perrin[106] recommended urgent decompression (less than 24 hours) following isolated acute cervical SCI in hemodynamically stable patients. Of note, they site a lack of level I evidence, concluding that there are no standards on the optimal timing of surgical intervention. In an effort to establish definitive guidelines on the role and timing of decompression in acute SCI, a large, multicenter prospective trial is currently underway.

Early Decompression

Clohisy et al[104] reported results of early versus late anterior decompression in 22 patients with thoracolumbar burst fractures. Surgery performed within 48 hours of injury resulted in a mean improvement of two Frankel grades and complete resolution of bowel and bladder function in 44% of patients, while surgery after 48 hours improved Frankel scoring by only one grade, with no patient recovering complete bowel or bladder function. Although the study was not randomized, these data offer some evidence that early anterior decompressive surgery might benefit neurologic outcome in patients with thoracolumbar fractures.

Late Decompression

For a variety of reasons, decompression may not be performed at the time of initial injury resulting in residual canal stenosis for extended periods of time (weeks to years). Considering this specific situation, Transfeldt et al[107] examined the effects of late decompression after burst fracture. In 49 patients with conus medullaris or cauda equina level injuries, statistically significant neurologic improvement was observed in patients decompressed within 2 years after injury. The overall rate of bladder improvement was 50% for fractures at or below T12. These data suggest that substantial improvements in Frankel grade and bladder/bowel function can be achieved in patients with even long-standing neural compression after burst fracture.

Anterior Reconstruction and Stabilization

Structural Allograft and Cages

By the nature of anterior decompression, the spine is iatrogenically destabilized. To remedy this, the vertebral body defect must be replaced with a supportive strut that will also lead to bony fusion. Structural autograft can be harvested from rib, fibula, or the iliac crest. The use of autogenous bone grafts as the sole means of anterior column support in the setting of thoracolumbar trauma is somewhat limited by the morbidity associated with the harvesting of these relatively large grafts.[108] Allograft bone, typically femoral or humeral shafts, can be used alternatively. In recent years, the widespread availability of expandable and nonexpandable cages has increased the number of options available for anterior reconstruction.[109] Such devices can be filled with harvested morcellized autograft or allograft. Anterior and/or posterior instrumentation is recommended to add further stability.

Anterior Instrumentation

Numerous constructs can be used for anterior stabilization. Several in vitro biomechanical studies have compared various anterior devices.[96,110-112] Among the more rigid devices are plates with fixed-angle vertebral body screws and cross-linked rod-screw-staple designs, such as the Kaneda system (DePuy Spine, Raynham, MA).

Kostuik[91] performed anterior surgery for thoracolumbar burst fractures in 35 patients with neurologic injury. Iliac crest autograft struts were used to reconstruct the anterior column, which was stabilized with a modified Harrington rod-screw system spanning from the vertebral bodies above and below the fractured segment. High rates of neurologic recovery were documented with incomplete injuries; complete neural damage showed no improvement. Nineteen of 21 patients with initial incomplete loss of bowel or bladder function showed some improvement at final follow-up. Twelve of 13 patients who were treated within 10 days of injury recovered useful bladder function, while only 5 of 8 patients treated more than 10 days after injury gained useful bladder function without incontinence.

To our knowledge, Kaneda et al[22] have reported the largest series of surgical stabilization for burst fractures. This included 150 consecutive patients with thoracolumbar burst fractures with neurologic deficits treated with a single-stage anterior decompression, strut grafting, and instrumentation using a rod-screw-staple device. The average canal clearance was nearly 100%, while the fusion rate was 93%. Anterior pseudarthroses were successfully treated by posterior instrumentation and fusion. One-hundred forty-two patients (95%) improved at least one Frankel grade.

The use of plate fixation has also been reported. Haas et al[113] documented excellent rates of neural recovery and maintenance of alignment using anterior decompression, strut grafting, and an anterior plate for a variety of thoracolumbar fractures. Ghanayem and Zdeblick[90] reported their results using an anterior plate in 12 patients with thoracolumbar burst fractures. In ten cases, postoperative kyphosis correction was maintained at 1-year follow-up. The other two patients had 10° to 20° of correction loss. Both of these patients had preoperative kyphosis angles greater than 50°, suggesting that anterior surgery alone may not be sufficient to stabilize the injuries with substantial posterior ligamentous disruption.

Comparison of Anterior and Posterior Surgery

Only a few studies have compared anterior and posterior surgery for burst fractures. Bradford and McBride[114] studied a group of 59 patients with thoracolumbar fractures and an incomplete neurologic deficit treated with either anterior or posterior surgery. Posterior surgery included posterolateral decompression through a transpedicular approach and stabilization, while anterior surgery entailed a full corpectomy at the level of injury. The posterior group was treated an average of 6.4 days from injury, while no case in the anterior group was operated on less than a month from injury. While not all had burst fractures, they found that neurologic recovery was related to the completeness of canal clearance. Motor, sensory, and bladder improvement was statistically better in the anterior group. Regarding bladder function specifically for conus level lesions, 70% of patients in the anterior group improved, while only 12% in the posterior group showed improvement. In contrast, motor recovery was not statistically affected by the choice of approach.

Stancić et al[115] compared the results of anterior and posterior surgery for what they deemed mechanically unstable thoracolumbar burst fractures in patients without neurologic deficit. While less blood loss and shorter operative times were documented for the posterior approach, anterior and posterior surgery resulted in equivalent clinical results. In a well-designed randomized prospective study, Wood et al[116] found equivalent clinical and radiographic results with anterior and posterior surgery.

Combined Anterior and Posterior Surgery

Combined anterior and posterior surgery can be performed to treat thoracolumbar burst fractures. The specific indications and benefits of this maneuver remain unclear; however, many surgeons feel that evidence of posterior ligamentous disruption is an important factor. The theoretical advantages of a combined approach include maximization of canal clearance, immediate circumferential stability, and optimized fusion rates. The added morbidity of two separate procedures is a potential disadvantage.

In a retrospective review, the results of combined anterior-posterior surgery were compared to those of posterior surgery alone for the treatment of thoracolumbar burst fractures.[20] Although the method of treatment had no effect on neurologic recovery, combined surgery resulted in better maintenance of kyphosis correction. Similar to nonsurgical series, loss of correction was not associated with a higher rate of back pain.

Less Invasive Surgery

Less invasive methods of thoracolumbar fracture surgery have been advocated; however, only a few published reports exist. One group examined their results using a thoracoscopic approach to perform corpectomy, anterior column reconstruction, and anterior instrumentation.[117] While the investigators considered it low, they had higher rates of vascular injury and neurologic deterioration than those reported for open surgery. Recognizing the steep learning curve, the efficacy and advantages of the thoracoscopic approach to spinal fractures remain to be seen.

Authors' Preferred Techniques

Indications for Posterior Surgery

In the our practices, posterior surgery is indicated primarily for kyphosis correction and stabilization, not decompression, of burst fractures (**Figure 14**). For thoracic level injuries associated with a truly complete SCI, there is probably little neurologic benefit to direct anterior decompression. In patients who have an incomplete neurologic injury, an anterior approach is generally preferred. Exceptions are injuries at the T3 and T4 level, which can be difficult to approach anteriorly. In these uncommon cases, direct decompression through an all-posterior approach, as described by Silvestro et al,[101] might be optimal.

In cases with a concomitant lamina fracture and neurologic deficit, a posterior approach is preferred to address the possibility of entrapped neural elements and posterior dural tear. The posterior approach (with or without an anterior decompression and fusion) is also preferred in cases with major PLC disruption, and certainly if the burst fracture is associated with a fracture-dislocation.

When the spinal canal has been decompressed posterolaterally, we recommend obtaining a postoperative CT scan to assess the adequacy of the decompression and integrity of the anterior column. A supplementary anterior decompression and fusion may be required if the neural elements are still compressed or the anterior column is markedly disrupted (especially when short-segment posterior fixation has been employed).[92,98]

Posterior instrumentation and fusion is ideal for those fractures with PLC disruption in neurologically intact patients. In cases of vertebral body height loss greater than 50% or extensive comminution, pedicle screws are placed two levels above and below the fractured vertebra. If there is minimal anterior column disruption, then short-segment stabilization is considered.[92,98]

Surgical Technique for Posterior Surgery

The neurologically intact patient is carefully positioned on a Jackson spine table. By nature of the location of the transverse chest pad and the iliac/thigh pads, an extension moment is delivered to the thoracolumbar junction. Gentle pressure can be applied to the apex of the kyphus to achieve further correction.

A standard midline approach is used to expose the vertebrae. If a lamina fracture is present, the dissection is performed carefully in search of entrapped neural elements. Under fluoroscopic guidance, pedicle screws are inserted into the desired levels. Rods should then be cut 1 cm to 1.5 cm longer than the measured distance between the upper and lower screws. We prefer to use monoaxial pedicle screws for maximum strength, lower profile, and to assist in the reduction. When inserting the screws, the sections above and below the fracture can be instrumented separately, placing the screws perpendicular to the long axis of the spine, and aligned similarly in the axial plane. The rod is contoured into physiologic sagittal alignment and when it is introduced into the screws, a harmonious contour results as the deformity is reduced. The rods should be fixed to the top screws first. They can then be delivered to the lower screw heads by cantilever bending to reduce the kyphotic deformity. At the thoracolumbar junction, the rod is not contoured. In the middle and upper thoracic spine, the rod should be contoured to approximate a normal degree of kyphosis.

The lock nuts should then be placed into the lower screws, but not tightened. A vise-grip rod holder can then be placed above the lower screws to act as an anchoring point. A distractor is then used to restore intervertebral height. The lower screws can then be tightened. Cross-links are added to provide additional torsional stability. The posterior elements, including the lateral spinous processes, laminae, facets, and transverse processes, should then be decorticated. Care should be taken not to disrupt the posterior ligaments or facets of unfused segments. Autologous bone graft is then placed over the bleeding bony surfaces. The wound is closed in layers.

Pitfalls and Bailouts

If short pedicle screws have been placed at the injured level, the screw heads may lie slightly lateral to the rod before distraction. This is a result of interpedicular widening, which can be reduced with longitudinal distraction. These screws should not be fixed to the rod until distraction has been used to restore height, which should help reduce lateral pedicular displacement.

Postoperative Care

Internal fixation usually obviates the need for postoperative bracing. However, this decision is made on a case-by-case basis. A lower threshold for bracing is held for patients who have undergone short-segment stabilization; those who seem likely to be noncompliant with postoperative restrictions, such as avoiding bending and heavy lifting; patients at higher risk for nonunion, such as smokers or diabetics; and those with osteopenic bone.

One of the major advantages of internal fixation in multiple-trauma patients is the avoidance of bracing. This facilitates nursing care, hygiene, skin care, and mobilization. Unless otherwise contraindicated, pharmacologic prophylaxis for venous thromboembolism can be cautiously initiated on postoperative day 4 or 5. Lower extremity sequential compression devices are placed immediately after surgery.

Radiographs should be obtained immediately postoperatively and at 3 months, 6 months, and 1 year or until solid bony fusion is evident. Activity is limited to walking and other activities of

FIGURE 14

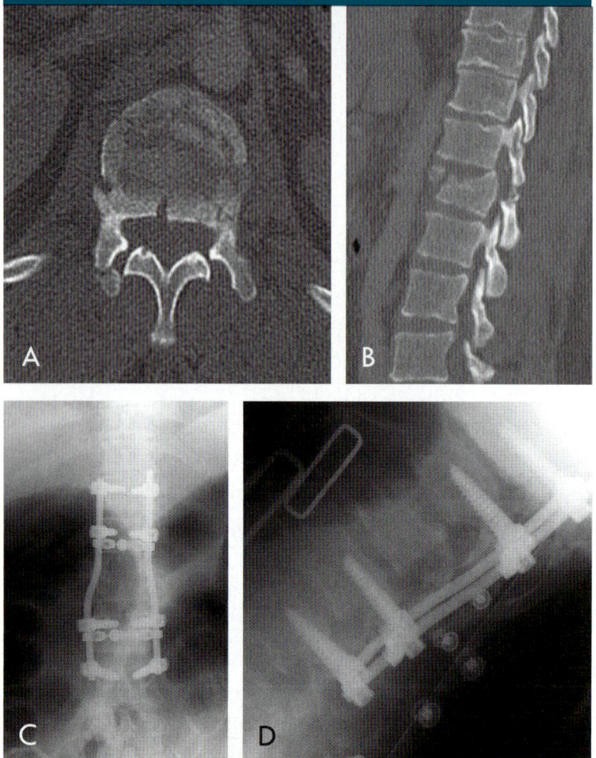

Figure 14 Case example of a 41-year-old male involved in a motor vehicle accident sustaining an L1 burst fracture-dislocation with complete neurologic injury (ASIA A) at that level. Patient underwent open reduction and T11-L3 instrumented fusion with autogenous iliac crest bone graft through a posterior approach. The patient was treated in a TLSO for 3 months postoperatively and went on to achieve successful fusion. **A** and **B,** Preoperative axial and sagittal CT imaging demonstrating retropulsion of posterior vertebral body and dislocation of T12-L1 facet. **C** and **D,** Immediate postoperative AP and lateral radiographs demonstrating pedicle screw fixation.

daily living until the fusion is solid. Return to a manual labor occupation or sports should be postponed until the patient is relatively pain-free and has acceptable functional return of strength and mobility.

Illustrative Cases

Case 1

Indications for Anterior Surgery

In a review of the literature, it appears that anterior surgery results in the most effective decompression of the spinal canal after burst fracture.[22,43,114] In our practices, anterior surgery is chosen for patients with either thoracic fractures associated with an incomplete SCI or thoracolumbar fractures associated with any neurologic deficit. Upper thoracic levels (above T5) can be difficult to access through an anterior approach, as discussed above, and may be better treated by posterior methods of decompression and fusion.

Anterior surgery for patients without a neurologic deficit has less clear indications. In our opinion, it may be indicated in cases of severe kyphotic deformity with high percentages of vertebral body height loss (greater than 70% to 80%). The rationale for this recommendation is that posterior short-segment constructs can have a high rate of failure in this situation.[92,98] If anterior surgery is elected in a neurologically intact patient, the surgeon must decide whether or not the spinal canal will be decompressed. If the canal is not decompressed, care must be taken to not push the bony fragments further into the neural elements during placement of an interbody device. On the other hand, if the spinal canal is decompressed, meticulous removal of the retropulsed bone fragments should be focused on avoiding any iatrogenic neurologic injury or dural tear.

Stand-alone anterior stabilization can be performed in most cases. Our preference is to use a rod-staple-screw construct at the thoracolumbar junction, as it provides excellent biomechanical stability compared with most plate-screw designs. At more cranial levels, the lower profile of a plate is desirable. Newer locking-plate designs may offer mechanical benefits over nonlocking plates. Supplemental posterior fixation is elected in those cases associated with massive posterior ligamentous disruption, particularly if facet joint gapping or posterior interspinous widening persists after anterior surgery. Anterior surgery is usually deferred in cases of retroperitoneal or intrathoracic injuries.

Surgical Technique for Anterior Surgery

The patient is placed in the lateral decubitus position with the left side up on a standard operating table. The approximate level of the injury should be positioned over the break of the table to facilitate intraoperative exposure. The preparation and draping of the skin should include the iliac crest. The intercostal interval approached should be one or two levels above the level of the fracture. For example, a T11 burst fracture should be approached by a thoracotomy between the T9 and T10 ribs.

The segmental vessels at the injured level, as well as the infra- and superjacent vessels, are ligated at the midvertebral body. This can preserve important arterial anastomotic branches that supply the artery of Adamkiewicz. The borders of the disk spaces above and below the fracture are then delineated via subperiosteal dissection. Posterior bony exposure should include the base of the pedicle.

After complete diskectomy, the majority of fractured bone is removed with a large rongeur. This bone can be saved for subsequent grafting. The remainder of the anterior, posterior, and lateral vertebral body can then be removed with a high-speed burr. A shell of anterior and lateral vertebral body is left to enhance healing of the interbody graft. Finally, the posterior vertebral body fragments are removed with straight and angled curets. When surgery is performed early, these fragments are usually quite mobile and are easily removed.

At this point, the first stage of instrumentation is begun. Our preference is a rod-screw-staple construct, such as the Kaneda device (**Figure 15**). First, the staple is tamped into place along the midlateral aspect of the vertebral body. The posterior holes should lie over the posterior aspect of the vertebral body. Next, drill holes are made. Bicortical screws may improve fixation. The posterior screws are placed parallel to the posterior vertebral body. The anterior screws are angled slightly posterior to triangulate with the anterior screw (**Figure 15,** *D*). Once the screws are in place, a distractor can then be used to finalize height restoration, kyphotic correction, and facilitate smooth placement of the interbody device. The deformity can also be reduced by manually pushing on the posterior elements with an anteriorly directed force. This maneuver is especially useful in patients with poor bone quality because the distractor may cause screw loosening when used for deformity correction.

Our preference is to use allograft bone or a titanium mesh cage (**Figure 16**). Either can be filled with salvaged corpectomy bone in addition to harvested iliac crest graft (if necessary). If the operating table was flexed to facilitate exposure, it is leveled before placing the interbody cage or graft. With gentle overdistraction applied through the screw-staple device and/or manual reduction, the cage or bone is tamped into place. Optimally, it should be centered along the end plates of the cranial and caudal vertebrae. Once the strut is in place, the distractor is removed. If a gap persists at the strut/end-plate interface, gentle compression may be applied through the screws. Rods are then cut to the appropriate length and inserted into the screw holes. A single cross-connector is then applied to increase the torsional rigidity of the construct.

Postoperative Care

With rigid fixation, postoperative bracing is usually not necessary and may be difficult when a chest tube has been placed. The patient should be mobilized as soon as possible. The chest tube is removed once drainage has diminished, and a follow-up chest radiograph obtained to rule out pneumothorax. Radiographic follow-up and return to work or sports is the same as that following posterior surgery.

Case 2

Indications for Combined Surgery

In most cases, either anterior or posterior surgery alone is adequate. However, there are several situations in which combined anterior and posterior approaches may be elected (**Figure 17**).

If the primary approach was posterior stabilization, anterior surgery may be performed in a staged fashion when a new or persistent neurologic deficit is present that is associated with residual canal compromise from retropulsed bony fragments, or progressive loss of correction ensues or is expected related to continued collapse of the fractured vertebral body.

If the primary approach was anterior surgery, posterior stabilization may be performed in a staged fashion when there is substantial residual posterior element gapping or disruption that may place added stress on the anterior construct, or substantial coronal or kyphotic deformity persists that might significantly affect overall spinal balance.

Initial combined anterior/posterior surgery may be planned for patients with a neurologic deficit with retropulsed bony fragments in addition to a lamina fracture with suspected entrapped nerve roots. Circumferential surgery is our treatment of choice for senile osteoporotic burst fractures that require surgical decompression and stabilization.[118]

Surgical Technique for Combined Surgery

Our techniques for anterior and posterior surgery have been detailed above. In most cases, the anterior procedure is performed first unless the patient has a fracture-dislocation, in which case the posterior approach is done first to realign the spine. Posterior surgery can be performed during the same anesthetic period or in a delayed second stage. Our preference is to use both anterior and posterior instrumentation. With combined surgery, instrumentation can be limited to the level above and below the fracture.

Pitfalls and Bailouts

Placing pedicle screws into a level that has been instrumented anteriorly can be challenging. The screw oftentimes must be inserted between the

FIGURE 15

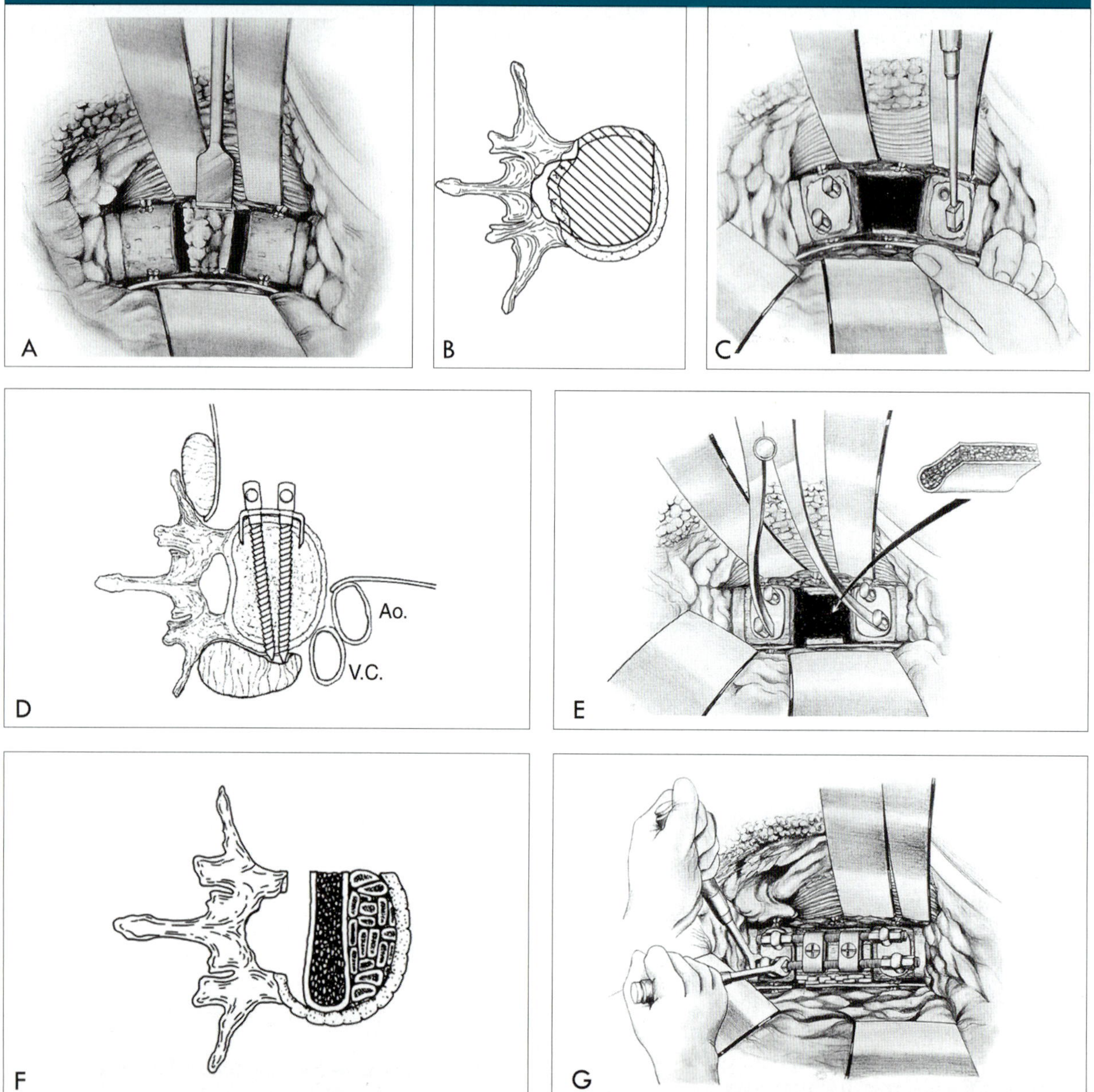

Figure 15 Drawings showing the technique of anterior corpectomy, strut grafting, and application of the Kaneda device. **A,** After excision of the intervertebral disks cephalad and caudad to the injured level, the fractured vertebral body is excised with use of a chisel, leaving the anterior longitudinal ligament intact. The displaced fragments of the vertebral body are removed from the anterior aspect of the PLL or thecal sac with use of long, sharp curets. **B,** Anterior decompression must be performed until the base of the contralateral pedicle is well visualized. **C,** After complete decompression, the vertebral plates of the Kaneda device are gently attached to the lateral aspect of the vertebral bodies cephalad and caudad to the vertebrectomy. Then, two screws are inserted into each vertebral body. A finger is passed across the vertebral body to feel the tip of the penetrated screw and to make sure that it does not protrude more than 3 or 4 mm beyond the vertebral body. **D,** The relation of the direction of the screws and the vertebral plate should be triangular, and the screws must penetrate the contralateral cortex. V.C. = vena cava; Ao. = aorta. **E,** Kyphosis is corrected with use of a spreader device applied to the heads of the two anterior screws. The tricortical iliac-crest graft and two or three pieces of rib are placed as a strut into the vertebrectomy gap. **F,** The tricortical portion of the iliac crest graft is inserted in the frontal plane beyond the contralateral pedicles. Bone chips from the resected vertebral body are packed into the gap between the iliac crest graft and the anterior vertebral wall. **G,** After bone grafting, threaded rods and two sets of the rod couplers are applied. (Reproduced with permission from Kaneda K, Taneichi H, Abumi K, Hashimoto T, Satoh S, Fujiya M: Anterior decompression and stabilization with the Kaneda device for thoracolumbar burst fractures associated with neurological deficits. *J Bone Joint Surg Am* 1997;79(1):69-83.)

FIGURE 16

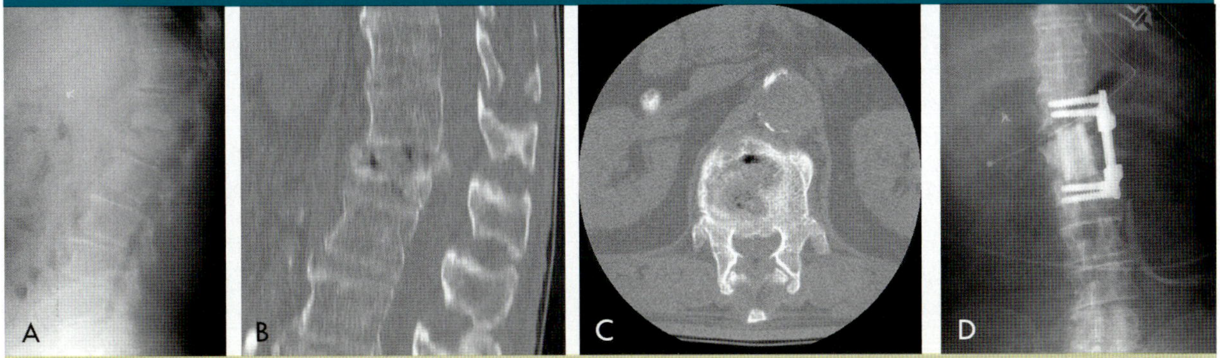

Figure 16 Case example of a 76-year-old male seen 9 months following a T12 burst fracture secondary to an 8-foot fall from a tree. The patient was intitially managed nonsurgically but presented with progressive pain and kyphotic deformity. Patient underwent T12 corpectomy with anterior fusion from T11 to L1 with a plate-and-rod construct with tibial allograft and autogenous bone graft from the vertebrectomy through a left-sided retroperitoneal approach. **A-C,** Preoperative lateral radiograph and CT scans demonstrating significant anterior column collapse and minimal canal encroachment. The patient was neurologically intact and therefore did not require decompression. **D,** Postoperative AP radiograph showing satisfactory coronal alignment with rod-and-screw construct.

FIGURE 17

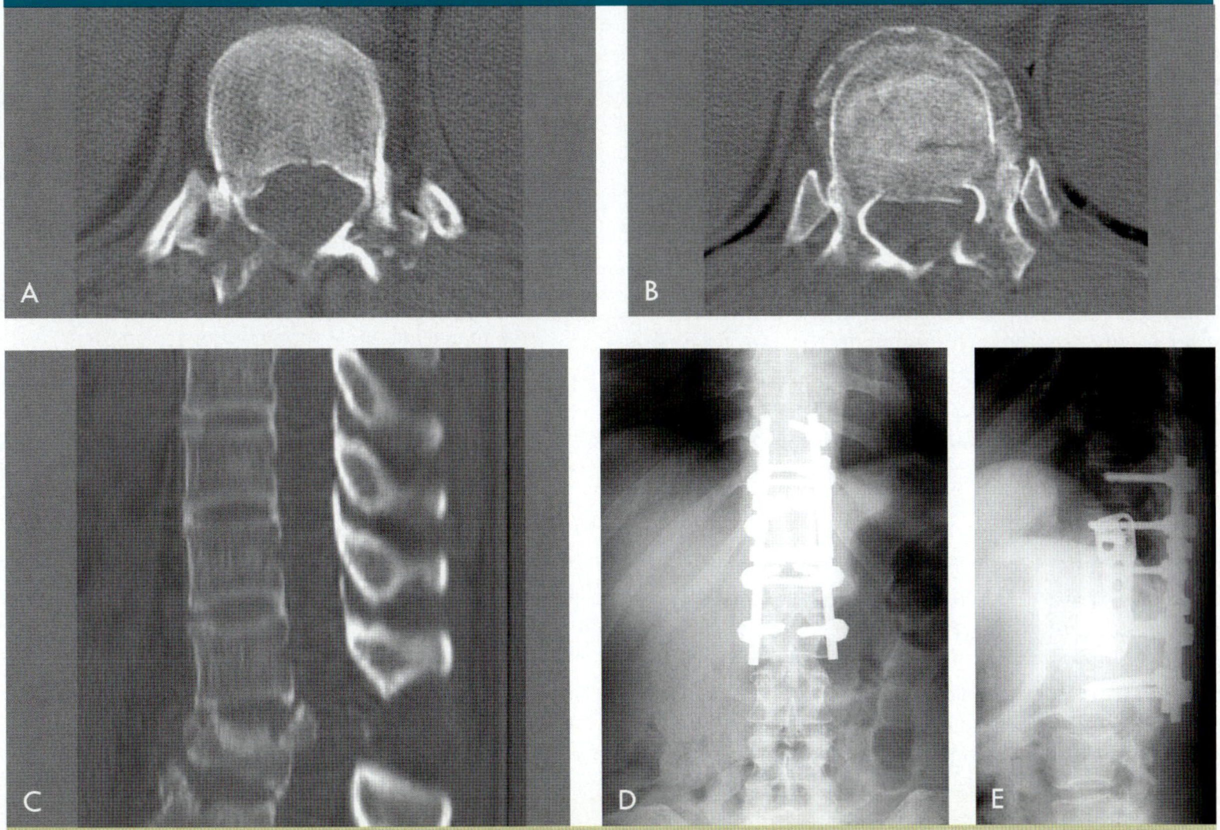

Figure 17 Case example of a 45-year-old female who sustained T12 burst and L1 compression fractures resulting from blunt trauma. The patient was neurologically intact and underwent posterior instrumented fusion with autogenous bone grafting from T10 to L2 followed by anterior corpectomy and tibial strut allograft at T12, with lateral sideplate fixation from T11 to L1 1 week later. The patient was treated in a TLSO for 3 months postoperatively and went on to achieve successful fusion. **A** and **B,** Preoperative axial CT images showing burst fracture of vertebral body with fracture extending into left pedicle and posterior arch of T12. **C,** Preoperative sagittal CT image showing subjacent compression fracture of L1 and significant widening of the T12-L1 interspinous processes, consistent with disrupted PLC. **D** and **E,** AP and lateral radiographs taken 3 months postoperatively demonstrating excellent coronal and sagittal alignment.

anterior vertebral body screws. In addition, AP fluoroscopic localization of the pedicle is often obscured by the screws. Intimate knowledge of the anatomic landmarks of the pedicle screw insertion site is crucial to proper screw placement. Altering the location of the anterior screws or using a device that is designed to be used in combination with pedicle screws may facilitate anterior/posterior instrumentation.

Postoperative Care

Postoperative care should proceed as it would for the other techniques. Because of the superior biomechanical stability of combined anterior and posterior instrumentation, postoperative orthoses are rarely used except in osteopenic patients.

Case 3

Surgical Timing and Complications

Surgical timing is an important consideration. This is particularly true when treating polytraumatized patients. In a retrospective review of patients with spinal fractures (including cervical, thoracic, and lumbar injuries), patients with injuries that were fixed within 3 days of injury had a lower rate of pneumonia and shorter hospital stay than those fixed more than 3 days after injury.[119] The two groups were not randomized, suggesting that the late fixation group could have included patients that were more severely injured. The average age, admission Glasgow coma scale, and chest injury scores were significantly higher in the late fixation group, although the injury severity scores were not statistically significantly different.[119]

It has been suggested that postoperative wound infections are more likely after fracture surgery than elective spine surgery. Rechtine et al[75] retrospectively reported a 10% incidence of wound infections after surgical stabilization of thoracolumbar fractures. While the study did not include a control group, the authors stated that this rate was higher than those previously reported in the literature for elective procedures. More importantly, a complete neurologic deficit was a statistically significant risk factor for infection. Other possible risk factors, including concomitant distant site infections or potential bacteremic sources such as open fractures, were not included in the analysis.

Summary

Although the optimal treatment of thoracolumbar burst fractures remains unclear, several treatment methods appear to be effective as long as neurologic and biomechanical principles are followed. Continued research is needed to determine the optimal treatment method for each injury pattern.

References

1. Bensch FV, Kiuru MJ, Koivikko MP, Koskinen SK: Spine fractures in falling accidents: Analysis of multidetector CT findings. *Eur Radiol* 2004; 14(4):618-624.
2. Alanay A, Acaroglu E, Yazici M, Surat A: Thoracolumbar spine fractures. *Spine (Phila Pa 1976)* 2001;26(7):840-841.
3. Andress HJ, Braun H, Helmberger T, Schürmann M, Hertlein H, Hartl WH: Long-term results after posterior fixation of thoraco-lumbar burst fractures. *Injury* 2002;33(4):357-365.
4. Arino VL: Our experience in 33 cases of thoracolumbar fracture treated by transpedicle instrument. *Chir Organi Mov* 2000;85(2):161-165.
5. Belmont PJ Jr, Taylor KF, Mason KT, Shawen SB, Polly DW Jr, Klemme WR: Incidence, epidemiology, and occupational outcomes of thoracolumbar fractures among U.S. Army aviators. *J Trauma* 2001;50(5):855-861.
6. Cotler JM: Introduction to thoracolumbar fractures. *Instr Course Lect* 1999;48:427-428.
7. Denis F, Burkus JK: Shear fracture-dislocations of the thoracic and lumbar spine associated with forceful hyperextension (lumberjack paraplegia). *Spine (Phila Pa 1976)* 1992;17(2):156-161.
8. Folman Y, Gepstein R: Late outcome of nonoperative management of thoracolumbar vertebral wedge fractures. *J Orthop Trauma* 2003;17(3): 190-192.
9. Louis CA, Gauthier VY, Louis RP: Posterior approach with Louis plates for fractures of the thoracolumbar and lumbar spine with and without neurologic deficits. *Spine (Phila Pa 1976)* 1998; 23(18):2030-2040.
10. Starr JK, Hanley EN Jr: Junctional burst fractures. *Spine (Phila Pa 1976)* 1992;17(5):551-557.
11. Holdsworth FW: Fractures, dislocations, and fracture-dislocations of the spine. *J Bone Joint Surg Br* 1963;45-B(1):6-20.
12. Cotterill PC, Kostuik JP, Wilson JA, Fernie GR, Maki BE: Production of a reproducible spinal burst fracture for use in biomechanical testing. *J Orthop Res* 1987;5(3):462-465.
13. White A, Panjabi M, eds: *Clinical Biomechanics of the Spine*, ed 2. Philadephia, PA, Lippincott-Raven, 1990.
14. Shen WJ, Liu TJ, Shen YS: Nonoperative treatment versus posterior fixation for thoracolumbar junction burst fractures without neurologic deficit. *Spine (Phila Pa 1976)* 2001;26(9):1038-1045.

15. Weinstein JN, Collalto P, Lehmann TR: Thoracolumbar "burst" fractures treated conservatively: A long-term follow-up. *Spine (Phila Pa 1976)* 1988;13(1):33-38.
16. Wood K, Buttermann G, Mehbod A, et al: Operative compared with nonoperative treatment of a thoracolumbar burst fracture without neurological deficit: A prospective, randomized study. *J Bone Joint Surg Am* 2003;85(5):773-781.
17. Alanay A, Acaroğlu E, Yazici M, Aksoy C, Surat A: The effect of transpedicular intracorporeal grafting in the treatment of thoracolumbar burst fractures on canal remodeling. *Eur Spine J* 2001;10(6): 512-516.
18. Alanay A, Acaroglu E, Yazici M, Oznur A, Surat A: Short-segment pedicle instrumentation of thoracolumbar burst fractures: Does transpedicular intracorporeal grafting prevent early failure? *Spine (Phila Pa 1976)* 2001;26(2):213-217.
19. Annicchiarico N: Internal A-O fixator for the reduction and stabilization of thoracolumbar fractures. *Chir Organi Mov* 2000;85(2):167-175.
20. Been HD, Bouma GJ: Comparison of two types of surgery for thoraco-lumbar burst fractures: Combined anterior and posterior stabilisation vs. posterior instrumentation only. *Acta Neurochir (Wien)* 1999;141(4):349-357.
21. Davies WE, Morris JH, Hill V: An analysis of conservative (non-surgical) management of thoracolumbar fractures and fracture-dislocations with neural damage. *J Bone Joint Surg Am* 1980;62(8): 1324-1328.
22. Kaneda K, Taneichi H, Abumi K, Hashimoto T, Satoh S, Fujiya M: Anterior decompression and stabilization with the Kaneda device for thoracolumbar burst fractures associated with neurological deficits. *J Bone Joint Surg Am* 1997;79(1): 69-83.
23. Katonis PG, Kontakis GM, Loupasis GA, Aligizakis AC, Christoforakis JI, Velivassakis EG: Treatment of unstable thoracolumbar and lumbar spine injuries using Cotrel-Dubousset instrumentation. *Spine (Phila Pa 1976)* 1999;24(22): 2352-2357.
24. McAfee PC, Bohlman HH, Yuan HA: Anterior decompression of traumatic thoracolumbar fractures with incomplete neurological deficit using a retroperitoneal approach. *J Bone Joint Surg Am* 1985; 67(1):89-104.
25. Müller U, Berlemann U, Sledge J, Schwarzenbach O: Treatment of thoracolumbar burst fractures without neurologic deficit by indirect reduction and posterior instrumentation: Bisegmental stabilization with monosegmental fusion. *Eur Spine J* 1999;8(4):284-289.
26. Sanderson PL, Fraser RD, Hall DJ, Cain CM, Osti OL, Potter GR: Short segment fixation of thoracolumbar burst fractures without fusion. *Eur Spine J* 1999;8(6):495-500.
27. Bernhardt M, Bridwell KH: Segmental analysis of the sagittal plane alignment of the normal thoracic and lumbar spines and thoracolumbar junction. *Spine (Phila Pa 1976)* 1989;14(7):717-721.
28. Vaz G, Roussouly P, Berthonnaud E, Dimnet J: Sagittal morphology and equilibrium of pelvis and spine. *Eur Spine J* 2002;11(1):80-87.
29. Gelb DE, Lenke LG, Bridwell KH, Blanke K, McEnery KW: An analysis of sagittal spinal alignment in 100 asymptomatic middle and older aged volunteers. *Spine (Phila Pa 1976)* 1995;20(12): 1351-1358.
30. Berry JL, Moran JM, Berg WS, Steffee AD: A morphometric study of human lumbar and selected thoracic vertebrae. *Spine (Phila Pa 1976)* 1987; 12(4):362-367.
31. Tan SH, Teo EC, Chua HC: Quantitative three-dimensional anatomy of cervical, thoracic and lumbar vertebrae of Chinese Singaporeans. *Eur Spine J* 2004;13(2):137-146.
32. Panjabi MM, Takata K, Goel V, et al: Thoracic human vertebrae: Quantitative three-dimensional anatomy. *Spine (Phila Pa 1976)* 1991;16(8): 888-901.
33. Oda I, Abumi K, Lü D, Shono Y, Kaneda K: Biomechanical role of the posterior elements, costovertebral joints, and rib cage in the stability of the thoracic spine. *Spine (Phila Pa 1976)* 1996;21(12): 1423-1429.
34. Magerl F, Aebi M, Gertzbein SD, Harms J, Nazarian S: A comprehensive classification of thoracic and lumbar injuries. *Eur Spine J* 1994;3(4): 184-201.
35. Denis F: The three column spine and its significance in the classification of acute thoracolumbar spinal injuries. *Spine (Phila Pa 1976)* 1983;8(8): 817-831.
36. Marino RJ, Ditunno JF Jr, Donovan WH, Maynard F Jr: Neurologic recovery after traumatic spinal cord injury: Data from the Model Spinal Cord Injury Systems. *Arch Phys Med Rehabil* 1999; 80(11):1391-1396.
37. Ko HY, Ditunno JF Jr, Graziani V, Little JW: The pattern of reflex recovery during spinal shock. *Spinal Cord* 1999;37(6):402-409.
38. Ertekin C, Reel F, Mutlu R, Kerküklü I: Bulbocavernosus reflex in patients with conus medullaris and cauda equina lesions. *J Neurol Sci* 1979;41(2): 175-181.
39. Vaccaro AR, An HS, Lin S, Sun S, Balderston RA, Cotler JM: Noncontiguous injuries of the spine. *J Spinal Disord* 1992;5(3):320-329.
40. Kuklo TR, Polly DW, Owens BD, Zeidman SM, Chang AS, Klemme WR: Measurement of thoracic

and lumbar fracture kyphosis: Evaluation of intraobserver, interobserver, and technique variability. *Spine (Phila Pa 1976)* 2001;26(1):61-66.

41. Petersilge CA, Emery SE: Thoracolumbar burst fracture: Evaluating stability. *Semin Ultrasound CT MR* 1996;17(2):105-113.

42. Hauser CJ, Visvikis G, Hinrichs C, et al: Prospective validation of computed tomographic screening of the thoracolumbar spine in trauma. *J Trauma* 2003;55(2):228-235.

43. McAfee PC, Yuan HA, Fredrickson BE, Lubicky JP: The value of computed tomography in thoracolumbar fractures: An analysis of one hundred consecutive cases and a new classification. *J Bone Joint Surg Am* 1983;65(4):461-473.

44. Frank E, Bonsell S: The accuracy of anterior-posterior measurements in the assessment of spinal canal compromise in burst fractures. *Neurol Res* 1994;16(6):410-412.

45. Cammisa FP Jr, Eismont FJ, Green BA: Dural laceration occurring with burst fractures and associated laminar fractures. *J Bone Joint Surg Am* 1989; 71(7):1044-1052.

46. Denis F, Burkus JK: Diagnosis and treatment of cauda equina entrapment in the vertical lamina fracture of lumbar burst fractures. *Spine (Phila Pa 1976)* 1991;16(8, Suppl):S433-S439.

47. Hashimoto T, Kaneda K, Abumi K: Relationship between traumatic spinal canal stenosis and neurologic deficits in thoracolumbar burst fractures. *Spine (Phila Pa 1976)* 1988;13(11):1268-1272.

48. Schönström N, Hansson T: Pressure changes following constriction of the cauda equine: An experimental study in situ. *Spine (Phila Pa 1976)* 1988;13(4):385-388.

49. Flanders AE, Spettell CM, Friedman DP, Marino RJ, Herbison GJ: The relationship between the functional abilities of patients with cervical spinal cord injury and the severity of damage revealed by MR imaging. *AJNR Am J Neuroradiol* 1999; 20(5):926-934.

50. Ohta K, Fujimura Y, Nakamura M, Watanabe M, Yato Y: Experimental study on MRI evaluation of the course of cervical spinal cord injury. *Spinal Cord* 1999;37(8):580-584.

51. Ramón S, Domínguez R, Ramírez L, et al: Clinical and magnetic resonance imaging correlation in acute spinal cord injury. *Spinal Cord* 1997;35(10): 664-673.

52. Selden NR, Quint DJ, Patel N, d'Arcy HS, Papadopoulos SM: Emergency magnetic resonance imaging of cervical spinal cord injuries: Clinical correlation and prognosis. *Neurosurgery* 1999; 44(4):785-793.

53. Shepard MJ, Bracken MB: Magnetic resonance imaging and neurological recovery in acute spinal cord injury: Observations from the National Acute Spinal Cord Injury Study 3. *Spinal Cord* 1999; 37(12):833-837.

54. Brightman RP, Miller CA, Rea GL, Chakeres DW, Hunt WE: Magnetic resonance imaging of trauma to the thoracic and lumbar spine: The importance of the posterior longitudinal ligament. *Spine (Phila Pa 1976)* 1992;17(5):541-550.

55. Petersilge CA, Pathria MN, Emery SE, Masaryk TJ: Thoracolumbar burst fractures: Evaluation with MR imaging. *Radiology* 1995;194(1):49-54.

56. Oner FC, van Gils AP, Faber JA, Dhert WJ, Verbout AJ: Some complications of common treatment schemes of thoracolumbar spine fractures can be predicted with magnetic resonance imaging: Prospective study of 53 patients with 71 fractures. *Spine (Phila Pa 1976)* 2002;27(6):629-636.

57. Nicoll EA: Fractures of the dorso-lumbar spine. *J Bone Joint Surg Br* 1949;31(3):376-394.

58. Holdsworth F: Fractures, dislocations, and fracture-dislocations of the spine. *J Bone Joint Surg Am* 1970;52(8):1534-1551.

59. Kelly RP, Whitesides TE Jr: Treatment of lumbodorsal fracture-dislocations. *Ann Surg* 1968; 167(5):705-717.

60. Whitesides TE Jr: Traumatic kyphosis of the thoracolumbar spine. *Clin Orthop Relat Res* 1977;128: 78-92.

61. Denis F: Spinal instability as defined by the three-column spine concept in acute spinal trauma. *Clin Orthop Relat Res* 1984;189:65-76.

62. White AA, Panjabi MM: Clinical instability of the spine, in Evarts CM, ed: *Surgery of the Musculoskeletal System*, ed 2. New York, NY, Churchill Livingstone, 1990, p 2151.

63. Shen WJ, Shen YS: Nonsurgical treatment of three-column thoracolumbar junction burst fractures without neurologic deficit. *Spine (Phila Pa 1976)* 1999;24(4):412-415.

64. Vaccaro AR, Lehman RA Jr, Hurlbert RJ, et al: A new classification of thoracolumbar injuries: The importance of injury morphology, the integrity of the posterior ligamentous complex, and neurologic status. *Spine (Phila Pa 1976)* 2005;30(20): 2325-2333.

65. Vaccaro AR, Baron EM, Sanfilippo J, et al: Reliability of a novel classification system for thoracolumbar injuries: The Thoracolumbar Injury Severity Score. *Spine (Phila Pa 1976)* 2006; 31(11, Suppl):S62-S69.

66. Cantor JB, Lebwohl NH, Garvey T, Eismont FJ: Nonoperative management of stable thoracolumbar burst fractures with early ambulation and bracing. *Spine (Phila Pa 1976)* 1993;18(8): 971-976.

67. Chow GH, Nelson BJ, Gebhard JS, Brugman JL, Brown CW, Donaldson DH: Functional outcome

of thoracolumbar burst fractures managed with hyperextension casting or bracing and early mobilization. *Spine (Phila Pa 1976)* 1996;21(18): 2170-2175.

68. Mumford J, Weinstein JN, Spratt KF, Goel VK: Thoracolumbar burst fractures: The clinical efficacy and outcome of nonoperative management. *Spine (Phila Pa 1976)* 1993;18(8):955-970.
69. Reid DC, Hu R, Davis LA, Saboe LA: The nonoperative treatment of burst fractures of the thoracolumbar junction. *J Trauma* 1988;28(8): 1188-1194.
70. Hartman MB, Chrin AM, Rechtine GR: Nonoperative treatment of thoracolumbar fractures. *Paraplegia* 1995;33(2):73-76.
71. Rechtine GR: Nonsurgical treatment of thoracic and lumbar fractures. *Instr Course Lect* 1999;48: 413-416.
72. Fidler MW, Plasmans CM: The effect of four types of support on the segmental mobility of the lumbosacral spine. *J Bone Joint Surg Am* 1983;65(7): 943-947.
73. Lumsden RM II, Morris JM: An in vivo study of axial rotation and immobilization at the lumbosacral joint. *J Bone Joint Surg Am* 1968;50(8): 1591-1602.
74. Brown T, Norton PL: The immobilizing efficacy of back braces; their effect on the posture and motion of the lumbosacral spine. *J Bone Joint Surg Am* 1957;39-A(1):111-139.
75. Rechtine GR II, Cahill D, Chrin AM: Treatment of thoracolumbar trauma: Comparison of complications of operative versus nonoperative treatment. *J Spinal Disord* 1999;12(5):406-409.
76. Burke DC, Murray DD: The management of thoracic and thoraco-lumbar injuries of the spine with neurological involvement. *J Bone Joint Surg Br* 1976;58(1):72-78.
77. Dendrinos GK, Halikias JG, Krallis PN, Asimakopoulos A: Factors influencing neurological recovery in burst thoracolumbar fractures. *Acta Orthop Belg* 1995;61(3):226-234.
78. Aligizakis A, Katonis P, Stergiopoulos K, Galanakis I, Karabekios S, Hadjipavlou A: Functional outcome of burst fractures of the thoracolumbar spine managed non-operatively, with early ambulation, evaluated using the load sharing classification. *Acta Orthop Belg* 2002;68(3): 279-287.
79. Willén J, Lindahl S, Nordwall A: Unstable thoracolumbar fractures: A comparative clinical study of conservative treatment and Harrington instrumentation. *Spine (Phila Pa 1976)* 1985;10(2): 111-122.
80. Panjabi MM, Kifune M, Wen L, et al: Dynamic canal encroachment during thoracolumbar burst fractures. *J Spinal Disord* 1995;8(1):39-48.
81. Wessberg P, Wang Y, Irstam L, Nordwall A: The effect of surgery and remodelling on spinal canal measurements after thoracolumbar burst fractures. *Eur Spine J* 2001;10(1):55-63.
82. Dai LY: Remodeling of the spinal canal after thoracolumbar burst fractures. *Clin Orthop Relat Res* 2001;382:119-123.
83. Kim NH, Lee HM, Chun IM: Neurologic injury and recovery in patients with burst fracture of the thoracolumbar spine. *Spine (Phila Pa 1976)* 1999; 24(3):290-294.
84. Vaccaro AR, Nachwalter RS, Klein GR, Sewards JM, Albert TJ, Garfin SR: The significance of thoracolumbar spinal canal size in spinal cord injury patients. *Spine (Phila Pa 1976)* 2001;26(4): 371-376.
85. Fontijne WP, de Klerk LW, Braakman R, et al: CT scan prediction of neurological deficit in thoracolumbar burst fractures. *J Bone Joint Surg Br* 1992;74(5):683-685.
86. Rasmussen PA, Rabin MH, Mann DC, Perl JR II, Lorenz MA, Vrbos LA: Reduced transverse spinal area secondary to burst fractures: Is there a relationship to neurologic injury? *J Neurotrauma* 1994;11(6):711-720.
87. Aydin E, Solak AS, Tuzuner MM, Benli IT, Kis M: Z-plate instrumentation in thoracolumbar spinal fractures. *Bull Hosp Jt Dis* 1999;58(2):92-97.
88. Bhat AL, Lowery GL, Sei A: The use of titanium surgical mesh-bone graft composite in the anterior thoracic or lumbar spine after complete or partial corpectomy. *Eur Spine J* 1999;8(4): 304-309.
89. Calista F, Gualtieri I, Conti P, Frontali P, Bianco T, Gualtieri G: The results of the surgical treatment of 64 patients with thoracic and lumbar fracture. *Chir Organi Mov* 2002;87(2):109-116.
90. Ghanayem AJ, Zdeblick TA: Anterior instrumentation in the management of thoracolumbar burst fractures. *Clin Orthop Relat Res* 1997;335:89-100.
91. Kostuik JP: Anterior fixation for fractures of the thoracic and lumbar spine with or without neurologic involvement. *Clin Orthop Relat Res* 1984; 189:103-115.
92. Parker JW, Lane JR, Karaikovic EE, Gaines RW: Successful short-segment instrumentation and fusion for thoracolumbar spine fractures: A consecutive 41/2-year series. *Spine (Phila Pa 1976)* 2000;25(9):1157-1170.
93. Gertzbein SD, Crowe PJ, Fazl M, Schwartz M, Rowed D: Canal clearance in burst fractures using the AO internal fixator. *Spine (Phila Pa 1976)* 1992;17(5):558-560.
94. Oda T, Panjabi MM: Pedicle screw adjustments affect stability of thoracolumbar burst fracture. *Spine (Phila Pa 1976)* 2001;26(21):2328-2333.

95. Oda T, Panjabi MM, Kato Y: The effects of pedicle screw adjustments on the anatomical reduction of thoracolumbar burst fractures. *Eur Spine J* 2001; 10(6):505-511.
96. Brodke DS, Gollogly S, Bachus KN, Alexander Mohr R, Nguyen BK: Anterior thoracolumbar instrumentation: Stiffness and load sharing characteristics of plate and rod systems. *Spine (Phila Pa 1976)* 2003;28(16):1794-1801.
97. Knop C, Fabian HF, Bastian L, Blauth M: Late results of thoracolumbar fractures after posterior instrumentation and transpedicular bone grafting. *Spine (Phila Pa 1976)* 2001;26(1):88-99.
98. McCormack T, Karaikovic E, Gaines RW: The load sharing classification of spine fractures. *Spine (Phila Pa 1976)* 1994;19(15):1741-1744.
99. Isomi T, Panjabi MM, Kato Y, Wang JL: Radiographic parameters for evaluating the neurological spaces in experimental thoracolumbar burst fractures. *J Spinal Disord* 2000;13(5):404-411.
100. Chang KW: A reduction-fixation system for unstable thoracolumbar burst fractures. *Spine (Phila Pa 1976)* 1992;17(8):879-886.
101. Silvestro C, Francaviglia N, Bragazzi R, Viale GL: Near-anatomical reduction and stabilization of burst fractures of the lower thoracic or lumbar spine. *Acta Neurochir (Wien)* 1992;116(1):53-59.
102. Eismont FJ, Green BA, Berkowitz BM, Montalvo BM, Quencer RM, Brown MJ: The role of intraoperative ultrasonography in the treatment of thoracic and lumbar spine fractures. *Spine (Phila Pa 1976)* 1984;9(8):782-787.
103. Vincent KA, Benson DR, McGahan JP: Intraoperative ultrasonography for reduction of thoracolumbar burst fractures. *Spine (Phila Pa 1976)* 1989; 14(4):387-390.
104. Clohisy JC, Akbarnia BA, Bucholz RD, Burkus JK, Backer RJ: Neurologic recovery associated with anterior decompression of spine fractures at the thoracolumbar junction (T12-L1). *Spine (Phila Pa 1976)* 1992;17(8, Suppl)S325-S330.
105. Vaccaro AR, Daugherty RJ, Sheehan TP, et al: Neurologic outcome of early versus late surgery for cervical spinal cord injury. *Spine (Phila Pa 1976)* 1997;22(22):2609-2613.
106. Fehlings MG, Perrin RG: The timing of surgical intervention in the treatment of spinal cord injury: A systematic review of recent clinical evidence. *Spine (Phila Pa 1976)* 2006;31(11, Suppl): S28-S36.
107. Transfeldt EE, White D, Bradford DS, Roche B: Delayed anterior decompression in patients with spinal cord and cauda equina injuries of the thoracolumbar spine. *Spine (Phila Pa 1976)* 1990; 15(9):953-957.
108. Vaccaro AR, Cirello J: The use of allograft bone and cages in fractures of the cervical, thoracic, and lumbar spine. *Clin Orthop Relat Res* 2002; 394:19-26.
109. Dvorak MF, Kwon BK, Fisher CG, Eiserloh HL III, Boyd M, Wing PC: Effectiveness of titanium mesh cylindrical cages in anterior column reconstruction after thoracic and lumbar vertebral body resection. *Spine (Phila Pa 1976)* 2003;28(9): 902-908.
110. Hitchon PW, Goel VK, Rogge T, Grosland NM, Torner J: Biomechanical studies on two anterior thoracolumbar implants in cadaveric spines. *Spine (Phila Pa 1976)* 1999;24(3):213-218.
111. Oda I, Cunningham BW, Abumi K, Kaneda K, McAfee PC: The stability of reconstruction methods after thoracolumbar total spondylectomy: An in vitro investigation. *Spine (Phila Pa 1976)* 1999; 24(16):1634-1638.
112. Shono Y, McAfee PC, Cunningham BW: Experimental study of thoracolumbar burst fractures: A radiographic and biomechanical analysis of anterior and posterior instrumentation systems. *Spine (Phila Pa 1976)* 1994;19(15):1711-1722.
113. Haas N, Blauth M, Tscherne H: Anterior plating in thoracolumbar spine injuries: Indication, technique, and results. *Spine (Phila Pa 1976)* 1991; 16(3, Suppl)S100-S111.
114. Bradford DS, McBride GG: Surgical management of thoracolumbar spine fractures with incomplete neurologic deficits. *Clin Orthop Relat Res* 1987; 218:201-216.
115. Stancić MF, Gregorović E, Nozica E, Penezić L: Anterior decompression and fixation versus posterior reposition and semirigid fixation in the treatment of unstable burst thoracolumbar fracture: Prospective clinical trial. *Croat Med J* 2001;42(1): 49-53.
116. Wood KB, Bohn D, Mehbod A: Anterior versus posterior treatment of stable thoracolumbar burst fractures without neurologic deficit: A prospective, randomized study. *J Spinal Disord Tech* 2005; 18 Suppl:S15-S23.
117. Khoo LT, Beisse R, Potulski M: Thoracoscopic-assisted treatment of thoracic and lumbar fractures: A series of 371 consecutive cases. *Neurosurgery* 2002;51(5 Suppl):S104-S117.
118. Bono CM, Garfin SR: Spinal osteoporosis. American Academy of Orthopaedic Surgeons Web site: *Orthopaedic Knowledge Online* 2002. http://www5.aaos.org/oko/description.cfm?topic=SPI008&referringPage= http://www5.aaos.org/oko/menus/topicAuthors.cfm. Accessed Sept 7, 2010.
119. Croce MA, Bee TK, Pritchard E, Miller PR, Fabian TC: Does optimal timing for spine fracture fixation exist? *Ann Surg* 2001;233(6):851-858.

CHAPTER 33
Low Lumbar Spine Trauma

Kris Radcliff, MD Todd Rubin, BS Lawrence Delasotta, MD, MPH Mohammad Reza Rasouli, MD
James Harrop, MD Alan M. Levine, MD Alexander R. Vaccaro, MD, PhD

Introduction

Treatment of injuries to the lower lumbar spine requires consideration of the unique mechanical and anatomic factors distinct from the thoracic and thoracolumbar spine.[1] Such features separate fractures of the lower lumbar spine from those that occur more frequently at the thoracolumbar junction. The treatment goals for spine trauma are (1) protection of the neural elements, (2) restoration and maintenance of normal sagittal and coronal balance, (3) early mobilization to prevent sequelae of immobilization, (4) conservation of motion segments, (5) prevention of degenerative disease, and (6) prevention of significant deformity.

Dr. Harrop or an immediate family member is a member of a speakers' bureau or has made paid presentations on behalf of DePuy, a Johnson & Johnson company, Stryker, and NeuroStem; serves as a paid consultant to or is an employee of DePuy, a Johnson & Johnson company; serves as an unpaid consultant to Geron and AScubio; and owns stock or stock options in AxioMed. Dr. Levine is deceased. At the time this chapter was written, Dr. Levine or an immediate family member had received royalties from Elsevier and US Spine; was a member of a speakers' bureau or had made paid presentations on behalf of Accuray; served as a paid consultant to or was an employee of US Spine; and had received research or institutional support from Accuray, Amgen Co., and Medtronic Sofamor Danek. Dr. Vaccaro or an immediate family member serves as a board member, owner, officer, or committee member of the North American Spine Society, American Spinal Injury Association, and the Cervical Spine Research Society; has received royalties from Aesculap/B. Braun, DePuy, a Johnson & Johnson company, Globus Medical, Medtronic Sofamor Danek, K2M, Stout Medical, Progressive Spinal Technologies, and Applied Spinal Intellectual Properties; serves as a paid consultant to or is an employee of K2M; has received research or institutional support from AO North America, DePuy, a Johnson & Johnson company, Medtronic Sofamor Danek, and Stryker; and owns stock or stock options in Globus Medical, Disk Motion Technology, Progressive Spinal Technologies, Advanced Spinal Intellectual Properties, Computational Biodynamics, Stout Medical, Paradigm Spine, K2M, Replication Medical, Spinology, SpineMedica, Orthovita, Vertiflex, Small Bone Technologies, NeuCore, Crosscurrent, Syndicom, In Vivo, Flagship Surgical, Pearl Diver, Location Based Intelligence, and Gamma Spine. None of the following or any immediate family member has received anything of value from or owns stock in a commercial company or institution related directly or indirectly to the subject of this chapter: Dr. Radcliff, Mr. Rubin, Dr. Delasotta, and Dr. Rasouli.

Historical Perspective

Historically, the high rate of pseudarthrosis, implant failure, and flat-back deformity made the low lumbar region less suitable for long instrumentation despite the advantage of earlier ambulation and anatomic reduction.[2,3] During the 1970s and 1980s, the lack of satisfactory techniques for reduction and stabilization of such injuries resulted in suboptimal outcomes, leading some authors to espouse nonsurgical management as a more appropriate alternative to surgery.[4,5] Furthermore, poorly conceptualized surgical approaches led to early failure, despite the more widely accepted use of pedicle screw fixation in the lumbar spine.[2,6-8] This caused some surgeons to accept chronic pain and failure to return to preinjury occupation as the natural history in this subset of patients.[9-11] Eventually, reports surfaced demonstrating better anatomic and functional reports with a surgical approach.[12,13]

Anatomy and Pathophysiology

Anatomically, the low lumbar spine's proximal extent is considered to start at L3. Biomechanically, the normal center of gravity intersects the spinal column on average at L3. Therefore, physiologic lordosis of the lumbar spine results from the relatively greater anterior height of the intervertebral disks at L3-L4, L4-L5, and L5-S1.[14] The typical kyphosis of the thoracic spines range from 15° to 49°,[15,16] whereas mean normal lumbar lordosis is approximately 60°. Indeed, almost 50° of lumbar lordosis is accounted for by the lower two segments of the lumbar spine, L4-L5 and L5-S1, with 24° and 25° of lordosis in asymptomatic standing volunteers. This alignment creates an overall sagittal balance of the spine in which a "plumb line" from C7 intersects the posterior corner of the S1 vertebral body. Given normal spinal alignment, there is a greater tendency for fractures identified at or proximal to L2 to result in kyphotic defor-

FIGURE 1

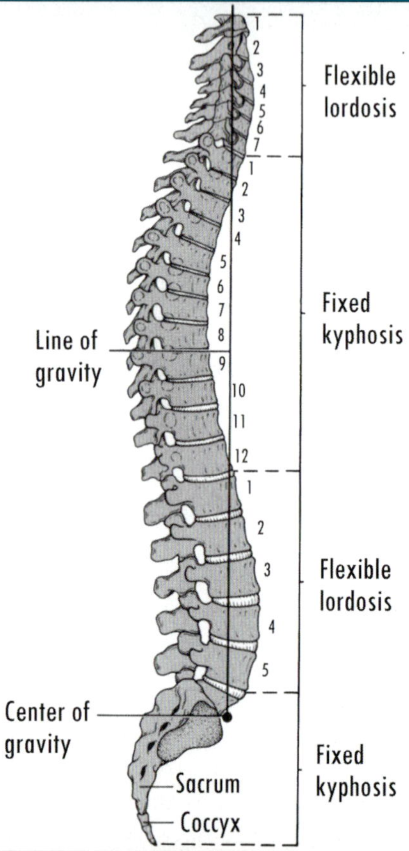

Figure 1 The spine is divided into four segments: two with relatively fixed kyphosis (the sacral and thoracic spine), and two with relatively flexible lordosis (the cervical and lumbar spine). The weight-bearing axis is anterior to the thoracic spine and thoracolumbar junction. It falls posterior to the vertebral bodies of the lumbar spine, making the pattern of fracture with axial-loading injuries significantly different in the lumbar spine compared with the thoracic and thoracolumbar spine. (Reproduced with permission from Levine AM: Lumbar and sacral spine trauma, in Browner BD, Jupiter JB, Levine AM, Trafton PG, eds: *Skeletal Trauma: Fractures, Dislocations, Ligamentous Injuries*, ed 2. Philadelphia, PA, WB Saunders, 1998, vol 1, pp 1035-1093.)

mation of the spine and for those below L3 to result in lordotic deformity.[15]

Pelvic alignment is also closely related to lumbar sagittal alignment. Sacral slope is defined as the inclination of the sacral base from the horizontal. Normal is approximately 45°. This angle is critical in determining the amount of shear force[17] to which the lumbosacral junction is subjected (**Figure 1**).

Additionally, there are anatomic features that result in different patterns of neurologic injury in the low lumbar spine. The nerves of the cauda equina are anatomically more similar to peripheral nerves as compared with the spinal cord or conus medullaris, and are much more resilient to traumatic injury. The dimensions of the spinal canal are wider caudally compared with more rostral levels. The thoracic spinal cord measures approximately 86.5 mm² and the thoracic spinal canal measures on average 17.2 mm × 16.8 mm². Thus, in the thoracic region, the cord occupies approximately 50% of the canal area. In the low lumbar region, the spinal canal enlarges relative to the size of the neural elements. In the lumbar region, the canal is typically large (23.4 mm × 17.4 mm).[18,19] At this level, the roots of the cauda equina are the only neural elements. In the distal portion of the canal, the cauda equina occupies less than one-third of the cross-sectional area. Consequently, increasing canal compromise can be tolerated in the low lumbar spine relative to the thoracic spine.

There are unique features of the bony anatomy of the low lumbar spine. The size and shape of the laminae change configuration at the various levels of the spine. The laminae in the thoracic and thoracolumbar region are rectangular in shape, longer in length than in width. In the midlumbar spine, the width and length of the laminae equalize. At L5, the lamina is considerably wider than it is long (**Figure 2**). The dural sac ends at S1 in approximately 15% of patients and at S2 in the remainder. The cross-sectional area diminishes from 90 mm² at the S1 level to approximately 15 mm² at S5.[20] In addition, the sacrum has the apex of its kyphosis at S3 and the roots are tightly tethered within the canal. As the spinal canal widens in the caudal region of the low lumbar spine, it is possible to access the anterior regions of the spine from a posterolateral approach.

The low lumbar vertebrae have several unique bony features that influence the morphology and treatment of injuries. Anatomically, these vertebrae are the largest and strongest in the body. The initial anatomic description of lumbar pedicle morphology and pedicle screw fixation was done by Saillant[21] in 1976 and was confirmed by two later studies performed in North America.[22,23] Critical features included sagittal and transverse widths of the pedicles, pedicle length, pedicle angle, and chord length (depth to the anterior cortex along a fixed orientation). The mean pedicle diameter increases from 8.5 mm at L3 to 10mm at L5. These dimensions vary within regions of the spine (thoracic versus lumbar) as well as within the lumbar spine itself. The mean transverse diameter measured on CT scan or anatomic specimen is approximately 9 mm at L1 and as high as 18 mm at

FIGURE 2

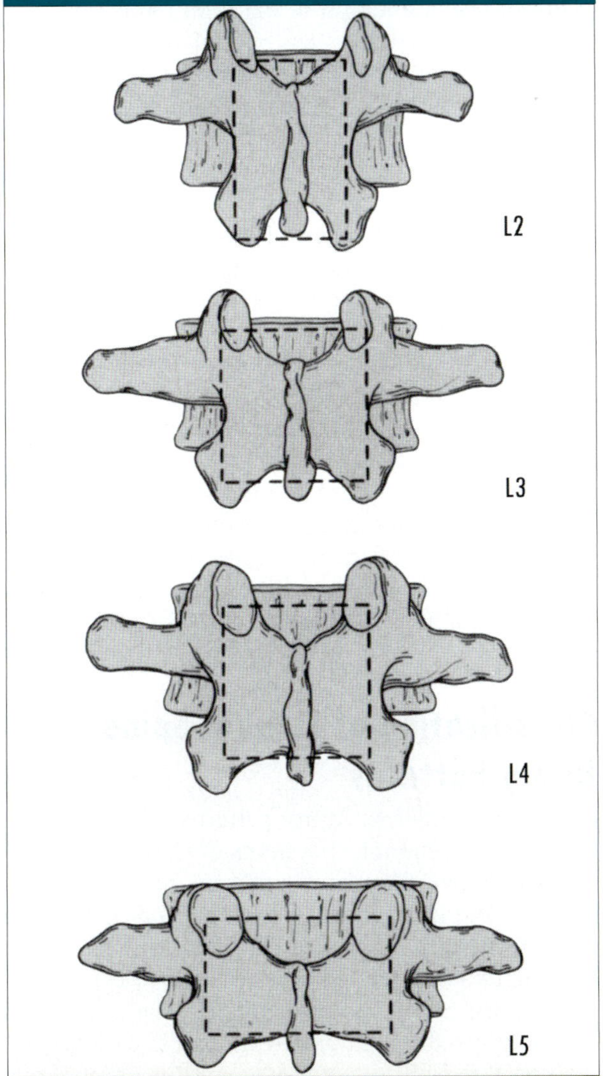

Figure 2 The shape of the lumbar laminae and relative size of the pedicles dramatically influence our ability to position hardware. From L2 to L5, the length of the laminae becomes less and the width becomes greater. Pedicle fixation is easier distally with the larger pedicle size. (Reproduced with permission from Levine AM: Lumbar and sacral spine trauma, in Browner BD, Jupiter JB, Levine AM, Trafton PG, eds: *Skeletal Trauma: Fractures, Dislocations, Ligamentous Injuries*. Philadelphia, PA, WB Saunders, 1992, vol 1, pp 805-848.)

FIGURE 3

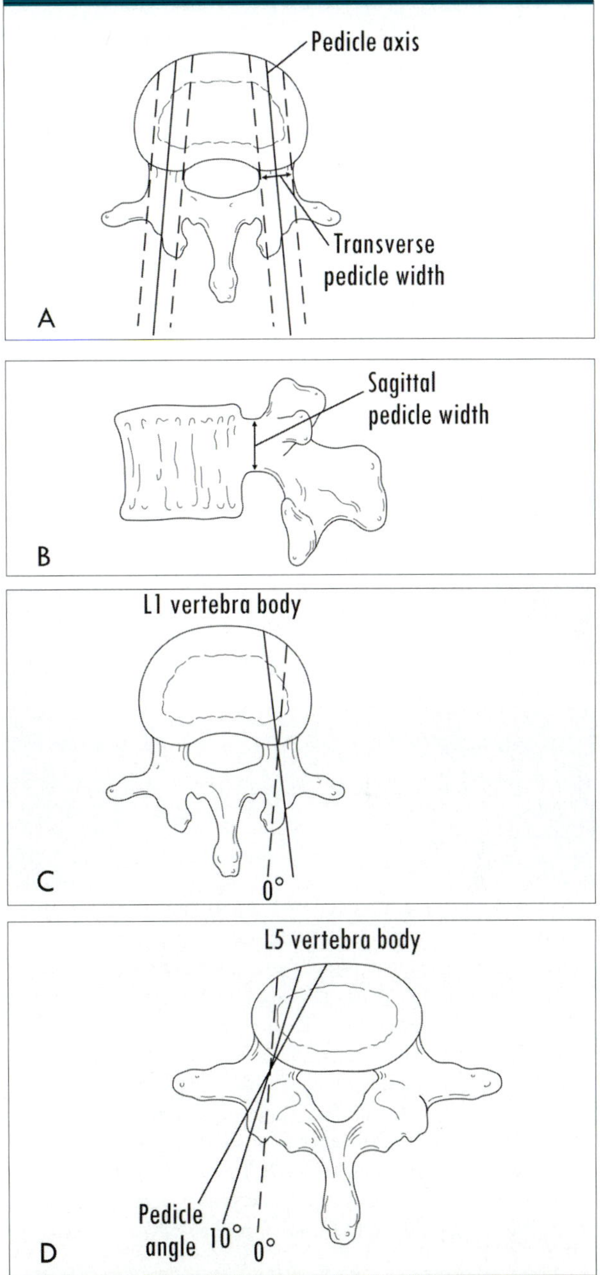

Figure 3 **A,** This axial view of a lumbar vertebral body shows the transverse pedicle width, which increases from L1 to L5. It also demonstrates the pedicle axis that likewise increases from L1 to L5. **B,** The sagittal view of the vertebral body shows the sagittal pedicle, which is relatively constant in the lumbar spine. **C,** This diagram shows an L1 axial view with the axis of the pedicle demonstrating the larger cortex-to-cortex distance. **D,** The axial view of L5 demonstrates how the anteroposterior length can increase with increasing angle. (Redrawn with permission from Levine AM: Lumbar and sacral spine trauma, in Browner BD, Jupiter JB, Levine AM, Trafton PG, eds: *Skeletal Trauma: Fractures, Dislocations, Ligamentous Injuries*. Philadelphia, PA, WB Saunders, 1992, vol 1, pp 805-848.)

L5 (**Figure 3,** *A*). The sagittal width in the lumbar spine is relatively constant with a mean of 14 mm to 15 mm at all levels (**Figure 3,** *B*). The angle of the pedicle axis generally increases in the lumbar spine with a mean of about 11° at L1, 15° at L3, and over 20° at L5 (**Figure 3,** *A*). Because the distance between the pedicles is greatest at L5 and the anteroposterior diameter of the vertebral body

FIGURE 4

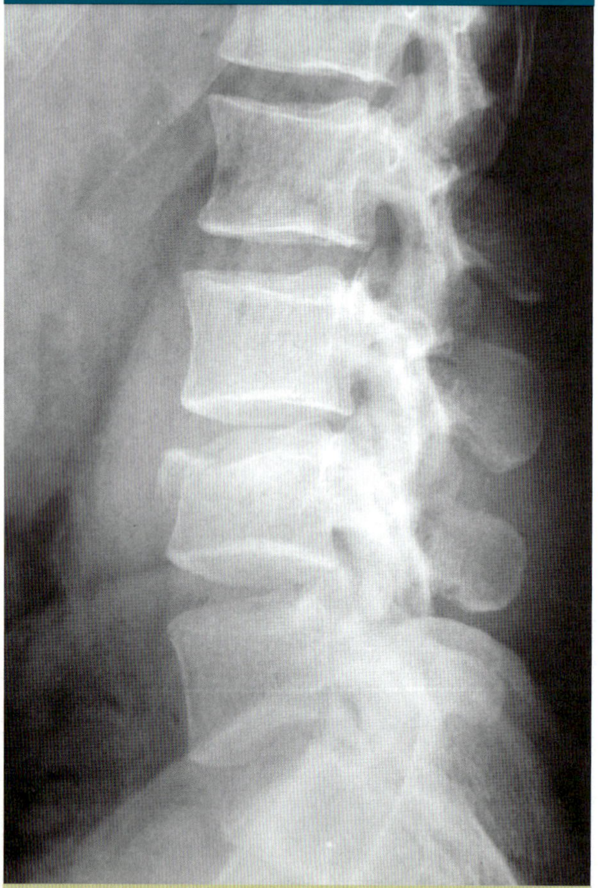

Figure 4 This lateral radiograph of the lumbar spine demonstrates an L4 compression fracture sustained during a motor vehicle accident. Note the compression of the anterior portion of the vertebral body. However, the posterior wall of the L4 body remains intact with its normal biconcave appearance. There is no widening of the interspinous distance. Overall alignment of the lumbar spine remains within physiologic norms. (Reproduced with permission from Levine AM: Lumbar and sacral spine trauma, in Browner BD, Jupiter JB, Levine AM, Trafton PG, eds: *Skeletal Trauma: Fractures, Dislocations, Ligamentous Injuries*. Philadelphia, PA, WB Saunders, 1992, vol 1, pp 805-848.)

is least at this location, the chord length (distance from posterior cortex to anterior cortex) can vary with the angle of insertion (**Figure 3**, *C* and *D*). Originally described by Roy-Camille et al,[13] if screws are inserted perpendicular to the posterior cortex along a zero-degree axis, the mean depth at L1 is approximately 40 mm and only 35 mm at L5. Increasing the angle of insertion to 10° to 15°, or increasing the angle of the axis of the pedicle, can increase the cortex-to-cortex distance by as much as 5 mm at L1 (to 50 mm) and 15 mm at L5 (to about 50 mm).

The low lumbar spine has increased flexion-extension mobility compared to other regions of the spine. The thoracic spine is relatively rigid as a result of the orientation of the facet joints and associated thoracic ribs and articulations. At the thoracolumbar junction, flexion-extension increases, whereas both lateral bending and rotation decrease. The facet joint orientation in the lumbar spine becomes oblique to the sagittal plane and therefore affords some sagittal and coronal stability. Therefore, from L1 to L5 there is a progressive increase in the degree of flexion-extension and a subsequent decrease in rotation. Flexion-extension increases from approximately 12° at the L1-L2 level to 20° at the L5-S1 level, with lateral bending remaining similar at about 6°.[15,25] The low lumbar spinal segments are mobile enough to form a relative hyperlordosis to compensate for the kyphosis in other spinal regions as well as maintain upright posture.[26] The iliolumbar ligaments, located below the pelvic brim, are significant stabilizers of the lumbosacral junction that are also unique to low lumbar fractures.[1]

Classification of Lumbar Spine Injury Patterns

A variety of different injury patterns can occur in the lumbar spine. Most systems of thoracolumbar trauma classification have either an anatomic reference[27,28] or a mechanistic reference,[29] but fail to achieve the desired goal of classifying injuries according to subsequent treatment categories. The ideal classification should define the nature of the potential instability and provide a treatment regimen or algorithm to counteract and/or prevent instability.[30] Although many classification systems exist, none have been entirely successful in achieving these goals.[31]

Traditional classification systems were based on mechanism of injury, direction of force vectors applied to the spine, and severity of neurologic injury. Accordingly, such injuries are grouped and described by both radiologic criteria as well as their major deforming forces. The major forces contributing to injuries are flexion and extension, compression, lateral bending, rotation, distraction, and shear. Most injuries are not caused by a single force, but by a major force with minor components from other, different types of forces. Recently, a focus on morphology of vertebral injuries over mechanism of injury has shown improved intra-observer and inter-observer reliability.[32] This classification identified three types of injury morphology: compression, distraction, and translation/rotation.

FIGURE 5

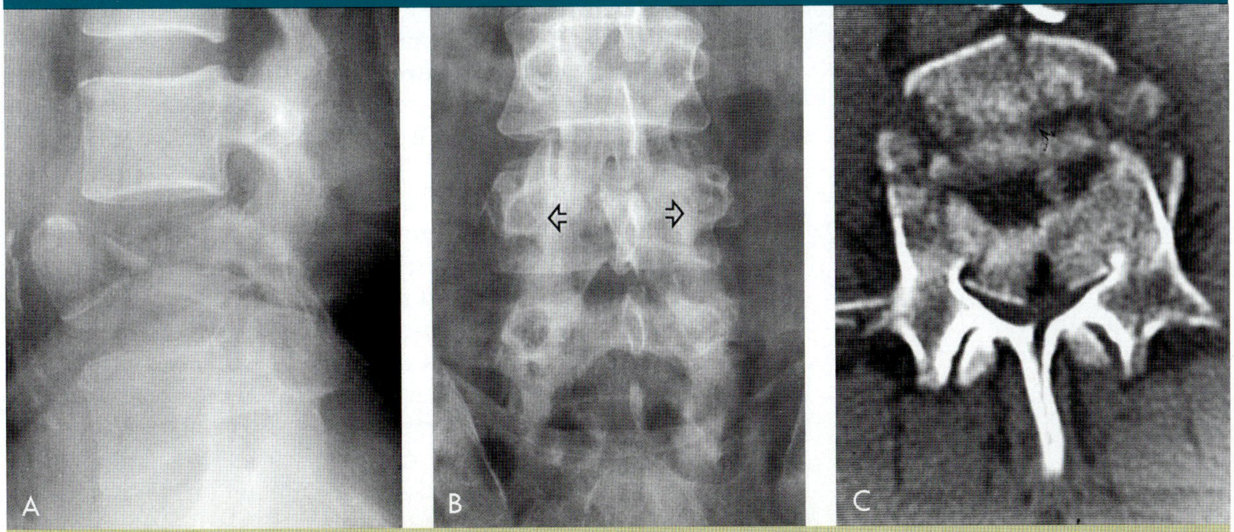

Figure 5 This is the classic burst fracture pattern with comminution of the vertebral body and the pedicles. This 46-year-old man represents a typical example after a fall. **A,** On the lateral radiograph, the patient demonstrates complete destruction of the L4 body with comminution of the pedicles and vertebral body. There is little kyphosis but simply loss of height in a symmetric fashion. The overall sagittal configuration of the spine remains relatively normal. **B,** The AP view demonstrates splaying of the pedicles (arrows). There is loss of height at the vertebral body noted as well. **C,** The CT scan demonstrates severe comminution of the vertebral body with marked retropulsion of bone into the neural canal. There is a disruption of the body at the pedicle junction and, in fact, comminution of the pedicles. This patient demonstrates a sagittal split of the spinous process at L4 as well. (Reproduced with permission from Levine AM: Lumbar and sacral spine trauma, in Browner BD, Jupiter JB, Levine AM, Trafton PG, eds: *Skeletal Trauma: Fractures, Dislocations, Ligamentous Injuries*. Philadelphia, PA, WB Saunders, 1992, vol 1, pp 805-848.)

Compressive injuries from axial loading may result in destruction of the anterior aspect of the vertebral body without loss of competence of the posterior vertebral cortex (**Figure 4**). They can vary from mild anterior compression with little to no instability to gross instability with significant posterior ligamentous disruption. Burst fractures are caused by a combined mechanism of flexion and axial loading. The pattern is characterized by marked widening of the pedicles on the AP radiograph with possible comminution of the pedicles, disruption of the body-pedicle junction, and disruption of the anterior and posterior vertebral body cortices (**Figure 5**). There is frequently a large retropulsed fragment of bone from the posterior portion of the vertebral body (**Figure 5, *C***). It is also possible to develop lateral compression fractures from asymmetric axial loading (**Figure 6**). Burst fractures may display varying degrees of kyphosis, height loss, and retropulsion. Fractures at L4 and L5 demonstrate little kyphosis, but may develop significant canal impingement. Reports by Levine and Edwards[12,33] indicated that most of these injuries occur in young patients, with slightly more than 50% younger than 20 years of age.[12,33,34] The mean canal compromise was only 47%, but in 5 of 22 patients, the retropulsed bone was so severe that it made contact with the undersurface of the lamina. The mean loss of vertebral height was approximately 25%. The measured kyphosis across the fracture level was only 8°. However, the loss of physiological lordosis from the collapsed vertebral body may significantly reduce global lumbar lordosis.

Distraction injury morphology is classically described as the result of use of a lap belt alone by a passenger in a motor vehicle accident, which predisposes to flexion-distraction injuries of the lumbar spine.[35,36] Distraction morphology fractures comprise less than 10% of all major fractures of the lumbar spine.[37] Three major types of distraction injuries occur: complete bony injury (Chance fracture), complete ligamentous injury, or ligamentous and part bony injury.[38] These injuries are usually the result of the pelvis and lower spine being anchored in a fixed position (eg, by an automobile lap belt).[35] On impact, the upper portion of the spine accelerates, and thus distracts and flexes away from the fixed lower portion.[39] In a bony injury pattern, the spinous process splits horizontally (**Figure 7**). Although the system is somewhat complex, the principle of differentiating

FIGURE 6

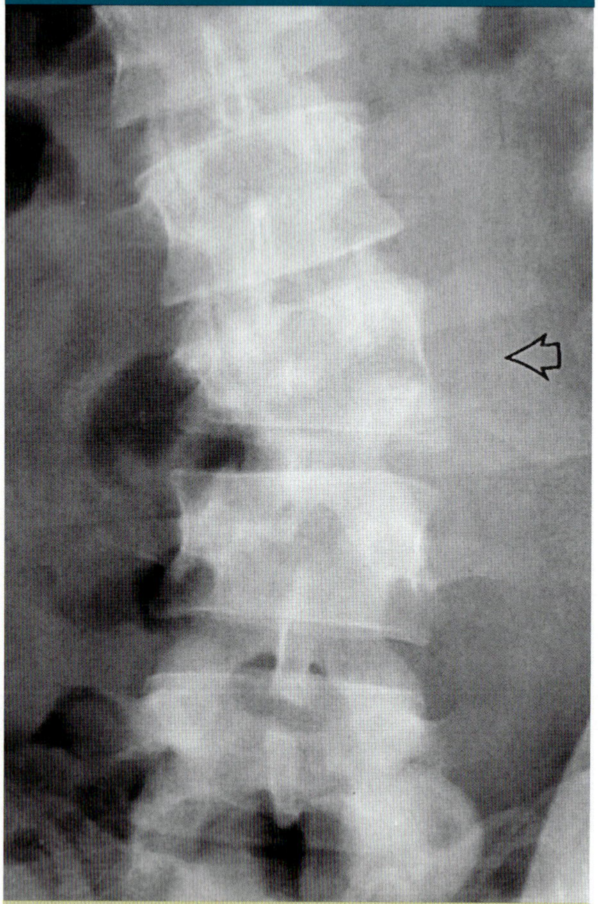

Figure 6 This 17-year-old boy sustained a burst fracture at the L3 level with severe lateral compression. The AP radiograph demonstrates the major deformity: severe lateral wedging to the left side with severe compression of the left lateral side of the vertebral body. In addition, there is a split of the transverse process and lamina of L3 on the right side (arrow). (Reproduced with permission from Levine AM: Lumbar and sacral spine trauma, in Browner BD, Jupiter JB, Levine AM, Trafton PG, eds: *Skeletal Trauma: Fractures, Dislocations, Ligamentous Injuries*. Philadelphia, PA, WB Saunders, 1992, vol 1, pp 805-848.)

the ligamentous from the bony component of the injury is critical. Injuries with a fracture line traversing the spinous process, pedicles, and body are likely to achieve satisfactory union and stability if appropriate sagittal alignment can be achieved. If the line of injury goes through the interspinous ligament and facets into the pedicle and body, nonunion may occur resulting in late complex residual instability (**Figure 8**). Isolated disruption of the posterior ligamentous complex (PLC; ie, supraspinous ligament, intraspinous ligament, facet capsules, ligamentum flavum) constitutes a continuum of injuries that occur in concert with other bony flexion injuries.[40,41]

The PLC is an important stabilizer of the lumbar spine. **Figure 9** illustrates a PLC injury in association with a lumbar burst fracture, compared to **Figure 10**, *E* and *F*, which illustrates an intact PLC.

Translation and rotation injuries are grossly unstable and compromise the surgeon's ability to obtain an anatomically stable reduction.[42] If the force is applied asymmetrically, or if the patient twists during impact, a rotational or lateral bending component of the injury may be involved. Translation injuries may result in complete disruption of the interspinous ligaments, facet capsules, and the involved disk. Shear injuries can result in severe vertebral body comminution (**Figure 11**). This injury is described in detail in chapter 31, Facet Fractures and Dislocations of the Thoracolumbar Spine. Radiographs of bilateral facet dislocations are usually diagnostic.[43,44] They demonstrate intact posterior walls of the vertebral bodies with significant translation (36%) and lesser degrees of anterior compression and loss of disk height (**Figure 12**). Although unilateral facet injuries and fracture-dislocations are rare in the thoracic/lumbar spine, facet fracture-dislocations occur at the thoracolumbar junction due to a combination of flexion, distraction, and rotational forces.[45-52]

Unclassified injuries involving soft tissue, avulsion fractures, and isolated ligamentous disruption may in fact prove challenging to treat because they constitute a large and highly variable group of injuries. The advent of the multidirectional CT scan as a screening modality following blunt trauma increased the identification of these injuries. For example, fractures of the transverse processes of the lumbar spine may represent several different injuries depending on the mechanism. The significance of an L5 transverse process fracture associated with a vertical shearing injury to the pelvis is different from that of multiple transverse process fractures resulting from indirect muscle forces causing avulsion fractures. Significant muscular forces produced by the paraspinous musculature at the time of impact can result in an avulsion fracture of the transverse process. End-plate avulsions[53] are a recognized phenomenon in the adolescent patient and are analogous to disk herniations in the adult patient. In the child, the ligamentous attachments are stronger than the bony attachment of the end plate (**Figure 13**). End-plate fractures can be visualized by a combination of CT and MRI, and should be

FIGURE 7

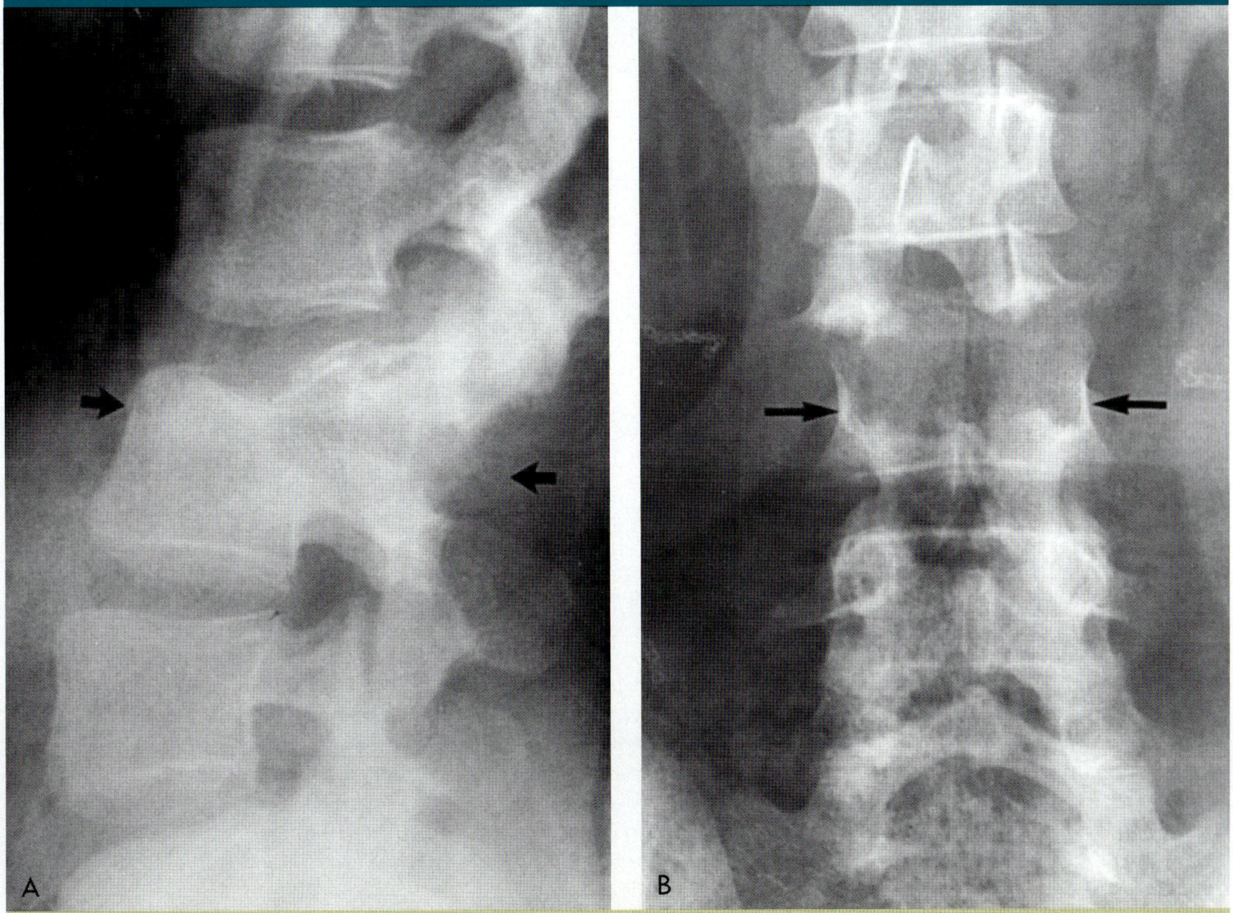

Figure 7 Flexion-distraction injury. This 11-year-old boy was a passenger restrained only by a lap belt (without a shoulder harness) in a motor vehicle accident. He sustained a flexion-distraction injury with paraplegia at the T12 level. **A,** The lateral radiograph demonstrates a Chance fracture with the fracture line proceeding through the pedicles and the vertebral body in a line between the two arrows. **B,** The AP view shows both the transverse processes and the pedicle to be split in an axial plane as marked by the arrows. Because this is strictly a bony injury, adequate bone-to-bone contact can be maintained and healing achieved without ligamentous instability. (Reproduced with permission from Levine AM: Lumbar and sacral spine trauma, in Browner BD, Jupiter JB, Levine AM, Trafton PG, eds: *Skeletal Trauma: Fractures, Dislocations, Ligamentous Injuries.* Philadelphia, PA, WB Saunders, 1992, vol 1, pp 805-848.)

treated by excision of the end-plate fragment, which usually resolves the neurologic symptoms completely. These are most frequently seen in the adolescent and young adult at the L4-L5 and L5-S1 level.[54] In the younger child, this may occur only with avulsion of the cartilaginous ring apophysis. In adolescents and young adults, an isolated portion of the limbus or the entire bony end plate can fracture.[54] The neural impingement associated with an end-plate avulsion fracture is the result of both the bony fragment and the disk herniation.[54-56]

Neurologic Deficit

In lumbar and sacral fractures, the presence of neurologic deficit often indicates instability of the spine or pelvis. With a large canal-to-neural element ratio, significant translation or angulation must take place to have neural injury, which typically requires a significant amount of energy. This is not a universal rule, however, because transverse process fractures and avulsions can be accompanied by nerve root avulsions. Also, neurologic injury in children can occur at a level above that of the actual bony injury because of the elastic nature of the cord and associated spinal elements.

FIGURE 8

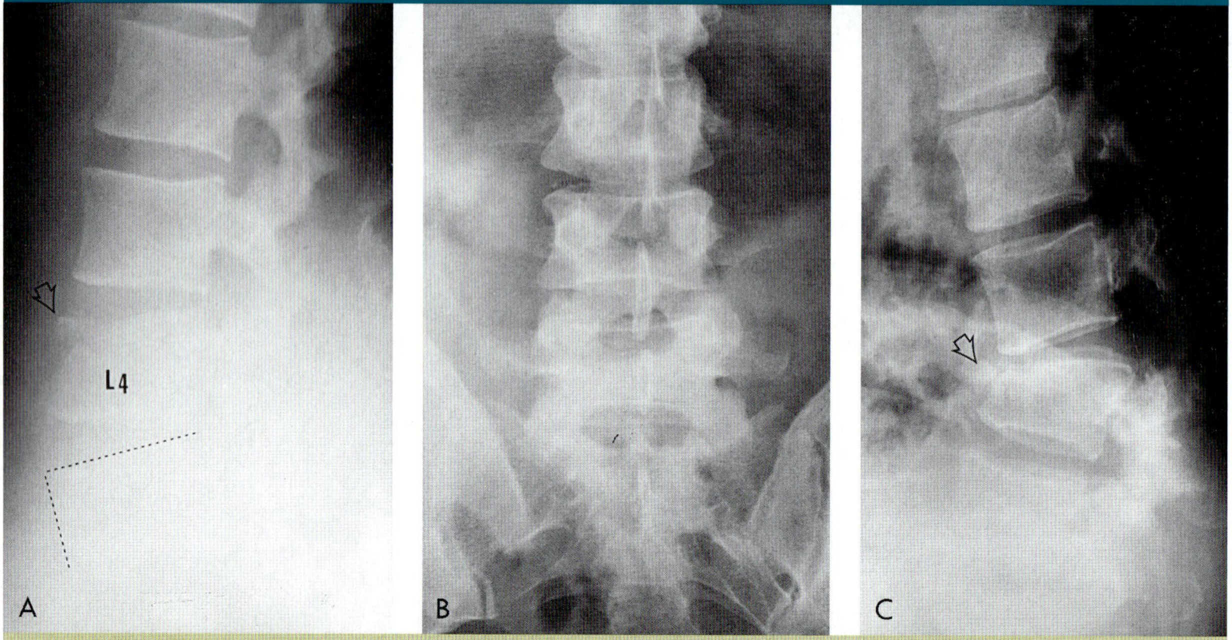

Figure 8 This 44-year-old woman was involved in a motor vehicle accident and sustained bilateral tibia fractures in addition to a fracture of L4. **A,** The lateral radiograph on admission demonstrates alignment of her low lumbar spine taken at the time of the acute evaluation. She had anterior compression (open arrow) with satisfactory alignment in the sagittal plane. **B,** The AP radiograph does not show any apparent disruption of the posterior elements. She was therefore placed in an orthosis. **C,** At 5 months after injury, the patient had significant back pain after being out of the orthosis for 2 months. A lateral view showed not only the anterior compression (open arrow) but also a disruption of the ligamentous restraints posteriorly, with subluxation of the facets and apparent disruption of the interspinous ligament. (Reproduced with permission from Levine AM: Lumbar and sacral spine trauma, in Browner BD, Jupiter JB, Levine AM, Trafton PG, eds: *Skeletal Trauma: Fractures, Dislocations, Ligamentous Injuries*. Philadelphia, PA, WB Saunders, 1992, vol 1, pp 805-848.)

FIGURE 9

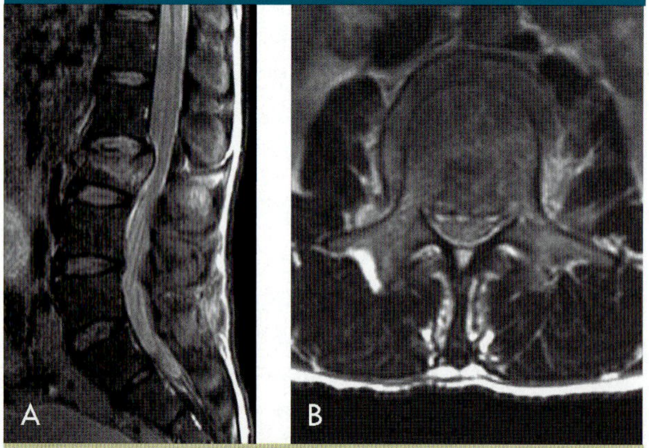

Figure 9 PLC injury. **A,** Short tau inversion recovery (STIR) midsagittal MRI scan indicates disruption of the supraspinous and interspinous ligaments off of the caudal aspect of L2 and an L3 burst fracture. **B,** Axial MRI scan demonstrates facet capsule effusions and disruption of the musculotendinous junction on the spinous process tip.

Neurologic injuries related to low lumbar spine injuries are usually of two types. The first is a complete cauda equina syndrome. This is often seen in severe burst fractures with canal retropulsion and large amounts of bone within the neural canal. The second type of injury is the isolated root injury or combination of root injuries. Studies by Cammisa et al[57] and Denis and Burkus[58] emphasize this clinically significant feature of low lumbar burst fractures. A small portion of the patients were noted to have a longitudinal laminar fracture, seemingly associated with traumatic dural lacerations.[57,58] In patients with lumbar burst fractures, a sagittal split in the spinous process may occur. When combined with a burst fracture and neurologic deficit, it is likely that a dural tear has occurred (**Figure 14**).

When evaluating these fractures, care should be taken to distinguish this feature, so that appropriate surgical intervention may be undertaken. Nerve roots can be outside the dural sac, and may be trapped within the split in the lamina. These may be nonrecoverable root avulsions, which can

FIGURE 10

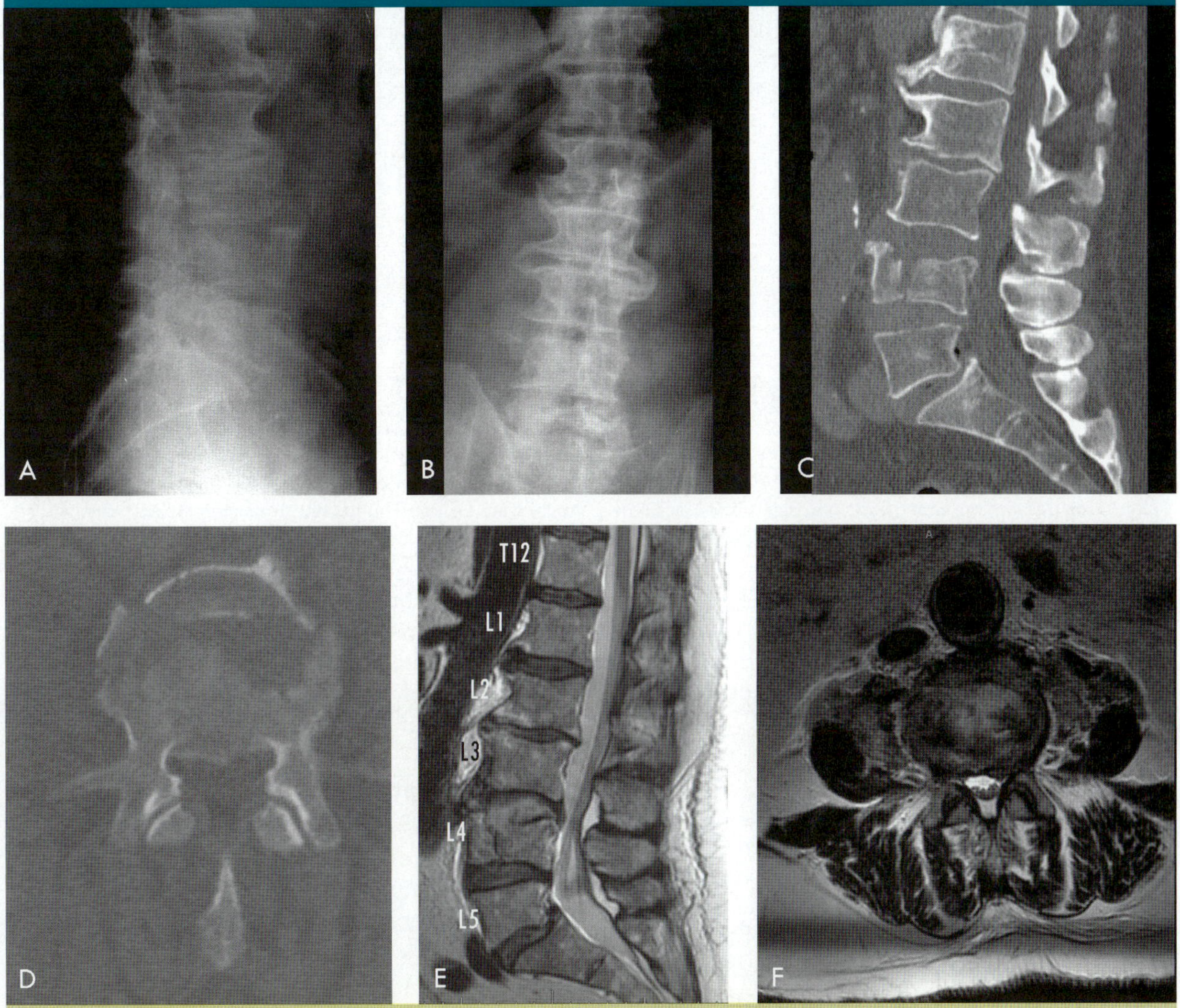

Figure 10 Nonsurgical management of a low lumbar burst fracture. **A,** Lateral lumbar radiograph demonstrates a burst fracture at L4. **B,** AP radiograph demonstrates no involvement of the pedicles or diastasis of the PLC. **C,** Sagittal CT scan demonstrates a coronal fracture plane through L4. **D,** Axial CT scan demonstrates minimal bony retropulsion. **E** and **F,** Midsagittal and axial MRI scans show moderate lumbar stenosis at L4-L5 with no disruption of the PLC.

occur in combination with transverse process avulsions. Lesser degrees of root injury occur with canal impingement. Isolated root injury is common with a retropulsed fragment of bone that catches the exiting root between itself and the undersurface of the lamina. Canal narrowing by translational deformity, as in bilateral facet dislocation, is less likely to cause severe neurologic deficit in the low lumbar spine than at the thoracolumbar junction.

Management

Indications

In the neurologically intact patient with any degree of body comminution and retropulsion, the goals of treatment are to maintain optimal reduction of alignment and allow the fracture to go on to union. In general terms, the indications for surgery in lumbar injuries are (1) the presence of progressive neurologic deficit, (2) significant deformity, and (3) potential for development of significant deformity.

The prognosis and management of neurologic deficits in the low lumbar spine from root injury is different from neurologic deficits in the thoracic spine from spinal cord injury.[48,59-64] There is general agreement regarding the benefit of nonsurgical care for low lumbar fractures as the majority involve root injuries.[57,62,65] Because the canal-to-neural element ratio is very large, a small degree of canal compromise (< 30%) in the absence of

FIGURE 10 ***(CONTINUED)***

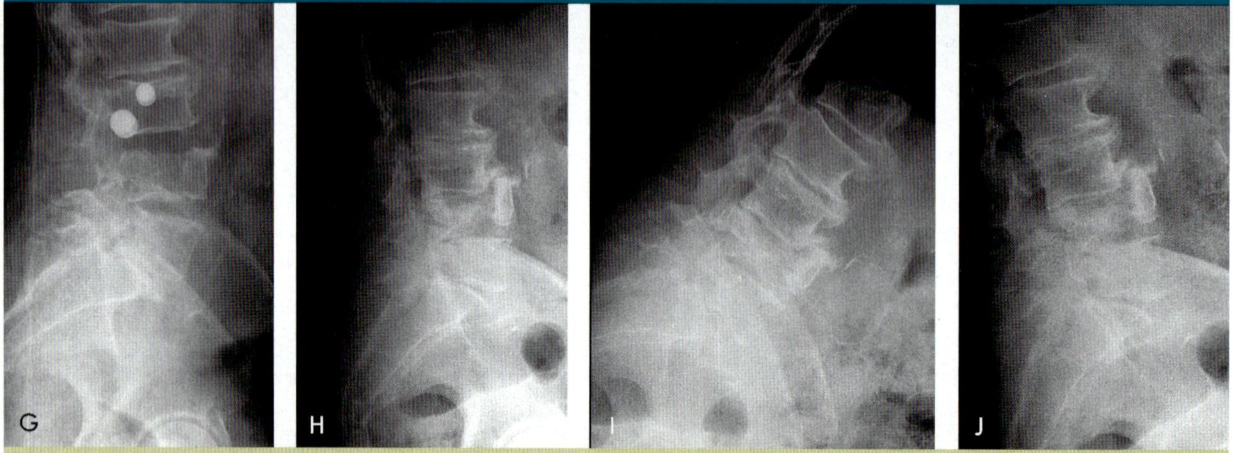

Figure 10 *(continued)* **G,** Upright lateral radiograph of patient in a lumbosacral orthosis with leg extension. Excellent alignment is observed. **H-J,** Lateral, flexion, and extension radiographs after 6 months of brace wear show chronic nonunion, L3-L4 disk desiccation, spondylosis, and subluxation of L3 into the L4 fracture site. The patient developed chronic pain and instability and ultimately required a corpectomy and grafting on the nonunion site.

severe deformity (kyphosis) tends not to significantly alter neural recovery. Therefore, even burst fractures with mild canal compromise may be regarded as stable and appropriate for nonsurgical treatment.

Severe neurologic deficit in the presence of a large degree of canal compromise is an indication for surgery. For example, cauda equina syndrome can often be treated successfully by direct neural decompression.[66] In addition, specific root involvement with localized compression of the root may be improved with direct exploration of the root and decompression. Patients with sagittal spinous process fractures, neurologic deficit, and dural tears with roots outside the dural sac may also benefit from direct decompression and dural repair.[57,58,67]

In lumbar fractures, certain patterns of injury can be defined as unstable. Those patients with severe PLC disruption and disk disruption from a flexion-distraction injury are considered to have unstable injuries. Surgical treatment is generally indicated. Most authors believe that nonsurgical treatment of severe ligamentous injuries does not restore stability, and prefer limited surgical stabilization.

Maintenance of sagittal balance (ie, lordosis) is critical for the normal weight-bearing axis of the body and, therefore, for optimal function of the paraspinous musculature. Accordingly, restoration to as normal an alignment as is feasible is desirable to obtain long-term pain-free functional results. Clinically stable fractures that do not have significant associated kyphosis or scoliosis can be optimally treated with external immobilization.

Some authors argue, however, that fractures with significant deformity cannot be successfully reduced and maintained with external immobilization and that they need surgical intervention for reestablishment of normal spinal alignment.

Treatment Options

Several options exist for the management of low lumbar fractures. Nonsurgical treatment consists mainly of postural reduction in combination with external immobilization by cast or orthosis. With the possible exception of pelvic and sacral fractures, the role of traction or external fixation is limited. Nonsurgical treatment may be indicated for stable injuries of the lumbar region.[68] The current trend is nonsurgical treatment of those patients who are neurologically intact with minimal to moderate deformity. For those with significant deformity or neurologic deficit, surgical treatment may offer improved long term results.

Surgical Principles and Approaches

The major goals of surgical treatment of lumbar spine and sacral injuries are anatomic reduction of the injury deformity, rigid fixation, neural decompression (when indicated), maintenance of sagittal alignment, minimization of fixation length, and minimization of the potential for perioperative complications. Surgical intervention can involve various procedures, including (1) reduction, stabilization, and fusion of spinal fractures from a posterior approach; (2) indirect or direct decompression of neural elements from a posterior or posterolateral (transpedicular) approach;

FIGURE 11

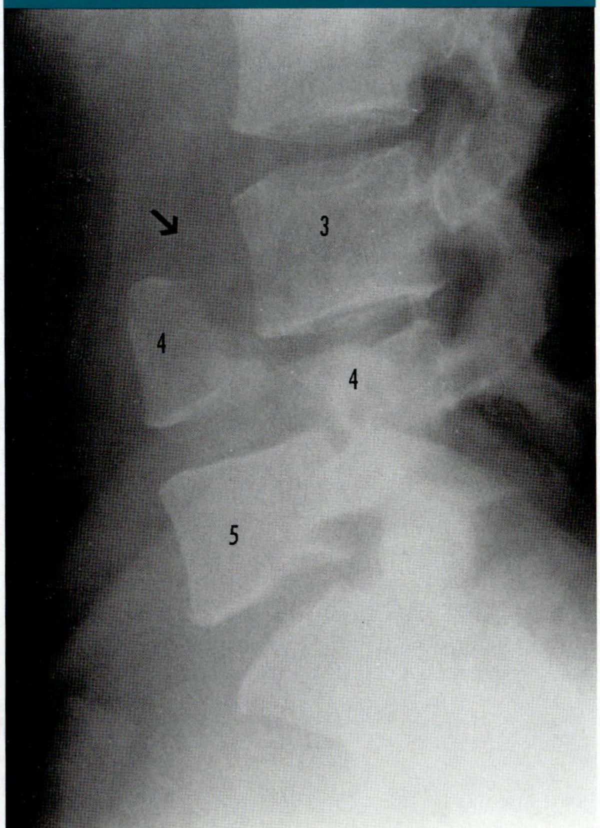

Figure 11 This lateral lumbar radiograph demonstrates a severe shear injury in a 26-year-old man ejected from a motor vehicle. There is total disruption of the spinal column, with a fracture line that passes obliquely from anterosuperior to posteroinferior through the body of L4. (Reproduced with permission from Levine AM: Lumbar and sacral spine trauma, in Browner BD, Jupiter JB, Levine AM, Trafton PG, eds: *Skeletal Trauma: Fractures, Dislocations, Ligamentous Injuries*. Philadelphia, PA, WB Saunders, 1992, vol 1, pp 805-848.)

(3) decompression/reduction, stabilization, fusion, and fixation from an anterior approach; and (4) a combined (anterior-posterior) surgical decompression and fusion. Considerations in selecting the surgical approach include the deforming forces, the acuity of the injury, and the need for neurologic decompression.

A general principle of achieving anatomic reduction is that the deforming forces that have caused the injury must be directly counteracted by the instrumentation system used to maintain the reduction. In addition, in the low lumbar spine, the deforming influence of normal physiologic forces must also be counteracted, specifically the shear force acting at the lumbosacral junction. The fixation procedure used should have an element of distraction and lordosis to restore the normal alignment. If a shorter construct can achieve the same degree of reduction and rigid fixation, it should be used preferentially to maintain as many mobile levels as possible in the lumbar spine. Minimizing fixation length to maintain the maximal number of mobile lumbar segments is the next important treatment goal and consideration in instrumentation of fractures of the lumbar spine. However, there must be a satisfactory balance between the number of levels requiring instrumentation to achieve satisfactory reduction and stabilization and the preservation of important lumbar motion segments. The final treatment goal for lumbar and sacral fractures is to minimize the extremely high complication rate associated with instrumentation of these injuries. Potential surgical complications include iatrogenic neural injury, infection, pseudarthrosis, instrumentation malplacement, dislodgment, or failure,[69] and iatrogenic flat back.[70]

The posterior approach allows circumferential reduction, posterior decompression, and rigid instrumentation with pedicle screws. Pedicle screw systems have a major advantage in the reduction and fixation of lumbar injuries because they reduce the number of levels that need instrumentation to achieve an adequate reduction and rigid stabilization. Rod-based pedicle fixation devices[71-75] are modular and allow progressive reduction of deformities after screw fixation with maintenance of correction. In addition, this form of internal fixation can achieve rigid fixation and maintenance of lordosis. Biomechanical analysis shows that in comparison with the intact spine, posterior instrumentation alone is 76% less stiff axially, posterior instrumentation with an anterior strut graft is 3% more stiff, and anterior instrumentation with an anterior strut graft is 15% more stiff.[76] The rate of failure of posterior instrumentation ranges from 9% to 54%.[77] Short-segment fixation one vertebral level above and below the fractured level is associated with a higher rate of failure compared to long segment instrumentation in one retrospective series.[78]

Anterior procedures for decompression, reduction of deformity (sagittal alignment), and stabilization may be used as a stand-alone procedure, especially in L3 burst injuries due to the difficulty of vessel mobilization near the bifurcation of the great vessels.[66] Results of clinical studies assessing the long-term outcomes of anteriorly treated lumbar fractures[79-81] have indicated satisfactory achievement and maintenance of reduction. The ability to slightly compress an interbody graft is

FIGURE 12

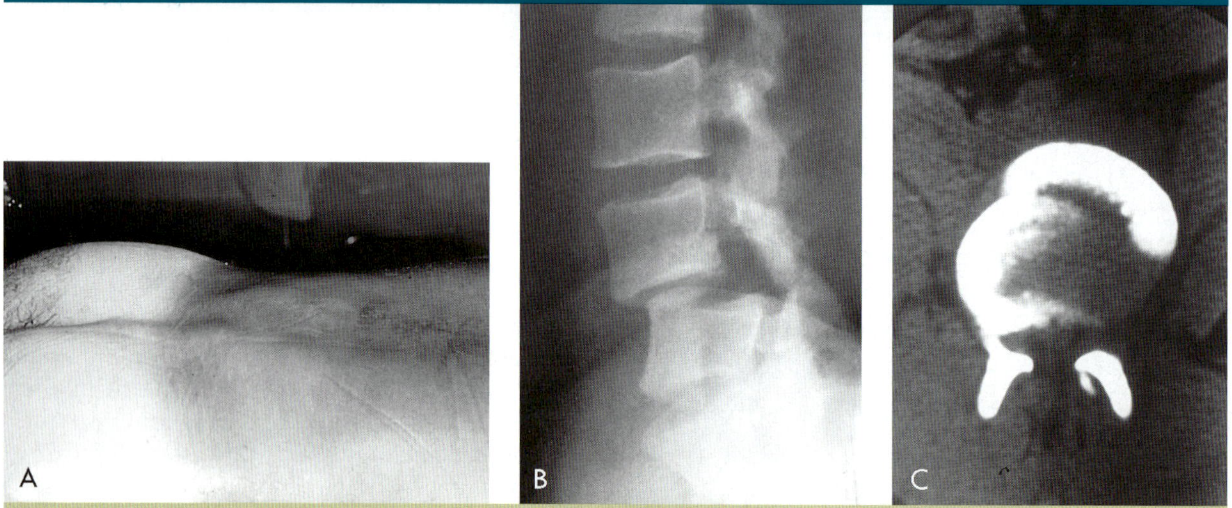

Figure 12 This patient sustained a bilateral facet dislocation at L4-L5. He presented with severe back pain, diffuse weakness below L4, and a severe kyphosis as seen in this preoperative photograph (**A**). **B,** The lateral radiograph showed severe translation of L4 over L5 with maintenance of height of the vertebral bodies. There were no fractures of the posterior wall, although slight comminution of the anterosuperior portion of L5 occurred. **C,** The CT scan shows an empty facet sign. In addition, the translational and slight rotational deformities are apparent on this cut of the CT scan. (Reproduced with permission from Levine AM: Lumbar and sacral spine trauma, in Browner BD, Jupiter JB, Levine AM, Trafton PG, eds: *Skeletal Trauma: Fractures, Dislocations, Ligamentous Injuries*. Philadelphia, PA, WB Saunders, 1992, vol 1, pp 805-848.)

easily performed with contemporary internal fixation systems. This is an improvement over previous plating systems, which simply functioned as neutralization devices.

Subacute deformities more than 6 weeks old may require posterior or combined anterior-posterior surgical approaches (**Figure 15**). Total reduction from an anterior approach alone can prove to be difficult in cases of subacute fractures as posterior scarring or healing of posterior element fractures may have occurred. In addition, most anterior spinal devices lack sufficient lever arms and rigidity of fixation points to be able to apply forces adequate for achieving total reduction.

Decompression of neural elements is not uniformly required after surgical treatment of lumbar burst fractures. It has been demonstrated that resorption of residual bone within the canal predictably occurs both with and without surgery.[64,82,83] Neural decompression can be achieved in several different ways, both directly and indirectly; the optimal method is dependent on the specific clinical situation. In acute lumbar spine injuries, there is significant experimental[84,85] and clinical evidence[61,86-90] that immediate indirect decompression by ligamentotaxis and complete correction of the deformity can provide adequate decompression of the neural elements. This technique has been shown to be most effective in the first 48 hours after injury. In the low lumbar spine and sacrum, however, indirect decompression is not as successful because the technique depends on distraction and tension through Sharpey's fibers. It is therefore less effective in an area of extreme lordosis or kyphosis.

Direct decompression via laminectomy and transpedicular decompression can be effective in revealing the area of compression and allowing for the decompression by removal of the bone fragments that are impinging upon the dural sac or nerve roots. Transpedicular or "egg-shell" decompression is a direct posterior technique that allows partial anterior decompression of the thecal sac, particularly below the conus level.[91,92] There are several studies that support the egg-shell procedure as a reliable and safe technique to achieve anterior decompression of the spinal canal and posterior stabilization through a single approach in the upper lumbar spine.[93] Limited retraction of the dural sac to achieve exposure is possible at the low lumbar levels.[94] However, this technique is only recommended for those areas of the spine involving the cauda equina or roots of the sacrum. Transpedicular decompression is technically easier within the first 2 weeks of injury, because the fragments are more mobile and more easily resected.

FIGURE 13

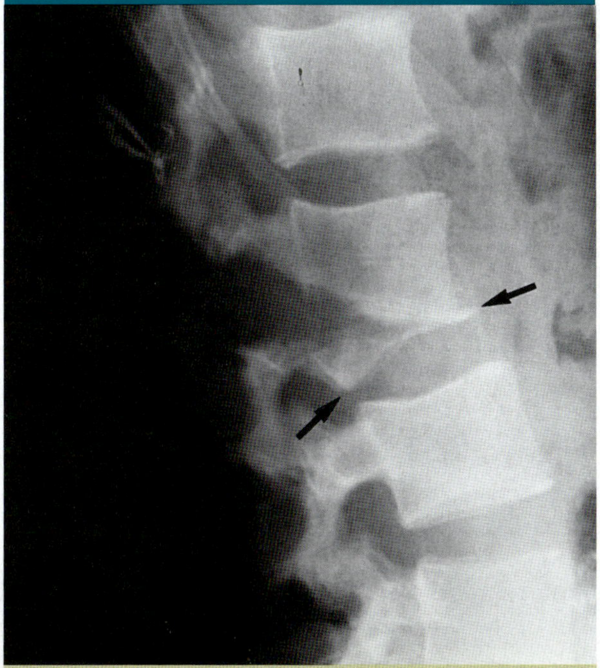

Figure 13 This lateral radiograph of the lumbar spine of a 16-year-old girl demonstrates an end-plate avulsion. She was involved in a motor vehicle accident and sustained complete paraplegia from the flexion-distraction injury several levels above the area of bony injury. Note the avulsion of the end plate of the vertebral body (arrows) with translation of the end plate anteriorly in addition to the flexion and distraction of the posterior portion of the end plate. (Reproduced with permission from Levine AM: Lumbar and sacral spine trauma, in Browner BD, Jupiter JB, Levine AM, Trafton PG, eds: *Skeletal Trauma: Fractures, Dislocations, Ligamentous Injuries*. Philadelphia, PA, WB Saunders, 1992, vol 1, pp 805-848.)

FIGURE 14

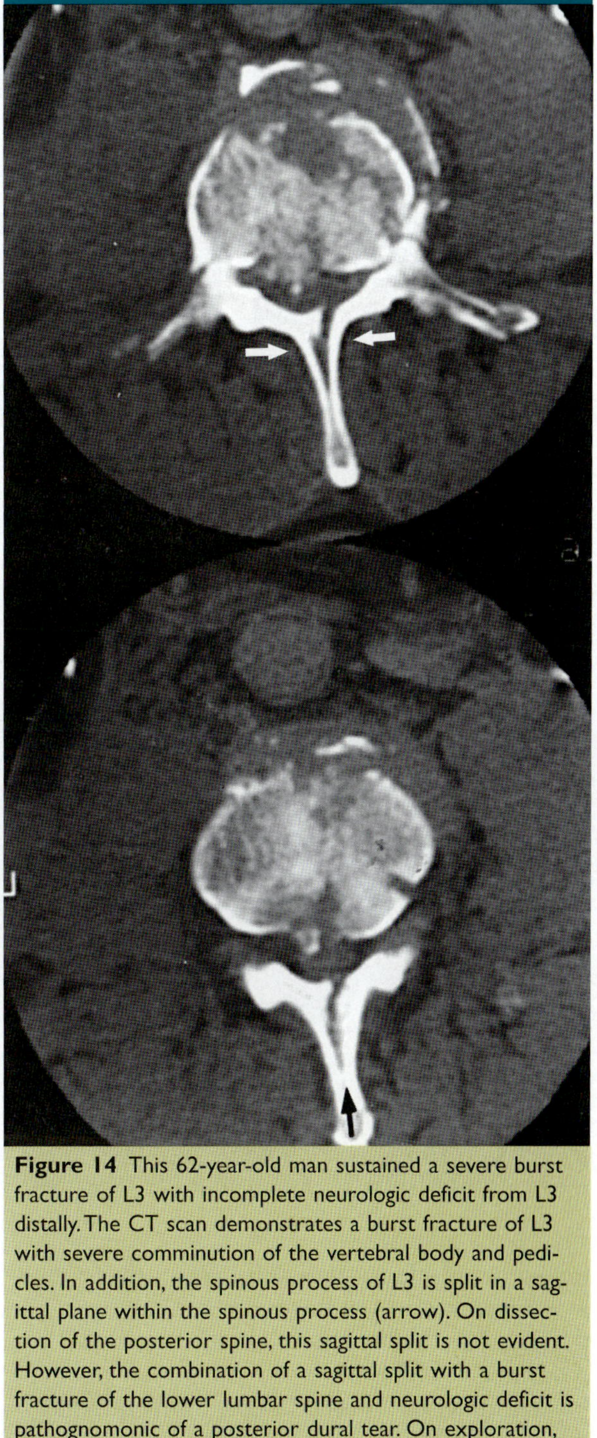

Figure 14 This 62-year-old man sustained a severe burst fracture of L3 with incomplete neurologic deficit from L3 distally. The CT scan demonstrates a burst fracture of L3 with severe comminution of the vertebral body and pedicles. In addition, the spinous process of L3 is split in a sagittal plane within the spinous process (arrow). On dissection of the posterior spine, this sagittal split is not evident. However, the combination of a sagittal split with a burst fracture of the lower lumbar spine and neurologic deficit is pathognomonic of a posterior dural tear. On exploration, the patient was found to have a 3-cm laceration of the posterior aspect of the dural sac with herniation of nerve roots through the sac and entrapment of the roots within the sagittal split of the spinous process. (Reproduced with permission from Levine AM: Lumbar and sacral spine trauma, in Browner BD, Jupiter JB, Levine AM, Trafton PG, eds: *Skeletal Trauma: Fractures, Dislocations, Ligamentous Injuries*. Philadelphia, PA, WB Saunders, 1992, vol 1, pp 805-848.)

Posterior Surgical Approach for Burst Fracture: Pearls and Pitfalls

The posterior approach for instrumentation of low lumbar burst fractures has become a more common technique. Pedicle fixation has the advantage of allowing fixation across short levels (three segments, two interspaces). The most common instrumentation schematic in the low lumbar spine is one level above and one level below the fractured vertebra body level. McLain et al[78] describe a high rate of failure with this short-segment fixation construct in the treatment of thoracolumbar burst fractures. In cases of severe vertebral body comminution, consideration should be given to anterior-posterior fixation. Reduction of kyphosis is effected with a radiolucent operating table with the abdomen hanging free, hip supports on the iliac crests, and the chest supported by pads posi-

FIGURE 15

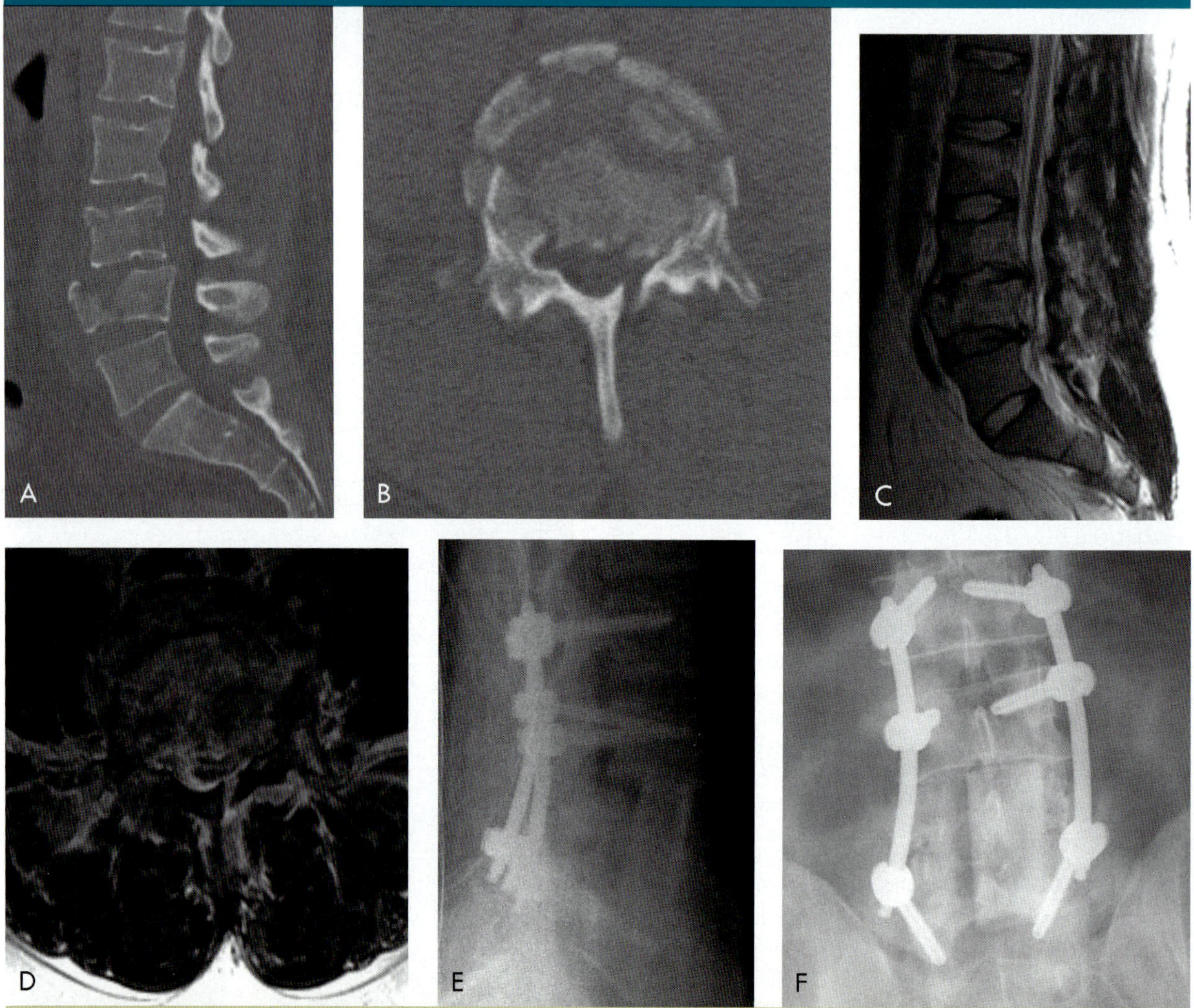

Figure 15 Anteroposterior reconstruction. **A,** Midsagittal CT scan illustrates L4 burst fracture with retropulsion of the vertebral body. **B,** Axial CT scan demonstrates severe canal compression and left lamina fracture. **C,** Midsagittal MRI scan demonstrates spinal stenosis and PLC destruction. **D,** Axial MRI scan at the level of the fracture shows severe nerve root compression. The patient clinically presented with cauda equina syndrome. **E** and **F,** Lateral and AP radiographs demonstrate L4 corpectomy and posterior L2 to L5 fusion with instrumentation.

tioned on a Jackson-type table. This position creates a three-point bending moment. Positioning the iliac crest holders more distally would effect more lordosis from postural reduction. A midline posterior incision is used. Dissection is carefully performed to avoid excess motion of the injured spine. Frequently, spinous process and posterior element fractures are encountered with posterior exposure. Care must be taken to prevent accidental durotomy during surgical exposure if the posterior elements are damaged. Furthermore, the capsule of the cephalad level facet joint that remains unfused should not be disturbed (**Figure 16**, *A*). Facet capsule violation increases segmental instability compared to laminectomy alone.[95] A traumatic dural tear may be encountered as well, which should be repaired or patched as necessary.

Pedicle screw orientation may be affected by deformity, the positioning of the patient on the operating table, the amount of kyphotic deformity of the fracture, and the shape of the vertebra. The orientation of the intraoperative marker can be used to guide the sagittal plane angle for pedicle screw placement. Pedicle screw starting points are determined by surface landmarks based on the location of the transverse process, pars interarticularis, and superior articular facet. (**Figure 16**, *B*).

FIGURE 16

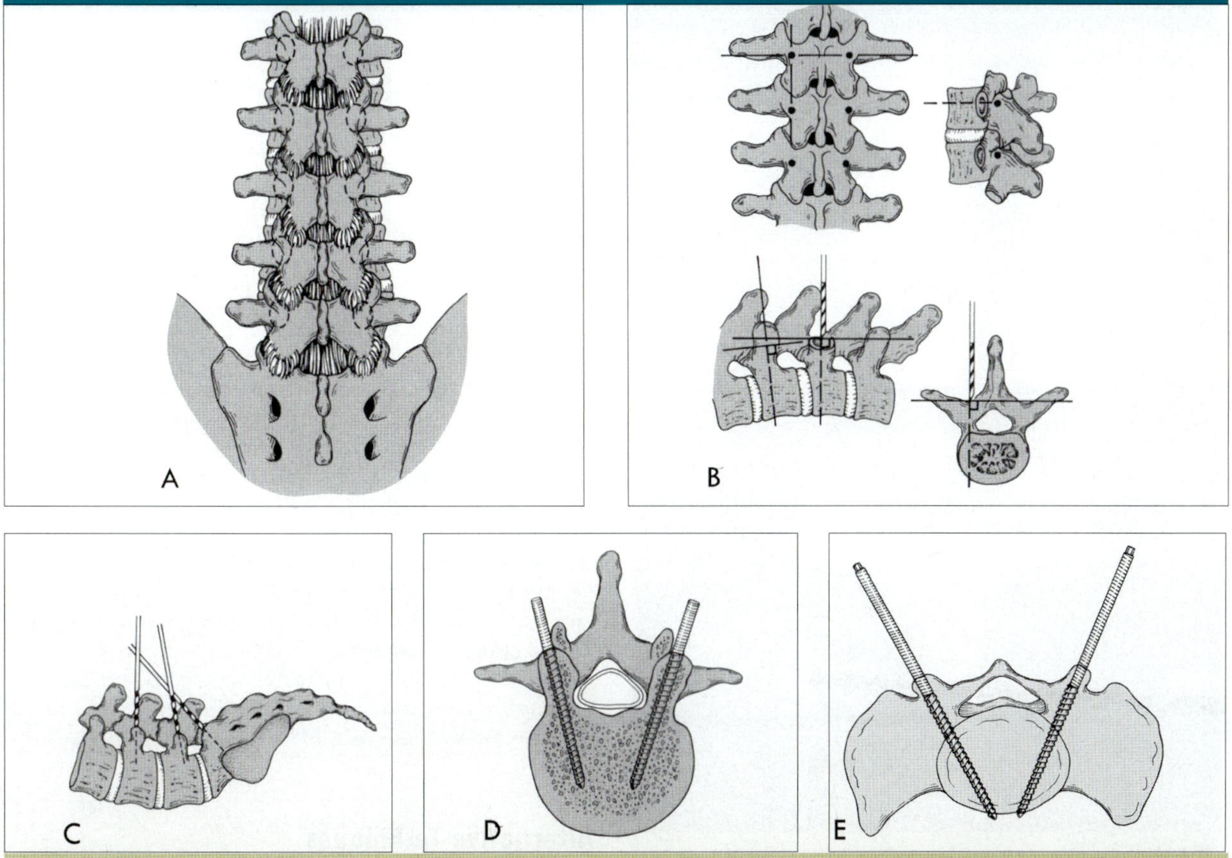

Figure 16 The surgical technique for pedicular fixation of low lumbar burst fractures. The technique shown emphasizes the critical features. **A,** When exposing the spine, care must be taken not to disrupt the interspinous ligament or the facet capsules proximal to the level of instrumentation. In exposing the transverse process opposite the superior pedicle, it is critical that the facet capsule not be disrupted. In view of the location of the pedicle and its proximity to the capsule, great care should be taken in this dissection. The technique of Roy-Camille (**B**) positions the entry point at the intersection of a line through the transverse processes and a line through the inferolateral edge of the facet joint. At L5, the lateral aspect of the pars interarticularis will be at the medial wall of the pedicle projection, whereas at more cephalad levels it will be at the midpoint of the pedicle projection. Entry into the pedicle can be facilitated by using a high-speed burr to remove the cortical bone at the location of the suggested entry point. A small probe, sound, or curet can be used to easily traverse the cancellous bone of the pedicle. This technique prevents inadvertent perforation of the pedicle walls. **C,** Drill bits can then be placed into pedicles so that the use of intraoperative image intensification or radiographs will allow identification of the position of the drill bits within the pedicles. The sagittal orientation of the drill bits within the vertebral bodies changes with the level. **D,** In view of the angle of the side wall of L5, the screws should be oriented approximately 25° medial and 15° caudal to accommodate the lordosis of L5. **E,** Fixation in the S1 vertebral body typically aims approximately 30° medially and 20° caudally. Bicortical purchase can be achieved because the anterior aspect of the S1 vertebral body is a safe zone for neurologic or vascular structures. (Reproduced with permission from Levine AM: Lumbar and sacral spine trauma, in Browner BD, Jupiter JB, Levine AM, Trafton PG, eds: *Skeletal Trauma: Fractures, Dislocations, Ligamentous Injuries*, ed 2. Philadelphia, PA, WB Saunders, 1998, vol 1, pp 1035-1093.)

Axial plane angulation is approximately 30° medial for S1, 25° medial for L5, 20° medial for L4, and 15° medial for L3 (**Figure 16,** *C* and *D*).[2] Laminoforaminotomies may be performed as necessary to determine the orientation of the pedicle.

Fixation in the fractured body may be considered depending on fracture morphology. The configuration of the fractured body must be clearly delineated on the CT scan before attempting screw placement. The most common pattern for L4 and L5 burst fractures is that the superior portion of the body and the pedicle are comminuted, but the inferior portion of the pedicle remains attached to the inferior portion of the vertebral body. This can be accompanied by a sagittal split in the body, in which the two halves of the vertebra are dissoci-

FIGURE 17

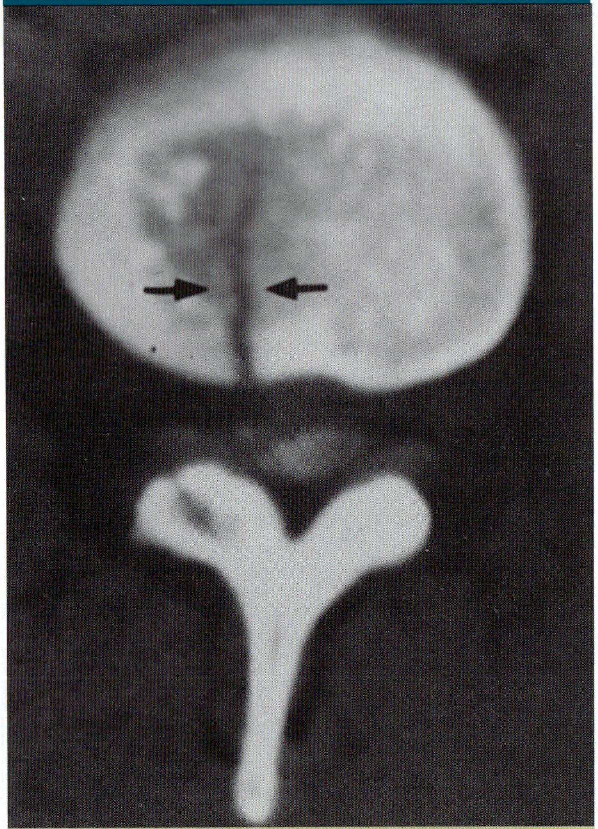

Figure 17 In this low lumbar burst fracture, there is a sagittal split in the lumbar vertebral body and one pedicle remaining attached to each of the lower halves of the body. This fracture will be rotationally unstable, particularly after laminectomy, and fixation will be required bilaterally. (Reproduced with permission from Levine AM: Lumbar and sacral spine trauma, in Browner BD, Jupiter JB, Levine AM, Trafton PG, eds: *Skeletal Trauma: Fractures, Dislocations, Ligamentous Injuries*, ed 2. Philadelphia, PA, WB Saunders, 1992, vol 1, pp 1035-1093.)

FIGURE 18

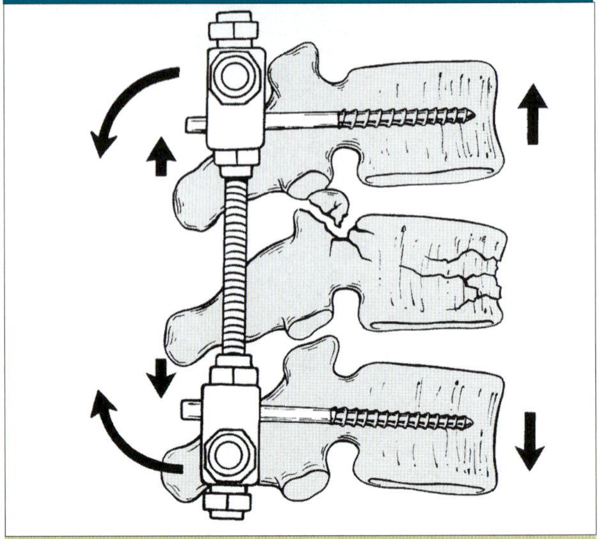

Figure 18 Lordosis of the fractured level can be achieved via application of cantilever bending forces on the cephalad and caudal vertebral bodies. (Reproduced with permission from Levine AM: Lumbar and sacral spine trauma, in Browner BD, Jupiter JB, Levine AM, Trafton PG, eds: *Skeletal Trauma: Fractures, Dislocations, Ligamentous Injuries*, ed 2. Philadelphia, PA, WB Saunders, 1998, vol 1, pp 1035-1093.)

ated (**Figure 17**). Bicortical purchase may be required if the two halves are sagittally split to prevent screws from entering into the fracture site.

After the screws are placed, then a longitudinal component (rod) can be introduced and reduction accomplished by application of lordosis and distraction. Lordosis should be effected before distraction because ligamentotaxis reduction will not be possible after ligaments are tensioned in distraction (**Figure 18**). Ligamentotaxis reduction may be difficult to effect in the low lumbar spine.[96] Care should be taken after screw insertion and before application of the rod to decorticate the transverse processes and sacral ala adequately, because the bulk of the devices could preclude adequate preparation for fusion after application.

Alternative Techniques

There are various other techniques that have their own advantages and disadvantages. They have been mainly used for the treatment of thoracic and thoracolumbar injuries, with a smaller percentage used for injuries of the upper lumbar area. Their applicability is limited when considered for low lumbar (L4 and L5) injuries alone.

Anterior Decompression and Fixation

Anterior surgical techniques are effective for direct decompression and stabilization of low lumbar fractures. The most commonly involved levels are the L2-L5. These can be accessed through a straightforward retroperitoneal approach, which allows excellent exposure of the vertebral bodies for adequate anterior decompression. Significant hemorrhage can be experienced in the anterior surgical treatment of acute lower lumbar fractures. The use of anterior internal fixation[6,79,80,97] for neutralization and stability achieves the goal of rigid fixation, and is adequate for long-term stabilization. Care must be taken that the devices do not protrude against the aorta, or vascular complications can arise. Dissection of L4, and especially of L5, requires extreme care in handling the iliac vein and iliolumbar vein.

Flexion-Distraction Injuries

These injuries most commonly occur at the thoracolumbar junction and were discussed in detail elsewhere in the text. The most common flexion-distraction injury in the thoracolumbar spine is the bilateral facet dislocation. This is distinctly rare in the lumbar spine, but requires special consideration. Such injuries can result in severe posterior ligamentous disruption and disk disruption. Prophylactic diskectomy should be considered before performing a compressive maneuver. This removes damaged disk material and prevents extrusion. Short-segment posterior instrumentation is an acceptable treatment option for these injuries.

Shear Injuries and Complex Deformities

The optimal stabilization construct for shear injuries and complex deformities generally involves a posterior approach for reduction of deformity followed by a posterior or staged anterior decompression.

Minor Bony, Disk, and Ligamentous Injuries

Avulsion fractures of the transverse processes can be treated symptomatically by external immobilization to support the severe muscular trauma associated with the more minor bony injury. Transverse process fractures associated with more severe bony injury can be treated secondarily by immobilization of the primary injury. End-plate avulsions in children simulating disk herniation in the acute injury setting require surgical intervention for direct decompression after appropriate diagnostic studies.[54,56,98] With a minor degree of disruption (sprain), external immobilization for 6 weeks to 2 months can allow sufficient healing to achieve symptomatic relief and stability.

Outcomes of Specific Types of Injuries

Anterior Wedge Compression Fractures

Compression fractures of the low lumbar spine are relatively frequent either as single or multiple injuries. Their outcome is usually favorable, with the possible exception of a patient with severe osteopenia. The most frequent problems are either failure to recognize accompanying pathologic bone or mistakenly identifying a burst fracture as a compression fracture. In evaluating these injuries, care must be taken to confirm that the posterior wall of the vertebral body remains intact. Comminution of the posterior wall converts the injury to the more significant burst pattern, which alters the prognosis and treatment program. The patient should also undergo a work-up for a pathologic fracture, including neoplasm or infection. The presence of a soft-tissue mass or involvement of the pedicles is concerning for pathologic bone. In addition, the surgeon must be certain that the compression fracture is not accompanied by ligamentous disruption.

The goal of treatment of compression fractures is prevention of further compression and residual kyphosis. Nonsurgical treatment, even in hyperextension, cannot restore vertebral height. Immobilization needs to be extended for a period of 1.5 to 3 months, until the vertebral body has consolidated. Increasing compression during the course of treatment interfering with the normal lordotic sagittal alignment of the spine may require a change in treatment.

Burst Fractures of the Lumbar Spine

For stable injuries in the low lumbar spine, external immobilization treatment options include extension casting, total contact casting orthosis (TCO), and thoracolumbosacral orthosis (TLSO). There are no studies that show a relative benefit of TCOs over TLSOs, although TCOs are likely associated with improved patient compliance because it is difficult to remove. For fractures of L2 through L4, a standard TCO is acceptable. For L5 burst fractures, a TLSO with leg extension (leg included) is recommended to immobilize the pelvis and prevent flexion at the fracture site. Immobilization by standard lumbar orthoses could potentially accentuate the motion at L4-L5 and L5-S1.[99,100] The optimal duration of bracing, usually 3 months, should allow adequate time for fracture healing. Regular follow-up is essential to evaluate fracture healing and spinal alignment.

The majority of the literature on the management of low lumbar burst fractures supports nonsurgical treatment. There is a paucity of literature regarding the long-term outcome of low lumbar burst fractures. Most of the burst fracture literature involves a mixed population of thoracolumbar and lumbar burst fractures. There are reports of successful nonsurgical treatment of thoracolumbar burst fractures.[76,101] Tropiano et al[93] concluded that reduction was better maintained in thoracolumbar fractures with nonsurgical treatment than in lumbar fractures and that posterior ligamentous instability was associated with poor functional outcomes.

Some reports suggest that patients with low lumbar burst fractures treated nonsurgically may experience poor outcomes. A clinical series determined a significant compensatory relationship between thoracic kyphosis, lumbar lordosis, and lumbopelvic alignment. In a long-term outcome study of nonsurgically treated low lumbar burst fractures,[95] focal kyphotic posture due to low lumbar burst fractures was associated with compensatory thoracic and pelvic changes and worse clinical outcome. An et al[2] found that surgical treatment, early rehabilitation, and improved lordosis of the lumbar spine were associated with improved outcome. **Figure 10** illustrates kyphotic collapse and failure of nonsurgical management of a thoracolumbar burst fracture in a lumbosacral orthosis with a leg extension.

There are several comparative studies that demonstrate improved results with surgical intervention. Dai[1] reported a clinical case series of 54 patients with low lumbar fractures with 1- to 12-year follow-up. Twenty-six patients were treated surgically and 28 were treated nonsurgically. There were no differences in final neurologic function between patients treated nonsurgically or surgically ($P > 0.05$). However, the patients treated surgically had significantly less pain compared to the patients treated nonsurgically ($P < 0.01$).[1] With relatively short follow-up (less than 4 years), trends in current studies suggest that those patients with neurologic deficit may have improved recovery with surgical intervention.[13,65] However, when the data are critically analyzed, the majority of patients have a significant degree of residual back pain and disability, even in the short term.[2,6,12,38] Posterior "short-segment" instrumentation and fusion for L3-L5 fractures has been demonstrated to maintain vertebral height and prevent kyphotic collapse with efficacy equal to that achieved with traditional posterior constructs (two fixation points above and below the fractured level) or anterior instrumentation and corpectomy. Some authors have suggested that short-segment posterior fixation involving only one spinal segment above and below the fractured level may be appropriate only when the vertebral body has mild loss of height, comminution, and fragment diastasis. The load-sharing classification of thoracolumbar burst fractures, based on these parameters, has also been applied to low lumbar fractures and found to be predictive of successful short-segment pedicle screw–based fixation in this region of the spine.[102,103] Additional anterior interbody support may be rendered in the osteopenic patient by percutaneous balloon-assisted vertebral body augmentation using cement.[2,104]

Complications of Surgical Treatment

Neurologic deterioration can occur intraoperatively and postoperatively. One possible cause of deterioration can be intraoperative displacement during patient positioning as the patient rolls from a supine to prone position. Intraoperative neurologic deterioration can be caused by applying distraction over a kyphotic segment of the lumbar spine and application of tension to neural elements over a prominent area of bone or discal tissue. Reduction of kyphosis should be accomplished before any distraction maneuver. In addition, passing sublaminar wires or any fixation device in the canal at the apical level of the kyphosis and deformity can involve increased neurologic deficit secondary to mass effect in the spinal canal. Hook placement at L5 and S1 can also result in neurologic deficit, because the very small canal and the severely lordotic lumbosacral junction can place the shoe of the hook in a position to compress the dural sac. Postoperative neurologic complications can also be caused by dislodgment of anterior grafts or by recurrence of deformity.

Hook dislodgment and rod disengagement can occur following surgical intervention. The incidence of hook dislodgment has ranged up to 20% in patients with lumbar spine trauma (**Figure 19**, *A*). This is the result of inadequate stabilization of the lumbar lordosis and the collapsing of the spine with loosening of the hardware when the patient is mobilized. Pedicle screw instrumentation can also be misplaced, resulting in impingement and compression of neural elements. (**Figure 19**, *B*).

Nonunion of lumbar spine fractures is a frequent complication. It has been reported in as many as 40% of fractures at the lumbosacral junction. More rigid fixation techniques with segmental fixation, as well as meticulous fusion techniques, are required to prevent this complication. Care must be taken with bulky posterior hardware so that the device does not obscure pertinent areas for bony fusion.

Most reports on spinal injury have noted loss of correction as well as residual kyphosis. This complication is related to the inability of the fixation system selected to achieve rigid fixation that does not change with patient mobilization. Proper selection of hardware and meticulous application with concern for counteracting deforming forces can minimize loss of correction.[105]

FIGURE 19

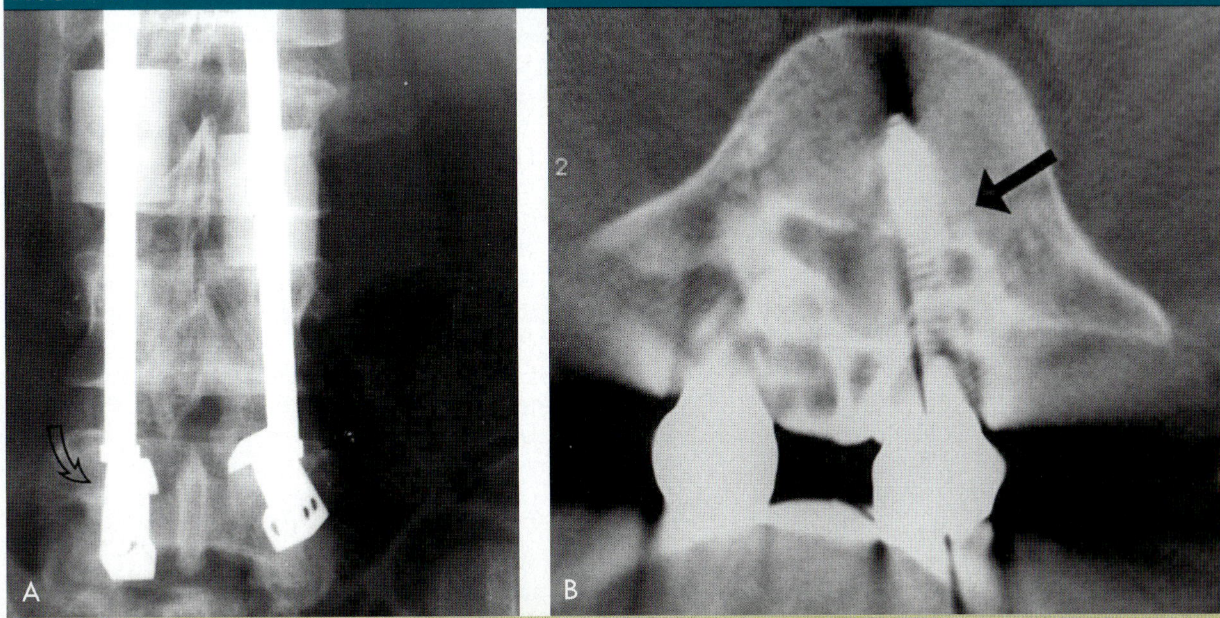

Figure 19 A, Dislodgment, a frequent complication with hook fixation to L4 or L5, is a result of the difficulty of adequately stabilizing the lumbar lordosis. The more segments of the lumbar spine that are spanned, the higher the rates of dislodgment. **B,** Although segmental fixation with pedicle screws can shorten the construct and more rigidly fix the lumbar lordosis, the surgical technique is more exacting. Especially in the traumatized spine where normal landmarks may be obscured, misplacement of screws is a potential complication. (Reproduced with permission from Levine AM: Lumbar and sacral spine trauma, in Browner BD, Jupiter JB, Levine AM, Trafton PG, eds: *Skeletal Trauma: Fractures, Dislocations, Ligamentous Injuries*, ed 2. Philadelphia, PA, WB Saunders, 1998, vol 1, pp 1035-1093.)

Conclusion

Treatment of lumbar and sacral fractures requires an understanding of the mechanics and normal functioning of the lumbar spine. Hardware selection depends on the goals to be achieved, the time to surgery, and the types of instabilities encountered. Appropriate consideration of the treatment goals for an individual patient and the injury leads to optimal results. The surgeon's selection of treatment should not be based on knowledge of a single technique, but rather on knowledge of the relative advantages and disadvantages of various nonsurgical and operative procedures for the treatment of lumbar spine fractures.

References

1. Dai LD: Low lumbar spinal fractures: Management options. *Injury* 2002;33(7):579-582.
2. An HS, Simpson JM, Ebraheim NA, Jackson WT, Moore J, O'Malley NP: Low lumbar burst fractures: Comparison between conservative and surgical treatments. *Orthopedics* 1992;15(3):367-373.
3. Stauffer ES, Neil JL: Biomechanical analysis of structural stability of internal fixation in fractures of the thoracolumbar spine. *Clin Orthop Relat Res* 1975;112:159-164.
4. Court-Brown CM, Gertzbein SD: The management of burst fractures of the fifth lumbar vertebra. *Spine (Phila Pa 1976)* 1987;12(3):308-312.
5. Fredrickson BE, Yuan HA, Miller H: Burst fractures of the fifth lumbar vertebra: A report of four cases. *J Bone Joint Surg Am* 1982;64(7):1088-1094.
6. An HS, Vaccaro A, Cotler JM, Lin S: Low lumbar burst fractures: Comparison among body cast, Harrington rod, Luque rod, and Steffee plate. *Spine (Phila Pa 1976)* 1991;16(8, Suppl): S440-S444.
7. Knight RQ, Stornelli DP, Chan DP, Devanny JR, Jackson KV: Comparison of operative versus nonoperative treatment of lumbar burst fractures. *Clin Orthop Relat Res* 1993;293:112-121.
8. Stephens GC, Devito DP, McNamara MJ: Segmental fixation of lumbar burst fractures with Cotrel-Dubousset instrumentation. *J Spinal Disord* 1992; 5(3):344-348.
9. Chan DP, Seng NK, Kaan KT: Nonoperative treatment in burst fractures of the lumbar spine (L2-L5) without neurologic deficits. *Spine (Phila Pa 1976)* 1993;18(3):320-325.

10. Finn CA, Stauffer ES: Burst fracture of the fifth lumbar vertebra. *J Bone Joint Surg Am* 1992;74(3): 398-403.
11. Mick CA, Carl A, Sachs B, Hresko MT, Pfeifer BA: Burst fractures of the fifth lumbar vertebra. *Spine (Phila Pa 1976)* 1993;18(13):1878-1884.
12. Levine AM, Edwards CC: Low lumbar burst fractures: Reduction and stabilization using the modular spine fixation system. *Orthopedics* 1988; 11(10):1427-1432.
13. Roy-Camille R, Saillant G, Mazel C: Plating of thoracic, thoracolumbar, and lumbar injuries with pedicle screw plates. *Orthop Clin North Am* 1986; 17(1):147-159.
14. Wambolt A, Spencer DL: A segmental analysis of the distribution of lumbar lordosis in the normal spine. *Orthop Trans* 1987;11:92-93.
15. Bernhardt M, Bridwell KH: Segmental analysis of the sagittal plane alignment of the normal thoracic and lumbar spines and thoracolumbar junction. *Spine (Phila Pa 1976)* 1989;14(7):717-721.
16. Winter RB: *Congenital Deformities of the Spine*. New York, NY, Thieme-Stratton, 1983.
17. Stagnara P, De Mauroy JC, Dran G, et al: Reciprocal angulation of vertebral bodies in a sagittal plane: Approach to references for the evaluation of kyphosis and lordosis. *Spine (Phila Pa 1976)* 1982;7(4):335-342.
18. Elliott HC: Cross-sectional diameters and areas of the human spinal cord. *Anat Rec* 1945;93: 287-293.
19. Rauschning W: Correlative multiplaner computed tomographic anatomy of the normal spine, in Post JD, ed: *Computed Tomography of the Spine*. Baltimore, MD, Williams & Wilkins, 1984, pp 20-67.
20. Denis F: Spinal instability as defined by the three-column spine concept in acute spinal trauma. *Clin Orthop Relat Res* 1984;189:65-76.
21. Saillant G: Anatomical study of the vertebral pedicles: Surgical application. *Rev Chir Orthop Reparatrice Appar Mot* 1976;62(2):151-160.
22. Krag MH, Weaver DL, Beynnon BD, Haugh LD: Morphometry of the thoracic and lumbar spine related to transpedicular screw placement for surgical spinal fixation. *Spine (Phila Pa 1976)* 1988; 13(1):27-32.
23. Zindrick MR, Wiltse LL, Doornik A, et al: Analysis of the morphometric characteristics of the thoracic and lumbar pedicles. *Spine (Phila Pa 1976)* 1987;12(2):160-166.
24. Scoles PV, Linton AE, Latimer B, Levy ME, Digiovanni BF: Vertebral body and posterior element morphology: The normal spine in middle life. *Spine (Phila Pa 1976)* 1988;13(10):1082-1086.
25. White AA III, Panjabi MM: The basic kinematics of the human spine: A review of past and current knowledge. *Spine (Phila Pa 1976)* 1978;3(1): 12-20.
26. Jackson RP, McManus AC: Radiographic analysis of sagittal plane alignment and balance in standing volunteers and patients with low back pain matched for age, sex, and size: A prospective controlled clinical study. *Spine (Phila Pa 1976)* 1994; 19(14):1611-1618.
27. Bucholz RW, Gill K: Classification of injuries to the thoracolumbar spine. *Orthop Clin North Am* 1986;17(1):67-73.
28. Holdsworth FW: Fractures, dislocations, and fracture-dislocations of the spine. *J Bone Joint Surg Am* 1970;52(8):1534-1551.
29. Ferguson RL, Allen BL Jr: A mechanistic classification of thoracolumbar spine fractures. *Clin Orthop Relat Res* 1984;189:77-88.
30. Whitesides TE Jr: Traumatic kyphosis of the thoracolumbar spine. *Clin Orthop Relat Res* 1977;128: 78-92.
31. McAfee PC, Yuan HA, Fredrickson BE, Lubicky JP: The value of computed tomography in thoracolumbar fractures: An analysis of one hundred consecutive cases and a new classification. *J Bone Joint Surg Am* 1983;65(4):461-473.
32. Vaccaro AR, Lehman RA Jr, Hurlbert RJ, et al: A new classification of thoracolumbar injuries: The importance of injury morphology, the integrity of the posterior ligamentous complex, and neurologic status. *Spine (Phila Pa 1976)* 2005;30(20): 2325-2333.
33. Levine AM, Edwards CC: Lumbar spine trauma, in Camins M, O'Leary P, eds: *The Lumbar Spine*. New York, NY, Raven Press, 1987, pp 185-212.
34. Levine AM: The surgical treatment of low lumbar fractures. *Semin Spine Surg* 1990;2:41-53.
35. Anderson PA, Rivara FP, Maier RV, Drake C: The epidemiology of seatbelt-associated injuries. *J Trauma* 1991;31(1):60-67.
36. Neumann P, Nordwall A, Osvalder AL: Traumatic instability of the lumbar spine: A dynamic in vitro study of flexion-distraction injury. *Spine (Phila Pa 1976)* 1995;20(10):1111-1121.
37. Rennie W, Mitchell N: Flexion distraction fractures of the thoracolumbar spine. *J Bone Joint Surg Am* 1973;55(2):386-390.
38. Chance GQ: Note on a type of flexion fracture of the spine. *Br J Radiol* 1948;21(249):452-453.
39. Haddad GH, Zickel RE: Intestinal perforation and fracture of the lumbar spine caused by lap-type seat belt. *NY State J Med* 1967;67(7):930-932.
40. Gertzbein SD, Court-Brown CM: Flexion-distraction injuries of the lumbar spine: Mechanisms of injury and classification. *Clin Orthop Relat Res* 1988;227:52-60.

41. Gumley G, Taylor TK, Ryan MD: Distraction fractures of the lumbar spine. *J Bone Joint Surg Br* 1982;64(5):520-525.
42. Lewis J, McKibbin B: The treatment of unstable fracture-dislocations of the thoraco-lumbar spine accompanied by paraplegia. *J Bone Joint Surg Br* 1974;56-B(4):603-612.
43. Levine AM, Bosse M, Edwards CC: Bilateral facet dislocations in the thoracolumbar spine. *Spine (Phila Pa 1976)* 1988;13(6):630-640.
44. O'Callaghan JP, Ullrich CG, Yuan HA, Kieffer SA: CT of facet distraction in flexion injuries of the thoracolumbar spine: The "naked" facet. *AJR Am J Roentgenol* 1980;134(3):563-568.
45. Carl A, Blair B: Unilateral lumbosacral facet fracture-dislocation. *Spine (Phila Pa 1976)* 1991;16(2):218-221.
46. Das De S, McCreath SW: Lumbosacral fracture-dislocations: A report of four cases. *J Bone Joint Surg Br* 1981;63-B(1):58-60.
47. Dewey P, Browne PS: Fracture-dislocation of the lumbo-sacral spine with cauda equina lesion: Report of two cases. *J Bone Joint Surg Br* 1968;50(3):635-638.
48. Herron LD, Williams RC: Fracture-dislocation of the lumbosacral spine: Report of a case and review of the literature. *Clin Orthop Relat Res* 1984;186:205-211.
49. Kramer KM, Levine AM: Unilateral facet dislocation of the lumbosacral junction: A case report and review of the literature. *J Bone Joint Surg Am* 1989;71(8):1258-1261.
50. Morris BD: Unilateral dislocation of a lumbosacral facet: A case report. *J Bone Joint Surg Am* 1981;63(1):164-165.
51. Samberg LC: Fracture-dislocation of the lumbosacral spine: A case report. *J Bone Joint Surg Am* 1975;57(7):1007-1008.
52. Zoltan JD, Gilula LA, Murphy WA: Unilateral facet dislocation between the fifth lumbar and first sacral vertebrae: Case report. *J Bone Joint Surg Am* 1979;61(5):767-769.
53. Micheli LJ: Low back pain in the adolescent: Differential diagnosis. *Am J Sports Med* 1979;7(6):362-364.
54. Epstein NE, Epstein JA: Limbus lumbar vertebral fractures in 27 adolescents and adults. *Spine (Phila Pa 1976)* 1991;16(8):962-966.
55. Handel SF, Twiford TW Jr, Reigel DH, Kaufman HH: Posterior lumbar apophyseal fractures. *Radiology* 1979;130(3):629-633.
56. Takata K, Inoue S, Takahashi K, Ohtsuka Y: Fracture of the posterior margin of a lumbar vertebral body. *J Bone Joint Surg Am* 1988;70(4):589-594.
57. Cammisa FP Jr, Eismont FJ, Green BA: Dural laceration occurring with burst fractures and associated laminar fractures. *J Bone Joint Surg Am* 1989;71(7):1044-1052.
58. Denis F, Burkus JK: Diagnosis and treatment of cauda equina entrapment in the vertical lamina fracture of lumbar burst fractures. *Spine (Phila Pa 1976)* 1991;16(8, Suppl):S433-S439.
59. Chapman JR, Anderson PA: Thoracolumbar spine fractures with neurologic deficit. *Orthop Clin North Am* 1994;25(4):595-612.
60. Clohisy JC, Akbarnia BA, Bucholz RD, Burkus JK, Backer RJ: Neurologic recovery associated with anterior decompression of spine fractures at the thoracolumbar junction (T12-L1). *Spine (Phila Pa 1976)* 1992;17(8, Suppl):S325-S330.
61. Crutcher JP Jr, Anderson PA, King HA, Montesano PX: Indirect spinal canal decompression in patients with thoracolumbar burst fractures treated by posterior distraction rods. *J Spinal Disord* 1991;4(1):39-48.
62. Lemons VR, Wagner FC Jr, Montesano PX: Management of thoracolumbar fractures with accompanying neurological injury. *Neurosurgery* 1992;30(5):667-671.
63. Mumford J, Weinstein JN, Spratt KF, Goel VK: Thoracolumbar burst fractures: The clinical efficacy and outcome of nonoperative management. *Spine (Phila Pa 1976)* 1993;18(8):955-970.
64. Sjöström L, Jacobsson O, Karlström G, Pech P, Rauschning W: Spinal canal remodelling after stabilization of thoracolumbar burst fractures. *Eur Spine J* 1994;3(6):312-317.
65. Hu SS, Capen DA, Rimoldi RL, Zigler JE: The effect of surgical decompression on neurologic outcome after lumbar fractures. *Clin Orthop Relat Res* 1993;288:166-173.
66. McAfee PC, Bohlman HH, Yuan HA: Anterior decompression of traumatic thoracolumbar fractures with incomplete neurological deficit using a retroperitoneal approach. *J Bone Joint Surg Am* 1985;67(1):89-104.
67. Aydınlı U, Karaeminoğullari O, Tişkaya K, Oztürk C: Dural tears in lumbar burst fractures with greenstick lamina fractures. *Spine (Phila Pa 1976)* 2001;26(18):E410-E415.
68. Holdsworth FW, Hardy A: Early treatment of paraplegia from fractures of the thoraco-lumbar spine. *J Bone Joint Surg Br* 1953;35-B(4):540-550.
69. Edwards CC, York JJ, Levine AM, et al: Determinants of spinal hook dislodgement. *Orthop Trans* 1986;10:8.
70. Lagrone MO, Bradford DS, Moe JH, Lonstein JE, Winter RB, Ogilvie JW: Treatment of symptomatic flatback after spinal fusion. *J Bone Joint Surg Am* 1988;70(4):569-580.
71. Dick W: The "fixateur interne" as a versatile implant for spine surgery. *Spine (Phila Pa 1976)* 1987;12(9):882-900.

72. Krag MH, Beynnon BD, Pope MH, Frymoyer JW, Haugh LD, Weaver DL: An internal fixator for posterior application to short segments of the thoracic, lumbar, or lumbosacral spine: Design and testing. *Clin Orthop Relat Res* 1986;203:75-98.
73. Magerl FP: External skeletal fixation of the lower thoracic and lumbar spine, in Uhthoff HK, ed: *Current Concepts of External Fixation of Fractures*. New York, NY, Springer-Verlag, 1982, pp 353-366.
74. Magerl FP: Stabilization of the lower thoracic and lumbar spine with external skeletal fixation. *Clin Orthop Relat Res* 1984;189:125-141.
75. Olerud S, Karlström G, Sjöström L: Transpedicular fixation of thoracolumbar vertebral fractures. *Clin Orthop Relat Res* 1988;227:44-51.
76. Butler JS, Fitzpatrick P, Ni Mhaolain AM, Synnott K, O'Byrne JM: The management and functional outcome of isolated burst fractures of the fifth lumbar vertebra. *Spine (Phila Pa 1976)* 2007;32(4):443-447.
77. Seybold EA, Sweeney CA, Fredrickson BE, Warhold LG, Bernini PM: Functional outcome of low lumbar burst fractures: A multicenter review of operative and nonoperative treatment of L3-L5. *Spine (Phila Pa 1976)* 1999;24(20):2154-2161.
78. McLain RF, Sparling E, Benson DR: Early failure of short-segment pedicle instrumentation for thoracolumbar fractures: A preliminary report. *J Bone Joint Surg Am* 1993;75(2):162-167.
79. Kaneda K, Abumi K, Fujiya M: Burst fractures with neurologic deficits of the thoracolumbar-lumbar spine: Results of anterior decompression and stabilization with anterior instrumentation. *Spine (Phila Pa 1976)* 1984;9(8):788-795.
80. Kirkpatrick JS, Wilber RG, Likavec M, Emery SE, Ghanayem A: Anterior stabilization of thoracolumbar burst fractures using the Kaneda device: A preliminary report. *Orthopedics* 1995;18(7):673-678.
81. Kostuik JP: Anterior fixation for fractures of the thoracic and lumbar spine with or without neurologic involvement. *Clin Orthop Relat Res* 1984;189:103-115.
82. Chakera TM, Bedbrook G, Bradley CM: Spontaneous resolution of spinal canal deformity after burst-dispersion fracture. *AJNR Am J Neuroradiol* 1988;9(4):779-785.
83. Krompinger WJ, Fredrickson BE, Mino DE, Yuan HA: Conservative management of fractures of the thoracic and lumbar spine. *Orthop Clin North Am* 1986;17(1):161-170.
84. Fredrickson BE, Edwards WT, Rauschning W, Bayley JC, Yuan HA: Vertebral burst fractures: An experimental, morphologic, and radiographic study. *Spine (Phila Pa 1976)* 1992;17(9):1012-1021.
85. Harrington RM, Budorick T, Hoyt J, Anderson PA, Tencer AF: Biomechanics of indirect reduction of bone retropulsed into the spinal canal in vertebral fracture. *Spine (Phila Pa 1976)* 1993;18(6):692-699.
86. Doerr TE, Montesano PX, Burkus JK, Benson DR: Spinal canal decompression in traumatic thoracolumbar burst fractures: Posterior distraction rods versus transpedicular screw fixation. *J Orthop Trauma* 1991;5(4):403-411.
87. Levine AM, Edwards CC, Gellad F: Indirect decompression of the spinal canal in the thoracolumbar spine. *American Spinal Injury Association, Abstracts Digest* Mar 20-22, 1987, pp 16-18.
88. Shuman WP, Rogers JV, Sickler ME, et al: Thoracolumbar burst fractures: CT dimensions of the spinal canal relative to postsurgical improvement. *AJR Am J Roentgenol* 1985;145(2):337-341.
89. Vornanen MJ, Böstman OM, Myllynen PJ: Reduction of bone retropulsed into the spinal canal in thoracolumbar vertebral body compression burst fractures: A prospective randomized comparative study between Harrington rods and two transpedicular devices. *Spine (Phila Pa 1976)* 1995;20(15):1699-1703.
90. Willén J, Lindahl S, Irstam L, Nordwall A: Unstable thoracolumbar fractures: A study by CT and conventional roentgenology of the reduction effect of Harrington instrumentation. *Spine (Phila Pa 1976)* 1984;9(2):214-219.
91. Hardaker WT Jr, Cook WA Jr, Friedman AH, Fitch RD: Bilateral transpedicular decompression and Harrington rod stabilization in the management of severe thoracolumbar burst fractures. *Spine (Phila Pa 1976)* 1992;17(2):162-171.
92. Viale GL, Silvestro C, Francaviglia N, et al: Transpedicular decompression and stabilization of burst fractures of the lumbar spine. *Surg Neurol* 1993;40(2):104-111.
93. Tropiano P, Huang RC, Louis CA, Poitout DG, Louis RP: Functional and radiographic outcome of thoracolumbar and lumbar burst fractures managed by closed orthopaedic reduction and casting. *Spine (Phila Pa 1976)* 2003;28(21):2459-2465.
94. Eismont FJ, Green BA, Berkowitz BM, Montalvo BM, Quencer RM, Brown MJ: The role of intraoperative ultrasonography in the treatment of thoracic and lumbar spine fractures. *Spine (Phila Pa 1976)* 1984;9(8):782-787.
95. Cardoso MJ, Dmitriev AE, Helgeson M, Lehman RA, Kuklo TR, Rosner MK: Does superior-segment facet violation or laminectomy destabilize the adjacent level in lumbar transpedicular fixation? An in vitro human cadaveric assessment. *Spine (Phila Pa 1976)* 2008;33(26):2868-2873.

96. Mueller LA, Mueller LP, Schmidt R, Forst R, Rudig L: The phenomenon and efficiency of ligamentotaxis after dorsal stabilization of thoracolumbar burst fractures. *Arch Orthop Trauma Surg* 2006;126(6):364-368.
97. Gardner VO, Thalgott JS, White JI, Lowery GL: The contoured anterior spinal plate system (CASP): Indications, techniques, and results. *Spine (Phila Pa 1976)* 1994;19(5):550-555.
98. Edwards CC, Levine AM: Early rod-sleeve stabilization of the injured thoracic and lumbar spine. *Orthop Clin North Am* 1986;17(1):121-145.
99. Fidler MW, Plasmans CM: The effect of four types of support on the segmental mobility of the lumbosacral spine. *J Bone Joint Surg Am* 1983;65(7): 943-947.
100. Brown T, Norton PL: The immobilizing efficiency of back braces; their effect on the posture and motion of the lumbosacral spine. *J Bone Joint Surg Am* 1957;39-A(1):111-139.
101. Blanco JF, De Pedro JA, Hernández PJ, Paniagua JC, Framiñán A: Conservative management of burst fractures of the fifth lumbar vertebra. *J Spinal Disord Tech* 2005;18(3):229-231.
102. Korovessis P, Baikousis A, Zacharatos S, Petsinis G, Koureas G, Iliopoulos P: Combined anterior plus posterior stabilization versus posterior short-segment instrumentation and fusion for mid-lumbar (L2-L4) burst fractures. *Spine (Phila Pa 1976)* 2006;31(8):859-868.
103. Parker JW, Lane JR, Karaikovic EE, Gaines RW: Successful short-segment instrumentation and fusion for thoracolumbar spine fractures: A consecutive 41/2-year series. *Spine (Phila Pa 1976)* 2000;25(9):1157-1170.
104. Marco RA, Kushwaha VP: Thoracolumbar burst fractures treated with posterior decompression and pedicle screw instrumentation supplemented with balloon-assisted vertebroplasty and calcium phosphate reconstruction. *J Bone Joint Surg Am* 2009;91(1):20-28.
105. Dekutoski MB, Conlan ES, Salciccioli GG: Spinal mobility and deformity after Harrington rod stabilization and limited arthrodesis of thoracolumbar fractures. *J Bone Joint Surg Am* 1993;75(2): 168-176.

CHAPTER 34
Fractures of the Sacrum

Kris Radcliff, MD Timothy DiIorio, MD Alvin Ong, MD Jordan Gruskay, BA
Alan M. Levine, MD Jeffrey A. Rihn, MD Alexander R. Vaccaro, MD, PhD

Introduction

Fractures of the sacrum are known to vary significantly in severity, ranging from the inconsequential buckle fracture to the grossly unstable injury with extensive neurologic deficit. Because of the unique position of the sacrum, surrounded by the relatively immobile sacroiliac joints and attached to the spine by a highly mobile disk space, the injuries encountered there vary widely depending on bone quality and the direction and amount of force applied. Within that continuum are avulsion fractures, buckle fractures, insufficiency fractures, pathologic fractures, isolated transverse and oblique fractures, and those sacral fractures associated with fractures of the pelvis. Despite increased recognition and imaging capabilities, sacral fractures, both with and without neural deficit, are often missed or their diagnosis is delayed. Thus, a systematic approach to the identification, assessment, classification, and treatment of these unusual injuries is necessary to minimize morbidity from neural deficit or the malunion or nonunion of sacral fractures.

Historical Perspective

In 1847, Malgaigne published his treatise on fractures, which contained a section devoted strictly to fractures of the sacrum. It is interesting to note that he credited Paul of Aegina (625-690) and Ambroise Paré (1510-1590) with the earliest writings on this subject. Malgaigne clearly distinguished between isolated sacral fractures and those that occurred in combination with pelvic injuries. He also gave a detailed description of injury biomechanics that included transverse, oblique, and vertical fracture patterns. Furthermore, his review of treatment methods provides insight into the earliest nonsurgical techniques.

Bonnin[1] published the next landmark article in 1945, presenting a series of 44 pelvic fractures with associated sacral injuries. He provided a detailed analysis of these fractures and proposed several classification schemes. In 1976, Gunterberg published his work on sacral resection, adding significant knowledge to both the neuroanatomy and bony biomechanics of the iliosacral region.[2] Schmidek et al[3] and Roy-Camille et al[4] both published notable reviews in the mid-1980s, with the latter work focusing specifically on transverse fractures. Later that decade, Denis et al[5] reported their comprehensive review of 776 pelvic fractures with 236 associated sacral injuries. The study presented a classification scheme that has gained widespread acceptance, and reviewed treatment protocols for each type of sacral fracture.

Dr. Ong or an immediate family member is a member of a speakers' bureau or has made paid presentations on behalf of Pfizer; serves as a paid consultant to or is an employee of Stryker; and has received research or institutional support from Pfizer and AK Pharma. Dr. Levine is deceased. At the time this chapter was written Dr. Levine or an immediate family member had received royalties from Elsevier and US Spine; was a member of a speakers' bureau or had made paid presentations on behalf of Accuray; served as a paid consultant to or was an employee of US Spine; and had received research or institutional support from Accuray, Amgen Co., and Medtronic Sofamor Danek. Dr. Rihn or an immediate family member has received research or institutional support from Medtronic Sofamor Danek. Dr. Vaccaro or an immediate family member serves as a board member, owner, officer, or committee member of the North American Spine Society, American Spinal Injury Association, and the Cervical Spine Research Society; has received royalties from Aesculap/B.Braun, DePuy, a Johnson & Johnson company, Globus Medical, Medtronic Sofamor Danek, K2M, Stout Medical, Progressive Spinal Technology, and Applied Spinal Intellectual Properties; serves as a paid consultant to or is an employee of K2M; has received research or institutional support from AO North America, DePuy, a Johnson & Johnson company, Medtronic Sofamor Danek, and Stryker; and owns stock or stock options in Globus Medical, Disk Motion Technology, Progressive Spinal Technologies, Advanced Spinal Intellectual Properties, Computational Biodynamics, Stout Medical, Paradigm Spine, K2M, Replication Medica, Spinology, Spine Medica, Orthovita, Vertiflex, Small Bone Technologies, NeuCore, Crosscurrent, Syndicom, In Vivo, Flagship Surgical, Pearl Driver, Location Based Intelligence, and Gamma Spine. None of the following authors or any immediate family member has received anything of value from or owns stock in a commercial company or institution related directly or indirectly to the subject of this chapter: Dr. Radcliff, Dr. DiIorio, and Mr. Gruskay.

Epidemiology

There is a bimodal distribution of sacral fractures in young and elderly patients. Low-velocity injuries (eg, falls) commonly result in compression fractures in the elderly. High-velocity injuries, such as falls from a height, suicide attempts, and motorcycle and other motor vehicle accidents, are common in young individuals. The majority of medium- to high-energy sacral fractures occur in conjunction with pelvic trauma. Sacral fractures have been reported to occur in association with 20% to 85% of pelvic fractures.[6,7] Although the quoted range of occurrence is wide (20% to 80%) because of constantly evolving methods of evaluation, the most realistic estimate is that approximately 40% to 45% of pelvic fractures occur in combination with a fracture of the sacrum. Isolated fractures of the sacrum are much less frequent, representing about 5% to 10% of all sacral injuries.[5,8]

Sacral fractures can be produced by both direct and indirect mechanisms. Direct injury mechanisms, such as blunt trauma to the sacrum and ilium, typically result in complex fracture patterns and low transverse fractures at the sacral apex of kyphosis (S3-S4).[3] Because the sacrum and pelvis make up a closed ring, forces imparted to the pelvic bones are transmitted to the sacrum laterally. Furthermore, force is also transmitted axially from the spinal column. The transmission of force to the sacrum from its connection to the pelvic ring or from the spinal column represents an indirect injury mechanism and typically results in a vertical fracture pattern or a high transverse fracture.

Anatomy/Biomechanics

The sacrum represents the terminal portion of the axial skeleton and typically consists of five fused vertebrae arranged in an overall kyphotic alignment with the apex at S3. The sacroiliac joint includes S1, S2, and part of S3, with the more caudal portion of the sacrum remaining free of the ilium. Methods of direct reduction and fixation of sacral fractures have been slow to evolve, in part because of the very difficult anatomic constraints of the sacrum. The sagittal contour of the sacrum is a gradual kyphosis of about 25° that extends from S1 to S5 with the apex between S2 and S3. At the lumbosacral junction (L5-S1), the weight of the torso is transmitted to the sacrum. The sacrum, in turn, transfers this load through the sacroiliac joint to the pelvis. The sacroiliac joint is therefore the connecting point between the axial and appendicular skeleton, and requires a stout ligamentous complex to stabilize this connection. The sacroiliac joint articulation occurs through the S1 and S2 vertebral bodies. The most significant stabilizers are the anterior and posterior sacroiliac ligaments, sacrotuberous ligaments, and sacrotransverse ligaments.

The sacral roots (S2-S4) are responsible for urinary continence and micturition, fecal continence and defecation, and sexual function. Input from the autonomic nervous system also plays an important role in all of these functions. The paired sacral nerve roots arise from the conus medullaris (at the level of the L1 vertebral body in an adult) and then course through the neural canal, exiting through the ventral and dorsal foramina.[9] Therefore, injury to the sacral roots can occur at the level of the conus medullaris, in the region of the sacral canal, or in the region of the foramina. The L5 roots exit the spinal canal posterior to the sacrum and then course anteriorly over the sacral ala as they traverse the pelvis. Fractures through the sacral ala can thus result in L5 root injury (**Figure 1**). The lumbosacral plexus and the internal iliac vein and artery cross the sacrum, coursing laterally at the S1 level (**Figure 2**). At their maximal thickness the sacral alae are frequently no more than 40 to 45 mm in their anteroposterior diameter. Denis et al[5] have studied in detail the sacral roots and foramina. They noted, on the basis of cross-sectional area, that root injury at the ventral foramen is less likely at S3 and S4 than at S1 and S2 of because the significant increase in the foramen-to-root ratio.[5] In assessing functional deficit from root injury, Gunterberg noted that unilateral disruption of the sacral roots does not result in loss of sphincter function; however, bilateral disruption results in loss of voluntary bowel and bladder control as well as in sexual dysfunction.[2] Previous studies on sacrectomy have found that the S3 nerve root is critical to the maintenance of bowel function and sexual function.[10,11]

Methods of direct reduction and fixation of sacral fractures have been slow to evolve, in part because of the very difficult anatomic constraints of the sacrum. The sagittal contour of the sacrum is a gradual kyphosis of about 25° that extends from S1 to S5 with the apex between S2 and S3. The effects of sacral resection on the biomechanical stability at the sacroiliac junction have been studied by Gunterberg.[2] His cadaveric studies revealed that the articulation between the sacrum and pelvis (at S1-S2) is the most critical for stability. Removal of the entire sacrum distal to the S1-2 "interspace" followed by testing with a vertical load to L5 resulted in weakening of the sacroiliac

FIGURE 1

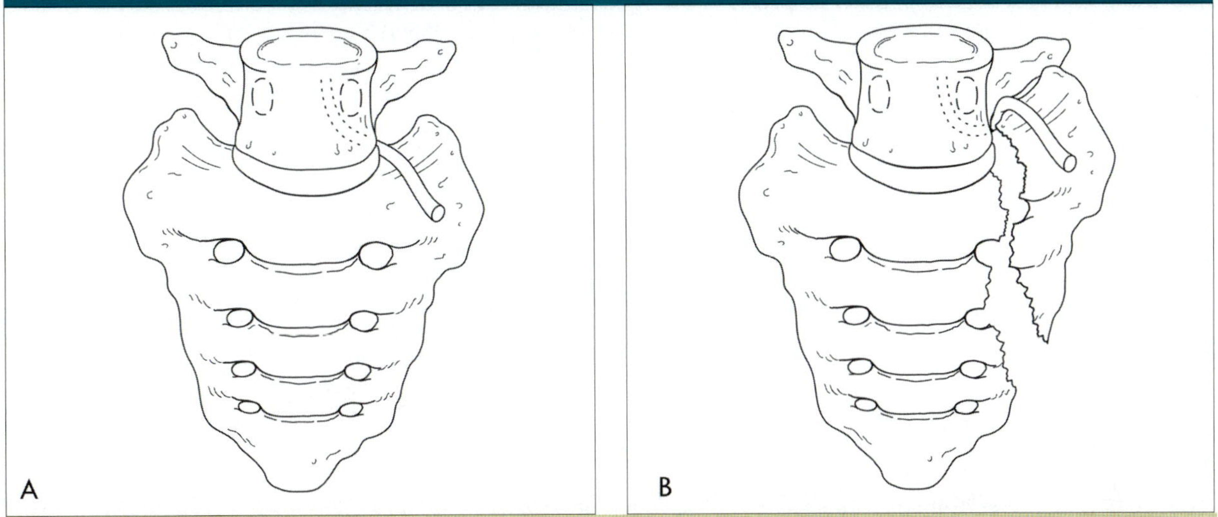

Figure 1 **A,** The L5 root courses proximally over the sacral ala to enter the lumbar plexus. In this location, it may be damaged by sacral fractures and by sacral fracture fixation. **B,** With vertical fractures of the sacrum in either zone 1 or 2, the L5 nerve root can be injured as it courses across the sacral ala. Mechanical damage or entrapment occurs as the L5 root is caught between the transverse process of L5 and the sacral ala as it migrates proximally; this has been termed the far-out syndrome. (Reproduced from Levine AM, Curcin A: Fractures of the sacrum, in Levine AM, Eismont FJ, Garfin SR, Zigler JE, eds: *Spine Trauma*. Philadelphia, PA, 1998, pp 506-524.)

junction by 30%. Extending the resection to include a major portion of S1, thereby removing half of the sacroiliac joint, weakened the junction by 50%. Using body weight and disk-loading calculations, Gunterberg postulated that adequate stability was retained at the sacroiliac joint after such resections to allow patients to safely stand and ambulate.[2]

Sacral anatomy creates a unique challenge for bony fixation. The area of maximal bone thickness occurs at the vestigial pedicle of each sacral segment and rapidly decreases with progression to distal sacral segments. At S3 or S4, the thickness may be as little as 15 mm to 20 mm. Pedicle screws at all levels penetrate from posterior to anterior and may be safely angled medially only at the S1 level. Pedicle screws directed medially through the anterior cortex of the body will safely avoid the neurovascular structures that lie on the lateral edge of the body and the medial edge of the ala. Angled properly along the vestigial pedicles of S1, pedicle screws will be 35 mm to 45 mm in length. In addition, at S1, "alar" screws can be angled laterally, parallel to the sacroiliac joint, and will enter a safe zone lateral to the neurovascular structures. Alar screws allow bicortical fixation with slightly longer screws of 40 mm to 50 mm, depending on the size of the patient. Therefore in most patients, both pedicle and alar screws can be simultaneously placed at S1. Pedicle screws can also be placed at S2 in most patients. However, on the left side, the sigmoid colon is in jeopardy with anterior screw penetration. The most secure bone fixation from S2 distally is with screws directed from medial to lateral. The entry point is on a line bisecting the dorsal foramina. The screws pass obliquely through the vestigial pedicle, traversing as much bone as possible without entering the sacroiliac joint. Placing successive screws in a convergent superoinferior direction can increase pullout strength. These anatomic considerations are of the most significance in transverse and oblique fractures.

Percutaneous lateral to medial sacroiliac joint screws can also be placed for treatment of sacral fractures. The concavity of the sacral alae may result in the false projection of the anterior aspect of the ala on a lateral view that may not accurately represent the entire bone. This may obscure the concavity of the ala and mislead the surgeon into thinking that a sacroiliac screw is intraosseous. With the use of image intensification, careful identification of both the superior and anterior aspects of the sacrum must occur to establish the safe zone for screw passage. This avoids the potential problem of exiting the ala anteriorly and then reentering it more medially.[12,13] At the S2 level, the body is usually identifiable, but it lies more posterior in the concavity of the sacrum. Passage of screws at that level is much more dangerous than at S1, and their use should be reserved for instances in which S1 is severely comminuted.

FIGURE 2

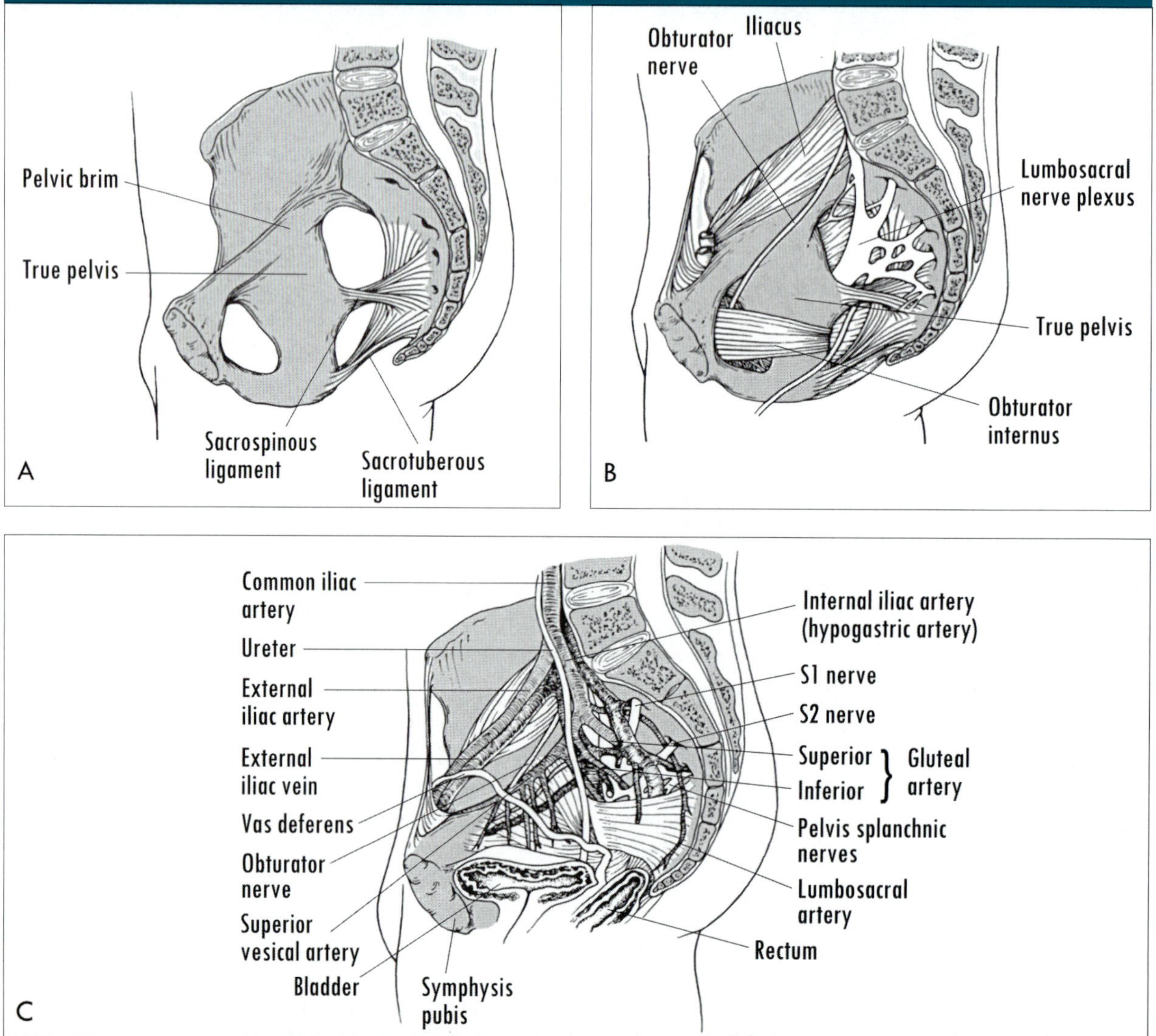

Figure 2 The anatomic relationship of the sacrum to the pelvis and sacral spine determines the nature of the fracture. **A,** The sacrum is secured to the pelvis by the sacrospinous and sacrotuberous ligaments. **B,** The major structures in the inner aspect of the pelvis are the lumbosacral plexus (as it originates from the L5 root and the sacral roots and leaves the pelvis through the greater sciatic notch at the sciatic nerve) and the superior gluteal artery. The internal obturator originates from the obturator membrane and loops out through the lesser sciatic notch. **C,** Anatomy of the internal aspect of the pelvis showing the relationship of the iliac vessels and lumbosacral plexus to the anterior surface of the sacral body and ala. (Reproduced with permission from Kellam JS, Browner BD: Fractures of the pelvic ring, in Browner BD, Jupiter JB, Levine AM, Trafton PG, eds: *Skeletal Trauma: Fractures, Dislocations, Ligamentous Injuries.* Philadelphia, PA, WB Saunders, 1992, pp 852-853.)

Evaluation

Following appropriate evaluation and stabilization of cardiovascular and pulmonary systems, the victim and the rescue personnel should be questioned about the details of the accident. Attention should be focused on high-energy deceleration mechanisms, such as jumps or falls from a height, motorcycle accidents, and roll-over motor vehicle accidents. These injury mechanisms should serve as warning signs to the evaluating physician to thoroughly evaluate the pelvic ring for injury. Physical examination should include palpation over the entire spinal column including the sacrum. Commonly, areas of localized tenderness and/or hematoma indicate the presence of a sacral fracture. Manual compression over the iliac crests, both anteroposteriorly and laterally, can also aid in identifying injury, although the examination may displace a fracture. As part of the routine examina-

FIGURE 3

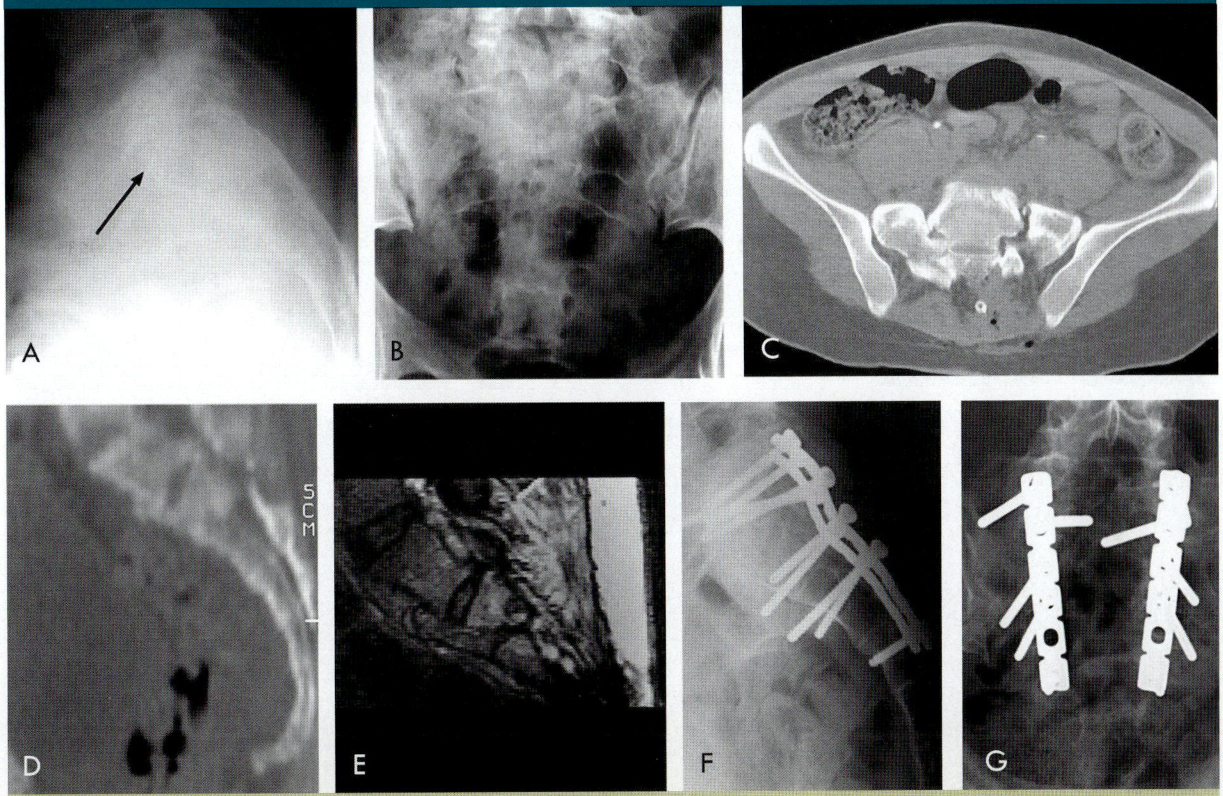

Figure 3 This 19-year-old woman was involved in a motor vehicle accident and sustained a transverse sacral fracture. The fracture was not well visualized on either the initial lateral (**A**) or AP (**B**) radiograph, and was therefore not recognized at first. The lateral radiograph only shows a slight break in the normal sagittal alignment (arrow). On the AP view, only the vertical component of the fracture is visible, because the fracture lines are obscured by overlying gas shadows. Although the patient had loss of bowel and bladder function, this also was not appreciated initially. However, when the localized neural deficit was recognized, a CT scan was obtained. **C,** The axial view does not reveal the transverse component of the fracture, but only the vertical portion. **D,** The midsagittal reconstruction does not clearly demonstrate the anatomy of the fracture. **E,** MRI, however, showed an angulated fracture in the S2 region. The fracture was in extreme kyphosis with the superior fragment displaced posterior to the inferior fragment. The patient underwent surgical reduction and decompression with plate fixation as shown on lateral (**F**) and AP (**G**) postoperative views. Note the double screw fixation in S1, which stabilizes the proximal fragment, with the most cephalad screw directed medially and the second screw directed laterally. The patient regained bowel and partial bladder function with return of perineal sensation. (Reproduced from Levine AM, Curcin A: Fractures of the sacrum, in Levine AM, Eismont FJ, Garfin SR, Zigler JE, eds: *Spine Trauma*. Philadelphia, PA, 1998, pp 506-524.)

tion, the external genitourinary system and the anus and rectum must be assessed for sensory, motor, and reflex function.[14-16] Perforations through the rectum and disruption of the bladder and ureter must be considered, as they are not uncommon with high-energy injuries to the pelvic ring. The patient with a sacral fracture associated with pelvic ring injury may require massive resuscitation efforts and very close monitoring as a result of disruption of sacral vasculature and associated catastrophic bleeding.[17] Mortality rates may be high despite optimal treatment[17,18] and may require measures such as military antishock trousers or a pelvic external fixator[19] to attain initial stability. Embolization may even be necessary to attain hemodynamic stability.[10] Particularly in the case of a sacral fracture associated with a lumbar spine fracture,[9] careful neurologic examination is critical to proper correlation of neurologic deficit with the appropriate level of injury.

After a general radiologic assessment appropriate for a polytrauma victim is completed, a more specialized evaluation of the sacrum and pelvis can be undertaken. Injuries to the sacrum may not be obvious on an AP pelvic radiograph because of the 45° posterior inclination of the sacrum. On both the AP and lateral views of the sacrum, detail is often obscured by overlying soft tissue and gas shadows (**Figure 3**, *A* and *B*). In addition, the overlying iliac wing makes precise definition of

FIGURE 4

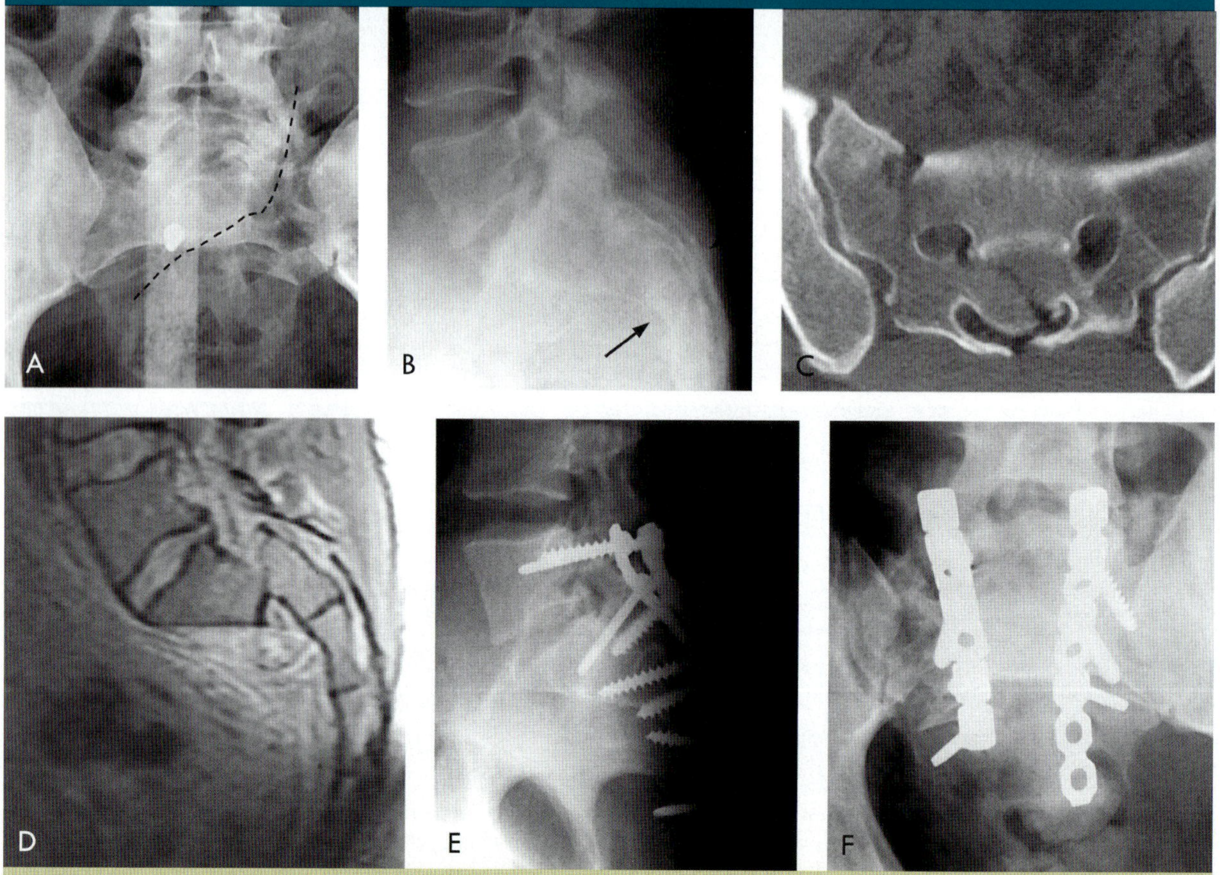

Figure 4 The patient, a 30-year-old-man, fell from a height of 35 ft, landing on both feet and falling backward onto his buttocks. He sustained multiple injuries to both feet and an oblique sacral fracture with a complete neural injury at the S2 level. **A,** The AP radiograph did not clearly demonstrate the oblique nature of the fracture line (dashed line) with extension into the L5-S1 articulation on one side. **B,** The lateral view shows the increase in kyphosis apparent at the fracture site (arrow). **C,** The axial CT scan clearly shows the oblique nature of the zone 3 line as it courses through the floor of the canal into the neuroforamen and into the ventral surface of the sacrum. **D,** The nature of the displacement is better seen on MRI, with the proximal fragment displaced anteriorly and the distal fragment posteriorly. The fracture traversed the base of the S1 facet on the right and therefore required plating to the L5 pedicle (**E** and **F**) to achieve reduction and stabilization. (Reproduced from Levine AM, Curcin A: Fractures of the sacrum, in Levine AM, Eismont FJ, Garfin SR, Zigler JE, eds: *Spine Trauma*. Philadelphia, PA, 1998, pp 506-524.)

the injury more difficult.[20-22] The exception to this rule is a vertical fracture of the sacrum, in which unilateral proximal migration of the hemipelvis and/or a transverse process fracture at L5 is usually apparent. A Ferguson AP view using a 30° cranial projection makes visualization of the upper sacrum easier, but it does not improve the view of the lower sacrum.[5] Coned-down sacral lateral, inlet, and outlet views should be obtained in every case of suspected sacral injury. Recognizing that these fractures are easily missed on plain radiographs, the films should be closely scrutinized with attention to the bony anatomy as described by Bonnin.[1] The thoracolumbar spine should be assessed carefully for evidence of burst fractures, L5 transverse process fracture, or lumbosacral facet dislocation, which are common associated injuries.[1,4,5,23]

CT scan has become the standard of care for the evaluation of both pelvic and sacral fractures[5,23-25] (**Figure 3**, *C*). CT scans with narrow sections (2-mm maximum sections) and appropriate orientation of the sagittal and coronal reconstructions, can provide detailed information about the fracture.[26] Attention to plane orientation is necessary, because even if the plane of the axial section is perpendicular to the two proximal segments of the sacrum, the orientation of the distal portion of the sacrum changes by 20° to 30°. Thus, as the images are taken through the area of the fracture, the reconstruction plane may not be appropriately aligned, resulting in distortion of the clarity of the fracture lines[27] (**Figure 3,** *D*).

For sacral fractures with severe neurologic deficit, the use of MRI may be considered in the work-up of these injuries (**Figure 3,** *E*). The combination of myelography and CT scan is of less value in this region, because flow of dye into the root sleeves in this area is limited.[14-16,26,28] MRI is now the study of choice as it has been found to be extremely helpful in the diagnosis and treatment planning of these injuries. The advantages of MRI include the ability to routinely obtain clear sagittal and axial views of the entire sacrum and neural elements (**Figure 4**). Neural element compression by displaced fracture fragments or hematoma within the canal can also be readily identified.

In patients with bowel and bladder functional deficit, additional studies (eg, cystometrograms[5,20,29] and electromyograms) should also be considered. Dynamic triggered electromyography, motor-evoked potentials, and somatosensory-evoked potentials can likewise be used to assess the neural injury.[30] These studies are helpful in precisely documenting the extent of the injury (especially in noncommunicative patients) and may also provide a prognosis for recovery. These studies are typically obtained soon after the acute injury occurs and can be repeated to assess for functional recovery.

Classification

Up to this point, no comprehensive system of classification of sacropelvic injuries has been universally accepted, though several different classifications of sacral fractures have been proposed.[1,4,5,23,31-33] The earliest detailed analysis and categorization of sacral fractures was published by Bonnin[1] in 1945. He identified six different types of sacral fractures from a review of 44 pelvic injuries, 20 of which had sacral involvement. Furthermore, he provided an insightful discussion of biomechanical mechanisms, neurologic injury, and radiographic evaluation. In 1972, Huittinen[34] contributed an understanding of the relationship of nerve root injuries. He found that nerve root avulsions were found in 40% of the patients with vertical shear fractures of the sacrum and almost universally in transverse fractures of the sacrum.

Schmidek et al[3] reviewed the literature and their own case material and proposed a classification that begins by distinguishing between direct and indirect traumatic mechanisms. Based on this framework, four fractures are described (**Figure 5**). Low transverse fractures and penetrating injuries (eg, gunshot wounds) are classified as direct trauma mechanisms. Meanwhile, indirect traumatic mechanisms often result in vertical fractures (lateral mass, juxta-articular, cleaving, or avulsion) or a high transverse pattern. Subsequently, Sabiston and Wing reviewed 35 sacral fractures and proposed a similar, but much simpler, system[32] (**Figure 6**).

The most comprehensive analysis of sacral fractures has been reported by Denis et al,[5] consisting of 235 sacral fractures in a series of 776 patients with pelvic injuries. To assist in the analysis of their data, these authors also performed anatomic cadaveric studies of the sacral roots and foramina. Their classification system is based on identifying three vertical zones through the sacrum (**Figure 7**). Zone 1 is in the region of the sacral ala and ends immediately lateral to the sacral foramina. Zone 2 encompasses the region of the foramina, and zone 3 covers the region of the central

FIGURE 5

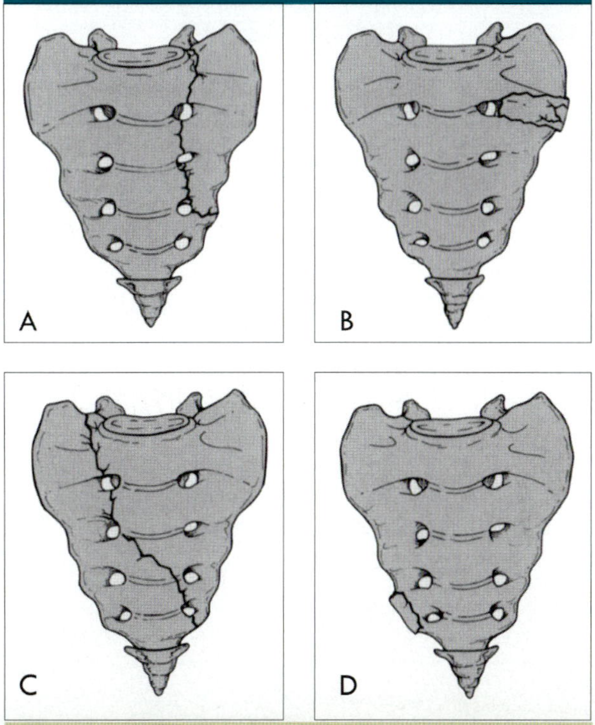

Figure 5 Schmidek classified vertical fractures into four patterns. These include lateral mass fractures (**A**), juxta-articular fractures (**B**), cleaving fractures (**C**), and avulsion fractures (**D**). (Redrawn with permission from Schmidek HH, Smith DA, Kristiansen TK: Sacral fractures. *Neurosurgery* 1984;15(5):735.)

5: Thoracolumbar Injuries

FIGURE 6

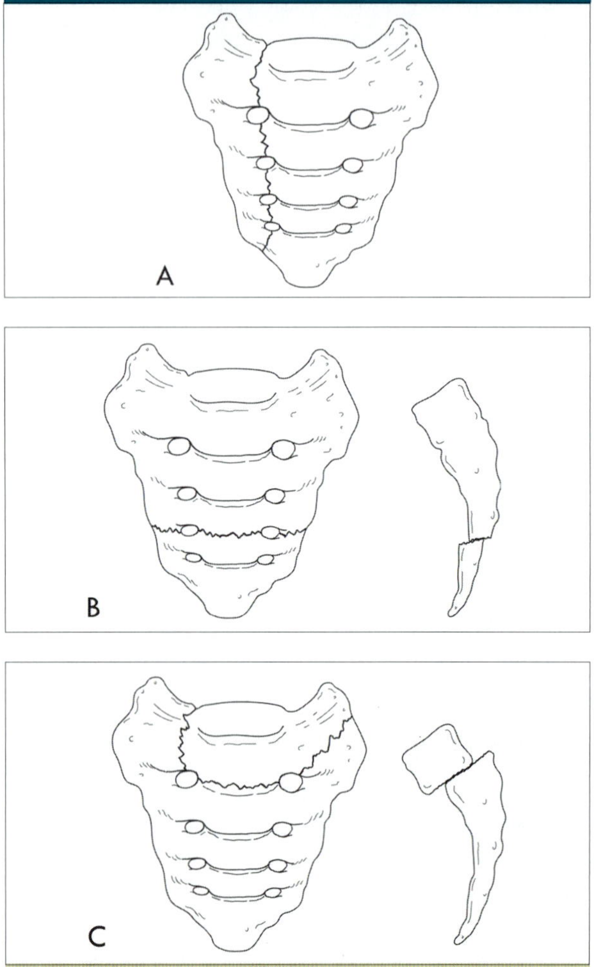

Figure 6 Sabiston's classification of sacral fractures had three main types: type **A,** vertical fractures; type **B,** transverse below the level of the sacroiliac joint; and type **C,** transverse at the level of the sacroiliac joints with vertical components. (Redrawn with permission from Sabiston CP, Wing PC: Sacral fractures: Classification and neurologic implications. *J Trauma* 1986;26(12):1114.)

FIGURE 7

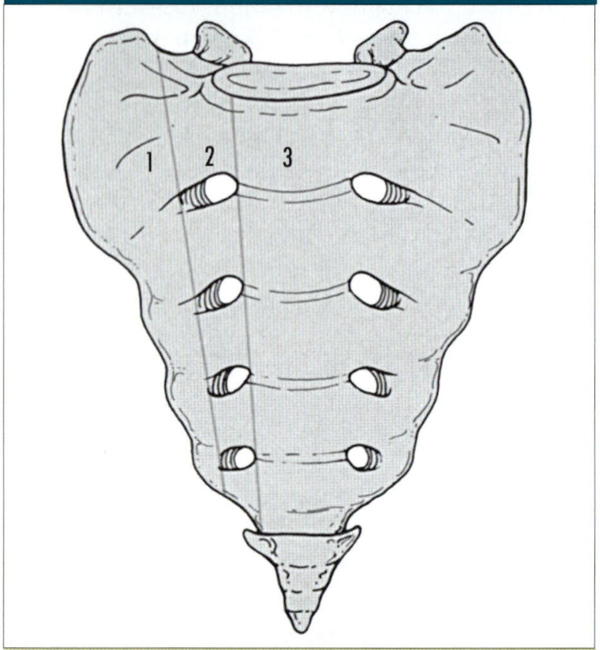

Figure 7 Denis et al classified 238 fractures of the sacrum according to zones. Zone I was the sacral ala and comprised 118 patients, with only 5.9% having neural deficit. Zone 2 was through the neural foramina and comprised 81 patients, of whom 28.4% had neural deficits. Zone 3 was through the central canal and was seen in only 21 patients, of whom 56.7% had deficits. (Redrawn with permission from Denis F, Davis S, Comfort T: Sacral fractures: An important problem: Retrospective analysis of 236 cases. *Clin Orthop Relat Res* 1988;227:67.)

sacral canal. Injuries are assigned to the highest zone that the fracture line transgresses. Therefore, a fracture that passes through all three zones would be classified as a zone 3 injury (**Figure 7**).

Zone 1 injuries ranged from minor avulsion fractures to unstable vertical shear mechanisms with fractures lateral to the sacral foramina. These injuries rarely presented with neurologic deficit (6%) other than sciatic nerve or L5 root involvement.[5] Zone 2 fractures passed through one or more foramina and carried a 28% incidence of neurologic injury. Because these fractures are usually unilateral and do not involve the central canal, bowel and bladder deficits are not expected. The L5 root, however, may be involved by entrapment in the alar fracture, leading to a "traumatic far-out syndrome" (**Figure 1**). Zone 3 fractures, by definition, transgress the central canal and carry an overall 57% incidence of neurologic injury; 76% of patients presented with bowel, bladder, and sexual function deficit.

Other than vertical fractures, oblique or transverse fractures can occur (**Figure 8**).[1,6,35,36] Transverse fractures were initially classified as a separate group by Roy-Camille et al[4] and then modified by Strange-Vognsen (**Figure 9**).[33,37] Roy-Camille et al reviewed 13 cases of transverse sacral fractures and also conducted cadaveric experiments to study the fracture mechanism. They noted that 11 of the 13 cases resulted from suicide jumps, implicating axial loading as the predominant force of injury. From their clinical and biomechanical data, three distinct fracture types were described. The type I injury is a flexion injury without significant displacement or deformity. The type II fracture is a flexion injury with posterior displacement of the cephalad fragment. Type III fractures are caused by

FIGURE 8

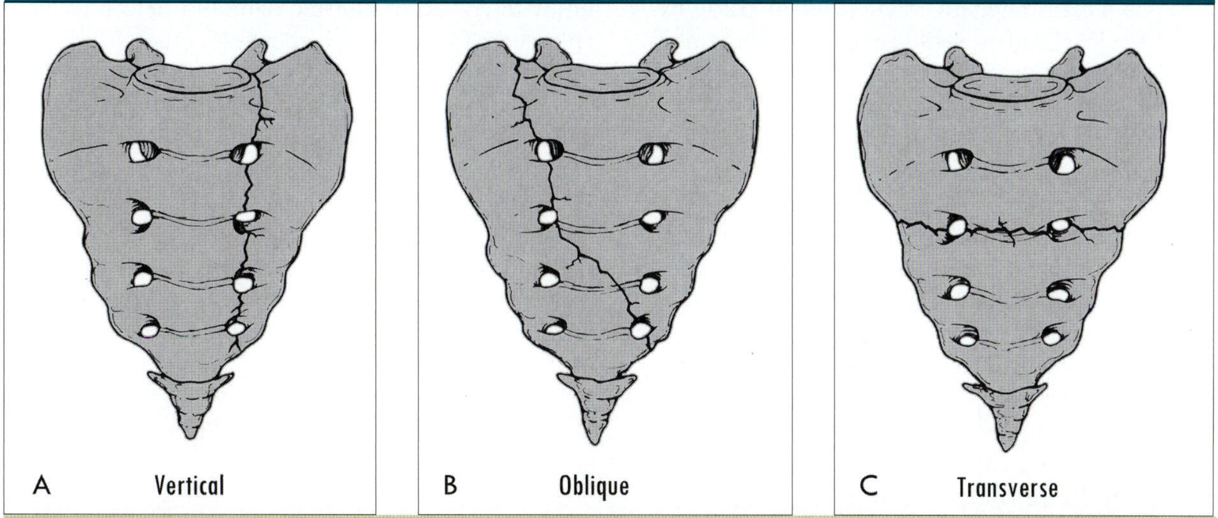

Figure 8 Classification of sacral fractures. Fractures of the sacrum can be classified in several different ways. One of the most common is according to the direction of the fracture line within the sacrum. Therefore, fractures can either be vertical (**A**), oblique (**B**), or transverse (**C**). These fractures can occur at any level in the sacrum. Vertical fractures may occur in the ala or through the foramina. Similarly, oblique fractures can occur at any location. Transverse fractures are less common and more frequently occur at the apex of the sacral kyphosis between S2 and S3, but they may occur as a high transverse fracture at S1 or S2. (Reproduced with permission from Levine AM: Lumbar and sacral trauma, in Browner BD, Jupiter JB, Levine AM, Trafton PG, eds: *Skeletal Trauma: Fractures, Dislocations, Ligamentous Injuries*. Philadelphia, PA, WB Saunders, 1992, p 818.)

FIGURE 9

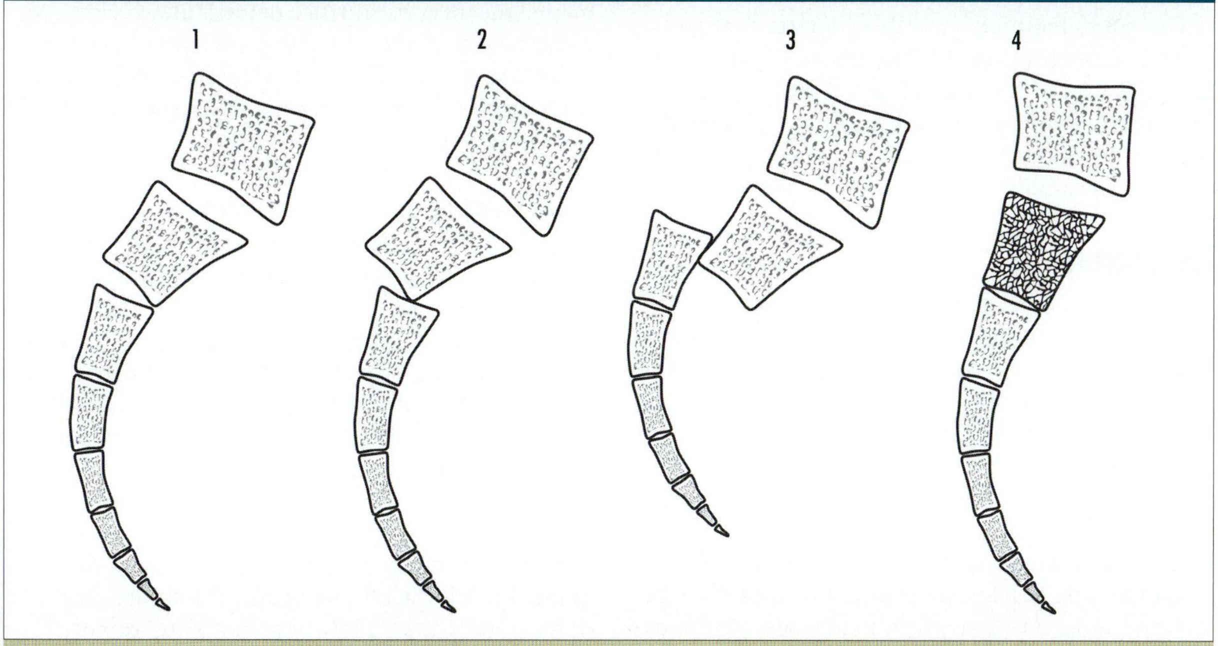

Figure 9 Subclassification of Denis zone 3 fractures as suggested by Strange-Vognsen and Lebech.[33] Type 1 fractures are flexion injuries with angulation and no translation. Type 2 fractures are combination flexion and translation injuries. Type 3 fractures are pure translation injuries in flexion or extension (flexion illustrated here). Type 4 fractures are axial loading injuries that result in comminuted fractures of the S1 and possibly S2 vertebral bodies. This classification is not mutually exclusive with that of Denis et al. (Redrawn with permission from Schildhauer TA, Bellabarba C, Nork SE, Barei DP, Routt ML Jr, Chapman JR: Decompression and lumbopelvic fixation for sacral fracture-dislocations with spino-pelvic dissociation. *J Orthop Trauma* 2006;20(7):447-457.)

an extension moment with anterior displacement of the cephalad fragment. A subsequent study by Kaehr et al[25] classified 140 fractures with the aid of CT scanning and emphasized the importance of that radiographic tool for complete understanding of the injury. Six types of injuries were visualized. Type I consisted of avulsion injuries. Type II injuries were through the ala and were the most common (45%). Type III injuries were transforaminal (23.6%) and type IV injuries were medial to the foramina. Type V fractures were transverse (5%) and type VI injuries were complex variations. Some of the fractures that are considered transverse are in fact oblique, a fact emphasized by Isler[23] but noted previously by Roy-Camille. The L5-S1 articulation can be disrupted by an oblique fracture of the sacrum. Extra-articular fracture of the base of the superior S1 facet may cause instability and spondylolisthesis at that level or, alternatively, the fracture may disrupt the joint integrity directly.

Treatment decisions are based on three criteria. First, it is important to know whether the sacral injury is isolated or is accompanied by a pelvic injury. Second, the fracture line must be identified as either vertical or transverse. Finally, if the fracture is oblique, it is important to ascertain whether it involves the L5-S1 articulation.

The combination of multiple longitudinal and transverse fractures in the sacrum may result in a disconnection of the axial skeleton from the pelvis, termed a spinopelvic dissociation.[38] These injuries may result in severe cauda equina compression and instability.[37]

Treatment

The three principal goals in managing sacral fractures are (1) reestablishment of stability of the pelvic ring and lumbosacral junction, (2) correction and prevention of angular (kyphotic) and translational (shear) deformities of both the pelvic ring–sacrum and lumbosacral junction, and (3) prevention of further neural deficit and treatment of existing neurologic injury with appropriate decompressive and stabilizing procedures.

Maintaining pelvic ring stability is important in both the acute and long-term management phases. In the immediate posttraumatic period, unstable pelvic injuries may be associated with significant and sometimes life-threatening hemorrhage. The application of external fixators can help to bring such hemorrhage under control.[39] Likewise, acute stabilization of the pelvic ring may also prevent further neurologic injury. For long-term management, reestablishing pelvic ring stability should ultimately prevent chronic pain and deformity and enhance patient care by allowing earlier mobilization.

The angular (kyphotic) and translational (shear) deformities associated with sacral fractures may be factors in both instability and neurologic injury. The presence of major angular or translational deformity often heralds an unstable injury, and correction of the deformity should accompany stabilization. Furthermore, correction of such deformities may relieve some of the compression of neural elements. Angular and translational deformities should also be corrected to prevent chronic skin problems (eg, over a sacral gibbus) or difficulty with sitting balance and lumbosacral biomechanics.

Neurologic injury can be caused directly as a result of compression of the sacral roots by fracture fragments, nerve entrapment at the level of the foramina or ala (L5 root), avulsion or laceration of the roots, or indirectly by traction on the cauda equina. Depending on the fracture pattern, the neurologic deficit can present as an isolated root deficit, radiculopathy, multiple root deficits, or complete cauda equina syndrome. Reestablishing pelvic ring stability and correcting the deformity may alleviate compression of the neural elements and prevent further deterioration. However, if the neural elements remain entrapped despite reduction and stabilization, direct decompression is required as well to prevent significant deficit or neuropathic pain.

Treatment of Specific Fractures

Because of the unique anatomic relationship of the spine and pelvis to the sacrum, treatment methods need to be tailored to four clinical situations: a vertical sacral fracture, a transverse sacral fracture, a sacral fracture in combination with a pelvic fracture, and a sacral insufficiency or iatrogenic fracture. Although some authors have recommended conservative treatment of these injuries,[1,32,40] a growing consensus supports surgical management.[3-5,29,41]

Patients with intact neurologic function and minimally displaced or angulated fractures (eg, stable zone 1 and 2 injuries) may only require 6 to 12 weeks of non–weight bearing followed by progressive mobilization in a cast or brace (**Figure 10**) and then ambulatory status as tolerated.[1,8,9,42-44] During this period, the patient's neurologic function is carefully monitored and the fracture is assessed with serial radiographs. Given the typically well-vascularized fracture site, these

FIGURE 10

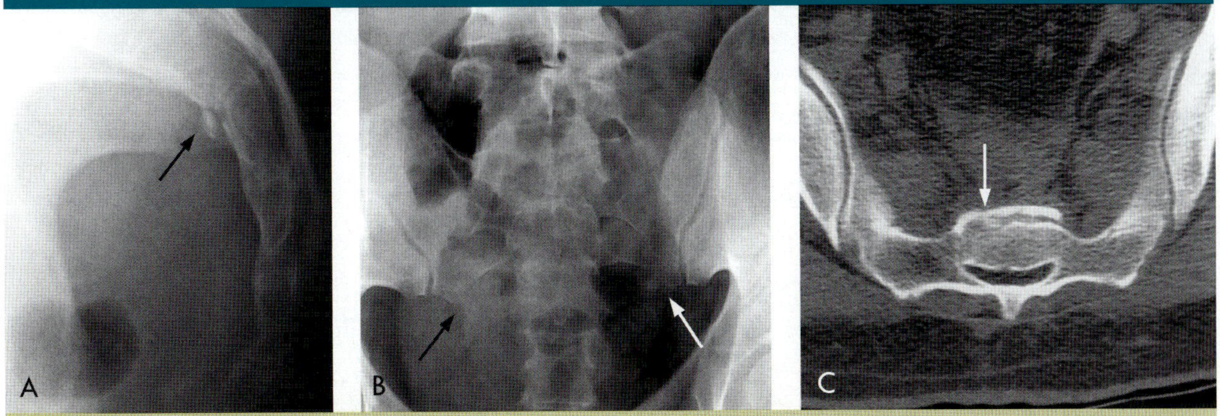

Figure 10 This patient fell from a height and landed on his buttocks. **A,** The lateral radiograph shows an increase in kyphosis and comminution of the anterior cortex (arrow). **B,** On the AP view, the fracture line occurred at the level of the termination of the sacroiliac joint and its attachment to the sacrum (arrows). **C,** The CT scan shows minimal comminution with only fracturing of the anterior cortex (arrow). (Reproduced from Levine AM, Curcin A: Fractures of the sacrum, in Levine AM, Eismont FJ, Garfin SR, Zigler JE, eds: *Spine Trauma*. Philadelphia, PA, 1998, pp 506-524.)

injuries should be fully united by 3 months.

Displaced vertical fractures, especially in zones 2 and 3, with or without other pelvic involvement, may be treated with fixation with percutaneous compression across the posterior aspect of the ilium and sacrum. Fully threaded screws may be used for direct screw fixation, which can be done with little or no compression. Recent biomechanical studies[34,45] evaluating fixation for transforaminal fractures have shown little difference between one or two iliosacral screws in combination with posterior tension bands or posterior transiliac bar devices. The technique of iliosacral screw placement, in either the prone or supine operative positions, has been well described (**Figure 11**). Occasionally, bowel preparation is indicated to improve image accuracy in the pelvis. Additionally, nitrous oxide anesthetic may be associated with extensive bowel gas and should not be used. Whether the patient is in a prone or supine position, the operation must be done on a radiolucent table to allow fluoroscopy[12,13] or CT scan guidance.[46] With a supine position, a radiolucent bolster is placed under the lumbosacral spine to allow sufficient access. The image intensifier is placed on the opposite side from the surgeon. Initial calibration of the angles is performed to determine the ideal position to obtain sacral inlet and outlet views. On a true pelvic inlet view, the S1 and S2 vertebral bodies are superimposed. The inlet view will be used to confirm the anteroposterior position of the screw in the S1 vertebral body (**Figure 11,** *A*). On a true pelvic outlet view, the S1 end plate is linear because the x-ray beam is

FIGURE 11

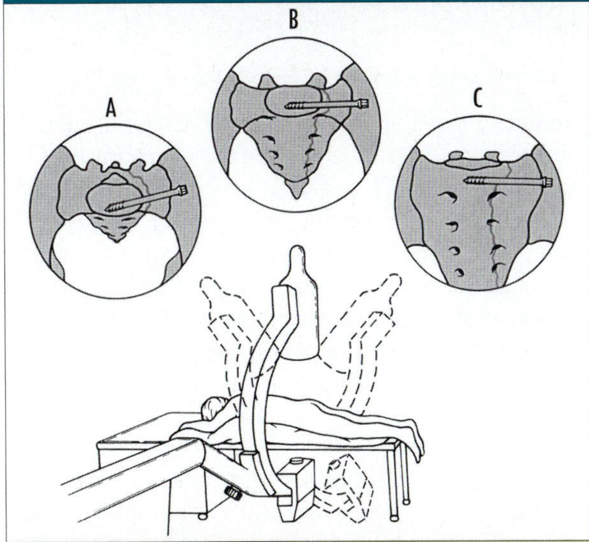

Figure 11 Iliosacral screw fixation. To be certain that iliosacral screw fixation into the sacrum is accurate, some type of monitoring is necessary, which in most cases is image intensification. The image must be placed so that 40° caudal and 40° cephalad views can be obtained. A partially threaded screw can be used for fractures in zone 1, although a fully threaded screw should be used in zone 2 (transforaminal) fractures so that compression is not applied to the comminuted bone, causing further impingement on the exiting roots. **A,** True pelvic inlet view. The S1 and S2 vertebral bodies are superimposed. **B,** Postoperative AP image. **C,** True pelvic outlet view. The S1 end plate is linear, indicating that the beam is parallel to the L5-S1 interspace. (Reproduced with permission from Kellam JS, Browner BD: Fractures of the pelvic ring, in Browner BD, Jupiter JB, Levine AM, Trafton PG, eds: *Skeletal Trauma: Fractures, Dislocations, Ligamentous Injuries*. Philadelphia, PA, WB Saunders, 1992, p 888.)

FIGURE 12

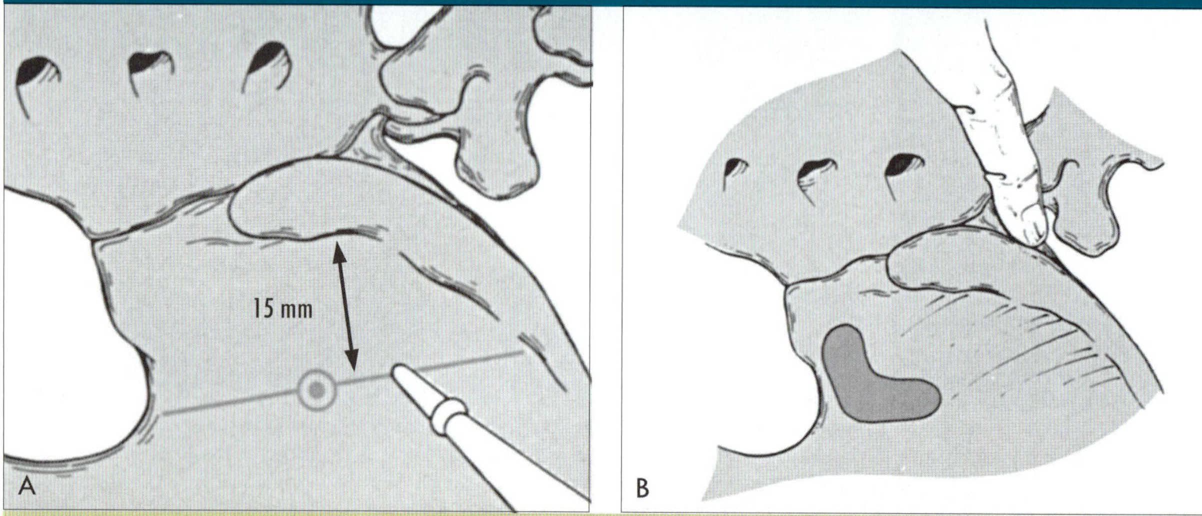

Figure 12 This figure shows the starting position for screw fixation of vertical sacral fractures. **A,** The proper position is 15 mm anterior to the gluteal attachments at the posterior superior iliac crest on a line drawn at the midportion of the greater sciatic notch. **B,** This point is also approximately 2.5 cm from the top of the posterior superior iliac crest and 2.5 cm superior to the greater sciatic notch. (Reproduced with permission from Kellam JS, Browner BD: Fractures of the pelvic ring, in Browner BD, Jupiter JB, Levine AM, Trafton PG, eds: *Skeletal Trauma: Fractures, Dislocations, Ligamentous Injuries.* Philadelphia, PA, WB Saunders, 1992, p 888.)

parallel to the L5-S1 disk space. The outlet view is used to confirm the cephalad-caudal position of the screw in the S1 vertebral body (**Figure 11,** *B*).

Next, care is taken that an anatomic reduction is achieved either by positioning or traction, and the reduction is verified by image intensification. The position of the starting hole is another critical aspect of obtaining adequate screw position. Several different techniques exist for determining the starting hole, but most are based on the intersection of single lines emanating from both the sciatic notch and the posterior superior iliac crest (**Figure 12**). If two screws are used, one screw should be as posterior and superior as possible in the S1 vertebral body and the other screw should be anterior and inferiorly placed. For unilateral involvement of the ala, penetration needs to be at least to the midline for zone 1 injuries and across the midline for zone 2 injuries. Penetration should cross the midline into the contralateral ala for zone 3 fractures with an oblique or vertical component. It is preferable to use a 6.5-mm fully threaded cannulated cancellous screw for vertical sacral fractures. This prevents further compression across the comminuted fracture site, which decreases the chance for impingement of roots in transforaminal fractures. Screw length generally averages between 60 mm and 90 mm, but a screw as long as 130 mm may be required to reach the contralateral ala. Use of the calibrated direct measurement on the image intensifier makes the choice of screw length easier. Washers should be used to prevent penetration of the screw head into the ilium.

For patients with either isolated oblique or transverse fractures of the sacrum, the technique of bilateral plating of the posterior surface of the sacrum is applicable (**Figures 3, 4,** and **13**). Minimally displaced fractures should not be considered for this technique. This procedure is done with the patient in the prone position, with slight flexion of the table in its midportion. A radiolucent operating table is necessary, with image intensification available for screw placement. A wide exposure of the spine is done from L5 down to S4 through a midline exposure. During posterior dissection in the area of the fracture line, care is taken to avoid motion of the comminuted fragments to prevent root damage or incidental durotomy. Dissection is performed laterally beyond the dorsal foramen at all levels from S1 to S4. The L5-S1 facet joint capsules are preserved if there is no involvement at L5-S1. Otherwise, the L5-S1 facet joint capsules are removed. Once exposure of the posterior aspect of the sacrum is achieved from S1 to S4, then the posterior aspect of the fracture line can be fully identified. Exposure of the posterior aspect of the sacrum can be facilitated by removing the distal attachment of the paraspinous musculature subperiosteally from the

FIGURE 13

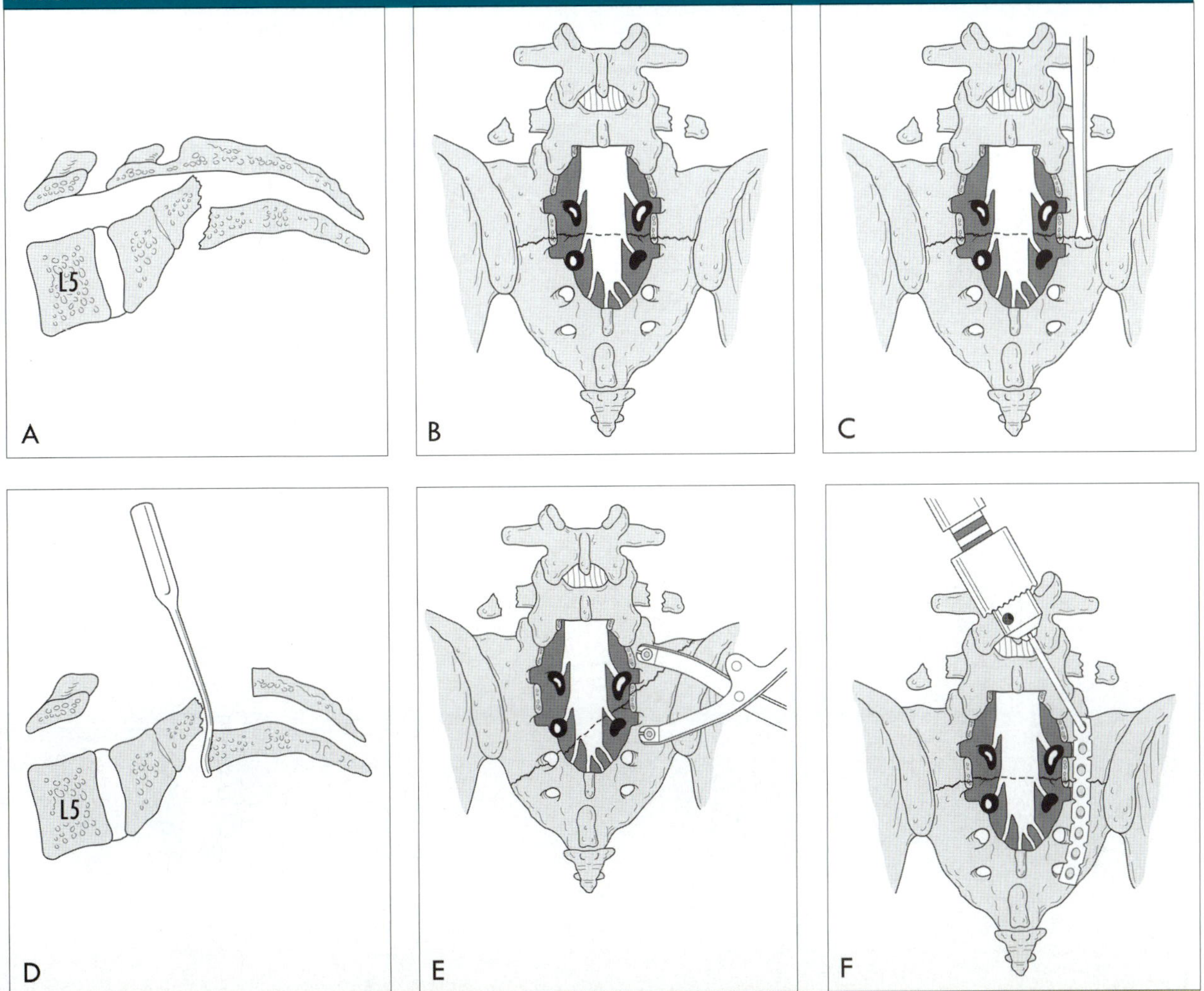

Figure 13 Technique of reduction and plate fixation of transverse sacral fractures. The transverse fracture line in the sacrum usually occurs at the region of the second or third dorsal foramen. **A,** The lateral view of the model demonstrates the kyphosis of the fracture as well as the translational deformity. The majority of transverse sacral fractures occur in the most kyphotic area of the sacrum, S2-S3. After appropriate work-up to delineate the direction of the fracture and the area of maximal sacral root compression, the patient is placed in the prone position with the hips flexed 45°. The incision runs from the inferior tip of the L4 spinous process to the region of S4. Although the sacrum is approached through a midline incision and the posterior aspect is stripped subperiosteally, exposure is often insufficient. The exposure can be broadened by detaching the inferiormost attachment of the paraspinal musculature from the sacrum posterior to S3 and S4. **B,** The first step in reduction is to expose the complete fracture line and then do a laminectomy approximately 2.5 cm in length, centered on the fracture line, to clearly visualize the neural elements. It should be carried far enough laterally to extend out into the dorsal foramen. **C,** After the nerve roots are clearly delineated, the fracture line is opened on both sides of the sacrum, first using a small curet and then gently inserting a small Cobb elevator in each side to pry apart the impacted fracture. By using the elevators to gently lever the fracture, the kyphosis and translation can be at least partially reduced. If the proximal fragment is posteriorly displaced (**D**), then the instrument should be placed under the ventral surface of the distal fragment. Separation of the fracture fragments and at least partial reduction are critical steps before plate fixation can begin. A 3.5-mm or 4.5-mm pelvic reconstruction plate is selected on the basis of hole spacing and the size of the sacrum. If the anatomic position is achieved manually, then the plate is contoured to directly match the contour of the posterior aspect of the sacrum; if the position is less than anatomic, then the plate is slightly undercontoured. If the fracture is more oblique and shortened, then a temporary screw can be placed in both the proximal and distal fragments and a distraction tool can be applied to achieve length while the final plate is being positioned. **E,** With the exception of the S1 segment, plate placement and screw starting points lie on a line along the dorsal foramen with the screw directed laterally into the residual pedicle. At S1, two screws are placed, with the more proximal screw directed laterally from the dimple at the base of the S1 facet. **F,** The proximal S1 screw is drilled bicortically and tapped and then inserted.

FIGURE 13 (CONTINUED)

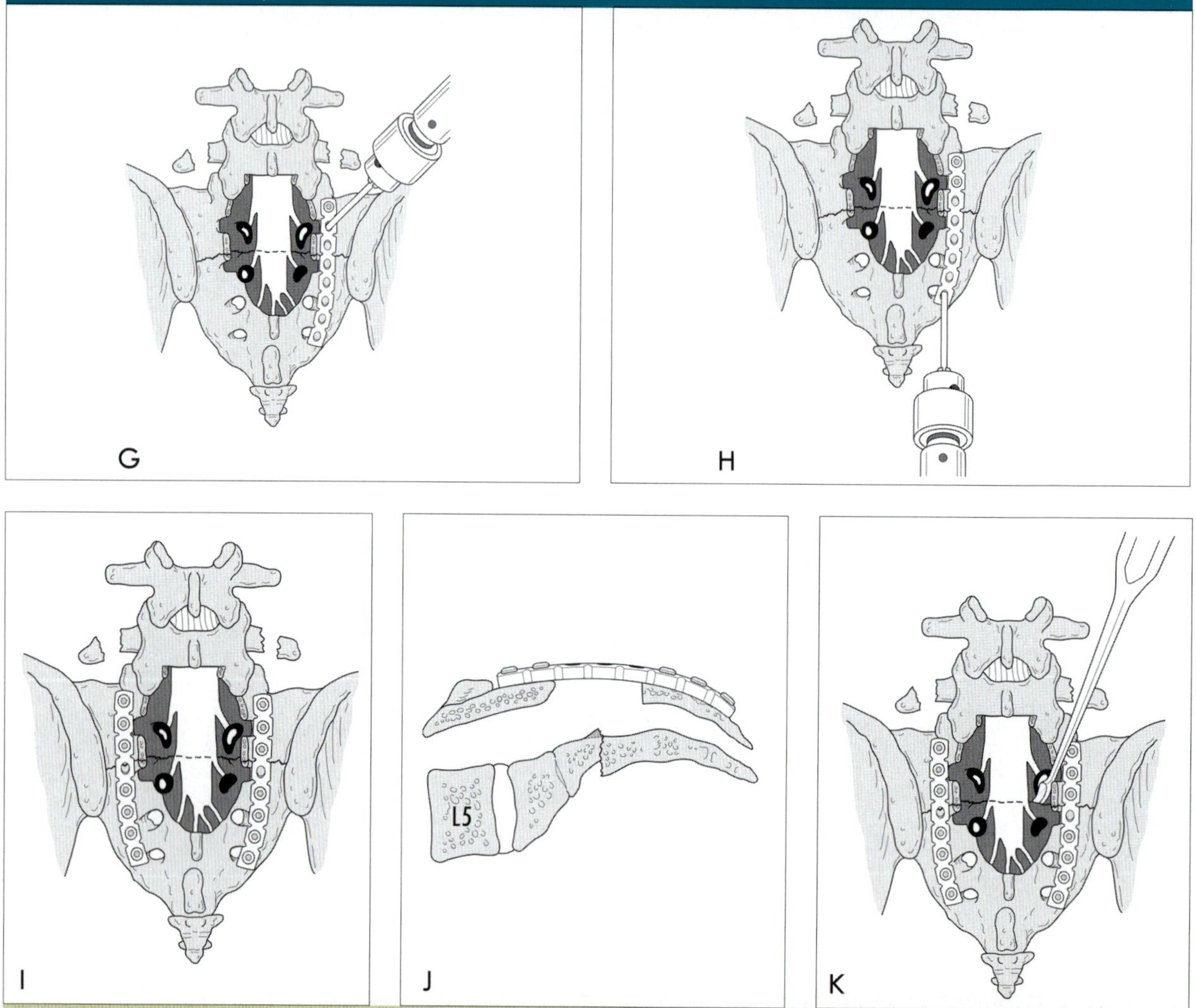

Figure 13 (*continued*) **G,** The second screw in S1 is inserted and directed medially into the body. It likewise is tapped and inserted either to the full depth of the body or bicortically. **H,** The starting site for the most distal screw is selected. A minimum of two and preferably three points of fixation need to be present distal to the fracture line. These screws are angled obliquely, parallel to the sacroiliac joint for maximal length and fixation. An attempt should be made to place pairs of adjacent screws to converge in the caudocephalad direction for maximal pull-out strength. The most distal screws will rarely exceed 20 mm, whereas the more proximal screws will average between 35 mm and 45 mm. The screw is tightened into position but is not used to achieve fracture reduction. If the reduction is not complete and the plate is completely in contact with the posterior aspect of the sacrum, further manual reduction is done before final tightening of all screws. Screws are then placed in every hole that does not fall directly over a dorsal foramen. **I,** The contralateral side is plated in a similar fashion. **J** and **K,** Decompression of the sacral roots is checked by gently retracting the roots toward the midline, and any residual impinging bone is removed with a curet or pituitary rongeur. Tamping the fragments down into the sacrum is much less effective. The contralateral side is also checked and, if reduction was incomplete, decompression is still possible by resecting the residual bone of the displaced portion of the floor of the canal. Decompression should not be attempted without stabilization, as shifting of the fracture alignment can easily cause compression to recur. (Modified with permission from Levine AM: Lumbar and sacral trauma, in Browner BD, Jupiter JB, Levine AM, Trafton PG, eds: *Skeletal Trauma: Fractures, Dislocations, Ligamentous Injuries.* Philadelphia, PA, WB Saunders, 1992, p 845.)

posterior aspect of the sacrum at its terminal portion, which generally occurs in the region of S3-S4. The next step is to perform a sacral laminectomy to accurately identify the sacral roots and the area of maximal deformity and compression. The laminectomy is begun proximal to the fracture and the level of deficit, and extended distally because the canal is larger proximally than distally. A small Kerrison rongeur and spinal curets are used to complete the laminectomy to the level of the sacral pedicles on both sides. The lateral decompression must extend laterally enough to identify the take-off point of the ventral root sleeves and the bone of the vestigial sacral pedicles. Once the deformity is identified and the laminectomy is completed, enabling direct visualization of the roots, attention is turned to reduction of the fracture. Care should be taken, however, to ascertain that the ventral surfaces of the roots at the level of the maximal fracture angulation are not trapped in the fracture site. Because the sacral roots are freely visible after the decompression, a Cobb elevator can be safely placed within the fracture to lever the fragments, or bone clamps may be used to apply corrective translational forces to reduce the fracture.[3,4] Complex multiplanar fractures would be reduced in similar fashion, with the possible addition of intraoperative skeletal traction to reduce the vertical shear. Plate placement is generally in a line directly over the dorsal foramina. Commonly 3.5-mm or 4.5-mm pelvic reconstruction plates are used to achieve stabilization. For transverse or transverse/oblique fractures within the body of the sacrum that do not involve the L5-S1 articulation, a minimum of two sets of screws proximal and distal to the fracture line is preferable. Because bone stock and screw fixation points are limited in the sacrum, reduction should not be achieved while levering on the plate. If the fracture configuration permits, we prefer to insert both medial and lateral screws into the sacrum at S1, thereby achieving optimum fixation into the superior fragment. The most proximal screw, at the lateral border of the S1 superior facet, is directed approximately 30° medially into the S1 body through the pedicle, aiming at the sacral promontory. The next screw, at the inferior edge of the S1 facet, is directed 35° laterally into the sacral ala and parallel to the sacral end plate. In the remainder of the levels, a single or double screw traversing the pedicle laterally and parallel to the sacroiliac joint is preferred. The average proximal screw inserted at the level of the medial border of the S1 facet is usually directed about 30° medially, entering into the S1 body; the screw length generally averages 35 to 45 mm. The next screw is inserted below the inferior edge of the S1 facet and is directed laterally approximately 35° into the sacral ala and parallel into the plane of the sacroiliac joint. The proximal screws average approximately 30 mm to 45 mm in length. The screws at S2, S3, and S4 are shorter (approximately 20 mm at the most distal point). The trajectory is between 20° and 35° laterally.

Fixation two levels above and below the fracture may require pedicle screw fixation into L4, L5, S1, or iliac bolts. Rods are connected to the screws, and cross-locking is suggested.[33] Plating constructs include 3.5-mm or 4.5-mm pelvic reconstruction plates. Bone grafting is usually not necessary for fractures contained totally within the sacrum, although any residual graft can be used to fill in the defects. However, for those that traverse the L5-S1 articulation, standard transverse process sacral alar grafting should be done with autologous cancellous bone. Reapproximation of the paraspinous musculature over the hardware and fracture is critical. These wounds are extremely fragile, particularly in the presence of a soft-tissue degloving injury (Morel-Lavellée lesion), which often accompanies high energy pelvic trauma. Additionally, patients can develop sacral decubiti that can compromise wound integrity. Careful monitoring and considering of gluteal rotational flaps with the assistance of a plastic surgeon is essential. Postoperatively, the patient is placed into a custom-molded total-contact orthosis, with one thigh incorporated into the brace. Once in the brace, the patient progresses to ambulation as tolerated. Bracing is typically continued on a full-time basis for 10 to 12 weeks. Plate removal is not advocated unless it is causing soft tissue irritation.

For a fracture with a pelvic ring disruption, in addition to preserving neural function, the goal is a stable, pain-free pelvic ring. Unstable pelvic injuries should be treated with emergent application of an external fixator as has been described.[34,39] If vertical displacement is present, then skeletal traction should be added. Several methods have been described for surgical management of pelvic injuries with sacral components including indirect reduction with either anterior external fixation or anterior surgical stabilization.[5,12,18,35,45,47-58] Finally, direct reduction and stabilization of vertical sacral fractures has been described[12,45,47-51] using both anterior and posterior sacroiliac plating, sacral bar techniques, and tension band plates across the ilium.[47,52] Most recently, the percutaneous stabilization technique with sacroiliac screws has been described.[9,12,13,39]

Sacral insufficiency fractures may be idiopathic or secondary to segmental posterior lumbosacral fixation in elderly, osteoporotic patients. These injuries are usually initially treated nonsurgically.[59] Surgery is indicated, however, for patients who have nonunions, persistent pain, neurologic deficits, or gross displacement.[60] Relapse of lower back or buttock pain and leg pain after thoracolumbar fusion to the sacrum may be related to a sacral fracture. Surgery should be considered in the presence of a concomitant L5-S1 pseudarthrosis and when symptoms do not improve with nonsurgical treatment.[61] Also, stabilization of the sacrum and pelvis may be required when a kyphotic deformity develops from the fracture, resulting in an acute loss in sagittal balance as well as an increase in pain.[62] In such cases, one of several surgical procedures described previously may be recommended. Percutaneous sacroplasty may be used to treat sacral fractures as long as the surgeon avoids polymethylmethacrylate (PMMA) cement injection into the actual fracture line.[63] This method appears to be a safe and effective treatment of painful osteoporotic sacral insufficiency fractures, resulting in rapid symptomatic improvement. However, the long-term sequelae of this procedure are unknown. Lumbopelvic fixation, a useful salvage treatment modality for patients who fail nonsurgical treatment, may also be recommended.[59] If this salvage treatment also fails, fibular grafting may be successfully used to treat sacral insufficiency fractures.[60] An approach that may be considered to remedy a fracture sustained from a previous surgery for multilevel instrumented fusion healed in a kyphotic position is the use of a sacral pedicle subtraction osteotomy, with multiple sacral alar osteotomies to correct the sacral kyphosis and pelvic incidence.[62]

Results

The majority of the literature about sacral fractures includes case reports and other anecdotal reports[1,4,14,21,22,43,44,55,56,64-67] and very few substantial and well-documented series. Denis et al[5] published the most extensive series and found that zone 1 stable injuries were well treated by bed rest and early mobilization. The incidence of neurologic injury and recovery seems to be highly dependent on fracture pattern and severity of neural tissue damage. Zone 1 and 2 fractures typically present with unilateral L5 or S1 root deficit in approximately 6% to 30% of patients.[5,7] Recovery from deficits caused by root avulsion or transection, which have been found to occur in as many as 40% of autopsy specimens studied,[34] cannot be expected. Recovery from deficits caused by root compression at the level of the sacral foramen, or traumatic far-out lesions of L5, occurs reliably after either closed reduction or decompression accompanied by open reduction and internal fixation.

Zone 3 injuries result in a greater than 50% incidence of neurologic deficit.[5,7] Transverse zone 3 fractures above the S4 foramen are almost invariably accompanied by severe sacral root deficit, including bowel, bladder, and sexual dysfunction.[28,64] Recovery from such a deficit is enhanced by direct decompression and stabilization and ranges from 50% to 100%.[5,7,20] Root avulsions are common in transverse fracture patterns, which often occur in the region of the dorsal root ganglion.[34] As shown by Gunterberg,[2] patients with unilateral sacral root disruption retain the potential for voluntary sphincter control, although recovery may take 6 months or longer. In the series of Denis et al,[5] five patients had loss of bowel and bladder function, were treated surgically, and had return of function in all cases, whereas in the three treated nonsurgically, two of three had partial return of function and one had no return. Denis et al[5] also noted neural fibrosis forming around the roots in cases of decompression following fracture healing. This observation further strengthens the argument for early surgical intervention. Gibbons et al[7] found either partial or complete recovery in 7 of 8 patients treated surgically and in only 3 of 15 treated nonsurgically. Furthermore, in the series of Albert et al,[9] surgically treated cases showed more consistent return of function than did nonsurgically treated cases. Because these are all root injuries, residual compression due to the kyphotic nature of the injury deformity is at least partially responsible for the failure of recovery seen with nonsurgical treatment. However, Sabiston and Wing[32] had nine patients with neural deficits, all of whom were treated conservatively with bed rest and traction. All but one showed some improvement.

Conclusions

Sacral fractures are potentially devastating injuries that occur most frequently in conjunction with pelvic ring trauma. A high index of suspicion is required when evaluating trauma patients to identify the injuries, as they are difficult to recognize and are frequently overlooked; however, a detailed clinical examination and careful scrutiny of the radiographs often uncover a sacral fracture. In many cases, with unstable injuries and dense neural deficit, aggressive decompression and stabilization can lead to early mobilization and good functional results. Surgical techniques vary on the basis of the constellation of injuries and the direction of the fracture line. Although they have been classified as zone 1 to 3 injuries, considering the direction of the fracture line is most helpful in deciding on the surgical treatment. Vertical fracture lines are best treated with iliosacral screw fixation. However, for purely transverse and oblique fractures through zone 3, with or without neurologic deficit, fixation techniques have dramatically evolved. In patients with neural deficit, early recognition, accurate imaging, and surgical stabilization and decompression are essential for optimal recovery of bowel and bladder function in cases of severely displaced fractures.

References

1. Bonnin JG: Sacral fractures and injuries to the cauda equina. *J Bone Joint Surg* 1945;27:113-127.
2. Gunterberg B: Effects of major resection of the sacrum: Clinical studies on urogenital and anorectal function and a biomechanical study on pelvic strength. *Acta Orthop Scand Suppl* 1976;162:1-38.
3. Schmidek HH, Smith DA, Kristiansen TK: Sacral fractures. *Neurosurgery* 1984;15(5):735-746.
4. Roy-Camille R, Saillant G, Gagna G, Mazel C: Transverse fracture of the upper sacrum. *Spine (Phila Pa 1976)* 1985;10(9):838-845.
5. Denis F, Davis S, Comfort T: Sacral fractures: An important problem. Retrospective analysis of 236 cases. *Clin Orthop Relat Res* 1988;227:67-81.
6. Bucknill TM, Blackburne JS: Fracture-dislocations of the sacrum: Report of three cases. *J Bone Joint Surg Br* 1976;58-B(4):467-470.
7. Gibbons KJ, Soloniuk DS, Razack N: Neurological injury and patterns of sacral fractures. *J Neurosurg* 1990;72(6):889-893.
8. Levine AM: Lumbar and sacral spine trauma, in Browner BD, Jupiter JB, Levine AM, Trafton PG, eds: *Skeletal Trauma*. Philadelphia, PA, WB Saunders, 1992.
9. Albert TJ, Levine MJ, An HS, Cotler JM, Balderston RA: Concomitant noncontiguous thoracolumbar and sacral fractures. *Spine (Phila Pa 1976)* 1993;18(10):1285-1291.
10. Ben-Menachem Y, Handel SF, Ray R, Childs TL: Embolization procedures in trauma: The pelvis. *Semin Intervent Radiol* 1985;2:158-181.
11. Guo Y, Palmer JL, Shen L, et al: Bowel and bladder continence, wound healing, and functional outcomes in patients who underwent sacrectomy. *J Neurosurg Spine* 2005;3(2):106-110.
12. Routt ML Jr, Meier MC, Kregor PK, Mayo KA: Percutaneous iliosacral screws with the patient supine technique. *Oper Tech Orthop* 1993;3:35-45.
13. Routt ML Jr, Simonian PT, Inaba J: Iliosacral screw complication. *Oper Tech Orthop* 1997;7(3): 206-220.
14. Dowling T, Epstein JA, Epstein NE: S1-S2 sacral fracture involving neural elements of the cauda equine: A case report and review of the literature. *Spine (Phila Pa 1976)* 1985;10(9):851-853.
15. Guidera KJ, Raney E, Ogden JA, Highhouse M, Habal M: Caudal regression: A review of seven cases, including the mermaid syndrome. *J Pediatr Orthop* 1991;11(6):743-747.
16. Schnaid E, Eisenstein SM, Drummond-Webb J: Delayed post-traumatic cauda equina compression syndrome. *J Trauma* 1985;25(11):1099-1101.
17. Hesp WL, van der Werken C, Keunen RW, Goris RJ: Unstable fractures and dislocations of the pelvic ring—results of treatment in relation to the severity of injury. *Neth J Surg* 1985;37(5): 148-152.
18. Goldstein A, Phillips T, Sclafani SJ, et al: Early open reduction and internal fixation of the disrupted pelvic ring. *J Trauma* 1986;26(4):325-333.
19. Ganz R, Krushell RJ, Jakob RP, Küffer J: The antishock pelvic clamp. *Clin Orthop Relat Res* 1991; 267:71-78.
20. Fountain SS, Hamilton RD, Jameson RM: Transverse fractures of the sacrum: A report of six cases. *J Bone Joint Surg Am* 1977;59(4):486-489.
21. van der Werken C, van Tets WF: Intrapelvic intrusion of the lumbosacral spine. *Acta Orthop Belg* 1992;58(3):336-338.
22. Yasuda T, Shikata J, Iida H, Yamamuro T: Upper sacral transverse fracture: A case report. *Spine (Phila Pa 1976)* 1990;15(6):589-591.
23. Isler B: Lumbosacral lesions associated with pelvic ring injuries. *J Orthop Trauma* 1990;4(1):1-6.
24. Gill K, Bucholz RW: The role of computerized tomographic scanning in the evaluation of major pelvic fractures. *J Bone Joint Surg Am* 1984;66(1): 34-39.
25. Kaehr DM, Anderson PA, Mayo KA, Benca PJ, Benirschke SK: Classification of sacral fractures based on CT imaging. *J Orthop Trauma* 1989; 3(2):163.
26. Rommens PM, Vanderschot PM, Broos PL: Conventional radiography and CT examination of pelvic ring fractures: A comparative study of 90 patients. *Unfallchirurg* 1992;95(8):387-392.
27. Savolaine ER, Ebraheim NA, Rusin JJ, Jackson WT: Limitations of radiography and computed tomography in the diagnosis of transverse sacral fracture from a high fall: A case report. *Clin Orthop Relat Res* 1991;272:122-126.
28. Ehrensperger J: Fractures of the sacrum and disk herniation: Rare lesions in the pediatric surgical patient? *Eur J Pediatr Surg* 1992;2(3):173-176.
29. Pohlemann T, Angst M, Schneider E, Ganz R, Tscherne H: Fixation of transforaminal sacrum fractures: A biomechanical study. *J Orthop Trauma* 1993;7(2):107-117.
30. Schrader SC, Sloan TB, Toleikis JR: Detection of sacral sparing in acute spinal cord injury. *Spine (Phila Pa 1976)* 1987;12(6):533-535.

31. Medelmann JP: Fractures of the sacrum: Their incidence in fractures of the pelvis. *Am J Roentgenol Radium Ther Nucl Med* 1939;42:100-103.
32. Sabiston CP, Wing PC: Sacral fractures: Classification and neurologic implications. *J Trauma* 1986; 26(12):1113-1115.
33. Strange-Vognsen HH, Lebech A: An unusual type of fracture in the upper sacrum. *J Orthop Trauma* 1991;5(2):200-203.
34. Huittinen VM: Lumbosacral nerve injury in fracture of the pelvis: A postmortem radiographic and patho-anatomical study. *Acta Chir Scand Suppl* 1972;429:3-43.
35. Browner BD, Cole JD, Graham JM, Bondurant FJ, Nunchuck-Burns SK, Colter HB: Delayed posterior internal fixation of unstable pelvic fractures. *J Trauma* 1987;27(9):998-1006.
36. Carl A, Blair B: Unilateral lumbosacral facet fracture-dislocation. *Spine (Phila Pa 1976)* 1991; 16(2):218-221.
37. Bellabarba C, Schildhauer TA, Vaccaro AR, Chapman JR: Complications associated with surgical stabilization of high-grade sacral fracture dislocations with spino-pelvic instability. *Spine (Phila Pa 1976)* 2006;31(11, Suppl)S80-S88.
38. Schildhauer TA, Bellabarba C, Nork SE, Barei DP, Routt ML Jr, Chapman JR: Decompression and lumbopelvic fixation for sacral fracture-dislocations with spino-pelvic dissociation. *J Orthop Trauma* 2006;20(7):447-457.
39. Kellam JF, Browner BD: Fractures of the pelvic ring, in Browner BD, Jupiter JB, Levine AM, Trafton PG, eds: *Skeletal Trauma*. Philadelphia, PA, WB Saunders, 1992.
40. Phelan ST, Jones DA, Bishay M: Conservative management of transverse fractures of the sacrum with neurological features: A report of four cases. *J Bone Joint Surg Br* 1991;73(6):969-971.
41. Fisher RG: Sacral fracture with compression of cauda equina: Surgical treatment. *J Trauma* 1988; 28(12):1678-1680.
42. Das De S, McCreath SW: Lumbosacral fracture-dislocations: A report of four cases. *J Bone Joint Surg Br* 1981;63-B(1):58-60.
43. Lee KS, Bae WK, Bae HG, Yun IG: Natural course of spontaneously reduced lumbo-sacral fracture-dislocation—a case report. *J Korean Med Sci* 1993; 8(5):390-393.
44. Purser DW: Displaced fracture of the sacrum: Report of a case. *J Bone Joint Surg Br* 1969;51(2): 346-347.
45. Simonian PT, Routt C Jr, Harrington RM, Tencer AF: Internal fixation for the transforaminal sacral fracture. *Clin Orthop Relat Res* 1996;323:202-209.
46. Nelson DW, Duwelius PJ: CT-guided fixation of sacral fractures and sacroiliac joint disruptions. *Radiology* 1991;180(2):527-532.
47. Ebraheim NA, Coombs R, Hoeflinger MJ, Zeman C, Jackson WT: Anatomical and radiological considerations in compressive bar technique for posterior pelvic disruptions. *J Orthop Trauma* 1991; 5(4):434-438.
48. Matta JM, Saucedo T: Internal fixation of pelvic ring fractures. *Clin Orthop Relat Res* 1989;242: 83-97.
49. Miller MD, Cain JE, Lauerman WC, Littlefield WG, Platenberg RC, Wilson MR: Posterior sacroiliac fixation using a sacral pedicle targeting device: an anatomical study. *J Orthop Trauma* 1993;7(6): 514-520.
50. Stocks GW, Gabel GT, Noble PC, Hanson GW, Tullos HS: Anterior and posterior internal fixation of vertical shear fractures of the pelvis. *J Orthop Res* 1991;9(2):237-245.
51. Tile M: Pelvic ring fractures: Should they be fixed? *J Bone Joint Surg Br* 1988;70(1):1-12.
52. Dietrich J, Mears DC: Surgical reconstruction of 121 unstable sacral fractures. *J Orthop Trauma* 1989;3(2):180.
53. Carter TR, Lambert K: Pubic diastasis with longitudinal fracture of the sacral body: Case report. *J Trauma* 1990;30(5):627-629.
54. Daum WJ, Patterson RM, Cartwright TJ, Viegas SF: Comparison of cortical and cancellous screw pull-out strengths about the posterior column and sacroiliac joint. *J Orthop Trauma* 1991;5(1):34-37.
55. Fredrickson BE, Yuan HA, Miller HE: Treatment of painful long-standing displaced fracture-dislocations of the sacrum: A case report. *Clin Orthop Relat Res* 1982;166:93-95.
56. Hanley EN Jr, Knox BD, Ramasastry S, Moossy JJ: Traumatic lumbopelvic spondyloptosis: A case report. *J Bone Joint Surg Am* 1993;75(11): 1695-1698.
57. Kristiansen TK: Fractures of the sacrum and coccygodynia, in Frymoyer JW, ed: *The Adult Spine: Principles and Practice*. New York, NY, Raven Press, 1991.
58. Leighton RK, Waddell JP, Bray TJ, et al: Biomechanical testing of new and old fixation devices for vertical shear fractures of the pelvis. *J Orthop Trauma* 1991;5(3):313-317.
59. Klineberg E, McHenry T, Bellabarba C, Wagner T, Chapman J: Sacral insufficiency fractures caudal to instrumented posterior lumbosacral arthrodesis. *Spine (Phila Pa 1976)* 2008;33(16):1806-1811.
60. Khanna AJ, Kebaish KM, Ozdemir HM, Cohen DB, Gonzales RA, Kostuik JP: Sacral insufficiency fracture surgically treated by fibular allograft. *J Spinal Disord Tech* 2004;17(3):167-173.
61. Papadopoulos EC, O'Leary PF, Pappou IP, Girardi

FP: Spontaneous posterior iliac crest regeneration enabling second bone graft harvest; a case report. *HSS J* 2009;5(2):114-116.

62. Hsieh PC, Ondra SL, Wienecke RJ, O'Shaughnessy BA, Koski TR: A novel approach to sagittal balance restoration following iatrogenic sacral fracture and resulting sacral kyphotic deformity: Technical note. *J Neurosurg Spine* 2007;6(4): 368-372.

63. Douis H, James SL: CT-guided sacroplasty for the treatment of zone II sacral insufficiency fractures. *Clin Radiol* 2009;64(10):1037-1040.

64. Davis AA, Carragee EJ: Bilateral facet dislocation at the lumbosacral joint: A report of a case and review of literature. *Spine (Phila Pa 1976)* 1993; 18(16):2540-2544.

65. Gertzbein SD: Posterior dislocation of the lumbosacral joint: A case report. *J Spinal Disord* 1990; 3(2):174-178.

66. Nagi ON, Dhillon MS, Gill SS: Bilateral fracture dislocation of the sacrum without injury to the anterior pelvis. *Orthopedics* 1993;16(2):215-217.

67. Strange-Vognsen HH, Kiaer T, Tøndevold E: The Cotrel-Dubousset instrumentation for unstable sacral fractures: Report of 3 patients. *Acta Orthop Scand* 1994;65(2):219-220.

CHAPTER 35
Gunshot Wounds of the Spine

Robert P. Norton, MD Jonathan G. Roper, MD Sebastian Lattuga, MD
Frank J. Eismont, MD

Key Points

- Because of the wide variation in bullet speed, bullet characteristics, and wound cavities, the treating physician must have a basic understanding of ballistics.
- Most low-velocity gunshot wounds to the spine are stable, and only rarely is it necessary to operate on such a wound to establish stability.
- Spinal infections are rare following a gunshot wound to the spine.
- The use of steroids is contraindicated in gunshot injuries to the spine.
- For uncontaminated cases, we recommend treatment with prophylactic parenteral antibiotics for 72 hours after injury and for 7 to 14 days after injury of a contaminated viscus.
- Complications such as chronic dysesthetic pain, cerebrospinal fluid–cutaneous fistulas, migration of the bullet within the spinal canal, and plumbism have all been reported as sequelae associated with gunshot wounds of the spine.

Introduction

It is important for treating physicians to understand wound ballistics and to formulate plans for patient evaluation and treatment based on sound medical principles to achieve optimal patient care and outcomes following gunshot wounds to the spine. Other penetrating injuries of the spine also have the potential for structural and neurologic injury. The incidence and severity of gunshot wounds of the spine will probably continue to increase in the civilian population in the future, and although some of the details may change, the principles of evaluation and treatment will remain the same.

Demographics and Epidemiology

With global escalation in firearm use, it should be no surprise that gunshot wounds to the spine account for 13% to 17% of all spinal cord injuries (SCIs) each year.[1-3] Bahebeck et al[4] evaluated the incidence, case fatality rate, and clinical patterns of firearm injuries in two cities in which firearms are forbidden. They found the incidence of firearm injuries to be 1.14 cases per 100,000 population per year, which is 5 to 50 times lower than the incidence in other cities of similar size in which firearms are legal.

In 1993, the Major Trauma Outcome Study[5] published information regarding the severity and outcome of 114,510 trauma patients in the United States and Canada from 1982 through 1989. The overall incidence of SCI was 2.6%, and 13.6% of the SCIs were caused by gunshot wounds. The study found that 79% of the victims were male and 21% were female; this same distribution was seen for SCI cases in general and for penetrating wounds of the spine. The average age of the patient was 33.5 years. In 1999, McKinley et al[6] reviewed 217 traumatic SCI rehabilitation admissions over a 5-year period and found patients with gunshot wound–induced SCIs were significantly younger and more frequently nonCaucasian, unmarried, and unemployed when compared to nonviolence-related traumatic SCI patients. In another study,[7] only 9% of penetrating wounds of the spine were classified as job-related injuries (presumably occurring to security guards, policemen, employees shot during robberies, etc). One study demonstrated that the likelihood of SCIs from a gunshot wound was higher among those who had previous gunshot wounds (30%) or who had prior involvement in the criminal justice system (52%).[8] Unlike sports injuries, which peak

Dr. Roper or an immediate family member owns stock or stock options in NuVasive. Dr. Eismont or an immediate family member has received royalties from Alphatec Spine; serves as a paid consultant to or is an employee of Alphatech Spine; and owns stock or stock options in Alphatech Spine. Neither of the following authors or any immediate family member has received anything of value from or owns stock in a commercial company or institution related directly or indirectly to the subject of this chapter: Dr. Norton and Dr. Lattuga.

This is an update of a chapter that was published as Eismont FJ, Lattuga S: Gunshot wounds of the spine, in Browner BD, Jupiter JB, Levine AM, Trafton PG, eds: Skeletal Trauma, *ed 3. Philadelphia, PA, Saunders/Elsevier, 2003, pp 983-1003. Some of the material appears in similar form in* Skeletal Trauma, *ed 4 (2009). The adaptations of the material and figures from earlier editions of* Skeletal Trauma *are reproduced with permission from Elsevier.*

FIGURE 1

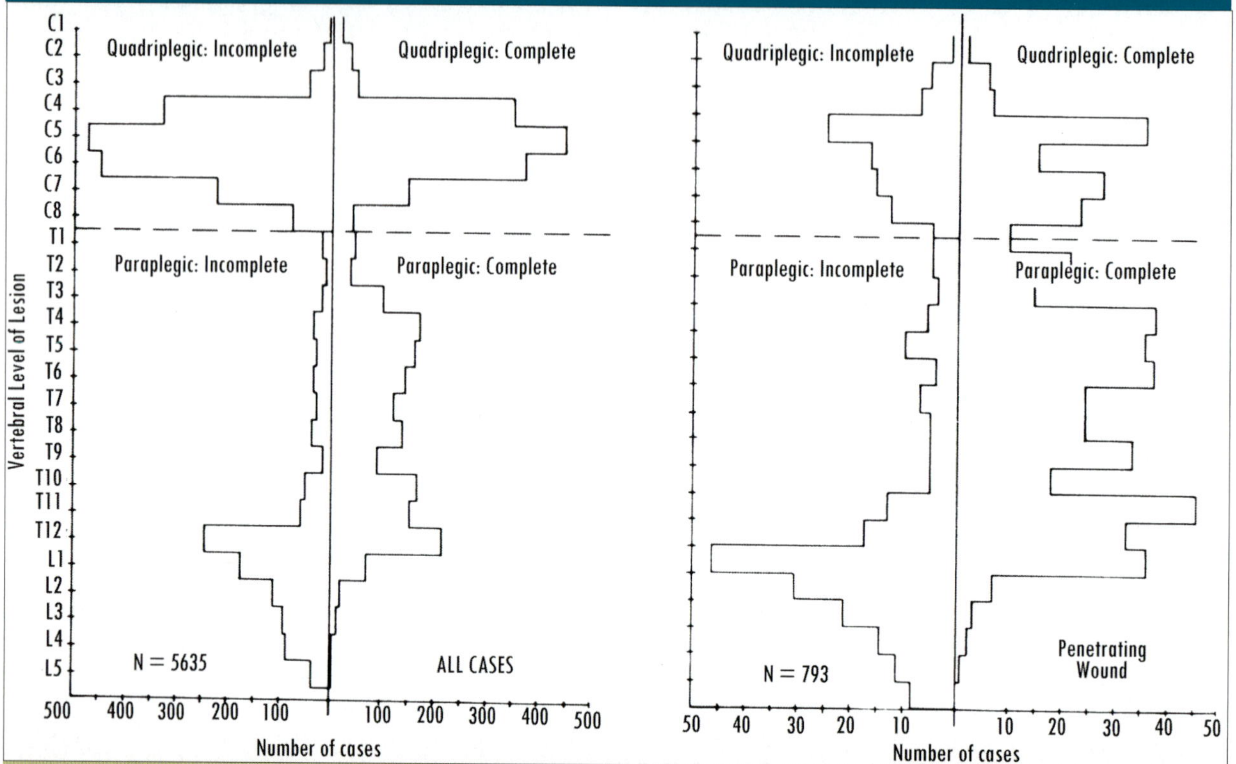

Figure 1 The bar graphs on the left represent the distribution of the levels of injury for all incomplete and complete SCIs. The bar graph on the right shows the distribution for penetrating wounds of the spine. Penetrating wounds constitute a higher percentage of complete injuries and, as is evident, a proportionately higher number of thoracic injuries. (Reproduced with permission from Young JA, Burns PE, McCutchen R, eds: *Spinal Cord Injury Statistics: Experience of the Regional Spinal Cord Injury Systems*. Phoenix, AZ, Good Samaritan Medical Center, 1982, pp 1-152.)

nationwide during the summer months, the incidence of penetrating wounds of the spine remained the same throughout the year, with 40% of them occurring on a weekend. Approximately 47% of all persons with SCIs are paraplegics, and 53% are quadriplegics. Sixty percent of all thoracic and lumbar injuries are complete lesions, as are 48% of the cervical injuries. For penetrating wounds of the spine, however, a significantly greater proportion are complete, and there is a much greater shift toward thoracic spinal injuries as compared with injuries of the neck or lumbar spine (**Figure 1**).

Using these older data, it would appear that approximately 1,400 new SCIs occur each year as a result of gunshot wounds of the spine. However, in many areas of the United States, the number of SCIs caused by gunshot wounds of the spine doubled during the 10-year period from 1981 through 1991,[9] and this estimate therefore may be an optimistically low number. The data from the Regional Spinal Cord Injury Center of the Delaware Valley suggest a similar trend.[1] Even more difficult to estimate is the number of patients with minor gunshot injuries to the spine (ie, those that cause no paralysis) because nationwide numbers are not available for this type of injury. Based on what is seen at our own medical center and SCI unit in Miami, the number of gunshot wounds of the spine without paralysis is similar to the number with associated paralysis. To add perspective, in 1989, it was estimated that 48,700 people would be killed in motor vehicle accidents in the United States and that slightly more than 30,000 civilians would be killed with firearms.[10] Five times as many people are wounded as are killed by gunshots.

Wound Ballistics

The term ballistics is defined in *Webster's New Universal Dictionary* as "the modern science dealing with the motion and impact of projectiles, especially those discharged from firearms." In a medical sense, ballistics is described as "the study of effects on the body produced by penetrating projectiles."[11]

FIGURE 2

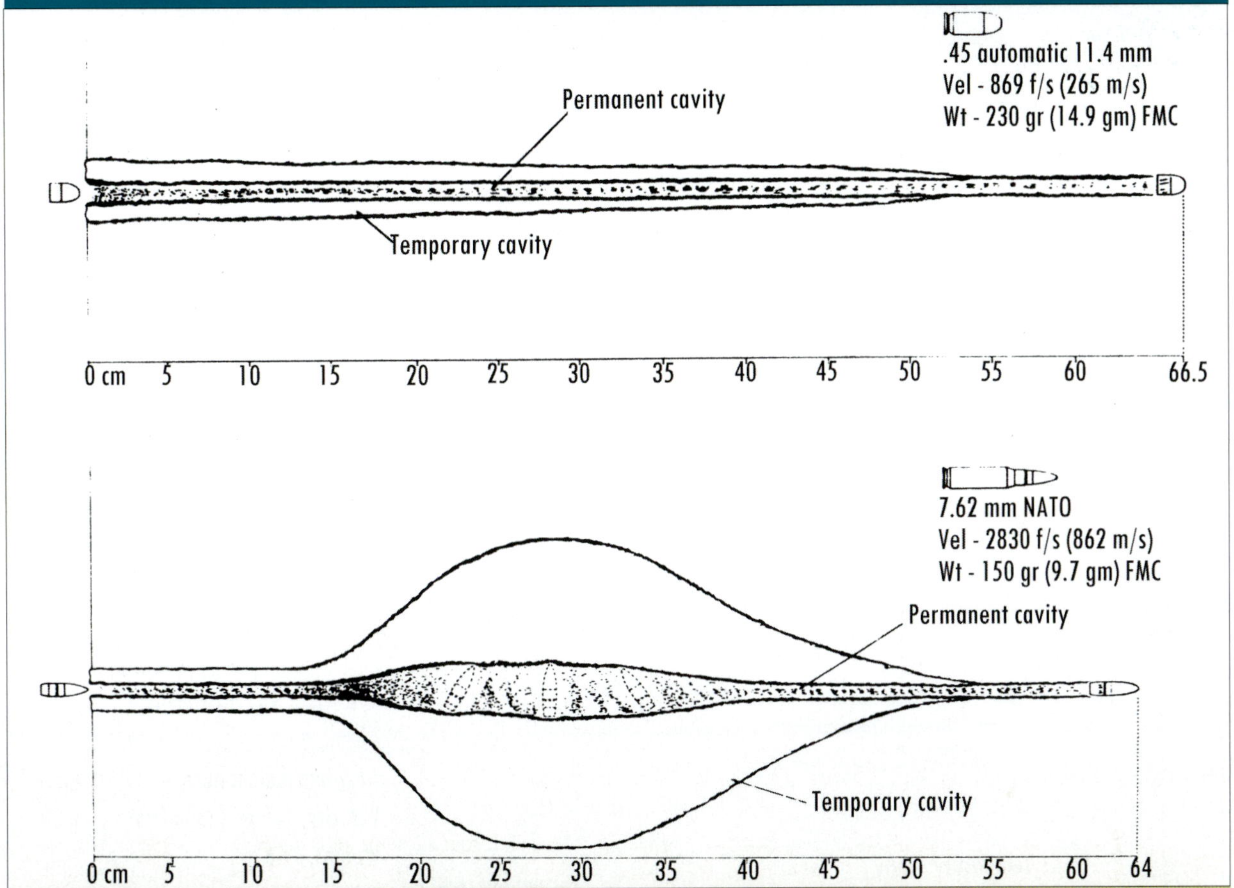

Figure 2 These figures represent the injury profile as seen after discharging weapons through a gelatin medium. Note that for the first 15 cm of travel through tissue, the injury patterns are extremely similar despite a significant difference in bullet velocity. It is not until the bullet yaws that the permanent cavity becomes significantly larger for a rifle injury as opposed to a handgun injury. (Reproduced with permission from Fackler ML, Bellamy RF, Malinowski JA: The wound profile: Illustration of the missile-tissue interaction. *J Trauma* 1988;28(suppl 1):S21-S29.)

To understand the basic concepts of ballistics, it is important to define several other relevant terms.

Mass: The weight of the bullet is usually measured in grams; most range in weight from 2 g to 10 g.

Velocity: The velocity of the bullet can be given in feet per second (ft/s) or in meters per second (m/s). A 0.45-caliber automatic handgun, for example, has a velocity of 869 ft/s (265 m/s), a 0.357-caliber Magnum has a velocity of 1,393 ft/s (425 m/s), and an AK-47 has a velocity of 2,340 ft/s (713 m/s).

Fragmentation: Fragmentation refers to the extent to which a bullet disintegrates into multiple pieces as it courses through tissue. This is often described by comparing the largest final bullet fragment to its original weight and is one of the most important factors in determining the extent of final tissue injury.

FIGURE 3

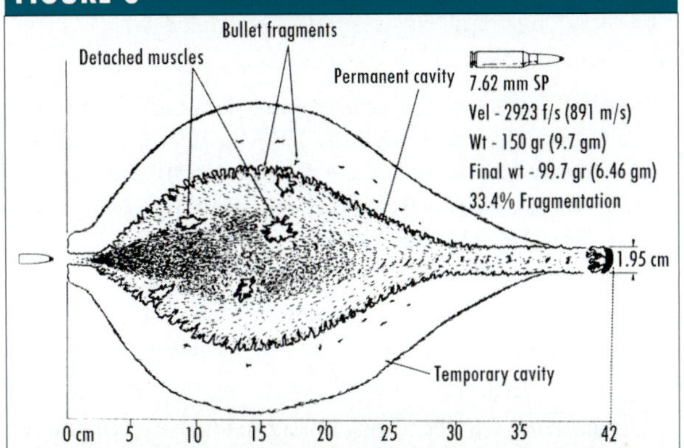

Figure 3 This wound profile is from the same rifle represented by the lower graph in **Figure 2**. The permanent cavity is significantly larger in this case and is entirely due to the use of a soft-point bullet, which leads to significant bullet fragmentation. (Reproduced with permission from Fackler ML, Bellamy RF, Malinowski JA: The wound profile: Illustration of the missile-tissue interaction. *J Trauma* 1988; 28(suppl 1):S21-S29.)

FIGURE 4

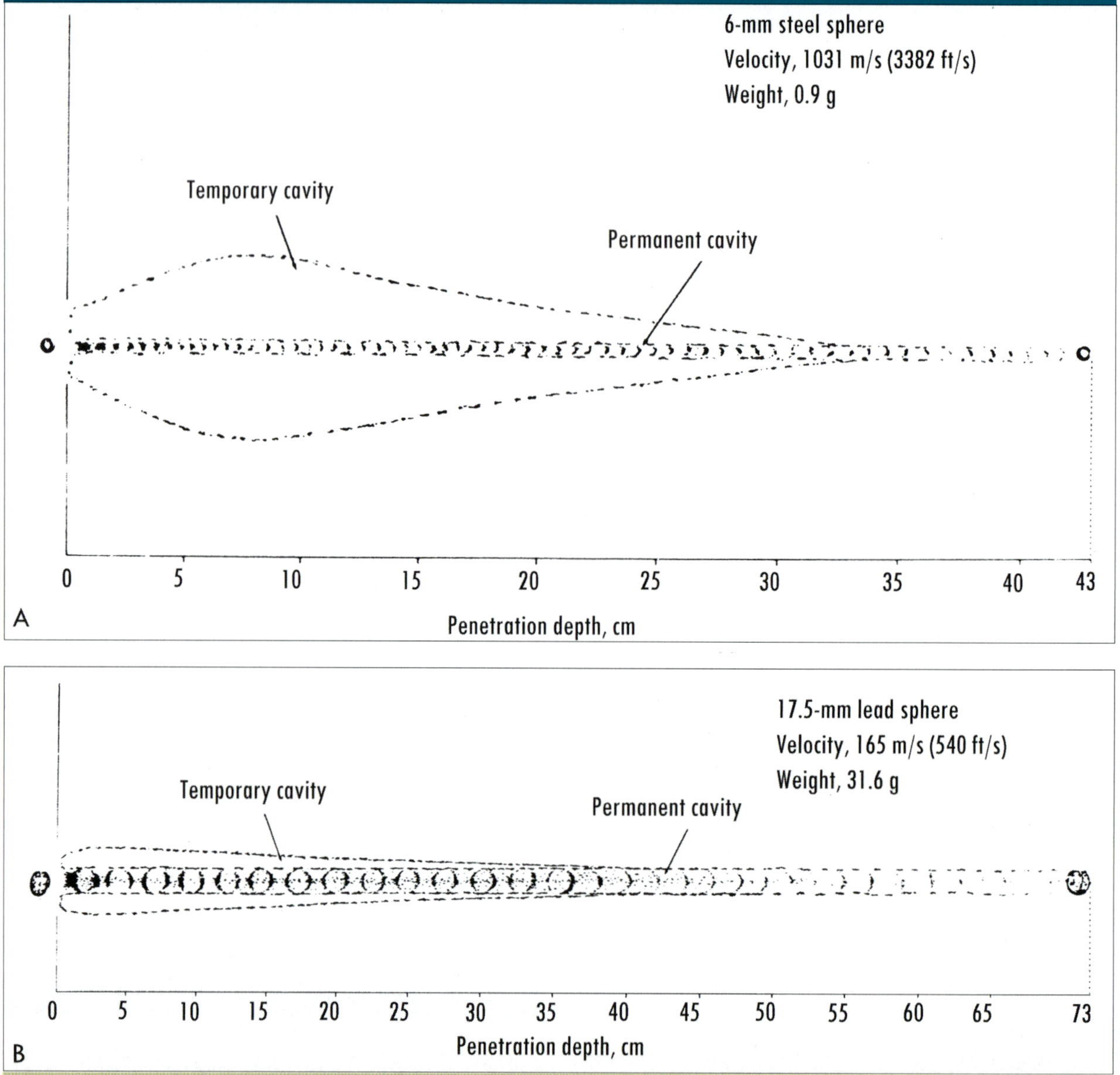

Figure 4 These wound profiles were obtained using a small sphere at a high velocity (**A**) to compare the injury with a large sphere at a slower velocity (**B**). The kinetic energy ($E = mv^2$) is the same in each of the two examples. However, the larger sphere penetrates 30 cm deeper and produces a permanent cavity more than 50 times the volume of that produced by the smaller sphere. (Reproduced with permission from Fackler ML: Wound ballistics: A review of common misconceptions. *JAMA* 1988;259(18):2730-2736.)

Permanent Cavity: This term refers to the permanent crushing of tissue resulting from the passage of the bullet.

Temporary Cavity: This is the stretching of tissue as a result of the passage of the bullet. Elastic tissue, such as muscle, is relatively resistant to damage from this type of stretching, whereas more solid tissue is more significantly damaged under the same circumstances.

To better understand the mechanism of tissue injury with gunshot wounds, surgeons may find it helpful to study the course of bullets in tissue or in gelatin tissue simulants.[12,13] Several such illustrations are shown in **Figures 2** through **4**. The cross-sectional area of the permanent cavity varies widely despite significant similarities in the velocities. The tissue effects of bullet fragmentation and yaw (the end-over-end rotation of the bullet) can be appreciated in these illustrations.

In a review of common misconceptions about wound ballistics, Fackler[11] makes the transition from the mechanical science of projectiles to the clinical art of patient care. Among the major misconceptions, he lists an overemphasis on bullet velocity and an exaggeration of tissue damage due to the effects of the temporary cavity. He also states that many of the positive effects of the administration of systemic antibiotics have been incorrectly attributed to the surgical débridement of tissue. He points out that the incidence of clostridial myositis decreased from 5% in World War I to 0.08% in the Korean War, even though the débridement techniques remained relatively unchanged during that period. This improvement can be more appropriately attributed to the increasing use of antibiotics on the battlefield. Fackler emphasizes the importance of evaluating the patient both clinically, with a hands-on physical examination, and radiographically, with standard radiographs to look for bullet fragmentation. Fackler's classic article gives an excellent explanation of ballistics and outlines sound principles regarding patient treatment and wound assessment.[11]

Composition of Bullets

The bullet projectile is most commonly composed of lead, but a portion of the bullet may consist of copper or brass. It is known that systemic toxicity may occur with lead that leaches out of a bullet, and this has been well described when bullets are bathed in synovial joint fluid[14-16] or lodged in the intervertebral disk space.[17] The exact incidence of this problem with gunshot wounds of the spine is unknown, but it is thought to be quite uncommon. In a series of 12 patients found to have bullet fragments lodged within the intervertebral disk and an average follow-up of 7.8 years, one patient developed plumbism.[18] Clinical manifestations of lead toxicity include encephalopathy, peripheral neuritis, and colic. Signs and symptoms may include anemia, pallor, basophilic stippling on peripheral smears, and a "lead line" along gingival margins. If lead toxicity is suspected, serum lead levels are diagnostic; if lead levels are significantly elevated, a bone-marrow aspiration may be required to assess hematopoietic toxicity. If lead toxicity can indeed be proved, then surgical excision of the bullet is indicated.

The toxicity of lead, copper, and brass at a more local level has been investigated in brain tissue.[19-21] It has been found that copper, when evaluated in the monkey brain, causes a severe necrotic local reaction, which is minimally evident with lead and nickel-coated pellets. The necrotic reaction can be so severe as to allow significant migration of the copper-coated pellet through the brain, whereas the other metal pellets remain in place.[21] This is also seen when a copper powder is sprayed on monkey brain, which causes a severe necrotizing foreign-body reaction that results in death of the animal.[19]

A study of the effects of bullet fragments on the spinal cord in a rabbit model has been published that shows a great variation depending on the intraspinal location and the fragment's metallic composition. Three types of fragments were tested, including aluminum ("silver-tipped" bullets), lead, and copper. If these were placed directly on the dura, none had any effect on the microscopic appearance of the spinal cord other than minor effects of a local spinal cord compression. If the fragments were placed intradurally and in contact with the spinal cord, there was a tremendous variation in local effect on the spinal cord. The aluminum fragment had minimal effect (**Figure 5**), the lead produced moderate local myelin and axon destruction (**Figure 6**), and the copper fragment produced severe local myelin and axon destruction (**Figure 7**). The rabbits with implanted copper fragments were the only group with elevated serum levels of the metal.[22]

On the basis of this animal research, it is recommended that copper-jacketed bullets be removed from the spinal canal, regardless of other considerations, to avoid the local toxicity effects on the neural tissue. Most often, however, it is not known if a bullet is copper-jacketed.

The presence of wadding in the back of a shotgun cartridge must be addressed for clinical reasons. Shotgun pellets are easily seen on plain radiographs, but the wadding of the shotgun is not apparent on plain radiographs, and it often acts as a significant foreign body unless it is removed. If a patient is shot with a shotgun at close range (6 m or less), the shotgun wadding should be sought within the wounds (**Figure 8**).[23,24]

Pathology of Spinal Gunshot Wounds

Pathologic specimens were collected and described following World War I. The War Office Collection contains 50 specimens, and these have been described in the literature by Keith and Hall.[25] They show considerable variation, from relatively mild bone or ligament injuries to severe disruptions of the spinal column. The spinal cord was often intact, even though the patient had sustained a complete SCI, presumably due to contusion of the spinal cord. The authors also noted that with injuries to the posterior arch or pedicles, associated

FIGURE 5

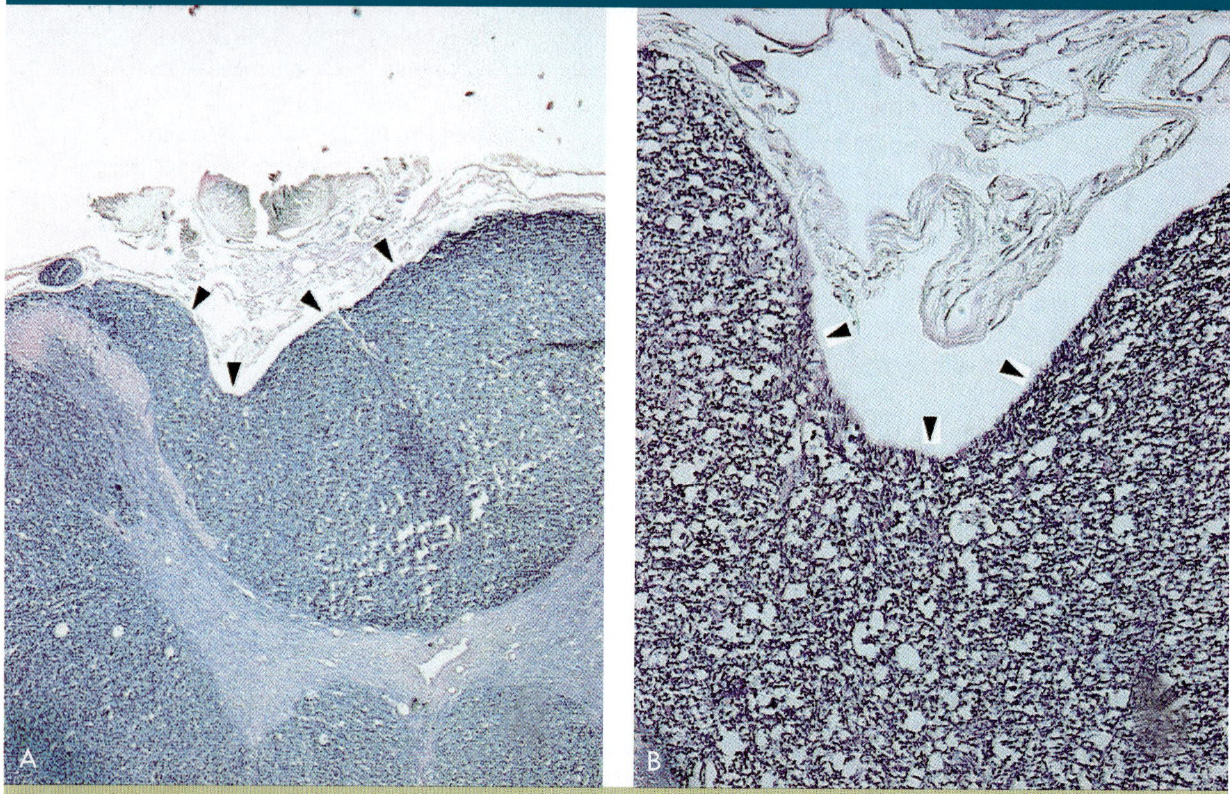

Figure 5 Axial cross sections through a rabbit spinal cord with an implanted intradural aluminum fragment. **A,** Image showing some indentation of the spinal cord (arrowheads) (solochrome-cyanin, ×5). **B,** Image showing minimal to no gliosis of the underlying spinal cord tissue. The surrounding connective-tissue matrix remains well organized (solochrome-cyanin, ×20). (Reproduced with permission from Tindel NL, Marcillo AE, Tay BK, Bunge RP, Eismont FJ: The effect of surgically implanted bullet fragments on the spinal cord in a rabbit model. *J Bone Joint Surg Am* 2001;83(6):884-890.)

secondary fractures of the vertebral body were common. However, when the vertebral body was the primary site of gunshot injury, secondary injury to the posterior elements seldom occurred. The reason for this contrast was presumably due to the vertebral body being composed primarily of cancellous bone, which is more easily deformed and hence transmits less energy to adjacent structures.

Klemperer et al[26] investigated the pathology of indirect injuries to the spinal cord in an animal model. They produced gunshot injuries to the posterior spinous processes or interspinous ligaments in anesthetized animals and found great variation among species in the presence and degree of SCI. This most likely correlated with the size of the spinal canal relative to the size of the spinal cord. In animals with extremely small canals, the incidence of SCI was extremely high. The pathologic sections of the spinal cord varied, as would be expected, but it was interesting that significant pathologic changes often were noted within the spinal cord even in some animals that had not sustained any paralysis.

Mirovsky et al[27] retrospectively reviewed all patients with neurologic deficit following gunshot wounds that did not penetrate the spinal canal. They identified 26 cases with either complete or incomplete paraplegia that were managed from 1977 to 2003. They found three patients with complete paraplegia at the thoracic level who did not indicate any sign of canal compromise. They did not comment on the size of the spinal canal; however, all injuries were at the thoracic level, where the ratio of spinal cord to canal size is the highest. They concluded that neurologic deficit following gunshot wounds is possible without violation of the spinal canal, most likely the result of emitted kinetic energy from the bullet. Their results were similar to those of Stauffer et al,[28] who reported on 185 patients with gunshot wounds of the spine. They had 106 patients with a complete lesion and 79 with an incomplete lesion. A total of 101 patients underwent laminec-

FIGURE 6

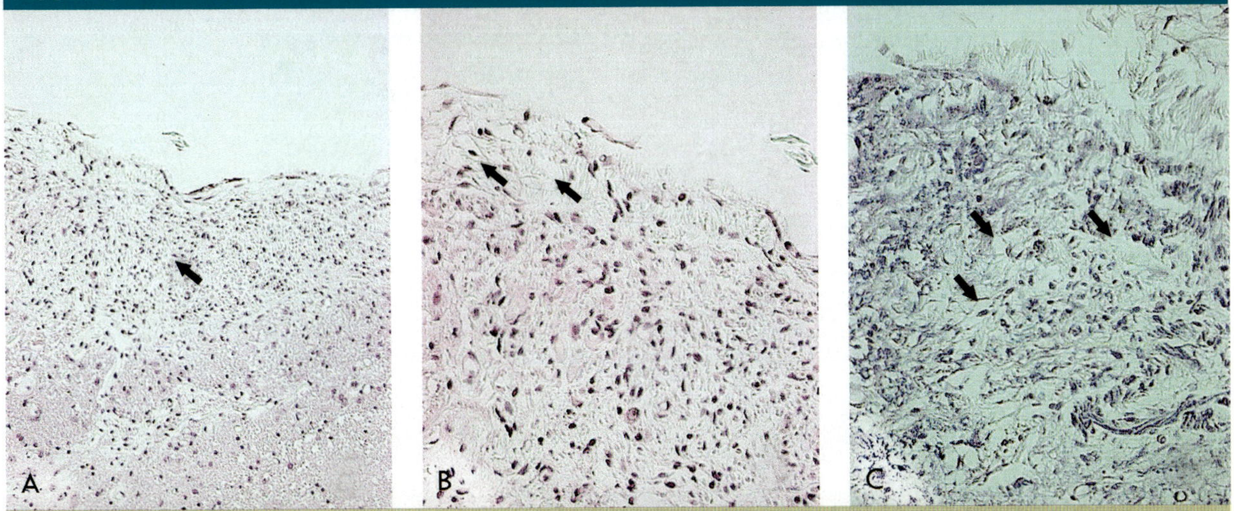

Figure 6 Axial cross sections through a rabbit spinal cord with an implanted intradural lead fragment. **A,** Image showing indentation of the dorsal column with a small area of gliosis adjacent to the area of depression (arrow) (hematoxylin and eosin, ×20). **B,** Image showing areas of gliosis and breakdown of supporting matrix (arrows) (hematoxylin and eosin, ×40). **C,** Image demonstrating loss of axonal elements with disorganization of the surrounding connective tissue adjacent to the area of fragment implantation (arrows) (solochrome-cyanin, ×40). (Reproduced with permission from Tindel NL, Marcillo AE, Tay BK, Bunge RP, Eismont FJ: The effect of surgically implanted bullet fragments on the spinal cord in a rabbit model. *J Bone Joint Surg Am* 2001;83(6):884-890.)

tomy. They found that the spinal cord appeared normal in six patients with complete injury and in five patients with an incomplete injury. The most likely mechanism is that the kinetic energy of the passing bullet imparts a concussive injury to the spinal cord. In addition, this energy may also disrupt or cause thrombosis of the vascular supply to the spinal cord. Stauffer et al[28] were the first to emphasize that emergent laminectomies for gunshot wounds of the spine did not improve neural function and markedly increased the risks of cerebrospinal fluid (CSF)-cutaneous fistulas, wound infections, and spinal instability.

Patient Evaluation

The evaluation of patients with gunshot wounds of the spine should include the same detailed history, physical examination, and radiographic evaluation as would be performed for patients with other suspected spine injuries. Attention is first given to the ABCs (airway, breathing, and circulation) of emergency treatment protocols.

The history should include a general description of the weapon (eg, handgun, rifle, assault weapon). Typically, this information is not available, but it can be helpful if known. The patient should be questioned as to whether any paralysis or paresthesias occurred immediately following the injury. If the patient did indeed have an episode of transient paralysis, a more detailed neurologic follow-up is indicated.

The importance of the physical examination cannot be overemphasized. This should include examination of the entrance and exit wounds, and the tissue should be palpated to assess the presence of crepitation and the general turgor of the tissue. The presence of a very large exit wound with crepitation and increased tissue turgor is consistent with wounds that have a large permanent cavity and may very well have significant tissue necrosis.[12] The physical examination should also include a good, detailed neurologic examination. The presence of paralysis or any abnormal reflexes should be documented.

The radiographic evaluation of the patient is also extremely important. Attention should be paid to the fracture type and the degree of bone comminution. The radiograph should be scrutinized to determine if the bullet remains in the torso and to assess the extent of bullet fragmentation. The wound is more likely to have a significant permanent cavity if there is increased bone comminution and bullet fragmentation. Such a case may be one of the few instances in which significant wound débridement is required.[12]

Klein et al[29] performed a retrospective analysis of 2,450 patients who were treated for gunshot wounds at the Ryder Trauma Center in Miami

FIGURE 7

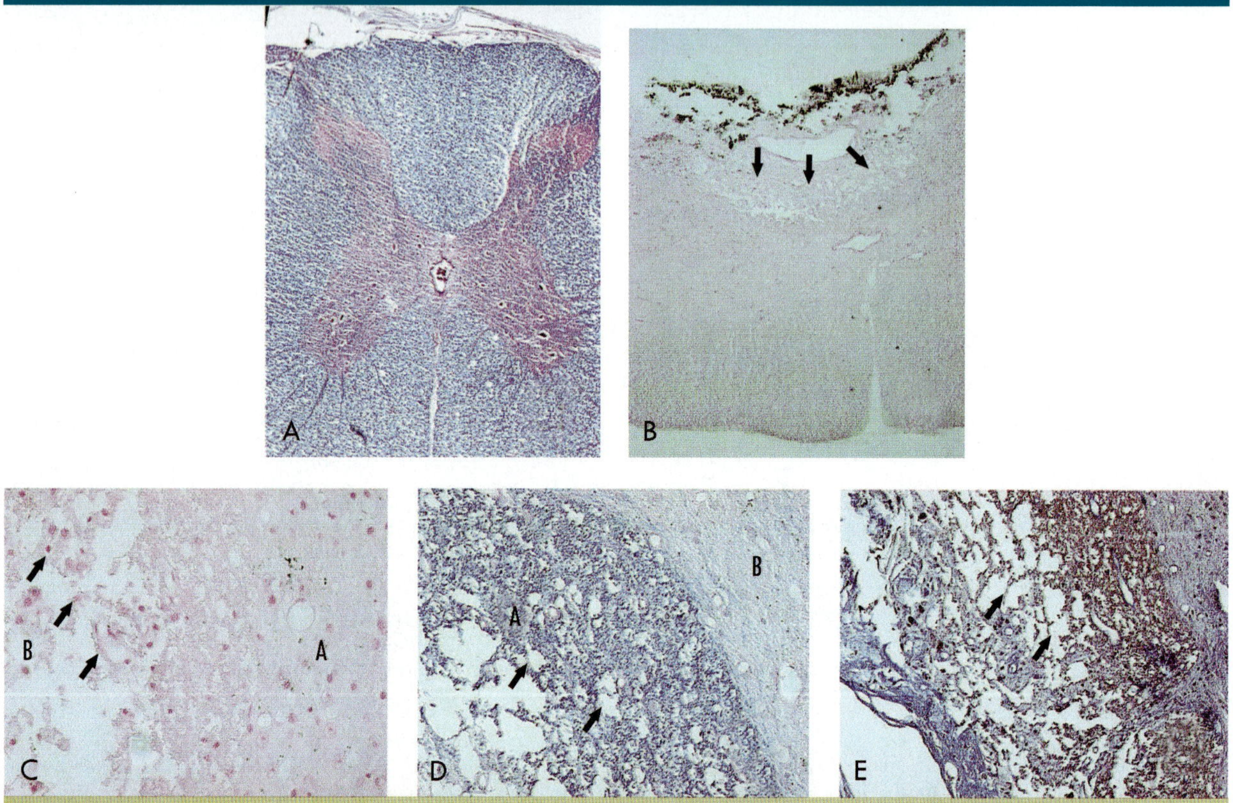

Figure 7 Axial cross sections through the spinal cords of rabbits with an implanted copper bullet fragment. **A,** An extradurally placed fragment caused no deformation or injury to the underlying spinal cord (trichrome, ×5). **B,** Image showing indentation and injury to the underlying spinal cord tissue from an intradurally placed copper fragment (arrows) (×5). **C,** Image showing destruction of the spinal cord parenchyma (arrows). The damage is confined to the white matter (A); the gray matter (B) is preserved (hematoxylin and eosin, ×40). **D,** Image showing vacuolization of the adjacent spinal cord tissue (arrows) with damage localized to the white matter (A); there is no damage to the gray matter (B) (solochrome-cyanin, ×40). **E,** Image showing disruption of the connective-tissue matrix adjacent to the site of implantation of the bullet fragment (arrows) (trichrome, ×40). (Reproduced with permission from Tindel NL, Marcillo AE, Tay BK, Bunge RP, Eismont FJ: The effect of surgically implanted bullet fragments on the spinal cord in a rabbit model. *J Bone Joint Surg Am* 2001;83(6):884-890.)

from 1991 to 2001. They found that 10% of patients with gunshot wounds had associated spine injuries, 13% of whom had significant spinal injuries but were without any neurologic symptoms. They concluded that a complete radiographic spine evaluation is mandatory after gunshot wounds to the face, neck, or trunk even without neurologic deficit.

CT may help to further assess the extent of the spine injury and the extent of spinal canal encroachment by bone or bullet fragments. The stability of the spine can also be better assessed with the help of CT; this is addressed later in greater detail in the section on Spine Stability.

The use of MRI in the evaluation of wounds with retained metallic ballistic fragments remains controversial. Radiologists are reluctant to perform MRI for patients with retained metallic bullet fragments, especially if the retained fragments are near vital and susceptible anatomic structures such as the spinal cord, for fear of further neurologic or soft-tissue damage secondary to bullet migration from the magnetic pull.[30-32] The most common complaint from patients undergoing MRI is that of a heat sensation in the area of the bullet. A report by Finitsis et al[33] evaluated the spine using MRI in 19 patients with metallic bullet fragments. Eighteen of the 19 patients had a previously acquired quadriplegia or paraplegia. The MRI scans were obtained within 3 weeks of injury in 6 patients with gunshot injuries, and in 13 patients who were from 1 month to 6 years from their injury. Ten had bullet fragments within the spinal canal. No patient reported untoward effects of the MRI scan. The results of the MRI scans led to surgical treatment of 3 of the 19 patients. The authors

FIGURE 8

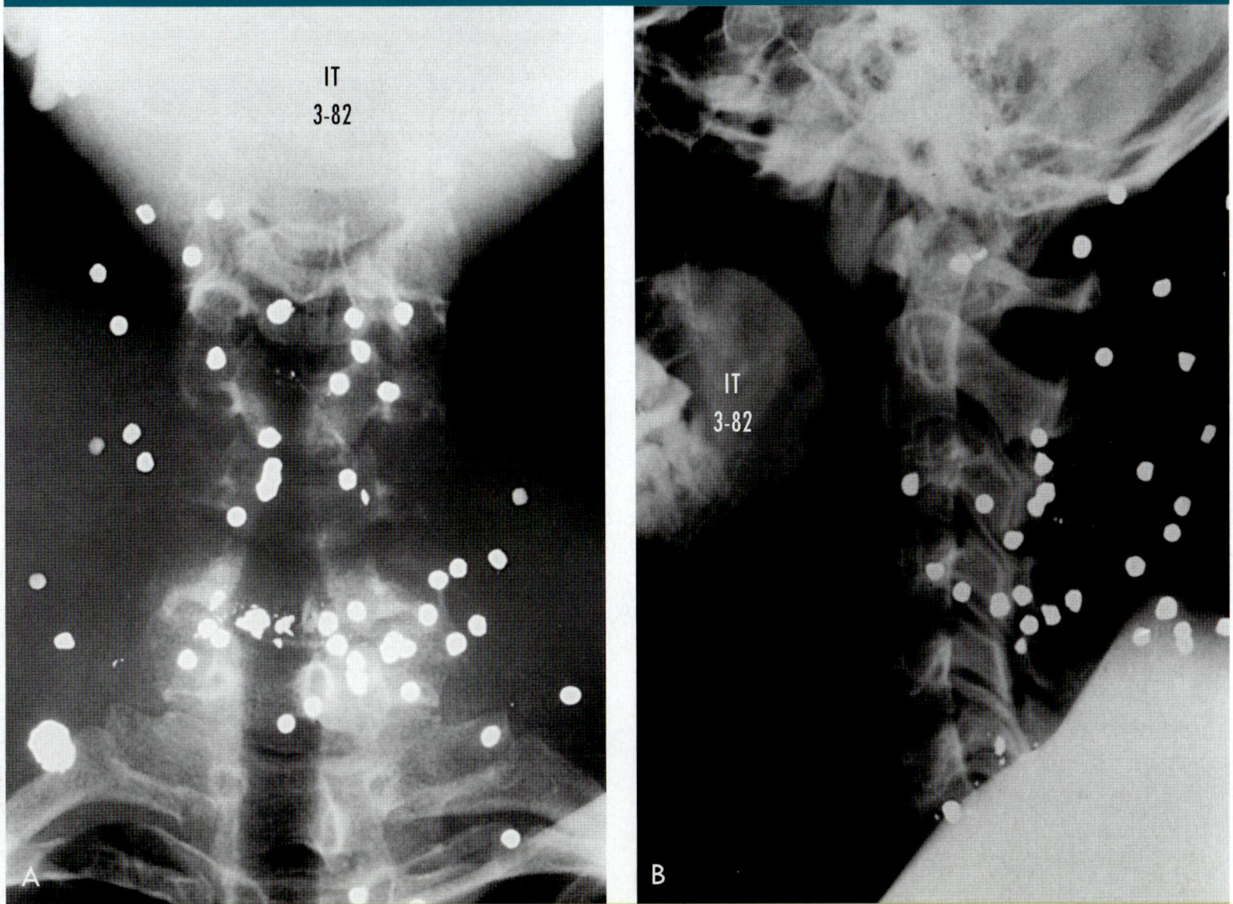

Figure 8 A and B, This patient was shot in the back of the neck with a pellet shotgun. He sustained complete quadriplegia as a result of the injury. It is important to recognize that removal of the pellets is not indicated, but surgical débridement, and especially a removal of the shotgun wadding, is necessary to prevent infection as this was a close-range injury. (Reproduced with permission from Eismont FJ, Lattuga S: Gunshot wounds of the spine, in Browner BD, Jupiter JB, Levine AM, Trafton PG, eds: *Skeletal Trauma*, ed 2. Philadelphia, PA, WB Saunders, 1997, p 1100.)

noted that patients with fragments known to be strongly ferromagnetic, such as the ball-bearing or Prometheus-type of air gun pellets,[34] were not included. Finitsis et al[33] support the use of MRI for patients with retained metallic ballistic fragments in the region of the spine if more information is needed to effectively treat the patient.[33] The treating physician must understand that this is an area of controversy and that there are at least potential risks with this diagnostic approach. If the projectile is ferromagnetic, there may be further local tissue damage. A myelogram followed by immediate CT and a 4-hour delayed CT scan remain the traditional method of assessing the spinal neural elements following a gunshot injury of the spine and may obtain the same information as MRI more safely.

The general surgical team that is helping to assess the patient may recommend other studies, such as a barium swallow, arteriography, and intravenous pyelogram, to evaluate the extent of soft-tissue injuries to structures adjacent to the spine.[35]

Treatment

Wound Care

Local wound care should be administered in the emergency department or in the formal operating room, depending on the severity of the injury. The operating room is more appropriate for treating large exit wounds and when physical and radiographic findings suggest the presence of large permanent cavities. Although this type of wound is uncommon in civilian practice, it is important to recognize that such cases exist.

Some investigators have suggested that physical examination alone may be sufficient in the evaluation of hemodynamically stable patients with

FIGURE 9

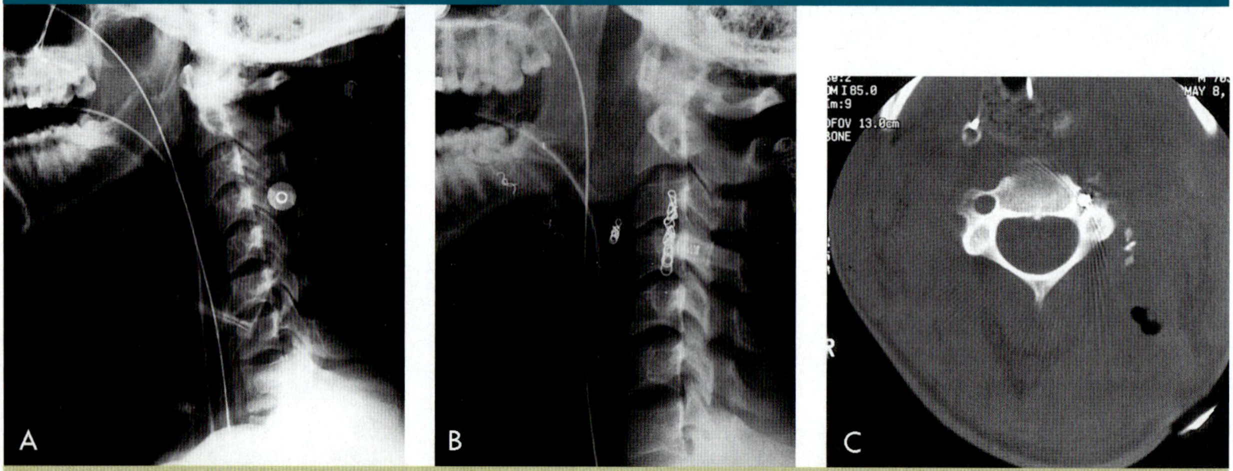

Figure 9 **A,** A lateral radiograph following a gunshot wound to the neck at the level of C3-C4. The patient's primary problem was significant bleeding. Angiography revealed an injury to the left vertebral artery. **B,** This lateral film was taken following insertion of a hemostatic coil into the left vertebral artery. This achieved complete hemostasis. **C,** This CT scan shows the location of the hemostatic coil within the left vertebral artery. (Reproduced with permission from Eismont FJ, Lattuga S: Gunshot wounds of the spine, in Browner BD, Jupiter JB, Levine AM, Trafton PG, eds: *Skeletal Trauma*, ed 2. Philadelphia, PA, WB Saunders, 1997, p 1100.)

gunshot wounds to the neck. However, in a prospective study of 59 patients with gunshot wounds to the neck, Mohammed et al[36] found that physical examination alone was not a good predictor of vascular injury in stable patients. They suggest that angiography and ultrasound may be needed to identify vascular injuries even in hemodynamically stable patients. Because of the proximity of the esophagus, the major blood vessels,[37,38] and the larynx and trachea in wounds of the neck, general surgeons in the past were extremely aggressive with recommending surgical exploration and traditionally recommended exploring all penetrating neck wounds.[38,39] Now, it is more often advocated that only those neck wounds with specific warning signs of serious injury be explored and those without such signs should be observed.[40-42] The same is true for penetrating injuries of the chest and abdomen.[35] The availability of emergency arteriography coupled with the use of intravascular hemostatic coils has also changed the indications for emergency exploratory surgery. Many cases previously requiring surgery to achieve hemostasis can now be managed with minimally invasive techniques (**Figure 9**).

Wound cultures should always be taken from the bullet tract. If the wound has been contaminated by the passage of the bullet through the pharynx,[43,44] esophagus, or colon,[45] or if the wound has been contaminated following injury, it is even more essential that appropriate cultures be taken. For routine uncontaminated cases, we would recommend 3 days of treatment with parenteral antibiotics, such as a second-generation cephalosporin, at maximal intravenous dosage, suggested by Heary et al.[46] Heary et al[46] showed that using steroids after gunshot wounds to the spine with neurologic deficit did not improve the chance of neurologic improvement and did increase the risk of adverse events, including gastrointestinal complications and pancreatitis.

If the bullet first penetrated the pharynx, the esophagus, or the colon, or if the wound was otherwise contaminated, a different antibiotic regimen is recommended (see discussion below in the section on Associated Injuries).[2,45,47,48]

Spine Stability: Assessment and Treatment

The majority of civilian gunshot wounds of the spine are stable.[28,49-54] In the cervical spine, 36% of the weight of the head is carried by the anterior vertebral bodies and disks, and 32% by each of the two posterolateral columns (ie, facet joints and lateral masses).[55]

If none of the three columns is compromised, then no immobilization is recommended. If one of the three columns is disrupted, a rigid cervical collar is recommended. If two or three of the three columns are disrupted, halo-vest immobilization is recommended. In the thoracic and lumbar spine, the three-column concept of Denis can be applied, but the mechanism of destruction is considerably different from that in the closed injuries for which this classification was designed.[56] If destruction is limited to one of the three columns, then no particular immobilization is needed. If two or three columns are compromised by the gunshot wound, then use of a thoracolumbosacral orthosis is recommended whenever the patient is out of bed. In a review of 36 gunshot wounds to the spine by Isiklar et al,[49] 12 patients had cervical spinal injuries and only 4 were unstable, requiring a halo vest and then a rigid brace. Of the 24 patients with thoracic and lumbar injuries, only 1 was unstable and was treated successfully in a brace; none required surgery for instability. Similarly, Medzon et al[53] identified 81 patients over a 13-year period with a gunshot wound to the head or neck and found 19 to have cervical spine fractures. Of the awake and alert patients without a neurologic deficit, only 5% had a fracture, and none were unstable. The authors concluded that spinal precautions and/or a hard cervical collar should not be maintained at the expense of delaying or hindering emergent life-saving airway or hemodynamic stabilization procedures in awake and neurologically intact persons.[53]

Unlike for closed SCIs, it is only rarely necessary to operate on a gunshot wound of the spine for purposes of establishing stability. Immobilization for these injuries of the cervical, thoracic, or lumbar spine is normally 6 to 8 weeks. At that time, flexion and extension plain radiographs of the affected region are performed to establish whether the spine has adequately healed and is stable.

The most unstable injuries are seen in small children, in whom the size of the vertebrae is small relative to the size of the bullet. Other factors predisposing to a significant instability of the spine include injuries with severe bone comminution and bullet fragmentation and previous laminectomy.[28] Even in these cases, although the instability may be significant, surgical treatment is seldom indicated. The temporary use of skull-tong traction for severe instability of cervical spine injuries or oscillating hospital bed treatment of severe thoracic or lumbar injuries may be indicated for 2 to 3 weeks; this allows early healing before routine mobilization, using braces as described previously.

In the experience of the senior author (F.J.E.), it is quite uncommon for patients with gunshot wounds of the thoracic or lumbar spine, even those with paralysis, to require any bracing after these injuries. Each patient should be carefully evaluated, however, because a few patients will be unstable.

Associated Injuries

It is important to consider associated viscus injuries in patients with gunshot wounds of the spine. If the bullet has first penetrated the pharynx,[43,44] esophagus, or colon,[45] then extra precautions should be taken to prevent spine infection. This is essential only when the bullet has first penetrated the viscus and then penetrated the spine, and it does not seem to be clinically important if the bullet first traversed the spine before perforating the viscus. The heat generated by the firing of the bullet does not autosterilize it.[57] The general surgical team normally performs emergency surgery to repair the viscus,[35] place adequate drains, and recommend broad-spectrum antibiotics to cover organisms normally found in the viscus. This is especially important for injuries of the pharynx, esophagus, and colon. It is less important for injuries of the stomach, duodenum, and small intestine, the contents of which are normally sterile; however, spine sepsis has also been rarely reported with gunshot wounds to the other segments of the gastrointestinal tract.[58] In contrast to recommendations of 25 years ago, which promoted radical spine débridement,[59] the best results have been reported by Roffi et al,[45] who recommended minimal or no spine débridement and protection with 1 to 2 weeks of parenteral antibiotics. Roffi et al[45] were the first to recommend not débriding the spine for patients with gunshot wounds through a contaminated viscus (ie, colon) and then through or into the spine. They recommended increasing the length of antibiotics to 7 to 14 days. This approach markedly decreased the chance of persistent spine infection after these injuries. The parenteral antibiotics should be broad-spectrum agents directed at the particular bacteria normally associated with injury of the particular viscus. If complications accompany the viscus repair, the length of time of antibiotic coverage may need to be extended. With this treatment protocol, the incidence of spine infection has been dramatically decreased, and it is now in the range of 5% to 15% for severe injuries involving the pharynx, esophagus, or colon. It is important to remember that spine infections after a gunshot wound can be insidious and that follow-up of at least 6 months is necessary before a patient can be considered free of spinal infection.[46,59]

Treatment of these transperitoneal colon injuries with a 2-day course of antibiotics plus irrigation of the missile tract at surgery has been recommended

FIGURE 10

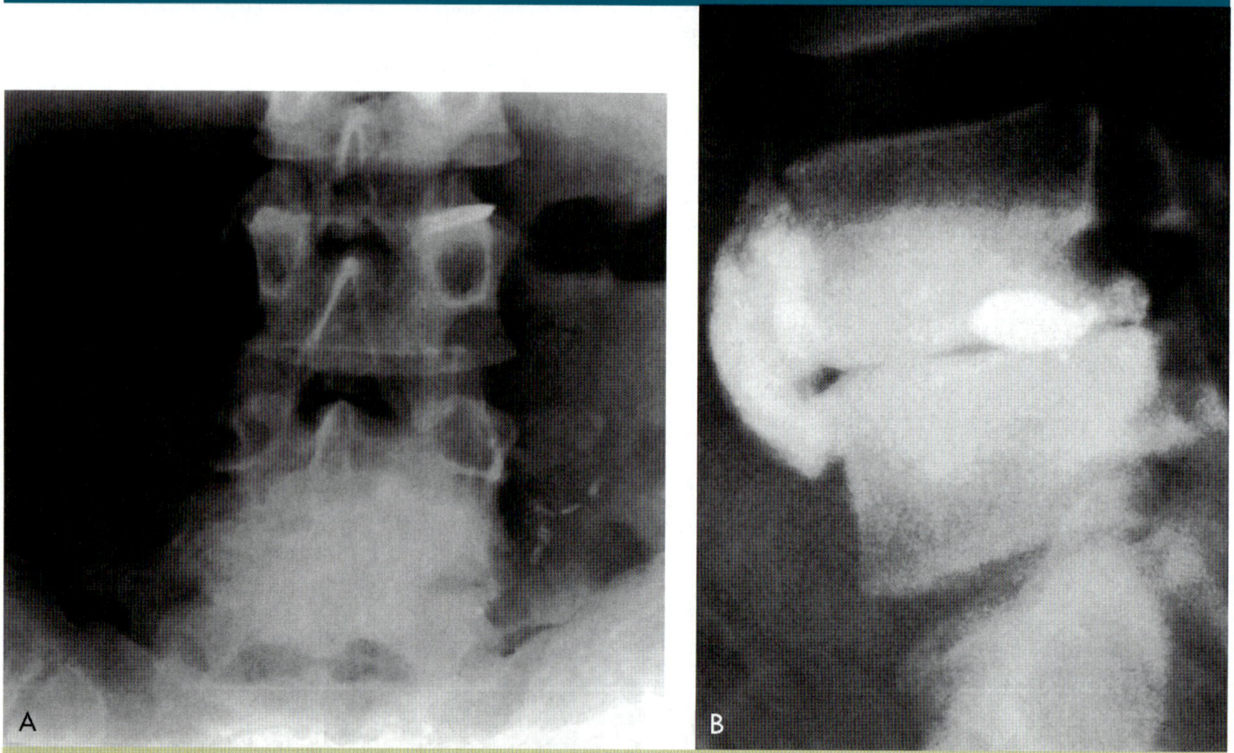

Figure 10 These AP (**A**) and lateral (**B**) radiographs of the lumbar spine were taken 9 years after the patient sustained a gunshot wound to the lumbar spine with the bullet lodged in the L4-L5 disk. The radiographs demonstrate elution of lead into the disk space. The patient had clinical evidence of plumbism with a serum lead level of 136 mgm/dL (reference, 0-24.9 mgm/dL). (Reproduced with permission from Scuderi GJ, Vaccaro AR, Fitzhenry LN, Greenberg S, Eismont F: Long-term clinical manifestations of retained bullet fragments within the intervertebral disc space. *J Spinal Disord Tech* 2004; 17(2):108-111.)

in the past.[47] However, considering both the findings of Roffi et al and the small number of patients with colon injuries in this particular series, we would recommend the longer 1- to 2-week course of antibiotics.

Bullet in the Disk Space

Three factors must be considered in deciding whether surgery is indicated when the bullet is located in the disk space. The first consideration is whether the patient is likely to develop lead poisoning. There is evidence in the literature suggesting that when a lead bullet is bathed in synovial fluid, the lead is leached out and can cause lead poisoning.[14-16] One article in the literature has suggested that this may also be the case with a lead bullet located within the disk space.[17] At our institution, we studied 12 patients who had bullets or bullet fragments within the intervertebral disk space.[18] One of the 12 patients did show clinical evidence of plumbism (**Figure 10**). She presented 9 years after her injury with reports of fatigue and constipation. Her serum lead level was 136 mg/dL. A normal blood lead level is 0; however, toxicity usually does not develop until the blood serum lead level exceeds 24 mg/dL (reference, 0-24.9 mg/dL). A peripheral blood smear revealed basophilic stippling. Plain radiographs revealed elution of the lead into the disk space at the L4-L5 level. The patient subsequently underwent a partial L4 and L5 laminectomy and diskectomy with excision of the bullet fragment. The patient's serum lead level normalized 6 months following bullet removal, and her complaints completely resolved 2 months postoperatively.

A review of the literature does not indicate what percentage of patients with bullets in the disk space will develop lead poisoning in the future; hence, it is not possible to make a sound scientific decision about whether surgery should be recommended routinely. An alternative to routine surgical removal would be to obtain serum lead measurements in patients who are suspected of having signs of lead toxicity. If there is a rise of

FIGURE 11

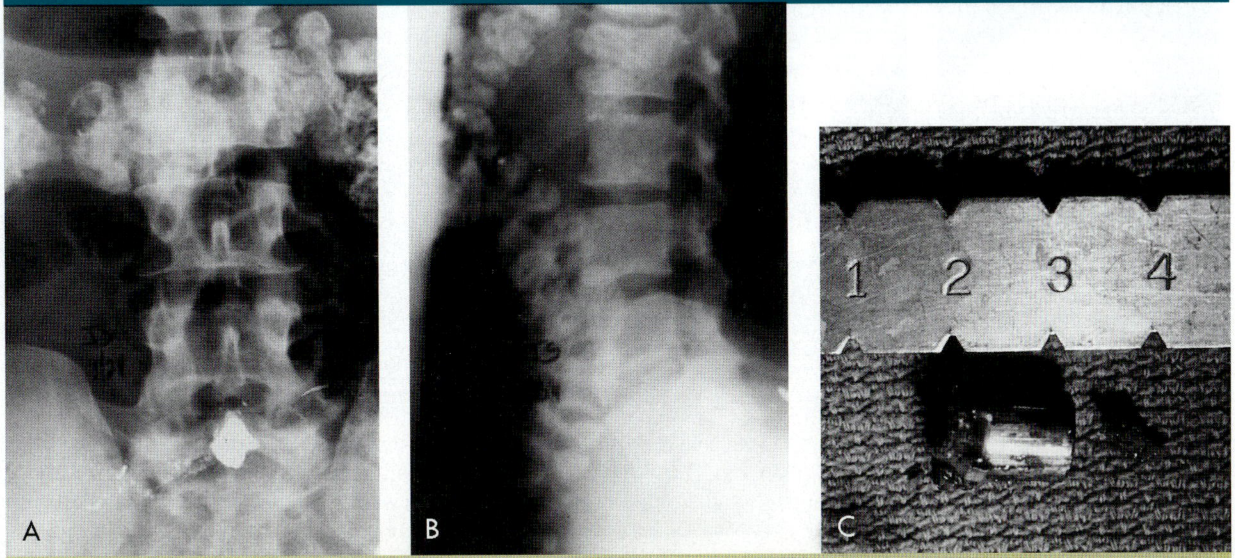

Figure 11 **A** though **C,** This young man was shot through the flank, and the bullet lodged within the spinal canal at the L5-S1 level. He had normal motor function in his legs but some dysesthesia in the S1 nerve root distribution, and he had some urinary dysfunction with elevated postvoid residual volumes. He was taken to surgery 8 days after the injury was inflicted, and the bullet was easily removed. A small dural laceration was easily repaired. The patient had return of normal urologic function. (Reproduced with permission from Eismont FJ, Lattuga S: Gunshot wounds of the spine, in Browner BD, Jupiter JB, Levine AM, Trafton PG, eds: *Skeletal Trauma*, ed 2. Philadelphia, PA, WB Saunders, 1997, p 1104.)

the serum lead to an abnormal level, removal of the bullet would be recommended.

The second consideration includes the mechanical disruption of the motion segment by the presence of a bullet within the disk space. Medical experience for this problem is also anecdotal. The patient can be monitored clinically, and if new symptoms of a mechanical problem develop (eg, worsening of local pain with upright posture and activity and decrease in local pain with recumbency), then consideration could be given to removal of the bullet with local fusion.

The third consideration regarding surgery is whether disk extrusion resulted from a gunshot wound of the spine. If this has occurred, and if the disk extrusion is causing significant symptomatic neural compression, then surgery is indicated for removal of the disk fragments to achieve neural decompression. This occurrence is extremely uncommon, but it has been reported in the literature.[60]

Bullet in the Spinal Canal

Many articles have been written concerning removal of bullets from the spinal canal;[28,61-68] however, until recently, this problem had not been reviewed in a scientific fashion. For conclusions to be valid, the two groups must have equivalent pathology, with one group having bullets removed and the other group having bullets left in place. It is also important that this study be done on a prospective basis, recording adequate neurologic information as well as quantitative assessment of reports of pain, for example. Such a review was performed by Waters and Adkins.[69] They reviewed records of 90 patients, of whom 32 had bullet removals and 58 had bullets left in place. They were able to conclude that at the T12-L5 levels, statistically significant neurologic motor improvement occurred with removal of the bullet from the spinal canal (**Figure 11**). However, there was no difference in improvement in the two groups with regard to sensation or pain experienced by the patients. In the thoracic spine (T1 through T11), no statistical difference was seen for either complete or incomplete injuries, whether or not the bullet was removed. Similarly, no difference was seen with bullet removal in the cervical spine; however, the authors suggest that the patient numbers were too small to be able to draw statistical conclusions about the cervical spine. This was the first review to show the benefits of removing intraspinal bullets from T12 to L5.

Adding our own subjective opinion to these data, we recommend that patients with cervical injuries undergo bullet removal, as this

FIGURE 12

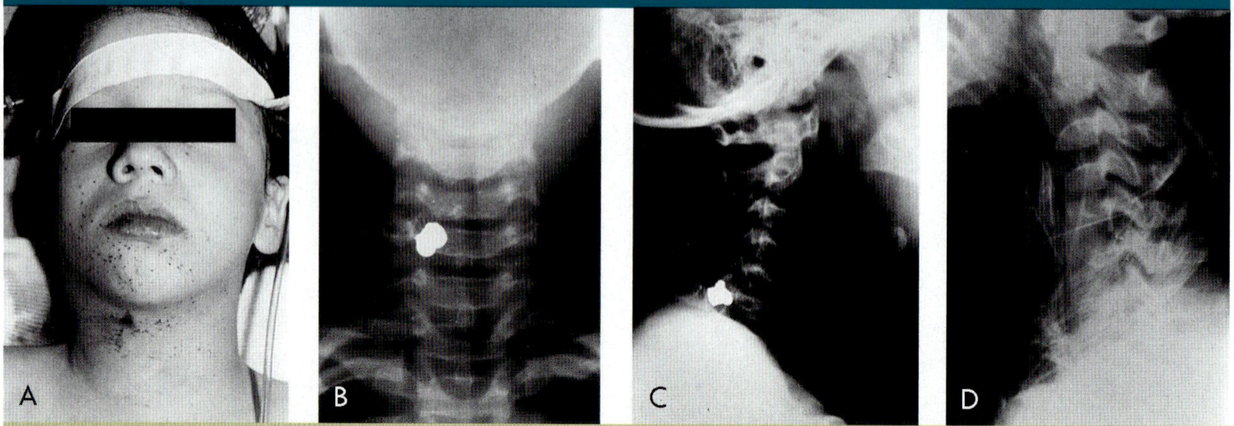

Figure 12 A through **D,** This young boy was accidentally shot in the neck and had progressive quadriparesis. At 24 hours after injury, he had lost all motor function in his legs. The plain films revealed that the bullet was filling the right side of the spinal canal. He was taken to surgery emergently and an anterior cervical procedure was performed. The trachea and esophagus were found to be intact. A corpectomy of C5 and C6 was performed to remove the bullet. An anterior cervical fusion was then performed using autologous iliac crest bone graft. The patient regained ambulation, and the only residual weakness involved the arms. (Reproduced with permission from Eismont FJ, Lattuga S: Gunshot wounds of the spine, in Browner BD, Jupiter JB, Levine AM, Trafton PG, eds: *Skeletal Trauma*, ed 2. Philadelphia, PA, WB Saunders, 1997, p 1106.)

significantly decreases the degree of spinal cord compression.[70] We recommend this approach even in cervical complete injuries, with the expectation not of cord function return, but rather for nerve root improvement at the adjacent level over a period of time. The rationale for doing this is the same as that for closed SCIs of the cervical spine accompanied by significant residual neural compression by bone or disk fragments, which can show nerve root improvement after elective decompression.[71,72]

It is generally accepted that surgery is indicated in patients with bullets in the spinal canal who are experiencing neurologic deterioration. We emphasize, however, that surgery should be performed only in patients in whom compression of the neural elements by bone, disk, bullet, or hematoma has been documented. Such deterioration is extremely uncommon but is occasionally seen (**Figure 12**). We emphasize that surgery is indicated only with demonstrated compression, as it is also known that neurologic deterioration can occur on the basis of ascending spinal cord necrosis with no residual neural compression and that this particular pathology is not helped by surgery; in fact, it may be worsened.

There have been a few reports of late neurologic sequelae after gunshot wounds to the spine.[73-76] These particular reports describe an epidural chronic inflammatory mass as a result of the retained bullet fragment. Most of these cases were caused by a retained bullet in a disk space. Late onset of neurologic symptoms is extremely rare, and we do not recommend removal of retained foreign bodies near or in the spinal canal to prevent a possible neurologic deterioration at a later date.

Once the decision has been made to surgically remove the bullet from the spinal canal, it is essential that a scout radiograph be taken in the operating room before the incision is made. The bullet can occasionally migrate within the spinal canal, depending on the position of the patient.[77-84] This is especially true for patients with large spinal canals and relatively small bullets. Various techniques have been described regarding minimally invasive bullet extraction from the spinal canal[85,86] and sacroiliac joint.[87,88]

Regarding the timing of surgery for removal of bullets from the spinal canal, we normally recommend that this surgery be performed at 7 to 10 days following the injury, because at this time such problems as CSF leakage and dural repair are simplified considerably (**Figure 13**). This obviously does not apply in cases of significant neurologic deterioration, which, as stated previously, require immediate surgery.

Rate of Neurologic Recovery

Most SCIs improve to some extent over time. Complete SCIs usually demonstrate root improvement at one or two levels, and incomplete SCIs have a chance for dramatic improvement in spinal

FIGURE 13

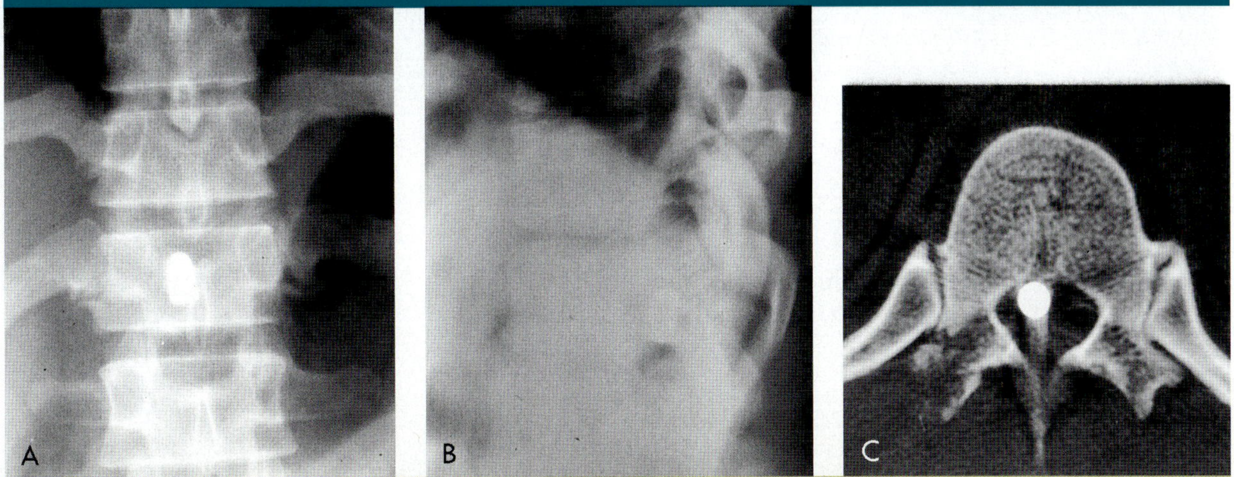

Figure 13 A through **C,** This patient, who had been shot, presented to the emergency department with complete paraplegia, no bowel or bladder function, and no motor or sensory function below L1. His neurologic condition was unchanged for 1 week. He was taken to surgery for removal of the bullet, which was located within the dura. The goal of surgery was not to improve the function of the conus medullaris, but rather to maximize the chance for improvement of the L1-L4 nerve rootlets that traveled past the level of injury. (Reproduced with permission from Eismont FJ, Lattuga S: Gunshot wounds of the spine, in Browner BD, Jupiter JB, Levine AM, Trafton PG, eds: *Skeletal Trauma*, ed 2. Philadelphia, PA, WB Saunders, 1997, p 1107.)

cord function and local root function over time. An early review of closed and open SCIs at the University of Miami showed statistically significant neurologic improvement at 6-month follow-up in patients with complete or incomplete open spinal cord injuries (most of which were caused by gunshot wounds), but the improvements started slightly later than in those with closed injuries (**Figure 14**).[89]

FIGURE 14

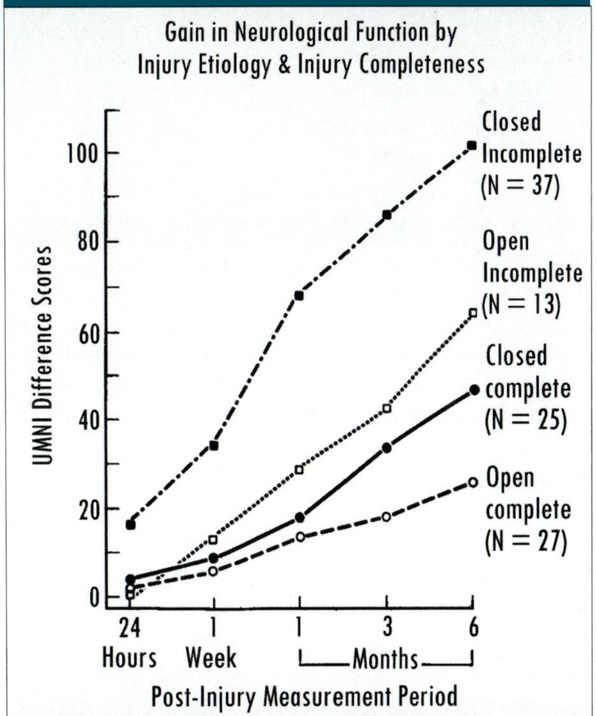

Figure 14 This graph shows that the prognosis for recovery in penetrating injuries of the spine is worse than that for closed injuries. This is true for both complete and incomplete injuries. (Reproduced with permission from Green BA, Eismont FJ, Klose KJ: A comparison of open versus closed spinal cord injuries during the first year post injury. *Annual Meeting of the American Spinal Injury Association*. New Orleans, LA, 1981.)

Complications

Neurologic Injury

The use of steroids is contraindicated in the treatment of patients with spinal cord injury from gunshot wounds. The results of the second National Acute Spinal Cord Injury Study (NASCIS II) was published in 1990.[90] This study demonstrated statistically significant improvements in both motor and sensory function at 6 weeks and 6 months after acute blunt SCI in patients treated with high-dose methylprednisolone. This randomized, double-blind, placebo-controlled trial found no statistically significant increased risk in the complication rates among patients with SCI who received methylprednisolone. Although the NASCIS II study excluded all gunshot wound victims,[90] some have extrapolated from the results of the study to justify administering steroids to these patients.

FIGURE 15

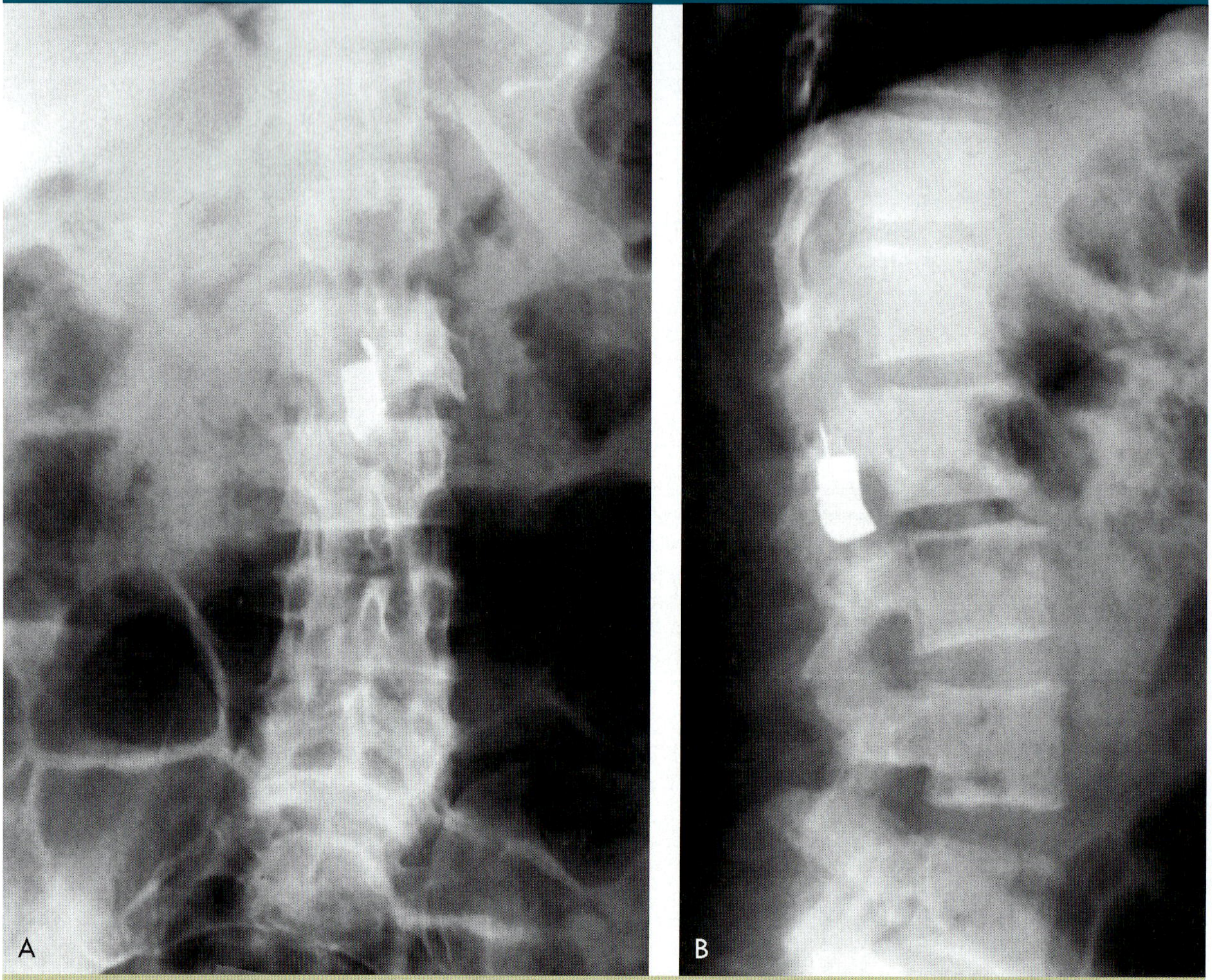

Figure 15 A and **B,** This patient had incomplete paraplegia following a gunshot wound to the spine. He had some function in almost every muscle group below the level of injury, but the main problem was severe pain radiating into the extremities. Passage of time and medical treatment with amitriptyline were unsuccessful. Following removal of the bullet, the patient had significant improvement of pain. Unfortunately, this type of positive response cannot be predicted with bullet removal. (Reproduced with permission from Eismont FJ, Lattuga S: Gunshot wounds of the spine, in Browner BD, Jupiter JB, Levine AM, Trafton PG, eds: *Skeletal Trauma*, ed 2. Philadelphia, PA, WB Saunders, 1997, p 1108.)

Heary et al[91] performed a retrospective review of 254 patients who were treated for gunshot wounds to the spine. Three subgroups were established: methylprednisolone (NASCIS II protocol), dexamethasone (initial dose, 10 mg to 100 mg), and no steroids. No statistically significant neurologic benefits were demonstrable from the use of steroids as measured using the motor scales recommended by the American Spinal Injury Association (ASIA) and the Frankel grading system. However, infectious complications were increased in both groups receiving steroids (not statistically significant). Gastrointestinal complications were significantly increased in the dexamethasone group, and pancreatitis was significantly increased in the methylprednisolone group. The mean duration of follow-up was 56.3 months.

A second retrospective review by Levy et al[92] found similar results in their analysis of 236 patients. They had 181 patients who did not receive steroids and 55 patients who were treated according to the NASCIS II protocol. No difference in neurologic function was found using Frankel scores. In contrast to the previous study, however, no significant difference in complications between the two groups was appreciated. Based on these

FIGURE 16

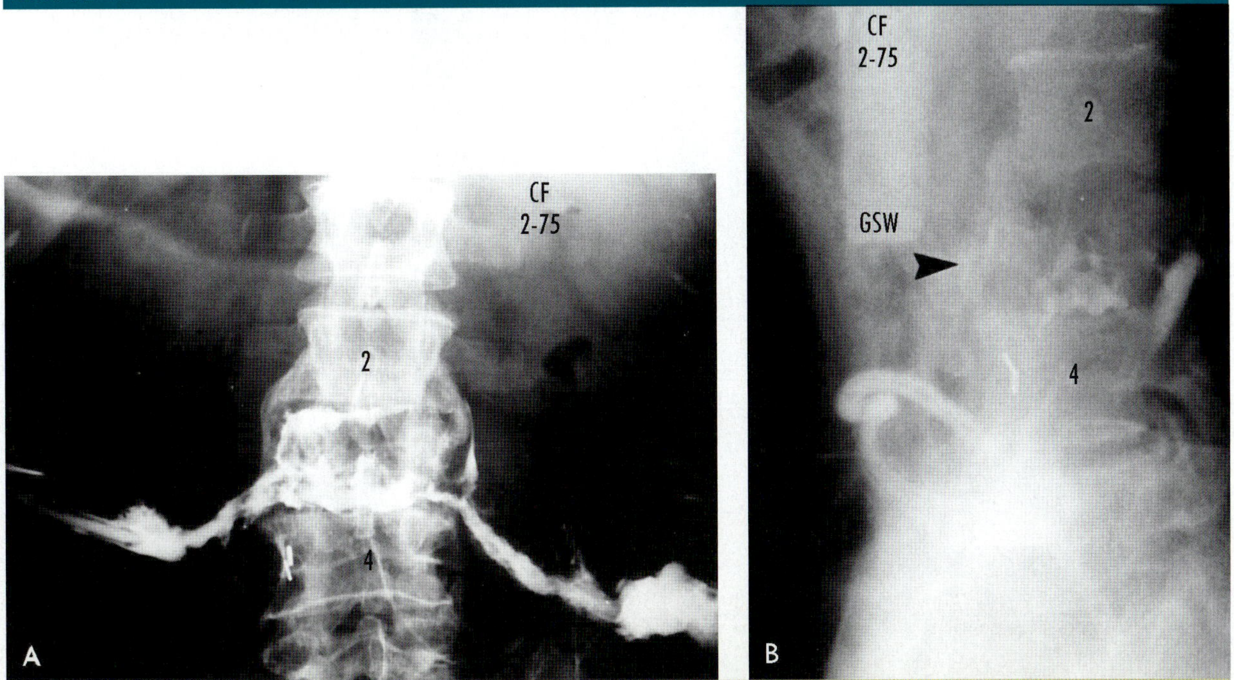

Figure 16 A and **B,** This patient sustained a gunshot wound with perforation of the colon, and the bullet traversed the L3 vertebral body. Chronic vertebral osteomyelitis developed, with a sinus draining through each flank. The sinogram reveals the significant vertebral destruction. Treatment of this problem requires assessment of the gastrointestinal tract to rule out any remaining bowel fistula. This should be followed by vigorous spine débridement and packing of the cavity with cancellous bone or viable soft tissue, followed by a protracted course of antibiotics. (Reproduced with permission from Eismont FJ, Lattuga S: Gunshot wounds of the spine, in Browner BD, Jupiter JB, Levine AM, Trafton PG eds: *Skeletal Trauma*, ed 2. Philadelphia, PA, WB Saunders, 1997, p 1111.)

two studies, we do not recommend treatment of these patients with steroids until the efficacy of such treatment is proven in a controlled study.

The clinical outcomes of paralysis resulting from gunshot wounds to the spine has been well studied and reported by Waters et al.[93] Motor and sensory evaluations were performed on patients with neurologic injuries resulting from gunshot wounds. The study found that 57% of the injuries were complete and 43% were incomplete. At the 1-year follow-up examination, 67% of the patients with complete lesions and 64% of those with incomplete lesions had no improvement in the neurologic level of injury (ie, the most caudal intact motor and sensory level did not change). Overall, however, the patients had a statistically significant improvement in the ASIA motor index score at 1 year after injury ($P < 0.0001$), and more improvement was seen with incomplete injuries than with complete injuries.

Harrop et al[94] set out to identify patients at risk for secondary neurologic deterioration after complete cervical SCI. In a retrospective review of 186 patients, 12 patients (6.0%) with ASIA grade A complete SCIs were found to have neurologic deterioration during the first 30 days after injury; however, none of the patients found to have a penetrating injury had deterioration.

Late neurologic deterioration in patients with an existing neurologic deficit caused by a gunshot wound to the spine has been reported by Gellad et al.[95] Eleven such patients were prospectively evaluated clinically, radiologically, and surgically. The study found a syringomyelic cavity in seven patients, an arachnoid cyst in three, and osteomyelitis in one. Similarly, Shahlaie et al[96] reported on a case of acute neurologic deterioration in a 16-year-old girl found to have occult Chiari malformation following a gunshot wound to the lumbosacral spine.

Patients initially intact following gunshot wounds to the spine who then develop late neurologic deterioration is uncommon, but it has occurred, even many years after the injury.[73,75,78,97-99] Instances of bullet migration within the spinal canal and the subsequent development of a neurologic deficit have been reported.[78] There are also cases of late development of spinal stenosis[75,98] or

FIGURE 17

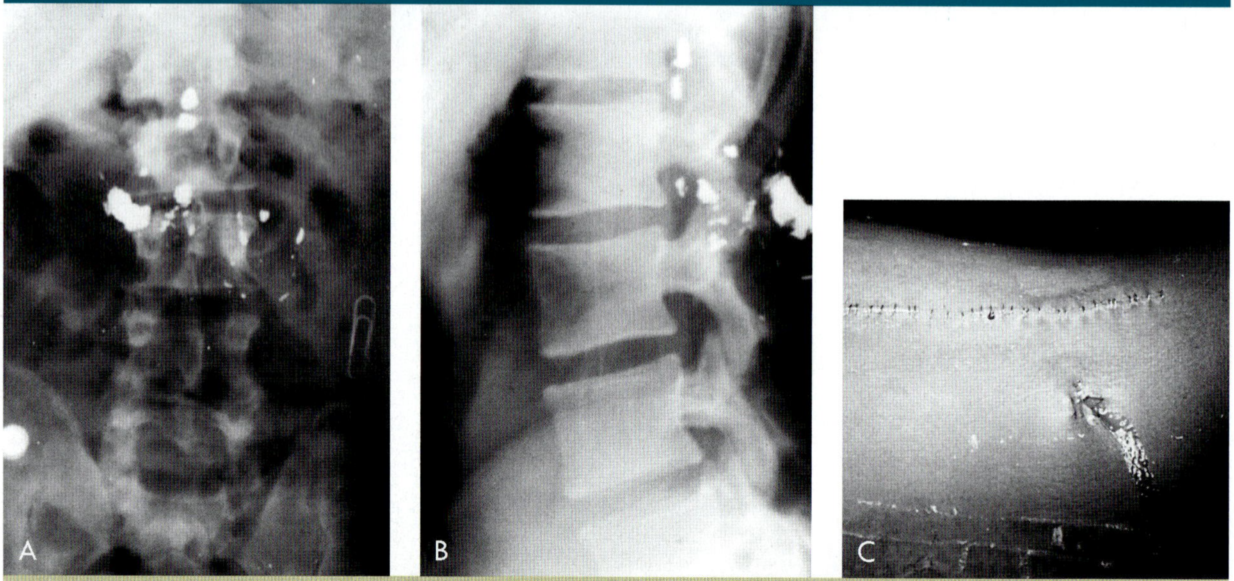

Figure 17 A through **C,** This patient was shot in the back and presented with complete paraplegia at the L1 level. He was taken to surgery emergently where a laminectomy was performed. Postoperatively, the patient developed a CSF-cutaneous fistula through the site of the bullet wound. It is now appreciated that this type of surgery is ineffectual, because no major bullet fragment is present within the spinal canal. The chance of developing the CSF-cutaneous fistula was also heightened by performing the surgery immediately. Treatment now requires placement of a subarachnoid CSF shunt and revision surgery to treat the CSF-cutaneous fistula, the postoperative infection, and the secondary meningitis. (Reproduced with permission from Eismont FJ, Lattuga S: Gunshot wounds of the spine, in Browner BD, Jupiter JB, Levine AM, et al, eds: *Skeletal Trauma*, ed 2. Philadelphia, PA, WB Saunders, 1997, p 1109.)

cauda equine syndrome.[73] Late deterioration may be caused by an intraspinal bullet fragment causing local spinal canal narrowing[75,98] or a combination of neural compression and local neurotoxic effects resulting from the type of metal in the bullet fragment.[22,73,75] These problems of late neurologic deterioration can often be successfully treated surgically. Although the algorithm for treatment of neurologic deficits associated with gunshot wounds to the spine has already been described, these cases suggest a cautious approach to the management of patients with retained bullets in the spinal canal.

Pain With Associated SCI

Chronic dysesthetic pain has been reported as a complication of gunshot injuries to the spinal cord.[95] Most commonly, this pain is described as a searing, burning type of pain that radiates into the paralyzed extremities. This deafferent pain often persists and may be completely disabling; however, in many cases, it improves with the passage of time and the use of conservative measures. Medical management often includes an aggressive course of nonsteroidal anti-inflammatory drugs in combination with amitriptyline or gabapentin.[99-101]

If the deafferent type of pain is still present and disabling, decompressive procedures are unlikely to significantly improve the symptoms (**Figure 15**). Studies show that surgical removal of the bullet from the spinal canal is not helpful in reducing pain early after the injury or at 1 year.[69,102] If surgery is contemplated for this type of deafferent pain, then use of a dorsal root entry zone (DREZ) lesioning procedure with intraoperative computer assessment can offer significant pain relief in some patients.[103,104] This technique is best used in patients without useful distal motor function because of the procedure-related risk of worsening the distal neurologic deficit.

Persistent severe local pain and aching that seems out of proportion to what would normally be expected should be evaluated to rule out underlying infection.

Spine Infections Following Gunshot Wounds

Spine infections occur infrequently following gunshot wounds of the spine. Most of those that do occur follow injuries to the pharynx,[43,44] esophagus, or colon.[45] They seldom occur after injury to any other organs, including the stomach or small bowel. Kumar et al[48] reported on 33 patients with

FIGURE 18

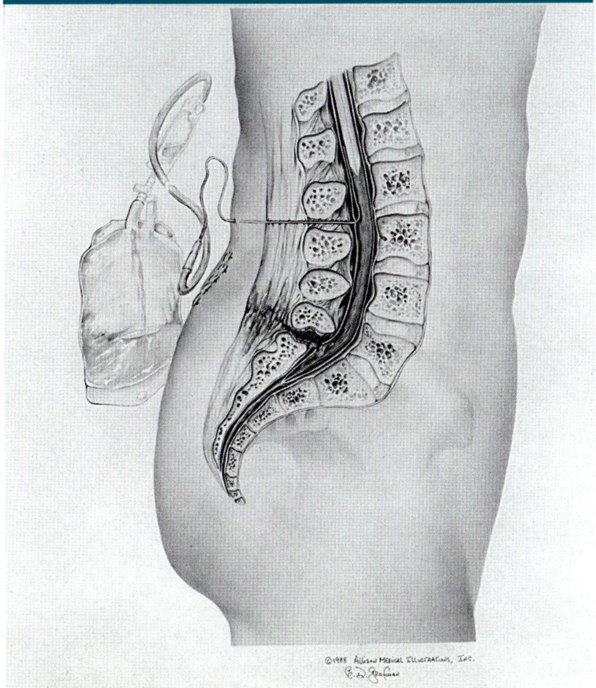

Figure 18 This drawing shows the use of a CSF subarachnoid cutaneous shunt, which allows decompression of the dura and healing of the original CSF-cutaneous fistula. (Reproduced with permission from Kitchell SH, Eismont FJ, Green BA: Closed subarachnoid drainage for management of cerebrospinal fluid leakage after an operation on the spine. *J Bone Joint Surg Am* 1989;71(7):984-989.)

gunshot wounds to the spine and associated viscus injury, with an average follow-up of 29 months. In 13 of their patients, the bullet passed through the colon or rectum before damaging the spine. All patients had immediate exploratory laparotomy, but none had immediate laminectomy, débridement of the missile tract, or bullet removal. A colostomy was performed in three patients, and primary repair or resection and anastomosis was performed in ten patients. The total duration of antibiotic treatment ranged from 2 to 43 days. Six patients received a single antibiotic (cefotetan) and seven received multiple antibiotics. Antibiotic coverage was extended depending on the complications encountered with the viscus repair or resection. Three patients developed peritonitis that required repeated wash-outs. There were no complications related to disk-space infection, osteomyelitis, or retained bullet fragments. The preceding sections have discussed methods of treatment to minimize this complication, including the routine use of prophylactic antibiotics for 72 hours after injury and for 7 to 14 days after injury of a contaminated viscus.[43-45]

The other common cause of infection following gunshot wounds of the spine is iatrogenic infection following surgery. Stauffer et al,[28] in their review of patients treated with laminectomy for bullet removal, found that 4% of patients developed a postoperative wound infection. These infections can be treated like any other postoperative infection of the spine.[105]

Significant fistula formation may be seen in patients with spine infections (**Figure 16**). In patients with a contaminated viscus injury, a fistula may occur from the viscus to the spine. In these cases, it is not possible to resolve the infection without adequate correction of the pharyngeal, esophageal, or bowel fistula. This may require tactics such as diversionary drainage and prolonged hyperalimentation. Some patients are seen with cutaneous fistulas leading to a vertebral osteomyelitis or disk-space infection, but it is much more common for this to occur in patients with a viscus fistula, as described earlier.

In general, extraspinal infections are much more common than spinal infections following a gunshot wound to the spine.[46] Additionally, military (high-velocity) gunshot wounds are distinctly different from civilian (low-velocity) handgun wounds and may benefit from surgical management because of the much greater degree of wound contamination and tissue destruction seen with military assault weapons.[46,106,107]

The indications for surgical treatment of patients with spine infections following gunshot wounds of the spine are the same as for patients with spine infection from other causes. They include progressive paralysis associated with the infection, progressive deformity, lack of a known organism, suspected foreign body associated with the infection, and failure of conservative treatment. In most cases, the spine infection is not identified until several weeks after the injury, and at that time, we normally recommend a CT-guided needle biopsy of the spine followed by a 6-week course of maximum-dose parenteral antibiotics. Open surgery would be reserved for the cases described previously.

CSF-Cutaneous Fistulas

CSF-cutaneous fistulas have been described after gunshot wounds to the spine. The fistula can connect with skin or with other body cavities. Occasionally they are seen as a direct result of the gunshot wound to the spine,[54] but they occur most commonly after acute surgical treatment with laminectomy (**Figure 17**). Stauffer et al[28] described their experience with 185 patients and

5: Thoracolumbar Injuries

FIGURE 19

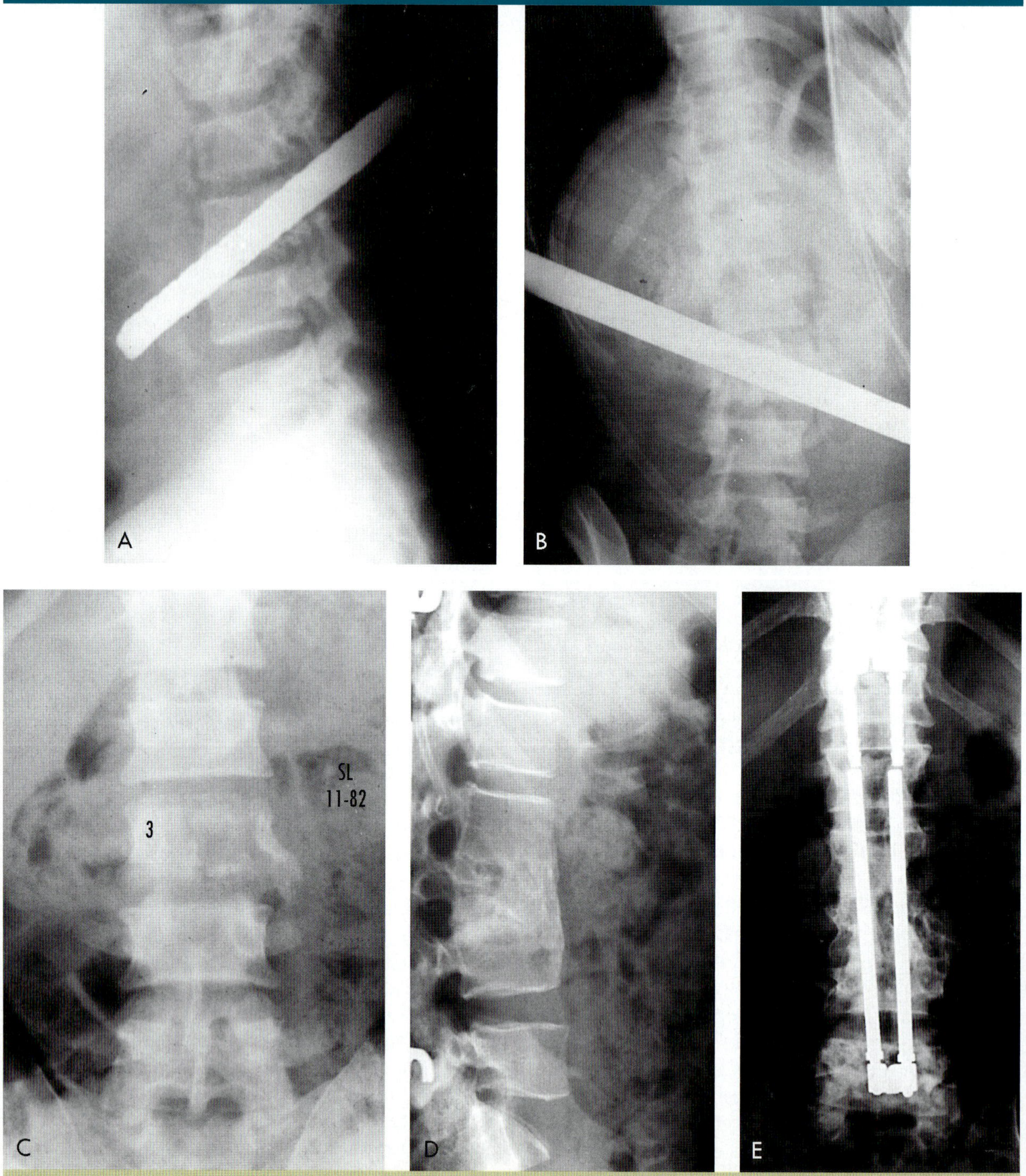

Figure 19 **A** and **B,** This patient was impaled on a reinforcing rod following a motorcycle accident. The rod was removed in the operating room with both anterior and posterior exposure of the spine provided. The spine was cultured and vigorously débrided at the time of initial emergency surgery. Despite 3 weeks of administration of broad-spectrum antibiotics, persistent vertebral osteomyelitis and pain developed and vertebral destruction continued (**C**). At 6 weeks after injury, the patient was returned to surgery for simultaneous anterior and posterior débridement, fusion, and stabilization. Pieces of clothing were found within the vertebral body, and cultures at surgery revealed standard pyogenic organisms as well as a fungus infection. **D** and **E,** Radiographs taken 10 years after injury reveal complete resolution of the infection. Broken rods and a flat-back deformity are now appreciated, but the patient is asymptomatic and able to participate in full wheelchair activities with no pain. (Reproduced with permission from Eismont FJ, Lattuga S: Gunshot wounds of the spine, in Browner BD, Jupiter JB, Levine AM, Trafton PG, eds: *Skeletal Trauma*, ed 2. Philadelphia, PA, WB Saunders, 1997, p 1112.)

FIGURE 20

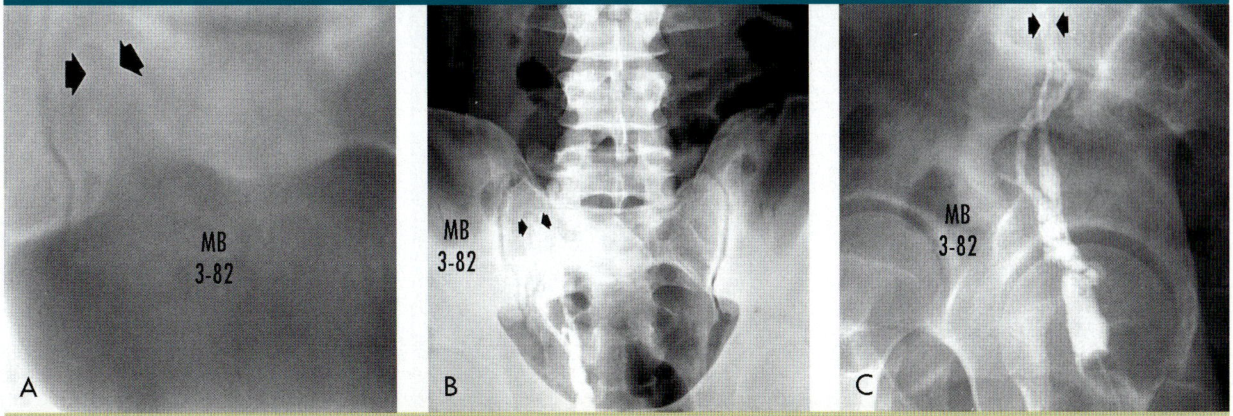

Figure 20 This man fell at a construction site and landed on a reinforcing rod, which pierced the perineum and transverse colon and penetrated the sacral ala. He presented to us many months after injury with a persistent perineal fistula, after several courses of antibiotics and anterior abdominal operations failed. **A,** AP tomogram of the sacrum shows the lytic tract in the ala caused by the penetrating rod and persistent infection (arrows). **B,** AP view of the pelvis immediately after the sinogram shows that the fistulous tract ends in the right ala (arrows). **C,** The lateral sinogram also confirms the source of the infection in the sacral ala. This patient was successfully treated with a posterior lateral muscle-splitting approach and wide débridement of the sacral ala, followed by a 6-week course of antibiotics for all organisms cultured from the alar bone debris. (Reproduced with permission from Eismont FJ, Lattuga S: Gunshot wounds of the spine, in Browner BD, Jupiter JB, Levine AM, Trafton PG, eds: *Skeletal Trauma*, ed 2. Philadelphia, PA, WB Saunders, 1997, p 1113.)

observed that CSF-cutaneous fistulas did not occur in patients who had not had laminectomies. In those treated with laminectomy, "spinal débridement," and bullet removal, the incidence was 6%.

Considering that most of the CSF-cutaneous fistulas are seen following acute surgical treatment is another reason for delaying removal of the bullet for 7 to 10 days except when emergency surgical decompression is needed. When surgery is performed to remove the bullet, meticulous dural repair and closure of the paraspinous muscles, deep fascia, and skin are necessary to minimize the chance of a postoperative CSF-cutaneous fistula.[108] At the time of repair of the dura, the seal should be checked with a Valsalva maneuver to make certain that it is indeed watertight. If a watertight closure cannot be achieved, then a lumbar subarachnoid cutaneous drain (**Figure 18**) should be placed to adequately decompress the dural sac by diverting spinal fluid, to promote proper healing and to prevent such problems as CSF-cutaneous fistulas and subsequent meningitis.[109]

Other Penetrating Injuries of the Spine

Impalement Injuries

Impalement injuries of the spine are uncommon. The trauma is usually massive, and there is usually more gross wound contamination than in other injuries to the spine.[110] Patients with impalement injuries to the spine should be taken to surgery for spine débridement. Cultures for aerobes, anaerobes, and fungus should be carefully obtained. Unlike the relatively clean gunshot wounds described earlier, these injuries require a minimum of 3 weeks of parenteral therapy with broad-spectrum antibiotics to cover the organisms found at the original débridement. It is also extremely important to rule out significant presence of foreign bodies (eg, pieces of clothing), which may have been driven into the spine at the time of the impalement injury (**Figure 19**).

Patients who have sustained an impalement injury to the spine often have recurrent spine infections and spontaneous drainage from sinus tracts. Successful treatment often requires sinography to define the course of the sinus, tomography or CT immediately after sinography to define the bone or disk pathology, and then surgery to débride the spinal source of infection as well as to excise the chronic sinus tract. The injection of methylene blue into the sinus tract helps to identify the tissue that requires excision (**Figure 20**). However, methylene blue should never be used if there is a possibility of a dural cutaneous fistula because intrathecal injection of methylene blue is fatal.

FIGURE 21

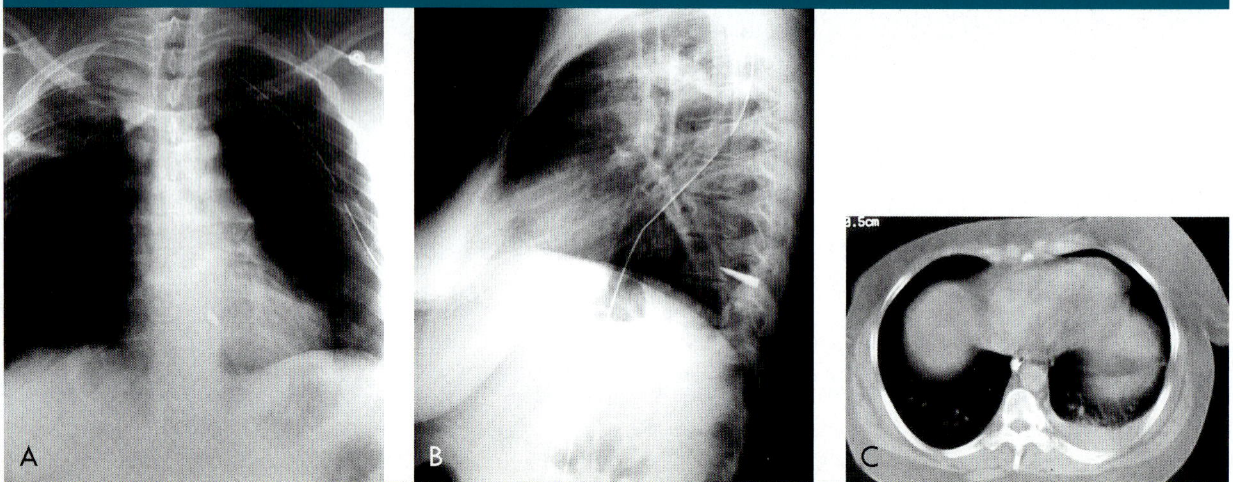

Figure 21 This patient presented to the emergency department after being stabbed with a pair of scissors. After emergency treatment of a pneumothorax, AP (**A**) and lateral (**B**) chest films reveal a metallic foreign body adjacent to the thoracic spine. **C,** CT verifies the location of the foreign body. This patient was taken to surgery for removal of the foreign body to minimize the chance of development of a persistent infection. (Reproduced with permission from Eismont FJ, Lattuga S: Gunshot wounds of the spine, in Browner BD, Jupiter JB, Levine AM, Trafton PG, eds: *Skeletal Trauma*, ed 2. Philadelphia, PA, WB Saunders, 1997, p 1114.)

Stabbing Injuries

Stabbing injuries of the spine are seen much less commonly than gunshot wounds of the spine in the United States, but in some countries, these are the most common type of penetrating injury of the spine. Radiographs should be taken immediately to make certain that no foreign bodies remain. Any remaining foreign bodies (**Figure 21**) should be surgically removed. These foreign bodies are not sterile and can be the source of persistent late infections. Stab wounds are very often associated with Brown-Séquard–type paralysis; hence, they have the best prognosis of incomplete spinal injuries. The general prognosis for patients with stab injuries to the spine is significantly better than for patients with gunshot wounds of the spine with the same extent of incomplete paralysis.

Conclusion

Unfortunately, the incidence of SCIs secondary to gunshot wounds of the spine is rising. Physicians must be familiar with the evaluation and treatment of these injuries. The importance of a good history, physical examination, and radiographic evaluation cannot be overemphasized. Most gunshot wounds of the spine can be treated nonsurgically, but it is important not to miss the rare injury that behaves clinically more like a typical war injury.

References

1. Farmer JC, Vaccaro AR, Balderston RA, Albert TJ, Cotler J: The changing nature of admissions to a spinal cord injury center: Violence on the rise. *J Spinal Disord* 1998;11(5):400-403.
2. Lin SS, Vaccaro AR, Reisch S, Devine M, Cotler JM: Low-velocity gunshot wounds to the spine with an associated transperitoneal injury. *J Spinal Disord* 1995;8(2):136-144.
3. Bono CM, Heary RF: Gunshot wounds to the spine. *Spine J* 2004;4(2):230-240.
4. Bahebeck J, Atangana R, Mboudou E, Nonga BN, Sosso M, Malonga E: Incidence, case-fatality rate and clinical pattern of firearm injuries in two cities where arm owning is forbidden. *Injury* 2005; 36(6):714-717.
5. Burney RE, Maio RF, Maynard F, Karunas R: Incidence, characteristics, and outcome of spinal cord injury at trauma centers in North America. *Arch Surg* 1993;128(5):596-599.
6. McKinley WO, Johns JS, Musgrove JJ: Clinical presentations, medical complications, and functional outcomes of individuals with gunshot wound-induced spinal cord injury. *Am J Phys Med Rehabil* 1999;78(2):102-107.
7. Young JA, Burns PE, McCutchen R, eds: *Spinal Cord Injury Statistics: Experience of the Regional Spinal Cord Injury Systems*. Phoenix, AZ, Good Samaritan Medical Center, 1982, pp 1-152.
8. Ragucci MV, Gittler MM, Balfanz-Vertiz K, Hunter A: Societal risk factors associated with spinal cord

injury secondary to gunshot wound. *Arch Phys Med Rehabil* 2001;82(12):1720-1723.

9. Capen D: Etiology of spinal cord injuries: Significant changes over ten years. *Annual Meeting of the American Academy of Orthopaedic Surgeons*. San Francisco, CA, February, 1993.
10. Magnuson E, Leviton J, Riley M: Seven deadly days. *Time* July 17, 1989, pp 30-61.
11. Fackler ML: Wound ballistics: A review of common misconceptions. *JAMA* 1988;259(18):2730-2736.
12. Fackler ML, Bellamy RF, Malinowski JA: The wound profile: Illustration of the missile-tissue interaction. *J Trauma* 1988;28(1 Suppl):S21-S29.
13. Fackler ML, Malinowski JA: The wound profile: A visual method for quantifying gunshot wound components. *J Trauma* 1985;25(6):522-529.
14. Leonard MH: The solution of lead by synovial fluid. *Clin Orthop Relat Res* 1969;64:255-261.
15. Switz DM, Elmorshidy ME, Deyerle WM: Bullets, joints, and lead intoxication: A remarkable and instructive case. *Arch Intern Med* 1976;136(8):939-941.
16. Windler EC, Smith RB, Bryan WJ, Woods GW: Lead intoxication and traumatic arthritis of the hip secondary to retained bullet fragments: A case report. *J Bone Joint Surg Am* 1978;60(2):254-255.
17. Grogan DP, Bucholz RW: Acute lead intoxication from a bullet in an intervertebral disc space: A case report. *J Bone Joint Surg Am* 1981;63(7):1180-1182.
18. Scuderi GJ, Vaccaro AR, Fitzhenry LN, Greenberg S, Eismont FJ: Long-term clinical manifestations of retained bullet fragments within the intervertebral disk space. *J Spinal Disord Tech* 2004;17(2):108-111.
19. Cushid JG, Kopeloff LM: Epileptogenic effects of metal powder implants in the motor cortex in monkeys. *Int J Neuropsychiatr* 1968;3:24-28.
20. Sherman IJ: Brass foreign body in the brain stem: A case report. *J Neurosurg* 1960;17:483-485.
21. Sights WP, Bye RJ: The fate of retained intracerebral shotgun pellets: An experimental study. *J Neurosurg* 1970;33(6):646-653.
22. Tindel NL, Marcillo AE, Tay BK, Bunge RP, Eismont FJ: The effect of surgically implanted bullet fragments on the spinal cord in a rabbit model. *J Bone Joint Surg Am* 2001;83(6):884-890.
23. Breitenecker R: Shotgun wound patterns. *Am J Clin Pathol* 1969;52(3):258-269.
24. May M, West JW, Heeneman H, Gowda CK, Ogura JH: Proceedings: Shotgun wounds to the head and neck. *Arch Otolaryngol* 1973;98(6):373-376.
25. Keith A, Hall ME: Specimens of gunshot injuries of the face and spine, contained in the army medical collection now on exhibition in the Museum of Royal College of Surgeons of England. *Br J Surg* 1919;7(25):55-71.
26. Klemperer WW, Fulton JF, Lamport H, Schorr MG: Indirect spinal cord injuries due to gunshot wounds of the spinal column in animal and man. *Mil Surg* 1954;114(4):253-265.
27. Mirovsky Y, Shalmon E, Blankstein A, Halperin N: Complete paraplegia following gunshot injury without direct trauma to the cord. *Spine (Phila Pa 1976)* 2005;30(21):2436-2438.
28. Stauffer ES, Wood RW, Kelly EG: Gunshot wounds of the spine: The effects of laminectomy. *J Bone Joint Surg Am* 1979;61(3):389-392.
29. Klein Y, Cohn SM, Soffer D, Lynn M, Shaw CM, Hasharoni A: Spine injuries are common among asymptomatic patients after gunshot wounds. *J Trauma* 2005;58(4):833-836.
30. Pohost GM, Blackwell GG, Shellock FG: Safety of patients with medical devices during application of magnetic resonance methods. *Ann N Y Acad Sci* 1992;649:302-312.
31. Shellock FG, Curtis JS: MR imaging and biomedical implants, materials, and devices: An updated review. *Radiology* 1991;180(2):541-550.
32. Teitelbaum GP, Yee CA, Van Horn DD, Kim HS, Colletti PM: Metallic ballistic fragments: MR imaging safety and artifacts. *Radiology* 1990;175(3):855-859.
33. Finitsis SN, Falcone S, Green BA: MR of the spine in the presence of metallic bullet fragments: Is the benefit worth the risk? *AJNR Am J Neuroradiol* 1999;20(2):354-356.
34. Oliver C, Kabala J: Air gun pellet injuries: The safety of MR imaging. *Clin Radiol* 1997;52(4):299-300.
35. Bishop M, Shoemaker WC, Avakian S, et al: Evaluation of a comprehensive algorithm for blunt and penetrating thoracic and abdominal trauma. *Am Surg* 1991;57(12):737-746.
36. Mohammed GS, Pillay WR, Barker P, Robbs JV: The role of clinical examination in excluding vascular injury in haemodynamically stable patients with gunshot wounds to the neck: A prospective study of 59 patients. *Eur J Vasc Endovasc Surg* 2004;28(4):425-430.
37. Fitzgerald LF, Simpson RK, Trask T: Locked-in syndrome resulting from cervical spine gunshot wound. *J Trauma* 1997;42(1):147-149.
38. Golueke P, Sclafani S, Phillips T, Goldstein A, Scalea T, Duncan A: Vertebral artery injury—diagnosis and management. *J Trauma* 1987;27(8):856-865.

39. Saletta JD, Lowe RJ, Lim LT, Thornton J, Delk S, Moss GS: Penetrating trauma of the neck. *J Trauma* 1976;16(7):579-587.

40. Menawat SS, Dennis JW, Laneve LM, Frykberg ER: Are arteriograms necessary in penetrating zone II neck injuries? *J Vasc Surg* 1992;16(3): 397-401.

41. Ordog GJ, Albin D, Wasserberger J, Schlater TL, Balasubramaniam S: 110 bullet wounds to the neck. *J Trauma* 1985;25(3):238-246.

42. Sheely CH II, Mattox KL, Reul GJ Jr, Beall AC Jr, DeBakey ME: Current concepts in the management of penetrating neck trauma. *J Trauma* 1975; 15(10):895-900.

43. Schaefer SD, Bucholz RW, Jones RE, Anderson RG, Carder HM: "How I do it"—head and neck: A targeted problem and its solution. Treatment of transpharyngeal missile wounds to the cervical spine. *Laryngoscope* 1981;91(1):146-148.

44. Schaefer SD, Bucholz RW, Jones RE, Carder HM: The management of transpharyngeal gunshot wounds to the cervical spine. *Surg Gynecol Obstet* 1981;152(1):27-29.

45. Roffi RP, Waters RL, Adkins RH: Gunshot wounds to the spine associated with a perforated viscus. *Spine (Phila Pa 1976)* 1989;14(8):808-811.

46. Heary RF, Vaccaro AR, Mesa JJ, Balderston RA: Thoracolumbar infections in penetrating injuries to the spine. *Orthop Clin North Am* 1996;27(1): 69-81.

47. Kihtir T, Ivatury RR, Simon R, Stahl WM: Management of transperitoneal gunshot wounds of the spine. *J Trauma* 1991;31(12):1579-1583.

48. Kumar A, Wood GW II, Whittle AP: Low-velocity gunshot injuries of the spine with abdominal viscus trauma. *J Orthop Trauma* 1998;12(7):514-517.

49. Isiklar ZU, Lindsey RW: Low-velocity civilian gunshot wounds of the spine. *Orthopedics* 1997; 20(10):967-972.

50. Yoshida GM, Garland D, Waters RL: Gunshot wounds to the spine. *Orthop Clin North Am* 1995; 26(1):109-116.

51. Ramasamy A, Midwinter M, Mahoney P, Clasper J: Learning the lessons from conflict: Pre-hospital cervical spine stabilisation following ballistic neck trauma. *Injury* 2009;40(12):1342-1345.

52. DuBose J, Teixeira PG, Hadjizacharia P, et al: The role of routine spinal imaging and immobilisation in asymptomatic patients after gunshot wounds. *Injury* 2009;40(8):860-863.

53. Medzon R, Rothenhaus T, Bono CM, Grindlinger G, Rathlev NK: Stability of cervical spine fractures after gunshot wounds to the head and neck. *Spine (Phila Pa 1976)* 2005;30(20):2274-2279.

54. Waters RL, Sie IH: Spinal cord injuries from gunshot wounds to the spine. *Clin Orthop Relat Res* 2003;408:120-125.

55. Pal GP, Sherk HH: The vertical stability of the cervical spine. *Spine (Phila Pa 1976)* 1988;13(5): 447-449.

56. Denis F: The three column spine and its significance in the classification of acute thoracolumbar spinal injuries. *Spine (Phila Pa 1976)* 1983;8(8): 817-831.

57. Wolf AW, Benson DR, Shoji H, Hoeprich P, Gilmore A: Autosterilization in low-velocity bullets. *J Trauma* 1978;18(1):63.

58. Hales DD, Duffy K, Dawson EG, Delamarter R: Lumbar osteomyelitis and epidural and paraspinous abscesses: Case report of an unusual source of contamination from a gunshot wound to the abdomen. *Spine (Phila Pa 1976)* 1991;16(3): 380-383.

59. Romanick PC, Smith TK, Kopaniky DR, Oldfield D: Infection about the spine associated with low-velocity-missile injury to the abdomen. *J Bone Joint Surg Am* 1985;67(8):1195-1201.

60. Robertson DP, Simpson RK, Narayan RK: Lumbar disc herniation from a gunshot wound to the spine: A report of two cases. *Spine (Phila Pa 1976)* 1991;16(8):994-995.

61. Cybulski GR, Stone JL, Kant R: Outcome of laminectomy for civilian gunshot injuries of the terminal spinal cord and cauda equina: Review of 88 cases. *Neurosurgery* 1989;24(3):392-397.

62. Heiden JS, Weiss MH, Rosenberg AW, Kurze T, Apuzzo ML: Penetrating gunshot wounds of the cervical spine in civilians: Review of 38 cases. *J Neurosurg* 1975;42(5):575-579.

63. Jacobson SA, Bors E: Spinal cord injury in Vietnamese combat. *Paraplegia* 1970;7(4):263-281.

64. Kupcha PC, An HS, Cotler JM: Gunshot wounds to the cervical spine. *Spine (Phila Pa 1976)* 1990; 15(10):1058-1063.

65. Pool JL: Gunshot wounds of the spine: Observations from an evacuation hospital. *Surg Gynecol Obstet* 1945;81:617-622.

66. Simpson RK Jr, Venger BH, Narayan RK: Treatment of acute penetrating injuries of the spine: A retrospective analysis. *J Trauma* 1989;29(1):42-46.

67. Simpson RL, Venager BH, Narayan RK: Penetrating spinal cord injury in a civilian population: A retrospective analysis. *Surg Forum* 1986;37: 494-496.

68. Yashon D, Jane JA, White RJ: Prognosis and management of spinal cord and cauda equina bullet injuries in sixty-five civilians. *J Neurosurg* 1970; 32(2):163-170.

69. Waters RL, Adkins RH: The effects of removal of bullet fragments retained in the spinal canal: A collaborative study by the National Spinal Cord Injury Model Systems. *Spine (Phila Pa 1976)* 1991; 16(8):934-939.

70. Cammisa FP, Eismont FJ, Tolli T: Penetrating injuries of the cervical spine, in Camins MB, O'Leary P, eds: *Disorders of the Cervical Spine*. Williams & Wilkins, Baltimore, MD, 1992, pp 317-322.
71. Anderson PA, Bohlman HH: Anterior decompression and arthrodesis of the cervical spine: Long-term motor improvement. Part II—Improvement in complete traumatic quadriplegia. *J Bone Joint Surg Am* 1992;74(5):683-692.
72. Bohlman HH, Anderson PA: Anterior decompression and arthrodesis of the cervical spine: Long-term motor improvement. Part I—Improvement in incomplete traumatic quadriparesis. *J Bone Joint Surg Am* 1992;74(5):671-682.
73. Kuijlen JM, Herpers MJ, Beuls EA: Neurogenic claudication, a delayed complication of a retained bullet. *Spine (Phila Pa 1976)* 1997;22(8):910-914.
74. Nino HE, Leppik IE, Lai C, Martin S: Progressive sensory loss one year after bullet injury of spinal cord. *JAMA* 1978;240(11):1173-1174.
75. Staniforth P, Watt I: Extradural "plumboma": A rare cause of acquired spinal stenosis. *Br J Radiol* 1982;55(658):772-774.
76. Wu WQ: Delayed effects from retained foreign bodies in the spine and spinal cord. *Surg Neurol* 1986;25(3):214-218.
77. Gupta S, Senger RL: Wandering intraspinal bullet. *Br J Neurosurg* 1999;13(6):606-607.
78. Karim NO, Nabors MW, Golocovsky M, Cooney FD: Spontaneous migration of a bullet in the spinal subarachnoid space causing delayed radicular symptoms. *Neurosurgery* 1986;18(1):97-100.
79. Ledgerwood AM: The wandering bullet. *Surg Clin North Am* 1977;57(1):97-109.
80. Rajan DK, Alcantara AL, Michael DB: Where's the bullet? A migration in two acts. *J Trauma* 1997;43(4):716-718.
81. Yip L, Sweeny PJ, McCarroll KA: Spontaneous migration of an intraspinal bullet following a gunshot wound. *Am J Emerg Med* 1990;8(6):569-570.
82. Moon E, Kondrashov D, Hannibal M, Hsu K, Zucherman J: Gunshot wounds to the spine: Literature review and report on a migratory intrathecal bullet. *Am J Orthop (Belle Mead NJ)* 2008;37(3):E47-E51.
83. Ceylan D, Cosar M: Migration of a bullet in the lumbar intervertebral disc space causing back pain: Case report. *Neurol Med Chir (Tokyo)* 2008;48(4):188-190.
84. Ben-Galim P, Reitman CA: Intrathecal migratory foreign body without neurological deficit after a gunshot wound. *Spine J* 2008;8(2):404-407.
85. Tumialán LM, Walkup RR, Gupta SK: Minimally invasive retrieval of a bullet from the L5-S1 neural foramina after transperitoneal gunshot wound. *Spine J* 2009;9(2):169-173.
86. Spakauskas B, Ambrozaitis KV, Kontautas E: The bullet in the dural sac: How to catch it? A report of two cases. *Medicina (Kaunas)* 2007;43(6):478-481.
87. Borra V, Serra MJ, Rubel IF: Trans-iliac removal of bullet fragments from the sacroiliac joint. *J Orthop Trauma* 2006;20(1):52-55.
88. Lee GH, Virkus WW, Kapotas JS: Arthroscopically assisted minimally invasive intraarticular bullet extraction: Technique, indications, and results. *J Trauma* 2008;64(2):512-516.
89. Green BA, Eismont FJ, Close KJ: A comparison of open versus closed spinal cord injuries during the first year post injury. *Annual Meeting of the American Spinal Injury Association*. New Orleans, LA, 1981.
90. Bracken MB, Shepard MJ, Collins WF, et al: A randomized, controlled trial of methylprednisolone or naloxone in the treatment of acute spinal-cord injury: Results of the Second National Acute Spinal Cord Injury Study. *N Engl J Med* 1990;322(20):1405-1411.
91. Heary RF, Vaccaro AR, Mesa JJ, et al: Steroids and gunshot wounds to the spine. *Neurosurgery* 1997;41(3):576-584.
92. Levy ML, Gans W, Wijesinghe HS, SooHoo WE, Adkins RH, Stillerman CB: Use of methylprednisolone as an adjunct in the management of patients with penetrating spinal cord injury: Outcome analysis. *Neurosurgery* 1996;39(6):1141-1149.
93. Waters RL, Adkins RH, Yakura J, Sie I: Profiles of spinal cord injury and recovery after gunshot injury. *Clin Orthop Relat Res* 1991;267:14-21.
94. Harrop JS, Sharan AD, Vaccaro AR, Przybylski GJ: The cause of neurologic deterioration after acute cervical spinal cord injury. *Spine (Phila Pa 1976)* 2001;26(4):340-346.
95. Gellad FE, Paul KS, Geisler FH: Early sequelae of gunshot wounds to the spine: Radiologic diagnosis. *Radiology* 1988;167(2):523-526.
96. Shahlaie K, Hartman J, Utter GH, Schrot RJ: Acute deterioration in occult Chiari malformation following missile spinal trauma: Case report. *J Neurosurg Spine* 2008;8(4):385-389.
97. Conway JE, Crofford TW, Terry AF, Protzman RR: Cauda equina syndrome occurring nine years after a gunshot injury to the spine: A case report. *J Bone Joint Surg Am* 1993;75(5):760-763.
98. Jeffery JA, Borgstein R: Case report of a retained bullet in the lumbar spinal canal with preservation of cauda equina function. *Injury* 1998;29(9):724-726.
99. Kvinesdal B, Molin J, Frøland A, Gram LF: Imipramine treatment of painful diabetic neuropathy. *JAMA* 1984;251(13):1727-1730.

100. Richards JS: Pain secondary to gunshot wounds during the initial rehabilitation process in spinal cord injury patients. *J Rehabil Res Dev* 1988;(25 Suppl):75.

101. Watson CP, Evans RJ, Reed K, Merskey H, Goldsmith L, Warsh J: Amitriptyline versus placebo in postherpetic neuralgia. *Neurology* 1982; 32(6): 671-673.

102. Richards JS, Stover SL, Jaworski T: Effect of bullet removal on subsequent pain in persons with spinal cord injury secondary to gunshot wound. *J Neurosurg* 1990;73(3):401-404.

103. Nashold BS Jr, Ostdahl RH: Dorsal root entry zone lesions for pain relief. *J Neurosurg* 1979; 51(1):59-69.

104. Spaić M, Petković S, Tadić R, Minić L: DREZ surgery on conus medullaris (after failed implantation of vascular omental graft) for treating chronic pain due to spine (gunshot) injuries. *Acta Neurochir (Wien)* 1999;141(12):1309-1312.

105. Gepstein R, Eismont FJ: Postoperative spine infections, in Garfin SR, ed: *Complications of Spine Surgery*. Williams & Wilkins, Baltimore, MD, 1989, pp 302-322.

106. Splavski B, Vranković D, Sarić G, Blagus G, Mursić B, Rukovanjski M: Early management of war missile spine and spinal cord injuries: Experience with 21 cases. *Injury* 1996;27(10):699-702.

107. Alaca R, Yilmaz B, Goktepe AS, Yazicioglu K, Gunduz S: Military gunshot wound-induced spinal cord injuries. *Mil Med* 2002;167(11):926-928.

108. Eismont FJ, Wiesel SW, Rothman RH: Treatment of dural tears associated with spinal surgery. *J Bone Joint Surg Am* 1981;63(7):1132-1136.

109. Kitchel SH, Eismont FJ, Green BA: Closed subarachnoid drainage for management of cerebrospinal fluid leakage after an operation on the spine. *J Bone Joint Surg Am* 1989;71(7):984-987.

110. Horowitz MD, Dove DB, Eismont FJ, Green BA: Impalement injuries. *J Trauma* 1985;25(9): 914-916.

CHAPTER 36
Immediate Postoperative Care

Reynold Rimoldi, MD   Jack E. Zigler, MD

Introduction

The rehabilitation course for the patient with an unstable spinal cord injury can be dramatically improved with appropriate surgical intervention. The care of these patients, however, differs significantly from the typical orthopaedic population in postoperative management. This chapter will review the principles of postoperative management of the patient with a spinal cord injury.

Respiratory Care

In addition to understanding the effects of general anesthesia, the surgeon needs to be aware of the respiratory changes common after spinal surgery. The effect of a general anesthetic is to decrease the lung vital capacity as well as facilitate compliance. Frequent position change and allowing the patient to assume a sitting position on postoperative day 1 (if the method of stabilization will allow it) will facilitate respiratory care. Smoking in the postoperative period should be prohibited. Incentive spirometry may prevent further postoperative atelectasis. Low-dose analgesics administered postoperatively at frequent intervals may improve respiratory function by decreasing pain and improving incentive respiratory therapy. Higher analgesic doses may promote respiratory dysfunction by decreasing the respiratory rate and tidal volume.

Oxygen should be used only if necessary, as prolonged administration may promote atelectasis by the nitrogen washout effect. This may in turn lead to oxygen toxicity. Patients with chronic hypercapnia may have a lowering of their respiratory drive if given oxygen. Patients with preexisting pulmonary disease should be considered for a planned 24-hour period of postoperative ventilator support. In those patients with associated posttraumatic pulmonary injury, close monitoring of arterial blood gases is mandatory.

Associated injuries to the chest occur in 18% of patients with thoracolumbar injuries.[1] Many of these injuries are not appreciated until the postoperative period. Early diagnosis and treatment of associated pulmonary contusions and pneumothorax are important to facilitate the acute postoperative respiratory course.

Deep Vein Thrombosis and Pulmonary Embolism

Knowledge pertaining to deep vein thrombosis (DVT) and the secondary complication of pulmonary embolism in the field of orthopaedics has stemmed from observations and research pertaining to lower extremity reconstruction and fracture work. Ninety percent of clinically important pulmonary emboli arise from proximally located deep vein thromboses. Up to 10% of hospital deaths per year are secondary to pulmonary embolism. Furthermore, approximately 60% of these fatal pulmonary embolus cases failed to receive prophylaxis against DVT.[2]

The diagnosis of pulmonary embolus is sometimes difficult. Therefore, it is important to maintain clinical awareness of this condition, which can be rapidly fatal; the majority of pulmonary emboli that result in death do so less than 1 hour from onset.[3]

Clinically significant DVT occurs in 7% of patients who have undergone spine surgery. Other risk factors observed in patients with spinal cord injury include associated trauma and paralysis that may increase the risk of DVT to 40%. Delay in mobilization of these patients also increases the risk of DVT. Patients who are immobilized in bed for less than 1 week have a 50% incidence of DVT, where periods of bed rest greater than 1 week increase the incidence to 80%.[4]

Many patients with traumatic spinal cord injury have other associated conditions including fractures of the long bones or pelvis. This further increases the risk, as fractures of the pelvis are associated with a 61% incidence of DVT and fractures

---

Dr. Rimoldi or an immediate family member is a member of a speakers' bureau or has made paid presentations on behalf of Stryker. Dr. Zigler or an immediate family member serves as a board member, owner, officer, or committee member of Cervical Spine Research Society; has received royalties from Zimmer, K2M, and Osprey; serves as a paid consultant to or is an employee of Alphatec Spine and Synthes; owns stock or stock options in Flexuspine; and has received nonincome support (such as equipment or services), commercially derived honoraria, or other non-research-related funding (such as paid travel) from AO and Synthes.

of the long bones are known to have an 80% associated incidence of DVT. Based on these statistics, routine prophylaxis should be considered in the postoperative patient with a spinal cord injury.

Understanding that thoracolumbar spine injuries are associated with increased risk of developing DVT that is highly associated with fatal pulmonary emboli, in the face of clinical difficulty in making that diagnosis, strong consideration should be given to prophylactic measures. All patients in the acute postoperative period should undergo basic prophylaxis such as the use of elastic hose or intermittent compressive devices. The institution of early lower extremity range-of-motion exercises and mobilization is important to reduce the incidence of symptomatic DVT. It is important to obtain baseline measurements of lower extremity girth because the more common physical findings of calf pain and positive Homans test are not usually apparent in a patient with neurologic sequela following a spinal cord injury. Therefore, in the postoperative patient who requires an extended period of bed rest, one should consider routine screening with the use of Doppler ultrasonography or plethysmography. These studies are more accurate for detecting clots in large veins of the thigh and are highly unreliable for detecting DVT in smaller calf veins; however, as mentioned above, the majority of clinically significant pulmonary emboli arise from proximal venous thromboses. If the suspicion remains high despite negative, noninvasive tests, invasive venography should be performed. Treatment of documented venous thrombosis includes administration of intravenous heparin, maintaining the activated partial thromboplastin time (PTT) at 1.5 to 2.0 times normal for approximately 1 to 2 weeks.

The most controversial aspect of prophylaxis within the acute postoperative period pertains to the use of anticoagulation. Intraoperative decision making may reduce the incidence of DVT. The use of epidural anesthesia can increase peripheral venous flow by decreasing blood flow within the skeletal musculature. The duration of surgery also has a correlative effect in the formation of DVT. Therefore, consideration of staging an anterior posterior procedure may reduce the incidence of thrombotic events in the acute postoperative patient undergoing decompression and/or stabilization for spinal cord injury. The use of anticoagulants, such as low molecular-weight heparin or warfarin, has the potential devastating complication of an epidural bleed, even when administration is delayed until the fourth postoperative day.[5]

Patients with complete spinal cord injuries that will result in no neurologic return cephalad to the area of injury should be considered for anticoagulation therapy, as the results of an epidural bleed are generally not going to cause further neurologic compromise. However, patients with no neurologic deficits or incomplete spinal cord injuries should not undergo routine prophylaxis with anticoagulants such as low molecular-weight heparin or warfarin because the complication of an epidural bleed or hematoma could further compromise their neurologic status. These patients should be treated with lower extremity compression devices and early mobilization.

In summary, our recommendation regarding the prevention of DVT in the acute postoperative period in a patient with spinal cord injury is to always use lower extremity compression hose or intermittent compressive devices. In patients with complete spinal cord injuries and no chance of regaining neurologic function, we recommend prophylaxis with anticoagulation therapy in addition to the above. In patients who are neurologically intact or who have incomplete spinal cord injuries, we recommend the use of anticoagulation therapy when a DVT is confirmed with noninvasive or invasive studies.

Hemodynamics

The sympathetic division of the autonomic nervous system contains preganglionic fibers that arise from the thoracic and upper lumbar segments of the spinal cord. Spinal cord trauma above T6 may compromise sympathetic outflow, resulting in neurogenic shock, hypotension, and bradycardia. Neurogenic shock is rarely seen in injuries at the thoracolumbar junction. Postoperative management should consist of fluid replacement and maintenance of mean blood pressure above 75 mm Hg and a urine output above 30 mL/hour. Postoperative bradycardia often does not require pharmacologic treatment and will stabilize in the first 72 hours after surgery.

Orthostatic hypotension can be a significant problem limiting early mobilization of the postoperative patient. Progressive position change allowing the vascular tree to acclimate is helpful. One should begin by elevating the head of the bed; progression to a tilt table or reclining wheelchair is followed by wheelchair mobilization or preliminary ambulation. Autonomic hyperreflexia, the uncontrolled increase in sympathectomy activity that is not inhibited by the damaged vasomotor center, is usually not a problem with injuries of the thoracolumbar junction.

Renal System

Postoperatively, long-term indwelling Foley catheterization should be avoided, as this leads to chronic bacteriuria. Intermittent catheterization should be instituted as soon as possible as the patient's hemodynamic status is stabilized, and postoperative volume accumulation is mobilized. We recommend maintaining Foley catheter drainage until urine output decreases to 400 to 600 mL every 8 hours. This is to prevent bladder distention and possible proximal reflux of urine. Overdistention may also lead to bladder diverticula, with an associated chronic urine reservoir encouraging bacterial infection. On occasion, fluid restriction of 2 L per 24-hour period may be necessary to prevent bladder overdistention when initiating intermittent catheterization.

Intermittent catheterization is begun every 6 hours. Patients with incomplete lesions are allowed to void voluntarily, and postresidual volumes are measured. If these are greater than 75 mL to 100 mL, these patients, too, are maintained on the catheterization protocol. Volumes above 600 mL of urine per catheterization should alert the clinician to increase the frequency of catheterization to every 4 hours.

Gastrointestinal Care

Postoperatively, patients are kept nil per os (NPO, meaning nothing by mouth), as ileus is common secondary to any spinal cord procedure involving nerve mobilization and vertebral stabilization. Retroperitoneal hematoma may also cause transient ileus. Maintenance fluids are administered intravenously. Daily postoperative evaluation should consist of abdominal monitoring by auscultation and palpitation to reveal distention and to determine the presence of bowel sounds. We prefer to begin oral liquids as bowel sounds return, usually on the second postoperative day. The appearance of flatus or stool allows the physician to advance the patient to a regular diet. Patients with neurologic injury require the institution of a bowel care program within days of injury. The choice of bowel program depends on the location of the cord injury. Patients exhibiting upper motor neuron lesions with intact bulbocavernosus reflexes may be regulated by taking advantage of the gastrocolic reflex. In this way, digital stimulation produces colonic peristalsis. Suppositories and stool softeners are important adjuncts in maintaining a consistent bowel program. We generally recommend choosing a convenient time to institute the program, usually after the evening meal. Glycerine suppositories are administered. Twenty minutes later, digital stimulation is begun. Docusate sodium is given on a daily basis, and the maintenance of a high-fiber diet is mandatory. Patients with flaccid paralysis often require manual evacuation of stool from the rectal vault. The most important part of bowel rehabilitation in these patients is the maintenance of soft stool by implementing a high-fiber diet.

Skin Care

Patients with neurologic deficits require meticulous attention to skin care. Log-rolling from side to back to side every 2 hours will generally provide adequate pressure relief. Areas of particular concern are the sacral prominence, the greater trochanters of the proximal femora, and the ischial tuberosities when the patient is in the seated position. Air-fluidized beds or air mattresses may provide pressure relief in patients who are difficult to transfer or who have developed early signs of skin breakdown (ie, redness or sloughing). Methods of internal spinal stabilization that still require postoperative brace support present an additional risk of skin breakdown. A Rancho Los Amigos Medical Center study, which included 147 patients with a 25-month follow-up, demonstrated a 4% incidence of pressure necrosis requiring surgical débridement when postoperative body jackets were used in patients with sensory deficits.[1] Meticulous skin inspection after brace use is vital to circumvent circumstances that may ultimately require myocutaneous flap coverage.

Wound Care

Surgical incisions are left dressed with the original postsurgical bandage until the third postoperative day. Infections secondary to contaminated incisions are not apparent until the fourth to sixth postoperative day. Drains should be left in place until output is less than 30 mL per 8 hours. Most will be discontinued on the second postoperative day. If the output remains high, requiring prolonged use of suction drainage, then the tubing from the skin toward the reservoir for a distance of 10 cm should be cleaned with a povidone-iodine or hexachlorophene solution. A first-generation cephalosporin is recommended during the initial 48 hours after surgery for prophylaxis against infection. Evaluation of antimicrobial concentrations in the blood, muscles, and hematomas of postoperative patients has demonstrated that first-generation cephalosporins reached levels twice that of any second- or third-generation cephalosporin.[6] There is a 10% to 20% incidence of cross-reactivity in patients with penicillin

TABLE 1

Hip Range of Motion (ROM) Related to the Use of Postoperative Immobilization[1]

	Degrees of Flexion
Body jacket	
Hip ROM, initial	93
Hip ROM, final	115
No body jacket	
Hip ROM, initial	117
Hip ROM, final	118

allergies who are administered cephalosporins. Manifestation of the allergic reaction include rash, urticaria, fever, eosinophilia, and anaphylaxis. A test dose of oral cephradine (250 mg) may be given to screen these patients before the first intravenous dose.

Postoperative Immobilization

The need for postoperative external immobilization depends on the method of stabilization used. Our series of 112 patients who underwent posterior stabilization for thoracolumbar (T11-L2) injuries has shown that a 17% incidence of hardware-related complications (failure, pseudarthrosis) accompanies the use of nonsegmental distraction rods alone.[1] An 8% incidence is associated with the use of posterior element wires.[1] Most of these consisted of failures at the bone-hook interface. Supplemental body-jacket immobilization is recommended for these patients for a period of 3 months postoperatively to reduce the risk of hardware-related complications. The use of more rigid and segmentally fixed implants using claw and pedicle screw constructs that stabilize at least two normal levels above and below the traumatized motion segment may not require postoperative external mobilization.

Body jackets (total-contact orthoses [TCOs]) should be manufactured from a negative plaster mold. These can be molded as early as the second postoperative day, if there is no abnormal distention, and applied to the patient by the fourth postoperative day. Off-the-shelf orthoses may apply abnormally high pressure on the skin, increasing the risk of breakdown. We recommend polypropylene jackets because they are durable and lightweight, thereby facilitating the early rehabilitation period. Jackets should consist of either anterior and posterior shells or one-piece shells for thoracolumbar fracture (T9-L3) with Velcro fasteners that will allow rapid application and removal. This is extremely important in patients with associated chest injuries who may require institution of cardiopulmonary resuscitation. A large anterior thoracic window is important to allow maximum chest expansion and optimize respiratory function. Jackets should be worn 24 hours per day, as repeated removal and reapplication may precipitate hardware dislodgment. An undergarment should be worn to cover all exposed skin and should be changed daily using meticulous hygiene. Daily changing and hygiene will allow careful skin inspection.

One must bear in mind that body jacket immobilization in patients with sensory deficits carries a risk of skin-related complications. Our series showed a 4% incidence of sacral decubitus ulcers requiring myocutaneous flap reconstruction.[1] Also, patients who require body jackets in the acute postoperative period require a longer time to achieve completion of their initial rehabilitation time (113 days [42 patients] versus 69 days [18 patients with no body jacket]). This is due in part to a significant decrease in the initial hip range of motion (**Table 1**). Internal fixation, which obviates the need for external immobilization, is obviously preferred to decrease the risk of brace-related complications as well as to improve early rehabilitation potential.

Jackets used in patients with intact upper lumbar dermatomes may experience numbness over the anterior thigh caused by pressure on the lateral femoral cutaneous nerve. This should not be confused with neurologic progression secondary to the spinal cord injury. It is treated by providing anteroinferior relief to the orthosis or restricting hip flexion when jacket immobilization is required.

Another rare complication of jacket immobilization is due to compression of the superior mesenteric artery and the third part of the duodenum.[7-11] Patients will exhibit nausea and vomiting. Abdominal distention is not a hallmark feature because the obstruction is in the proximal portion of the gastrointestinal tract. Bowel sounds are normal, and flatus and stool are still passed. Postoperative analgesics that also cause nausea and vomiting may delay the diagnosis. Prolonged delay in diagnosis can lead to hypovolemia and hypokalemic alkalosis. Treatment consists of nasogastric suction and intravenous fluid replacement. Electrolytes should be closely monitored as potassium replacement is often necessary. Positional changes such as foot elevation in the supine position may relieve the symptoms. Abdominal windows are usually not successful in alleviating the condition. Symptoms should improve in 48 to 72 hours; if they do not, then jacket removal is necessary.

Since its first description by Perry and Nickel in 1959,[12] halo immobilization has been an important adjunct in the care of the patient with cervical spine trauma. It may be occasionally used following surgical stabilization or applied in the surgical suite for nonsurgical treatment. The circumference of the skull is measured above the ears, and the appropriate-size ring is selected. Povidone-iodine preparation is used, and four halo pins are applied to fix the ring to the skull, allowing 1 cm of clearance between the skull and ring circumferentially. Pins are placed in the opposite fashion (left posterior and right anterior, then right posterior and left anterior). The posterior pins are placed above the tragus of the ear, taking care to avoid the more anterior temporal arteries. Correct anterior pin placement is over the lateral orbit to avoid the more medial supraorbital and supratrochlear nerves as well as the frontal sinus. All pins are tightened 1 in-lb at a time in opposite fashion using a torque screwdriver. The vest is applied and reduction is checked with a lateral radiograph. Halo pins may be tightened 2 days after initial application to 8 in-lb. It is critical to readjust the vest after mobility of the patient. We do not recommend further tightening to avoid penetration of the inner table of the skull if the pins are extremely loose. The pins may be retorqued at 7 and 30 days if less than two turns are necessary to achieve tightness. Twenty percent of patients will exhibit pin-tract infection. Pin care using povidone-iodine scrub is important to reduce the incidence of infection. Vests should be well padded to avoid skin breakdown. Use of a circumferential halo cast is discouraged because if the need for cardiopulmonary resuscitation arises, the patient's life may depend on the expeditious removal of the vest. The use of a vest with articulated anterior struts is suggested. Intubation of the patient with a halo vest may be difficult otherwise. A tracheostomy tray should be located on the ward where patients with halo casts are located to ensure prompt airway access in emergent situations.

Complications

Complications that occur in the acute postoperative period are listed in **Table 2**. The surgeon must be especially aware of progressive neurologic deterioration. This unfortunate complication and uncontrollable bleeding are the only two indications requiring emergent return to the surgical suite. Neurologic deterioration may be due to postoperative hematoma, which must be evacuated, or malposition of hardware or the bone graft, which must be removed or repositioned. Postoperative hematomas in patients who underwent anterior cervical exposure can cause life-threatening airway obstruction. For this reason, anterior cervical procedures require drainage postoperatively. We recommend a tracheostomy tray at the bedside to allow rapid evacuation of the hematoma if this should occur in the early postoperative period.

TABLE 2

Acute Postoperative Complications

Hematoma
Hardware failure
Hardware malposition
Infection
Displaced bone graft
Injury to viscera
Dural tears

(Reproduced from Rimoldi RL, Zigler JE: Immediate postoperative care, in Levine AM, Eismont FJ, Garfin SR, Zigler JE: *Spine Trauma*. Philadelphia, PA, WB Saunders, 1998, pp 562-566.)

Esophageal perforation may occur rarely during anterior cervical surgery but it is not usually recognized until the early postoperative period. Persistent dysphasia that does not improve by the fourth postoperative day should alert the surgeon to possible esophageal perforation. Patients should be studied with esophagoscopy or an esophagogram. Patients with perforations should be treated with nasogastric suction and intravenous fluids. Small perforations should resolve in 2 to 3 weeks. Patients should be restudied before resuming oral intake. Perforations that are refractory to conservative treatment may require sternocleidomastoid flap coverage.[13] Unrecognized esophageal perforation may cause septic mediastinitis, which has a high rate of morbidity and mortality.

Anterior decompression of the thoracic spine or thoracolumbar junction involves exposure of the chest cavity. A chest tube is placed in the eighth intercostal space postoperatively. Initial management consists of suction through a column of approximately 20 cm H_2O. Chest radiographs are checked daily. Forty-eight hours postoperatively, the suction is turned off and the patient is left to water-seal. If air leaks are observed, suction is continued. Chest tubes should never be discontinued if an air leak is present. This could lead to a tension pneumothorax, requiring reinsertion. Chest tubes are discontinued 24 hours after water seal, if no air leak is present. Removal is performed during maximum inspiration. A pressure dressing is applied and a chest radiograph is immediately taken to rule out pneumothorax. It is important to encourage aggressive respiratory therapy in the early postoperative period. Intercostal nerve blocks are occasionally used to assist respiration by preventing splinting of the chest wall secondary to postoperative incisional pain.

Inadvertent dural tears rarely go unrecognized until the postoperative period. However, some may be discovered by clear drainage exuding from the wound on the third to fourth postoperative day. These usually occur after late anterior decompression for a healed vertebral fracture. Recumbency and closed gravity drainage of 200 to 300 mL of cerebrospinal fluid per 24-hour period through an intradural puncture at the third lumbar motion segment for 3 days will usually stop the fluid leak.[14] If drainage does not cease, then reexploration with meticulous dural repair or a dural patch graft with sealant is indicated.[15]

Infections are usually due to *Staphylococcus aureus*. Prolonged antibiotics may be appropriate if the infection is recognized within the first 2 weeks after surgery. Late infection requires meticulous débridement of all nonviable tissue to remove the organism's protective environment, and prolonged use of culture-directed antibiotics. Many bacteria secrete a glycocalyx slime that adheres to foreign bodies and nonviable osseous tissue and protects them from systemic antibiotics. Superficial infections involving only soft tissue require a 2-week course, while deep infections involving graft or hardware require 4 to 6 weeks of intravenous antibiotics. In trauma patients, postoperative infections are more common in those who have additional risk factors such as obesity, diabetes, and debilitation, and in those who are immunocompromised.

The long-term mechanical result of the unstable low thoracic or lumbar fracture with neurologic compromise has not been altered by surgical intervention. However, surgical stabilization and the current standard of postoperative care in the paraplegic patient have been shown to shorten the initial rehabilitative period. Hospital costs to the patient and community may also be reduced.

References

1. Rimoldi RL, Zigler JE, Capen DA, Hu SS: The effect of surgical intervention on rehabilitation time in patients with thoracolumbar and lumbar spinal cord injuries. *Spine (Phila Pa 1976)* 1992; 17(12):1443-1449.
2. Gillies TE, Ruckley CV, Nixon SJ: Still missing the boat with fatal pulmonary embolism. *Br J Surg* 1996;83(10):1394-1395.
3. Donaldson GA, Williams C, Scannell JG, Shaw RS: A reappraisal of the application of the Trendelenburg operation to massive fatal embolism: Report of a successful pulmonary-artery thrombectomy using a cardiopulmonary bypass. *N Engl J Med* 1963;268:171-174.
4. Gibbs NM: Venous thrombosis of the lower limbs with particular reference to bed-rest. *Br J Surg* 1957;45(191):209-236.
5. Coventry MB, Nolan DR, Beckenbaugh RD: "Delayed" prophylactic anticoagulation: A study of results and complications in 2,012 total hip arthroplasties. *J Bone Joint Surg Am* 1973;55(7): 1487-1492.
6. Jones S, DiPiro JT, Nix DE, Bhatti NA: Cephalosporins for prophylaxis in operative repair of femoral fractures: Levels in serum, muscle, and hematoma. *J Bone Joint Surg Am* 1985;67(6): 921-924.
7. Evarts CM, Winter RB, Hall JE: Vascular compression of the duodenum associated with the treatment of scoliosis: Review of the literature and report of eighteen cases. *J Bone Joint Surg Am* 1971;53(3):431-444, passim.
8. Gray SW, Akin JT Jr, Milsap JH Jr, Skandalakis JE: Vascular compression of the duodenum (Part I). *Contemp Surg* 1976;9:37-39.
9. Hughes JP, McEntire JE, Setze TK: Cast syndrome: Duodenal dilation or obstruction in a patient in a body cast, with review of the literature. *Arch Surg* 1974;108(2):230-232.
10. Shandling B: The so-called superior mesenteric artery syndrome. *Am J Dis Child* 1976;130(12): 1371-1373.
11. Skandalakis JE, Akin JT Jr, Milsap JH Jr, Gray SW: Vascular compression of the duodenum (Part II). *Contemp Surg* 1977;10:33-36.
12. Perry J, Nickel VL: Total cervicalspine fusion for neck paralysis. *J Bone Joint Surg Am* 1959;41-A(1): 37-60.
13. Fuji T, Kuratsu S, Shirasaki N, et al: Esophagocutaneous fistula after anterior cervical spine surgery and successful treatment using a sternocleidomastoid muscle flap: A case report. *Clin Orthop Relat Res* 1991;267:8-13.
14. Kitchel SH, Eismont FJ, Green BA: Closed subarachnoid drainage for management of cerebrospinal fluid leakage after an operation on the spine. *J Bone Joint Surg Am* 1989;71(7):984-987.
15. Eismont FJ Jr, Wiesel SW, Rothman RH: Treatment of dural tears associated with spinal surgery. *J Bone Joint Surg Am* 1981;63(7):1132-1136.

CHAPTER 37
Rehabilitation

Jack E. Zigler, MD Cheryl Resnik, MS, DPT Lisa Carroll, PT
Adriana Ramirez, OTR/L, BS Michal Atkins, MA, OTR/L Lilli Thompson, PT, NCS, ATP

Rehabilitation Philosophy in the 21st Century

Spinal cord injury (SCI) is a catastrophic event that significantly alters every aspect of the patient's life. It is estimated that there are approximately 12,000 new cases of SCI each year and between 235,000 and 311,000 persons living with SCI in the United States. SCI primarily affects young adults. The average age at injury between the years 1973 and 1979 was 28.7 years. However, since 2005, the average age of injury is 40.2 years.[1] The individual, most often a healthy, relatively young person, is plunged into the bewildering world of emergency medical care, spinal immobilization apparatus, surgeries, and initial total dependency on others for all of the most basic human needs. The involved person is suddenly confronted with physical and functional problems such as motor and sensory deficits and/or bowel and bladder dysfunction. Along with maintaining their health and avoiding secondary conditions, individuals with SCI must learn to adjust to changed roles in their families, jobs, and communities.[2]

The acute care facility offers the first step on the long road to recovery, treating the most urgent medical problems and stabilizing the spine. Managed care and other cost-containment measures have dramatically changed the management of health problems in patients with SCI. Patients channeled through the acute care system with shortened lengths of stay require rehabilitation facilities and community resources to supplement the care continuum.[3] The role of rehabilitation is to assist the patient in regaining the emotional stability, physical strength, and daily life skills necessary to reintegrate, to whatever degree possible, into their previous roles and relationships.[4] The interdisciplinary team is involved with each patient in creating an environment in which the patient participates fully in community life, fulfilling social roles and making decisions that lead to self-determination, resulting in a sense of personal well-being and ultimately an improved quality of life.[5] The team consists of a physician (often a physiatrist), a nurse, a physical therapist, occupational therapist, a social worker, and a psychologist. Other professionals, such as communication disorders therapists, recreational therapists, dietitians, and respiratory therapists, are also available to the patient as needed.

Trends that emphasize cost containment through early discharge have by necessity altered the interdisciplinary team's approach not only upon admission but also throughout the rehabilitative process. Initial patient screening by the interdisciplinary team members are generally completed within 24 hours of admission, including getting the patient out of bed, if medically and orthopaedically stable. Initial assessments are completed within 3 to 7 days of admission. The assessments may be performed by members of more than one discipline working together to expedite the process and make it less repetitious to the patient. The American Spinal Injury Association (ASIA) evaluation standards are often used to establish the patient's level of injury (Appendix 1).

Rehabilitation in the next millennium will require a shift from a biomedical model, where appropriate treatment is determined by professional perceptions of need related to the causes and pathologies of disease or injury, to a model that places more emphasis on the consumer perspective and holistic models of care. It is generally agreed that rehabilitation should focus on: (1) function rather than disease or injury; (2) inclusion of the consumer in the identification of his or her own needs; (3) empowerment of the

Dr. Zigler or an immediate family member serves as a board member, owner, officer, or committee member of Cervical Spine Research Society; has received royalties from Zimmer, K2M, and Osprey; serves as a paid consultant to or is an employee of Alphatec Spine and Synthes; owns stock or stock options in Flexuspine; and has received nonincome support (such as equipment or services), commercially derived honoraria, or other non-research-related funding (such as paid travel) from AO and Synthes. None of the following authors or any immediate family member has received anything of value from or owns stock in a commercial company or institution related directly or indirectly to the subject of this chapter: Dr. Resnik, Dr. Carroll, Dr. Ramirez, Dr. Atkins, and Dr. Thompson.

TABLE 1

Hospital Length of Stay (LOS) (Acute Care and Rehabilitation in Model System)

Year of Injury	Acute LOS (days)	Rehab LOS (days)
1973-1979	24.0	98.0
1980-1984	23.0	86.0
1985-1989	19.0	73.0
1990-1994	15.0	58.0
1995-1999	13.0	44.0
2000-2004	13.0	42.0
2005-2009	12.0	38.0

(Adapted with permission from *2009 Annual Report for the Model Spinal Cord Injury Care Systems*. Birmingham, AL, National Spinal Cord Injury Statistical Center, 2010.)

consumer in the development, delivery, and evaluation of rehabilitation services; (4) recognition of the impact that environmental factors have in the creation and maintenance of disablement; and (5) individualized service delivery that considers the best rehabilitation options for that person's unique situation.[6]

Both acute care and rehabilitation hospitals are implementing self-management models to improve outcomes of patients at discharge. The self-management model requires a shift in the patient-caregiver relationship. Patients are no longer "told" what to do by the medical team to improve their health or improve their physical function. Instead, a partnership is built between the patient, family, caregivers, and interdisciplinary team, with a shared responsibility for making and carrying out health-related decisions.[7] Caregivers provide the patients expertise and tools, while patients are responsible for their day-to-day rehabilitative program and health decisions. It is the decision of the person with the SCI to determine what his or her life roles and activities will be. The family and/or significant others are involved early in the rehabilitation process.

Due to the shortened lengths of stay (**Table 1**), short-term goals are established following comprehensive team assessment in collaboration with the patient and potential caregivers. Long-term goals are addressed either by community reintegration programs or outpatient services provided by the rehabilitative facility. All identified goals must be realistic and meaningful to the patient. The thrust of treatment must be tailored toward maximizing the patient's potential as well as problem-solving situations that might arise once the patient returns home. It is imperative that the importance of the activity to the individual and the patient's level of confidence in being able to complete the goal are considered when establishing and creating action plans to achieve the goals. Strengthening a single wrist extensor muscle, for example, may superficially appear to be a trivial accomplishment, but it may allow a person with C5 tetraplegia with some C6 return to grasp a utensil and feed himself or herself with an appropriate setup. This small act may reaffirm some measure of independence in a person who has lost physical control over much of his or her body. Learning to change clothing while in a wheelchair allows a person with paraplegia the freedom and confidence to return to work or participate in leisure activities without the fear of being unable to change soiled clothing should a bladder or bowel accident occur while out in the community.

SCI patients are being transferred to rehabilitation institutions sooner after their injuries. One of the positive outcomes of earlier transfer of patients with SCI from acute care hospitals to rehabilitative model centers was a lower incidence of pressure sores and other preventable medical complications.[8] This is supported by information obtained from Rancho Los Amigos National Rehabilitation Center in Downey, California. Patients who enter the system within 24 hours of injury have significantly fewer pressure sores, respiratory complications, and urinary tract infections than those who enter the system more than 24 hours postinjury. Those patients admitted in the first 24 hours of injury spend approximately 30 fewer days hospitalized during initial acute care and rehabilitation than those who enter the system more than

24 hours after injury. It is not uncommon to admit to the rehabilitation facility patients who continue to require extensive acute medical attention. For example, a patient may have sustained multiple gunshot wounds to the body, including abdominal wounds. Along with conventional rehabilitation, such patients may require gastric feeding and wound care. These marginally medically stable patients require highly skilled physicians and nurses who are competent in general medical care, as well as in SCI acute complications such as orthostatic hypotension and autonomic dysreflexia. The entire interdisciplinary team is also expected to be highly competent across a broad spectrum of medical issues. Ongoing communication among team members is vital to ensure the patient's safety and appropriate medical management.

The rehabilitation staff has the difficult challenge of supporting the individual through an overwhelming emotional crisis, involving grieving at the loss of real physical abilities and the resultant adjustment to altered future hopes and expectations. At the same time, the staff must facilitate and motivate the patient to fully participate in rehabilitation. The health care team must allow for the natural course of each person's adaptation to injury, while encouraging activity versus passivity and optimism versus dwelling on losses as the rehabilitation process continues.

As the rehabilitation community has had decades to reflect on its past successes and failures, practice philosophies have been refined. This is particularly true in the shift toward carefully balancing issues relating to physical performance. Accounts and observations of patients with SCIs, now decades postrehabilitation, have focused on the fact that some postrehabilitation patients have experienced unanticipated damage to their musculoskeletal system. Overtasking weak muscles and using muscles and joints that are imbalanced have resulted in late pain and decreased function in some persons. Examples are shoulder and hand injuries, and pain caused by pushing a manual wheelchair with insufficient upper extremity strength.[9] Evidence also points to a higher risk of cardiovascular disease associated with the sedentary lifestyle and the inadequate physical activity of many patients with SCIs.[10] It is therefore vital to analyze each patient's daily routines and physical activities to educate the patient in choosing "smart activities." For example, a power, rather than a manual, wheelchair may be recommended for a patient with a weak shoulder girdle who is planning to return to school. This recommendation enhances functional mobility but decreases physical activity. This person must then compensate by incorporating a routine daily exercise program to maintain cardiovascular and respiratory conditioning for health. Conserving patients' energy to allow them to engage in those activities that are most meaningful to them is essential. Some people with tetraplegia, for example, may choose to have an attendant dress them in the morning to have sufficient energy to work later in the day.

Paradoxically, while rehabilitation prepares the patient to reenter the community, it may also hinder this process. The inpatient treatment phase fosters a dependency that must later be overcome if the patient is to attain the highest level of self-sufficiency.[11] The physical limitations of the newly injured patient, the encouragement to comply with hospital routines, and the hospital's provision of all basic needs through highly structured scheduling all foster dependency. Thus, the patient's ability to take active responsibility for day-to-day life is compromised. These well-described regressive aspects of the sick role—the "exemption from normal social role responsibilities"[12]—broaden, rather than narrow, the gap between the patient's former life and new posttraumatic adaptations.

This dependency, along with socioeconomic factors, complicates attempts to ease the transition from hospital to home environment. The rehabilitation team should seek to facilitate the patient's transition from the sick role to the role of an active consumer. Throughout the inpatient rehabilitation process, patients should assume responsibility for directing their care and selecting which activities are relevant to them in preparation for discharge back to their home and community. Good examples of self-directed patient care are (1) the patient performing self-intermittent catheterization or seeking out assistance at the scheduled times identified by the physician, and (2) using the Internet and other resources to line up interviews for personal attendants before, or upon, discharge.

Pressure to lower inpatient rehabilitation costs have resulted in trends toward shortening inpatient stay and enhancing outpatient and community health care services. Attempts to ease the transition to the home environment have included providing community outings for hospitalized patients, day treatment, home-care programs, and providing comprehensive ambulatory medical services through outpatient clinics. A highly specialized health care team is required to meet the patient's ongoing needs. Some rehabilitation centers provide lifelong follow-up by a spinal injury care clinic, in which a primary nurse screens patients who are then referred to the appropriate health-care providers. These programs all reflect the trend toward increasing outpatient and community health care services.

This chapter presents the key aspects of rehabilitation of the spinal cord-injured patient. First, the model system approach to SCI management is described, followed by the interdisciplinary treatment team concept. Finally, clinical aspects of care are described by discipline.

Model System Approach to Spinal Cord Injury

The federally sponsored model SCI system program began in 1970 with a system in Phoenix, Arizona. The initial funding and direction was under the Rehabilitation Services Administration. Within 4 years, the program was expanded to include six additional regional model SCI system projects. In 1983, the University of Alabama at Birmingham (UAB) Department of Rehabilitation Medicine received federal grant funds to establish a national SCI data center. The UAB manages the National Spinal Cord Injury Data Research Center that served the Model SCI Care Systems Project between 1973 and 1981. UAB's National SCI Statistical Center is known as the hub of the network of federally sponsored regional Model Spinal Cord Injury Care System facilities. The National Institute on Disability and Rehabilitation Research (NIDRR), Office of Special Education and Rehabilitative Services, and the US Department of Education sponsors the Model Spinal Cord Injury System.[1,13] Since 1970, as many as 21 model SCI systems have been designated, varying with each funding cycle.

The model system program was originally established as a research and demonstration project to evaluate the effectiveness of a systemized approach to the care and rehabilitation of patients with SCI. While most model systems vary according to differences in the region they serve (climate, physical and cultural geography, population characteristics, population density, governmental structures, and so forth), all are similar in their basic structure. They are designed to respond to the needs of those who become spinal cord-injured, from the time of injury through lifetime follow-up. In this regard, although some systems use the term "center" in their titles, they are distinguished in terms of the scope of their services and influence.

The term center, as it relates to SCI, may refer to a rehabilitation facility, to an acute care facility, or (less often) to a facility that provides both acute care and rehabilitation. A model SCI system, on the other hand, always includes acute care and rehabilitation, as well as more comprehensive services.

Although the mainstay of a system is typically the rehabilitation component, it may also oversee, among other things, the emergency medical services provided at the scene of the accident; the method of transport to the system's acute care unit; emergency triage of the patient; protocols employed in the acute management of the patient, such as the initiation of turning programs to prevent pressure sores and other complications; bladder management programs to ensure the best possible urologic status throughout the patient's life; early rehabilitation procedures; and the orderly movement from acute care to rehabilitation. In this regard, within a system, the formal rehabilitation component is usually made aware of a patient and his or her status within 24 hours of the injury, and is kept apprised of the patient's status until a transfer has been completed. Within a model SCI system, rehabilitation is addressed in a comprehensive team-oriented fashion. The system's efforts also embrace the spinal cord-injured person's reintegration into and maintenance within the community. In this regard, the system is concerned with the ongoing medical and emotional viability of the rehabilitated person and thus offers comprehensive outpatient services directed to the special needs of the spinal cord-injured. Additionally, the system monitors adequate and appropriate community services in the areas of employment, education, attendant services, housing, transportation, recreation, and other services necessary for return to community life.

In summary, a model SCI system is designed to address the needs of patients with SCIs in a coordinated manner, from the time of injury through lifetime follow-up. A system operates in a dynamic fashion to continually monitor the patient's movement through and beyond the system. Outcomes are continually being monitored to ensure that the services are being offered in the most productive and cost-effective manner. Accordingly, system efforts are directed toward the evaluation and development of new and better methods through ongoing research.

Finally, system efforts provide for the constant monitoring of SCI events—ie, who gets injured; and how, where, and why. From this perspective, model SCI system activities make a full circle in that the information is applied to efforts directed at prevention of the injury itself.

Team Approach to Rehabilitation

Rehabilitation of the person who has sustained an SCI requires a well-integrated care team consisting of, at a minimum, a physician, rehabilitation nursing staff, physical and occupational therapists, a social worker, and a psychologist. Speech therapy, sexual counseling, and recreational therapy may also be necessary. All rehabilitation programs are centered around the following key areas of concern: integumentary integrity, cardiopulmonary status and function, neurologic status, bowel and bladder function, self-care skills, mobility, and reintegration of the patient into the community. While each member of the team has primary responsibility for one or more of these key areas, all team members must be aware of the entire breadth of the rehabilitative process to help educate the patient and enhance the efficacy of the rehabilitation.

Use of the ASIA standards for evaluation is recommended (Appendix 1). These provide consistent data for communication between clinicians and centers regarding national SCI statistics. Evaluation of additional data is also recommended to provide the team members with a comprehensive picture of the patient. The evaluation can be conducted in a team format with each professional concentrating on his or her specific area of expertise. This improves the efficiency of the evaluation process and prevents the patient from having to undergo multiple repetitions of the same procedures.

The medical chart is reviewed for general information such as age, past injuries, and the general state of health before injury. Information regarding the mechanism of the spinal injury and the bony level of injury is pertinent. Other injuries sustained at the same time, such as brain injuries, internal injuries, or other fractures, are also identified. Spinal stability should be ascertained through the chart review or through direct consultation with the attending physician before initiating either an evaluation or a treatment session.

The comprehensive evaluation (with additional items added to the ASIA standards) consists of eight major areas of emphasis: (1) sensory testing, (2) motor control, (3) respiratory function, (4) joint range of motion, (5) muscle tone, (6) skin integrity, (7) functional level, and (8) bulbar function screening (detailed evaluation of patients on ventilator support or with suspected head injury).

Consulting Services

The consulting services required for the spinal cord rehabilitation team include orthopaedic surgery; urology; internal medicine; general surgery; ear, nose, and throat; plastic surgery; and dental services. Other subspecialty areas may be required as well, depending upon the patient's preinjury status or severity of trauma.

It is clearly important to screen for admission to the rehabilitation service if these services are not readily available. Some patients require a more extensive primary hospital stay so that their consulting services can institute management at an earlier stage. Prolongation of rehabilitation can commonly result from inappropriate early transfer to the rehabilitation facility.

The dental service can manage patient problems without delay of therapy by providing periodic care appointments. Inadequate dental care before SCI or concomitant dental trauma may interfere with the rehabilitation process. Dental problems may present difficulties with mouthstick use or adequate calorie intake.

A bulbar examination is of paramount importance when the patient has suffered concomitant head injury. The clinician should evaluate bulbar function if the patient exhibits any of the sequelae of brain injury (eg, memory loss, cognitive impairment, difficulty concentrating, etc). This is necessary as patients with brain injury frequently have difficulty swallowing and handling secretions. The problem is compounded if the patient is immobilized in a halo or tongs and cannot assist the swallow mechanism by head movement. The examination should evaluate the strength of the tongue muscles, the soft palate, the gag reflex, and the swallow, in addition to eye movement and visual fields. If impairment is found, consultation with a communication disorders specialist is recommended to test for cognitive deficits. Even subtle cognitive impairments may influence the patient's ability to meet functional goals. Soft palate weakness and an impaired ability to swallow affect the patient's ability to consume a regular diet.[14]

The plastic surgery service is used for coverage of the exposed areas about the pelvis, hips, and spine that may develop pressure sores. Orthopaedic management of bony infections, spasticity, and contractures is often required in conjunction with muscle pedicle flaps to cover defects. The entire staff focuses on prevention, but there is still a definite population of patients who develop open

FIGURE 1

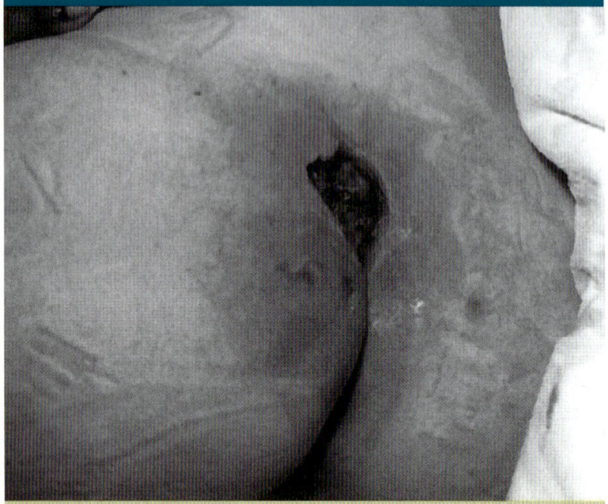

Figure 1 A full-thickness sacral decubitus ulcer may prolong hospitalization and cost up to $70,000 in additional health care for treatment. (Reproduced from Zigler JE, Atkins MS, Resnik CD, Thompson L: Rehabilitation, in Levine AM, Eismont FJ, Garfin SR, Zigler JE, eds: *Spine Trauma*. Philadelphia, PA, WB Saunders, 1998, pp 567-607.)

pressure ulcers that cannot close by primary healing.

An ancillary service that is important to the long-term management of persons with SCI is a seating clinic. In this clinic, appropriate wheelchair positioning and pressure relief are designed and fabricated for maintenance of skin integrity. Outpatient and inpatient consultation should be available to prevent the need for surgical flap coverage. Because the average cost of readmission for treatment of a single pressure sore averages $70,000, these preventive services are essential (**Figure 1**).

Surgical Considerations in the Rehabilitative Program

Proper management directed toward stabilizing the spine, preventing further injury, and facilitating mobilization allows the newly injured patient to begin the rehabilitation program soon after injury. Delayed rehabilitation can result from a single poor decision regarding patient management, be it in the field by an emergency medical technician, by an emergency department physician, or in planning and performing surgery by an orthopaedic or neurologic surgeon. Inappropriate decision making in the early postinjury period can lead to disastrous complications, or to multiple surgeries.[15]

Once care of the patient is assumed, the treating physician must initially provide spinal immobilization and assessment. Cervical injuries may be stabilized by use of a cervical collar, sandbags, or traction. Thoracic and thoracolumbar injuries may be stabilized by bed rest, with appropriate nursing care directed at log-rolling the patient to minimize rotational stresses on the spine.

Medical and neurologic assessment should be performed immediately, and serial neurologic evaluations should follow during the first 24 hours until it is clear that the neurologic injury is not progressive. Appropriate radiographic studies are obtained, and a treatment plan is devised. Patients with mechanically stable injuries may be mobilized when comfortable and started on their rehabilitation programs. Those with unstable spines may require treatment with traction and ultimately with internal fixation before they can be safely mobilized for therapy and skills training.

Early decision making should be based on viewing the spinal injury as having two separate components. Mechanical stability should be assessed independent of the quality of neurologic injury. Care of each portion of the injury often overlaps, but we find it useful to consider restoration of stability and potentiation of neurologic recovery individually.

Spinal injuries may be acutely stable or unstable. Gunshot wounds are typically stable injuries. They may be associated with either complete or incomplete cord injuries. Patients with gunshot wounds can usually be mobilized immediately after their injury with no external immobilization required other than for comfort. Ligamentous dislocations in all areas of the spine that are associated with neurologic deficit, typically flexion-distraction injuries, are almost always unstable. Bilateral facet dislocations without fracture, notoriously unstable injuries, demand reduction and immobilization before a patient can be placed in a wheelchair or other ambulatory device.

The extent of SCI is determined by clinical neurologic examination after the patient has emerged from the variable period of spinal shock. Complete cord injuries, by definition, have extremely poor potential for spinal cord functional recovery but may experience root escape. Incomplete injuries have variable recovery and must be treated as having theoretical potential for total return of function.

As a conceptual aid, we recommend formulating a Punnett square, with quadrants representing each of the possibilities discussed above (**Table 2**).

TABLE 2

Sample Punnett Square

	Mechanically stable	Mechanically unstable
Neurologically complete	A	B
Neurologically incomplete	C	D

Quadrant A, composed of mechanically stable and complete SCIs, is best represented by gunshot wounds that have traversed the spinal canal but have left enough bony elements intact to confer stability. Patients with this type of injury at any level may be mobilized and their rehabilitation program started as soon as they are medically stable and comfortable. Surgical stabilization, and even external bracing with halo vests or thoracolumbosacral orthoses (body jackets), is generally not necessary.

In quadrant B, consisting of complete cord injury with an unstable spine, we find the patient with very poor potential for spinal cord recovery. However, injudicious, unprotected mobilization may jeopardize root recovery at or above the level of injury, or may even conceivably injure the more proximal spinal cord by ascending epidural hematoma, or by direct cord trauma such as by tethering over a traumatic kyphosis. In these patients, the spine needs to be stabilized before mobilization for rehabilitation. In the cervical spine, bilateral facet dislocation is a good example of this injury type. The dislocation should be reduced, and the spine stabilized by instrumented fusion. Internal fixation allows fuller participation in a rehabilitation program without the restrictions of a prolonged external immobilization device. Additionally, pure ligamentous injuries have a considerably lower healing rate than do surgical fusions, and may ultimately necessitate surgery if the initial 12 weeks of nonsurgical treatment results in nonunion. For these reasons, we generally recommend early internal fixation for our complete, unstable injuries. Only in the thoracic spine do we consider nonsurgical treatment, based on literature identifying increased morbidity and mortality with surgical intervention, although these cases are still considered on their individual merits.[16] This may require that the patient be temporarily placed in a skilled nursing facility and then readmitted once orthopaedically cleared to participate in the rehabilitative program.

Quadrant C represents incomplete SCIs that are mechanically stable. Stab wounds to the spine with Brown-Séquard syndrome and incomplete SCI, although relatively rare, are an excellent example of this injury type. These patients may be mobilized early, because their spines are stable, but should have their neurologic progress serially followed. Patients who have plateaued neurologically but demonstrate a persistent anatomic lesion causing cord compression, such as vertebral body or disk fragments, may benefit from late anterior decompression.

Quadrant D, incomplete cord lesions associated with mechanically unstable spines, represents the most challenging subgroup of patients. Their spines must be stabilized not only to facilitate early rehabilitation but also to protect the injured spinal cord from further damage and to allow the zones of edema surrounding the area of actual injury an opportunity to resolve. Critical decision making is essential in this subgroup to minimize the chance of further injury to the already traumatized spinal cord. Spinal immobilization and initial medical stabilization followed by surgical decompression and internal fixation is recommended. Early internal fixation will protect the spinal cord from further injury, and will allow earlier participation in an appropriate rehabilitation program.[17]

When operating on acute cervical spine instability, where the most common mechanism of injury is flexion and compression, the posterior surgical approach is generally recommended. Posterior ligamentous structures are torn in tension as a result of the injury moment. The anterior structures are usually intact, although compressed. Anterior surgery, incising these last remaining stabilizers of the spine, may cause circumferential instability and must be accompanied by an appropriate anterior column fixation construct. Posterior stabilization and fusion allow dissection through the already injured tissue planes, and replace the torn posterior ligaments with a mechanically stable construct leading to a boney fusion. Both anterior and posterior fusion are sometimes necessary to offer both decompression as well as circumferential 360° stability.

Even for simple posterior fusion, a careful, well-planned surgical technique that is different than surgery for the degenerative spine is recommended. A large review of patients following posterior fusion after trauma has suggested that fusion extension beyond the intended levels may occur in a large percentage of cases.[18] Patients with complete tetraplegia need maximum cervical spine range of motion to operate mouthstick devices or

FIGURE 2

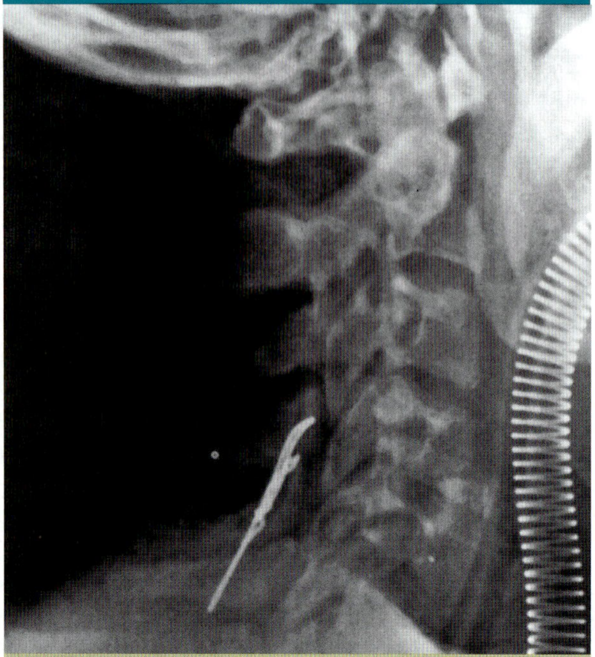

Figure 2 The simple wire loop has been demonstrated to be an effective internal tension band. Combined with appropriate external immobilization, the fusion rate with autologous iliac crest bone graft is almost 100%. (Reproduced from Zigler JE, Atkins MS, Resnik CD, Thompson L: Rehabilitation, in Levine AM, Eismont FJ, Garfin SR, Zigler JE, eds: *Spine Trauma*. Philadelphia, PA, WB Saunders, 1998, pp 567-607.)

to function with upper extremity assistive devices. Inadvertent fusion extension to adjacent uninjured levels may deny potential motion segments and may make the patient even more dependent on an aide. The surgeon should consider that any posterior elements exposed by soft-tissue stripping may fuse, regardless of where the fixation and bone graft are placed. Care should thus be taken to only expose those levels that are intended to be included in the fusion mass. Although many fixation techniques exist for posterior cervical fixation, the simple wire loop historically has been found to be effective and cost-effective in a busy public facility. The base of the superior spinous process is drilled through and the wire is passed through the interspinous ligament beneath the inferior spinous process, and then the loop is hand tightened (**Figure 2**). An autogenous iliac crest graft is placed along the exposed laminae. Decortication is minimized and local anesthesia can be used. The fusion rate with this technique approaches 100%.[19] Postoperative use of a Philadelphia collar for 6 weeks, followed by a soft collar for 6 weeks, allows upper extremity rehabilitation to proceed unimpaired by a halo vest. Lateral mass or even pedicular fixation are other options, particularly useful when the posterior arch is traumatized.

If future corpectomy is being considered, an additional segment is generally fused posteriorly; this will act as a tension band against which an anterior construct may be placed. For example, if a patient has a C5 burst fracture with retropulsed bone, the surgeon should strongly consider a posterior fusion from C4 to C6 if a later anterior corpectomy of C5 and an anterior column reconstruction from C4 to C6 are likely.

For injuries at thoracic, thoracolumbar, and lumbar levels that require surgical reduction and internal fixation, segmental pedicle screw fixation allows rehabilitation without the need for external support. A large historic review of instrumented posttrauma patients demonstrated a significant reduction in rehabilitation time when sublaminar or spinous process wires were used in conjunction with hook-rod constructs.[20] This early study was one of the first to demonstrate the advantages of segmental fixation, allowing patients to be rehabilitated without external immobilization, facilitating wheelchair and transfer skills. Pedicular fixation is now generally used for segmental constructs.

Pedicle fixation devices offer an additional advantage by decreasing construct length minimizing the number of motion segments involved in fixation. Anterior approaches for decompression and stabilization may allow intervention to involve the shortest segment fusion. Any construct that limits the span of fused segments in the paraplegic patient should be given strong consideration by the surgeon, as long as it confers mechanical stability.

Patient Evaluation

The rehabilitation team needs to create a patient-centered and collaborative problem-solving relationship in which the patient gets both inpatient and outpatient practice at medical self-management (eg, managing medications, diet, exercise) and participation management (ie, returning to his or her full roles and important life activities) (R Lewthwaite, unpublished data, 2006).

A self-management model is in use at Rancho Los Amigos National Rehabilitation Center for patients with SCI. An interview is conducted before the evaluation to identify activities important to that individual. Health and medical needs that are identified, and self-confidence regarding self-management and participation are assessed. The patient and family are educated as needed to the rehabilitation process (active learner versus passive recipient) and the patient is encouraged to collaborate, problem solve, and ask questions (R Lewthwaite, unpublished data, 2006).

Determination of Level of Injury

A comprehensive evaluation of the neurologic status, including thorough assessment of the musculoskeletal system, is essential before initiating treatment. This evaluation provides the team with information necessary to determine the patient's functional level of neurologic injury. This functional level is the basis for development of a treatment plan to achieve short- and long-term goals with the patient.

A spinal cord-injured patient is usually described by level of injury. In the literature, the term level may refer to the bony level of fracture, the neurologic level of injury, or the functional level. For the purposes of this discussion, the term functional level is used. Functional level is determined by the lowest level at which sensation is bilaterally intact and muscles supplied by nerves innervating that segment have a manual muscle test grade of 3+/5 or better. This level is used by the entire team when establishing a diagnosis and prognosis for the patient's functional outcome. A muscle grade below 3+/5 reflects a muscle that is generally too weak or lacks the endurance to perform primary functions.

Patients are further described as having complete or incomplete injuries. The patients described in this chapter are labeled incomplete only if sacral sparing is present. To be considered to have sacral sparing, the patient may only have perianal sensation or the ability to flex the great toe. This indicates that some communication exists between the motor cortex and the most distal portion of the spinal cord. An incomplete injury may have a better prognosis for potential return of function below the level of injury.[21]

A patient with a complete injury has no volitional muscle control or sensation in S4-S5. A zone of partial preservation of muscle function may exist below the functional level of injury. Generally, the greater the initial sparing and the faster the neurologic recovery, the better the prognosis.[22,23]

Systems Evaluation

All patients, regardless of level of injury, are evaluated from a systems perspective that assists the team in early identification of the general health status of the patient and potential areas of concern. Following is a brief discussion of the systems that should be evaluated and the relevance to the spinal-injured population.

Integumentary System

Nearly all persons suffering an SCI have sensory deficits that place them at high risk for skin breakdown. Complications of poor skin care can be extremely expensive, requiring use of specialized support beds and plastic surgical flap procedures. Complications can be prevented by the patient and interdisciplinary team through instruction in and practice of lying prone in bed and performing wheelchair pressure raises. Monitoring and assessing the patient's comprehension of methods to prevent pressures sores is a vital part of the rehabilitation education process. When a pressure sore occurs in the acute rehabilitation phase, hospitalization is often extended, and surgery may be required to manage open pressure ulcers that cannot close by primary healing.

Cardiopulmonary System

Patients frequently present to the rehabilitation unit with a compromised cardiopulmonary system resulting from either the level of injury, soft-tissue injuries from gunshot wounds, or bony injuries such as rib fractures. Additionally, premorbid medical conditions (diabetes, peripheral vascular disease) may also impact the cardiopulmonary system and may impact rehabilitation.

Persons with tetraplegia are especially susceptible to acute pulmonary obstruction. The loss of accessory respiratory musculature predisposes these patients to mucous plugs and secretion buildup. Airway maintenance and avoidance of further respiratory complications are prime concerns. Observation for distress and frequent suctioning are needed. These patients often have limited chest expansion, which decreases their ability to cough and mobilize secretions. Treatment includes frequent position changes, postural drainage, percussion, intermittent positive pressure breathing, incentive spirometry, or manual assistance in coughing, depending on the stability of the injury. Vigilance by the staff in detecting early respiratory distress can be life-saving.

Respiratory function is tested to determine ventilatory capacity, diaphragm strength, and chest-wall mobility. Patients with functionally complete injuries at C3 and above usually require ventilatory support. Patients with functional C4 complete injuries may require ventilatory support initially. Patients with functional injuries from C4 to C8 will have diaphragm strength intact but no control of the intercostal or abdominal muscles. Patients with injuries from T1 to T12 will have varying degrees of chest wall and abdominal weakness that may interfere with respiration.

The respiratory evaluation should include (1) breathing pattern, (2) chest excursion, (3) cough function, (4) vital capacity, and (5) forced expiratory volume in 1 second (FEV_1).[24] The breathing pattern is established by observation and palpation of the patient's chest and abdomen during quiet breathing in the supine position. In normal respiration, the chest and abdomen rise and fall at the same time. Patients with significant chest-wall paralysis will be able to use only their diaphragm. This is identified by the rise and fall of the abdomen and either no chest-wall movement or paradoxical motion. Patients with chest-wall paralysis may also begin to use their neck accessory muscles to supplement their diaphragm.

Chest excursion is measured at the level of the xiphoid process with a cloth tape measure placed around the patient's chest. The difference in circumference between maximal inspiration and maximal expiration is noted. Normal excursion in a young adult is 3.25 in. This measurement can be affected by the degree of chest-wall paralysis.[25]

Cough function is tested to evaluate the patient's ability to clear lung secretions. The test is rather subjective, but provides necessary information. The FEV_1 is closely tied to the patient's ability to cough. Vital capacity is measured in the supine position using a spirometer. The percentage of normal for a given age, sex, and height is determined. This test should be repeated in the upright position to evaluate the influence of gravity on the patient's ability to breathe.[26] Patients with chest wall and abdominal paralysis should wear an abdominal binder and compressive stockings when coming to sitting position in the early stages of rehabilitation to minimize the effects of gravity on the abdominal contents and venous pooling. In the absence of sufficient abdominal wall strength to maintain the position of the internal organs, the diaphragm is pulled down when the patient sits up and the diaphragm's normal excursion is compromised. The corset substitutes for the abdominal wall muscles by pressing on the abdomen. The proper position of the internal organs is maintained, allowing the diaphragm to function more normally.[27]

Neurologic System

A complete sensory examination includes testing of light touch (posterior columns, anterior spinothalamic tract), pain (lateral spinothalamic tract), and proprioception (posterior columns). All dermatomes are tested using the ASIA standards for location of preferred testing sites, because individual variations may exist in dermatomes. This information is critical to determining a functional level for the patient as well as to identifying the presence or absence of sacral sparing. All sensory examinations are performed distal to proximal. Pain sensation testing is performed with a sterilized pin; light touch is assessed with a piece of cotton or a light touch of the examiner's finger. Proprioception is tested at all joints and is considered intact only when the patient responds 100% accurately to small arcs of motion.

Other autonomic functions, such as blood pressure and pulse rate, may be altered following SCI. The average person with tetraplegia has a heart rate of 60 beats/min and a blood pressure of 100/60 mm Hg. Patients with high thoracic paraplegia may experience similar changes. Patients who have been on prolonged bed rest may experience limited compensatory vasoconstriction and reduced sympathetic activity, resulting in orthostatic hypotension. Treatment of this condition includes use of an abdominal binder or corset, snug-fitting support hose, or wrapping the lower extremities in elastic bandages. Patients are encouraged to practice sitting up in bed and slowly raising the head off the bed 10° to 20° at a time, stopping frequently if dizziness occurs. Patients who experience dizziness while sitting in a wheelchair may be treated by reclining the wheelchair and/ or elevating the lower extremities.

Autonomic dysreflexia is caused by stimulation of the sympathetic and parasympathetic systems, causing a reflex rise in blood pressure that, due to the SCI, cannot be relieved by normal compensatory mechanisms. If not controlled, the precipitous rise in blood pressure may lead to a cerebrovascular accident or other vascular injury. Symptoms of autonomic dysreflexia include headache, sweating above the level of injury, facial flushing, urticaria (hives) above the level of injury, or nasal congestion. Common causes of dysreflexia include bladder distention, kidney stones, bladder infection, spasms, too-rapid emptying of the bladder, or blocked catheter tubing. Colonic distention can also cause dysreflexia secondary to hard stool, excessive gas, stretching the rectum, or rough digital removal of stool. Skin may also be irritated from sunburn or frostbite, pressure sores, or even an excessively tightened leg bag.

The occurrence of autonomic dysreflexia demands immediate action. Intervention includes sitting the patient up in an attempt to positionally lower the blood pressure. Blood pressure should be monitored immediately. Any tight clothing should be loosened. Catheter tubing should be checked to be sure there is no kink or other drainage problem, and the patient's catheter bag should be emptied. The catheter should be gently irrigated with 30 mL of irrigating solution, and if there are no results, the catheter should be quickly changed. Only 500 mL of urine should be removed following recatheterization. After several minutes, additional urine can be drained from the bladder. Rapid bladder drainage may lead to bladder spasm, which could once again elevate the blood pressure. If a patient voids reflexively, the bladder should be stimulated to empty by tapping in the suprapubic region, pulling the pubic hair, or stroking the inside of the thigh.

Persons with SCI who are at risk of developing autonomic dysreflexia must be taught to manage the condition themselves or how to instruct family members or care providers should they be physically incapable of performing the necessary intervention themselves.

Bowel and Bladder Function

All spinal-injured patients are at risk of developing medical problems as a result of the impact of the injury on bowel and bladder function. Bowel programs are instituted on admission after accurate neurologic diagnosis has been established. Manual evacuation and suppository programs are provided and taught to the patient or a person the patient has identified to be involved in his or her care. Dietary guidance is also a vital part of the bowel program education process. Patients tailor their bowel programs according to their personal lifestyles (eg, choosing AM or PM evacuation programs). Clean intermittent catheterization training is provided by nursing services to the patients, family members, and/or caregivers.

Urology oversees bladder management and medical treatment of frequently seen problems such as urinary tract infections and calculi. The service is also essential to long-term outpatient management of neurogenic bladder problems. Patients with SCI often require cystoscopic evaluation of the lower urinary tract as well as bladder neck incision to facilitate complete drainage of the bladder. These procedures are done while the patient is in the rehabilitation service with minimal delay in total therapy time.

The major genitourinary management problem for the acute spinal cord-injured patient is urinary tract sepsis. Despite early removal of indwelling catheters and the practice of clean, self-administered intermittent catheterization, some patients have persistent urinary tract infections. An acute febrile illness with shaking chills and some decrease in blood pressure is the hallmark of the urinary tract infection. Prompt recognition by the nursing staff and immediate attention by the physician and urologic consultant are required. Often a cause of delay in rehabilitation, this potentially life-threatening problem is, in general, successfully treated by intravenous antimicrobial therapy. Appropriate diagnostic and therapeutic measures can then be taken for stone removal or improved bladder drainage.

Musculoskeletal System

The muscle testing procedure outlined by the ASIA standards identifies key muscles corresponding to each neurologic level. These muscles are tested with the patient supine. To obtain a functional motor control evaluation, additional muscle testing is essential. A manual muscle test to determine muscle strength provides the clinician with a basis for the patient's functional motor status. ASIA defines a functional muscle as a grade of 3/5, or the ability to move the joint through its full range against gravity, but not hold against resistance. However, many clinicians identify a 3+/5 as a minimal functional muscle grade, defining it as the ability of the muscle to move the joint through the full range against gravity and hold against some resistance. A manual muscle grade below this means the patient will not have the endurance to perform functional tasks and will not have the strength to move an object against gravity. Therefore it is not considered "functional." At all times during the evaluation and treatment the stability status of the spine must be considered. In the presence of an unstable cervical fracture, no resistance is given to the muscles of the neck and shoulder girdle. An unstable lumbar fracture precludes resistance being given to the muscles at or around the hips (Appendices 2 and 3).

Joint range of motion is determined for all joints. As in muscle testing, hip flexion and shoulder range are limited to 90° in the presence of unstable spine fractures. Specific joint ranges are necessary for a patient to meet functional goals in the rehabilitation process. Evaluation of joint range of motion identifies premorbid muscle tightness and areas that will require early intervention.

Muscle tone is evaluated by applying a passive quick stretch to a muscle group, so that the clinician can determine a baseline of muscle reactivity. On initial evaluation, a patient may be areflexic,

reflexic, or hyperreflexic in responding to a quick musculotendinous stretch. A patient demonstrating areflexia may still be in the spinal shock phase of injury or may be displaying the signs of a cauda equina injury, a peripheral nerve injury, or a cord infarct. Significant increases in the responses to quick stretch (hyperreflexia) may prevent a patient from meeting functional goals and may cause restrictions on free joint motion in the future.

Functional Evaluation

Activities of Daily Living (ADLs)

Assessment of the patient's daily routine is performed through both interview and observation. In the interview, details are gathered regarding the patient's daily routines just before his or her injury as well as the patient's current ability to perform ADLs. Self-care skills are routine activities necessary to maintain a healthy body. They include eating, hygiene, grooming, bathing, dressing, and toilet functions. The Functional Independence Measure is widely used to assess functional outcomes; however, the Quadriplegia Index of Function and the Modified Barthel Index are instruments designed especially for patients with SCI.[28-30] The interview is followed by observations of function.

Mobility

Most SCIs that require admission to a rehabilitation center will affect a person's ability to move their bodies. The majority of patients will need to learn how to move themselves around on the bed, from bed to chair and back, and how to move from place to place, usually in a wheelchair. Detailed discussion of these mobility issues will be addressed later in the chapter.

Goal Setting

As with the evaluation process, goal setting involves a continuous process of reexamination for the purpose of meeting the individual patient's needs and functional desires. To meet these needs, short-term and long-term goals are established. Short-term goals may address functional performance areas and tasks, underlying problems, or the component skills necessary to perform an ADL.[28] The functional level established by the team during the evaluation serves as a useful guideline in forming long-term goals. It assists in guiding patients toward realistic, attainable goals, thus minimizing failure. Another tool useful for clinicians is the Expected Functional Outcomes chart developed by the Consortium for Spinal Cord Medicine and published in 1999.[31] This chart predicts the degree of functional independence for a particular level of spinal cord injury (excerpts from this chart are provided in Appendix 4). Note that the classic ASIA muscle testing may differ from the Consortium guidelines. For example, the Consortium describes a patient with C6 tetraplegia as having a functionally innervated serratus anterior, clavicular pectoralis, and latissimus dorsi, where the ASIA scoring for that patient would be based on examination of the functional wrist extensors (extensor carpi radialis brevus and longus).

Treatment

The following material is organized by functional level as described earlier in this chapter, beginning at the highest level of injury, to promote understanding of the functional capacity gained as the injury moves distally. The treatment that is required to assist the patient in becoming competent in achieving the functional goal is integrated into the discussion.

Ventilator-Dependent Tetraplegia (C1-C4)

Special Evaluation Needs

Patients with high cervical lesions (C1-C4) have absent to minimal functional use of their upper extremities and require ventilatory support in the initial stages of rehabilitation. Not all patients are able to use alternative methods such as glossopharyngeal breathing, neck breathing, or phrenic nerve pacing to remain off the ventilator. These patients will then require full-time ventilatory support, possibly for the rest of their lives. To evaluate the patient's neck accessory muscles, the patient must be removed momentarily from the ventilator. This is often anxiety-producing for the patient. The therapist should establish the patient's trust before attempting this examination.

The examination is performed by observation and palpation of both the neck accessory muscles and the diaphragm. Patients must be predominantly diaphragmatic breathers to support themselves off the ventilator. Patients injured at C2 or higher have nonfunctional diaphragms. These patients may be able to ventilate themselves using their neck muscles to expand the chest cavity. Increased body weight and size may have a negative effect on success. Children and persons with small body size have demonstrated greater success, but some have lost the ability to adequately ventilate themselves with neck breathing as they grow.

Treatment

Even the most efficient neck breather will require time to build the endurance needed for support off the ventilator. The neck muscles, although potentially strong, usually have not functioned as primary respiratory muscles other than during periods of heavy exertion. Like any other muscle, they fatigue. Neck muscle strengthening is conducted using general principles of muscle strengthening. Specific strengthening activities for respiratory function involve removing the patient from the ventilator for slowly increasing periods of time. The first session may result in the patient being able to support himself or herself off the ventilator for only 10 to 15 seconds.

The diaphragm is also a muscle that responds to strengthening. Strengthening may be performed using manual resistance to the diaphragm, or through the use of resisted inspiratory trainers. It is important to preserve the patient's chest expansion during this early period through manual stretching until the patient reaches the maximal respiratory capability. Insufficient range of motion in the costal joints will act as a mechanical block to the patient's ability to expand the chest wall for breathing and coughing.

It is strongly recommended that all ventilator-dependent patients be trained in some alternative method of breathing that could sustain them for a minimum of 10 minutes. This enables the patient to ventilate in case of equipment failure or power outage. The ability to do so may mean the difference between life and death. This capacity also facilitates easier transfers in more difficult situations such as going into a car or bathing. It is recommended that the patient's family or caregiver be included in this training. When the patient leaves the hospital, all involved with care should feel capable of handling emergency situations that will undoubtedly arise. Ten minutes of unassisted breathing provide both the patient and caregivers with time to handle most situations.

Glossopharyngeal breathing is a specialized technique of gulping air into the lungs using oral, pharyngeal, and laryngeal structures. The technique was first used for the poliomyelitis patient population having respiratory paralysis. It is used today for the spinal cord-injured patient in conjunction with a Passy-Muir valve to enable time off the ventilator. A detailed description of the technique can be found in the manual *Glossopharyngeal Breathing*.[32]

Other mechanisms that supply ventilatory support include surgically implanted diaphragmatic pacers and the pneumobelt. Implanted pacers require specialized surgical intervention. Use of the pneumobelt can be initiated by the therapist. Patients have noted that certain advantages exist with use of these alternative breathing methods. Cosmesis is improved when the tubing from the tracheostomy to the ventilator is discontinued, and the ability to speak is improved because the tracheostomy can be plugged. The patient must return to a ventilator at night when on the pneumobelt because it will not function effectively when the wearer is in the supine position.

It is recommended that physical, respiratory, and communication disorders therapists work closely as a team when treating the ventilator-dependent patient. Blood gases or pulse oximetry is necessary to verify the patient's ability to achieve satisfactory gas exchange when off the ventilator and using one of the alternative methods of breathing. An automatic alarm system and a head or cheek control switch must also be available for the patient to summon help if a mechanical failure should occur.

Treatment Goals

After ventilation has been addressed, treatment goals are directed at preventing upper extremity complications such as development of edema, pain, or range-of-motion limitations. Prevention of upper extremity complications is necessary to maximize function in the event of possible motor recovery, to ensure the patient's comfort, and to preserve the aesthetic appearance of the arm and hand. Thus, treatment must include upper extremity positioning in bed and in the wheelchair, daily range-of-motion exercises, and patient and attendant education in routine upper extremity care. Correct bed positioning is established as soon as possible. It focuses on eliminating direct pressure over the glenohumeral joint and positioning the shoulder in external rotation. Additionally, preventing elbow flexion and supination contractures is achieved by positioning the elbow in extension and the forearm in pronation whenever possible. To assist in managing correct positioning, a schedule is posted on a communication board at the patient's bedside.

To preserve the functional position of the hand, temporary prefabricated soft resting hand splints or long opponens splints are issued to the patient. In cases where a more permanent hand orthosis is warranted, the static wrist-hand orthosis (WHO) is fabricated by an orthotist to replace the temporary prefabricated splint previously used.[33] The WHO is a dorsal hand splint that maintains the functional position of the hand. The wrist is supported at 20° to 30° of extension. A palmar bar preserves the transverse palmar arch of the hand. The thumb is abducted and all fingers are left free to assume a functional position with some interphalangeal flexion. Upper extremity range-of-motion exercises are performed daily and the patient and significant others are instructed in motion principles and execution.

Functional Goals

Persons who have sustained an injury resulting in tetraplegia at the level of C1 through C4 are expected to attain the ability to drive their own motorized wheelchair and perform tabletop activities such as writing, using a computer, painting, and reading. Most will need assistance with set-up for these activities. They will remain dependent in other ADLs. The expected functional goals of patients with high-level tetraplegia are limited. Thus, a critical element in their rehabilitation process involves enhancing independence through the use of attendants and community resources.

Group discussions are designed to enable patients to feel confident in exercising control over their environment. Because all patients with high-level tetraplegia injuries require attendant care, special emphasis is placed on education in the use of attendants. Discussions focus on hiring, training, and optimally using the limited time they may have with their attendants. Assertiveness training in which patients role-play realistic scenarios helps them to focus on effective communication as a means of gaining control of their lives. Patients are also empowered by learning and gaining knowledge about community resources and rights provided by the American with Disabilities Act (ADA), which bans discrimination on the basis of disability. The ADA guarantees equal opportunity for individuals with disabilities in public and private sector services and employment. Other group discussions cover subjects such as returning to school and work, and pursuing leisure activities.

The vocational opportunities of the patients with high-level tetraplegia injuries have expanded markedly with the advent of computer technology. The patient with tetraplegia can execute all business activities such as networking, directing employees, and managing office work with an adapted computer terminal. These technological advances are of special significance to a person with tetraplegia who either must be or chooses to be homebound, as it enables him or her to work at home. The occupational therapist explores with the patient his or her interests as well as vocational aptitudes. The therapist provides the patient with a simulated work setting in which the patient can become aware of capabilities and limitations. All prevocational data are given both to the patient and to a vocational rehabilitation counselor to further prepare the patient for work and to aid in vocational placement. It must be noted, however, that only a few patients with high tetraplegia are currently employed. Most lack the education, resources, and appropriate environment to become employed.

Some individuals with the financial resources and familial or caregiver support are referred to the driver's program for a passenger evaluation. In these circumstances, patients are given individualized information regarding possible van modifications that would best meet their needs and are given appropriate specifications for their wheelchair.

Specialized Equipment Needs

The most reliable and basic orthosis used by patients with high tetraplegia is the mouthstick, a mouth-controlled, 12-in to 18-in–long rigid rod with specialized tips for the performance of various activities. The mouthpiece is Y-shaped to permit speech and swallowing. Patients are trained to use mouthsticks by performing graded activities, starting with simple activities such as pushing checkers on a checkerboard and then gradually going on to more complex tasks such as writing. They progress to functional activities such as turning pages, writing, filing, typing, and using a calculator, tape recorder, and telephone. Some leisure activities that are performed with mouthsticks include operating a radio and television, drawing, painting, and playing board and electronic games. To accomplish these versatile tasks, specialized mouthsticks are used.

Mouthsticks may be static or dynamic. A static mouthstick includes a rigid rod with an end piece specific to performing an activity such as writing or turning pages. Interchangeable tips are available for other activities. A dynamic mouthstick has a moving component activated by the tongue that brings about the distal movement of the tip. The pincer mouthstick, for example, aids in picking up light objects with a tongue-activated clamp. The docking station is the device that holds the mouthstick when it is not in use.

Neck strength graded at 3+/5 and above enables the patient with C4 tetraplegia to manipulate most mouthsticks. Patients with C1 through C3 tetraplegia who are ventilator-dependent with absent or weak neck muscles are much more limited in function. These patients have greater difficulty in manipulating mouthsticks as well as in docking them to switch or complete an activity. The patient with C1 tetraplegia may achieve partial head flexion by using the platysma muscle. Neck flexion coupled with lip and tongue movement may enable the person to use a mouthstick for simple activities. The patient, however, is fully dependent on others to arrange the set-up of all activities. Additional functional compensation is achieved through specialized equipment. An example of such equipment is the dynamic protractable mouthstick. This mouthstick allows for elongation of the distal end, thus aiding the patient in manipulating objects.

With ongoing, rapid advances in technology, new options become available for persons with tetraplegia. Independence and the ability to participate more fully in home, school, and work environments are just a few of the benefits realized through use of new technologies. The computer is now a common tool in our society and is used for numerous activities including writing, personal finances, networking, inventory, and so forth. There are many ways in which persons with tetraplegia can operate a computer. These include using mouthsticks or other pointing devices on a keyboard, head movement to control the cursor on the screen with an on-screen keyboard, a pneumatic sip-and-puff switch to operate a computer with Morse code or a scanning array, or even voice input. For more detailed information about computer access, a book written specifically for persons with SCI is available from the Bay Area and Western Chapter of the Paralyzed Veterans of America, Palo Alto, CA.[34]

Environmental control units (ECUs) have also had a great impact on the independence of persons with tetraplegia. ECUs allow control of lights, appliances, and other electrical devices when the usual method of operation is difficult or impossible. By pressing a button or switch, or giving voice commands, a person has the ability to answer the telephone, unlock and open a door, change the television channel, turn a light on and off, activate a call alarm, and much more. Many persons with SCI benefit from simple adaptations and low-cost ECUs. Others may need more sophisticated and complex ECUs.

As technology advances, the number of possible solutions to meet the needs of patients with disabilities increases. These range from low-cost, low-tech solutions to more sophisticated and complex high-tech solutions with their associated higher costs. Multiple technology needs are best met by an interdisciplinary team specializing in assistive technology, including the client and care providers. An evaluation is conducted to determine solutions that will best meet the individual's needs and abilities, and the constraints of costs and environments in which the technology is to be used. When technological recommendations are made, they must be compatible with other equipment used to assist the individual in the performance of necessary and desired activities within his or her environment(s). For example, the technology now exists to operate a power wheelchair, communication device, computer, and ECU with the same power wheelchair controller, the whole a neat and aesthetically pleasing package. Even though this technology exists, it may or may not be the most beneficial solution for a particular patient. A team approach is needed to determine if it would actually be beneficial for mobility, communication, and other functional needs

Some functional use of the upper extremities can be seen in the patient with C4 tetraplegia with some C5 root escape. While for most patients at this functional level driving a wheelchair with hand controls may be the highest functional goal, stronger patients may be able to engage in light self-care and selected tabletop activities. With deltoid and biceps strength of 2–/5 or better, and with maximum assistance in setting up an activity, the patient with tetraplegia may be able to feed, brush teeth, wash the face, shave, and write, type, and perform other desktop activities. These tasks are accomplished with the aid of orthoses. To support the weight of the arm and to enhance proximal strength, a mobile arm support (MAS) is fitted. This excellent mechanical device, which is also called a ball-bearing feeder, "supports the weight of the arm and provides assistance to shoulder and elbow motions through a linkage of ball-bearing joints."[35]

To achieve prehension, the person with C4 tetraplegia with weak C5 muscles (deltoids and biceps, 2–/5 to 3/5) requires an additional orthosis because of lack of wrist or hand function. The universal cuff, also known as the utensil holder, is the most common device used for feeding. This cuff fits around the palm of the hand and has a pocket for inserting utensils. To change from feeding to another activity, the patient or an aide changes the tool inserted into the pocket. Other activities that can be performed with a universal cuff include brushing teeth and performing light hygiene and grooming. The universal cuff is very light and therefore appropriate for patients who have weak deltoids and biceps strength of 2–/5 to

FIGURE 3

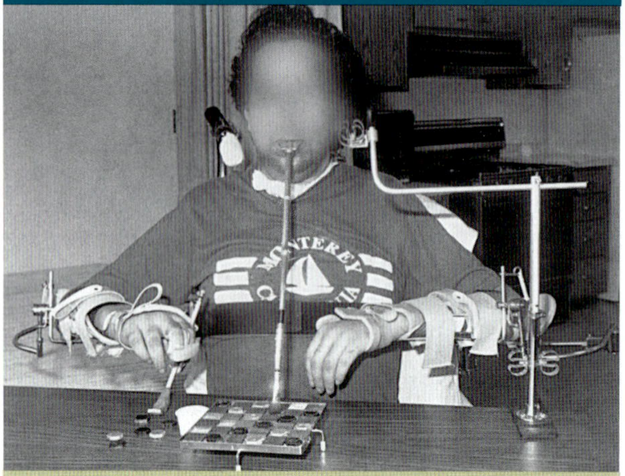

Figure 3 A patient participating in occupational therapy using mobile arm supports, upper extremity orthoses, and a mouthstick.

3/5. Although it is inexpensive and easy to fabricate, it lacks versatility. A more versatile and durable functional metal orthosis is the ratchet WHO, a mechanical device which enables a person with wrist and hand paralysis to manipulate objects. The ratchet WHO is positioned on the forearm, wrist, thumb, index, and middle fingers. To pick up an object, orthosis closure is achieved by manual pressure on the finger pieces to approximate the thumb. To release objects, a button is pressed. The ratchet, although versatile and durable, is expensive, heavy, and more noticeable on the patient's hand than the universal cuff.

The patient should experiment with all available orthoses. The therapist assists the patient in selecting the best orthosis to meet his or her functional needs. Thorough training is critical for the patient to derive maximal functional benefit from orthoses. (Orthosis training is discussed later in this chapter.)

Some patients with weak C5 muscles benefit from combining the upper extremity orthosis and a mouthstick. This is especially advantageous when one arm is too weak to assist the more functional upper extremity. In this case, the mouthstick is used to stabilize objects (**Figure 3**).

C5 Cervical Injuries

Treatment Goals

As with patients with high-level tetraplegia, upper extremity deformity, edema, and pain must be prevented and managed. Functional joint range of motion is maintained through bed and wheelchair positioning, daily exercises, and educating the patient and caregivers. While the patient is lying in bed, emphasis is placed on avoiding direct pressure on the glenohumeral joint and on maintaining shoulder external rotation. Patients with C5 tetraplegia may develop elbow flexion and forearm supination contractures due to unopposed biceps activity. To avoid such deformities, the elbow must be maintained in extension and the forearm in full pronation. If limitations develop, serial casting with long-arm casts is most effective. The patient is also issued a prefabricated WHO to protect the wrist against excessive stretch of the weak or absent wrist extensors.[33]

Strengthening of the upper extremities begins as soon as the patient's neck is stabilized and medical clearance is provided by the physicians. It is recommended that strengthening begin as soon after the injury as possible. With the aid of an overhead frame and springs and slings, the patient can begin upper extremity active assistive exercises while still in bed.[36] Neuromuscular electrical stimulation, an electric current that brings about muscle excitation and induces motor response, provides for additional muscle activation when the patient is lying in bed.[33] In the wheelchair, strengthening is achieved through the use of orthotic devices and weights, as well as through therapeutic and functional activities.

The MAS is often used during the initial period following bed rest to support the arms and enhance proximal shoulder movement. The MAS assists patients whose deltoid strength is 2–/5 or better to achieve shoulder flexion, thus enabling them to increase strength and endurance through repetitive motion. Additionally, it allows them to perform functional activities involving the head, such as feeding, hygiene, and grooming. When deltoids and biceps develop 3+/5 or better strength and when endurance improves, the MAS is no longer needed.

Strengthening is also achieved by a program of progressive exercises that begins with active assistive exercises through the use of the MAS and skateboards. Next, active exercises are performed against gravity. To further strengthen muscles, mechanical resistance is applied through the use of weights and exercise machines specially developed to meet the needs of the person with tetraplegia.[37]

Functional Goals

Persons with tetraplegia functioning at the C5 level (deltoids and biceps 3+/5 or above and intact pain sensation) may be able independently to don and doff their orthoses. Following assistance in set-up, they are able to feed themselves using

FIGURE 4

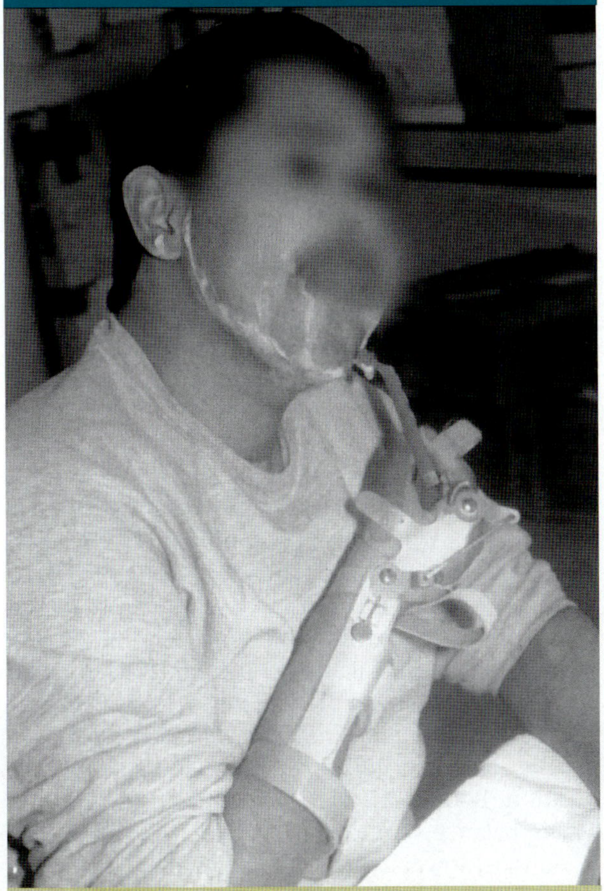

Figure 4 A patient shaving with a wrist-driven WHO.

adaptive equipment that is necessary due to the lack of wrist and finger muscle control. Patients at this level are able to accomplish self-care skills such as feeding, brushing teeth, and grooming; home skills such as cooking; and community skills such as shopping (**Figure 4**).[31] In addition, they are expected to be able to write, type, and execute more complex desktop vocational and leisure activities. However, patients at this functional level lack trunk control and muscles below the shoulders; therefore, they are mostly dependent or assisted in dressing and bathing.[33] Patients with C5 tetraplegia may also be able to drive a specially equipped van independently (Appendix 5).

These patients may be able to propel a manual wheelchair with adapted hand rims, but because of their muscle weakness and limited endurance, a power wheelchair with hand controls would be the most functional. The person with a C5 injury will require assistance for all transfers and bed mobility activities.

Prevocational training involves exploring with the patient his or her interests and vocational aptitudes. Exploring work skills, the therapist provides the patient with a simulated work setting in which the patient can become aware of capabilities and limitations. As in the case of persons with high tetraplegia, prevocational data are given to the patient and to an appropriate vocational counselor.

Driving training is performed in a specially adapted van. Steering wheel and other controls are fitted to meet individual needs and driving demands are gradually increased as the patient gains proficiency and confidence. Special emphasis must be placed on safety considerations. Factors that may interfere with safe driving, such as spasticity, spasms, and medication side effects, must be addressed before the patient is able to drive independently.[38]

As with patients with high-level tetraplegia, a critical element in the rehabilitation process of the patient with C5 tetraplegia involves enhancing independence through the effective use of attendants and community resources. A home visit is performed to ensure a barrier-free and safe home environment. Additionally, training in the community is performed and group discussions regarding attendant management, child care, transportation, and returning to school or work are held.

Specialized Equipment Needs

In order that patients sustaining injury at the C5 level may accomplish these many activities despite considerable upper extremity weakness, specialized devices are required. A primary concern is that the wrist must be stabilized with a splint or orthosis. To stabilize the wrist, a hand cock-up splint is worn.[33] Next, a device is attached to the hand to enable the person to perform activities. The universal cuff is a simple, light, inexpensive utensil holder that rests around the palm.[33] Other U-shaped clamps fit around the palm of the hand and may be attached to a device such as a shaver or telephone receiver. Devices are made for writing, typing, feeding, and performing hygiene and grooming. Some selected patients benefit from a more versatile piece of equipment such as the ratchet WHO mentioned previously. This orthosis eliminates the need for a variety of adaptive devices. With the ratchet WHO, the person is trained to pick up, hold, manipulate, and release objects. However, our experience is that therapists and patients prefer the use of orthoses and adaptive equipment other then the ratchet. This is partially because of its cumbersome operation, appearance, and excessive weight.[33]

The patient with C5 tetraplegia with functional return (3+/5 or above) of the extensor carpi radialis longus (C6 functional level in the ASIA classification) is significantly different from other patients with C5 tetraplegia as he or she can achieve a greater degree of independence. This is because of the very important role of wrist extensors in hand function through tenodesis (the functional finger closure of the hand when the wrist is extended and the opening of the fingers when the wrist is flexed). This motion, which is caused by long-finger flexor tendon tightness, is used by the patient with tetraplegia to grasp, release, and manipulate light objects.

To enhance functional tenodesis, maintenance of correct hand position and range, as well as strengthening of the wrist, is of critical importance. To maintain the functional finger tightness necessary for optimal tenodesis, care must be taken to maintain a correct relationship between the fingers and wrist at all times to avoid stretching the finger flexors and losing the tenodesis action. While ranging or pursuing functional activities, the wrist is maintained in extension when the fingers are flexed. When the fingers are extended, the wrist is flexed. Occasionally, spasticity may interfere with functional tenodesis. When medications and splinting do not improve hand function, percutaneous phenol blocks to motor points administered by the physician may decrease spasticity, improving hand opening and closure.[39] To increase wrist strength for those patients 6 months postinjury, the static WHO, used to maintain a functional hand position for C1 through C4 patients with tetraplegia, is replaced by a dynamic orthosis called the wrist-action WHO (WAWHO). The WAWHO is a transitional orthosis that allows for active-assistive wrist extension with the aid of a rubber band attached to a post above the wrist.

For prehension, and for maintaining strong tenodesis, the patient with tetraplegia with wrist extensors of at least 3+/5 or above can use the metal wrist-driven WHO (WDWHO), also called the wrist-driven flexor hinge hand splint or the tenodesis splint. To achieve closure, the patient extends the wrist, transferring mechanical force to the fingers. To open the hand, gravity assists in wrist flexion, causing finger extension. To assist weak 3+/5 wrist extensors, a vertical post with a rubber band is added. With the WDWHO, the patient learns to perform many activities.

The WDWHO is durable, yet expensive and heavy for some patients. It is fabricated by an orthotist and is custom-made. If orthotic services are not available to make a WDWHO and if a WDWHO is not an appropriate solution for the patient, alternative solutions for achieving functional tenodesis must be sought. Some therapists fabricate their own devices.[40] One such device is a thumb loop that attaches to a wrist band with a rubber band. As the patient flexes the wrist, the rubber band pulls the thumb against the index finger.

C6 Cervical Injuries

Treatment Goals

As with other levels of injury, treatment is initially focused on maintaining upper extremity joint range and on strengthening. Following instruction, the patient with C6 tetraplegia is able to perform range-of-motion exercises unassisted. The patient must learn the importance of tenodesis hand motion and range the fingers accordingly. Upper extremity strengthening is achieved by a progressive resistive exercise program.

To maximize use of the upper extremities, wheelchair sitting balance must be adequate. Good sitting balance allows the patient to use the arms without holding onto the chair, to reach the ground, resume a sitting position, and adjust body position. Both individual and group training in sitting balance should be provided.

As most lower body self-care skills are performed in bed and require prolonged sitting, the patient must be physically ready to begin these activities. The patient should have a hip flexion range of 0° to 110° to protect the back muscles from excessive stretching, good body-handling skills, and some ability to roll from side to side. To aid in donning pants, socks, and shoes, the patient may need assistive devices such as sewn loops to pull up clothing. Patients who cannot meet these physical requirements may need dressing sticks and reachers. To further simplify the task, training in buttoning a shirt or zippering pants can be practiced first as a tabletop activity. Similarly, practicing the application of an external catheter on a large plastic syringe and connecting the catheter to a leg bag on a table makes accomplishing the task later in bed easier.

Functional Goals

The functional outcome of rehabilitation of the person with C6 tetraplegia varies greatly (Appendix 6). This patient has only the minimal muscle strength required to achieve full independence. Full independence, therefore, can be mastered only with hard and, at times, frustrating work. Flexibility in setting and adjusting patients' goals is critical. Upon discharge from the hospital, most patients with C6 tetraplegia achieve modified independence in light self-care skills and community skills. However, they may require assistance in some light home skills, and self-care skills such as lower body dressing, bathing, and bowel management.[31] Interfering factors such as spasticity, spasms, obesity, or long extremities can further complicate accomplishing these tasks. The person with C6 tetraplegia may achieve full independence after leaving the hospital as the skills initially learned in therapy are practiced over a long period of time and muscles become stronger.

If the C6 level is intact, the patient's function improves greatly. In addition to normal shoulder girdle strength, the C6 level provides some function to the clavicular portion of the pectoralis major, the serratus anterior, and the extensor carpi radialis longus. The pectoralis enables the person to roll from side to side, and perform activities that require crossing the midline of the body such as dressing. Wrist extensors are fundamental to tenodesis hand motion. They allow the patient with tetraplegia to manipulate objects despite the absence of finger motion. In addition to these key muscles, added scapular stability brought about by function of the serratus anterior (3+/5 or above) and teres major muscles enables the patient to better propel a manual wheelchair, and partial innervation of the pronator teres assists in stabilizing and positioning the hand in pronation. A patient with an injury at this level may be able to perform sliding board transfers, roll from supine to prone in bed, and perform independent pressure relief when sitting by bending forward while in the wheelchair. Added sensation in the C6 dermatome allows the patient with C6 tetraplegia to manipulate objects with greater dexterity and eliminates some need for visual compensation.

Self-care skills involving the lower body, such as dressing and bladder and bowel care, are challenging and require patience and perseverance. To ensure success, a thorough understanding of the purpose and procedure used to accomplish each task is critical. Visual aids such as videotapes, slides, and pictures that describe an activity are helpful. A peer with a similar functional level who can demonstrate the tasks to the patient provides extra encouragement.

The patient with C6 tetraplegia may use the WDWHO to enhance hand function. Training with the WDWHO includes self-care skills such as feeding, brushing teeth, grooming, dressing, and managing the bladder; home skills such as cooking and laundering; and community skills such as shopping. Although writing can be achieved with a WDWHO, most patients prefer to use a smaller device for this activity. Writing devices, which can either be fabricated by the occupational therapist or purchased, attach to the hand alone, thereby providing greater wrist and forearm freedom of movement and allowing fine motor coordination.

Bowel management, a challenging task, is best accomplished on a commode chair above a toilet. The patient practices inserting a suppository and performing digital stimulation with special devices. To prevent injury to the rectal area, the therapist should alert the patient to all necessary precautions (such as the danger of damaging rectal tissues because of lack of sensation), practice this skill often, and adapt the equipment to meet the patient's needs.

As with patients with high-level tetraplegia, a critical element in the rehabilitation process of the patient with C6 tetraplegia involves enhancing independence through the effective use of community resources. A fundamental difference, however, is that unlike the patient with high-level tetraplegia, the patient with C6 tetraplegia may need the assistance of an attendant only temporarily and only for selected tasks. A home visit is made to assure a barrier-free and safe home environment. Training in the community is performed and group discussions regarding child care, transportation, and return to school or work are held.

Prevocational and driving training are also part of the program for the patient with C6 tetraplegia. The patient with C6 tetraplegia can drive a car with hand controls if he or she can transfer in and out of the car independently and if muscle power is sufficient to manipulate the wheelchair. However, most persons with C6 tetraplegia find driving a van more convenient and more energy-conserving, because a lift is used to get them in and out of the van. A detailed description of driving and of driving equipment can be found in the manual *A Driver Training Program for Persons with Physical Disabilities*.[38]

C7 Cervical Injuries

Treatment Goals

At the C7 level, the patient has full innervation to the clavicular portion of the pectoralis major, the serratus anterior, and the extensor carpi radialis brevis and longus muscles. In addition, the sternal pectoralis major, triceps, and latissimus dorsi are partially innervated. The presence of this additional nerve level greatly increases the patient's functional abilities. Most patients will be able to perform independent transfers to multiple surfaces and perform depression-type raises for pressure relief. The presence of the serratus anterior and latissimus dorsi provides the essential components of the force couple for shoulder girdle stability. This additional shoulder girdle stability will enable the person to propel a wheelchair on a variety of surfaces and on inclines.

While the techniques for how to perform transfers are provided and practiced during the inpatient rehabilitation stay, the majority of patients with tetraplegia will not be independent with transfers at discharge. The patient will learn by practicing at home, and seeking outpatient services or resources in their community.

Functional Goals

The key muscle that allows the person with C7 tetraplegia to perform ADLs with greater ease than the patient with C6 tetraplegia is the triceps. This muscle allows the patient to reach for objects. With the added aid of the innervated latissimus dorsi, the patient may now support the body in transfers and in activities such as bowel management.

The functional goals, treatment, and outcome of rehabilitation of the patient with C7 tetraplegia are similar to those for patients with C6 tetraplegia. Therefore, only treatment elements unique to the patients with C7 tetraplegia are mentioned here.

At C7, finger extensors are innervated. Thus, the extensor digitorum communis is functioning but is unopposed because the finger flexors are not functional. This added finger extension may interfere with tenodesis hand motion. To avoid the loss of functional tenodesis, metacarpophalangeal (MCP) and proximal interphalangeal joint range must be maintained. This is accomplished through range-of-motion exercises as well as through night splinting, which encourages adaptive shortening of the flexor digitorum profundus, superficialis, and flexor pollicis longus. The WDWHO reinforces tenodesis hand motion and provides substitution for a weak pinch and grasp.

C8 Cervical Injuries

Functional Goals

The upper extremity muscles of the patient with C8 tetraplegia are fully innervated except for some intrinsic muscles of the hand. Thus, the patient with C8 tetraplegia is expected to be independent in all self-care, light home skills, and community skills.[31] Lack of intrinsic finger muscles (called an intrinsic-minus hand) does, however, cause some difficulty with fine motor coordination as well as with stabilization of objects and with power grip and pinch. Additionally, due to lack of lumbricals, which contribute to the functional positioning of the hand by MCP joint flexion, the fingers assume a less functional tenodesis position as the MCP joints are extended. To compensate for the lack of intrinsic muscle power, extrinsic hand muscles are strengthened. This is achieved through a progressive resistive exercise program, through functional electrical stimulation, and other functional as well as therapeutic activities. Crafts such as woodworking and copper tooling are therapeutic activities. These crafts increase hand endurance through repetitive resistive motion.

Splints and orthoses are also available to provide functional hand position and enhance hand strength. To achieve functional hand position, a lumbrical bar (MCP joint extension stop) that flexes the MCP joints is used. It is important to note, however, that most patients with C8 tetraplegia prefer going without splints and orthoses as they can function independently without them with compensatory techniques.

Other treatment of the patient with C8 tetraplegia is similar to the treatment of paraplegics. For further details, see the following section.

Paraplegia

While each cervical nerve root that escaped injury has a great effect on a patient's functional abilities, the case is not quite the same for the paraplegic population. In general, a high thoracic injury (T1 through T8) leaves the patient with intact upper extremities, allowing the carrying out of all transfers, wheelchair activities, self-care, self-enhancement, and self-advancement roles independently. These patients do have significantly reduced trunk control compared to lower-level thoracic injuries (T9 through T12). The patient with an injury at T9 through T12 has sufficient trunk stability to perform high-level wheelchair skills. However, these patients require assistance with heavy housekeeping and physically demanding vocational pursuits.[28,31] For physically demanding home skills such as cleaning cupboards that are out of reach, performing heavy yard work, or putting out trash cans, assistance is advised to prevent unnecessary injuries and conserve energy. If the person has no available assistance or chooses to perform heavy home skills independently, these activities can be simplified to meet his or her needs.

Examples of high-level wheelchair skills are "wheelies" (popping up the front of the chair to jump curbs), and transfers out of the chair to the ground. The ability to transfer to the floor means the patient may need less equipment for daily activities, such as a tub bench for bathing. Because of the shortened lengths of stay, patients are unable to learn the advanced wheelchair skills as inpatients and require further training through community reintegration programs or outpatient therapy services.

When the level of injury is in the lumbar region, ambulation becomes a consideration. A patient with an injury at the L1 through L3 level may be able to ambulate at the household level with a knee-ankle-foot orthosis (KAFO) because of the motor function of the hip flexors and adductors. At the L4 level, the quadriceps should be functional. A manual muscle grade of 3+/5 may enable the patient to ambulate in an ankle-foot orthosis (AFO). The gluteus medius and tensor fascia lata receive partial innervation at L5. These muscles provide adequate hip stability that allows patients to walk with AFOs. At the sacral level, ambulation may be possible without the use of an orthosis. Gait training will be discussed in detail later in this chapter.

Each of the functional goals described is merely a guideline. Individual variation in functional outcomes must be considered. Age, body type, current health status, resources for therapy and equipment, and cognitive and motivational factors all have potential to influence the patient's ultimate functional outcome.

Treatment

A prerequisite for any functional activity is good wheelchair balance. It is optimal for the patient to be able to use both upper extremities without support. This task is especially challenging to the person with a high thoracic (T1 through T5) injury who lacks trunk musculature. To improve wheelchair balance, the patient receives both individual and group training. Group activities are especially helpful in facilitating spontaneous motion as the patient's attention is drawn to group interaction, thereby lessening fear of movement.

Upper extremity strengthening is frequently necessary following a long period of immobility. The progressive resistive program may begin in bed, using wrist weights and barbells, and progress to modified universal gym equipment in physical therapy.

Functionally, light self-care skills such as grooming and hygiene pose no difficulty for the paraplegic. However, self-care skills involving the lower body and demanding adequate body-handling skills require the therapist's intervention. Lower body dressing should begin when hip flexion range is 0° to 110°, to avoid stretching low back muscles in prolonged sitting. Optimally, the patient should also be able to come to a sitting position from supine, maintain balance in a prolonged sitting position, and roll from side to side. Because acquiring these skills takes time and much practice, it is often necessary to begin training with compensatory techniques. Initially, these techniques may involve bringing up the back of the hospital bed to maintain prolonged sitting and using assistive devices such as a dressing stick to reach the feet. When dressing in bed is mastered, the patient is trained to dress in the wheelchair.

Safety precautions must be of special consideration in showering and bathing training. Slippery surfaces make it difficult to maintain balance, especially when the arms are engaged in washing the body. The patient must be taught to have all needed supplies nearby to avoid precarious reaching. Patients must also learn to test the water temperature with their hands before entering. Simulating bathing conditions to resemble those at the patient's home is helpful.

Once the person with paraplegia has learned to perform self-care skills, treatment must focus on the challenges of home life. Most home skills, such as meal preparation, housekeeping, and laundry, remain realistic and require only minimal instruction to be performed from a wheelchair. Training must emphasize planning skills, energy conservation, and safety precautions. Knowledge of the patient's home floor plan assists in making instructions specific to the architectural barriers the patient will encounter. The final goal in home-skills training is to enable the patient to apply his or her knowledge to any situation that may arise. The patient must develop the ability to plan ahead, to organize efficiently, and to problem-solve effectively.

Day passes and overnight passes provide an excellent opportunity for the patient to test the skills learned in the hospital at home. Detailed discussion of information gathered on passes allows the patient to practice problem solving with the help of the therapist. Group discussions in which patients are encouraged to provide their own solutions to problems are helpful.

Incomplete Paraplegia

The patient with an incomplete injury may be unable to achieve goals higher than a patient with a complete injury of the same level. It is with these patients that the manual muscle test grade of

3+/5 becomes critical. Muscles that are graded below 3+/5 have insufficient strength to take on significant tasks. The patient should be made aware of the strength needed for specific functional activities. This will help the person gain a better understanding about future function without taking away all hope. Patients with muscle grades of 1/5 or 2/5 in the trunk and lower extremities are sometimes resistant to participating in therapy that stresses only the basic body-handling skills. Due to shortened lengths of stay, the emphasis of the inpatient program is directed toward maximizing the patient's functional independence as an inpatient and then continuing to follow their progression through community reintegration services and/or outpatient services.

Discharge Planning and Follow-up

A critical goal for the rehabilitation team is to facilitate the patient's smooth transition from hospital to home and community. To accomplish this goal, discharge planning must begin early in the rehabilitation process. The involvement of the patients' significant others must be encouraged early, especially with patients who require assistance with ADLs. Family members are encouraged to observe therapy, ask questions, and learn to perform the routine care they may need to provide at home, such as passive range-of-motion exercises.

An early visit to the patient's home will facilitate a successful transition from hospital to community. Unfortunately, many patients do not have a clear discharge destination until the end of their rehabilitation stay. With these patients, home visits are conducted at discharge. During home visits, the patient, physical therapist, and occupational therapist meet with the patient's family to discuss the patient's homecoming. Discussion is focused on the removal of architectural barriers that interfere with the patient's ability to perform daily routines independently, and to achieve maximal wheelchair accessibility and safety. To many families and patients, the home visit is a startling confrontation with the realities of disability. To reduce the anxiety often aroused during the visit, skills learned in rehabilitation should be practiced and used in the home setting.

Day passes and overnight passes are extremely useful in preparing the patient for community reentry. During these passes, the patient is encouraged to try out new skills learned in therapy. Following passes, the patient and therapist attempt to solve the problems the patient encountered and could not solve independently. On these passes, trial use of adaptive equipment is important in identifying the patient's specific needs.

To ensure that needed adaptive equipment and orthoses do not end up in the closet, the patient must have a good understanding of the function and routine maintenance of those devices. Supplementing discussions with written instructions on the care of equipment will help ensure their proper functioning. When such written information is given to the patient, the therapist needs to be certain that the material is understood. Often, therapists err by dispensing written instructions requiring college-level literacy, a level above that of most spinal cord–injured patients. The patient must also have tried alternative ways to achieve goals that are attained with equipment and fully appreciate their pros and cons. This will allow the patient to continue to independently assess the use of the equipment. Prior to discharge, the patient must also have a clear understanding of how to obtain repairs when equipment malfunctions.

Prior to discharge, the patient must also be instructed and well-practiced in a routine home strengthening program to maintain and increase functional ability and cardiovascular conditioning.

Lifelong follow-up by an SCI health-care team provides the SCI patient with specialized care to meet evolving problems and needs. If the patient and therapist identify new functional goals, further treatment is planned by the outpatient team to achieve these goals. Patients who are unable to come to the hospital's outpatient clinic are referred to other health-care providers.

Patients who are either homebound or require more extensive follow-up at home are referred to the Visiting Nurse Association.

Functional Evaluation

Activities of Daily Living and Instrumental ADLs

ADLs include self-care, home, and community skills. Self-care skills are routine activities necessary to maintain a healthy body. They include eating, hygiene, grooming, bathing, dressing, and toilet functions. Home skills are routine tasks performed to maintain an adequate living environment. Light home skills include preparing meals, washing dishes and clothes, ironing, sweeping floors, vacuuming, changing bed linens, and some aspects of child care. Heavy home skills include tasks such as emptying trash cans, scrubbing floors, and cleaning cupboards. Community skills are activities performed in one's neighborhood. These include shopping, accessing public transportation services, driving, attending school, working, and so forth.

Home and Community Evaluation

To evaluate the accessibility of the patient's postdischarge environment, a visit should be conducted as soon as possible. The home visit is an invaluable tool used to assess home accessibility and safety. The therapist is able to evaluate the capacity of the patients and their families to problem solve.[28] Equipment that will be needed and modifications that will increase independence or decrease the burden of care for the person and/or the family are recommended. This visit is also important in evaluating some of the self-care and home skills practiced during therapy. The evaluation should include the postdischarge community to determine, for example, if the patient will be able to go to the corner store unassisted or is able to verbally direct others when assistance is required.

Vocation and Leisure

Only 11.6% of patients resume work 1 year after injury.[1] The National SCI Database reported the employment rate was higher among patients with paraplegia than among patients with tetraplegia. Twenty years after injury, 35.4% of SCI patients are employed.[1] Rarely is a complete vocational evaluation administered during acute rehabilitation because patients are focused on more immediate challenges.[13,41] Therefore, the focus of the inpatient prevocational program is to gather information, explore vocational options with the patient, and refer patients to appropriate state vocational rehabilitation agencies.[42] Assessment of the patient's basic work skills includes collection of work-related data and physical capabilities, encompassing social, educational, and work history as well as observation of work habits and the ability to follow directions and observe safety rules. Vocational examinations are usually administered as an outpatient service. The vocational evaluations assess the patient's interests and aptitudes, both manually and cognitively. A battery of tests evaluating items such as interests, manual dexterity, mechanical comprehension, functional capacity, and academic knowledge, as well as job samples, are used to assist the therapist in providing the patient and vocational counselors with an assessment of the patient's overall work potential.

Because persons with SCI have a high rate of unemployment and more free time than their nondisabled counterparts, it is important to find past relevant and meaningful activities.[28,41] One study found leisure satisfaction to be the most significant predictor of life satisfaction following an SCI.[43]

Driving Evaluation

In our society, driving is the ultimate form of independence needed to carry out ADLs. According to one study, access to the environment is important in predicating satisfaction with life for a person with an SCI.[44]

A motor vehicle driving assessment, which is occasionally done at the end of the patient's inpatient rehabilitation hospital stay, evaluates the person's ability to drive a vehicle independently and safely. The evaluation, which includes sessions behind the wheel, also provides patients with information regarding adaptive equipment such as hand controls and vehicle modifications.[38]

Goal Setting

Self-management includes goal selection, information collection, decision-making action, and self-reaction.[45] Once the initial evaluation has been completed, the patient in collaboration with the team identifies the short- and long-term goals as well as action plans to practice the goals identified. During the inpatient rehabilitative program, the patient may have difficulty identifying goals because this is a new situation and the patient does not have a frame of reference from prior experience. For example, a patient with T4 ASIA A paraplegia may identify ambulation as a goal during the 3-week inpatient program. The team would acknowledge this goal and then ask questions to elicit other activities the patient identifies as important to learn before going to his or her discharge destination. The team member may identify the functional capabilities associated with key muscles at each segmental level (Appendix 6) to educate the patient on the functional outcomes at different levels of SCI. The therapist will also evaluate the other factors that may limit functional outcomes such as spasticity, inadequate range of motion at key joints, unsupportive social system, or a less-than-optimal living situation to which the patient will be returned. These factors will appear as problems to solve during the rehabilitation program and may carry over to the patient's return to the community. Secondary to the decrease in lengths of stay, patients and families begin learning information and practicing skills that will be necessary for successful outcomes at discharge.

Functional Skills

Transfers

The ability to move from one surface to another is called a transfer. Being able to perform this activity independently greatly increases a person's independence. There are two basic types of active transfers that can be performed: sliding board transfers and depression transfers.

The sliding board transfer is performed by placing a polished wooden or plastic board under the patient to bridge the gap between the surfaces the patient is transferring to and from. The patient then uses the low-friction board to slide from one surface to the other. Assistance in performing this transfer can range from total assistance, as may be required by a person with C4 tetraplegia, to the independent transfer performed by some persons with C6 tetraplegia provided they can place the board and have sufficient trunk balance to perform the maneuver safely.

To perform the depression transfer, the person must be able to lift the buttocks off one surface and shift over to the other surface using the upper extremities. Most paraplegics use this type of transfer. Some patients with tetraplegia are able to perform this more advanced transfer using the muscles of the shoulder girdle in conjunction with locked elbows to achieve the lift needed.

If a person has sufficient upper extremity strength and good trunk balance, transferring to surfaces of widely varying height increases independence. This ability allows people to transfer out of the wheelchair and down to the ground, to ascend and descend stairs in a sitting position, and access a car for easy transportation.

Wheelchair Skills

The person with an SCI achieving the best reintegration into society usually demonstrates the highest level of functional independence. Wheelchair skills are an integral part of this reintegration process. Propelling a wheelchair on a level hospital hallway does not indicate that the person will be able to function in the chair outside the hospital. True rehabilitation is not complete until the person has achieved higher-level wheelchair skills, if physically able. These skills include the ability to propel the chair on uneven surfaces such as grass, gravel, and dirt; safely propel up and down a 10° slope; handle curb cutouts; and perform wheelies, which enable the person to go over small obstacles and up and down curbs without curb cutouts.

Most patients with paraplegia are able to achieve independence in basic skills such as curb cutout and ramps during the inpatient rehabilitative program unless other factors are present. These factors include severe spasticity, obesity, medical complications, inappropriate equipment, or lack of self-confidence from inadequate practice or training. Advanced wheelchair skills are achieved by practicing curbs, sand, and stairs, in the outpatient services or on their own in the community. Persons with higher-level injuries (T2 through T5 and C6 through C8) may be unable to achieve adequate trunk balance in the initial phases of learning but many are able to become proficient in these advanced skills with concentrated practice over a longer period of time. The most difficult advanced skills are transferring from ground to wheelchair and wheelies.

Ambulation

Neuroplasticity after SCI and training is an emerging paradigm shift in rehabilitation and walking recovery. The nervous system is responsive to input and can learn even after injury.[46] Since Barbeau[47] first reported suspending a human over a treadmill to assess feasibility for walking training, clinicians have increasingly adopted the use of a body-weight support system in clinical practice.[46] This approach came from observations by neuroscientists that complete midthoracic spinalized cats could be trained to step with their hindlimbs on a treadmill when trained intensely and repetitively using a suspended sling for trunk support and manual assistance for stepping. Scientists attributed the stepping response to peripheral sensory input processed by the central nervous system.[47] It was demonstrated that specific sensory input associated with locomotion was integrated and interpreted by the spinal cord neural circuitry to generate a coordinated stepping pattern called "central pattern generation".[47] Current research has linked basic science with rehabilitation science to advance the development of effective and science-based rehabilitation for the recovery of walking after neurologic injury.[48,49]

Evidence indicates that people with chronic, incomplete motor SCI may recover or improve walking function after training without associated improvements in ASIA lower extremity motor scores.[48,50]

In the old model, the patient learns to compensate, using other abilities to complete a task or to modify the task or the environment to accomplish the goal.[46,51] Clinical decision making has been guided by expected outcomes based on degree of motor and sensory loss from total to partial. The emerging rehabilitation concepts include recovery based on intense practice of a specific task (locomotion); providing appropriate sensory input (loading and unloading, trunk posture, hip extension, limb kinematics) associated with the locomotor task to tap the intrinsic neural networks generating stepping activity; permissiveness of the training environment (treadmill speed, body-weight support) to enhance practice of the locomotor task; integration of postural control as a corequisite for locomotion; and minimizing compensation (load bearing through legs versus load bearing through arms, hip hiking for swing).[46] In conjunction with providing treatment to enhance recovery of walking, other factors must be considered that may influence such recovery. These factors include muscle weakness and dyscoordination, as well as postural problems related to bearing weight, maintaining balance, and developing propulsion. In addition, problems related to loss of sensory function and hyperactive spinal reflexes may interfere with coordination, balance, and other factors important to walking.[52]

Walking is one of the primary goals of many patients in the initial phases of rehabilitation. If the patient presents in the initial rehabilitation phase with a complete thoracic or higher-level injury, the treatment team must work together with the patient to focus on the body-handling, transfers, and wheelchair skills necessary to maximize independent function. A person presenting with an incomplete lesion and potentially functional lower extremities or a spinal injury of the lumbar or cauda equina region should initiate ambulation training during the initial rehabilitation, and then also continue as an outpatient. The functional needs, motivation, and potential must be evaluated individually in each case.

Within a recovery model, an evaluation is proposed that looks at walking from a different perspective.[53] Walking entails three neural control mechanisms: a reciprocal stepping pattern (for propulsion), balance (upright and dynamic equilibrium), and adaptability (the ability of the individual to respond to the demands of the environment and to meet his or her own behavioral goals). An evaluation of walking should assess each of these elements including subcomponents of each of the elements. This approach would serve as a framework for evaluation and developing outcome measures and treatment planning.[47,52]

The term locomotor training has emerged to describe a physiologically based approach to retraining walking after neurologic injury that capitalizes on the intrinsic mechanisms of the spinal cord to generate stepping in response to specific afferent input associated with the task of walking.[46,54,55]

Use of the body-weight support system and the treadmill may provide a permissive evaluation environment that will allow for assessment of stepping, balance, and adaptability. Walking over ground for people with compromised nervous system function after SCI requires significant neurophysiologic and biomechanical demand to support body weight, to balance, and to generate the necessary forces for walking.[46] The individual walks with an altered pattern overground, compensating for various motor and sensory deficits and using braces and assistive devices. Although walking capacity ultimately must be applied overground, the body-weight support and treadmill environment with manual assistance may provide an alternative means to discern the potential of the nervous system and a viable training environment.[56,57]

In one case study, a man with incomplete SCI at C5-C6 and an ASIA classification of D participated in 45 sessions of locomotor training. Upon completion of the program, his walking speed and independence improved from 0.19 m/s as a home ambulatory using a rolling walker and right AFO to a 1.01 m/s as a full-time ambulator using a cane only for community mobility.

However, a multicenter spinal cord injury locomotor trial compared 12 weeks of step training with body-weight support on a treadmill that included overground practice to a defined but more conventional overground mobility intervention in patients with incomplete traumatic SCI within 8 weeks of onset. The results found no difference in walking outcomes after 12 weeks of the assigned therapy as well as at the planned 6- and 12-month primary outcomes. Independence in walking based on the FIM-L (Functional Independence Measure Locomotor) Score and walking speed was consistently similar at 2-intervals and improved roughly in parallel to increases in lower extremity strength. For patients referred to inpatient rehabilitation who are still graded ASIA B at 4 to 8 weeks after injury, gains in the ability to walk are modest and few achieve functional ambulation. Functional ambulation for those graded ASIA C and D, however, is often achieved by 12 weeks of rehabilitation but less likely to be reached by only 6 weeks of therapy. Patients who are graded ASIA C and ASIA D on admission for rehabilitation are likely to recover the ability to walk at the leisurely velocities used by healthy individuals for the distances needed for community activities by 6 months.[58]

As technology advances, the use of electrical stimulation for ambulation becomes more feasible. Improvements in electrode design, the use of electrodes sewn into lower extremity garments, and compact stimulation units are currently in use. People still find limitations in the functional application of these devices and electrical stimulation is currently not appropriate for all persons with SCI.

While advances in research continue to drive a shift in the paradigm, patients may still choose to use an orthosis in the home and community as a matter of benefit, safety, and clinical judgment.[48]

In the spinal cord-injured population, lower extremity orthoses function as a replacement for totally paralyzed muscles or as an assist for weak muscles. This provides both stability and protection for the joints of the lower extremities. The selection of orthotic components influences the potential for successful ambulation. It is critically important to recognize the high physiologic cost of ambulation with paralysis in comparison to wheelchair propulsion. In a study of persons with paraplegia, the average walking speed was less than half of normal, while oxygen consumption increased 50% and the heart rate was elevated by 28%. In comparison, the same persons tested propelling wheelchairs demonstrated a mean heart rate decrease of 22%, while oxygen consumption per minute decreased 44% and velocity increased by two-thirds.[59]

If the level of injury requires walking with bilateral locked KAFOs and a swing-through gait, it is important to realize what a physically challenging task this is. In the absence of adequate quadriceps strength to stabilize the knee, locked KAFOs or other devices providing knee stability are required. The patient must have the ability to lift and swing the body forward in the swing phase and also maintain balance and lower body stability in the stance phase. Walking using this method is very slow and requires high energy expenditure. Despite slow velocities, oxygen is consumed at a high rate. Many persons choose this method of walking only as a form of exercise, for limited use on special occasions, or to access locations that are inaccessible from a wheelchair.[35]

A trial with temporary braces and preparation time to achieve the specific physical requirements necessary to walk successfully in the locked KAFO is recommended before permanent braces are ordered. The more challenging physical demands include sufficient upper extremity strength to repeatedly lift the entire body, adequate cardiorespiratory endurance, and adequate hamstring range to avoid injury if falling and permit the patient the range to get up from the floor. Patients should train to meet these physical requirements while simultaneously learning the basic skills of transfers to and from bed and wheelchair. The capacity to perform 50 to 100 continuous dips in the parallel bars, to achieve a minimum of 20% of predicted maximum oxygen consumption (VO_2max) on an exercise test, and to achieve full range of motion in all lower extremity joints is recommended for the patient planning to walk with locked KAFOs.

Ambulation with unlocked KAFOs, a combination of a KAFO and an AFO, or bilateral AFOs requires much less of an energy demand. People using bilateral AFOs have energy costs for ambulation approaching near-normal values. This has resulted in higher success rates for independent ambulation in patients requiring this form of bracing. Efficiency studies have demonstrated that wheelchair propulsion is still faster and more efficient than walking with a combination AFO and KAFO. Patients with this need should be encouraged to walk, but many may still prefer to use a chair for long-distance mobility.[35]

Bracing with AFOs is necessary for the patient exhibiting plantar flexor or dorsiflexor weakness. The AFO can provide stability and controlled forward progression in persons with calf weakness. Normal muscle strength in the calf is indicated by the ability to perform 20 continuous unilateral toe raises. This functional muscle test closely replicates the demand placed on the gastrocnemius-soleus complex during ambulation. The calf must function repeatedly to meet a high torque demand with each step of the gait cycle. A muscle grade of less than 4/5 will not provide the endurance needed to maintain stability and controlled forward progression for functional distances.[60] Unpublished data from Rancho Los Amigos Medical Center (1995) have demonstrated that the use of an AFO will not prevent the calf muscles from contracting during ambulation. Therefore, a muscle group with the capacity to gain strength will not be precluded from doing so by use of the brace. Walking function is enhanced, joint stability is maintained, and functional muscle strengthening occurs simultaneously with use of an appropriately adjusted AFO.[10]

Equipment

Items such as wheelchairs, cushions, braces, assistive ambulation devices, and bathing and toilet devices can significantly enhance a patient's function and increase independence. However, not all people view equipment from a positive perspective. Acceptance, use, or abandonment of equipment is a personal choice made by the individual. A clinician can do several things to reduce the likelihood of ordering inappropriate and costly items of equipment that will not be used. An open discussion with the patient and, if appropriate, the caregiver furnishes an opportunity to explore attitudes, uncover fears, and provide education about the pros and cons of specific equipment use. Giving the person an opportunity to use equipment, make choices, and provide feedback during the decision-making phase brings that individual into an active role. The more active the patient is in the identification of benefits, drawbacks, uses, and limitations of equipment, the more likely he or she is to feel comfortable with the ultimate choice.

The members of the rehabilitation team can make recommendations for home, school, or work modifications to improve accessibility. It is helpful for team members involved in decision making to visit the sites with the patient to determine actual needs. It is also important that the patient play an active role in the problem-solving process because he or she will ultimately be the one living with and using the equipment. Clinicians must remain current on the latest technology available and gain an understanding of the patient's individual lifestyle and needs. When necessary and possible, the therapist should make a visit to the home. If this is not possible, a detailed drawing with measurements of doorways and pertinent space, such as the bathroom design showing bathtub, sink, and commode distances, should be made available to the therapist. This is critical to ensure that the equipment will be feasible in the actual home environment.

Wheelchairs

A wheelchair is necessary when full-time walking is not a goal. As a result of technological advances in wheelchair design and wheelchair components, the selection of the most appropriate chair requires knowledge, expertise, and careful study. Wheelchairs vary in price from low-end economy chairs to extremely high-tech, high-priced models. In the era of third-party payment, the therapist must be able to justify the need for the specific chair chosen and its components. The following is a general discussion of the various types of wheelchairs available on the market today.

A manual wheelchair requires the patient to provide the motive power by pushing on the rims of the wheels. If the person does not have good grip strength, the rims can be plastic-coated to increase the friction and substitute for the patient's lack of grip. The type of wheelchair found in general hospitals or pharmacies is inappropriate for most persons with an SCI. It is critical to this population that a chair be lightweight, have a low center of gravity, have maneuverability, and be easily transported in a vehicle. A standard hospital wheelchair may weigh between 45 lb and 55 lb, but the ultralight models can weigh as little as 17 lb. The increase in price to obtain a lightweight chair is justified when potential trauma to the shoulder joint exists from repeated lifting of the wheelchair and full-time propulsion is considered. In addition, the low center of gravity and high maneuverability of these chairs allow the person to handle most architectural barriers with lower energy expenditure than needed in a standard-weight chair.

Power wheelchairs vary from a manual wheelchair with an add-on motor to a computer-operated chair controlled by breath or voice. Due to the need for continued maintenance and parts, a patient must have resources for long-term equipment support. Only the necessary components should be ordered. These include power recline systems that enable the person to obtain ischial pressure relief independently, custom seating systems for maintenance of proper positioning, and environmental control systems that allow independent action in specific surroundings. The most sophisticated and expensive wheelchairs are required by those who are ventilator-dependent. The physical limitations in mobility necessitate intricate power-activation methods such as head, breath, or tongue control switches.

Another consideration in selecting the appropriate wheelchair is the ability of the patient to transport the chair. Some models of power wheelchairs weigh more than 350 lb and are not transported easily without a van and lift or ramp accommodation. Other power models are designed for easier transport, but the patient will require assistance for disassembly, reassembly, loading, and unloading of the chair.

The most important consideration in wheelchair prescription is the functional capability the chair provides. Having a power wheelchair may enable a person with a high-level lesion to return to work. When prescribing a wheelchair, all the factors listed previously—injury level, physical requirements, resources for upkeep, and transportability—must be weighed to provide the patient with the most appropriate wheelchair.

Wheelchair Cushions

Of equal importance to the wheelchair is the wheelchair cushion. Skin breakdown over the ischial tuberosities, coccyx, greater trochanter, or sacrum is a frequent cause of rehospitalization in this population. The proper cushion is an important component in the prevention of this totally preventable and costly complication. A large variety and price range of cushions are available. Materials also vary. Cushions may be made of foam, air, gel, or other substances. They are available off the shelf or can be customized to provide pressure relief.

Capillary occlusion and tissue necrosis result from 13 mm to 34 mm of unrelieved pressure. The cushion should serve to prevent the person from bearing excessive weight on the bony prominences through one of two means: total relief of all contact over the high-risk areas, or dispersion of weight over a wider area via total contact with the buttocks and lower extremities. Worn and ineffective cushions must be replaced on a regular basis. Outpatient services should be provided to maintain proper seating throughout the patient's life span. An individual's needs will vary with functional, health, and age-related changes.

Bathroom Equipment

The first and most important bathroom accessory is the padded commode. If the patient is unable to assist in any aspect of the bowel program, or does not have the trunk balance to sit on a toilet, a commode chair should be considered. Many of the models available commercially can be wheeled directly over the toilet and provide more balance support than a toilet alone. While the bowel program can be performed in bed, the upright position allows gravity to aid in elimination and usually is more aesthetically acceptable to patient and caregiver.

If the patient can transfer to the toilet, a padded raised toilet seat with a side cutout allows access for suppository insertion, digital stimulation, and hygiene. The addition of grab bars or armrests may provide enough stability to carry out toileting functions independently.

A variety of bath benches are available for support of the patient while bathing. The patient's transfer skill and balance determine the specific needs. The benches range from a small seat or chair inside the tub to more elaborate benches that extend outside the tub and provide a cushioned surface for the patient to slide along. The greater the patient's skills, the smaller and simpler the equipment can be.

Grab bars, as mentioned earlier, are useful in most bathrooms near the commode and in the tub. They provide a sturdy handhold for patients who require some additional balance assist.

Orthoses for Ambulation

Lower extremity orthoses provide stability and assistance to those patients for whom walking is a functional goal, and those with lower extremity paralysis or proprioceptive loss.

Orthotic Components

Ankle-Foot Orthosis

The AFO extends from below the fibular head to the foot and is used to control motion and alignment of the ankle and foot. The AFO may be designed with two metal uprights attached to a shoe, as a combination of metal uprights with a custom-molded plastic footplate, or as a molded plastic shell (**Figure 5**).

Knee-Ankle-Foot Orthosis

The KAFO extends from thigh to foot and is used to control the motion and alignment of the knee, ankle, and foot. The KAFO is composed of metal uprights extending to the thigh, a knee joint, and a thigh band. KAFOs are generally fabricated from metal or metal and plastic combinations and either attach to a shoe or a custom-molded polypropylene footplate (**Figure 5**).

Ankle Joint

The ankle joint is a single-axis joint that controls mediolateral motion and dorsiflexion and plantar flexion by means of a stop or an assist. The use of a double-adjustable ankle joint is beneficial to persons with SCI. It provides the ability to adapt the orthosis to meet the changing needs of the patient experiencing neurologic recovery. The following are modifications to the typical double-adjustable ankle joint:

Ankle Stops

Stops limit range of motion to a specific arc or fixed position. Steel dowels and set-screws are placed in the channels of the joint. Placement of the stop in the anterior channel results in limitation of dorsiflexion. Placement in the posterior channel limits plantar flexion.

Ankle Joint Assists

Weak ankle musculature can be supplemented with springs in the channels of the ankle joints. A

FIGURE 5

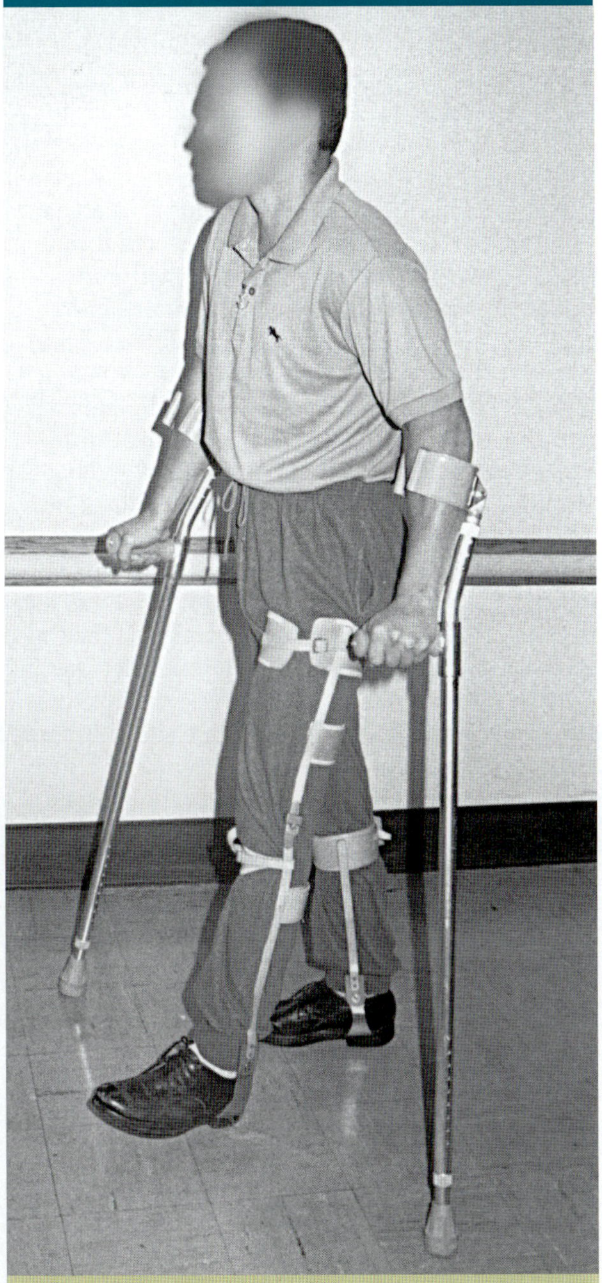

Figure 5 A patient ambulating in a knee-ankle-foot (KAFO)–ankle-foot orthosis combination. When quadriceps strength is fair and/or better, the knee joint of the KAFO is unlocked.

spring placed in the posterior channel allows controlled plantar flexion in loading and assists with dorsiflexion as the foot is unloaded during the start of the swing phase. As a general rule, although exceptions do exist, springs are not placed in anterior channels as they tend to force the foot into plantar flexion.

Knee Joint and Knee Joint Mechanisms

These are generally single-axis joints that either lock into extension or permit full or adjustable joint motion into knee flexion and extension. All knee joints can be unlocked to allow for flexion in sitting. KAFO stance stability is usually achieved through a knee-locking mechanism or offset knee hinges such as the following:

Drop Lock

The drop lock has a ring that drops over the mechanical joint when the knee is extended. The drop ring then maintains a fully extended knee joint until it is lifted manually out of place. This lock can be engaged either by gravity or manually.

Offset Hinge

The axis of the mechanical joint is posterior to the metal uprights. The posterior location of the axis in relation to the ground reaction force encourages extension in stance. This creates a relatively stable knee joint with the ability to flex in the swing phase of gait for clearance.

Free-Motion Knee Joint

This mechanical joint allows free flexion and extension but prevents hyperextension of the knee. Unlike the human knee joint, the mechanical joint has a fixed axis. This precludes the mechanical joint from moving in complete unison with the anatomic knee, which has a changing axis of rotation. Proper placement of the mechanical knee joint by an orthotist is critical to ensure proper alignment with the freely moving knee joint.[61]

Shoe Attachments

Appropriate shoes and their attachments are important orthotic components. A sturdy shoe is a prerequisite to orthoses that attach to the shoe by means of a stirrup. Leather shoes are recommended for the patient with impaired sensation or an altered vasomotor response because they allow for some aeration. The patient must remember to put the shoes on without curling under insensate toes and to check the skin regularly for pressure points.

Stirrups

A spinal injury orthosis is attached to the footwear with a solid steel stirrup riveted directly to the sole of the shoe under the anterior section of the heel. The stirrup, shaped like a U, provides a permanent attachment between the uprights and the shoe. The shank portion of the stirrup then can extend forward to the metatarsal heads of the foot. The extended shank provides a longer and more stable lever arm necessary for a patient walking with bilateral KAFOs. The shank is covered with a 0.5-in–thick covering of appropriate material to prolong wear and provide a nonslip surface for contact with the ground.

Orthotic Variations

Orthoses are undergoing continuous change as research and technology advances.

The reciprocating gait orthosis extends from the thoracic region to the feet. It provides not only support for the lower limbs and trunk, but also assists in reciprocal motions of the lower extremities for walking.[62] The resultant gait is frequently very slow, the orthosis is cumbersome to put on, and the patient frequently requires assistance to come to the standing position if electrical stimulation is not used in conjunction with it. Initial fabrication is expensive and maintenance of the cables is critical.

Modified KAFOs exist that consist of additional components: double uprights, offset knee joints, one posterior thigh band, a hinged anterior leg band, ankle joints with adjustable anterior and posterior pin stops, a cushioned heel, and specially designed footplates embedded in the sole of the shoe. The disadvantages are their weight and appearance.[63]

The hip-knee-ankle-foot orthosis (HKAFO) is similar to the KAFO but with the addition of a pelvic band and hip joints. The hip joints allow single-axis motion for flexion and extension. This orthosis is used more frequently in the pediatric population than with adults because of the considerable amount of support necessary to remain upright.

Special Populations and Procedures

Tendon Transfer Surgery for Improved Upper Extremity Function After Cervical Spine Injury

Upper extremity reconstructive surgery is considered for selected patients when maximum muscle return has occurred, generally no earlier than 1 year after injury because some of these procedures permanently alter the musculoskeletal structure and the biomechanics of the upper extremities. The goal of surgery is to improve functional use of the upper extremities for ADLs. Reconstructive surgery will not provide for a normal hand but rather restore pinch and grasp. The most common tendon transfers include transfer of the brachioradialis to the flexor pollicis longus, and of the posterior deltoid to the triceps. Less common procedures are transfer of the brachioradialis to the extensor carpi radialis brevis and rerouting of the biceps to allow pronation with elbow flexion.[64]

Transfer of the brachioradialis to the flexor pollicis longus allows patients with C6 and C7 tetraplegia to perform active lateral pinch.[65] The goal of the posterior deltoid-to-triceps transfer is to provide the patient with C6 tetraplegia with functional elbow extension, enabling him or her to reach for objects, and, if performed bilaterally, to assist with wheelchair transfers. These two surgeries are frequently combined to allow the patient to contract muscles at or around the elbow during functional hand use (lateral prehension).[60] This shortens the time of postoperative rehabilitation. The purpose of the brachioradialis-to-extensor carpi radialis brevis transfer is to augment wrist extension, enabling the patient with C5 tetraplegia to manipulate objects through tenodesis function.

To ensure the success of tendon transfer operations, a thorough evaluation is performed before surgery. In addition to the routine evaluation mentioned earlier, emphasis is placed on careful analysis of hand function with the aid of the Jebsen hand test.[66] An in-depth interview and discussion is aimed at identifying specific functional goals. Patient goals must be consistent with postoperative functional expectations, and the patient must have a clear understanding of the limitations of reconstructive surgery. The patient must understand the postoperative course, its duration, and the functional limitations imposed following surgery. He or she must have the resources to provide for additional assistance and transportation during the postoperative period.

Following surgery, the patient is discharged home with an arm cast. Four weeks postoperatively, an intensive inpatient or outpatient occupational therapy program is begun. Therapy includes positional and protective splinting, active and gentle passive range-of-motion exercises, reeducation of the transferred tendon through isometric and active exercise, biofeedback, neuromuscular electrical stimulation, and therapeutic activities.[64] Functional training begins with light therapeutic activities that require minimal prehensile force. Demand is gradually increased. Resumption of daily routines must be gradual to protect the transferred tendons from overstretching. At completion of the intensive 2- to 4-week occupational therapy program, the patient follows through with a detailed home exercise and activity program.

Progress is routinely monitored in the outpatient clinic.

Patients With Children

Child care poses unique challenges to the parent with SCI, especially if the care involves a baby or a toddler. After initial practice with a doll, training must involve the child. With practice, it has been demonstrated that the child, too, adapts to the new situation and assists the parent in his or her activities. Establishing a safe way to be carried on the parent's lap and climbing up to a higher surface to be picked up or diapered, are ways in which the child can be trained to assist the parent. People with SCI can benefit from books and videotapes concerning child rearing created specifically for the disabled population.

Transition to Home and the Community

To complete the transition from hospital to community, community living skills training is essential. Community outings provide an opportunity to enable the patient to begin finding ways to manage in the community from the wheelchair. These outings may include taking a bus, shopping, and dining out. As with home skills, emphasis is placed on thorough planning before the activity. Group discussions serve to educate patients about community resources and their rights to services.

Another crucial element in achieving independence is engaging in meaningful work. Following an in-depth evaluation of the patient's vocational interests, aptitudes, and physical abilities, the patient is encouraged to try out different vocational activities in a simulated work environment. Worksite evaluation may help prepare the patient to return to a previous job. Prevocational and vocational counselors assist in the process of vocational evaluation and continue training the patient after discharge from the hospital.

Avocational activities must also be explored to provide the patient with meaningful leisure time. This is especially important with the older patient who is forced to retire and is suddenly left with many hours of unstructured time.

As with other ADLs, driving training of patients with paraplegia requires less instruction than with patients with tetraplegia. Driving training must include behind-the-wheel practice sessions with hand controls and instruction in transferring the wheelchair in and out of the car. As with other activities, safety is the primary concern. Spasm patterns and spasticity are evaluated and the patient is alerted to the special considerations that must be attended to while driving.

Treatment of Patients with Spinal Cord and Mild Head Injuries

Approximately 40% of all SCIs are coupled with loss of consciousness.[67] Mild head injuries often go undetected because attention at the acute hospital is placed on emergency medical management, and cognitive deficits may be subtle. All new patients who have a history suggestive of possible head trauma, such as a period of unconsciousness following the injury, or who have exhibited cognitive deficits should be evaluated by a communication disorders specialist. If needed, these patients receive cognitive therapy as part of their rehabilitation process. The role of the occupational therapist is to evaluate and treat perceptual deficits as well as to guide the patient in ADLs, with emphasis on those cognitive areas that require special considerations.

Perceptual deficits are dysfunctions in the process of recognition and interpretation of sensory stimuli. Disturbances in the perception of spatial relations, body scheme, recognition of objects (gnosis), and motor planning (praxis) may interfere with the patient's ability to function. Treatment of these dysfunctions is approached with compensatory education, including the patient's understanding of the deficits, modifying the environment to simplify tasks, and experiential learning. Emphasis is placed on safety precautions in performing ADLs.

Often, spinal cord-injured patients with severe head injuries are treated on a brain injury ward. Only patients with minimal cognitive deficits are treated by the spinal injury service staff. Cognitive deficits are treated collaboratively by the team to provide a structured and predictable environment.

One of the roles of the communication disorders specialist is to guide the team, defining the most suitable approach to meet the individual patient's needs. These needs may include providing the patient with a noise-free treatment area to avoid distractions, simplifying tasks, or repeating instructions to facilitate memory retention.

Treatment of Children With Spinal Cord Injury

The treatment of children with SCI focuses on their developmental stage so as to plan appropriate treatment, provide for an appropriate physical, social, and emotional context for dealing with the losses from their injury, and gain their fullest cooperation and involvement in the process of rehabilitation.

Evaluation

In addition to the evaluations outlined earlier for the adult with SCI, children must be assessed within a developmental framework. An interview with the parents or primary caregivers provides information about the preonset occupational behavior of the child in the areas of self-care, play, school, home, and community skills.

Developmental tests are used to determine the age level at which the child is presently functioning. These results not only determine the goals according to age-appropriate expectations but guide the treatment process as well. In addition, they may reveal cognitive deficits that had not previously been noted in the child with combined SCI and brain injury. The Gesell developmental schedule for children 4 weeks to 6 years old is most commonly used.[68]

Another developmental assessment tool used to assess hand function in children is the Bruininks-Oseretsky test of motor proficiency.[69] This allows the therapist to compare scores with norms for ages 4 to 14 years on such tasks as visuomotor control, upper limb speed, and dexterity.

Perception is another area that requires specific testing with performance norms based on age. There are several instruments available to test perception, some of which cover as broad an age range as 2 to 15 years. There are nonmotor tests of visual perception that may be used for the child with tetraplegia.

Goal Setting

While the adult with SCI collaborates with the therapist to set goals, in pediatrics it is often the family or caregiver who is more involved in this process, depending on the age of the child. The youngster's former level of independence in various ADLs is a good framework from which to start, with progress guided by principles of normal development. For children without cognitive deficits, the goals are usually set to reestablish preexisting skills or to learn compensatory or adaptive techniques wherever possible. For those children with concomitant brain injuries who now function at a lower age level than premorbidly, goals are projected based on their current level of developmental performance rather than age-appropriate expectations.

Special Considerations

There are numerous special considerations in the treatment of the child with SCI. Key principles of normal development guide the selection of activities and various factors are weighted differently at different stages. Issues that are vital for the infant, such as sensorimotor experiences and exploratory behavior, change as the transition is made to the toddler who begins to acquire self-care skills and more actively manipulates objects in the environment. The need to master increasingly complex self-care, play, and academic skills is important for the preschool and school-age child. Issues that face the adolescent include school, prevocational, home, and community skills. All of this must be viewed within the sociocultural context of the individual and in light of where the child was on the continuum of development at the time of the injury.

Although the longer length of the extremities of some adults may interfere with their self-care, the immature extremities of children may pose problems for them. In growing children whose skeletal growth is not yet mature, the use of thoracolumbosacral orthoses to reduce the development of spinal deformities is common and affects self-care performance. Some children who are able to master basic dressing skills continue to require assistance only to don the body jacket.

Play is a critical area of occupational behavior and assisting the child to reestablish a repertoire of age-appropriate play activities is an important goal. Special attention needs to be given to play activities that the child with SCI can easily engage in with able-bodied peers to avert a tendency toward solitary play and isolation. Yasukawa writes: "Children will pass through several stages of play: sensorimotor play, symbolic play, and play with rules. At each stage, the child with SCI may require special adaptations and an atmosphere conducive to development and learning."[70]

Moreover, purposeful play is used as treatment to provide the child with fun, challenging, and successful experiences. Many of the traditional treatment techniques used for adults, such as progressive resistive exercises, cannot be used with children, and therapists must find creative ways to use or adapt play activities to meet these treatment needs.

With the advent of Public Law 94-142, which mandates that education be provided in the "least restrictive environment," many children in wheelchairs who were formerly assigned to segregated special education classrooms now have access to their preinjury classes. Just as work-site evaluations are required for the adult, school sites must also be assessed with the goal of determining workstations in the child's classroom. Training is required of teachers and classroom aides, especially for children with tetraplegia who may need a very specific set-up of their equipment to function at school. Classmates may also benefit from a session with the therapist to reintegrate the child back into an environment that has had no previous experience with persons in wheelchairs.

The home and community skills of the pediatric population vary widely with age, sex, cultural norms, and family expectations. The goals and treatment must be tailored specifically to the individual child and family to enable them to resume their former roles in these areas.

The treatment of perceptual dysfunction in the adult with SCI with brain injury is approached with compensatory education. Since perceptual processes are founded on a basis of normal sensorimotor experiences, which become denied or altered in the child with SCI (with or without brain injury), consideration must be given to providing those experiences in treatment to promote the ongoing maturation of perception in the younger child.

Children as Outpatients

Much of the education and training that is provided to the adult with a focus on self-responsibility is provided to the family or caregiver of the child who is not yet old enough for such responsibility. It is particularly critical that children receive routine follow-up as outpatients to keep pace with the many changes that result from physical growth and developmental maturation. Ongoing therapy on an outpatient basis is indicated to address the child's changing needs.

Aging With a Spinal Cord Injury

The percentage of persons older than 60 years of age at injury has increased substantially since 1980.[1] As the life expectancy for individuals living with an SCI continues to increase, physical therapy will need to establish services that address the needs of the physical, personal, and environmental factors that are specific to this patient population.

Cardiopulmonary Systems

The current leading causes of death after SCI for persons surviving at least 1 year after injury are respiratory complications: pneumonia, septicemia, and pulmonary emboli.[1] Morbidity and mortality in persons with an SCI are related to the neurologic level of the SCI. Patients with tetraplegia and high paraplegia have the greatest risk due to paralysis of intercostal and abdominal muscles resulting in a decreased cough function. Diaphragm weakness or paralysis also occurs with higher-level lesions. Other conditions that have a negative impact on respiratory function include spinal deformity with its increased risk of pulmonary infections. Age-associated changes increase respiratory system risk as well. These include the natural decrease in lung compliance or elasticity and the decreasing vital capacity with age.[26,71]

The rate of cardiovascular disease in people with SCI has been reported as high as 228% of the rate of the able-bodied population. Additionally, cardiovascular disease is occurring at an earlier age in people with SCIs.[72] The SCI population is susceptible to all known risk factors associated with cardiovascular disease, worsened by (1) a potential for progressive inactivity leading to deconditioning, (2) continued high rates of smoking, (3) susceptibility to hypertension and hypotension, (4) evidence of elevated cholesterol levels, and (5) the potential for a progressive increase in the total body mass with a decreasing lean body or muscle mass.

Musculoskeletal Dysfunction

As people age with SCI, an increased susceptibility to musculoskeletal dysfunction has been reported. This may be a result of increased or abnormal stress placed on the upper extremities while engaging in wheelchair propulsion and transfers, an increased need to engage in overhead activities because of seating height, and in some situations prolonged crutch-walking.[73] Data from a large population of patients averaging 12 years postinjury demonstrated a 55% incidence of upper extremity pain in subjects with tetraplegia, with the shoulder being the primary location. In subjects with paraplegia, 64% had upper extremity pain. The most common site was the wrist, presenting with carpal tunnel symptoms.[67]

Potential causes of the high incidence of upper extremity pain may relate to overuse, underuse, or less than optimal biomechanical use of the arms. For example, increased stress may occur in joints not anatomically suited for a particular activity. Also, the increased life expectancy of people with SCIs results in greater time to accumulate stress and for clinicians to track it. The high incidence of upper extremity pain may also be the result of a musculoskeletal system that is undergoing normal aging changes and poor biomechanics over a long period of time, resulting in muscle strength and flexibility imbalances.[74]

These issues reinforce the need to focus the rehabilitative programs at every phase with a long-term perspective. Tailoring programs to meet specific needs aids in identification of individual areas of vulnerability early in rehabilitation. Clinicians must be educators of patients, family members, and caregivers. Educational interventions should focus on creating lasting knowledge and behavior that encourages and promotes the patient as a lifelong manager of his or her own health, wellness, and learning. The preliminary results of the Strengthening Optimal Movement Performance study conducted by the pathokinesiology laboratory at Rancho Los Amigos National Rehabilitation Center indicate that persons with paraplegia (from a chronic SCI) and shoulder pain, who received a standardized and individualized protocol for the shoulder that included strengthening for hypertrophy and endurance and stretching exercises, had statistically significantly less pain than those who received only education as a control. The patients also reported improved physical function, community activity and quality of life.[75]

Activity for Health

Physical activity and exercise convey substantial benefits for health, fitness, and function in all segments of the population, including people with SCI. Increased physical activity can positively affect several cardiovascular risk factors in people with SCI.[9] Links have been identified between activity and physiologic factors. A study of persons with paraplegia found those who were employed to be lighter in weight, leaner, and to possess greater aerobic power than their unemployed counterparts.[76] Short bouts of moderate-intensity activity scattered throughout the day may be sufficient to confer a positive health benefit in the prevention and risk reduction of inactivity-related diseases.

In the area of musculoskeletal dysfunction, therapists can have a substantial impact. Detailed evaluation of an individual with an SCI provides insight into muscle imbalances, joint restrictions, and musculotendinous tightness. The biomechanical analysis of activity performance conducted by clinicians can clearly reveal areas of current vulnerability or potential for future problems. Task analysis provides insight into specific issues such as the muscle energy system used, the type of muscle contraction required, and the position necessary for the function.

Therapy programs should then be tailored to address these issues with patients to target prevention or resolution. A specific strengthening or stretching program to restore muscle strength balance around joints may be possible. Other injuries or conditions existing in conjunction with the SCI have to be factored in to that lifetime equation. Changes in spasticity and the development of heterotopic ossification, spinal deformity, or pressure ulcers are conditions that may occur over a lifetime. Also, preexisting conditions such as diabetes and other health-related concerns must be taken into consideration when focusing on the development of a program for the lifetime of the patient.

Psychological Intervention

Psychological intervention plays an important role in addressing the various issues related to the complicated process of recovery and adjustment.

SCI results in many changes in the individual's life that he or she is forced to deal with. There are changes in social status as the individual instantly becomes a member of a minority that has a generally socially devalued role and one in which he or she is seen as less desirable and less capable. Socioeconomic status and interpersonal relationships may be dramatically altered. The inability to perform certain functions affects the individual's vocational, social, and familial roles. Being unable to carry out job-related tasks may result in economic dependence, and places pressure on other family members to alter their roles. Friendships and family relationships often suffer from the stress and may deteriorate or completely dissolve.

Rehabilitation occurs while the patient is undergoing an extremely complex and individualized process of adjustment and adaptation. The patient is learning how to maintain health and avoid medical complications and is adjusting to changed roles in the family, job, and community.[77] Intervention may begin with assessment of premorbid personality characteristics, and emotional, social, and occupational functioning. As lengths of stay decrease, identification and treatment of patients with depression is essential to maximizing the participation of the patient throughout the rehabilitation process. Furthermore, many of the patients may be discharged home depressed and may require outpatient psychological services. The rehabilitation team needs to have an understanding of the total process the patient is going through. One way of viewing the adjustment process is analogous to the stages of grieving: denial, anger, bargaining, depression, and acceptance, as put forth by Kübler-Ross.[78] Patients think, feel, and act in ways that function to reduce the pain they are experiencing. No "stages" theory purports an ordered passage through each stage. The utility of such theories is in generating an understanding and sensitivity to the individual responses in a way that facilitates positive growth. The stages of grieving apply to the rehabilitation process in the way they manifest in corresponding physical aspects of rehabilitation. The stage of denial broadly relates to the period of acute care and early rehabilitation when there is a greater need for total care. As the patient begins to relearn basic ADLs and attempts to establish control, anger becomes the predominant emotion. Bargaining may replace or accompany anger as progress in the treatment program begins to slow down. When the reality of the situation is more fully appreciated by the patient, generally accompanied by a plateau in the rehabilitation program, depression is the predominant response. Acceptance, in this theory, is the final stage, when the individual experiences a renewed growth in abilities.

During the course of rehabilitation, it is important for the team to be provided with a forum in which to address patient behaviors that may interfere with progress in the treatment program. Increased levels of depression, decreased frustration tolerance, a premorbid drug and alcohol abuse history, control issues, and so forth, may all produce behaviors that prevent the patient from maximum participation in the program. The patient and family along with the team need to identify the optimal strategies that facilitate learning and participation in the rehabilitative program. As an example, a patient with paraplegia normally is in rehabilitation for 21 days; however, in one case the patient has his own business and a young child at home and wants to be discharged in 1 week. The patient and interdisciplinary team must work together to ensure all education is completed and basic skills are learned. It is determined that the program can be completed in 10 days, which is acceptable to both the patient and the team to facilitate a safe discharge home.

The area of sexual function or dysfunction is of prime concern to this patient population. The psychologist plays an important role in addressing the area of sexuality. Sexual function is managed in the same fashion as other areas of functioning in an attempt to establish a pattern of life as close to that of premorbid functioning as possible. A formal sexual function program has two components: an educational group series designed to address the issues at a general level, and an individual sexual function evaluation designed to address individual specific sexual function issues with a physician and the psychologist present. The program provides an opportunity to address the areas of sexual dysfunction, alternative behaviors, precautions, and other areas related to sexual counseling.

References

1. *Spinal Cord Injury Facts and Figures at a Glance*. Birmingham, AL, National Spinal Cord Injury Statistical Center, 2010. Available at https://www.nscisc.uab.edu/public_content/pdf/Facts%20and%20Figures%20at%20a%20Glance%202010.pdf. Accessed August 13, 2010.
2. Forchheimer M, Tate DG: Enhancing community re-integration following spinal cord injury. *NeruoRehabilitation* 2004;19(2):103-113.
3. Fiedler IG, Laud PW, Maiman DJ, Apple DF: Economics of managed care in spinal cord injury. *Arch Phys Med Rehabil* 1999;80(11):1441-1449.
4. Dijkers MP: Community integration: Conceptual issues and measurement approaches in rehabilitation research. *Topics in Spinal Cord Injury Rehabilitation: Community Reintegration* 1998;4(Part I): 1-16.
5. Tate DG: Forward: Community reintegration . *Topics in Spinal Cord Injury Rehabilitation: Community Reintegration* 1998;4(Part I):vi-vii.
6. Kendall MB, Ungerer G, Dorsett P: Bridging the gap: Transitional rehabilitation services for people with spinal cord injury. *Disabil Rehabil* 2003; 25(17):1008-1015.
7. Bodenheimer T, MacGregor K, Sharifi C: *Helping Patients Manage Their Chronic Conditions*. Oakland, CA, California HealthCare Foundation. June 2005. Available at http://www.chcf.org/publications/2005/06/helping-patients-manage-their-chronic-conditions.
8. Oaks DD, Wilmot CB, Hall KM, Sherek JP: Benefit of early admission to a comprehensive trauma center for patients with spinal cord injury. *Arch Phys Med Rehabil* 1990;71(9):637-643.
9. Waters RL, Adkins RH: The musculoskeletal system, in Whiteneck G, ed: *Aging with Spinal Cord Injury*. New York, NY, Demos, 1993, pp 53-71.
10. Perry J: Spinal cord injury reciprocal gait, in Perry J, ed: *Gait Analysis: Normal and Pathologic Function*. Thorofare, NJ, Slack, 1992, p 463.
11. Atkins MS: A descriptive study: *The Occupational Therapy Predischarge Home Visit Program for Spinal Cord Injured Adults*. Los Angeles, CA, University of Southern California, 1989. Thesis.
12. Twaddle AC: The concepts of the sick role and illness behavior. *Adv Psychosom Med* 1972;8: 162-179.
13. *Spinal Cord Injury Information Network*, at http://www.spinalcord.uab.edu/show.asp?durki=21392. Accessed August 25, 2010.
14. *Guide for the Physical Therapy Bulbar Evaluation*. Downey, CA, Rancho Los Amigos Medical Center Physical Therapy Department, 1989.

15. Zigler J, Capen D: Management of unstable cervical spine injuries. *Complications Orthop* 1989; July/Aug:124-128.

16. Capen DA, Gordon ML, Zigler JE, Garland DE, Nelson RW, Nagelberg S: Nonoperative management of upper thoracic spine fractures. *Orthop Rev* 1994;23(10):818-821.

17. Capen D, Zigler J, Garland D: Surgical stabilization in cervical spine trauma. *Contemp Orthop* 1987;14:25-32.

18. Capen DA, Garland DE, Waters RL: Surgical stabilization of the cervical spine: A comparative analysis of anterior and posterior spine fusions. *Clin Orthop Relat Res* 1985;196:229-237.

19. Zigler J, Rockowitz N, Capen D, Nelson R, Waters R: Posterior cervical fusion with local anesthesia. The awake patient as the ultimate spinal cord monitor. *Spine (Phila Pa 1976)* 1987;12(3): 206-208.

20. Rimoldi RL, Zigler JE, Capen DA, Hu SS: The effect of surgical intervention on rehabilitation time in patients with thoracolumbar and lumbar spinal cord injuries. *Spine (Phila Pa 1976)* 1992; 17(12):1443-1449.

21. Waters RL, Adkins RH, Yakura JS, Sie I: Motor and sensory recovery following incomplete paraplegia. *Arch Phys Med Rehabil* 1994;75(1):67-72.

22. Rieser T, Mudiyam R, Waters R: Orthopedic evaluation of spinal cord injury and management of vertebral fractures, in Adkins HV, ed: *Spinal Cord Injury*. New York, NY, Churchill Livingston, 1985.

23. Waters RL, Adkins RH, Yakura JS, Sie I: Motor and sensory recovery following incomplete tetraplegia. *Arch Phys Med Rehabil* 1994;75(3): 306-311.

24. Wetzel J: Respiratory evaluation and treatment, in Adkins RH, ed: *Spinal Cord Injury*. New York, NY, Churchill Livingstone, 1985.

25. Carlson B: Normal chest excursion. *Phys Ther* 1973;53(1):10-14.

26. Wilmot CB, Hall KM: The respiratory system, in Whiteneck G, ed: *Aging with Spinal Cord Injury*. New York, NY, Demos, 1993, pp 93-104.

27. Alvarez SE, Peterson M, Lunsford BR: Respiratory treatment of the adult patient with spinal cord injury. *Phys Ther* 1981;61(12):1737-1745.

28. Atkins M, Clark D, Waters R: Upper limb orthoses, in Lin V, ed: *Spinal Cord Medicine: Principles and Practice*. New York, NY, Demos Medical Publishing, 2003, pp 663-674.

29. Gersham GE, Labi MI, Dittmar SS, et al: The Quadraplegia Index of Function (QIF): Sensitivity and reliability demonstrated in a study of thirty quadriplegia patients. *Paraplegia* 1986;24(1): 38-44.

30. Yarkony GM, Roth EJ, Heinemann AW, Wu YC, Katz RT, Lovell L: Benefits of rehabilitation for traumatic spinal cord injury: Multivariate analysis in 711 patients. *Arch Neurol* 1987;44(1):93-96.

31. Consortium for Spinal Cord Medicine: *Outcomes Following Traumatic Spinal Cord Injury: Clinical Practice Guidelines for Health-Care Professionals*. Washington, DC, Paralyzed Veterans of America, 1999. Available at http://www.pva.org/site/DocServer/OUT.pdf?docID=686. Accessed October 6, 2010.

32. Dail C, Rodgers GM, Adkins H: *Glossopharyngeal Breathing*. Downey, CA, Professional Staff Association of Rancho Los Amigos Medical Center, 1979.

33. Atkins M: Spinal cord injury, in Trombly C, Vining Radomsky M, eds: *Occupational Therapy for Physical Dysfunction*, ed 5. Philadelphia, PA, Lippincott Williams & Wilkins, 2002, pp 965-999.

34. O'Leary S: *Computer Bits '95: Computer Access for Persons with Spinal Cord Injury*. Palo Alto, CA, Bay Area and Western Chapter, Paralyzed Veterans of America, 1995.

35. Waters RL: Energy expenditure, in Perry J, ed: *Gait Analysis: Normal and Pathologic Function*. Thorofare, NJ, Slack, 1992, p 464.

36. Benton LA, Baker L, Bowman BR, et al : *Functional Electric Stimulation—A Practical Clinical Guide*. Downey, CA, Professional Staff Association of Rancho Los Amigos Medical Center, 1981.

37. Hill JP: *Spinal Cord Injury: A Guide to Functional Outcome in Occupational Therapy*. Rockville, MD, Aspen, 1986.

38. Gowland C, Simoes N: *A Driver Training Program for Persons with Physical Disabilities*, ed 2. Downey, CA, Professional Staff Association of Rancho Los Amigos Medical Center, 1984.

39. Garland DE, Lilling M, Keenan MA: Percutaneous phenol blocks to motor points or spastic forearm muscles in head-injured adults. *Arch Phys Med Rehabil* 1984;68(5):243-245.

40. Garber SL, Gregorio TL: Upper extremity assistive devices: Assessment of use by spinal cord-injured patients with quadriplegia. *Am J Occup Ther* 1990; 44(2):126-131.

41. Yerxa EJ, Locker SB: Quality of time use by adults with spinal cord injuries. *Am J Occup Ther* 1990; 44(4):318-326.

42. Alfred WG, Fuhrer MJ, Rossi CD: Vocational development following severe spinal cord injury: A longitudinal study. *Arch Phys Med Rehabil* 1987; 68(12):854-857.

43. Coyle CP, Lesnik-Emas S, Kinney WB: Predicting life satisfaction among adults with spinal cord injuries. *Rehabil Psychol* 1994;39:95-111.

44. Richards JS, Bombardier CH, Tate D, et al: Access to the environment and life satisfaction after spi-

nal cord injury. *Arch Phys Med Rehabil* 1999; 80(11):1501-1506.

45. Jones F: Strategies to enhance chronic disease self-management: How can we apply this to stroke? *Disabil Rehabil* 2006;28(13-14):841-847.
46. Behrman AL, Bowden MG, Nair PM: Neuroplasticity after spinal cord injury and training: An emerging paradigm shift in rehabilitation and walking recovery. *Phys Ther* 2006;86(10): 1406-1425.
47. Barbeau H: Locomotor training in neurorehabilitation: Emerging rehabilitation concepts. *Neurorehabil Neural Repair* 2003;17(1):3-11.
48. Behrman AL, Lawless-Dixon AR, Davis SB, et al: Locomotor training progression and outcomes after incomplete spinal cord injury. *Phys Ther* 2005;85(12):1356-1371.
49. Edgerton VR, Roy RR, Hodgson JA, Prober RJ, de Guzman CP, de Leon R: A physiological basis for the development of rehabilitative strategies for spinally injured patients. *J Am Paraplegia Soc* 1991;14(4):150-157.
50. Behrman AL, Harkema SJ: Locomotor training after human spinal cord injury: A series of case studies. *Phys Ther* 2000;80(7):688-700.
51. American Physical Therapy Association: Guide to Physical Therapist Practice: Second edition. American Physical Therapy Association. *Phys Ther* 2001;81(1):9-746.
52. Barbeau H, Ladouceur M, Norman KE, Pépin A, Leroux A: Walking after spinal cord injury: Evaluation, treatment, and functional recovery. *Arch Phys Med Rehabil* 1999;80(2):225-235.
53. Ladouceur M, Pépin A, Norman KE, Barbeau H: Recovery of walking after spinal cord injury. *Adv Neurol* 1997;72:249-255.
54. Barbeau H, Visintin M: Optimal outcomes obtained with body-weight support combined with treadmill training in stroke subjects. *Arch Phys Med Rehabil* 2003;84(10):1458-1465.
55. Wernig A, Müller S, Nanassy A, Cagol E: Laufband therapy based on 'rules of spinal locomotion' is effective in spinal cord injured persons. *Eur J Neurosci* 1995;7(4):823-829.
56. Edgerton VR, Leon RD, Harkema SJ, et al: Retraining the injured spinal cord. *J Physiol* 2001; 533(Pt 1):15-22.
57. Visintin M, Barbeau H: The effects of parallel bars, body weight support and speed on the modulation of the locomotor pattern of spastic paretic gait: A preliminary communication. *Paraplegia* 1994;32(8):540-553.
58. Dobkin B, Barbeau H, Deforge D, et al: The evolution of walking-related outcomes over the first 12 weeks of rehabilitation for incomplete traumatic spinal cord injury: The multicenter randomized Spinal Cord Injury Locomotor Trial. *Neurorehabil Neural Repair* 2007;21(1):25-35.
59. Cerny D, Waters R, Hislop H, Perry J: Walking and wheelchair energetics in persons with paraplegia. *Phys Ther* 1980;60(9):1133-1139.
60. Paul SD, Gellman H, Waters R, Willstein G, Tognella M: Single-stage reconstruction of key pinch and extension of the elbow in tetraplegic patients. *J Bone Joint Surg Am* 1994;76(10):1451-1456.
61. *Lower-Limb Orthotics*. New York, NY, New York University Medical Center Post-Graduate Medical School of Prosthetics and Orthotics, 1986.
62. Fishman S, Berger N, Edelstein JE, Springer WP: Lower-limb orthoses, in Bunch WH, ed: *Atlas of Orthotics: Biomechanical Principles and Application*. St Louis, MO, Mosby–Year Book, 1985.
63. Roemer M: *An Introduction to the US Health Care System*. New York, NY, Springer-Verlag, 1982.
64. Green BA, Callahan RA, Klose KJ, de la Torre J: Acute spinal cord injury: Current concepts. *Clin Orthop Relat Res* 1981;154:125-135.
65. Waters R, Moore KR, Graboff SR, Paris K: Brachioradialis to flexor pollicis longus tendon transfer for active lateral pinch in the tetraplegic. *J Hand Surg Am* 1985;10(3):385-391.
66. Hentz VR, House J, McDowell C, Moberg E: Rehabilitation and surgical reconstruction of the upper limb in the tetraplegia: An update. *J Hand Surg Am* 1992;17(5):964-967.
67. Sie IH, Waters RL, Adkins RH, Gellman H: Upper extremity pain in the postrehabilitation spinal cord injured patient. *Arch Phys Med Rehabil* 1992; 73(1):44-48.
68. Gesell A: *Developmental Diagnosis: Normal and Abnormal Child Development, Clinical Methods and Pediatric Application*. Hagerstown, MD, Harper & Row, 1969.
69. Bruininks RH: *Bruininks-Oseretsky Test of Motor Proficiency Examiner's Manual*. Circle Pines, MN, American Guidance Service, 1978.
70. Yasukawa A: Spinal cord injury, in Hill JP, ed: *A Guide to Functional Outcomes in Occupational Therapy*. Rockville, MD, Aspen, 1986.
71. DeVivo MJ, Stover SL: Long-term survival and causes of death, in Stover SL, Dehisa JA, Whiteneck G, eds: *Spinal Cord Injury: Clinical Outcomes from the Model Systems*. Gaithersburg, MD, Aspen, 1995, pp 289-316.
72. Le CT, Price M: Survival from spinal cord injury. *J Chronic Dis* 1982;35(6):487-492.
73. Hooker SP, Wells CL: Aerobic power of competitive paraplegic road racers. *Paraplegia* 1992;30(6): 428-436.
74. Lewthwaite R, Thompson L, Boyd LA, et al: Reconceptualizing physical therapy for spinal injury

rehabilitation: Physical activity for long-term health and function, in *Infusions: Research into Practice*. Downey, CA, Center for Research in Clinical Biokinesiology, Physical Therapy Department, Rancho Los Amigos Medical Center, 1994, pp 1-9.

75. Mulroy SJ, Thompson L, Kemp B, et al: Strengthening and optimal movements for painful shoulders (STOMPS) in chronic spinal cord injury: A randomized, controlled trial. *Phys Ther* 2011; 91(3):305-324.

76. Noreau L, Shephard RJ: Return to work after spinal cord injury: The potential contribution of physical fitness. *Paraplegia* 1992;30(8):563-572.

77. Thompson NJ, Coker J, Krause JS, Henry E: Purpose in life as a mediator of adjustment after spinal cord injury. *Rehabil Psychol* 2003;48(2):100-108.

78. Kübler-Ross E: *On Death and Dying*. London, United Kingdom, Routledge, 1973.

Appendix 1 Standard Neurological Classification of Spinal Cord Injury

A, The American Spinal Injury Association (ASIA) neurologic classification of SCI form is composed of several sections. The initial portion grades five muscle groups in the upper extremities and five muscle groups in the lower extremities on a score of 1 to 5. A composite motor score is then obtained. The next section grades light touch and pin prick. The final section on the first page of the form specifies the level of injury. B, Functional independence is compared at admission and discharge. Finally, an impairment scale is specified from A to E and a clinical spinal syndrome is identified, if present.

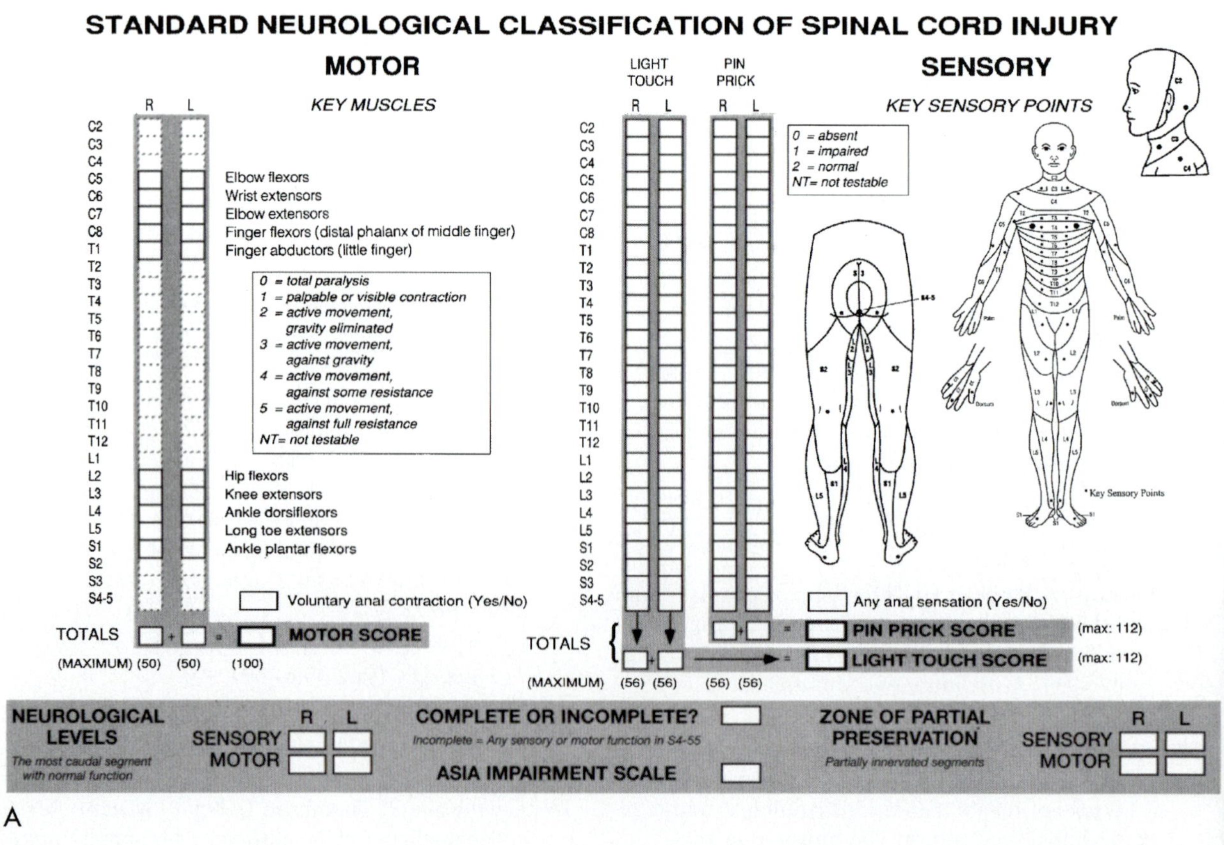

STANDARD NEUROLOGICAL CLASSIFICATION OF SPINAL CORD INJURY

MOTOR — KEY MUSCLES (R, L)

C2, C3, C4
C5 Elbow flexors
C6 Wrist extensors
C7 Elbow extensors
C8 Finger flexors (distal phalanx of middle finger)
T1 Finger abductors (little finger)
T2–T12, L1
L2 Hip flexors
L3 Knee extensors
L4 Ankle dorsiflexors
L5 Long toe extensors
S1 Ankle plantar flexors
S2, S3
S4-5 Voluntary anal contraction (Yes/No)

0 = total paralysis
1 = palpable or visible contraction
2 = active movement, gravity eliminated
3 = active movement, against gravity
4 = active movement, against some resistance
5 = active movement, against full resistance
NT= not testable

TOTALS ☐ + ☐ = ☐ MOTOR SCORE
(MAXIMUM) (50) (50) (100)

SENSORY — LIGHT TOUCH (R, L), PIN PRICK (R, L) — KEY SENSORY POINTS

C2 … S4-5

0 = absent
1 = impaired
2 = normal
NT= not testable

Any anal sensation (Yes/No)

TOTALS ☐ + ☐ = PIN PRICK SCORE (max: 112)
☐ + ☐ = LIGHT TOUCH SCORE (max: 112)
(MAXIMUM) (56) (56) (56) (56)

* Key Sensory Points

NEUROLOGICAL LEVELS — The most caudal segment with normal function — SENSORY R L, MOTOR R L

COMPLETE OR INCOMPLETE? ☐ — Incomplete = Any sensory or motor function in S4-S5

ASIA IMPAIRMENT SCALE ☐

ZONE OF PARTIAL PRESERVATION — Partially innervated segments — SENSORY R L, MOTOR R L

A

Functional Independence Measure (FIM)

LEVELS		
	7 Complete Independence (Timely, Safely) 6 Modified Independence (Device)	No Helper
	Modified Dependence 5 Supervision 4 Minimal Assist (Subject = 75%+) 3 Moderate Assist (Subject = 50%+) **Complete Dependence** 2 Maximal Assist (Subject = 25%+) 1 Total Assist (Subject = 0%+)	Helper

	ADMIT	DISCH
Self-Care		
A. Eating	☐	☐
B. Grooming	☐	☐
C. Bathing	☐	☐
D. Dressing-Upper Body	☐	☐
E. Dressing-Lower Body	☐	☐
F. Toileting	☐	☐
Sphincter Control		
G. Bladder Management	☐	☐
H. Bowel Management	☐	☐
Mobility		
Transfer:		
I. Bed, Chair, Wheelchair	☐	☐
J. Toilet	☐	☐
K. Tub, Shower	☐	☐
Locomotion	W☐ C☐	W☐ C☐
L. Walk/Wheelchair	☐	☐
M. Stairs	☐	☐
Communication	A☐ V☐ V☐ N☐	A☐ V☐ V☐ N☐
N. Comprehension	☐	☐
O. Expression	☐	☐
Social Cognition		
P. Social Interaction	☐	☐
Q. Problem Solving	☐	☐
R. Memory	☐	☐
Total FIM	☐	☐

NOTE: Leave no blanks; enter 1 if patient not testable due to risk.

COPY FREELY - DO NOT CHANGE
RESEARCH FOUNDATION OF THE STATE UNIVERSITY OF NEW YORK

B

ASIA IMPAIRMENT SCALE

☐ **A = Complete:** No motor or sensory function is preserved in the sacral segments S4-S5.

☐ **B = Incomplete:** Sensory but not motor function is preserved below the neurological level and extends through the sacral segments S4-S5.

☐ **C = Incomplete:** Motor function is preserved below the neurological level, and the majority of key muscles below the neurological level have a muscle grade less than 3.

☐ **D = Incomplete:** Motor function is preserved below the neurological level, and the majority of key muscles below the neurological level have a muscle grade greater than or equal to 3.

☐ **E = Normal:** Motor and sensory function is normal.

CLINICAL SYNDROMES

☐ Central Cord
☐ Brown-Séquard
☐ Anterior Cord
☐ Conus Medullaris
☐ Cauda Equina

Appendix 2 Treatment Guidelines for Patients with Quadriplegia[a]

Time	Orthopaedic Treatment	Program	Considerations/Precautions
Onset or first 3 weeks postoperatively	Radiographs: AP and lateral neck in flexion and extension to determine stability Patient in halo or hard collar Hard collar to remain on at all times	• 3-person turn • WC tolerance • Self-raise • UE resistive exercises, bilaterally • Light unilateral UE activities, ie, self-feeding and light hygiene • Light tabletop activities • UE ROM exercises—easy available exercises • Neck strengthening—isometric, symmetric only • Respiratory program • Dependent sliding board transfers • WC propulsion • LE ROM exercises • Walking only if safe and able without UE aids	Stability must be confirmed by physician before upright activities All postoperative patients must avoid neck extension and rotation; patients with PSF should avoid neck flexion Minimal resistance only to shoulders during manual muscle testing No reciprocal activities Log-roll before stabilization and when patient is out of collar UE resistive exercises, unilaterally, for elbows, wrists, fingers
3-6 weeks	Radiographs: not needed to progress program	• 2-person turn • UE resistive exercises, unilaterally • UE reciprocal pulleys • UE ROM exercises—no limitations • Manual muscle testing—no limitations • Neck strengthening—isometric, unilateral • Assisted sliding board transfers • Active sitting balance • Walking with UE aids for balance only • UE self-ROM exercises bilaterally	Avoid head, neck, and trunk rotation during activities; allow straight depression only Maintain head in neutral
6-12 weeks	**ASD**	**ASD**	**ASD**
	Radiographs: AP and lateral neck Hard collar to remain on at all times	• Turn with patient assist as able • Prone • Pedestal bath with one side of collar on • UE dressing • UE self-ROM exercises • Driver training	No change

Time	Orthopaedic Treatment	Program	Considerations/Precautions
6-12 weeks	**PSF**	**PSF**	**PSF**
	Radiographs: AP and lateral neck in flexion and extension to determine stability D/C hard collar if stable Soft collar as needed for patient comfort	• Turn with patient assist as able • Prone • Self-bowel program • Self-intermittent catheterization and self-application of external catheter • Self-positioning • Dressing • UE self-ROM exercises • Driving • Home and community skills • Bathing • Neck strengthening–isotonic • All mat activities • LE self-ROM exercises • Independent transfers WC into car • Advanced WC skills • Walking with UE aids as needed	Program begun only after patient is determined to be stable and hard collar is removed If patient is unstable and hard collar is continued, advance program only as stated for ASD
12 weeks	**ASD**	**ASD**	**ASD**
	Radiographs: AP and lateral neck in flexion and extension to determine stability D/C hard collar if stable	• Refer to PSF 6-12 weeks for program	Program begun only after patient is determined to be stable and hard collar is removed

[a]These are treatment guidelines only. Alterations in the program may be initiated with physician approval. The time periods above are approximate and the program depends on the medical and physical status of the patient. Pain, decreases in muscle strength, or sensory changes are indications to modify the patient program. Treatment should be initiated only in those patients with stable spines. Patients with gunshot wounds generally have spinal stability; however, this must be confirmed by radiograph. Once stability is confirmed, patients with gunshot wounds may be on an unrestricted program.

Patients with unstable spines requiring uncommon procedures are progressed on an individual basis. Common procedures are ASD with diskectomy or corpectomy and PSF with wires.

ASD = anterior spinal decompression; PSF = posterior spinal fusion; D/C = discontinue; WC = wheelchair; UE = upper extremity; ROM = range of motion; LE = lower extremity.

(From Rancho Los Amigos Medical Center, spinal injury service, physical therapy, occupational therapy, and nursing departments.)

Appendix 3 Treatment Guidelines for Patients with Paraplegia[a]

Time	Orthopaedic Treatment	Program	Considerations/Precautions
Phase 1 (onset or first 3 weeks postoperatively)	Radiographs: AP and lateral spine to determine stability T1-T2 fx: BJ with neck ring T3-T4 fx: BJ with shoulder straps T5 fx and below: BJ only	• 2-person turn • WC tolerance • Self-raise • T4 fx and above: UE resistive exercises, bilaterally • T5 fx and below: unrestricted UE activity • Respiratory program • WC propulsion • Dependent sliding board transfers • L2 fx and above: unrestricted LE ROM exercises except when hooks are below fx • L3 fx and below or when hooks are used at L3, L4, or L5: hip flexion limited to 90° • UE dressing with BJ	Stability must be confirmed by physician before upright activities All postoperative patients must avoid back extension and rotation No resistance to trunk and hips during manual muscle testing Log-roll before stabilization and when patient is out of BJ
Phase 2 (3-6 weeks)	Radiographs: AP and lateral spine 1. CD instrumentation 2. Harrington rods with segmental wires Begin guidelines at 3-6 weeks	• Prone • Males: self-application of external catheter side-lying or upright with BJ and self-IC • UE dressing, LE dress, bathing with BJ • LE resistive exercises, bilaterally • Hamstring stretch • Abdominal and back strengthening—isometric, symmetric only • Straight depression transfers—assisted with legs • Walking with UE aids for balance only • Active sitting balance activities • Advanced WC skills if no BJ	Minimal resistance only to trunk and hips during manual muscle testing Avoid excessive torque

Time	Orthopaedic Treatment	Program	Considerations/Precautions
Phase 3 (6-12 weeks)	Radiographs not needed to progress program	• Turn with patient assistance • Self-bowel program in BJ • Pedestal bath with back of BJ on • LE dressing in BJ • UE activities—unrestricted for all levels of injury including power building • Independent transfers to bed, toilet, and car • LE resistive exercises, unilaterally • Self-ROM exercises • Walking with UE aids as needed • Manual muscle testing—no limitations	No change
Phase 4 (12 weeks)	Radiographs: AP and lateral spine in flexion and extension to determine stability Discontinue orthosis if stable	• Unrestricted program • Self-positioning and prone • Self-skin inspection • Self IC—females • Abdominal and back strengthening—isotonic • All mat activities • All advanced transfers • All advanced WC skills	Program begun only after patient is determined to be stable and orthosis is removed

[a]These are treatment guidelines only. Alterations in the program may be initiated with physician approval. The time periods above are approximate and the program depends on the medical and physical status of the patient. Pain, decreases in muscle strength, or sensory changes are indications to modify the patient program. Treatment should be initiated only in those patients with stable spines. Patients with gunshot wounds generally have spinal stability; however, this must be confirmed by radiograph. Once stability is confirmed, patients with gunshot wounds may be on an unrestricted program.

Patients with unstable spines requiring uncommon procedures are progressed on an individual basis.

fx = fracture; BJ = body jacket; CD = Cotrel-Dubousset; WC = wheelchair; UE = upper extremity; LE = lower extremity; ROM = range of motion; IC = intermittent catheterization; .

(From Rancho Los Amigos Medical Center, spinal injury service, physical therapy, occupational therapy, and nursing departments.)

Appendix 4 Expected Functional Outcomes

Expected Functional Outcomes for Level C6 Injury[a]

Functionally relevant muscles innervated: Clavicular pectoralis supinator, extensor carpi radialis longus and brevis, serratus anterior, latissimus dorsi

Movement possible: Scapular protractor, some horizontal adduction, forearm supination, radial wrist extension

Patterns of weakness: Absence of wrist flexion, elbow extension, hand movement, total paralysis of trunk and lower extremities

			FIM/Assistance Data[b]		
	Expected Functional Outcomes	**Equipment**	**Exp**	**Med**	**IR**
Respiratory	Low endurance and vital capacity secondary to paralysis of intercostals; may require assist to clear secretions				
Bowel	Some to total assist	Padded tub bench with commode cutout or padded shower/commode chair Other adaptive devices as indicated	1-2	1	1
Bladder	Some to total assist with equipment; may be independent with leg bag emptying	Adaptive devices as indicated	1-2	1	1
Bed mobility	Some assist	Full electric hospital bed Side rails Full to king standard bed may be indicated			
Bed/wheelchair transfers	Level: Some assist to independent Uneven: Some to total assist	Transfer board Mechanical lift	3	1	1-3
Pressure relief/ positioning	Independent with equipment and/or adapted techniques	Power recline wheelchair Wheelchair pressure relief cushion Postural support devices Pressure-relief mattress or overlay may be indicated			
Eating	Independent with or without equipment; except cutting, which is total assist	Adaptive devices as indicated (eg, U-cuff, tendinosis splint, adapted utensils, plate guard)	5-6	5	4-6
Dressing	Independent upper extremity; some assist to total assist for lower extremities	Adaptive devices as indicated (eg, buttons, hooks, loops on zippers, pants, socks; velcro on shoes)	1-3	2	1-5
Grooming	Some assist to independent with equipment	Adaptive devices as indicated (eg, U-cuff, adapted handles)	3-6	4	2-6
Bathing	Upper body: independent Lower body: some to total assist	Padded tub transfer bench or shower/commode chair Adaptive devices as needed Handheld shower	1-3	1	1-3

	Expected Functional Outcomes	Equipment	FIM/Assistance Data[b] Exp	Med	IR
Wheelchair propulsion	Power: independent with standard arm drive on all surfaces Manual: independent indoors; some to total assist outdoors	Power: may require power recline or standard upright power wheelchair Manual: lightweight rigid or folding frame with modified rims	6	6	4-6
Standing/ambulation	Standing: total assist Ambulation: not indicated	Hydraulic standing frame			
Communication	Independent with or without equipment	Adaptive devices as indicated (eg, tendinosis splint; writing splint for keyboard use, button pushing, page turning, object manipulation)			
Transportation	Independent driving from wheelchair	Modified van with lift Sensitized hand controls Tie-downs			
Homemaking	Some assist with light meal preparation; total assist for all other homemaking	Adaptive devices as indicated			
Assist required	Personal care: 6 h/day Homecare: 4 h/day		10[c]	17[c]	8-24[c]

Expected Functional Outcomes for Level L2-S5 Injury[a]

Functionally relevant muscles innervated: Fully intact abdominals and all other trunk muscles; depending on level, some degree of hip flexors, extensors, abductors, adductors; knee flexors, extensors; ankle dorsi, flexors, plantar flexors

Movement possible: Good trunk stability; partial to full control of lower extremities

Patterns of weakness: Partial paralysis of lower extremities, hips, knees, ankle, foot

	Expected Functional Outcomes	Equipment	FIM/Assistance Data[b] Exp	Med	IR
Respiratory	Intact function				
Bowel	Independent	Padded toilet seat	6-7	6	6-7
Bladder	Independent		6	6	6-7
Bed mobility	Independent				
Bed/wheelchair transfers	Independent	Full to king standard bed	7	7	7
Pressure relief/positioning	Independent	Wheelchair pressure relief cushion Postural support devices as indicated			
Eating	Independent		7	7	7
Dressing	Independent		7	7	7
Grooming	Independent		7	7	7

	Expected Functional Outcomes	Equipment	FIM/Assistance Data[b] Exp	Med	IR
Bathing	Independent	Padded tub bench Handheld shower	7	7	6-7
Wheelchair propulsion	Independent on all indoor and outdoor surfaces	Manual rigid or folding lightweight wheelchair	6	6	6
Standing/ ambulation	Standing: independent Ambulation: functional, independent to some assist	Standing frame Knee-ankle-foot orthosis or ankle-foot orthosis Forearm crutches or cane as indicated			
Communication	Independent				
Transportation	Independent in car, including loading and unloading wheelchair	Hand controls			
Homemaking	Independent complex cooking and light housekeeping; some assist with heavy housekeeping				
Assist required	Homemaking: 0-1 h/day		0-1[c]	0[c]	0-2[c]

[a]Excerpted with permission from Consortium for Spinal Cord Medicine: *Outcomes Following Traumatic Spinal Cord Injury: Clinical Practice Guidelines for Health Care Professionals*. Washington, DC, Paralyzed Veterans of America, 1999. A total of eight similar charts on different spinal cord injury levels are available at http://www.pva.org/site/DocServer/OUT.pdf?docID=686.

[b]Functional Independence Measure (FIM)/Assistance Data: Exp = expected FIM score; Med = National Spinal Cord Injury Statistical Center (NSCISC) median; IR = NSCISC interquartile range. The NSCISC sample size for Level C6 was FIM = 43, Assist = 35. The sample size for Level L2-S5 was FIM = 20, Assist = 16.

[c]Hours per day.

Appendix 5 Functional Goals for Patients With Quadriplegia (Consider Age, Sex, Weight, Body Type, Motivation)[a]

Functional Level[a] of Key Muscles[b] (Manual Muscle Test Grade)	Wheelchair	Feeding	Hygiene and Grooming	Bowel and Bladder Care	Dressing Skills	Desktop	Home Skills	Driving
C4 Neck accessories *Diaphragm* *Trapezius*	Electronic with chin control	*Dependent*	*Dependent*	*Dependent*	*Dependent*	*Assisted* with equipment	*Dependent*	*Dependent*
C4 with weak C5 muscles Muscles above and *deltoids* (2/5 to 3/5)[a] *Biceps* (2/5 to 3/5)[c]	Electric with hand control and mobile arm support	*Assisted* with equipment	*Assisted* with equipment	*Dependent*	*Dependent*	*Assisted* with equipment	*Dependent*	*Dependent*
C5 Muscles above and *deltoids* *Biceps*	Electric with hand control	*Assisted* with equipment	*Assisted* with equipment	*Dependent*	*Dependent*	*Assisted* with equipment	*Dependent*	*Independent* Van with lift sensitized controls
C6 Muscles above and *wrist extensors* *Clavicular* *Pectoralis* *Serratus anterior* Other important muscle: pronator teres	*Manual*	*Independent* May require equipment	*Independent* May require equipment	*Independent* with equipment	*Independent* Upper body *Assisted-independent* Lower body	*Independent* May require equipment	*Independent* Light *Assisted* Heavy	*Independent* Hand controls *Dependent* Wheelchair loading
C7 Muscles above and *triceps* Other important muscle: latissimus dorsi	Manual	*Independent* May require equipment	*Independent* May require equipment	*Assisted-independent* with equipment	*Independent* Both upper and lower body	*Independent* May require equipment	*Independent* Light *Assisted* Heavy	*Independent* Wheelchair loading Hand controls
C8 Muscles above and *extrinsic finger flexors*	Manual	*Independent*	*Independent*	*Independent*	*Independent*	*Independent*	*Independent*	*Independent* Hand controls
T1 Normal hand muscles above and *intrinsic finger muscles*	Manual	*Independent*	*Independent*	*Independent*	*Independent*	*Independent*	*Independent*	*Independent* Hand controls

[a]The lowest segment at which muscle strength of key motors is 3+/5 or better and pain sensation is intact.

[b]A muscle that significantly changes functional outcome (*italic*).

[c]Note that key muscles' strength for this functional level is 2/5 to 3/5.

(From Rancho Los Amigos Medical Center, occupational therapy department.)

Appendix 6 Functional Goals for Patients With Complete SCI (Consider Age, Sex, Weight, Body Type, Motivation)[a]

Quadriplegics					Paraplegics			
C1-C4 Neck Upper Trapezius	**C5 Deltoids Biceps**	**C6 Wrist Extensors**	**C7-C8 Triceps Weak Hand**		**T1-T8 Chest Extension**	**T9-12 Trunk Extension**	**L1-2 Hip Extensors**	**L3-5 Knee Extensors**
				Relief of skin pressure				
X	X			(I) With electric recliner				
	*	*	*	(I) Forward loop or lean				
		X	X	(I) Depression raises	X	X	X	X
				Wheelchair propulsion				
X	X	*	*	Electric				
	*	*		Manual with projection rims				
		X	*	Manual with friction rims				
		*	X	Manual with standard rims	X	X	X	X
				Bed transfers				
X	*			Mechanical/ manual lift				
*	X	*		(A) Sliding board				
		X	*	(I) Sliding board				
		*	X	(I) Depression	X	X	X	X
				Car transfers				
X	X	*		Mechanical lift/ independent				
	*	*		(A) Sliding board				
		X	*	(I) Sliding board	*			
		*	X	(I) Depression	X	X	X	X
				Toilet transfers				
X	X			Mechanical lift to commode				
	*	*		(A) Sliding board to commode				
		X	*	(I) Sliding board to raised seat				

Quadriplegics					Paraplegics			
C1-C4 Neck Upper Trapezius	**C5 Deltoids Biceps**	**C6 Wrist Extensors**	**C7-C8 Triceps Weak Hand**		**T1-T8 Chest Extension**	**T9-12 Trunk Extension**	**L1-2 Hip Extensors**	**L3-5 Knee Extensors**
		*	X	(I) Depression to raised seat	X	X	X	X
				Tub transfers				
	*	*		(A) Sliding board to tub bench				
		X	*	(I) Sliding board to tub bench				
		*	X	(I) Depression to tub bench	X	X	X	X
				(I) To bottom of tub		*	*	*
				Cough				
X	X			Dependent manual				
	*	X	*	Self-manual	*			
		*	X	Independent	X	X	X	X
				Curb management				
		*	X	(I) 2-in curbs				
			*	(I) 4- and 6-in curbs	X	X	X	X
				Wheelchair into car				
		*		(A) Dependent/unable				
		*		(I) With loop on wheelchair				
		X	X	Independent	X	X	X	X
				Ambulation				
			*	Physiologic	*	*	X	
				Household			X	
				Limited community			*	X
				Community			*	X

[a]X = most patients; * = some patients; I = independent; A = assisted.

(From Rancho Los Amigos Medical Center, spinal injury service and physical therapy departments.)

CHAPTER 38
Posttraumatic Syringomyelia

Andrew Jea, MD David M. Benglis Jr, MD Steven Falcone, MD, MBA
Barth A. Green, MD, FACS

Introduction

Syringomyelia, or cavitation within the substance of the spinal cord without an ependymal lining, has been recognized for over 300 years as a pathologic entity. Charles Estienne is credited for the first pathologic description in 1564, in *La dissection des parties du corps humain*;[1] he described a cystic lesion in the spinal cord that contained a "fluid, reddish, like the fluidity of that of the ventricles."

Portal, in 1804, first appreciated and connected the clinical syndrome of an intramedullary cyst with the pathologic changes of the spinal cord.[2] Ollivier d'Angers then coined the term syringomyelia, combining the Greek words for tube or pipe and marrow. He documented a connection between the fourth ventricle and this cystic structure, which he believed to be a congenital anomaly.[1,3,4]

The classic clinical description of syringomyelia is that of a dissociated, suspended segmental sensory loss, consisting of loss of sensation to pain and temperature and preservation of sensation to proprioception and light touch. Slowly progressive distal motor dysfunction may also occur. A syrinx may extend to the medulla and cause lower brainstem dysfunction; in this case, the pathologic lesion is termed syringobulbia.

Those ependymal-lined cavities that appeared to be pathologic dilatations of the central canal were termed hydromyelia. Some authors viewed hydromyelia, in which the central canal was dilated but preserved, and syringomyelia, with or without a connection to the central canal, as stages of a common process (**Figure 1**). Hence, unification of the terms resulted in the concept of syringohydromyelia or hydrosyringomyelia.[1,3,5,6]

Dr. Benglis or an immediate family member has received nonincome support (such as equipment or services), commercially derived honoraria, or other non-research-related funding (such as paid travel) from Medtronic Sofamor Danek and DePuy, a Johnson & Johnson company. None of the following authors or any immediate family member has received anything of value from or owns stock in a commercial company or institution related directly or indirectly to the subject of this chapter: Dr. Jea, Dr. Falcone, and Dr. Green.

Barnett,[7] in the first English-language monograph on syringomyelia, published in 1973, proposed a classification based on a variety of clinical and experimental observations and studies, broadly classified into communicating (associated with Chiari I malformation, Chiari II malformation, basilar arachnoiditis) and noncommunicating (associated with occult spinal dysraphism, spinal cord trauma, spinal cord tumor, spinal arachnoiditis) syringomyelia (**Table 1**).

Recent experimental and clinical work, including that of Milhorat et al[8-13] and Oldfield et al,[14] has helped to clarify pathophysiology and treatment of this syndrome.

Etiology, Pathology, and Pathophysiology

Historical Perspective

Although the pathogenesis of syringomyelia has not yet been completely defined, the association

FIGURE 1

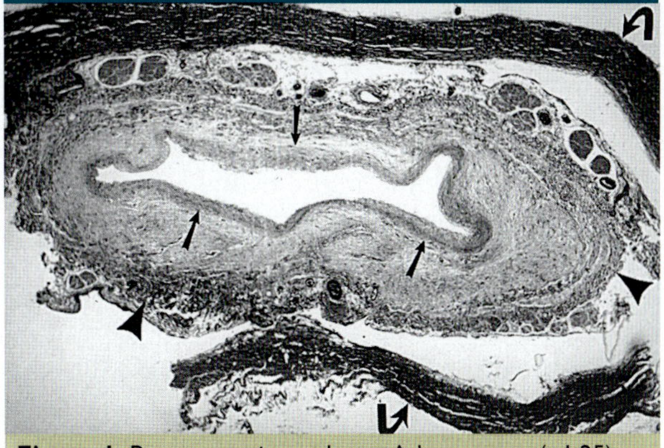

Figure 1 Posttraumatic cord cyst. A low-power (×1.25) microscopic section image of a posttraumatic syringomyelia. There is a large, centrally located syrinx in the parenchyma of the spinal cord, which is surrounded by a thick wall of reactive astrocytes (arrows). The pia is thickened, and there are tissue changes that involve the spinal roots (arrowheads). The dura is also thickened (curved arrows). (Reproduced from Madsen PW III, Falcone S, Bowen BC, Green BA: Post-traumatic syringomyelia, in Levine AM, Eismont FJ, Garfin SR, Zigler JE, eds: *Spine Trauma*. Philadelphia, PA, WB Saunders, 1998, pp 608-629.)

TABLE 1

Types of Syringomyelia and Associated Abnormalities

Communicating	Chiari I malformation Chiari II malformation Basilar arachnoiditis
Noncommunicating	Occult spinal dysraphism Spinal cord trauma Spinal cord tumor Spinal arachnoiditis

between syringomyelia and congenital abnormalities was appreciated long ago. Tamaki and Lubin[15] credited Baumler with establishing this relationship in 1887. Poser[16] remarked that Schlesinger's 1895 monograph indicated an associated congenital abnormality in one-third of the cases of syringomyelia that he had reviewed.

Ollivier d'Angers formulated, and Leyden further refined, the developmental theory of syringomyelia formation.[16,17] These investigators stated that syringomyelia must be considered a congenital disorder and believed that the syrinx was a result of incomplete occlusion of the primitive fold. Improper fusion of the two folds of the primitive medullary groove allowed the groove to become lined with germinal cells, resulting in simple hydromyelia.

In 1879, Kahler and Pick theorized that chronic intrauterine inflammation resulted in gliosis and aberrant development of the spinal cord, leading to syrinx formation.[16] In 1910, Haener speculated that birth trauma may arouse neural activity in abnormally enclosed tissue, with resultant syrinx formation.[16]

In a series of landmark papers, W.J. Gardner expounded his hydrodynamic theory of the pathogenesis of syringomyelia.[18-23] He based this theory on three observations: (1) dye injected into the ventricular system was recovered from the syrinx at operation, (2) fluid withdrawn from the syrinx at operation strongly resembled cerebrospinal fluid (CSF) found in the ventricular system, and (3) experimental hydrocephalus produced by obstruction of the normal outflow of CSF from the fourth ventricle resulted in the formation of syringomyelia that was in communication with the ventricular system.[24] His contention was that syringomyelia resulted from a failure of the embryonic rhombic roof to achieve fenestration during a critical period of development. The inabilty of CSF in the fourth ventricle to gain the usual access to the subarachnoid space during the sixth to eighth week of embryogenesis forced the hindbrain to herniate through the foramen magnum. A Chiari malformation was thereby created, and the failure of the CSF to expand the subarachnoid space resulted in communicating hydrocephalus. Gardner believed that the effect of the hindbrain malformation was to increase the obstruction to outflow at the foramen of Magendie and deflect the pulse wave of CSF into the opening of the central canal at the obex. The pulse wave effect of the diverted CSF acted as a water-hammer, gradually dilating the central canal or dissecting the substance of the spinal cord around the canal and creating a syrinx. From the perspective of Gardner, a congenital hindbrain defect that obstructed the CSF flow from the fourth ventricle to the subarachnoid space was the sine qua non of syringomyelia, and the concept of noncommunicating syringomyelia was nonexistent. West and Williams[25] and Ball and Dayan[26] questioned the necessity of a direct communication to the fourth ventricle for production of a syrinx. Milhorat et al[8,11] demonstrated in large autopsy studies that the majority of syringes did not communicate with the fourth ventricle and that the central canal was not patent in most normal adult patients.

Williams[27,28] proposed an alternative theory to explain syrinx formation, speculating that a partial block of the spinal subarachnoid space produced a pressure differential between the ventricular system and the spinal subdural space during Valsalva-type maneuvers. He explained that venous distention associated with these maneuvers produced an increased intracranial pressure that was not evenly distributed to the lumbar subarachnoid space because of a more proximal complete or partial subarachnoid block. This pressure difference was labeled craniospinal pressure dissociation, and the lower pressure in the lumbar theca caused fluid to be drawn into the syrinx. This phenomenon was termed suck. Williams also believed that the cavity enlarged after its initial formation as the result of compression of the lower end of the cavity with the rapid filling of the epidural venous plexus during a cough or sneeze. The fluid in the syrinx was then propelled rostrally, dissecting the central canal or pericentral parenchyma of the spinal cord. Williams applied the term slosh to this part of his theory to explain syrinx extension.[29]

Oldfield et al[14] used MRI with and without cardiac gating, intraoperative ultrasonography, and direct intraoperative observation of the exposed hindbrain and documented the downward movement of the cerebellar tonsils during systole. This group interpreted the data as obviating the necessity of a direct communication with the fourth ventricle, as advocated by Gardner. Moreover, they observed that the syringomyelic cord did not enlarge with Valsalva maneuver and that venous pressure had little to do with syrinx elongation, disputing the Williams "suck and slosh" theory. The authors proposed that the abnormal pulse wave in the spinal subarachnoid space, caused by the partial obstruction by the hindbrain, placed pressure on the spinal cord and dissected the central canal, causing the cyst to enlarge.

Milhorat et al[13] proposed that normal CSF flow was from the spinal subarachnoid space through the parenchyma of the spinal cord into the central canal. The CSF then flowed into the fourth ventricle outlet at the obex. By injecting kaolin into the central canal of rats, the resulting inflammatory reaction caused stenosis of the proximal central canal, and a syrinx was formed. The authors suggested that the disruption of normal CSF flow by the inflammatory stenosis caused the syrinx to form and was a model of syringes associated with the majority of hindbrain malformations that pressed on the proximal spinal cord, obstructing the central canal and blocking communication of the syrinx and the fourth ventricle.

Communicating Syringomyelia

In 1896, Chiari published an addendum to an earlier work in which he described anomalies associated with hydrocephalus; this addendum included descriptions of patients with hydromyelia. Gardner and Goodall[30] found that most patients undergoing surgical decompression for symptomatic Chiari I malformation had a concurrent syringomyelia. Gardner et al[31] later demonstrated, in surgery, communication between the syrinx of the upper cervical cord and the ventricles in patients undergoing suboccipital craniectomy and cervical laminectomy for decompression. Indigo-carmine was injected into the patient's lateral ventricle, and colored CSF was recovered by direct puncture of the cervical syrinx.

Appleby et al[32] established that a "communicating" type of syringomyelia could be acquired from chronic arachnoiditis involving the basal cisterns and obstructing the outflow of CSF from the fourth ventricle (**Figure 2**).

Noncommunicating Syringomyelia

Syringomyelia Associated With Spinal Arachnoiditis

The association between spinal arachnoiditis and syringomyelia was first reported by Vulpian in 1861 and later by Charcot and Joffroy in 1869. Some authors believed the occlusion of blood vessels supplying the cord by the arachnoid scarring to be the underlying pathophysiologic process for intramedullary cavitation.[33-35]

Williams[27] implicated craniospinal pressure dissociation, secondary to obstruction of the subarachnoid space, as the factor responsible for cyst formation and extension. An analysis published in 2004 went on to explain that blockage of the spinal subarachnoid CSF pathway produces a relative increase in the pressure inside the spinal cord distal to the blockage point.[36] Repetitive formation of this pressure gradient then induces CSF leakage into the spinal parenchyma, leading to the formation of syringomyelia.

Barnett[37] and Milhorat et al[8] considered this type of syrinomyelia to be of the "noncommunicating" type, as no connection between the cyst and the fourth ventricle could be demonstrated.

Syringomyelia Associated With Spinal Cord Tumors

The association between syringomyelia and spinal cord tumors has been well established. Simon's paper in 1875 was the first to report the simultaneous occurrence of syringomyelia and tumors.[38]

A variety of pathophysiologic mechanisms for the creation of syringes associated with neoplasms have been proposed. Edema, blockage of the perivascular spaces with resultant tissue fluid stasis, cavitation secondary to disturbance of blood supply to the cord, and spontaneous hemorrhage into or autolysis of the mass have been implicated as causal or sustaining events of syrinx formation.[33,39,40] Other authors contend that syringomyelia associated with a spinal cord tumor is itself a true neoplastic growth.[16,38,41-43] A number of authors believed that this disordered gliosis was the underlying pathophysiologic disorder even in syringomyelia that was not associated with an intramedullary neoplasm;[1,44-46] this led some clinicians to recommend radiation therapy as a rational but extreme form of primary therapy. Today, the use of radiation therapy should be restricted to the primary therapy of a known neoplasm or as an adjunct to surgical resection of a tumor.

Total or subtotal obstruction of CSF flow by an intramedullary tumor may be a significant factor

FIGURE 2

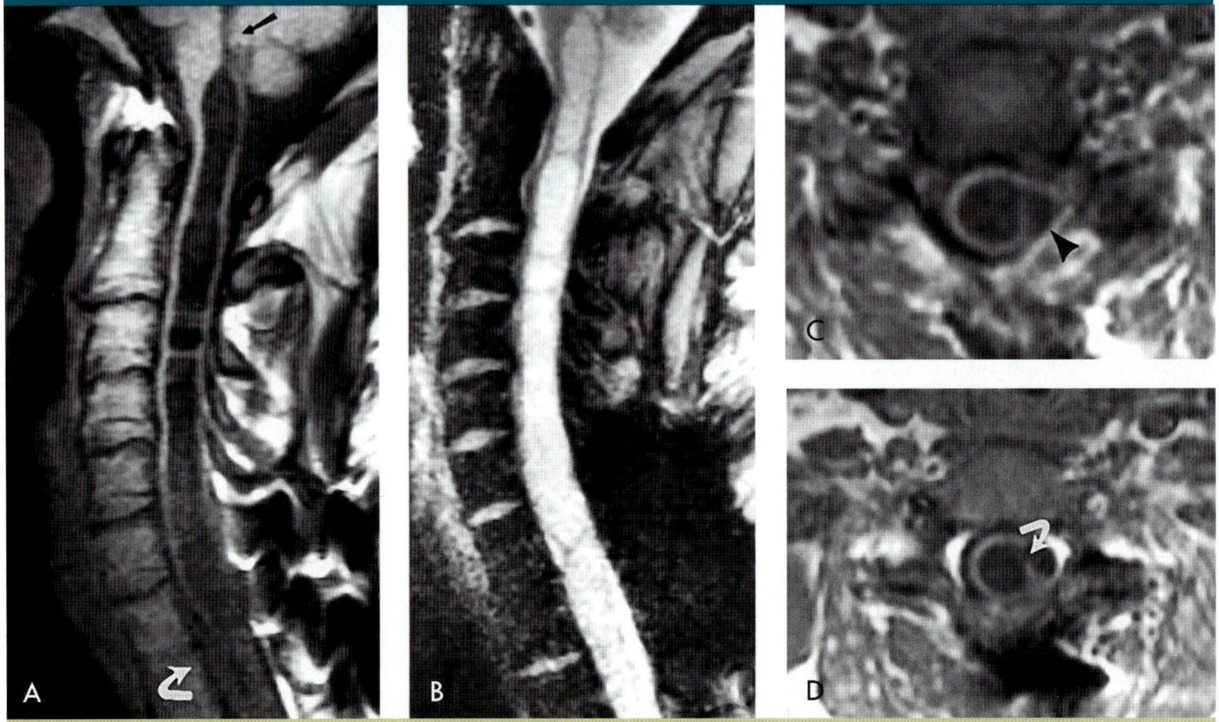

Figure 2 Posttraumatic cord cyst. **A,** A T1-weighted sagittal image of the cervical spine demonstrates a septated syrinx of the spinal cord that extends to the obex (arrow). Myelomalacia is seen in the upper thoracic spinal cord (curved arrow). **B,** The gradient echo sagittal image shows the abnormally expanded spinal cord, with increased signal intensity. The septations are less apparent. **C,** The T1-weighted axial image at the C6-C7 level demonstrates a fluid loculation (arrowhead), which has characteristics of either an extramedullary collection or an intramedullary component of the cyst. **D,** The T1-weighted axial image at C7-T1 more clearly reveals a rent or fissure on the left side of the cord surface communicating with the subarachnoid space (curved arrow). Note metallic artifact from prior posterior fusion (**A-D**). (Reproduced from Madsen PW III, Falcone S, Bowen BC, Green BA: Post-traumatic syringomyelia, in Levine AM, Eismont FJ, Garfin SR, Zigler JE, eds: *Spine Trauma*. Philadelphia, PA, WB Saunders, 1998, pp 608-629.)

for the development of syringomyelia. The subarachnoid and the extracellular space of the central nervous system may be considered as a single-fluid compartment with no barrier to fluid movement between them. Interference with CSF flow must influence extracellular fluid flow of the spinal cord. The high ratio of syrinx cavities associated with intramedullary tumors may be attributable to their simultaneous influence on the subarachnoid and extracellular spaces. On one side, transudation from tumor vessels, breakdown products of tumor cells, or even active secretion raise the protein content and thus the viscosity of the extracellular fluid. On the other side, the interference with CSF flow leads to an increase of extracellular fluid flow inside the spinal cord. If the tumor displaces and compresses spinal cord tissue, this combination of mechanisms may exceed the capacity of the extracellular space and may explain the high proportion of syrinx cavities associated with intramedullar tumors.[47]

Less commonly, intramedullary cysts present in association with an extramedullary neurofibroma or meningioma. The removal of the extramedullary mass lesion is usually followed by a spontaneous collapse of the associated syrinx.

In a surgical series of 100 intramedullary tumors, 45% presented with associated syringes.[47] A syrinx was more likely to be found above than below the tumor level. Ependymomas and hemangioblastomas were the most common tumor types to be associated with syringes. Astrocytomas tended to demonstrate syringes less often. The higher the spinal level, the more likely a syrinx was encountered.

Syringomyelia Associated With Spinal Cord Trauma

The pathophysiologic basis for the formation and extension of syringes of the injured spinal cord remains the subject of considerable debate. The onset of signs and symptoms of progressive posttraumatic cystic myelopathy ranges from as early as 2 to 3 months following injury to as long as 30 years after injury.[48] Approximately 4% to 10% of patients suffering a traumatic spinal cord injury develop progressive spinal cord dysfunction associated with an expanding syrinx.[49-51]

FIGURE 3

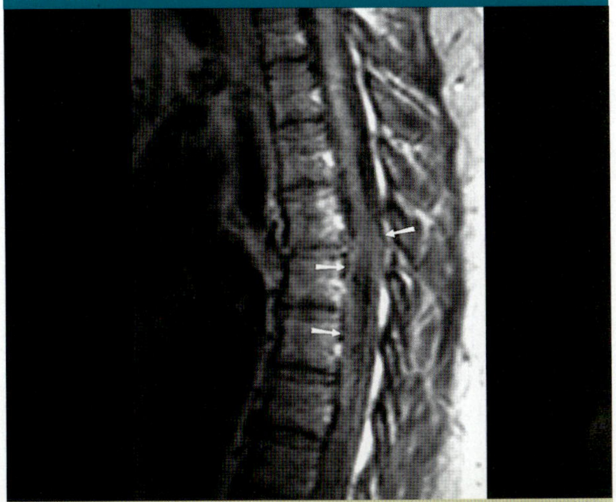

Figure 3 Cystic changes in the posttraumatic cord. Postgadolinium T1-weighted sagittal image demonstrates a kyphotic deformity with apex at T4-T5. There is abrupt cord enlargement at T5 and enhancement of the cord surface from T5 to T6-T7. At surgery, dural adhesions were identified. (Reproduced from Madsen PW III, Falcone S, Bowen BC, Green BA: Post-traumatic syringomyelia, in Levine AM, Eismont FJ, Garfin SR, Zigler JE, eds: *Spine Trauma*. Philadelphia, PA, WB Saunders, 1998, pp 608-629.)

Milhorat's large autopsy study demonstrated that syringes associated with trauma had distinctly different histopathologic findings and were associated with different clinical symptoms when compared with those lesions that were in communication with the fourth ventricle or those cavities that appeared to be isolated dilatations of the central canal.[8,49] The syringes associated with spinal cord injury involved the parenchyma of the cord asymmetrically. They were not associated with the central canal and often extended to the pial surface (**Figures 3** and **4**). Examination of pathologic specimens revealed nonreversible damage to spinal nuclei and tracts, including focal necrosis, central chromatolysis, and Wallerian degeneration.

The possible factors implicated in the production of the initial cystic lesions in posttraumatic spinal cords included ischemia secondary to arterial and/or venous obstruction, lysosomes and other intracellular enzymes, liquefaction of a prior hematoma, mechanical damage from compression of the substance of the cord at the time of initial injury, or tethering by delayed formation of extensive subarachnoid adhesions and/or a bony gibbus.[52-60]

Similarly, the mechanism for the extension of the syringomyelia remains a matter of controversy, and several mechanisms have been proposed. Several authors felt strongly that the mechanism of both rostral and caudal extension of the syrinx, which produced late neurologic symptoms, was a one-way valve-like connection of the subarachnoid space into the cavity.[12,61-64] Less frequently

FIGURE 4

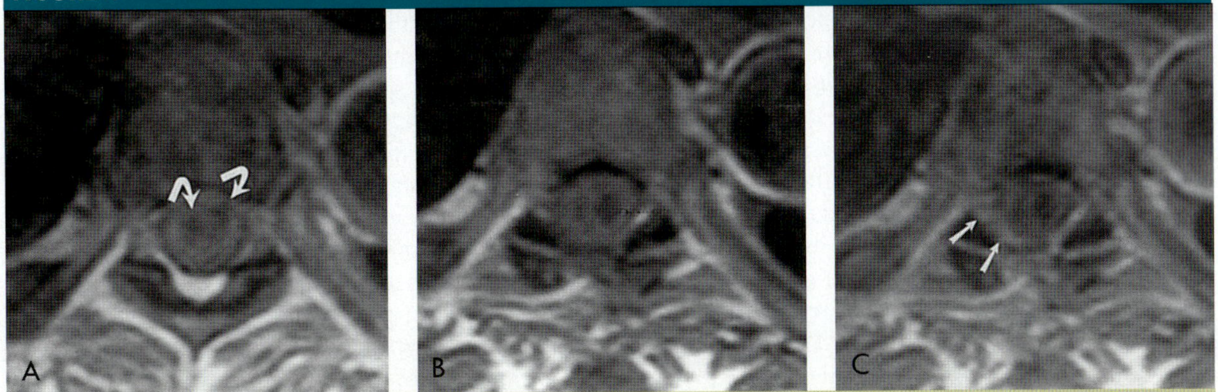

Figure 4 Cystic changes in the posttraumatic cord in the same patient as in Figure 3. Preoperative (**A**) and postoperative (**B**) T1-weighted axial images at the T5-T6 level were obtained without gadolinium. In **A,** there are poorly defined intramedullary regions (curved arrows) of slightly decreased signal. In **B,** the same regions are more sharply defined, have a lower signal, and greater cephalocaudad extent. **C,** The postoperative and postgadolinium T1-weighted image demonstrates linear enhancement (arrows) consistent with scarring and probable recurrence of adhesions postoperatively. (Reproduced from Madsen PW III, Falcone S, Bowen BC, Green BA: Post-traumatic syringomyelia, in Levine AM, Eismont FJ, Garfin SR, Zigler JE, eds: *Spine Trauma*. Philadelphia, PA, WB Saunders, 1998, pp 608-629.)

observed presentations of posttraumatic cysts include patients with a history of herniated cervical or thoracic disks and individuals with a history of a therapeutic spinal puncture that results in the introduction of an irritative chemical substance into the thecal sac. This substance may cause a lumbar arachnoiditis that can ascend to involve the thoracic spine and may be associated with subarachnoid and/or intramedullary cysts.

Posttraumatic syringomyelia may be classified into two types. A preoperative distinction could be made based on the presence (high-pressure type) or absence (low-pressure type) of the flow-void sign on a T2-weighted magnetic resonance image. With midline myelotomy, fluid within a high-pressure syrinx would spout out, resulting in sustained neurologic improvement. In the low-pressure type, drainage of the syrinx would not collapse the expanded spinal cord, and the surgical outcome would be modest at best.[65]

Clinical Features

The onset of this disorder is commonly between the ages of 25 to 40 years. Males are somewhat more affected than females. Syringomyelia most often affects the cervical or thoracic spinal cord, sometimes extending rostrally into the medulla.

Hydrocephalus may be found in 10% to 33% of patients but is more likely related to an associated Chiari malformation.[25] This frequent association supports the concept of a hydrodynamic mechanism for the formation of syringomyelia.

Clinical features are variable and dependent on the anatomic structures involved in a cross-sectional area as well as longitudinally. Anterior horn involvement results in weakness and wasting, especially in the upper extremities, and fasciculations. Posterior horn and decussating spinothalamic fiber involvement results in loss of pain and temperature sensation, usually in a suspended, segmental distribution, involving the arms and trunk and sparing the legs. Patients may occasionally feel pain that is characterized as boring or lancinating. The large fibers of the dorsal columns are usually unaffected and therefore proprioception and light touch is preserved. The autonomic pathways of the interomediolateral column may be affected, resulting in a Horner syndrome, trophic changes of the skin, a neurogenic bladder, and dyshidrosis. Corticospinal tract involvement may result in spastic paraparesis. Patients experience a loss of deep tendon reflexes in the upper extremities. A skeletal survey may reveal congenital anomalies including basilar impression and invagination, Klippel-Feil deformity, and spina bifida occurring primarily at C1.[66] Developmental scoliosis may occur as a result of cord cavitation and is probably not an unassociated congenital lesion.[67] Although discussed extensively in the literature, painless joint destruction (Charcot joints) occurs in less than 5% of patients with syringomyelia.[68]

Cranial nerve (CN) involvement is seen with syringobulbia. Most often signs and symptoms are unilateral. CN XII involvement results in tongue weakness and atrophy. CN XI dysfunction can result in weakness and wasting of the sternocleidomastoid and trapezius muscles. CN IX and X involvement produces dysphagia and dysarthria. CN VII involvement results in a facial palsy. Involvement of the spinal tract of CN V produces sensory loss of pain and temperature of the face in an "onion-skin" distribution, and reduced corneal sensation and reflex.

The clinical course of syringomyelia is usually insidious, worsening over several years to decades. Alternatively, the patient may worsen in an abrupt stepwise fashion punctuated by intervals of clinical stability.[69] The prognosis of untreated syringomyelia is compatible with modified but productive survival for decades in 50% of surviving patients.[70] The remainder become incapacitated and die as a direct result of the pathologic process.

Presentation of Progressive Posttraumatic Cystic Myelopathy

Progressive posttraumatic cystic myelopathy (PPCM)[51,71,72] is associated with single or multiple connected or separated spinal cord cysts or cystic cavities that may be located with their connections in the intramedullary or subarachnoid compartments, or in some cases in both, and even may be associated with spinal cord fissure. Cysts may result from a variety of causes, ranging from a very significant high-velocity injury from a penetrating missile wound causing quadriplegia or paraplegia, to a relatively minor trauma characteristically associated with transient or minimal neurologic deficit. Postsurgery patients form the second most common category of posttraumatic spinal cord cysts; these patients typically have undergone an integral spinal procedure that results in local tethering of the spinal cord or more diffuse blockage of flow in the subarachnoid space. Most patients in this group present with a history of surgery for an intraspinal mass, although patients with a history of arachnoiditis can also present with lesions.

The onset of signs and symptoms of PPCM have ranged from as early as 2 to 3 months fol-

FIGURE 5

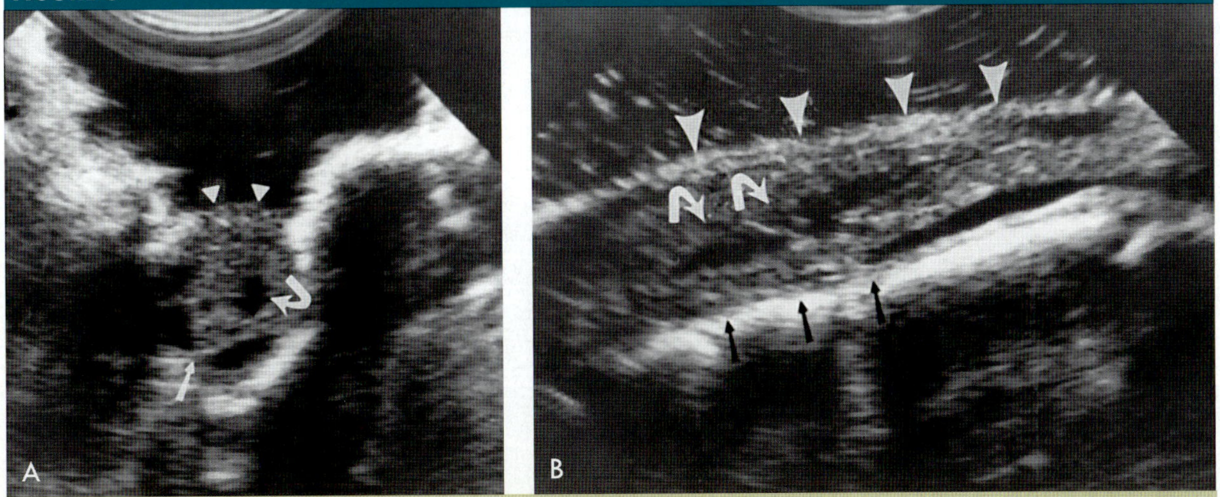

Figure 5 Microcystic myelomalacia in a 56-year-old patient with radicular pain and a history of spine trauma. Intraoperative sonogram via laminectomy at T6: axial (**A**) and sagittal (**B**) images. The spinal cord is tethered both dorsally to the dura (arrowheads), with loss of normal hypoechoic space, and ventrally (arrows). As a result of the tethering, the spinal cord is enlarged. The echo pattern of the spinal cord parenchyma is heterogenous, with absence of a normal central echo and the presence of microcysts (curved arrows). A confluent cyst is not present and after the spinal cord was surgically untethered, the cysts collapsed. (Reproduced from Madsen PW III, Falcone S, Bowen BC, Green BA: Post-traumatic syringomyelia, in Levine AM, Eismont FJ, Garfin SR, Zigler JE, eds: *Spine Trauma*. Philadelphia, PA, WB Saunders, 1998, pp 608-629.)

lowing the initial traumatic event to as long as 30 years postinjury. The signs and symptoms, in order of decreasing frequency, are: (1) motor loss, (2) sensory loss, (3) local or radicular pain (non-deafferentiated, neurogenic, "burning" pain), (4) increased spasticity and tone, (5) hyperhidrosis (above level of lesion), (6) autonomic dysreflexia, (7) sphincter loss or sexual dysfunction, (8) Horner syndrome (may be alternating), (9) respiratory insufficiency (usually related to changes in position), and (10) change in motor "tone" (increased or decreased).

At presentation, the signs and symptoms may be unilateral or bilateral, and may alternate from side to side with changes in position. They may also present as a solitary sign or symptom, or in any combination. The increased utilization of noninvasive MRI has more frequently identified asymptomatic cases compared with the previously employed imaging techniques.

This descriptive situation has been compounded by the clinical entity progressive posttraumatic myelomalacic myelopathy (PPMM),[73] which can clinically and radiographically mimic PPCM. Unlike PPCM, patients found to have PPMM do not have an associated cavitary lesion in the spinal cord. Rather than a confluent cyst, microcystic changes within a zone of myelomalacia predominate, most often associated with widening and posterior or lateral tethering of the spinal cord. Although MRI can provide clues to the correct diagnosis because areas of myelomalacia have irregular, ill-defined margins and do not follow CSF signal intensity, intraoperative ultrasound or myelotomy has been required to unequivocally establish the absence of a cyst (**Figures 5** through **10**). Recognition of this entity can assist the surgeon in planning for the correct surgical therapy.

Diagnosis

Diagnosis of syringomyelia was based on clinical presentation and course in the late 19th and early 20th centuries. This clinical diagnosis represented a difficult task for the medical or surgical neurologist of that time, as the disorder had an insidious onset and a variable clinical course. Intramedullary neoplasms,[1] as well as demyelinating diseases (multiple sclerosis, amyotrophic lateral sclerosis), disorders of metabolism and nutrition (subacute combined degeneration in vitamin B12 deficiency), infectious causes of spinal cord dysfunction (tabes dorsalis from syphilis), and degenerative disease (cervical spondylosis leading to stenosis and cervical myelopathy), were most troublesome to differentiate from a syringomyelic process. In most patients, the classic clinical finding of segmental weakness and atrophy of the hands and arms, with loss of tendon reflexes and

FIGURE 6

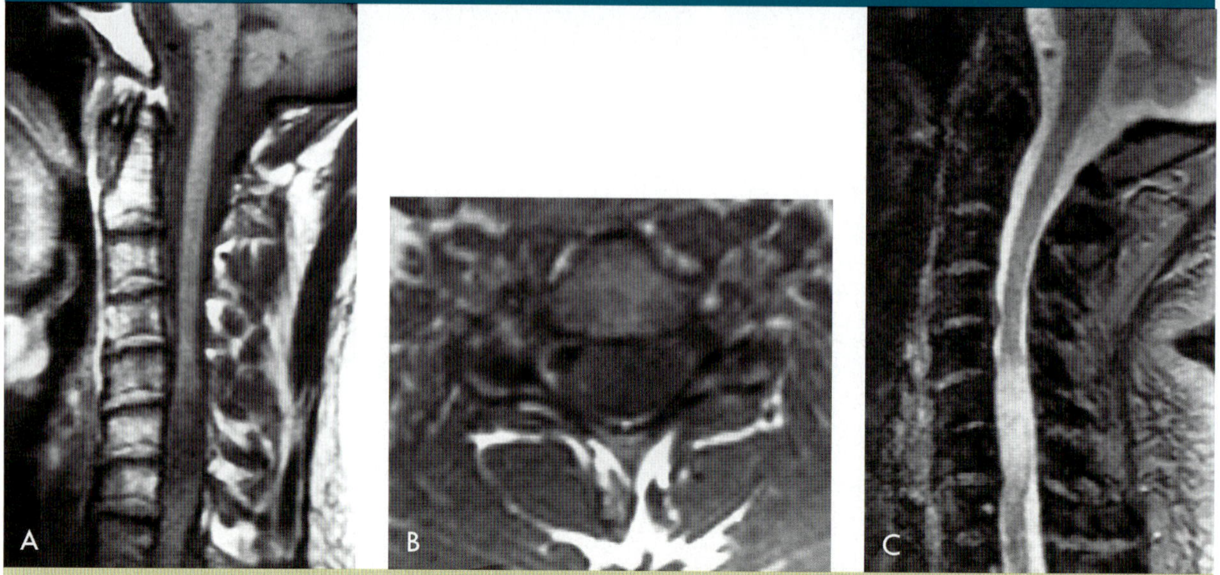

Figure 6 Posttraumatic, expansile myelomalacia. T1-weighted sagittal (**A**) and axial (**B**) images of the cervical spine. There is expansion of the spinal cord with an abnormal, decreased signal within the spinal cord parenchyma at C6-C7 (**B**). The signal intensity of the expanded spinal cord is greater than that of CSF and its borders are ill-defined. **C,** On the gradient echo sagittal image, the myelomalacic segment of the spinal cord has increased signal intensity. (Reproduced from Madsen PW III, Falcone S, Bowen BC, Green BA: Post-traumatic syringomyelia, in Levine AM, Eismont FJ, Garfin SR, Zigler JE, eds: *Spine Trauma*. Philadelphia, PA, WB Saunders, 1998, pp 608-629.)

segmental dissociated sensory loss, could not be found.[74]

Currently, the diagnostic test of choice for syringomyelia is MRI.[75] The initial MRI examination includes, as a minimum, sagittal and transverse views of the lesion plus the adjacent spinal cord and/or brainstem in T1-weighted images (**Figure 11**). The addition of T2-weighted and/or mixed proton-density images can complement the T1-weighted images. Gadolinium-enhanced images are considered an essential part of the work-up to detect tumors and differentiate between scar and disk material, especially in postoperative or posttraumatic cases.[76] Inclusion of the entire rostrocaudal extent of each cyst is important.

In addition to conventional MRI, a new generation of MRI software technology is currently available, including cine MRI, which is a real-time, motion picture-like analysis of spinal fluid flow dynamics in and around the spinal cord cyst.[77] Magnetic resonance angiography is another technological advance that can be helpful in cases of syringomyelia associated with vascular lesions.

Spinal instrumentation, bullet fragments, or the inability of the patient to tolerate the enclosed space of the scanner degrades the ability of the MRI to provide adequate anatomic assessment. In these cases, a myelogram in combination with immediate and delayed high-resolution CT is performed. Difficulty in differentiating myelomalacia or an intramedullary tumor from a confluent syrinx represents a limitation of this technique.[78]

Treatment

The treatment of syringomyelia continues to be controversial. There is no universally accepted method of intervention or consensus on the benefit of therapy.

The first report of successful surgical therapy of syringomyelia was that of Abbe and Coley in 1892.[79] They performed a three-level laminectomy and opened the dura to expose the cyst. They aspirated clear fluid from the spinal cord cyst, which collapsed with aspiration. This report was significant not because of clinical improvement with cyst drainage but because it showed that syringomyelia could be approached surgically without morbidity.

Direct Approaches to Noncommunicating Syringomyelia

Methods

If surgery for syringomyelia-associated spinal arachnoiditis and deteriorating neurologic status is attempted, then the reconstruction of an alternative subarachnoid pathway around the area of ad-

FIGURE 7

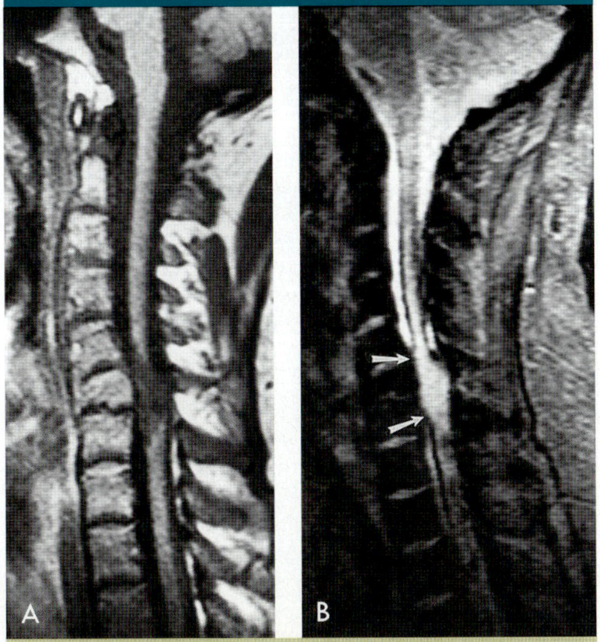

Figure 7 Expansile myelomalacia in a patient with a history of burst fracture of C6. **A,** T1-weighted sagittal image of the cervical spine demonstrates focal narrowing of the spinal canal at C6. There is abnormal, decreased signal of the spinal cord from C5-C6 to mid-C7, with focal cord expansion at C6. The area of abnormal cord signal has irregular borders, and the signal intensity is greater than that of the CSF. The spinal cord is atrophic above and below the level of injury. **B,** Midline gradient echo image from a cardiac gated cine acquisition shows the absence of CSF flow in the ventral aspect of the canal at C6-C7 (arrows). (Reproduced from Madsen PW III, Falcone S, Bowen BC, Green BA: Post-traumatic syringomyelia, in Levine AM, Eismont FJ, Garfin SR, Zigler JE, eds: *Spine Trauma*. Philadelphia, PA, WB Saunders, 1998, pp 608-629.)

FIGURE 8

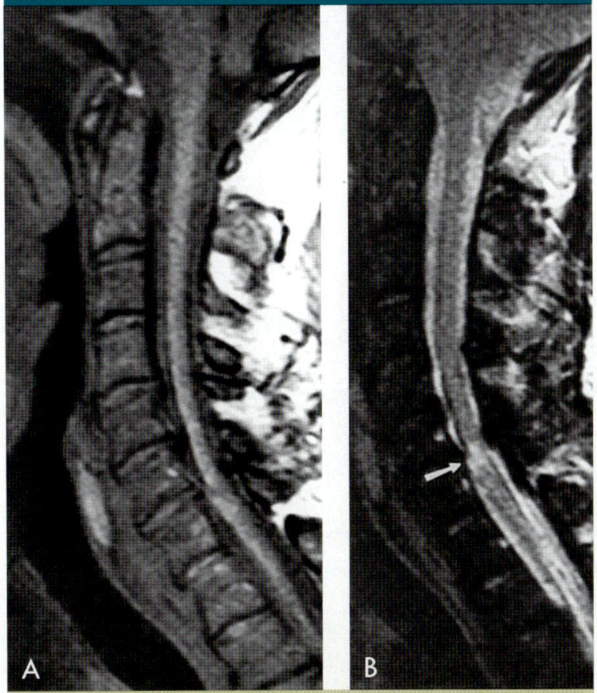

Figure 8 Compressive myelomalacia. Proton density (**A**) and T2-weighted (**B**) sagittal images of the cervical spine. Ventral and dorsal osteophytes compress the spinal cord at C6-C7. This is associated with a focal area of increased signal (arrow) on the T2-weighted image. The proton density image shows that the majority of the abnormal signal is greater than CSF. (Reproduced from Madsen PW III, Falcone S, Bowen BC, Green BA: Post-traumatic syringomyelia, in Levine AM, Eismont FJ, Garfin SR, Zigler JE, eds: *Spine Trauma*. Philadelphia, PA, WB Saunders, 1998, pp 608-629.)

hesion is essential.[51] A wide laminectomy, intradural exploration with limited dissection of adhesions to establish free communication with the subarachnoid space above and below the area of adhesion, and an expansile duraplasty are performed.

Preoperative drainage of an intramedullary cyst may be accompanied by rapid neurologic improvment, and surgical removal of the tumor almost always decompresses the syrinx.[42] However, delayed development of syringomyelia after spinal surgery may account for postoperative neurologic deterioration in some patients.[80]

Surgical intervention for a posttraumatic cyst was apparently first undertaken with good results, as reported by Freeman[81] in 1959; he advocated surgical drainage as the treatment of posttraumatic syringomyelia. An essential component of the surgery is untethering of the spinal cord and nerve root adhesions, as well as reduction of any bony gibbus or soft-tissue mass at the site of injury. This may first require a posterior approach for intradural exploration and untethering of the cord and root adhesions, followed by an anterior approach to remove any bony gibbus or soft-tissue mass. Others included reconstruction of the subarachnoid space with a surgical meningocele and the addition of a syringosubarachnoid shunt in maintaining the patency of the cyst into the subarachnoid space;[82,83] however, a shunt failure rate of 5% to 50% should be anticipated (**Table 2**).[48,61,65,82,84-88] The introduction of a foreign body in the form of a shunt tube and the surgical procedure may result in fixation of the cord to the dura by scar tissue and neurologic deterioration.[89]

Poussepp and Elsberg have been given credit for development of the midline myelotomy (the Elsberg-Poussepp operation) for treatment of

FIGURE 9

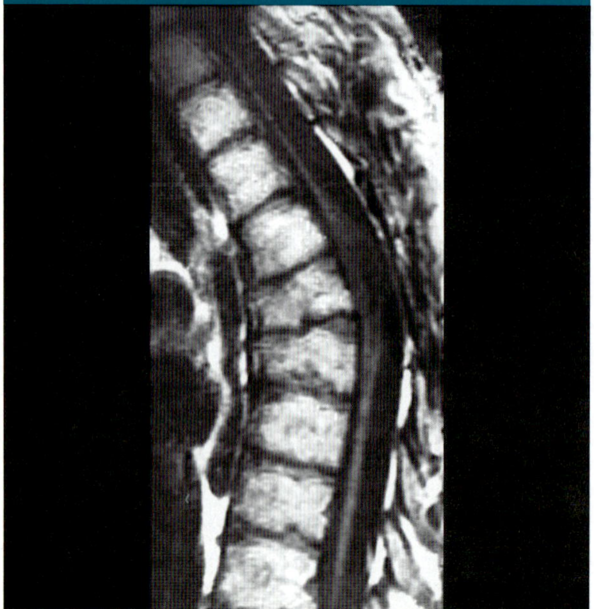

Figure 9 Expansile myelomalacia. The T1-weighted sagittal image of the lower thoracic cord demonstrates traumatic wedge deformities in two lower thoracic bodies, and an associated kyphotic deformity of the bony spinal column. At the level of the bony injury, the spinal cord is focally expanded and there is an abnormal, decreased signal in the cord parenchyma that is not as low as CSF signal intensity. The spinal cord is markedly atrophic above and below the injury level. (Reproduced from Madsen PW III, Falcone S, Bowen BC, Green BA: Post-traumatic syringomyelia, in Levine AM, Eismont FJ, Garfin SR, Zigler JE, eds: *Spine Trauma*. Philadelphia, PA, WB Saunders, 1998, pp 608-629.)

FIGURE 10

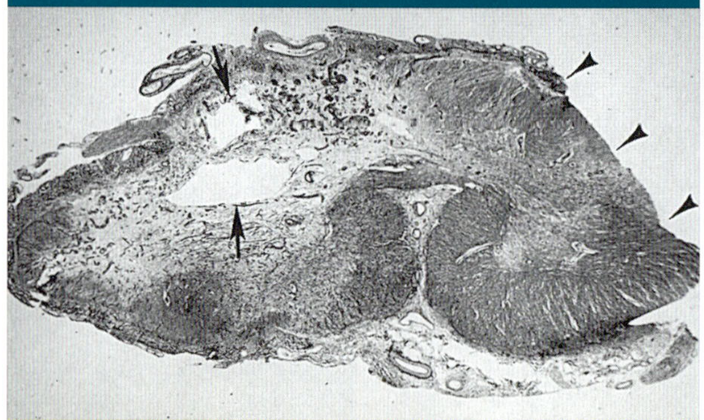

Figure 10 Microcystic myelomalacia in a 74-year-old man with ankylosing spondylitis who suffered a midcervical fracture-distraction injury and survived only 4 days after injury. Low-power (×1.25) microscopic section. (Reproduced from Madsen PW III, Falcone S, Bowen BC, Green BA: Post-traumatic syringomyelia, in Levine AM, Eismont FJ, Garfin SR, Zigler JE, eds: *Spine Trauma*. Philadelphia, PA, WB Saunders, 1998, pp 608-629.)

FIGURE 11

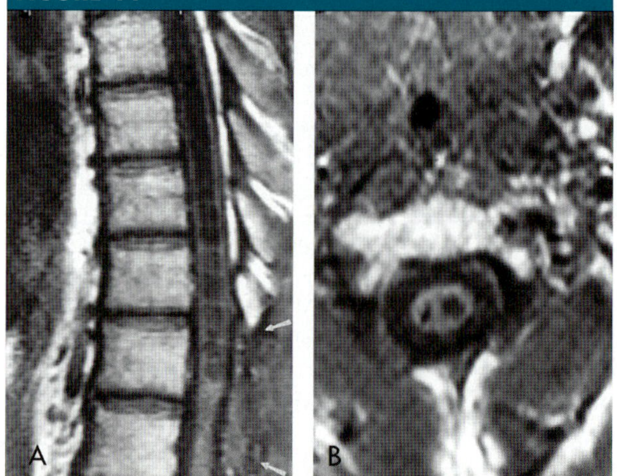

Figure 11 Posttraumatic cord cyst. A T1-weighted sagittal image (**A**) of the lower thoracic spinal cord and a T1-weighted axial image (**B**) at the C2 level. There is an expansile septated cyst of the spinal cord. The axial image demonstrates the "double-barrel" appearance of the cyst. There have been lower thoracic laminectomies (**A,** arrows). (Reproduced from Madsen PW III, Falcone S, Bowen BC, Green BA: Post-traumatic syringomyelia, in Levine AM, Eismont FJ, Garfin SR, Zigler JE, eds: *Spine Trauma*. Philadelphia, PA, WB Saunders, 1998, pp 608-629.)

spinal cord cysts.[71,90] Unlike Poussepp and Elsberg, Frazier[91] performed a paramedian myelotomy and attempted to marsupialize the syrinx into the subarachnoid space. A small 2-mm vertical myelotomy is usually performed in the midline at the dorsal median raphe. In the case of an eccentrically located cyst, the myelotomy is placed at the dorsal root entry zone rather than in the midline. In patients with double-barreled or multiloculated cysts (**Figure 11**), more than one myelotomy and shunt tube may be required. Whenever a syringosubarachnoid shunt is placed, several centimeters of shunt tubing should protrude from the myelotomy opening and into the distal subarachnoid space. If severe scarring with tethering of the spinal cord or obliteration of the subarachnoid space from a previous trauma or surgery is encountered, placement of a subarachnoid shunt tube in the conventional dorsal position is not adequate because of increased vulnerability to obstruction by scar tissue. In this situation, the distal shunt catheter may need to be placed in the ventral subarachnoid space by passing the shunt tubing laterally and caudally between the nerve roots. Syringosubarachnoid shunts work best when oriented so that fluid drains dependently in the upright position.

TABLE 2

Surgical Series Reporting Results of Syringomyelia Shunting Procedures

Authors (Year)	No. of Patients	Procedure Performed	Follow-up	Clinical Results
Tator et al (1982)[84]	20	Syringosubarachnoid shunting	Mean 5 y	75% excellent; 25% deterioration
Barbaro et al (1984)[61]	34	15 syringoperitoneal shunting; 19 syringosubarachnoid shunting	1.5-12 y	Syringoperitoneal shunt: 53% good, 27% fair, 20% poor; Syringosubarachnoid shunt: 32% good, 26% fair, 42% poor
Suzuki et al (1985)[85]	29	Syringoperitoneal shunt	Mean 1 y	76% improved; 17% unchanged; 7% deteriorated
Padovani et al (1989)[86]	29	Syringosubarachnoid shunting	Mean 5 y	31% improved; 59% stabilized; 10% deteriorated
Hida et al (1994)[48]	10	Syringosubarachnoid shunting; Syringoperitoneal shunting	NA	30% shunt malfunction
Sgouros and Williams (1995)[83]	73	56 syringoperitoneal shunting; 14 syringosubarachnoid shunting	NA	Only 53.5% of syringoperitoneal and 50% of syringosubarachnoid patients stable at 10 years; 15.7% complication rate; 5% shunt obstruction
Asano et al (1996)[65]	5	Syringosubarachnoid shunting	NA	40% obstruction; 20% deterioration
Batzdorf et al (1998)[87]	42	Syringosubarachnoid, syringoperitoneal, syringopleural shunting	NA	50% shunt failure
Schaller et al (1999)[88]	10	Syringoperitoneal shunting	Mean 44 mo	30% shunt obstruction or infection

NA = not available.

Meticulous hemostasis is important because blood at the surgical site may result in accelerated scarring and obstruction of the shunt tubing postoperatively.

After the initial shunting procedure, intraoperative ultrasonography is important to ensure that the entire cystic cavity is collapsed and that the shunt tubing is in good position.

Electromyographic monitoring complements motor- and somatosensory-evoked response monitoring to warn of compromise of the spinal cord or nerve roots.

Results

A recent review of surgery for syringomyelia through various approaches and techniques found that the reported effectiveness of surgical intervention had not changed in the past 100 years, with 67% to 76% patients improving neurologically postoperatively.[92] Only the mortality rate had decreased, from 5% to 1% in recent surgical series.

Barnett[37] reported that management of patients with arachnoiditis was unrewarding, whether medical or surgical therapy was attempted. He considered both steroids and lysis of adhesions to be ineffective in the treatment of this disorder.

Although effective in several small surgical series,[3,25,61,85,86] the placement of a syringoperitoneal or syringosubarachnoid shunt is of questionable value.[37,82,83] The optimal treatment and determination of the indications for surgery await further research with relevant experimental models and a well-designed, multicenter clinical trial.[92]

Tables 2[48,61,82,84-88] and **3**[72,93-96] list some of the major surgical series in treating noncommunicating syringomyelia, represented most prominently by posttraumatic syringomyelia, with lysis of adhesions and/or shunting of the syrinx. Overall, they show surgical treatment of posttraumatic syringomyelia to be of modest reward. Many

TABLE 3

Surgical Series Reporting Results of Procedures on Noncommunicating Syringes

Author(s) (Year)	No. of Patients	Procedure(s) Performed	Follow-up	Clinical Results
Adelstein (1938)[93]	86	Laminectomy; myelotomy	NA	76% improved; 12% worsened
Pitts and Groff (1964)[94]	33 (46 procedures)	Laminectomy; laminectomy + myelotomy; laminectomy + drainage	2-31 y	16% good; 49% fair; 36% poor
Love and Olafson (1966)[95]	35	Laminectomy; laminectomy + syrinx aspiration; laminectomy + syringosubarachnoid shunt	1-10 y	29% excellent; 34% good or unchanged; 23% poor; 14% lost to follow-up
Anderson et al (1985)[96]	11	7 laminectomy + syrinx aspiration; 4 laminectomy + syringostomy	Mean 11.8 y (1.3-18.5 y)	18% improvement; 9% no progression; 73% deterioration
Lee et al (2001)[72]	45	Laminectomy + untethering + duraplasty; laminectomy + syringosubarachnoid shunting + duraplasty	Mean 22.5 mo (12-84 mo)	73% satisfactory; 20% unchanged; 7% deteriorated

NA = not available.

patients show short-term recovery of neurologic function, only to deteriorate again in long-term follow-up.

Authors' Preferred Approach to the Diagnosis and Treatment of Progressive Posttraumatic Cystic Myelopathy

The initial evaluation of patients suspected of having a spinal cord syrinx or cyst should include a comprehensive history and physical and neurologic examination. The neurologic examination should always include a detailed motor assessment, using the standard 0 to 5 scale and a multimodality sensory evaluation, testing either pain or temperature for the anterolateral columns and either vibration or position sense for the dorsal columns. A rectal examination should be carefully performed and should include an evaluation of volitional sphincter control and a multimodality sensory assessment of the perianal area. Reflexes are the least reliable part of neurologic assessment, but side-to-side asymmetries or the presence of a pathologic sign such as Babinski reflex is important to document. Because some spinal cord cysts are continuous rostrally past the foramen magnum and into the brainstem, a careful examination of cerebral, cerebellar, and cranial nerve function should be part of the initial neurologic examination.

Once a detailed history and physical and neurologic assessment are complete and documented, the information obtained will guide the imaging studies. Imaging tests should always include a plain radiographic series of the involved spinal levels and flexion and extension views to rule out any mechanical instability. A high-resolution CT scan with thin slices and bone and soft-tissue windows provides valuable information in planning surgical management. These studies are enhanced with sagittal, coronal, and three-dimensional reconstructions.

Currently, the most sensitive imaging test for soft tissue is the new-generation high-resolution MRI. Initial MRI examination should include, as a minimum, sagittal and transverse views of the lesion plus the adjacent spinal cord and brainstem tissue in T1-weighted images. Administration of gadolinium can be quite beneficial in defining scar, infected, or neoplastic tissue. The addition of either T2-weighted or mixed proton-density scans can complement but not replace the T1-weighted views. Fast spin-echo techniques increase the amount of T2-weighted information in the presence of metallic artifact, seen frequently after an instrumented fusion, because they decrease magnetic susceptibility effects.[97,98] Inclusion of the entire rostrocaudal extent of each cyst is important. Gadolinium-enhanced images are helpful in defining scar tissue associated with a syrinx in posttraumatic cases.

Although certain institutions continue to use air myelography or conventional myelography with delayed CT-enhanced images,[99] we believe that MRI techniques are the test of choice for the initial evaluation and postoperative follow-up of cystic spinal cord lesions. The only exception to this generalization concerns cases where metal wires, rods, plates, screws or other instrumentation, or bullet fragments degrade the MRI sufficiently to prevent adequate anatomic assessment. In these cases, a myelogram in combination with immediate and delayed high-resolution CT, which cuts through the area of the syrinx, is performed. The delayed CT scans are obtained anywhere from 4 to 8 hours to as long as 12 to 24 hours in some institutions, but we find a 6- to 8-hour period after the initial myelogram and CT study to be adequate. Difficulty in the differentiation of myelomalacia from a confluent syrinx represents a significant limitation of this technique and may lead to unnecessary surgical intervention. Myelography does, however, allow diagnosis of a fissure, as the associated intramedullary cyst fills rapidly compared to a cyst not associated with a fissure. The latter lesion depends upon transependymal migration of the contrast agent over a period of several hours before becoming visible. The patients with a fissure will typically develop symptoms from the cystic lesion within weeks of the initial trauma, in contrast to PPCM without a fissure or PPMM, which most often becomes symptomatic a minimum of 3 months after injury.

Real-time ultrasound may be useful for postoperative follow-up studies of patients undergoing a laminectomy. This procedure is much more effective and feasible in young children or thinner patients than in patients with a large soft-tissue mass over the lesion. The evolution of MRI has decreased the need for ultrasound for postoperative evaluation of these patients.

Multimodality neurophysiologic assessment includes an electromyography (EMG) study and both somatosensory-evoked potentials (SSEPs) and motor-evoked potentials (MEPs) for evaluation of the afferent and efferent spinal cord pathways plus the local H-reflex.[100] Electrical cortical stimulation is used for intraoperative MEP monitoring, whereas magnetic transcortical stimulation[101] is more appropriate for awake patients as an outpatient or inpatient assessment tool. Real-time EMG is the most useful intraoperative monitoring technique in the cervical and lumbar levels as it affords immediate feedback and does not require the computer averaging on which SSEP and MEP monitoring depend. Urodynamics can add invaluable information regarding the status of the patient's bladder and sphincter function. The combination of physical and neurologic examination findings plus imaging studies supplemented by the neurophysiologic assessment battery provides an important database for the clinician to consult when planning therapy.

Up to 10% of patients suffering a traumatic spinal cord injury experience a progressive spinal cord dysfunction associated with an expanding syrinx.[49,72] Symptoms are usually accompanied by rostral extension of the cyst from the lesion site but may also accompany a caudal extension. The majority of these patients have the spinal cord tethered by either soft-tissue scar, a bony gibbus, or a combination of both. Scar tissue tethering is most frequently dorsal because the majority of these patients spend several days in the supine position, and the spinal cord assumes a dependent position abutting the dorsal dura. As blood congeals and scar tissue forms, the pulped spinal cord is tethered to the dura. In the majority of cases where a bony gibbus or herniated disk material tethers the cord locally, the ventral aspect of the spinal column is involved. Ventral tethering presents an extraordinary technical challenge. An anterior approach with corpectomy is required for safe and effective untethering; blind attempts to untether the spinal cord from a posterior approach can lead to devastating cord injury from damage to the anterior spinal artery complex. Although the majority of intramedullary cysts are localized in the dorsal central area of the spinal cord (ie, the dorsal gray matter and adjacent white matter), a significant number present as eccentric unilateral cysts or even double- or triple-barreled complex lesions. These cysts may be connected at the rostral or caudal end of the lesion, although they sometimes remain totally independent of each other.

The subarachnoid cysts associated with posttraumatic cysts, in contrast to congenital subarachnoid cysts, have a thinner wall and contain the same clear CSF as found in the adjacent subarachnoid space. They also are more firmly anchored to the adjacent dura and do not present with the same gallbladder or balloon-type configuration characteristic of congenital lesions. A rare variation of this lesion is a traumatic pseudomeningocele, which can create an epidural compressive lesion on the spinal cord and may be difficult to identify on routine MRI.

There is little consensus among clinicians regarding the surgical management of posttraumatic syringomyelia, and many neurosurgeons contend that there is no effective surgical treatment. These practitioners believe that patients should ultimately resign themselves to accepting their fate—a progressive neurologic deterioration to complete paralysis or even death. Less controversial is the doctrine that the asymptomatic syringes should not be treated.

Our basic criteria for surgical treatment of posttraumatic cysts has been the presence of one or more signs and symptoms of PPCM. Normally, cysts less than 1 cm in rostrocaudal extent are not considered to be of an adequate size for successful shunting and are, therefore, followed with serial MRI and clinical observation. Surgical management of a posttraumatic syrinx requires preoperative assessment of several factors, including the rostrocaudal extent of the cyst(s), the exact location in the spinal cord parenchyma, the relationship of associated intramedullary or subarachnoid cysts, and the presence of a fissure. An essential component of the surgery is the untethering of the spinal cord and nerve root adhesions, as well as reduction of any bony gibbus or soft-tissue mass at the site of injury. This may first require a posterior approach for intradural exploration and untethering the cord and root adhesions, followed by an anterior approach for removing any bony gibbus or soft-tissue mass. The second essential component of a surgical treatment protocol should be shunting of the spinal cord cyst(s) to the subarachnoid space or fenestration or resection of any associated subarachnoid cyst to allow unrestricted communication with an adjacent patent subarachnoid space. The senior author (B.A.G.) favors spinal cord cysts-to-subarachnoid space shunts over cyst-to-peritoneal or cyst-to-pleural shunts. With aggressive lysis of adhesions in the subarachnoid space and the addition of an expansile duraplasty, the need for extraspinal shunts have all but been eliminated except in those rare cases associated with acute arachnoiditis. This should be done using illumination and magnification either from loupes and headlight or the operating microscope under real-time ultrasonography guidance.

Exploration and shunting of the intramedullary cyst should always proceed from the caudal end, with the tube being directed up toward the rostral extent of the cyst. If the tube will not traverse the entire length of the cyst, the possibility exists that the rostral part of the cyst will become loculated and symptomatic. Some syringes extend from the conus up into the brainstem and one shunt tube may not be adequate to drain the lesion. Passage of the shunt tube may be obstructed by the thoracic kyphosis. In this instance, a single-level laminectomy is performed at the caudal end of the cyst and a second laminectomy is performed just below the innervation of the hands (ie, at approximately T2). Cyst-to-peritoneal or cyst-to-pleural shunts are performed via myelotomies at both levels and the upper shunt is guided into the most rostral extent of the lesion under intraoperative radiographic control to avoid kinking of the tube and to verify proper tube placement.

A small 2-mm vertical myelotomy is usually performed in the midline, avoiding the loops of the dorsal central vein of the spinal cord. The myelotomy is usually performed with a No. 11 blade, which we have found to be more accurate and less destructive than a microlaser. In the case of an eccentrically placed cyst, the myelotomy is placed in the dorsal root entry zone rather than in the midline. In cases with double-barreled or multiloculated cysts, more than one myelotomy and shunt tube may be required. Ventricular, peritoneal, or lumboperitoneal shunt tubing is modified for shunting spinal cord cysts. Extra holes are cut in the proximal and distal ends to enhance free CSF flow.

The incorporation of a freeze-dried dural allograft or fascia lata autograft is recommended to create a locally enlarged subarachnoid space and an environment less likely to scar and posteriorly retether to the spinal cord. Patients should be positioned in the prone position for shunt placement so as to optimize real-time ultrasound assessment, which is mandatory to ensure successful cyst collapse and obliteration intraoperatively.

The maintenance of meticulous intradural hemostasis is important, because blood in the surgical site can result in accelerated scarring and retethering of the spinal cord postoperatively. Spinal cord bleeding is best managed with a piece of thrombin-soaked absorbable gelatin sponge, microbipolar coagulation, or both. Perioperative intravenous antibiotics, steroids, and mild hypothermia are routinely used in our institution. After the initial shunting procedure, it is essential to repeat real-time ultrasound with sagittal and transverse images to ensure that the entire cystic cavity is collapsed and the shunt tube is in good position. This imaging technique is particularly useful to verify successful treatment of both parts of a confluent double-barreled cystic lesion when attempting to use a single catheter.

While subarachnoid cysts may be adequately treated by resection and removal of the cyst wall, some cases require a subarachnoid cyst-to-subarachnoid space shunt tube for adequate drainage. Some patients with a combination of subarachnoid and intramedullary cysts connected by a fistula have been adequately treated with a wide removal of the subarachnoid cyst wall. In these cases, it is not necessary to stent the fissure, but when the fissure is less apparent, a shunt needs to be placed.

All cases of PPCM are preceded by percutaneous placement of a lumbar, thoracic, or C1-C2 CSF drain placement. The CSF drain is continued for 5 to 7 days postoperatively to allow for healing of the suture line for the duraplasty. During this period, the patient is kept with the head of the bed at 0° and turned semiprone to semiprone every 2 hours to prevent CSF leak, pseudomeningocele formation, and retethering in this immediate postoperative period.

We have not had any obvious success with medical management that uses steroids or nonsteroidal anti-inflammatory agents in preventing retethering. We have had some early, intriguing responses with interferon and immunosuppressive agents, usually reserved for patients with keloid and hypertrophic scar formation.[102] However, more work in the laboratory and long-term clinical follow-up is needed.

Conclusions

Although technologic advances in noninvasive imaging methods have improved the ability to diagnose syringomyelia, effective therapy for these lesions has not similarly evolved. The accumulated experience of surgical therapy for these lesions has affirmed that the use of a foreign body (shunt tube) is not optimal and that reinsertion of the shunt or the lysis of adhesions frequently causes the production of additional scar tissue. On the other hand, surgical treatment of communicating syringomyelia associated with Chiari malformations, like its pathophysiology, is more established and better understood, leading to more rewarding surgical results and clinical outcomes. The research laboratory, particularly in pharmacologic treatment, holds the key to the ultimate solution for the problem of syringomyelia.

References

1. Finlayson AI: Syringomyelia and related conditions, in Joynt RJ, ed: *Clinical Neurology*. Phildelphia, PA, JB Lippincott, 1989, vol 3, pp 1-17.
2. Wilson SA: Syringomyelia: Syringobulbia, in Bruce AN, ed: *Neurology*. Baltimore, MD, Williams & Wilkins, 1955, vol 2, pp 1187-1202.
3. Ballantine HT, Ojemann RG, Drew JH: Syringomyelia, in Kraybuhl H, Maspes PE, Sweet WH, eds: *Progress in Neurological Surgery*. New York, NY, S Karger, 1971, vol 4, pp 227-245.
4. Foster JB, Hudgson P: Historical introduction, in Barnett HJM, Foster JB, Hudgson P, eds: *Syringomyelia*. London, United Kingdom, WB Saunders Co, 1973, pp 3-10.
5. Hoffman HJ, Neill J, Crone KR, Hendrick EB, Humphreys RP: Hydrosyringomyelia and its management in childhood. *Neurosurgery* 1987;21(3): 347-351.
6. Williams B: Progress in syringomyelia. *Neurol Res* 1986;8(3):130-145.
7. Barnett HJ: The epilogue, in Barnett HJM, Foster JB, Hudgson P, eds: *Syringomyelia*. London, United Kingdom, WB Saunders Co, 1973, pp 302-313.
8. Milhorat TH, Capocelli AL Jr, Anzil AP, Kotzen RM, Milhorat RH: Pathological basis of spinal cord cavitation in syringomyelia: Analysis of 105 autopsy cases. *J Neurosurg* 1995;82(5):802-812.
9. Milhorat TH, Johnson RW, Milhorat RH, Capocelli AL Jr, Pevsner PH: Clinicopathological correlations in syringomyelia using axial magnetic resonance imaging. *Neurosurgery* 1995;37(2): 206-213.
10. Milhorat TH, Johnson WD, Miller JI, Bergland RM, Hollenberg-Sher J: Surgical treatment of syringomyelia based on magnetic resonance imaging criteria. *Neurosurgery* 1992;31(2):231-245.
11. Milhorat TH, Kotzen RM, Anzil AP: Stenosis of central canal of spinal cord in man: Incidence and pathological findings in 232 autopsy cases. *J Neurosurg* 1994;80(4):716-722.
12. Milhorat TH, Miller JI, Johnson WD, Adler DE, Heger IM: Anatomical basis of syringomyelia occurring with hindbrain lesions. *Neurosurgery* 1993;32(5):748-754.
13. Milhorat TH, Nobandegani F, Miller JI, Rao C: Noncommunicating syringomyelia following occlusion of central canal in rats: Experimental model and histological findings. *J Neurosurg* 1993; 78(2):274-279.
14. Oldfield EH, Muraszko K, Shawker TH, Patronas NJ: Pathophysiology of syringomyelia associated with Chiari I malformation of the cerebellar tonsils: Implications for diagnosis and treatment. *J Neurosurg* 1994;80(1):3-15.

15. Tamaki K, Lubin AJ: Pathogenesis of syringomyelia: Case illustrating the process of cavity formation from embryonic cell rests. *Arch Neurol Psychiatry* 1938;40(4):748-761.

16. Poser CM: *The Relationship Between Syringomyelia and Neoplasm*. Springfield, IL, Charles C. Thomas, 1956.

17. MacKay RP, Favill J: Syringomyelia and intramedullary tumor of the spinal cord. *Arch Neurol Psychiatry* 1935;33:1255-1278.

18. Gardner WJ: Anatomic anomalies common to myelomeningocele of infancy and syringomyelia of adulthood suggest a common origin. *Cleve Clin Q* 1959;26:118-133.

19. Gardner WJ: Diastematomyelia and the Klippel-Feil syndrome. *Cleve Clin Q* 1964;31:19-44.

20. Gardner WJ: Hydrodynamic mechanism of syringomyelia: Its relationship to myelocele. *J Neurol Neurosurg Psychiatry* 1965;28:247-259.

21. Gardner WJ: Myelocele: Rupture of the neural tube? in Ojemann RG, ed: *Clinical Neurosurgery*. Baltimore, MD, Waverly Press, 1968, vol 15, pp 57-79.

22. Gardner WJ, Angel J: The mechanism of syringomyelia and its surgical correction, in Fisher RG, ed: *Clinical Neurosurgery*. Baltimore, MD, Waverly Press, 1959, vol 6, pp 131-140.

23. Gardner WJ, McMurray FG: "Non-communicating" syringomyelia: A non-existent entity. *Surg Neurol* 1976;6(4):251-256.

24. McLaurin RL, Bailey OT, Schurr PH, Ingraham FD: Myelomalacia and multiple cavitations of spinal cord secondary to adhesive arachnoiditis: An experimental study. *AMA Arch Pathol* 1954;57(2):138-146.

25. West RJ, Williams B: Radiographic studies of the ventricles in syringomyelia. *Neuroradiology* 1980;20(1):5-16.

26. Ball MJ, Dayan AD: Pathogenesis of syringomyelia. *Lancet* 1972;2(7781):799-801.

27. Williams B: The distending force in the production of "communicating syringomyelia." *Lancet* 1969;2(7613):189-193.

28. Williams B: Cerebrospinal fluid pressure changes in response to coughing. *Brain* 1976;99(2):331-346.

29. Williams B: On the pathogenesis of syringomyelia: A review. *J R Soc Med* 1980;73(11):798-806.

30. Gardner WJ, Goodall RJ: The surgical treatment of Arnold-Chiari malformation in adults: An explanation of its mechanism and importance of encephalography in diagnosis. *J Neurosurg* 1950;7(3):199-206.

31. Gardner WJ, Abdullah AF, McCormack LJ: The varying expressions of embryonal atresia of the fourth ventricle in adults: Arnold-Chiari malformation, Dandy-Walker syndrome, arachnoid cyst of the cerebellum, and syringomyelia. *J Neurosurg* 1957;14(6):591-605.

32. Appleby A, Bradley WG, Foster JB, Hankinson J, Hudgson P: Syringomyelia due to chronic arachnoiditis at the foramen magnum. *J Neurol Sci* 1969;8(3):451-464.

33. Liber AF, Lisa JR: Rosenthal fibers in non-neoplastic syringomyelia: A note on the pathogenesis of syringomyelia. *J Nerv Ment Dis* 1937;86:549-559.

34. Nelson J: Intramedullary cavitation resulting from adhesive spinal arachnoiditis. *AMA Arch Neurol Psychiatry* 1943;50(1):1-7.

35. Caplan LR, Norohna AB, Amico LL: Syringomyelia and arachnoiditis. *J Neurol Neurosurg Psychiatry* 1990;53(2):106-113.

36. Chang HS, Nakagawa H: Theoretical analysis of the pathophysiology of syringomyelia associated with adhesive arachnoiditis. *J Neurol Neurosurg Psychiatry* 2004;75(5):754-757.

37. Barnett HJ: Syringomyelia associated with spinal arachnoiditism, in Barnett HJM, Foster JB, Hudgson P, eds: *Syringomyelia*. London, United Kingdom, WB Saunders Co, 1973, pp 220-244.

38. Barnett HJ, Rewcastle NB: Syringomyelia and tumours of the nervous system, in Barnett HJM, Foster JB, Hudgson P, eds: *Syringomyelia*. London, United Kingdom, WB Saunders Co, 1973, pp 261-301.

39. Feigin I, Ogata J, Budzilovich G: Syringomyelia: The role of edema in its pathogenesis. *J Neuropathol Exp Neurol* 1971;30(2):216-232.

40. Russell DS: Capillary haemangeioma of spinal cord associated with syringomyelia. *J Pathol Bacteriol* 1932;35:103-112.

41. Ferry DJ, Hardman JM, Earle KM: Syringomyelia and intramedullary neoplasms. *Med Ann Dist Columbia* 1969;38(7):363-365.

42. Peerless SJ, Durward QJ: Management of syringomyelia: A pathophysiological approach, in Weiss MH, ed: *Clinical Neurosurgery*. Baltimore, MD, Williams & Wilkins, 1983, vol 30, pp 531-576.

43. Slooff JL, Kernohan JW, MacCarty CS: *Primary Intramedullary Tumors of the Spinal Cord and Filum Terminale*. Philadelphia, PA, WB Saunders Co, 1964.

44. Conway LW: Hydrodynamic studies in syringomyelia. *J Neurosurg* 1967;27(6):501-514.

45. Putnam TJ: Syringomyelia–diagnosis and treatment. *Med Clin North Am* 1936;19:1571-1582.

46. Wechsler IS: Syringomyelia (including spinal gliosis), in *A Textbook of Clinical Neurology*. Philadelphia, PA, WB Saunders Co, 1927, pp 159-164.

47. Samii M, Klekamp J: Surgical results of 100 intramedullary tumors in relation to accompanying syringomyelia. *Neurosurgery* 1994;35(5):865-873.
48. Hida K, Iwasaki Y, Imamura H, Abe H: Posttraumatic syringomyelia: Its characteristic magnetic resonance imaging findings and surgical management. *Neurosurgery* 1994;35(5):886-891.
49. Griffiths ER, McCormick CC: Post-traumatic syringomyelia (cystic myelopathy). *Paraplegia* 1981; 19(2):81-88.
50. Rossier AB, Foo D, Shillito J, Dyro FM: Posttraumatic cervical syringomyelia: Incidence, clinical presentation, electrophysiological studies, syrinx protein and results of conservative and operative treatment. *Brain* 1985;108(Pt 2):439-461.
51. Schurch B, Wichmann W, Rossier AB: Post-traumatic syringomyelia (cystic myelopathy): A prospective study of 449 patients with spinal cord injury. *J Neurol Neurosurg Psychiatry* 1996;60(1): 61-67.
52. Cushing HW: Haematomyelia from gunshot wounds of the spine: A report of two cases, with recovery following symptoms of hemilesion of the cord. *Am J Med Sci* 1898;115:654-683.
53. Fairholm DJ, Turnbull IM: Microangiographic study of experimental spinal cord injuries. *J Neurosurg* 1971;35:277-286.
54. Holmes G: The Goulstonian lectures on spinal injuries of warfare: Part I. The pathology of acute spinal injury. *BMJ* 1915;2:769-774.
55. Kao TCC, Chang LW: The mechanism of spinal cord cavitation following spinal cord transection. *J Neurosurg* 1977;46(2):197-209.
56. Kao CC, Chang LW, Bloodworth JM Jr: The mechanism of spinal cord cavitation following spinal cord transection: Part 2. Electron microscope observations. *J Neurosurg* 1977;46(6): 745-756.
57. Mair WG, Druckman R: The pathology of spinal cord lesions and their relation to the clinical features in protrusion of cervical intervertebral discs; a report of four cases. *Brain* 1953;76(1):70-91.
58. McVeigh JF: Experimental cord crushes: With special reference to the mechanical factors involved and subsequent changes in the areas of the cord affected. *Arch Surg* 1923;7:573-600.
59. Wolman L: The disturbance of circulation in traumatic paraplegia in acute and late stages: A pathological study. *Paraplegia* 1965;2:213-226.
60. Woodard JS, Freeman LW: Ischemia of the spinal cord; an experimental study. *J Neurosurg* 1956; 13(1):63-72.
61. Barbaro NM, Wilson CB, Gutin PH, Edwards MS: Surgical treatment of syringomyelia: Favorable results with syringoperitoneal shunting. *J Neurosurg* 1984;61(3):531-538.
62. Hughes JT: Pathological changes after spinal cord injury, in Illis LS, ed: *Spinal Cord Dysfunction: Assessment*. Oxford, United Kingdom, Oxford University Press, 1988, pp 34-44
63. Stoodley MA, Jones NR, Brown CJ: Evidence for rapid fluid flow from the subarachnoid space into the spinal cord central canal in the rat. *Brain Res* 1996;707(2):155-164.
64. Williams B: Simultaneous cerebral and spinal fluid pressure recordings: 2. Cerebrospinal dissociation with lesions at the foramen magnum. *Acta Neurochir (Wien)* 1981;59(1-2):123-142.
65. Asano M, Fujiwara K, Yonenobu K, Hiroshima K: Post-traumatic syringomyelia. *Spine (Phila Pa 1976)* 1996;21(12):1446-1453.
66. Dyste GN, Menezes AH, VanGilder JC: Symptomatic Chiari malformations: An analysis of presentation, management, and long-term outcome. *J Neurosurg* 1989;71(2):159-168.
67. Hall PV, Lindseth RE, Campbell RL, Kallsbeck JE: Myelodysplasia and developmental scoliosis: A manifestation of syringomyelia. *Spine (Phila Pa 1976)* 1976;1:48-56.
68. Schlesinger EB, Antunes JL, Michelsen WJ, Louis KM: Hydromyelia: Clinical presentation and comparison of modalities of treatment. *Neurosurgery* 1981;9(4):356-365.
69. Zager EL, Ojemann RG, Poletti CE: Acute presentations of syringomyelia: Report of three cases. *J Neurosurg* 1990;72(1):133-138.
70. Boman K, Iivanainen M: Prognosis of syringomyelia. *Acta Neurol Scand* 1967;43(1):61-68.
71. Edgar R, Quail P: Progressive post-traumatic cystic and non-cystic myelopathy. *Br J Neurosurg* 1994;8(1):7-22.
72. Lee TT, Alameda GJ, Camilo E, Green BA: Surgical treatment of post-traumatic myelopathy associated with syringomyelia. *Spine (Phila Pa 1976)* 2001;26(24, Suppl):S119-S127.
73. Falcone S, Quencer RM, Green BA, Patchen SJ, Post MJ: Progressive posttraumatic myelomalacic myelopathy: Imaging and clinical features. *AJNR Am J Neuroradiol* 1994;15(4):747-754.
74. Honan WP, Williams B: Sensory loss in syringomyelia: Not necessarily dissociated. *J R Soc Med* 1993;86(9):519-520.
75. Pojunas K, Williams AL, Daniels DL, Haughton VM: Syringomyelia and hydromyelia: Magnetic resonance evaluation. *Radiology* 1984;153(3): 679-683.
76. Slasky BS, Bydder GM, Niendorf HP, Young IR: MR imaging with gadolinium-DTPA in the differentiation of tumor, syrinx, and cyst of the spinal cord. *J Comput Assist Tomogr* 1987;11(5):845-850.
77. Quencer RM, Post MJ, Hinks RS: Cine MR in the evaluation of normal and abnormal CSF flow:

Intracranial and intraspinal studies. *Neuroradiology* 1990;32(5):371-391.

78. Sotaniemi KA, Pyhtinen J, Myllylä VV: Computed tomography in the diagnosis of syringomyelia. *Acta Neurol Scand* 1983;68(2):121 127.
79. Abbe R, Coley W: Syringomyelia, operation exploration of cord, withdrawal of fluid, exhibition of patient. *J Nerv Ment Dis* 1892;19:512-520.
80. Quencer RM, Morse BM, Green GA, Eismont FJ, Brost P: Intraoperative spinal sonography: Adjunct to metrizamide CT in the assessment and surgical decompression of posttraumatic spinal cord cysts. *ARJ Am J Roentgenol* 1984;142(3): 593-601.
81. Freeman LW: Ascending spinal paralysis; case presentation. *J Neurosurg* 1959;16(1):120-122.
82. Sgouros S, Williams B: Management and outcome of posttraumatic syringomyelia. *J Neurosurg* 1996; 85(2):197-205.
83. Sgouros S, Williams B: A critical appraisal of drainage in syringomyelia. *J Neurosurg* 1995; 82(1):1-10.
84. Tator CH, Meguro K, Rowed DW: Favorable results with syringosubarachnoid shunts for treatment of syringomyelia. *J Neurosurg* 1982;56(4): 517-523.
85. Suzuki M, Davis C, Symon L, Gentili F: Syringoperitoneal shunt for treatment of cord cavitation. *J Neurol Neurosurg Psychiatry* 1985;48(7):620-627.
86. Padovani R, Cavallo M, Gaist G: Surgical treatment of syringomyelia: Favorable results with syringosubarachnoid shunting. *Surg Neurol* 1989; 32(3):173-180.
87. Batzdorf U, Klekamp J, Johnson JP: A critical appraisal of syrinx cavity shunting procedures. *J Neurosurg* 1998;89(3):382-388.
88. Schaller B, Mindermann T, Gratzl O: Treatment of syringomyelia after posttraumatic paraparesis or tetraparesis. *J Spinal Disord* 1999;12(6):485-488.
89. Steinmetz A, Aschoff A, Kunze S: The iatrogenic tethering of the cord. *Acta Neurochir (Wien)* 1993; 123:219-220.
90. Elsberg CA: *Surgical Diseases of the Spinal Cord.* New York, NY, PB Hoeber, 1941, pp 551-553.
91. Frazier CH: Shall syringomyelia be added to the lesions appropriate for surgical intervention? *JAMA* 1930;95:1911-1912.
92. Aschoff A, Donauer E, Huwel N, et al: Evaluation of syrinx-surgery: A critical comment on requirements for reliable follow-up studies. *Acta Neurochir (Wien)* 1993;123:224-225.
93. Adelstein LJ. The surgical treatment of syringomyelia. *Am J Surg* 1938;40:384-395.
94. Pitts FW, Groff RA: Syringomyelia: Current status of surgical therapy. *Surgery* 1964;56:806-809.
95. Love JG, Olafson RA: Syringomyelia: A look at surgical therapy. *J Neurosurg* 1966;24(4):714-718.
96. Anderson NE, Willoughby EW, Wrightson P: The natural history and the influence of surgical treatment in syringomyelia. *Acta Neurol Scand* 1985; 71(6):472-479.
97. Rudisch A, Kremser C, Peer S, Kathrein A, Judmaier W, Daniaux H: Metallic artifacts in magnetic resonance imaging of patients with spinal fusion: A comparison of implant materials and imaging sequences. *Spine (Phila Pa 1976)* 1998; 23(6):692-699.
98. Tartaglino LM, Flanders AE, Vinitski S, Friedman DP: Metallic artifacts on MR images of the postoperative spine: Reduction with fast spin-echo techniques. *Radiology* 1994;190(2):565-569.
99. Stevens JM, Olney JS, Kendall BE: Post-traumatic cystic and non-cystic myelopathy. *Neuroradiology* 1985;27(1):48-56.
100. Calancie B, Harris W, Broton JG, Alexeeva N, Green BA: "Threshold-level" multipulse transcranial electrical stimulation of motor cortex for intraoperative monitoring of spinal motor tracts: Description of method and comparison to somatosensory evoked potential monitoring. *J Neurosurg* 1998;88(3):457-470.
101. Eisen AA, Shtybel W: AAEM minimonograph #35: Clinical experience with transcranial magnetic stimulation. *Muscle Nerve* 1990;13(11): 995-1011.
102. Berman B, Villa AM, Ramirez CC: Novel opportunities in the treatment and prevention of scarring. *J Cutan Med Surg* 2004;8(Suppl 3):32-36.

CHAPTER 39
Complications of the Musculoskeletal System Following Spinal Cord Injury

Michael J. Botte, MD   William J. Peace, MD   Lorenzo L. Pacelli, MD

Acute spinal cord injury (SCI) results in the well-recognized disability from limb dysfunction.[1-3] However, other associated extremity problems commonly occur, resulting in further functional loss, interference with patients' independence, and additional emotional stress. Anson and Shepherd[4] noted that of 348 patients with postacute SCI, more that 95% of the patients reported at least one significant secondary problem, and more than half reported three or more. In a recent study, 8% required rehospitalization within 5 years of their original rehabilitation, with an average length of stay of 72 days.[5] Although many extremity problems are unavoidable or result from the initial SCI, many associated problems or complications may be avoided or minimized with preventive care and with prompt diagnosis and management.[5-20] This chapter reviews the additional musculoskeletal complications that can occur in the patient with an SCI. The complications are divided into the following sections: (1) complications involving the bones and joints, (2) complications involving muscle, (3) complications associated with overuse of the upper extremity for weight bearing in the paraplegic patient, and (4) miscellaneous complications (**Table 1**).

Complications Involving Bones and Joints

Two common complications involving bone and joints are fractures in the extremities and neurogenic heterotopic ossification.

Dr. Pacelli or an immediate family member has received royalties from Ascension Orthopedics; is a member of a speakers' bureau or has made paid presentations on behalf of Ascension Orthopedics; and serves as a paid consultant to or is an employee of Ascension Orthopedics. Neither of the following authors or any immediate family member has received anything of value from or owns stock in a commercial company or institution related directly or indirectly to the subject of this chapter: Dr. Botte and Dr. Peace.

Extremity Fractures

Fractures in the extremities of the SCI patient present unique problems with both diagnosis and treatment.[21-38] These fractures can be divided into two main types: (1) acute fractures sustained in normal bone at the time of SCI and (2) subsequent pathologic fractures sustained in osteoporotic bone in the patient with a long-standing paretic extremity.[35] In addition, a third type of fracture will be briefly discussed—a fracture sustained in a normal limb above the level of paralysis in a patient with long-standing SCI.[23,33]

Acute Fractures Sustained at the Time of SCI

Acute fractures sustained at the time of SCI occur in previously normal bone and usually involve high-speed injuries.[23,33] The pathomechanics, configuration, and anatomic location of the fractures are similar to those in patients without SCI. The reported incidence of extremity fractures occurring in the multiple-trauma SCI patient ranges from 6% to 20%,[23,27-31,33,35,39] with long-bone fractures accounting for 26% to 44% of these fractures. Eleven percent to 19% of long-bone fractures occur in the upper extremity and 19% to 47% occur in the lower extremity. Pelvic fractures occur in up to 28% of these patients.[23,33] Malunion and delayed union are common, occurring in 4% to 16%.[23,33] Overall complication rates may be as high as 40%.[35]

Clinical diagnosis of extremity fracture in the paretic extremity may not be initially apparent. Pain may be absent due to impaired sensibility. Deformity may be lacking in nondisplaced or stable fractures. Decreased cognition in the multiple-trauma patient adds to the difficulty in prompt diagnosis. The examiner is often misdirected toward more obvious injuries. Fractures in the carpus and tarsus often show little limb deformity, and swelling may be minimal. The presence of swelling, ecchymoses, increased warmth, lacerations, abrasions, and crepitus requires careful examination and appropriate radiographic evaluation. CT or MRI is often helpful in the elucidation of fractures of the carpus and tarsus. In addition,

TABLE 1

Extremity Problems and Complications Following SCI

I. Complications involving bones and joint
- A. Extremity fractures
  - Acute fractures sustained at the time of SCI
  - Pathologic fractures in long-standing SCI
  - Fractures sustained in a normal limb in long-standing paraplegia patients
- B. Neurogenic heterotopic ossification

II. Complications involving muscle
- A. Spasticity
- B. Joint contracture
- C. Paralysis: upper extremities
- D. Paralysis: lower extremities

III. Problems of upper extremity overuse (weight bearing)
- A. Upper extremity pain
  - Rotator cuff injury
  - Shoulder tendinitis, bursitis
- B. Carpal tunnel syndrome
- C. Cubital tunnel syndrome

IV. Miscellaneous complications
- A. Regional pain syndromes
- B. Venous thrombosis
- C. Gravitational edema
- D. Muscle atrophy
- E. Osteoporosis
- F. Skin ulceration and infection

the multiple-trauma patient deserves routine pelvis radiographs. Careful examination and a low threshold for radiographic examination will help diagnose these difficult fractures.

Treatment

Treatment of acute fractures in the SCI patient is directed toward early fracture stabilization to allow patient mobilization and early rehabilitation, and to minimize complications associated with prolonged bed rest. Surgical stabilization and early mobilization have been shown to decrease the frequency of deep venous thromboses and decubitus ulcers,[27-31] as well as general medical problems of atelectasis and pneumonia. Besides allowing early mobilization, internal fixation of fractures obviates the need for casts, splints, and traction, all of which are poorly tolerated in the neurologically involved extremity. Impaired sensibility increases the chances of skin ulceration with casts or splints. Spastic limbs with increased muscle tone or clonus are difficult to manage in traction or within splints. In addition, plaster immobilization prevents joint mobilization, interferes with self-care, and hinders wheelchair transfers. The physical weight of these devices can be difficult to manage for the patient with a paretic limb.

If the patient is medically stable and there are no contraindications, early open reduction and internal fixation of major long-bone fractures is desirable.[33] This procedure can often be performed at the time of initial spine stabilization. Most fractures are treated according to standard orthopaedic principles. Some fractures that might otherwise be treated with closed methods (such as the clavicle, humerus, distal radius, metacarpals, tibia, and metatarsals) may be difficult to manage if spasticity or paralytic muscle imbalance is present.[22] Rigid internal fixation remains the method of choice. Intramedullary nailing of humerus fractures will allow early upper extremity weight bearing for wheelchair transfers. If surgery for extremity fractures is contraindicated, the use of well-padded splints or bivalved casts may provide a reasonable alternative,[33] with consideration for performing internal fixation at a later date when the patient becomes medically stable.

External fixation systems may have application in specific fractures such as severely comminuted distal radius fractures; however, external fixators are often poorly tolerated in this patient population. Levine et al[32] have emphasized the difficulty in the use of external fixation in patents with SCI. External fixation systems interfere with patient positioning, can interfere with joint mobilization, and can predispose to trophic ulcers. Bulky fixators can hinder skin care and limit positioning to only supine or one lateral position. Wheelchair transfers and sitting may be more difficult. External fixators may present a hazard to the contralateral limb from injury from the external fixation pins or rods. In the rare circumstances when external fixation is used, the devices must be well padded and checked frequently for evidence of skin irritation or ischemia. In general, rigid internal fixation is preferred over external fixation systems in the SCI patient.

Pathologic Fractures in Long-Standing SCI

Pathologic fractures occur in osteoporotic bone in the patient with long-standing SCI. The incidence has been noted to be approximately 7%, ranging from 1% to 34%.[35,40] These fractures are usually low-energy injuries and result from minimal trauma to the osteoporotic paralytic limb. Falls from wheelchairs or during transfers, positioning in bed, or physical and manual mobilization of a joint have sufficient energy to cause fractures and are common causes of injury.[21,28] Severe spasticity of the lower limbs with an acute muscle contraction can propel a patient out of a wheelchair and result in long-bone fracture. Long-bone fractures occur more often in paraplegic patients than in quadriplegics, due to the paraplegics' increased activity level and participation in physical activities.[36] Most fractures are sustained in metaphyseal areas of the lower extremity, commonly near the knee involving the distal femur or proximal tibia (**Figure 1**). Other common sites for fracture include the distal tibia, intertrochanteric region of the femur, femoral neck, and diaphysis of the femur or tibia.[36] Fractures of the pelvis and small bones of the hands and feet are relatively rare. Because of impaired sensibility and the minimal trauma required to fracture an osteoporotic bone, the fracture can initially go unrecognized. If deformity is minimal, swelling, ecchymoses, and warmth may be the only clinical signs. Fractures occurring near joints can clinically mimic infection, joint effusion, heterotopic ossification, or phlebitis. A high index of suspicion will promote earlier radiographic evaluation and confirmation.

Osteoporosis in the SCI patient is a major risk factor for fractures and, in general, these fractures are considered pathologic. The development of osteoporosis with loss of bone mineral density is a complex and multifactorial problem. It develops from both metabolic changes and from stress deprivation in the paralytic limbs.[40-46] In the paraplegic patient, osteoporosis does not develop in the levels above the injury. In the quadriplegic patient, it can develop to an equal extent in the upper and lower extremities.[44] Lack of weight bearing plays a role in development of osteoporosis, but the effects of the lack of forces from muscle contraction and from spasticity remains controversial.[36,40,41,44,45] The loss of bone mass commences following SCI and is accompanied initially by a negative calcium balance. Calcium balance may become positive by the sixth month postinjury, but a steady state of bone loss may not occur until 2 years after SCI.[40,41] The degree of osteoporosis is variable, involves trabecular bone more than cortical bone, and involves long bones to a greater extent than the spine.[41,44] Trabecular bone loss was found to be between 15% and 25% at 1 year (radius, ulna, tibia),[44] and may be as high as 50% after 2 years (femoral neck).[41] The lumbar spine may be unaffected, even within the levels of paralysis. In some patients, osteoporosis occurs at a slower rate, and a year may be required before osteoporosis is sufficiently advanced to cause pathologic fractures.[47]

FIGURE 1

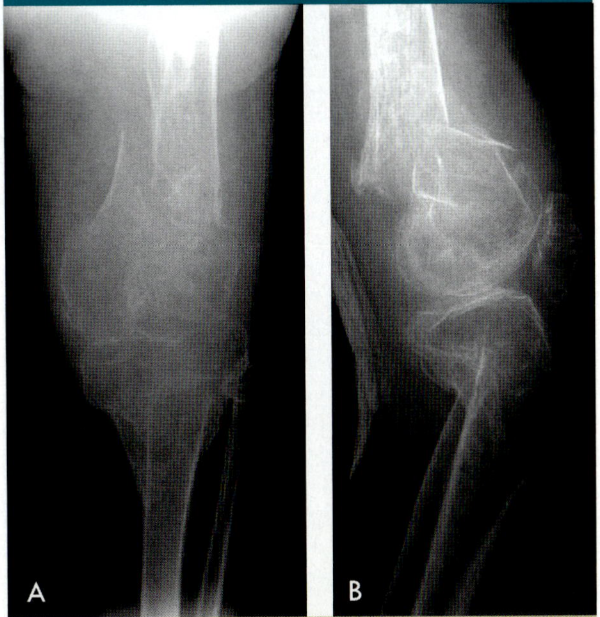

Figure 1 AP (**A**) and lateral (**B**) radiographs of the knee of an SCI patient, showing fracture of the distal femur and proximal tibia. The bone is osteoporotic and the fracture is considered pathologic. Most pathologic fractures in SCI patients occur near the knee.

Moynahan et al[48] have noted a higher fracture rate in SCI patients with the greater amount of bone density loss.

Treatment

Treatment of these pathologic fractures depends on the type of fracture and the degree of limb paresis or spasticity. In the paralytic nonfunctional extremity with little or no spasticity, pathologic fractures can usually be managed nonsurgically, using well-padded splints or bivalved casts[8,25,49] (**Figure 2**). The skin is checked on a weekly basis to avoid skin irritation or sores in these patients with loss of sensibility. Surgical stabilization has traditionally been avoided because fixation may be difficult to achieve or be easily lost in the osteoporotic bone. There is also an increased incidence of infection due to the atrophy of the surrounding muscle and skin. Fortunately, most of these pathologic fractures heal without surgery.[35] In nonambulatory patients, moderate degrees of fracture deformity may be acceptable, as long as previous functions are preserved and fracture deformity or callus do not result in areas of increased pressure on the skin. Ease of positioning, sitting, and transfers must be maintained. Fractures of the femoral neck treated nonsurgically can form a

FIGURE 2

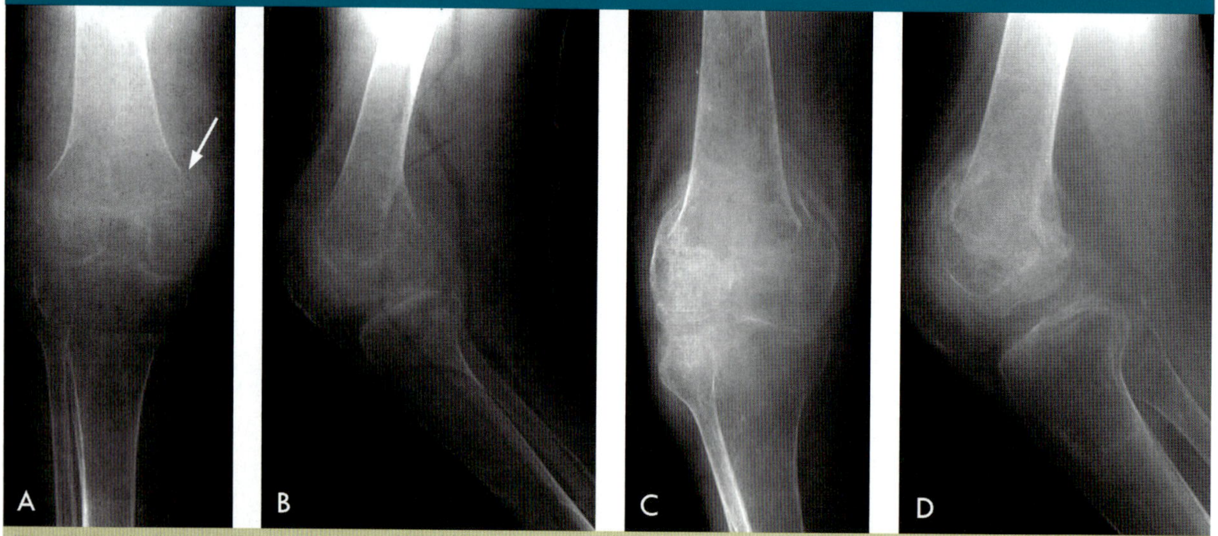

Figure 2 AP (**A**) and lateral (**B**) radiographs of the distal femur of an SCI patient with a fracture of the distal femur. **C** and **D,** Successful union was achieved using closed methods.

FIGURE 3

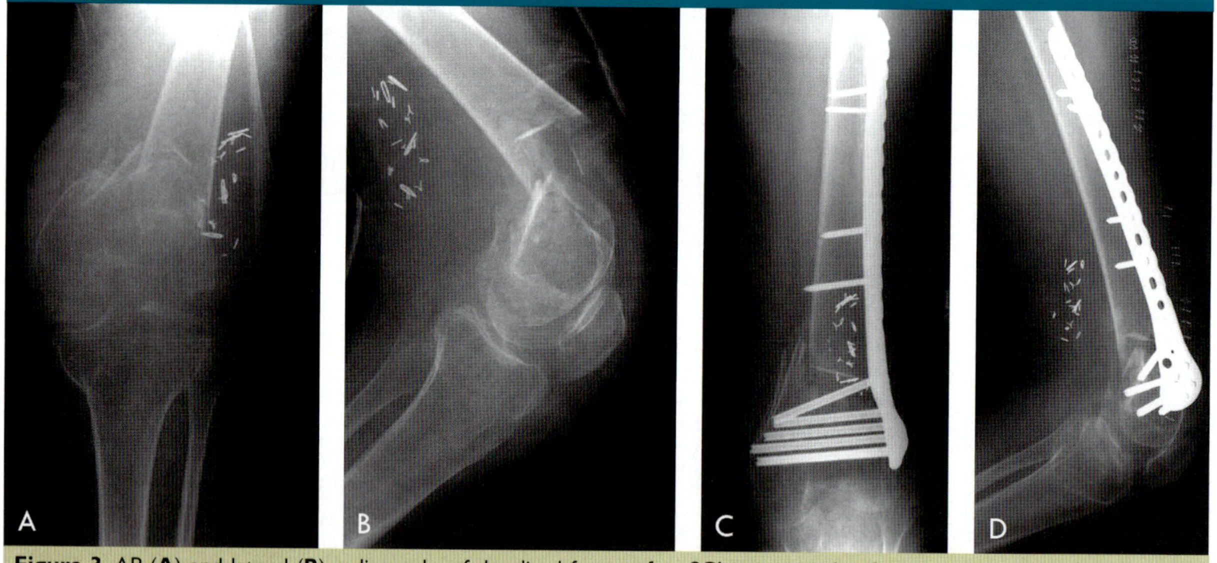

Figure 3 AP (**A**) and lateral (**B**) radiographs of the distal femur of an SCI patient with a fracture of the distal femur. Closed treatment was initially used. Because of delayed union, surgical fixation was performed 3 months after initial injury (**C** and **D**). Successful union was achieved.

pseudarthrosis. Pseudarthrosis of the femoral neck has been noted to cause no additional disability to the nonambulatory patient, provided there are no major rotational deformities. Stauffer[47] noted that in some patients, pseudarthrosis of the hip may actually allow an increased range of motion. Nonambulatory patients with fractures in paralytic limbs usually have little or no discomfort, so the fracture can usually be easily reduced and maintained in well-padded splints or bivalved casts.[47]

Delayed union or nonunion may occur in severely displaced fractures or those with soft-tissue interposition. Management of these fractures may require surgical stabilization (**Figure 3**).

Although closed management has traditionally been advocated for these pathologic fractures in a nonambulatory patient, the use of rigid internal fixation does have advantages. Internal fixation avoids the use of casts or splints and associated skin problems, and obviates the need for frequent

FIGURE 4

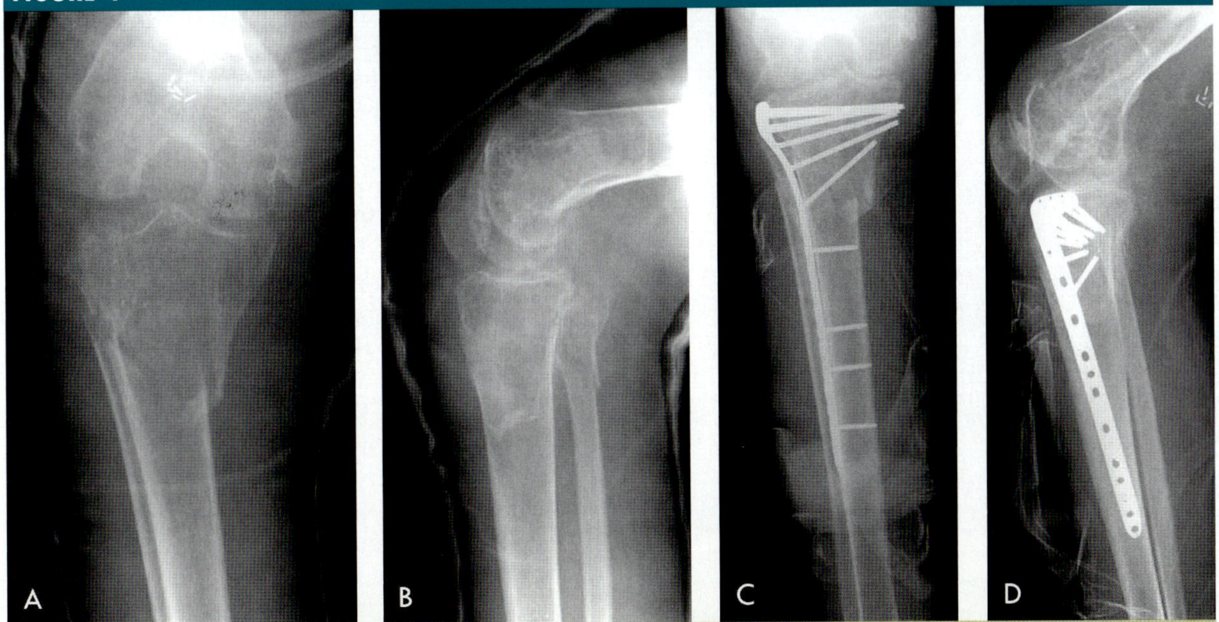

Figure 4 AP (**A**) and lateral (**B**) radiographs of the proximal tibia in an SCI patient who sustained bilateral lower extremity long-bone fractures. Because of the bilateral injuries, surgical fixation was chosen (**C** and **D**) to facilitate rehabilitation and positioning.

skin checks and recasting.[38] Internal fixation allows for earlier limb mobilization to avoid joint contractures. Wheelchair transfers, patient positioning, lifting, skin care, dressing, and hygiene are facilitated with internal fixation. Garland et al[31] have shown that upper extremity fractures treated surgically had a lower incidence of medical complications such as deep venous thromboses and decubitus ulcers (4%) compared with those treated nonsurgically (28%). New internal fixation devices and techniques allow smaller incisions and minimally invasive placement of internal fixation. In general, we have been tending to consider internal fixation more frequently, and will more aggressively internally fix a fracture that has developed a delayed union or nonunion (**Figures 3** and **4**).

In the paraparetic patient who has residual function of the lower extremities or who was ambulatory before fracture, treatment is directed toward restoring function, and is, in general, similar to treatment of patients in the general population. Open reduction and internal fixation of displaced femoral neck fractures minimizes the chances of nonunion or osteonecrosis of the femoral head. Open reduction and internal fixation of displaced intertrochanteric fractures or subtrochanteric fractures can prevent shortening or varus malunion. Internal fixation of severely shortened diaphyseal femur fractures will minimize limb-length discrepancy. Displaced intra-articular fractures in the ambulatory patient require surgical restoration of the articular surface. In severely displaced fractures or those with soft-tissue interposition, surgery is usually performed to achieve adequate reduction and union.

In the quadriparetic patient with an upper extremity fracture, goals of fracture care are to maintain preexisting function of the extremities. Therefore, fractures must be satisfactorily reduced, using internal fixation as necessary. If internal fixation is required in severely osteoporotic bone, additional external immobilization with splints may be necessary. Postoperative therapy for mobilization of the limb is individualized.

In any limb with severe spasticity, it may be difficult or impossible to manage a fracture with closed methods.[22,29-31,35] In these patients, open reduction and internal fixation is preferred. Alternatively, phenol nerve block or use of botulinum toxin (Botox) injections to the involved muscles will decrease spasticity and possibly facilitate closed treatment of the fracture. The phenol block will decrease spasticity, and lasts 3 to 6 months,[50-53] usually enough time to allow fracture healing. Phenol blocks and Botox are covered in more detail in the subsequent discussion of spasticity.

FIGURE 5

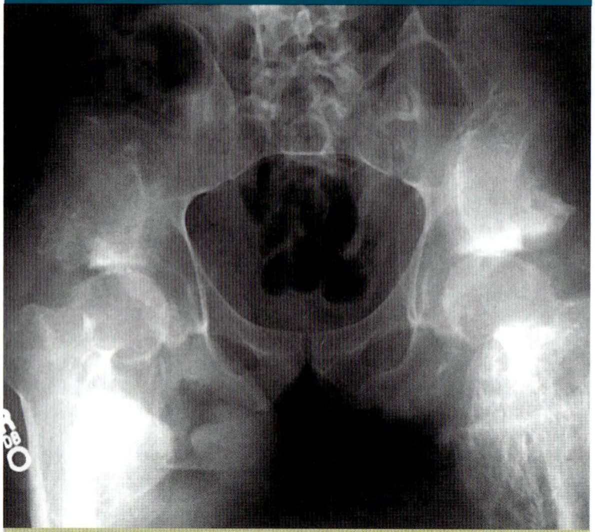

Figure 5 AP radiograph of pelvis of SCI patient with heterotopic ossification of the hip. Restricted motion leads to difficulty with wheelchair transfers and positioning. (Reproduced from Botte MJ: Complications of the musculoskeletal system following spinal cord injury, in Levine AM, Eismont FJ, Garfin SR, Zigler JE, eds: *Spine Trauma*. Philadelphia, PA, WB Saunders, 1998, pp 639-660.)

As already noted, external fixation devices are, in general, poorly tolerated in the SCI patient. External fixation systems interfere with patient positioning and turning, and predispose to pressure sores.[30-32] Wheelchair transfers, sitting, and joint mobilization may be more difficult. In the rare circumstance when external fixation is used, the devices must be well padded, checked frequently for skin irritation or ischemia, and meticulous pin care must be provided to prevent infection. In general, rigid internal fixation is preferred over external fixation systems in the SCI patient. If casts or splints are used, special attention must be paid to skin inspection and protection.[26]

Fracture Sustained in a Normal Extremity in the Long-Standing Paraplegic Patient

Fractures of this type consist of traumatic injuries that occur in normal bone above the level of long-standing paralysis. These injuries are often high-energy fractures, and are sustained in a group of patients who are vigorous and motivated to remain active.[33] Many of these patients drive motor vehicles. In the treatment of these fractures, an effort must be made to maintain the patient's independence. Most fractures can be treated much like those in the non-SCI patient, with similar indications for surgical stabilization. An aggressive surgical approach avoids the use of casts or splints, and thus allows earlier limb mobilization to promote rapid rehabilitation. In fractures of the diaphysis of the humerus, intramedullary nailing usually allows earlier weight bearing for wheelchair transfers.[22]

Neurogenic Heterotopic Ossification

Neurogenic heterotopic ossification is a spontaneous formation of bone that usually occurs near major synovial joints in a patient who has sustained an injury to the central nervous system (**Figure 5**).[27,54-72] It was first described as a complication following SCI by Riedel in 1883.[27] It occurs in the levels of paralysis and most commonly develops in the vicinity of the hip.[22,27,61-64,72] The elbow, shoulder, and knee are involved to a lesser extent, and the formation does not seem to occur in the hands or feet.[22,60] The exact etiology of this bone formation remains unknown. It is not a response to or result of local soft-tissue trauma or joint injury. Because the deposited bone in neurogenic heterotopic ossification usually occurs near or around joints, it is sometimes termed periarticular ossification.[73,74]

Associated Problems

The bone formation can result in mechanical restriction of motion or frank ankylosis. Secondary contractures of the soft tissues may form if mobilization of the joint is not maintained or is prevented by the heterotopic bone. Pain or discomfort may be initially present if limb sensibility is intact. The resultant loss of motion can severely impede function. Sitting, transfers, ambulation, dressing, and hygiene may be impaired or prevented. Restricted positioning can secondarily lead to pressure-sore formation and subsequent infection.[60,75-79] Lack of joint motion increases the likelihood of pathologic fracture of the osteoporotic bone during positioning or lifting. In the elbow region, heterotopic ossification can encroach on the cubital tunnel, resulting in ulnar nerve entrapment.[59]

Incidence and Joints Involved

The reported incidence of neurogenic heterotopic ossification in patients with SCIs is between 10% and 53%,[55,63,68] and seems to occur less in the pediatric population than in adults.[64] Loss of motion occurs in about one-third of patients developing heterotopic ossification.[63,80,81] In about 5%, complete ankylosis develops.[27,63] Heterotopic ossification is more common in quadriplegics than paraplegics, and forms in the neurologically impaired limbs. Both spastic or flaccid extremities may be affected, and ossification may occur in patients with either incomplete or complete spinal cord lesions.[80] Large amounts of bone can be formed adjacent to joints. The bone is usually deposited between the muscle planes; it does not develop within muscles or within joints. The bone can, however, distort or displace neighboring muscles or neurovascular structures. The ossification may completely encase nerves or vessels. It is unclear why the hip is most commonly involved.[22,27,61-64,72] When the hip is involved, bone is usually deposited anterior to the joint, extending from the anterosuperior iliac crest, anterior to the capsule, to the region of the lesser trochanter or anterior aspect of the proximal femur. It occasionally develops posteriorly, from the ischium to the posterior aspect of the lesser trochanter. When the knee is involved, heterotopic bone usually forms medially to the medial condyle and extends up the femur for variable lengths.[27] The shoulder and elbow are only occasionally involved. Involvement in wrists, hands, ankles, and feet is rare.

Time of Development

The time of initial occurrence of heterotopic bone is variable, and can occur from 12 weeks to 12 months after SCI. It is usually detected at approximately 2 months postinjury.[27] In the pediatric population, development or detection seems to occur much later, where the average time to detection of heterotopic ossification from spinal insult was 6.5 years.[64] Once diagnosed, its time of maturation is even more variable and often difficult to assess. "Maturation" generally refers to the time of cessation of bone growth, and is usually based on radiographic appearance (discussed later), stabilization of levels of serum alkaline phosphatase (although not always reliable), and decreasing or static activity on repeated technetium bone scans and sulfur colloid scans. The bone usually increases in size over a 6-month period, then shows progressive signs of maturation thereafter. Garland[27] has described two classes of heterotopic ossification based on clinical presentation and behavior. Class I (comprising about 90%) has its initial occurrence at about 2 months after SCI, has a peak of activity over the next 5 or 6 months, and is followed by maturation where ossification becomes relatively inert. In class II (comprising about 10%), the initial occurrence and peak of activity occur at similar times as class I; however, potential to form heterotopic ossification remains for months or years. Chances for recurrence following excision are higher in class II.[27] In the pediatric population, the heterotopic bone lesion has shown some potential to partially resorb spontaneously.[64]

Clinical Findings

An inflammatory response usually precedes or coincides with formation of heterotopic bone formation. Clinical findings during the development of neurogenic heterotopic ossification include tenderness (if sensibility is intact), swelling, warmth, redness, and stiffness or ankylosis of the involved joint. This clinical presentation can mimic infection, thrombophlebitis, arthritis, tumor, or trauma. Occasionally a palpable mass is initially detectable. Once mature, the swelling, warmth, and redness may subside, leaving only joint stiffness and a possible palpable bone mass. Secondary soft-tissue contractures of the joint can occur if the limb is not mobilized.

Radiographic, Ultrasound, and Laboratory Evaluation

Radiographs of heterotopic ossification may be difficult to interpret. Initial radiographs often fail to demonstrate the bone formation, despite positive clinical findings. The technetium bone scan, however, will usually show evidence of bone formation activity. It may take an additional few days to several weeks before the bone formation (and ossification) will become apparent on standard radiographs. In the early period of bone formation, the heterotopic ossification may appear radiographically as an indistinct, fluffy shadow of ossification around the joint, with poorly defined margins. It increases in size on subsequent radiographs and, as it matures, the bone becomes well-defined with distance margins and linear trabeculations, and the size of the bone mass stabilizes. Because both mature heterotopic ossification and immature heterotopic ossification may coexist, and the mature ossification can radiographically obscure the immature ossification, radiographic determination of maturity is not always reliable.[80] During active bone formation, serum alkaline phosphatase is usually elevated. It may remain elevated for years, reaching elevations as high as 500 IU.[27,56,63,64,80-83]

Sonographic diagnosis of heterotopic ossification has been investigated by Cassar-Pullicino,[58] and may prove valuable in the early detection of heterotopic ossification. More investigations are needed to establish its role in detection of early heterotopic ossification.

Microscopic Findings

Histologically, heterotopic ossification resembles that of woven bone formation, with areas of concurrent inflammation. Initially, it may appear as disorganized lamellar bone with osteoblastic activity (within the first 8 months). The immature bone demonstrates hypervascularity.[80] Eventually, the bone develops the appearance of mature cortical bone, with a decrease in osteoblastic activity, decrease in hypervascularity, and a more organized lamellar pattern. It may take 18 months before the bone appears histologically as mature bone.[80]

Treatment

Treatment includes management of associated pain, maintenance of joint motion, use of pharmacologic agents to decrease inflammation and bone production, and surgical resection of bone and release of associated contractures.[27,54,59-65,70-72,78] Radiation is an additional adjunct that can be used in the perioperative period. Other methods under investigation include use of warfarin and extracorporeal shock-wave treatment.[56,57]

Nonsteroidal anti-inflammatory medications are used to decrease the inflammation noted in the early stages, and hopefully help decrease bone production. Indomethacin 50 mg three times a day with meals is commonly used. Because inflammation is an early part of heterotopic ossification production, it is hoped that anti-inflammatory medications may help block the process.

Maintenance of motion by passive mobilization is one of the initial treatment methods for neurogenic heterotopic ossification. Maintenance of joint motion helps preserve function, and aids in positioning, dressing, hygiene, and prevention of pressure sores. Mobilization of the affected joint is instituted early, as soon as the diagnosis is made. Mobilization may not alter the formation of heterotopic ossification, but can prevent secondary soft-tissue contractures and maintain or increase motion by producing microfractures or pseudarthrosis through an ankylosing mass of bone.[28,78,80,81] Aggressive passive motion does not appear to aggravate the inflammatory response or adversely affect bone production.[78] However, in the patient with spared sensibility, mobilization may be difficult because of associated discomfort. Analgesics and anti-inflammatory medications may help. Allowing the joint to undergo prolonged immobilization must be avoided, as secondary soft-tissue fixed contractures develop. Forceful manipulation of the joint (under anesthesia if needed), is somewhat controversial, but has been shown to increase motion with some types of neurogenic heterotopic ossification.[28] Increased motion usually occurs by causing fracture or microfracture through the forming heterotopic bone. The indications and role of forceful manipulation in the SCI patient have not been well established, but hopefully this method will prove to be safe and effective. All manipulations must be done with caution to prevent undesired pathologic fracture of osteoporotic long bones.

Disodium etidronate has been shown to be effective in preventing the occurrence of heterotopic ossification or in reducing its extensiveness once it is clinically evident.[28,62,78,84] Disodium etidronate works by inhibition of the formation and growth of hydroxyapatite crystals. Recommended dose is 20 mg/kg/day for prophylaxis, initiated before clinical or radiographic evidence of heterotopic ossification and continued for 3 months. For established heterotopic ossification, treatment is initiated and continued for six months. Garland et al[28] have noted recurrence or rebound of heterotopic ossification in certain patients even after 6 months of treatment. Some feel that disodium etidronate does not prevent heterotopic ossification, but rather only delays its formation. Thus its role in heterotopic ossification remains controversial.

Warfarin has recently been evaluated as a treatment of heterotopic ossification.[57] Because one of the proteins in bone, osteocalcin, is produced by a vitamin K–dependent carboxylation, the investigators have raised the possibility that treatment with warfarin may prevent the formation of ectopic bone. Buschbacher et al[57] demonstrated early success with warfarin in the prevention of heterotopic bone. Although these early studies are promising, additional investigation is needed to establish the role of this method in the treatment or prevention of heterotopic ossification.

Surgical resection of heterotopic ossification can be performed in severe or refractory cases. Indications include limitation of motion with function loss, including difficulty in positioning, sitting, dressing, transfers, or hygiene.[28,61,63,80,81] Resection needs to be planned carefully, as this surgery is associated with high morbidity. Surgical complications or problems include hemorrhage, sepsis, and reankylosis.[63] Neurovascular structures may be displaced or encased in the bone mass, and thus cautious dissection, good visibility, and adequate exposure are required for resection. Computerized axial tomography or standard polytomography will help access the three-dimensional structure of the bone mass. The timing of resection of heterotopic ossification is controversial. It is generally accepted that early resection of immature bone has a higher incidence of recurrence and hemorrhage than resection of mature bone. The immature bone is usually highly vascular. However, delaying surgery until bone is mature may take years, and results in problems associated with prolonged joint immobilization (such as fixed soft-tissue contracture and cartilage erosions).[85-89] Evaluating the maturity of bone is difficult, and usually based on appearance of standard radiographs, stabilizing alkaline phosphatase levels, and decreasing activity on technetium bone scans. These parameters are not always reliable.[27] Therefore, specific recommendations for time of resection of heterotopic bone are difficult to determine. It has been recommended to wait a minimum of 14 months following diagnosis to achieve adequate bone maturity to minimize hemorrhage and reduce chance of recurrence. Resection should only involve removal of adequate bone to acquire desired motion. The entire mass does not always need to be resected, and often only a wedge of bone need be removed. Heterotopic bone removal produces dead space and bleeding surfaces of bone; therefore, placement of wound drains is recommended. Substantial postoperative blood loss can occur through drains, and should be carefully monitored.[80] Blood must be available for transfusion if needed when heterotopic bone is resected at the hip. Low-dose radiation may have an increasing role as an adjunct to surgical excision of neurogenic ossification. Similar to treatment as given in posttraumatic heterotopic ossification, the radiation is given at or near the time of excision, usually within the following day to be most effective. A dose can also be given preoperatively, the day of or just before surgery. Preoperative consultation with a radiation oncologist will facilitate radiation treatment to coincide with surgical excision. Low dose radiation treatment, (approximately 500 rad) has been show to impede the formation of new bone. A disadvantage of perioperative radiation is the increased risk of wound dehiscence or infection.

As an investigational preoperative treatment of heterotopic bone, Brissot et al[56] have used extracorporeal shock-wave treatment. In this investigational method, patients with heterotopic ossification received treatments once a week for 4 consecutive weeks. Their data indicate a decrease in pain, increase in motion (about 10°), and an increase in ambulation distance (1,126 m increased to 2,776 m). The authors conclude that extracorporeal shock-wave treatment might be a reasonable complement to usual medical treatment, physiotherapy, and before surgical resection.[56] Additional studies are needed to clarify the role of this method in the management of heterotopic ossification.

Following surgical resection, close follow-up and continued mobilization should be reinstituted early to maintain motion. Physical therapy for 6 months may be required to maintain gains in motion. In patients with restricted hip motion undergoing resection of heterotopic ossification, 74% have been shown to gain satisfactory motion to allow sitting, achieving an average gain of 30° in the arc of motion.[63] Preoperative range of motion seems to be an important predictor of final postoperative motion. Patients with ankylosed hips usually gain the least motion following resection. As noted earlier, complication rates are often high (infection or operative blood loss occurring in up to 79%), and bony recurrence is common (occurring, to some degree, in 92%). However, surgical resection remains an effective means of increasing motion, and with proper planning and realistic expectations, it offers a reasonable method for management of this difficult problem.

Complications Involving Muscle

Development of Spasticity Versus Paralysis

Injury to the spinal cord can produce different effects on muscle, including paralysis (which indicates no volitional muscle function), paresis (weak muscle function), or spasticity (which includes increased tone, hyperactive reflexes, clonus).[7,87,90-101] The effect on muscle depends on the type and level of cord injury, the involvement of nerve roots, and the time elapsed from injury. Immediately following a severe SCI, flaccid paralysis develops below the level of the lesion. Flaccidity usually lasts less than 24 hours, and is followed by development of spasticity.[47] Spasticity develops as a result of disruption of the upper motor neuron inhibitory pathways from the brain to the anterior horn cells of the spinal cord. Muscle control from the brain is impaired or eliminated. Primitive reflex action predominates from the uninjured cord below the level of injury. Thus, the period of flaccidity is followed by a period of increasing muscle tone, return of stretch reflexes, and a progression to hyperactive reflexes. In addition, sudden muscle contractions or spasms may become frequent and occur with minimal stimulus to the muscle or overlying skin. Clonus, rigidity, and the "clasp-knife" reflex can develop. At this point of increased tone and hyperactivity, the muscles are considered to be spastic.[87]

Spasticity develops in the muscles distal to the level of cord damage, mediated by primitive reflex activity from the intact cord distal to the injury. However, spasticity does not develop at the level of cord injury, because the spinal reflex arc is disrupted at this level by injury to the motor neuron cell body. Instead, flaccid paralysis (no function) or paresis (weakness) occurs at the level of injury. Nerve root injury may also contribute to or account for weakness at the level of injury, and is discussed later. If there is an incomplete SCI, some neurologic recovery may occur. Muscles that are spastic may improve (becoming less hypertonic) with time, and the muscles may return to a less hyperreflexic state. Gradual recovery of volitional control can occur as well (in the incomplete lesion), and contributes to improved extremity function. This recovery period is variable, and usually occurs over a 6- to 12-month period following the initial SCI. At approximately 1 year after injury, most patients with an incomplete SCI will have approached or reached the end of the period when spontaneous neurologic recovery usually occurs, and little or no further neurologic recovery can be expected.

In addition to injury to the spinal cord, nerve roots or anterior horn cells in the vicinity of the cord lesion may be injured. Trauma that injures the cervical cord often injures the neighboring nerve root, especially roots in the foramen between dislocated or fractured vertebrae. The nerve root may originate from the normal cord proximal to the injured cord and be damaged as it leaves the foramen,[47] thus resulting in some muscle function loss that is above the level of cord injury. When a nerve root is damaged, this is a peripheral nerve injury and is thus a lower motor neuron lesion. Paralysis or weakness (but not spasticity) of the corresponding muscles results. Therefore, there may be a group of flaccid or weak muscles (from nerve root injury) that are proximal to the level of spastic muscles (from cord injury). If the nerve root is only partially injured and remains structurally intact (neurapraxia or axonotmesis), the impaired function of the corresponding muscle may gradually return. This may explain why some patients with a complete SCI subsequently gain the function of one or two root levels over time (it is a peripheral nerve that is recovering, not the spinal cord). If the continuity of the nerve root is disrupted (neurotmesis), function will not spontaneously recover, and the affected muscles will remain weak or flaccid.

To summarize, depending on the type of injury to the spinal cord and nerve roots, different types of muscle impairment may ultimately occur at or below the level of injury: (1) paralysis, (2) paresis, and (3) spasticity. At the level of injury, muscles will be weak or flaccid, due to either damage to the cord at this level (thus disrupting both volitional control and spinal reflex activity) or to nerve root injury (resulting in a peripheral nerve injury and paresis). Below the level of SCI, the muscles will be paralyzed or paretic (depending on completeness of the cord injury), and spasticity will usually be present, due to loss of upper motor neuron inhibitory control.

In many complete cervical SCIs that involve the cord between the C5 and T1 root levels, muscles in the upper extremity are often predominantly weak or flaccid, with little or no spasticity. This occurs because the cord or nerve roots have been segmentally damaged over a few levels, and thus, as mentioned before, spinal reflex arcs at these levels are disrupted and spasticity cannot occur. Because spasticity only occurs in areas where the spinal reflex is intact, upper extremity spasticity, if present, usually develops at the more distally innervated muscles (innervated by roots C7, C8, or T1), because these levels are more apt to be distal to the injured segment of cord (and thus the spinal reflex arc is intact). Spasticity does, however, rarely occur in the more proximally innervated muscles in the upper extremity (such as C5 or C4) if the cord lesion is proximal to these levels. Many of these patients, though, do not survive because of paralysis of the diaphragm (C4 root level) and resulting respiratory failure. Therefore, spasticity is seen less often in the upper extremity than in the lower extremity, and paralysis or paresis becomes the predominant upper extremity problem.

Injuries in the lumbar spine can produce either upper motor neuron or lower motor neuron injuries. The cauda equina begins at about the L2 level. Injuries proximal to this level produce mostly upper motor neuron lesions (with varying degrees of lower motor neuron involvement if nerve roots are injured). These injuries usually result in muscle spasticity distal to the injury. Distal to the conus medullaris, only lower motor neurons exist, and injuries in these areas produce peripheral nerve injuries manifested by paralysis or paresis, without spasticity. In reality, many injuries in the vicinity of L2 injure both the cord above the conus and associated nerve roots or parts of the cauda equine; therefore, clinical presentations with both spasticity and flaccidity are possible.

In SCIs, the degree of spasticity is variable. In the incomplete cord lesion, some volitional control may be superimposed on either spastic or paretic muscles below the level of injury. Volitional control does not return in the true complete SCI.

Muscle strength in the SCI patient should not progressively decrease. Ascending or progressive loss of muscle function following the initial injury is worrisome. In the acute stages of spinal injury, this may indicate progressive nerve or cord compression (ie, from disk protrusion, hematoma, edema, loss of vertebral reduction). Loss of muscle function that occurs at a later time may indicate ascending syrinx formation within the cord or loss of spine stability. Progressive muscle loss in any of these settings requires immediate investigation.

In the following section, problems associated with spasticity and paralysis and their management will be discussed. Although these two topics will be discussed separately, one must keep in mind that they often occur in the same extremity simultaneously, hence the term spastic paralysis.

As explained above, weakness is often predominant in the upper extremity and spasticity is often predominant in the lower extremities. Management of these problems has evolved so that efforts in the upper extremity are usually directed mainly toward restoring function of weak muscles using reconstructive procedures such as tendon transfers and tenodeses. In the lower extremity, however, efforts are directed more toward the control of noxious spasticity, using muscle or tendon releases or lengthenings.

Spasticity

Following the initial period of flaccidity immediately following SCI, spasticity develops to varying degrees.[47,87,96] It occurs in both complete and incomplete SCI. The incidence of spasticity appears higher among cervical and upper thoracic level injuries than in the lower thoracic and lumbosacral levels.[102] In some patients, spasticity is mild, and the muscles remain predominantly weak or flaccid. In others, spasticity is so severe that minimal stimulation of muscle produces sudden violent muscle contractions. Severe increased muscle tone can prohibit adequate joint mobilization.

Nature of Spasticity and Muscle Patterning

Spasticity in the SCI patient differs in character from that in the brain injury, stroke, and cerebral palsy patient. In brain injury, stroke, and cerebral palsy, chronic increased tone or continuous static muscle contractions are usually seen. In the SCI patient, however, spasticity often manifests as periodic, distinct, sudden muscle contractions triggered by minimal stretch or cutaneous stimulation. Two patterns of muscle contraction often occur: (1) those in which the major limb flexors contract, thus withdrawing the limb toward the body (known as flexor patterning); and (2) those in which the extensor muscles contract, resulting in the limb extending away from the body (known as extensor patterning). Patients often have alternating flexor and extensor patterning. The type of patterning may be dependent in part on the type of stimulation initiating the response, or on the position of the limb at the time of stimulation.

Problems Associated With Spasticity

Joint mobilization in the spastic limb can be difficult. It can be painful, potentially harmful to the limbs, and time-consuming. If spasticity prevents or impairs limb mobilization, difficulty with positioning the extremity occurs. The feet may not be able to be positioned on the wheelchair platform. Sitting, transfers, and positioning in bed can be difficult. Dressing the patient becomes time-consuming. Proper hygiene may be prevented, especially in the axilla, groin, and antecubital fossa. Mobilization of the joint for articular cartilage and soft-tissue nutrition is prevented. Spasticity can interfere with joint mobilization used in the management of heterotopic ossification formation. If the joints cannot be adequately mobilized, stiffness of soft tissues can lead to fixed joint contracture.[22,103,104]

Occasionally, severely spastic muscles will produce sudden violent muscle contractions that are hazardous to the patient. These sudden contractions are able to propel an individual out of a wheelchair or bed, and can result in extremity fracture. Operation of a car or machinery can be dangerous or difficult. Wheelchair transfers are sometimes prevented.

In the patient with an incomplete SCI, spasticity may be superimposed on a limb with retained motor and sensory function. The spasticity can severely impair what residual function remains. If sensibility is intact, chronic increased muscle tone and sudden muscle contractions can be painful.

Spasticity as an Aid to the Patient

Occasionally, the hyperactive reflexes or increased muscle tone can be of use to the SCI patient, and this must be kept in mind before the surgical ablation of spasticity. By changing muscle position or touching the overlying skin, some patients are able to trigger an extension spinal reflex of the lower extremity, thereby facilitating standing or wheelchair transfers. Pinching the calf of the leg can cause a flexor reflex and thus can help in dressing the lower part of the body.[95] Reflex activity can also be used to provoke desired reflexes to assist with functional electrical stimulation during gait.[105]

Assessment of Spasticity

Measurement and quantification of spasticity is difficult, although new methods of accessing muscle tone and function are now being investigated.[91,100,106-116] Other conditions can contribute to joint stiffness and interfere with accurate assessment of spasticity. These include soft-tissue contracture, heterotopic ossification, undetected fracture or dislocation, and extremity pain.[51] Fracture or dislocation can be evaluated radiographically. Heterotopic ossification, as discussed earlier, is accompanied by an inflammatory reaction, increased alkaline phosphatase, increased activity on technetium bone scans, and radiographic changes. Differentiating between the relative contributions of pain, increased muscle tone, and contracture can be more difficult. Diagnostic lidocaine nerve blocks can help differentiate these by temporarily eliminating pain and muscle tone, thereby allowing the relative contributions of fixed soft-tissue contracture to be evaluated. Extremity nerve blocks in the evaluation of spasticity are outlined by Keenan.[51] These include blocks to the brachial plexus, musculocutaneous nerve, median nerve at the elbow, median and ulnar nerve blocks at the wrist, sciatic nerve, femoral nerve, obturator, and posterior tibial nerve.

It should be noted that a sudden increase in spasticity in the limbs may be a signal that an occult pathologic process is occurring, one that the patient is not aware of because of impaired sensibility. Possible problems include urinary tract infection, renal calculi, blockage of a catheter, or infected decubiti.[95] In the patient with a sudden increase of spasticity, these other problems should be suspected and appropriately evaluated.

Goals in Management

The main goals in the management of spasticity are to decrease muscle tone that interferes with function, retain limb motion to prevent contractures, and relieve pain that is often associated with spasticity. These are optimally accomplished by a multidisciplinary approach with a well-coordinated rehabilitation team. Management includes manual joint mobilization, limb splinting in a desirable position between therapy sessions, use of a standing frame, electrical stimulation of antagonist muscles to facilitate relaxation of the agonist, oral pharmacologic medications, serial lidocaine nerve blocks, phenol nerve blocks, surgical neurectomy, and surgical reconstruction. In the initial 12-month period of neurologic recovery (when spasticity may be decreasing), irreversible procedures such as neurectomy or tendon lengthenings should be avoided, because spontaneous recovery may obviate the need for these procedures, or result in an "overcorrection" deformity. In this 12-month period, mobilization, medications, and lidocaine or phenol nerve blocks should be used to their utmost effectiveness to avoid joint contractures.

Mobilization

Mobilization is performed by passive joint manipulation with proper splinting between mobilization sessions. The multiple benefits of joint mobilization include maintenance of lubrication efficiency of the joint, maintenance of the normal patterns of the soft-tissue matrix, assistance of orientation of new collagen fibers according to stresses, and prevention of increased cross links in the collagen matrix, thereby avoiding fixed contractures. Electrical stimulation can be used as an important adjuvant. Electrical stimulation of an agonist muscle not only provides a method of moving the joint, but also assists in the relaxation of the antagonist.

Oral Medications

Muscle tone can be decreased with several systemic pharmacologic agents.[117-124] Baclofen, diazepam, and dantrolene sodium are frequently used to help control sudden muscle contractions and to decrease increased tone.[22,125] Baclofen can be given orally or intrathecally (see below).[126-137] Baclofen blocks release of excitatory transmitters, thereby decreasing severity of sudden muscle spasms. Given in divided doses of 10 to 60 mg per day, it is well tolerated, has few side effects, and is less sedative than other medications used to decrease muscle tone. Diazepam enhances presynaptic inhibition, also resulting in reduction of painful spasms. It can be given in divided doses of 4 to 30 mg per day. The major side effect is sedation. It is also potentially habit-forming. Dantrolene sodium exerts inhibitive effect directly on muscle within the cell membrane and has no central nervous system depressant effect.[6] Side effects are minimal and there is no known tolerance. Hepatotoxicity is a potential side effect of all of these medications. Medications used less often or under investigation for treatment of spasticity include gabapentin, propranolol, thymoxamine, tizanidine, clonidine, divalproex sodium (Depakote), 4-aminopyridine, ziconotide, glycine, and intravenous orthenadrine citrate.[94,138-150]

Intrathecal Drug Delivery Systems

Over the last decade, the further development of intrathecal pumps has allowed the administration of medications with relative safety into the intrathecal space. Medications used to decrease both spasticity and associated pain include baclofen, clonidine, opiates, and local anesthetics.[151,152] By decreasing spasticity, a decrease in pain is often concomitantly achieved. The use of intrathecal opiates and local anesthetics can also be effective specifically in chronic pain syndromes.[153,154]

Baclofen currently seems to be the most successful and well-studied intrathecal medication for spasticity.[138,155-173] Baclofen delivered intrathecally has an advantage over the oral route because it applies a small concentration of baclofen directly to the target neural tissue. A smaller concentration is adequate to control spasticity while minimizing central side effects. The pump is placed in a subfascial pocket in the abdominal wall. A catheter is routed subcutaneously from the intrathecal space to the pump. The pump can be refilled by injection into the reservoir chamber. The dosage and rate of administration can be easily adjusted by using a laptop computer that sends wireless information to the pump. Continuous infusion of intrathecal baclofen has been shown to be effective in managing spasticity secondary to SCI. It has now become one of the more popular methods to control difficult spasticity.

Although the majority of investigations support the use and safety of intrathecal medication, especially baclofen, potential complications can occur. These include pump failure, catheter migration or failure, dehiscence of the suture line, infection or granuloma of the catheter, meningitis, medication overdose, seizure with the initial baclofen bolus, development of scar tissue around the device, pressure-sore formation, seroma accumulation, and withdrawal syndrome after discontinuance of the device.[49,174-183] Despite these complications, the benefits obtained seem to outweigh the potential problems.[184-188]

Lidocaine or Marcaine Nerve Blocks

Lidocaine or marcaine nerve blocks are effective temporary means of controlling or temporizing spasticity. As discussed above, regional lidocaine nerve blocks are helpful diagnostically to distinguish deformity caused by spasticity or by fixed contracture. Lidocaine nerve blocks can also be given in a serial fashion, before mobilization therapy. In some cases, daily nerve blocks will help alleviate spasticity. Lidocaine nerve block before serial casting will ease joint mobilization and cast application. Marcaine is much longer-acting than lidocaine, and can be used when a prolonged block is desired.

Phenol Nerve Block

Phenol nerve blocks have proven to be useful in the management of spasticity.[22,50,52,53,189-195] Phenol denatures the protein in a peripheral nerve, causing axonal degeneration. Because the continuity of the nerve sheath is not disrupted, the axons regenerate and nerve function returns.[51,194] These nerve injections, therefore, provide a much longer nerve block than lidocaine. A 5% solution can be injected in a closed or open (surgical) fashion. Five-percent aqueous solutions are used with closed blocks, and 3% to 5% solutions in glycerin are used with open blocks. Glycerin helps provide continued slow release of the phenol.[51] Phenol injection into a "mixed nerve" (containing both motor and sensory components) should not be performed in the patient with intact sensibility, as painful paresthesias may result. If sensibility is present, the phenol blocks should be reserved for nerves or nerve branches that carry predominantly motor fibers, such as pure motor nerves, the motor branches of the mixed nerve, or the motor points of the muscle. Injections into the motor branches are most accurately and safely performed by open block with direct visualization. When injected in a closed fashion, a Teflon-insulated needle with exposed tip guided by a nerve stimulator will assist with accurate placement of phenol. Closed phenol nerve blocks often provide relief from spasticity for up to 3 months. Open blocks, using a 5% solution of glycerin injected directly into the motor branches of the nerve, will provide longer relief, often up to 6 months. Phenol is not currently an approved substance by the US Food and Drug Administration, and proper patient consent is required. Phenol should not be autoclaved, as it can be denatured. Phenol is most optimally used in the period of neurologic recovery. It is hoped that as the nerve regenerates, the spasticity will decrease (if spontaneous recovery continues). If excessive spasticity remains when neurologic recovery has reached a plateau, then definitive surgery can be planned.[51,189]

Botulinum Toxin Nerve Blocks

In recent years, botulinum toxin has become a popular method to temporarily control spasticity in the extremities.[67,196-201] Botulinum toxin type A is a protein produced by *Clostridium botulinum* that inhibits the calcium-mediated release of acetylcholine at the neuromuscular junction. This block at the neuromuscular junction will stop the action potential from propagating down a motor nerve to reach the muscle, thus blocking muscle contraction. In the spastic muscle, this results in decreased hypertonic nature of the muscle, providing some degree of relaxation.

The botulinum toxin is injected directly into the muscle mass. Precise motor points do not need to be localized as in phenol blocks. The given dose varies, depending on the size of the muscle. Most dosing ranges between 10 and 200 units. Current practice is to wait at least 12 weeks before reinjection and not to administer a total of more that 400 units in a single treatment. It can be injected through a syringe attached to a hypodermic needle that doubles as a monopolar electromyographic recording electrode. In this way, muscle activity can be monitored during the injection procedure. This will assist in accurate injection of the botulinum toxin in the correct (spastic) muscle or portion of muscle with the maximal amount of hypertonicity.[67]

Botulinum toxin has been shown to be safe, effective, and well tolerated. Botulinum toxin has several advantages over phenol. Permanent scarring of the nerve, often seen from phenol or alcohol injections, does not occur. The onset of the effect of botulinum toxin occurs over a 2-week period. Its duration is variable, but can last up to 3 to 5 months.[67] Physical therapy is then instituted using both active and passive techniques to increase muscle range of motion. In a patient with an incomplete SCI, botulinum toxin blocks can be repeated as needed during the period of time in which neurologic recovery can be expected (usually within the first 12 months following the spinal injury).

Alcohol Nerve Block

In a patient with complete spinal injury with severe spasticity, alcohol peripheral nerve block can be used in a similar fashion as phenol. This method has never been as popular as phenol. The alcohol is toxic to the nerve and causes nerve damage, usually providing a permanent effect. The alcohol nerve block probably provides, in a sense, a nerve injury similar to a neurectomy. Sangwan et al[101] noted that use of alcohol peripheral nerve blocks in these patients is effective, safe, and simple. Alcohol nerve block is contraindicated in a patient with incomplete injury, where permanent undesirable weakness may develop. In addition, if the patient has some retained sensibility, the alcohol nerve block may result in painful paresthesias. An alcohol block is probably the safest when given in an open fashion, thus avoiding or minimizing damage to the surrounding muscles, tendons, or vessels. In this setting, one could also just consider neurectomy.

Motor Neurectomy

If a patient has persistent noxious spasticity and no further neurologic recovery is occurring or expected (ie, the patient is beyond the 12-month period of spontaneous recovery), open motor neurectomy can be performed. Prior to neurectomy, the effects of the neurectomy can be simulated with a lidocaine or phenol block. If the block produces the desired results, neurectomy may be feasible. One must realize that neurectomy alone will not correct a fixed contracture; it will only address the spastic component of the muscle. Prior lidocaine block will help differentiate the relative contributions of spasticity and fixed contracture causing the deformity. The spastic component will be obliterated with the block; the fixed contracture will remain.

Common neurectomies performed include muculocutaneous (for elbow flexion), motor branch to the brachioradialis (for elbow flexion), deep motor branch of the ulnar nerve (intrinsic plus deformity of the hand), superficial branch of the obturator nerve (adduction deformity of the thighs), motor branches of the femoral nerve (hip flexor or knee extensor spasticity), motor branches of the sciatic nerve (knee flexion spasticity), and motor branches of the posterior tibial nerve (equinovarus deformity). In performing a neurectomy, it is desirable to remove a segment of nerve to prevent spontaneous repair from axonal regeneration.

Intrathecal Injection of Alcohol or Phenol (Contraindicated)

Intrathecal injections using alcohol or phenol to control noxious spasticity have been reported; however, they are mentioned here only to discourage their use. Intrathecal injections should not be performed. These injections, using either alcohol or phenol, produce permanent lower motor neuron lesions. This results in a flaccid paralysis. The loss of all spasticity allows severe atrophy to occur, placing the lower extremities at higher risk for pressure sores. Any functionally useful extensor patterning is lost, such as that used for wheelchair transfers. The spastic bowel and bladder are converted to a flaccid bowel and bladder, resulting in loss of reflex evacuation and subsequent incontinence. There should never be a need or indication for alcohol or phenol intrathecal injection. The peripheral nerves or muscles should be addressed instead of the intrathecal space. Peripheral phenol nerve blocks, motor neurectomies, or muscle lengthening or release will control even the most noxious spastic muscles.

Rhizotomy, Cordotomy, and Cordectomy

Severance of the nerve roots or part or all of the cord has been performed to disrupt the reflex arc and convert a severely spastic extremity into a flaccid extremity. Similar complications as mentioned above with intrathecal injection may occur. Therefore, these procedures have lost popularity and in general should not be performed. Severe spasticity should be treated at the level of the peripheral nerve or muscle, as described above.

Electrical Stimulation

Electrical stimulation has several uses in the rehabilitation setting.[202-208] In spastic or contracted muscle, it is used as an adjunct to stimulate weak agonist muscle and relax strong antagonists. Specific types of electrical stimulation have application to control spasms or are used for pain management, such as the transcutaneous electrical nerve stimulation (TENS) units. When used as an adjunct for function, it is called functional electrical stimulation (see below). Peripheral repetitive magnetic stimulation has also been investigated as a method to reduce muscle tone in spasticity.[209]

Joint Contracture

One of the most disastrous and often preventable complications of spasticity is the formation of a fixed contracture.[85,87,210] If a joint is not mobilized, either actively or passively, a contracture will develop. Contractures develop following immobilization from spasticity, paralysis, heterotopic ossification, or following injury. A joint moved once daily through its full range of motion will not develop a contracture. Contractures occur from loss of elasticity or fixed shortening of soft tissues. Tissues involved include joint capsule, ligaments, muscle-tendon units, skin, nerves, and vascular structures. A fixed contracture often prevents any joint motion, and causes subsequent irreversible joint changes. Articular cartilage erosions, fatty infiltration, and intra-articular adhesion formation develop.[85-89] Contractures interfere with function and hygiene. A joint contracture restricts limb position, causes problems with wheelchair transfers, interferes with dressing and sitting, and secondarily increases the potential for pressure sore formation. Proper hygiene may be difficult to maintain, especially in the groin, axilla, antecubital fossa, and popliteal fossa. Skin maceration can lead to ulceration and infection. In addition, the contractures themselves are often painful, especially when the limb is forcibly manipulated or positioned. Therefore, one of the most important goals in the management of spasticity is to maintain joint motion to prevent fixed contracture.

Treatment

Contractures are difficult to treat, requiring considerable time and discomfort to the patient, and often requiring surgical intervention. The most important aspect in the treatment of contractures is prevention. Joint mobilization and proper splinting should be initiated early following SCI, commencing when the patient is still in the intensive care unit, as soon as medical stability permits. Once established, treatment of a contracture includes manual mobilization followed by well-padded serial casting as needed. Casts are changed weekly to inspect skin, allow further limb mobilization, and achieve further correction in a new cast. Serial drop-out casts are effective in the management of contracture. Dynamic splints may be attempted; however, these will not work if considerable spasticity coexists, especially if clonus is present.

Management of Specific Deformities

Shoulder

Involvement of the shoulder with spasticity is common in the SCI patient, as injuries that occur proximal to the C5 root level can result in paralysis of the diaphragm (C4) and often result in respiratory failure. However, in the survivors of these proximal cervical SCIs, spasticity can be severe. Function is usually minimal, and reconstruction difficult because of a lack of available donor muscles and the presence of limb spasticity throughout. Deformity of the shoulder with spasticity is usually manifested by adduction and internal rotation. Muscles responsible for the deformity include the pectoralis major, subscapularis, teres major, and latissimus dorsi. Problems with hygiene, positioning, and dressing can arise. Rehabilitation efforts are initially directed toward mobilization to prevent contracture. Orthoses are not practical to correct this deformity. Phenol nerve blocks to the motor points of the pectoralis can be performed if the patient is in the period of neurologic recovery of spasticity.[50] If the patient has reached a plateau in improvement and no further neurologic recovery is expected, a surgical release of spastic muscles can be performed to aid positioning and hygiene. Release of the pectoralis major and subscapularis are performed first, followed by the teres major and latissimus dorsi as needed.[211]

Elbow

Severe spasticity of the elbow is rare, as these muscles are innervated primarily by nerve roots from the C5 level; for spasticity to occur, the lesion must be proximal to this level. Many patients with more proximal lesions do not survive, as discussed previously. If spasticity is present, initial treatment is mobilization to prevent contracture, and well-padded splints between therapy sessions to maintain correction. During the period of neurologic recovery, closed phenol nerve block to the musculocutaneous nerve can aid with mobilization. If spasticity is severe, and there is no volitional control in the extremity of a patient who is beyond the period of spontaneous recovery, motor neurectomy or surgical release of the biceps, brachialis, and brachioradialis can be performed. These will facilitate hygiene, positioning, and dressing. If there is preservation of volitional control, then selective lengthening of the elbow flexors can be performed to augment function.[66]

Hand and Wrist

Spasticity of the hands and wrist can occur in the SCI patient, but is usually associated with proximal cord lesions with spasticity throughout the upper extremity. In the severely affected patients, there is usually flexion deformity at the wrist and the hand (combined with flexor patterning of the upper extremity, ie, elbow flexion, shoulder adduction and flexion). The hand can assume an intrinsic-plus position if the intrinsic muscles are spastic and the extrinsic muscles paretic or paralytic.[52] If contracture develops, fixed shortening of the flexor tendons of the wrist or digits can be treated with mobilization, serial casting, or tendon lengthening as needed. If lengthening is necessary, fractional lengthening is preferred when volitional control is present.[212] Fixed intrinsic contracture can be treated with intrinsic muscle lengthening.[66,189]

In the more distal cervical cord injuries (ie, C8, T1 root levels), an intrinsic-minus hand deformity may develop. This is due to loss of nerve root or cord disruption at the C8 or T1 level, resulting in paralysis of intrinsic muscles of the hand. If the extrinsic flexors and extensors are intact (because these are innervated by a more proximal spinal cord level), the imbalance will produce the intrinsic-minus or "claw-hand" deformity." This problem is discussed under Paralysis: Upper Extremities.

Hip

Flexor patterning of the lower extremity results in hip flexion and adduction. Hip flexion is usually caused by spasticity of the rectus femoris and the iliopsoas. The anterior portion of the tensor fascia lata may contribute to hip flexion. Hip adduction is usually caused by spasticity of the adductor longus, brevis, magnus, and the gracilis. Problems with hygiene in the groin are common. Difficulty in transfers, standing, and dressing also occur. There is no feasible orthosis to treat flexion and adduction deformities of the hip. Mobilization may be initiated and prone positioning attempted to prevent contracture. Serial femoral and obturator lidocaine nerve blocks or closed phenol nerve blocks can be given. Open phenol blocks to the motor branches of the obturator nerve or femoral nerve can be given if closed phenol blocks are not adequate. Nerve blocks to the quadriceps muscles will also decrease knee extension, which may or may not be desirable. It is difficult to block the motor nerve to the iliopsoas muscle. If the patient has reached a plateau in a physical therapy program providing mobilization and is beyond the period of expected neurologic recovery, muscle lengthenings or release can be performed. If the patient is a nonambulator, adduction deformity can be addressed with tenotomy of the adductor longus, brevis, gracilis, and possibly a portion of the adductor magnus. Alternately, obturator neurectomy can be performed; however, this may not alleviate a deformity caused by fixed muscle-tendon contracture. If the patient is an ambulator, the adductor magnus should be preserved to provide some adduction of the hip and prevent undesirable overcorrection manifested by hip abduction. In the nonambulator, chronic refractory hip flexion deformity can be managed with release of the rectus femoris, iliopsoas, sartorius, and anterior portion of the tensor fascia lata.

Whenever surgical lengthenings or releases are considered, care must be given in assessing the functional status of the limb. If the patient has functional lower extremities, muscle lengthenings should be performed in place of releases. At the hip, this might include Z-lengthening of the iliopsoas tendon, fractional lengthening or release of the rectus femoris, and partial release of the adductor muscles (release of the adductor longus, brevis, and gracilis, while preserving the adductor magnus). Fixed contractures of these muscles can be treated by lengthening or release, depending on functional status. Residual contracture of the joint capsule can usually be corrected with mobilization or prone positioning once the deforming spastic or contracted muscle forces are eliminated.

Knee

Knee flexion deformity is common in the SCI patient, caused by spasticity of the medial and lateral hamstring muscles.[213] This deformity increases the potential for pressure-sore development on the hindfoot, makes transfers difficult, and causes hygiene problems in the popliteal fossa. If sudden muscle spasms occur, the patient can be propelled from the wheelchair. Initial treatment of chronic knee flexion deformity from spasticity includes mobilization to prevent contracture and medications to control spasticity. Serial lidocaine nerve blocks to the sciatic nerve in the proximal thigh may help alleviate hamstring spasticity. Closed phenol nerve block to the sciatic nerve can be performed in the patient without sensibility. The sciatic nerve is blocked in a closed fashion by percutaneous injection at the distal margin of the gluteus maximus, guided with the nerve stimulator and insulated needle. If sensibility in the lower extremity is present, closed phenol block to the sciatic nerve should not be done because painful paresthesias can occur from the phenol injection into a nerve containing sensory fibers. In these patients, open phenol block to the motor branches of the sciatic nerve can be performed, thus avoiding phenol injection into sensory fibers. This requires a large surgical exposure to adequately identify and inject the motor branches to the hamstrings. It is difficult to inject many of the more distal branches in the thigh. In the ambulatory patient with knee flexor spasticity that interferes with function, and who has reached a plateau in neurologic recovery, surgical lengthening of the hamstring muscles can be performed. In the nonambulatory patient with noxious knee flexor spasticity that interferes with transfers, positioning, or hygiene, and who has reached a plateau in neurologic recovery, release of the distal hamstrings can be performed.[214]

Occasionally, knee extensor spasticity is present. This can be troublesome or beneficial. Sudden muscle spasms can propel the patient from a bed or chair. However, the patient may use knee extensor patterning to stabilize the limb during wheelchair transfers. When knee extensor spasticity is difficult to control or unsafe for the patient, a phenol block to the femoral nerve in the proximal thigh will help to temporarily control quadriceps spasms. If the patient is beyond the recovery period (1 year after SCI), selective release of the distal quadriceps or neurectomy of the motor branches of the femoral nerve may be performed. However, these procedures may accentuate knee flexion spasticity, and should be avoided or performed cautiously in the patient who also has alternating knee flexor spasticity or patterning.

Foot/Ankle

Equinus deformity of the foot is common, caused by spasticity of the gastrocnemius and soleus muscles.[213,215-218] Severe deformity causes difficulty with standing, transfers, wearing shoes, and placement of the feet on the wheelchair platform. Manual mobilization, splinting, and pharmacologic control of spasticity are initiated first. Serial lidocaine nerve blocks to the posterior tibial nerve in the popliteal fossa can help alleviate spasticity. Serial casting with well-padded casts can be performed for fixed contractures; however, frequent cast replacement is necessary to allowed skin inspection. If the patient is no longer improving in a therapy program and is beyond the period of expected neurologic recovery, tendo Achillis lengthening can be performed. If hindfoot varus is present, this can be addressed with lengthening of the tibialis posterior or tibialis anterior tendons. The split tibialis anterior tendon transfer (SPLATT procedure) is only rarely performed in the SCI patient, as this procedure does not address the commonly spastic tibialis posterior.[213,215-218]

Toes

Clawing of the toes (hyperextension at the metatarsophalangeal joint, flexion at the proximal interphalangeal joint) can cause skin irritation on the dorsum of the toes from pressure against the shoes. Clawing can be caused by intrinsic muscle weakness, muscle imbalance, or by spasticity of the extrinsic extensors and flexors. Correction of deformity can be performed with lengthening or release of the extensor tendons (and flexors as necessary). These can be combined with resection arthroplasty or arthrodesis of the proximal interphalangeal joint if fixed joint deformity exists. Phalangectomy should generally be avoided because the loss of bone and ligamentous stability can result in lateral deviation of the toes if spasticity is present.

Occasionally, only flexion deformities will be present, manifested by flexion at the metatarsophalangeal and interphalangeal joints. Painful skin irritation on the distal tip of the toe can result as the toes are flexed into the shoe or floor. Release

FIGURE 6

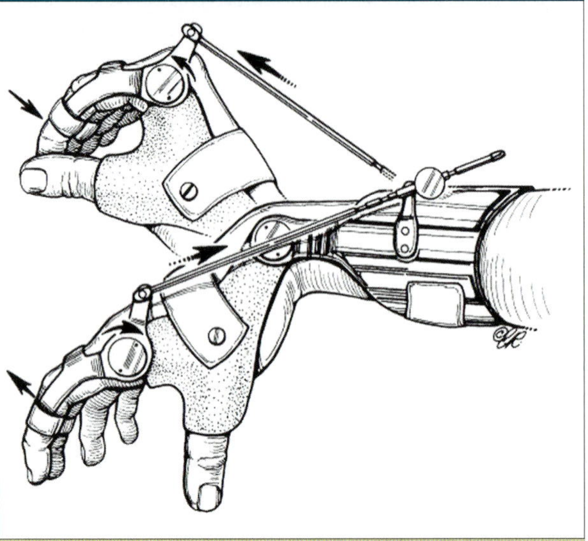

Figure 6 Wrist-driven orthosis. Active wrist extension with the orthosis in place provides a means of single-hand grip. This device is dependent on adequate wrist extensor strength. As the wrist is dorsiflexed, the fingers are flexed to bring them into contact with the thumb, which is fixed. As the wrist is palmar flexed, the fingers are extended. If wrist extensor strength is not adequate, tendon transfer to provide extensor strength can be considered. The brachioradialis is commonly used as a donor for this transfer. A similar but static ratchet-type of orthosis is available that will hold the fingers in pinch position if the wrist is passively extended into a locked mode. (Reproduced with permission from McDowell CL: Tetraplegia, in Green DP, ed: *Operative Hand Surgery*. New York, NY, Churchill Livingston, 1988, pp 1597-1618.)

of both the long and short flexor can be performed. Release of the toe flexors can be performed through incisions on the plantar aspect of the toes. Loss of active toe flexion is usually not a problem.[213,215-218]

If flexion deformity is present only at the proximal interphalangeal joint, without flexion at the distal phalangeal joint, the short toe flexors may be responsible. Involvement of these muscles can be verified with a posterior tibial nerve block at the ankle. This will selectively block the intrinsic flexors, leaving the extrinsic toe flexors functioning. If the deformity corrects with this block, then the short toe flexors are responsible, and these can be selectively released.[218]

Paralysis: Upper Extremities

Loss of upper limb function constitutes one of the most severe problems the quadriplegic patient faces. When surveyed by questionnaire, many quadriplegic patients indicated they would prefer restoration of hand function over restoration of walking capacity, bladder or bowel function, or even sexual function.[9] Orthoses and surgical reconstruction play an important role in the rehabilitation of the upper extremity. Recently, new techniques in functional electrical stimulation of the upper extremity have been shown to be promising in the restoration of function.

Principal Functions to Restore

It has been estimated that 70% of traumatic tetraplegic patients can be helped by surgical reconstruction.[219-221] Two of the most desirable functions to restore are: (1) active elbow extension, and (2) single-hand grip (usually provided by lateral pinch).[222-251] In addition, reconstruction of finger flexion has been emphasized.[223,249] Other desirable functions include forearm pronation and intrinsic augmentation (for claw deformity), but these should be considered only after restoration of elbow extension and single-hand grip, provided available donor muscles are available.[249,251-254]

Elbow extension can be reconstructed if a functional deltoid is present, using a deltoid-to-triceps tendon transfer. Restoration of elbow extension allows a patient to stabilize himself/herself in the wheelchair and improves control of self-help devices. Patients may gain the ability to hang up clothes or to take objects down from an overhead shelf. In rare cases, a patient may gain the ability to move from bed to wheelchair or to pivot without help (even though these bed-to-chair functions depend more on muscles that forwardly flex and depress the humerus such as the pectoralis). These motions allow locking of the elbow in extension, providing adequate elbow stability for transfers.

Single-hand grip can be accomplished by several different methods: (1) use of a wrist-driven flexor hinge orthosis, powered by volitional wrist extension to provide pinch (**Figure 6**); (2) tendon transfer (brachioradialis to extensor carpi radialis brevis) to provide or augment weak wrist extension to power a wrist-driven flexor hinged orthosis and provide pinch; (3) the Moberg tenodesis procedure to provide lateral pinch; and (4) opponensplasties to provide thumb-to-finger pinch.[223] These are discussed in more detail later.

Patient Selection and Classification

Patient selection for any type of surgical reconstruction in the tetraplegic patient can be difficult because of the complexity of the physical examination, the possibility of changing neurologic status (in the incomplete SCI) over the first

FIGURE 7

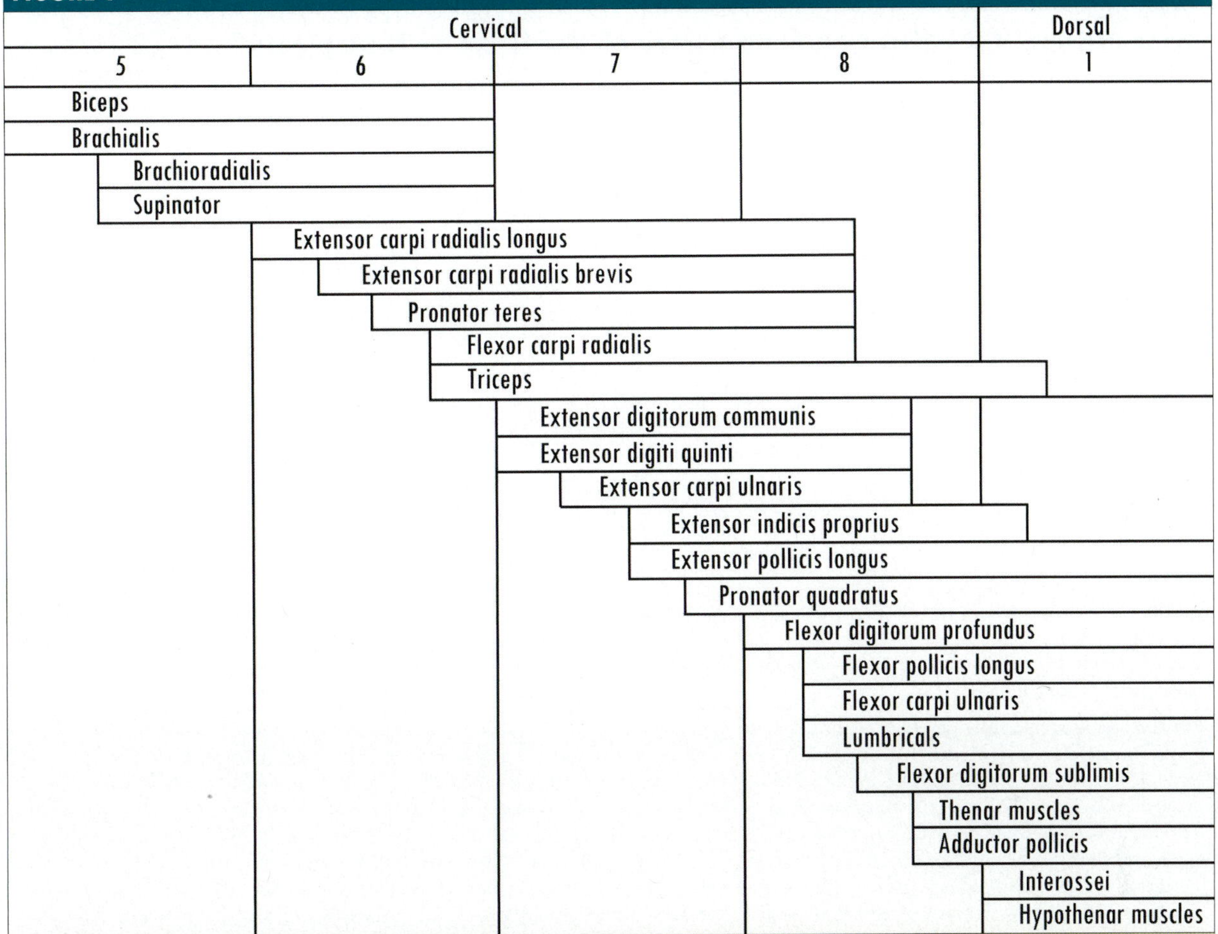

Figure 7 Segmental innervation of muscles of the elbow, forearm, and hand. (Reproduced with permission from Zancolli EA: *Structural and Dynamic Bases of Hand Surgery*, ed 2. Philadelphia, PA, JB Lippincott, 1979, p 231.)

12 months, and the multiple subjective factors that should be considered (patient age, occupation, interests, and expectations). Surgical reconstruction of each of the different functional levels will be discussed separately later. However, general considerations are overviewed first.

Selection for surgical reconstruction is dependent upon existing motor and sensory function. In the past, quadriplegic patients were classified by the cervical spine segment injured, assuming that the level of paralysis and sensory loss coincided with the bone injury (**Figure 7**).[254] However, this classification was not consistently accurate, because the level of boney injury may not coincide with the actual level of cord injury. In addition, spinal injury may not be symmetric and there may be unusual patterns of sparing of sensory or motor function. Nerve root injury from a higher spinal level may coexist with the cord lesion. Therefore, a more useful classification was developed by McDowell et al[242,243] and approved by an international group of surgeons working with tetraplegics. This classification is based on the most distal muscle available for transfer, and patients are grouped into nine groups. The groups are further subdivided according to sensibility (**Table 2**). In group 0 (the most severely affected group), only the deltoid is available for transfer; the rest of the upper extremity is paralytic or paretic. In group 9 (the least involved patient in this classification), the only weak muscles are the hand intrinsics, and multiple muscles are available for transfer. Specific transfers are discussed below.

Sensory Evaluation

Successful surgical reconstruction of the upper limbs is dependent on the presence of adequate sensibility. Sensory evaluation should include stereognosis and two-point discrimination. In most patients, stereognosis and two-point

TABLE 2

International Classification for Surgery of the Hand in Tetraplegia[a]

Sensibility	Motor Group	Characteristics	Function
O or Cu	0	No muscle below elbow suitable for transfer	Flexion, supination of elbow
	1	Brachioradialis	
	2	ECRL	Extension of wrist (weak or strong)
	3	ECRB[b]	Extension of wrist
	4	PT	Extension and pronation of wrist
	5	FCR	Flexion of wrist
	6	Finger extensors	Extrinsic extension of fingers (partial or complete)
	7	Thumb extensor	Extrinsic extension of thumb
	8	Partial digital flexors	Extrinsic flexion of fingers (weak)
	9	Lacks only intrinsics	Extrinsic flexion of fingers
	X	Exceptions	

ECRL = extensor carpi radialis longus; ECRB = extensor carpi radialis brevis; PT = pronator teres; FCR = flexor carpi radialis. O and Cu are explained below, in point (3).

[a](1) The classification does not include the shoulder. It is a guide to the forearm and hand only. Determination of patient suitability for posterior deltoid-to-triceps transfer of biceps-to-triceps transfer is considered separately. (2) The need for triceps reconstruction is stated separately. It may be required to make brachioradialis transfers function properly. (3) There is a sensory component to the classification. Afferent input is recorded using the method Moberg described and precedes the motor classification. Both ocular and cutaneous input should be documented. When vision is the only afferent available, the designation is "Occulo" (abbreviated O). Assuming there is 10 mm or less two-point discrimination in the thumb and index finger, the correct classification would be Cu, indicating that the patient has adequate cutaneous sensibility. If two-point discrimination is greater than 10 mm (meaning inadequate cutaneous sensibility), the designation O would precede the motor group (example O 2). (4) Motor grouping assumes that all listed muscles are grade 4 (Medical Research Council [MRC]) or better and a new muscle is added for each group; for example, a group 3 patient will have brachioradialis, ECRL, and ECRB rated at least grade 4 (MRC).

[b]It is not possible to determine the strength of the ECRB without surgical exposure.

(Adapted with permission from McDowell CL: Tetraplegia, in Green DP, ed: *Operative Hand Surgery*, ed 2. Churchill Livingstone, New York, NY, 1988, pp 1597-1618. Modified by McDowell CL, Moberg EA, House JH: The Second International Conference on Surgical Rehabilitation of the Upper Limb in Tetraplegia (Quadriplegia). *J Hand Surg Am* 1986;11:604-608.)

discrimination of at least 10 mm is required in order for pinch or grip to be useful.[74,220] If two-point discrimination of 10 mm or less is not present, grip needs to be guided or regulated by direct vision. Using direct vision to regulate grip can usually guide only one hand at a time.[248] Therefore, a prerequisite for surgical reconstruction of grip is the presence of two-point discrimination and stereognosis in at least one hand.

As mentioned, the motor group classifications are subdivided according to sensibility. When sensibility is adequate to regulate grip, the classification of "Cu" (cutaneous) is given, which indicates cutaneous afferents good enough to lead the grip. If sensibility is not adequate to lead grip, direct vision is required to regulate grip, and the sensory classification is 0. For example, a patient with the brachioradialis available for transfer and adequate sensibility in both hands is classified as CuCu 9.

Timing of Surgical Reconstruction

Surgical reconstruction in the quadriplegic upper extremity is usually not performed before 1 year postinjury. This usually provides adequate time for the neurologic recovery to reach a plateau, to allow the patient sufficient time to adjust psychologically to the paralysis, and to realize that there will be no further recovery. In addition, recovery from spasticity usually becomes static by 1 year after injury, thus providing a static clinical picture of limb function. If there is any evidence of continuing neurologic recovery or improvement in function in a therapy program, surgical reconstruction should be delayed until there is no longer any motor or sensory improvement.

FIGURE 8

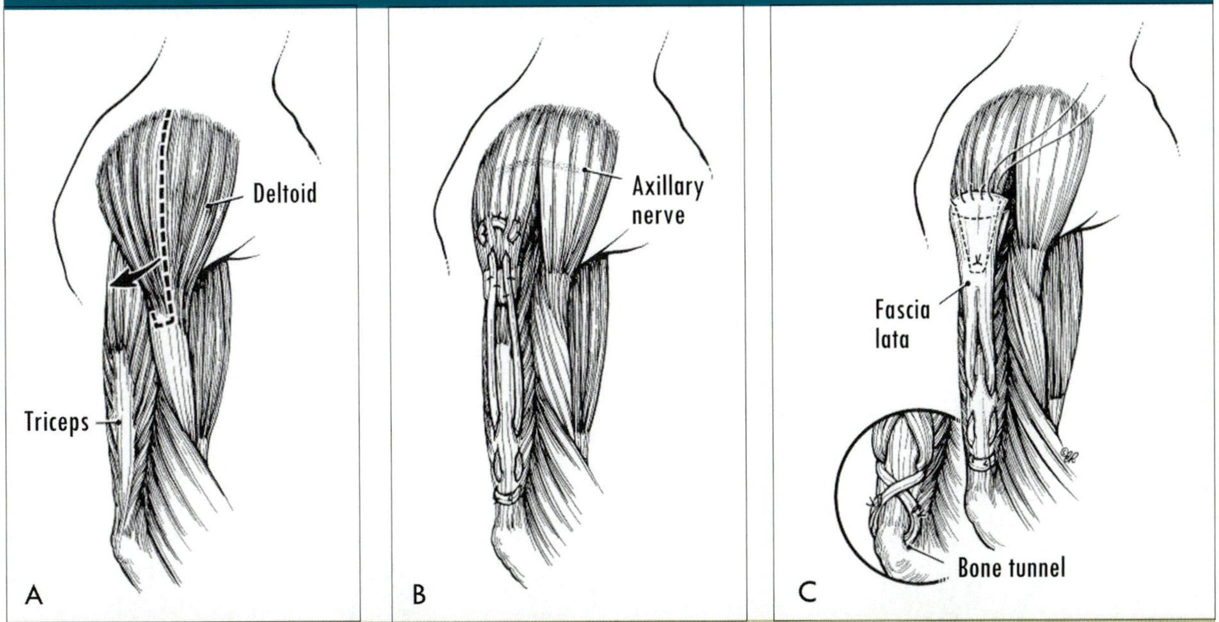

Figure 8 Posterior deltoid-to-triceps transfer (Moberg) can provide active elbow extension. **A,** The posterior border of the muscle belly is isolated, preserving as much of the tendinous insertion as possible. **B,** An intercalary tendon graft is required, usually obtained from toe extensors or fascia lata. The tendon grafts are laced into the distal end of the deltoid muscle belly and triceps aponeurosis. **C,** Fascia lata used for graft. (Reproduced with permission from McDowell CL: Tetraplegia, in Green DP, ed: *Operative Hand Surgery*. New York, NY, Churchill Livingston, 1988, pp 1597-1618.)

Basic Principles in Limb Reconstruction

Principles of limb reconstruction have been developed and illustrated by the excellent writings of Moberg, Zancolli, McDowell, Waters, House, Hentz, Fridén, Van Heest, and others.[222-251,253-259]

In general, the least affected limb should undergo reconstruction first. Surgery should be performed on the dominant extremity first (if both are similarly impaired.) If adequate cutaneous sensibility is not present, surgery should be done only on the side with the better residual motor function (using vision to guide the grip in this extremity). Only one surgical procedure should be performed at a time. Restoration of elbow extension should precede other procedures that restore pinch or grasp to the hand. Simplicity in surgery is the safest, using available muscles of the extremity to strive for one or two simple functions. True opposition in pinch is usually not necessary; lateral pinch (key pinch) is more useful. Severe spasticity or fixed contracture needs to be controlled or corrected before tendon transfers.

Surgical Procedures

Surgical procedures will be discussed according to motor classification. It must be reiterated that two-point discrimination of less than 10 mm and intact stereognosis must be present for useful hand function without guidance by direct vision, and that an individual can visually guide only one hand at a time. Therefore, at least one hand should have adequate cutaneous sensibility. Direct vision can guide the other.

Group 0

In general, patients in group 0 have functioning deltoids but no muscle function below the elbow suitable for transfer (**Table 2**). This corresponds roughly to a C5 functional level. If elbow flexion itself is lacking, this can be restored provided the deltoid is functional. The posterior portion of the deltoid is transferred to the triceps, using an intercalary tendon graft harvested from the fascia lata, toe extensor, or tibialis anterior (**Figure 8**). Patients in group 0 may be candidates for an externally powered orthosis. Most of these patients can use some assistive devices attached to one hand.

The biceps-to-triceps transfer is an alternative method used to restore elbow extension (**Figure 9**). Recent studies indicate superior results using the biceps to triceps compared to the deltoid transfer, with improved strength in antigravity use of the arm, overhead reaching, and in driving activities.[249] The biceps may also be used to

FIGURE 9

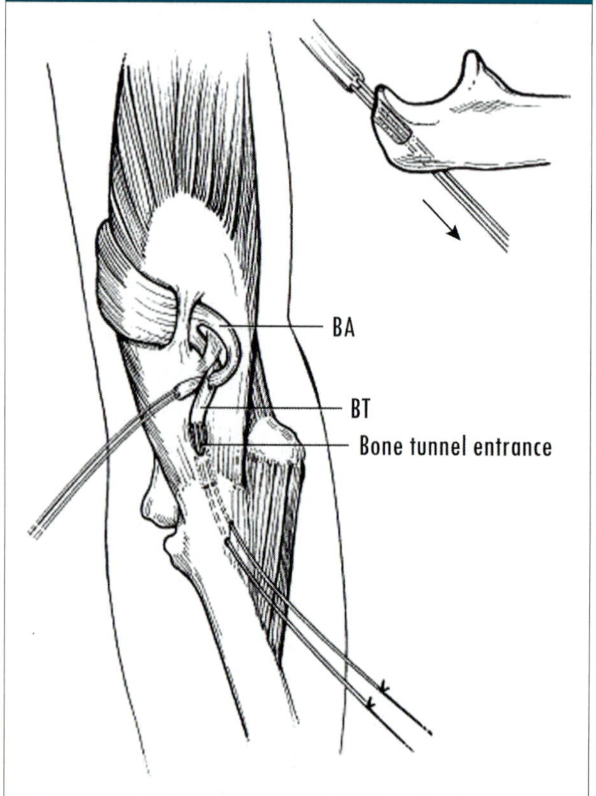

Figure 9 Biceps to triceps is an alternative method for establishing elbow extension. The biceps tendon (BT) and bicipital aponeurosis (BA) are released and the muscle is mobilized and rerouted medially around the arm. The tendon is inserted in a braiding technique into the triceps tendon and then directly interested to the olecranon with a bone tunnel. (Reproduced with permission from Van Heest A: Tetraplegia, in Green DP, ed: *Green's Operative Hand Surgery*, ed 5. Philadelphia, PA, Elsevier Churchill Livingstone, 2005, pp 1271-1295.)

FIGURE 10

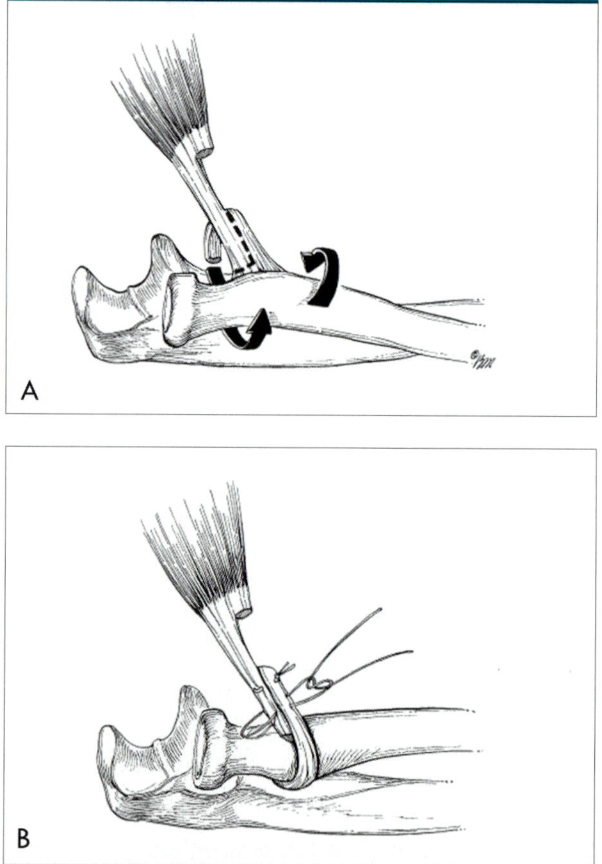

Figure 10 Zancolli's technique to improve pronation is performed by converting the biceps tendon into a forearm pronator. Half of the biceps tendon is rerouted behind the neck of the radius (**A**) and sutured to the remaining stump (**B**). (Reproduced with permission from Van Heest A: Tetraplegia, in Green DP, ed: *Green's Operative Hand Surgery*, ed 5. Philadelphia, PA, Elsevier Churchill Livingstone, 2005, pp 1271-1295.)

provide forearm pronation by rerouting its insertion (**Figure 10**) (discussed later). The need to achieve forearm pronation should be appreciated before using the biceps to achieve elbow extension.

Group 1

Patients in this group have a strong brachioradialis, but poor function distally, including poor wrist extensors. Transfer of the brachioradialis into the extensor carpi radialis brevis and/or longus can provide sufficient wrist extension to power a wrist-driven flexor hinge orthosis.[219,221,260] This can provide a type of single-hand grip (**Figure 11**). In addition, lateral pinch can be augmented or reconstructed with the Moberg reconstruction.[219-221] The Moberg reconstruction requires strong wrist extension as a prerequisite. Reconstruction of lateral pinch consists of: (1) tenodesis of the flexor pollicis longus to the distal palmar radius, to provide thumb flexion and create lateral pinch when the wrist is actively extended; (2) resection of the proximal annular pulley of the thumb to permit the tendon to bowstring and increase the strength of the key pinch; (3) internal fixation of the interphalangeal joint of the thumb to prevent flexion at the interphalangeal joint and maintain a broad contact surface; and (4) tenodesis of the extensor hood mechanism to the metacarpal of the thumb to prevent hyperflexion of the metacarpophalangeal joint (**Figure 12**). Many modifications of this procedure have been described.[231,248,261,262] An alternative reconstruction is the wrist-driven flexor hinge hand described by Nickel et al.[260] This in-

FIGURE 11

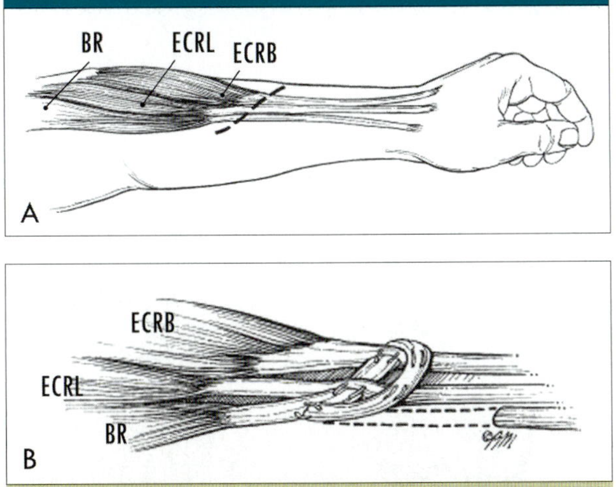

Figure 11 Brachioradialis (BR) to extensor carpi radialis longus (ECRL) and brevis (ECRB) can be used to provide wrist extension so that either a wrist-driven orthosis for grip or the Moberg tenodesis becomes feasible. **A,** Normal anatomy. **B,** Transfer of BR into the ECRL and ECRB. (Reproduced with permission from McDowell CL: Tetraplegia, in Green DP, ed: *Operative Hand Surgery*. New York, NY, Churchill Livingston, 1988, pp 1597-1618.)

FIGURE 12

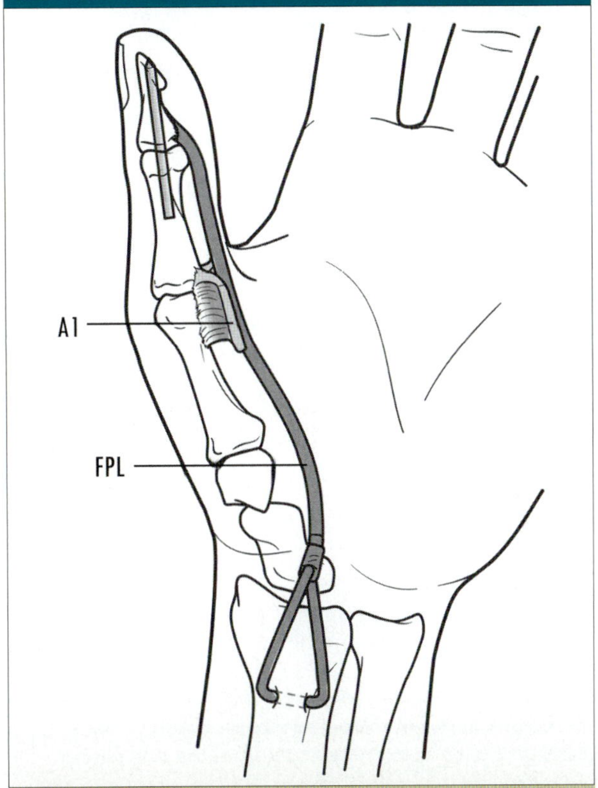

Figure 12 Moberg reconstruction to provide key pinch. Strong wrist extension is a prerequisite. If wrist extension is weak, the brachioradialis can be transferred to the extensor carpi radialis brevis to provide wrist extension. Salient features of this reconstruction include tenodesis of the flexor pollicis longus (FPL) to the distal palmar radius, to provide thumb flexion and create key pinch when the wrist is actively extended; resection of the proximal annular A1 pulley of the thumb to permit the tendon to bowstring and increase the strength of the key grip; internal fixation of the interphalangeal joint of the thumb to prevent interphalangeal joint flexion and maintain a broad contact surface; and tenodesis of the extensor hood mechanism to the metacarpal of the thumb to prevent hyperflexion of the metacarpophalangeal joint.

cludes stabilization of the thumb and interphalangeal joints of the index and long fingers with arthrodesis, and tenodesis of the profundus tendons of the index and long fingers to the distal radius so that the tips of those two fingers are brought into contact with the thumb during wrist extension.[260] Alternative methods of achieving pinch have been discussed by Freehafer, Kelly, House and Van Heest.[25,223,233-236,249] These methods include transfer of the brachioradialis to a rerouted flexor digitorum superficialis (from the ring finger, routed across the palm) and inserted into the abductor pollicis brevis tendon, or split and transferred into the dorsum of the thumb over the proximal phalanx.

Group 2

Patients in this group have function of the extensor carpi radialis longus. They are able to operate a wrist-driven orthosis for single-hand grip and are also candidates for single-hand grip or lateral pinch reconstruction as described earlier. Because the extensor carpi radialis brevis is such an effective wrist extensor and wrist extension is so valuable, this muscle should not be transferred.[25,223] However, the brachioradialis is available for transfer and can be used in different ways (because it is not needed to provide wrist extension, as in group 1 patients.) Possible options include transfer of the brachioradialis to the flexor pollicis longus to increase strength of pinch,[218,248] or to the extensor pollicis longus, extensor pollicis brevis, or abductor pollicis longus to open the thumb-index web space to improve the release phase of the grasp-release sequence. The usefulness of these procedures does not seem to be as promising as had been anticipated,[219,241] and transfer of the brachioradialis in group 2 patients is not recommended by McDowell.[241]

Some patients in group 2 (and group 3) have weak forearm pronation, but active wrist extension. These patients can use a tenodesis effect for grasp, but if the hand cannot be pronated, gravity cannot be used to provide a tenodesis effect.

FIGURE 13

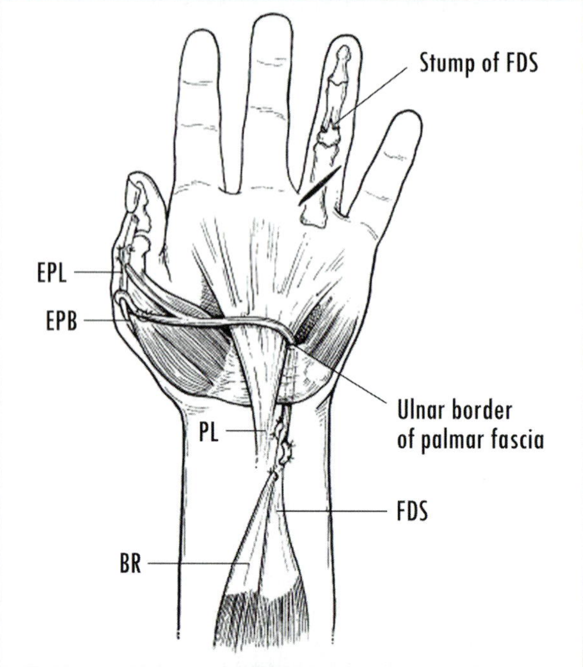

Figure 13 The thumb adduction-opponensplasty is produced by transfer of the brachioradialis (BR) (or flexor carpi ulnaris or flexor superficialis from the ring finger) rerouted around a palmar fascial pulley to a dual insertion that controls thumb rotation and stabilizes the metacarpophalangeal and interphalangeal joints for better lateral pinch. The brachioradialis can be used as the motor in group 5 and the flexor carpi ulnaris in groups 7 and 8. EPL = extensor pollicis longus; EPB = extensor pollicis brevis; FDS = flexor digitorum superficialis; PL = palmaris longus. (Reproduced with permission from Van Heest A: Tetraplegia, in Green DP, ed: *Green's Operative Hand Surgery*, ed 5. Philadelphia, PA, Elsevier Churchill Livingstone, 2005, pp 1271-1295.)

FIGURE 14

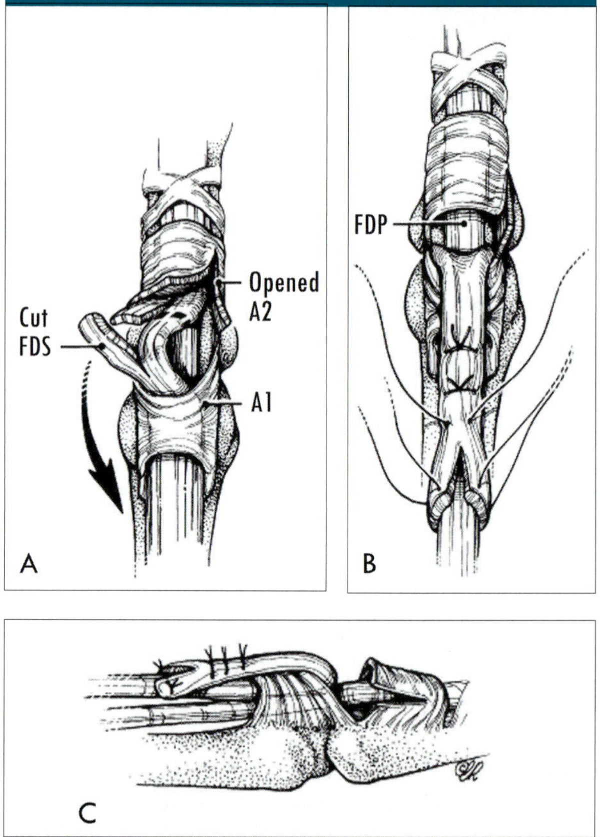

Figure 14 Zancolli's lasso intrinsic tenodesis procedure to restore intrinsic balance and improve metacarpophalangeal joint flexion, as well as decrease interphalangeal joint flexion deformities. **A,** Release of flexor digitorum superficialis (FDS). **B,** Tenodesis of the FDS to itself. **C,** Completed procedure. FDP = flexor digitorum profundus. (Reproduced with permission from Van Heest A: Tetraplegia, in Green DP, ed: *Green's Operative Hand Surgery*, ed 5. Philadelphia, PA, Elsevier Churchill Livingstone, 2005, pp 1271-1295.)

Zancolli described achieving forearm pronation by converting the biceps into a forearm pronator (**Figure 10**).[249,251,253,254] The tendon is rerouted around the radius, converting the biceps from a supinator to pulling in the opposite direction as a pronator.

Group 3

Patients in this group have function of both the extensor carpi radialis longus and brevis. This group is similar to the C6 functional level. Many patients are content with a wrist-driven flexor hinge splint to provide pinch. These patients are good candidates for surgical reconstruction of key pinch (**Figure 12**). Alternatively, using brachioradialis, an adduction-opponensplasty can be produced (**Figure 13**). With both wrist extensors functioning, the extensor carpi radialis longus also becomes available for transfer (leaving the extensor carpi radialis brevis as the remaining wrist extensor because of its more central insertion). In this group of patients, Zancolli has described a two-stage reconstruction to provide digital release, to prevent clawing, and to provide digital flexion.[241,251,253,254] In the first stage, digit and thumb extension tenodeses are performed to provide release during wrist palmar flexion. To prevent or reduce clawing, each flexor digitorum superficialis tendon is tenodesed to itself around the A1 pulley, maintaining slight flexion at the metacarpophalangeal joint (lasso procedure) (**Figure 14**). The thumb interphalangeal joint is fused to prevent hyperflexion. In the second stage of the reconstruction, digital flexion is established with transfer of the extensor carpi radialis longus to the flexor digitorum profundus and the brachioradialis is transferred to the flexor pollicis longus.[250,251,253,254] In many patients of groups 2 and 3, lack of forearm pronation may present an additional problem. These patients have active wrist extension and use the tenodesis effect for grasp and release. If the forearm cannot be pronated, however, gravity cannot be used to produce palmar flexion of the wrist and digital extension for release of grasp. In these patients, the biceps tendon can be transferred around the radial side of the radius, transforming it into a forearm pronator.[253,254]

Group 4

In this group, the pronator teres is intact. The pronator teres provides a useful antagonist to the supination provided by the biceps. Therefore, function of the pronator is valuable, and its use as a donor for transfer is controversial. Zancolli[253,254] has described its transfer to the flexor carpi radialis to strengthen wrist extension and augment wrist-activated tenodesis reconstructions.

Group 5

The flexor carpi radialis is intact in this group, and the patient has active flexion and extension of the wrist. These patients are similar to the C7 functional patient. Reconstruction efforts are directed to providing digital flexion and extension. Because wrist flexion is valuable, the flexor carpi radialis is usually not transferred, as long as the brachioradialis, extensor carpi radialis longus, and pronator teres are available for transfer. House has described a two-stage reconstruction that provides digital flexion and release.[235] The first stage (extensor phase) involves tenodesis of the common extensors and the extensor pollicis longus to the distal radius or a transfer of the brachioradialis to the common extensors and the extensor pollicis longus for digital extension. Stabilization of the thumb is accomplished by carpometacarpal joint arthrodesis or tenodesis of the abductor pollicis longus. In the second stage (flexor phase), the extensor carpi radialis longus is transferred to the profundus tendons to the index, long, ring, and little fingers. The pronator teres is transferred to the flexor pollicis longus. Intrinsic tenodeses as described by Zancolli (group 3) are also performed, as the intrinsics are not functioning.

Group 6

The extensor digitorum communis is strong in this group; however, the extensor pollicis longus is too weak to extend the thumb out of the palm. The extensor pollicis longus can be sutured to the common extensors so that active extension of the fingers will produce extension of the thumb.[105,249]

Group 7

In this group, the extensor pollicis longus is strong and need not be augmented. Attention is directed toward reconstruction of weak digital flexion and intrinsic augmentation, using the lasso procedure described by Zancolli.[241,242,249,251,253,254]

Group 8

Patients in this group lack strength in extrinsic finger flexion. Occasionally, the ulnar flexors have adequate strength, but flexor power to the radial flexors is weak. These can be balanced by suturing all four profundus tendons together.[105] Active flexion to the thumb can be provided with transfer of the brachioradialis to the flexor pollicis longus. Because intrinsics are also weak, intrinsic augmentation is usually required, using the lasso procedure as mentioned above.

Group 9

Patients in group 9 lack intrinsic strength, and clawing is usually present. Intrinsic augmentation can be performed to eliminate hyperextension deformity at the metacarpophalangeal joints.

Following most tendon transfers, the transferred tendon is immobilized for about 4 weeks, or mobilized in a protected range. A closely supervised hand therapy program follows, in which active and passive motion is initiated.

Paralysis: Lower Extremities

Patients with spinal cord lesions proximal to the proximal lumbar levels often develop severe spasticity. Severe noxious spasticity is often an overwhelming but treatable condition. In these patients, the problems with spasticity often overshadow problems of paresis. Tendon transfers for reconstruction are not generally feasible until severe spasticity is controlled and contractures eliminated.

Cord injuries proximal to the conus medullaris are upper motor neuron lesions, and thus severe spasticity is often present. Reconstructive efforts are directed mostly toward correction of deformity from spasticity using tendon lengthenings and releases. Less emphasis is placed on reconstruction to restore strength to weak muscles using tendon transfers. Management of deformity from spasticity was discussed previously under spasticity.

Injuries that occur distal to the level of the second lumbar vertebra injure the cauda equina, and produce lower motor neuron lesions that result in lower extremity weakness. These injuries, therefore, do not produce spasticity. Injury of varying severity to nerve roots may occur, and incomplete lesions causing different patterns of weakness may result. Therefore, clinical presentations of specific root-level injuries are often not seen. The affected muscles become flaccid or paretic. In these patients, reconstructive efforts are directed toward reconstruction of the flaccid or paretic paralytic limb, and many of the same concepts of bracing and tendon transfers developed for peripheral nerve injuries or anterior horn cell diseases are feasible. Use of functional electrical stimulation is gaining popularity, and is discussed in a subsequent section.

Weakness of the Hip and Knee

Requirements for ambulation include adequate balance, limb stability, and a means of hip advancement. Paraplegic patients with functional levels between T1 and T5 will lack trunk balance and are usually wheelchair-dependent. Patients with functional levels between T6 and T10 will have some trunk stability, and exercise ambulation with bilateral long-leg braces and crutches or parallel bars may be possible. Stability of the knee can be provided with a knee-ankle-foot orthosis. With functional levels between T11 and L1, trunk stability will be present; however, hip advancement is lacking, and limited, if any, household ambulation will be possible. In the patient with an L2 functional level, some hip flexion will be intact, and household ambulation may be possible. If L3 or L4 levels are intact, the quadriceps and hip adductors will be functioning, and community ambulation will be possible. Ankle stability can be provided with an ankle-foot orthosis.

Weakness of Ankle Plantar Flexion

Ambulatory patients may have weakness of the gastrocnemius-soleus complex that allows the ankle to collapse into dorsiflexion during stance. This results in excessive forward advancement of the tibia. Compensatory flexion at the knee occurs, which increases demands on the quadriceps during stance. This can result in loss of stability at both the knee and ankle. Many patients with gastrocnemius-soleus complex weakness subsequently develop a second gait pattern in which the knee is passively locked in extension at or immediately after floor contact. This prevents knee collapse during stance, and avoids the increased demand on the quadriceps if the knee is in flexion during stance. Although this gait pattern increases stability, the chronic hyperextension stresses on the knee can eventually lead to genu recurvatum and knee pain, especially in the active patient. Treatment of a weak gastrocnemius-soleus complex is aimed at providing ankle stability using a rigid ankle-foot orthosis. Double upright orthoses are the most stable and generally most effective. However, they are heavy, and can be difficult to use in the paretic limb. New designs in polypropylene orthoses may provide adequate stability and are much lighter.

Weakness of Ankle Dorsiflexion

Inadequate dorsiflexion strength with a "foot drop" is caused by weakness of the tibialis anterior, extensor hallucis longus, and extensor digitorum longus. The patients often drag the toes on the floor during swing-through. Treatment is stabilization with an ankle-foot orthosis. A flexible polypropylene orthosis allows a small amount of controlled ankle motion during stance and provides adequate dorsiflexion during swing. If foot drop is the only gait problem, a lightweight flexible polypropylene orthosis with posterior trim lines is sufficient to provide a neutral toe position during swing. Its flexibility allows some ankle motion during stance.

Weakness of Foot Eversion

A varus deformity may result either from spasticity of the inverters of the foot (tibialis posterior or tibialis anterior) or from weakness of the evertors (peroneus longus and peroneus brevis). Deformity caused by weakness of the foot evertors can usually be improved with an ankle-foot orthosis. Lightweight flexible polypropylene orthoses are usually adequate.

Use of Functional Electrical Stimulation in Paretic or Paralytic Extremities

Functional Electrical Simulation in the Upper Extremity

Electrical stimulation of muscle is a means of producing contraction of muscle when there is neuromuscular impairment. Electrical stimulation with muscle contraction can assist mobilization of the joint to prevent contractures, help relax spastic antagonist muscles, and, if timed or controlled carefully, can augment function of the limb.[105,263-271] In addition, there is evidence that electrical stimulation of muscle strengthens the muscle and improves endurance.[268] If the muscle is stimulated to provide a specific movement or function of the extremity (ie, digital flexion for grasp, ankle dorsiflexion during gait), then the stimulation is called functional electrical stimulation.[269-272] The muscles can be stimulated by surface electrodes placed on the skin, or by surgically implanted electrodes placed either on the epimyseal surface of the muscle or near the respective motor nerve.[270,271,273,274]

In the tetraplegic upper extremity, functional control by electrical stimulation has been studied by Peckham et al.[270,273,275] Restoration of key pinch, grasp, and release have been studied using a percutaneous electrode system. Patients have included those in groups 0 and 1 (functional C5 or C6) with cutaneous sensibility that was usually intact. At these levels of cord injury, there are few adequate muscles available for tendon transfer. Prerequisites for successful use include successful control of spasticity, adequate seated balance, and nearly full range of movement of the shoulder, elbow, and fingers. Intact lower motor neurons are required, and the muscle must be electrically excitable by stimulation of its peripheral nerve. The electrodes are strategically placed in the forearm to stimulate the digital and thumb flexors and extensor muscles. The electrodes are connected to a controller, which in turn is connected to a transducer placed on the contralateral shoulder. Firing the electrodes is controlled volitionally by the patient via contralateral shoulder movements through the transducer. The electrodes usually remain in place over a year. This system requires no voluntary control below the level of the elbow, yet yields adequate key grip or lateral pinch to handle small objects and palmar prehension to handle large objects. Many alternate methods of volitional control of muscle excitation have been developed, including potentiometers mounted on a fixed surface and moved by the patient's opposite extremity, potentiometers attached to an orthosis that measures position of the wrist, on-off switches that select a slowly increasing or decreasing command, and voice control.[273,275] Using two grasp patterns, the user can hold objects such as eating utensils and writing implements, and position the hand for functions such as the use of a keyboard or control of switches and knobs.[273,275]

Functional Electrical Stimulation in the Paraplegic Lower Extremity

Function in the lower extremity can be augmented with electrical stimulation. In paraplegic patients (and usually with preservation of some lower extremity function), functional electrical stimulation is able to improve standing or walking. These systems are promising to provide significant gains in function. However, the systems are not always practical. Patients must be carefully selected, goals must be realistic, and obstacles such as adapting to and maintaining equipment need to be overcome.

Kralj et al[271] have developed a successful system to augment standing and walking in the paraparetic patient. In their system, the patient incorporates as much preserved function as possible into the restoration of ambulation. Patient capabilities are used to the maximal extent, including remaining motor skills and preserved reflexes. A four-channel stimulation unit is used. The four-channel gait pattern is controlled by the patient via trigger switches built into the handles of walkers or crutches. Standing is accomplished by stimulation of the quadriceps, enabling the patient to stand with exaggerated lordotic posture. Gravity is used to stabilize the extended hips. Limb advancement is accomplished by stimulating a reflex synergistic flexion in the extremity, combined with the patient's shifting of body weight using the upper extremities and the walker or crutches. In their series, only 15% of all admitted patients were selected as candidates. Of these selected, 75% of patients with T4-T5 lesions were able to use the four-channel walking system. Only 60% continued to use the system at home because of time required to don the equipment.

Although relatively few well-documented studies in functional electrical stimulation have been performed, investigations by Kralj and others seem to support several conclusions: Functional electrical stimulation for standing is an important function, enabling patients to perform tasks in an upright position. Such standing may extend the transfer capabilities for patients and may be considered a therapeutic modality. Functional electrical stimulation used to augment walking seems to be able to provide useful but limited household ambulation.[105,276] The importance and role in the daily life of SCI patients needs to be determined. For long-term use, the time for donning and removing the device are important considerations. In addition, cosmesis and availability of the functional electrical stimulation-assisted devices are of prime importance. Surgically implantable systems have advantages over the surface-applied systems, and may prove superior for long-term use. Surface systems are useful for short-term use, such as therapeutic, training, and evaluation purposes to prepare and select patients for implantation.[105,271]

Complications Associated With Upper Extremity Weight Bearing in the Paraplegic Patient

The paraplegic patient relies on the upper extremities for activities of daily living, locomotion, and wheelchair transfers. These activities result in higher stresses on the shoulders, elbows, wrists, and hands, which can precipitate problems associated with overuse. Frequent problems include extremity pain (especially at the shoulder), and peripheral neuropathies.[7,277-283]

Upper Extremity Pain (Rotator Cuff Tears, Tendinitis, Bursitis)

Multiple studies have shown a high percentage (51% to 100%) of SCI patients eventually develop pain in their upper extremities. The pain is usually associated with or aggravated by wheelchair use or crutch walking. The reported incidence of extremity pain increases with time, from 52% to 78% during the first 5 years to 100% after 20 years.[7,279,281,283,284]

The shoulder joint has the highest incidence of pain. Silfverskiold and Waters[285] noted 78% of quadriplegic individuals and 35% of paraplegic individuals had nontraumatic shoulder pain in the first 6 months. One-third to one-half of all patients develop shoulder pain during wheelchair transfers within the first 5 years. This incidence of pain increases to 70% at 10 years. Implicated causes of chronic shoulder pain include rotator cuff tears, bicipital tendinitis, and bursitis. Arthrography performed in paraplegic patients with persistent shoulder pain revealed a 45% incidence of rotator cuff tears. Intra-articular pressures of the shoulder joint are elevated during active transfers, reaching pressures greater than 250 mm Hg. Although increased stresses and activity at the shoulder seem to contribute to soft-tissue injury, degenerative arthritis does not universally develop, even in long-standing paraplegic patients or those who have used crutches for swing-through gait for many years. Gait studies in paraplegic crutch-walkers imply occurrence of increased loads through the glenohumeral and acromiohumeral joints during upper extremity weight bearing.[283]

Subdeltoid (subacromial) bursitis of the shoulder is manifested by pain under the acromion. The pain is increased with activity and sometimes increased with abduction (as in rotator cuff injury). Diagnosis of bursitis is usually made by exclusion of other causes. Chronic rotator cuff attritional injuries can be excluded with arthrography or MRI. Tendinitis of the rotator cuff may be difficult to exclude. Radiographs may show calcifications in the supraspinatus tendon. Bicipital tendinitis causes pain along the biceps tendon in the bicipital groove on the anterior surface of the humeral head. Pain is well localized and increases with elbow flexion against resistance. Bursitis and tendinitis are usually self-limiting, and can often be controlled by rest, decreasing activity, and anti-inflammatory medications. Because the wheelchair patient requires use of the upper extremities for activities of daily living, decreasing activity may be difficult. Occasional and limited lidocaine and steroid injections can be useful in the treatment of bursitis and tendinitis. Treatment of rotator cuff tears depends on the extent of injury and limitations of the patient. Rarely have chronic attritional tears of the cuff been of sufficient magnitude to require surgical repair. In general, indications for surgical repair are the same as for patients in the general population.

Besides the shoulder, the hand is also commonly involved with pain. About 9% of patients report hand pain, usually in the palm. Pain in the palm is usually due to direct soft-tissue irritation from repeated trauma during wheelchair propulsion. A second source of hand pain is the development of carpal tunnel syndrome. Pain also occurs in the elbow and forearm, involving approximately 5% of patients.[279,280,283] Bone density in the forearm has been noted to be increased in paraparetic patients who rely on swing-through crutch-walking for ambulation.[283]

Carpal Tunnel Syndrome

Carpal tunnel syndrome has been associated with wheelchair use and transfers.[277,279,286] Up to 64% of paraplegic patients studied were noted to have signs or symptoms consistent with carpal tunnel syndrome, and the prevalence was noted to increase with the length of time from SCI. The high incidence has been attributed to both the frequent use of the wrist in an extended position during lifting and transfers, and to the repetitive trauma sustained to the palmar aspect of the wrist while propelling a wheelchair. Concurrent ulnar neuropathy at the elbow was noted in 40% of those with carpal tunnel syndrome.[277]

In the paraplegic patient with symptoms, signs, and electrodiagnostic confirmation of carpal tunnel syndrome, treatment should include standard initial treatment measures of rest, splinting, and anti-inflammatory medications. Splinting may not be practical in this population and persistent or severe symptoms usually require surgical decompression. Prolonged recovery of grip strength and persistent incisional discomfort are common, probably related to these patients being dependent on upper extremity function for activities of daily living.

Cubital Tunnel Syndrome

Besides carpal tunnel syndrome, an increased incidence of ulnar neuropathy has been associated with the upper extremity use in paraplegic patients.[277,283] Of those with carpal tunnel syndrome, concurrent cubital tunnel syndrome was noted in 40%.[277] An awareness of this problem and appropriate evaluation of nerve function will allow prompt detection and appropriate management.

Miscellaneous Complications

Additional problems of the musculoskeletal system that occur in the patient with SCI include regional pain syndromes, venous thrombosis, gravitational edema, muscle atrophy, osteoporosis, and pressure sores (**Table 1**).

Regional Pain Syndromes

Regional pain syndromes, including reflex sympathetic dystrophy, are recognized causes of extremity pain in the SCI patient.[284,287-290] In the tetraplegia patient, regional pain syndromes involve the upper extremity in about 10% of patients.[287,288] Common findings include diffuse hand or extremity pain, swelling, and stiffness. Less frequently, trophic changes of skin and hyperhydrosis are present. Radiographs often show periarticular osteopenia. Three-phase radionuclide scintigraphy (triple-phase bone scan) is a sensitive and specific diagnostic study to confirm the diagnosis. Management of this problem includes limb mobilization (if pain will permit), splinting to prevent contractures, peripheral nerve or stellate ganglion block, systemic medication (sympatholytic medications such as alpha blockers, and/or calcium channel blockers), and/or surgical sympathectomy. Early consultation with an anesthesia pain specialist will provide access for sympathetic blocks. Early diagnosis and treatment of sympathetically mediated pain seems to improve outcome.

There is an additional type of pain syndrome that is poorly understood, often referred to as pain of central origin.[93,282,289] Neuritic or neuropathic in nature, this pain is thought to involve, to some degree, up to 60% of patients with posttraumatic paraplegia or tetraplegia. The type and intensity of pain is variable, and many individuals describe it as severe, continuous burning, or lancinating.[289] It occurs in the absence of the usual skin color and temperature changes seen in sympathetically mediated pain. In addition, the patient may have contributing pain from other sources such as painful spasticity or spasms, heterotopic ossification, or joint stiffness and capsulitis.[98,291] Sjölund[289] has noted two types of this central neuropathic pain: (1) segmentally distributed pain at the lesion; and (2) pain in the body below the lesion, often with late onset. The segmental pain at the level of the lesion may be related to nerve root injury or entrapment, or by limb denervation referred to as "direct segmental deafferentation." The second type is thought to involve or contain several forms of central pain, evoked either by the original spinal lesion, by an expanding syrinx in the spinal cord, or by secondary changes at higher levels of the somatosensory systems. This second type of pain can be continuous or independent of any stimulus. Partial spinal lesions, especially those centrally located in the cervical spinal cord, may be more prone to produce pain than the complete spinal lesions. Treatment of these types of central pain syndromes is difficult, and they may be resistant to several methods of treatment. Medications used include oral and intrathecal opiates, serotonin reuptake inhibitors, sodium channel blockers, oral carbamazepine, gabapentin, and clonidine.[289] Neurostimulations and/or TENS units may give some relief, but response is variable. Neurodestructive procedures and central neurostimulation have generally not been successful. Biofeedback and cognitive-behavioral rehabilitation may be helpful. Overall, pain of central origin is poorly understood, and available treatments are limited. A multidisciplinary approach should be used, including participation with an anesthesia pain specialist, a neurologist and/or neurosurgeon, rehabilitation/physical medicine specialist, physical and occupational therapists, and rehabilitation nurses.

Venous Thrombosis

Venous thrombosis usually occurs within the first 40 days of hospitalization, and appears to be more common in SCI patients than in other hospitalized patients. Contributing factors include immobilization and the loss of pump action from active muscle contraction. If sensibility is not intact, diagnosis may be difficult.

Prophylactic anticoagulation is now standard practice in patients with sudden lower limb paralysis. Thromboprophylaxis is usually continued until the patient regains independent mobility. The duration of anticoagulation in long-term immobile patients is variable, but is usually discontinued after 4 months as the risk of venous thromboembolism seems to drop after 3 to 4 months. Development of muscle spasticity has been traditionally considered to be the reason for the lower risk after 3 to 4 months, because lower limb spasticity/spasm might be able to improve the calf muscle pump action. Others suggest, however, that there are vascular changes following long-term lower limb inactivity that are universal to all immobile patients, which is probably the main protecting factor against venous thrombosis. Overall recommendations for prophylactic anticoagulation usually include coverage over the first 4 months following the acute onset of immobility in all neurologically impaired immobile patients regardless of their muscle tone state.

If a venous thrombosis does develop in the SCI patient, diagnosis may be difficult. Findings include unilateral edema, warmth, and an increase in calf circumference. Minor edema may be the only presenting sign. Differential diagnosis includes heterotopic ossification, infection, tumor, gravitational edema, and pathologic fracture. Doppler evaluation or venography is usually diagnostic. Treatment is anticoagulation, usually beginning with intravenous heparin followed by oral long-term anticoagulant drugs such as warfarin. Physical therapy should cease temporarily during the acute stage. Late venous thrombosis can also occur, presenting in the second or third month after injury, but the risk overall is lower after 4 months.

Gravitational Edema

Gravitational edema is caused by extravascular fluid pooling from dependence of the limb and lack of active muscle action. It occurs mostly in the lower extremities, and may accompany a long session of sitting in a wheelchair with the lower limbs dependent. Gravitational edema usually subsides within a few hours with extremity elevation. It is mentioned here briefly because it can mimic or mask other more serious disorders, such as thrombophlebitis, infection, occult fracture, or heterotopic bone formation.

Muscle Atrophy

In the SCI patient, lean soft-tissue mass (muscle mass) in the affected levels decreases dramatically during the first months after injury, while fat content tends to increase. Lean muscle mass is better maintained in patients who develop spasticity, although the bone mineral mass seems to be unaffected by the spasticity. In the paraplegic patient, the lean mass of the upper limbs increases early after SCI because of increased muscle use of the upper extremities for transfers and due to positive effects of physical and occupational therapy. As opposed to the minimal effects of mobilization and exercise on bone mineral loss, exercises to prevent atrophy have been shown to maintain and even increase muscle mass.[45,46]

Osteoporosis

Osteoporosis is a recognized consequence of SCI and occurs in almost every SCI patient.[40-46] As noted earlier, it manifests itself as an increase in the incidence of long-bone fractures, especially in the lower extremity. The pattern of bone loss seen in SCI patients is different from that usually encountered with endocrine disorders and pure disuse osteoporosis.[40] There is, in general, no demineralization in the areas above the SCI level. Several factors that appear to have an influence on the bone mass in SCI patients include the degree (completeness) of the injury, muscle spasticity, age, sex, and duration after injury.[40,42,45] In the lumbar spine, bone demineralization remains relatively low compared to that of the long bones below the level of injury. In fact, Biering-Sørensen et al[41] noted the bone mineral content of the lumbar spine in quadriplegic individuals to be within normal range 2 to 25 years after SCI. The preservation of bone mineral content in these patients may be due to the maintenance of load on the spine while sitting in a wheelchair.

Bone mineral density loss begins early after SCI and continues for about 2 years until a steady state is reached.[40,42,44,45] The amount of bone loss is variable among patients, and data suggest that fractures occur more often in those with greater loss in bone density.[48] Wilmet et al[46] noted approximately 4% loss per month of trabecular bone and 2% loss per month of cortical bone during the first year. At 6 months, trabecular bone mineral density of the radius, ulna, and tibia was reduced in subjects with tetraplegia by 19%, 15%, and 5%, respectively. At 12 months, the trabecular loss in the radius, ulna, and tibia was found to be 25%, 15%, and 15%, respectively. Cortical bone density is less affected than trabucular bone, and was found to be reduced 12 months after SCI, with 3% loss in the radius, 4% loss in the ulna, and 7% loss in the tibia.[44] When comparing bone mineral density loss in the paraplegic to the quadriplegic individual, there was no significant difference in tibial bone loss in both cortical and trabecular bone in studies by Frey-Rindova et al.[44] However, others have noted lower bone mineral content values in the femoral neck in patients with cervical lesions compared to those with thoracic lesions.[41,48] In patients with long-standing SCI (between 2 and 25 years), Biering-Sørensen et al[41] noted an average bone mineral content loss of 25% in the femoral neck and 50% in the proximal tibia. A new steady-state level between bone resorption and formation seems to be reestablished about 2 years after the SCI, but may continue after this time. SCI may not only cause bone loss, but also alter bone structure and microstructure. As noted above, trabecular bone is more affected than cortical bone in the SCI population.

The pathogenesis of osteoporosis after SCI remains complex and perplexing.[40] Disuse may play an important role in the pathogenesis of osteoporosis, but neural factors also appear to be important. SCI leads to impaired calcium and phosphate metabolism and appears to involve the parathyroid hormone–vitamin D axis. Loss of weight bearing and muscle stress on bone probably remain significant factors in development of osteoporosis. Spasticity with its associated stress on bone has been noted to provide some protection from bone mineral loss.[42] However, recent studies have questioned the positive effects from spasticity, where spasticity had no influence on bone mineral loss.[41,44] The daily use of long-leg braces has also been studied and shows no significant influence on the bone mineral content loss.[41]

Treatment of osteoporosis in SCI includes pharmacologic intervention with calcium, phosphate, vitamin D, calcitonin, and bisphosphonates. Unfortunately, the routine use of bone-active drugs for the prevention and treatment of osteoporosis remains low, despite the availability of these effective therapies.[40]

Intensive long-bone loading exercise activity in early rehabilitation using a tilt table and standing exercises can possibly attenuate the decrease of bone mineral density.[44] Physical therapy with limb mobilization and functional stimulated exercises (electrically stimulated cycling or resistance training, walking exercises) has traditionally also been also used to attempt to prevent some bone loss. Recent studies seem to indicate that limb mobilization may not significantly influence the loss of bone mineral density,[44,45] and, overall, the impact of these exercises on bone remains poorly established. However, these exercises do have a positive effect on muscle atrophy, and appear to increase muscle mass and/or prevent atrophy.[45] Many unanswered questions remain about the pathogenesis of osteoporosis and its clinical management.[40,44]

TABLE 3

Physical and Social Factors Associated With Pressure Sores

Factors associated with increased risk of pressure sores	Severe spasticity Fixed contractures Obesity Smoking Chronic use of pain medications History of alcohol or drug abuse History of incarceration Attempted suicide
Factors associated with decrease risk of pressure sores	College degree Married Employed

(Adapted with permission from Krause JS, Vines CL, Farley TL: An exploratory study of pressure ulcers after spinal cord injury: Relationship to protective behaviors and risk factors. *Arch Phys Med Rehabil* 2001;82(1):107-113.)

Skin Ulceration and Infection

Pressure sores are one of the most serious and most preventable complications in the SCI patient.[11,292-294] Proper prophylactic care should completely eliminate this problem. However, pressure sores continue to be a problem in the SCI patient. A single indiscretion in care can lead to persistent, repeated ulceration with resultant hospitalization, loss of independence, and disruption of social adjustment. Subsequent osteomyelitis and sepsis can lead to the death of the patient.

Areas that are at high risk for ulceration are those where subcutaneous tissue is thin and skin overlies a bony prominence. These include the sacrum, ischial tuberosity, greater trochanter, malleoli, the os calcis, the base (styloid) of the fifth metatarsal, the dorsum of the proximal interphalangeal joints of the toes (if flexion contracture exists), and the distal end of the toes. Severe spasticity and flexion contractures increase the risk due to limited positioning. Additional physical and social risk factors associated with development of pressure sores include being overweight, chronic use of pain medications, positive smoking history, having undergone alcohol or drug treatment, or a history of incarceration.[295] Factors associated with lower risk of pressure sores include having completed a college degree, being married, and being currently employed[295] (**Table 3**).

FIGURE 15

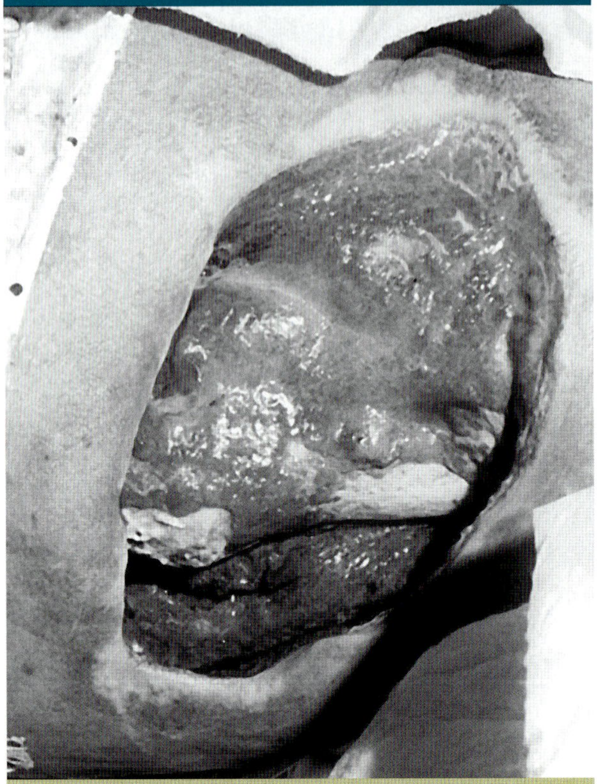

Figure 15 Pressure sore in hip region with exposed greater trochanter. Osteomyelitis commonly develops when bone is exposed. In the management of pressure sores, prevention is emphasized as the most important aspect of treatment. (Reproduced from Botte MJ: Complications of the musculoskeletal system following spinal cord injury, in Levine AM, Eismont FJ, Garfin SR, Zigler JE, eds: *Spine Trauma*. Philadelphia, PA, WB Saunders, 1998, pp 639-660.)

Etiology

Continuous pressure leads to ischemia of all tissues between the skin and underlying bone. Lack of sensibility and paralysis do not promote or allow the patient to reposition himself/herself to relieve the ischemic area. Necrosis follows, usually in the subcutaneous fat, which has a lesser blood supply than the dermis. With proper care, healing may occur, but the ulcer fills with dense nonresilient scar tissue covered with thin epithelial tissue. Thick cicatrix covered with thin epithelium has poor resistance to repeat breakdown, and repeated or chronic ulcers may result. Chronic ulcers also are at high risk for infection. Osteomyelitis can develop in areas of prominence, such as the greater trochanter, that becomes exposed in the ulcer (**Figure 15**). Pressure sores in the hip and pelvis region can result in a septic hip joint and osteomyelitis of the pelvis, leading to systemic sepsis.

Treatment

Treatment of pressure sores is prevention. Proper padding, frequent positioning, and constant surveillance for early evidence of skin ischemia need to be instituted. Established ulcers require unloading of the pressure, local wound care, control of infection, correction of nutritional deficiencies, correction of contractures or spasticity that may be contributing to pressure areas, and surgical reconstruction as needed.[292] A multidisciplinary approach is recommended for these difficult problems. Reconstruction can require serial surgical débridements followed by tissue coverage procedures.

For the sacral pressure sore, a gluteal flap can be transferred using several techniques according to the shape and size of the sore.[294] For large lesions, muscles flaps with overlying skin are transferred (musculocutaneous flaps). The gluteus maximus is anatomically comprised of two muscles, each with its own blood supply. The superior portion of the muscle is supplied by the superior gluteal artery, and the inferior portion is supplied by the inferior gluteal artery. Either or both are valuable as muscle or myocutaneous flaps for the sacral region. The gluteus maximus can be transferred either as a turnover flap or as a V-Y transposition. In the turnover flap, the superior gluteal artery is used as a base. Following débridement of infected soft tissue or bone, the superior portion of the gluteus maximus is detached distally from its distal insertion along the iliotibial tract. The distal portion is then turned over onto itself, so that the distal portion reaches and covers the sacral area. Alternatively, the muscle can be transferred using a V-Y advancement technique. Both the sacral and distal insertions are detached, and the muscle is translated proximally to cover the sacrum.

For the ischial pressure sore, ischiectomy can be performed with or without coverage using the gluteus maximus. The inferior portion of the gluteus muscle is detached distally from femur, creating a flap that is rotated medially to cover the ischial tuberosity. Alternatively, the hamstring muscles can be used either as a turnover flap or V-Y translational flap.

The trochanteric pressure sore can be managed with ostectomy with or without muscle coverage. The tenser fascia lata muscle, used as a fasciocutaneous flap, is located adjacent to the greater trochanter and a portion is easily detached distally and rotated to cover the greater trochanter. The vastus lateralis can be used to augment the tenser fascia lata flap.

Osteomyelitis underlying open pressures is a difficult problem. To attempt to cure the condition, the infected bone requires resection, and the open ulcer requires aggressive débridement and soft-tissue reconstruction.[292] Coverage is provided, as described above, by local pedicle or distant tissue flaps. If a healthy bed of granulation tissue is present, skin grafting may also be used; however, quality of the skin is less optimal than that accomplished with pedicle or free-tissue flaps. Trochanteric pressures sores that result in osteomyelitis of the proximal femur can advance to septic arthritis of the hip followed by osteomyelitis of the acetabulum. Osteomyelitis of the acetabulum can rapidly result in infection of the ileum, and the patient's prognosis may be grave. Osteomyelitis of the acetabulum can be treated with resection of the proximal femur and curettage of the acetabulum or, alternatively, amputation of the limb with acetabular resection or hemipelvectomy. These procedures may be needed for advancing refractory infections.[292]

Osteomyelitis from pressure sores can, at times be treated with chronic antibiotic suppression. This, combined with local wound care, will not eradicate the infection, but may be feasible to keep the infection controlled. Even with suppression, chronic osteomyelitis can lead to systemic sepsis, endocarditis, or septic emboli. SCI patients who develop osteomyelitis from pressure sores can ultimately die from sepsis or related complications. This underscores the importance of prevention of pressure sores.

Conclusion

The many problems and associated complications of the musculoskeletal system in the patient with SCI have been outlined. The numerous potential problems and the consequences of delay in diagnosis or proper management emphasize the need for vigilance and a constant high index of suspicion for complications. An aggressive prophylactic and treatment approach is necessary in the management of these patients. Although some of the problems presented here are unavoidable or are an unchangeable consequence of SCI, many can be prevented or minimized with awareness, the use of proper preventive measures, and a thorough evaluation when a problem is suspected.

References

1. Aito S, D'Andrea M, Werhagen L: Neurological and functional outcome in traumatic central cord syndrome. *Spinal Cord* 2007;45(4):292-297.
2. Chan SC, Chan AP: Rehabilitation outcomes following traumatic spinal cord injury in a tertiary spinal cord injury centre: A comparison with an international standard. *Spinal Cord* 2005;43(8):489-498.
3. Westgren N, Levi R: Quality of life and traumatic spinal cord injury. *Arch Phys Med Rehabil* 1998;79(11):1433-1439.
4. Anson CA, Shepherd C: Incidence of secondary complications in spinal cord injury. *Int J Rehabil Res* 1996;19(1):55-66.
5. Paker N, Soy D, Kesiktaş N, et al: Reasons for rehospitalization in patients with spinal cord injury: 5 years' experience. *Int J Rehabil Res* 2006;29(1):71-76.
6. Barat M, Dehail P, de Seze M: Fatigue after spinal cord injury. *Ann Readapt Med Phys* 2006;49(6):277-282, 365-369.
7. Davis R: Pain and suffering following spinal cord injury. *Clin Orthop Relat Res* 1975;112:76-80.
8. Drigotaite N, Krisciūnas A: Complications after spinal cord injuries and their influence on the effectiveness of rehabilitation. *Medicina (Kaunas)* 2006;42(11):877-880.
9. Hanson RW, Franklin MR: Sexual loss in relation to other functional losses for spinal cord injured males. *Arch Phys Med Rehabil* 1976;57(6):291-293.
10. Hjeltnes N, Jansen T: Physical endurance capacity, functional status and medical complications in spinal cord injured subjects with long-standing lesions. *Paraplegia* 1990;28(7):428-432.
11. Krause JS: Factors associated with risk for subsequent injuries after traumatic spinal cord injury. *Arch Phys Med Rehabil* 2004;85(9):1503-1508.
12. Levi R, Hultling C, Nash MS, Seiger A: The Stockholm spinal cord injury study: 1. Medical problems in a regional SCI population. *Paraplegia* 1995;33(6):308-315.
13. Levi R, Hultling C, Seiger A: The Stockholm Spinal Cord Injury Study: 2. Associations between clinical patient characteristics and post-acute medical problems. *Paraplegia* 1995;33(10):585-594.
14. McKinley WO, Tewksbury MA, Godbout CJ: Comparison of medical complications following nontraumatic and traumatic spinal cord injury. *J Spinal Cord Med* 2002;25(2):88-93.
15. McKinley WO, Gittler MS, Kirshblum SC, Stiens SA, Groah SL: Spinal cord injury medicine: 2. Medical complications after spinal cord injury: Identification and management. *Arch Phys Med Rehabil* 2002;83(3, Suppl 1):S58-S64, S90-S98.
16. Noreau L, Proulx P, Gagnon L, Drolet M, Laramée MT: Secondary impairments after spinal

cord injury: A population-based study. *Am J Phys Med Rehabil* 2000;79(6):526-535.

17. Unalan H, Gençosmanoğlu B, Akgün K, et al: Quality of life of primary caregivers of spinal cord injury survivors living in the community: Controlled study with short form-36 questionnaire. *Spinal Cord* 2001;39(6):318-322.
18. Walter JS, Sacks J, Othman R, et al: A database of self-reported secondary medical problems among VA spinal cord injury patients: Its role in clinical care and management. *J Rehabil Res Dev* 2002; 39(1):53-61.
19. Yarkony GM, Bass LM, Keenan V III, Meyer PR Jr: Contractures complicating spinal cord injury: Incidence and comparison between spinal cord centre and general hospital acute care. *Paraplegia* 1985;23(5):265-271.
20. Yarkony GM, Roth EJ, Cybulski GR, Jaeger RJ: Neuromuscular stimulation in spinal cord injury: II. Prevention of secondary complications. *Arch Phys Med Rehabil* 1992;73(2):195-200.
21. Barros Filho TE, Greve JM, Oliveira RP, Chiovatto J, Carneiro JF: Femoral fracture in patients with spinal cord injury. *Rev Hosp Clin Fac Med Sao Paulo* 1991;46(6):289-292.
22. Botte MJ, Moore TJ: The orthopaedic management of extremity injuries in head trauma. *J Head Trauma Rehabil* 1987;2:13-27.
23. Comarr AE, Hutchinson RH, Bors E: Extremity fractures of patients with spinal cord injuries. *Am J Surg* 1962;103:732-739.
24. Freehafer AA, Mast WA: Lower extremity fractures in patients with spinal-cord injury. *J Bone Joint Surg Am* 1965;47:683-694.
25. Freehafer AA: Long-term management of lumbar paraplegia, in Pierce DA, Nickel VL, eds: *The Total Care of the Spinal Cord Injuries*. Boston, MA, Little, Brown, and Company, 1977.
26. Freehafer AA, Hazel CM, Becker CL: Lower extremity fractures in patients with spinal cord injury. *Paraplegia* 1981;19(6):367-372.
27. Garland DE: Clinical observations on fractures and heterotopic ossification in the spinal cord and traumatic brain injured populations. *Clin Orthop Relat Res* 1988;233:86-101.
28. Garland DE, Razza BE, Waters RL: Forceful joint manipulation in head-injured adults with heterotopic ossification. *Clin Orthop Relat Res* 1982;169: 133-138.
29. Garland DE, Rieser TV, Singer DI: Treatment of femoral shaft fractures associated with acute spinal cord injuries. *Clin Orthop Relat Res* 1985;197: 191-195.
30. Garland DE, Saucedo T, Reiser TV: The management of tibial fractures in acute spinal cord injury patients. *Clin Orthop Relat Res* 1986;213:237-240.
31. Garland DE, Jones RC, Kunkle RW: Upper extremity fractures in the acute spinal cord injured patient. *Clin Orthop Relat Res* 1988;233:110-115.
32. Levine AM, Krebs M, Santos-Mendoza N: External fixation in quadriplegia. *Clin Orthop Relat Res* 1984;184:169-172.
33. McMaster WC, Stauffer ES: The management of long bone fracture in the spinal cord injured patient. *Clin Orthop Relat Res* 1975;112:44-52.
34. Mukand J, Sniger W, Kaufman J, Biener-Bergman S: Common causes of knee effusions in spinal cord injury: A random study. *Am J Phys Med Rehabil* 1998;77(2):113-117.
35. Nottage WM: A review of long-bone fractures in patients with spinal cord injuries. *Clin Orthop Relat Res* 1981;155:65-70.
36. Ragnarsson KT, Sell GH: Lower extremity fractures after spinal cord injury: A retrospective study. *Arch Phys Med Rehabil* 1981;62(9):418-423.
37. Retief PJ: Immobilisation of fractured limbs in the patient with spinal cord injury. *S Afr Med J* 1988; 73(7):442.
38. Sobel M, Lyden JP: Long bone fracture in a spinal-cord-injured patient: Complication of treatment—a case report and review of the literature. *J Trauma* 1991;31(10):1440-1444.
39. Tricot DA, Hallot R: Traumatic paraplegia and associated fractures. *Paraplegia* 1968;5(4): 211-215.
40. Jiang SD, Dai LY, Jiang LS: Osteoporosis after spinal cord injury. *Osteoporos Int* 2006;17(2): 180-192.
41. Biering-Sørensen F, Bohr H, Schaadt O: Bone mineral content of the lumbar spine and lower extremities years after spinal cord lesion. *Paraplegia* 1988;26(5):293-301.
42. Eser P, Schiessl H, Willnecker J: Bone loss and steady state after spinal cord injury: A cross-sectional study using pQCT. *J Musculoskelet Neuronal Interact* 2004;4(2):197-198.
43. Eser P, Frotzler A, Zehnder Y, Schiessl H, Denoth J: Assessment of anthropometric, systemic, and lifestyle factors influencing bone status in the legs of spinal cord injured individuals. *Osteoporos Int* 2005;16(1):26-34.
44. Frey-Rindova P, de Bruin ED, Stüssi E, Dambacher MA, Dietz V: Bone mineral density in upper and lower extremities during 12 months after spinal cord injury measured by peripheral quantitative computed tomography. *Spinal Cord* 2000;38(1):26-32.
45. Giangregorio L, McCartney N: Bone loss and muscle atrophy in spinal cord injury: Epidemiology, fracture prediction, and rehabilitation strategies. *J Spinal Cord Med* 2006;29(5):489-500.

46. Wilmet E, Ismail AA, Heilporn A, Welraeds D, Bergmann P: Longitudinal study of the bone mineral content and of soft tissue composition after spinal cord section. *Paraplegia* 1995;33(11): 674-677.
47. Stauffer ES: Long-term management of traumatic quadriplegia, in Pierce DS, Nickel VL, eds: *The Total Care of Spinal Cord Injuries*. Boston, MA, Little, Brown and Company, 1977.
48. Moynahan M, Betz RR, Triolo RJ, Maurer AH: Characterization of the bone mineral density of children with spinal cord injury. *J Spinal Cord Med* 1996;19(4):249-254.
49. Dario A, Tomei G: A benefit-risk assessment of baclofen in severe spinal spasticity. *Drug Saf* 2004; 27(11):799-818.
50. Botte MJ, Keenan MA: Percutaneous phenol blocks of the pectoralis major muscle to treat spastic deformities. *J Hand Surg Am* 1988;13(1): 147-149.
51. Keenan MA: The orthopaedic management of spasticity. *J Head Trauma Rehabil* 1987;2(2):62-71.
52. Keenan MA, Todderud EP, Henderson R, Botte M: Management of intrinsic spasticity in the hand with phenol injection or neurectomy of the motor branch of the ulnar nerve. *J Hand Surg Am* 1987; 12(5 Pt 1):734-739.
53. Keenan MA, Botte MJ: Technique of percutaneous phenol block to the recurrent motor branch of the median nerve. *J Hand Surg Am* 1987: 12(5 Pt 1):806-807.
54. Botte MJ, Keenan MA, Abrams RA, von Schroeder HP, Gellman H, Mooney V: Heterotopic ossification in neuromuscular disorders. *Orthopedics* 1997;20(4):335-341.
55. Bravo-Payno P, Esclarin A, Arzoz T, Arroyo O, Labarta C: Incidence and risk factors in the appearance of heterotopic ossification in spinal cord injury. *Paraplegia* 1992;30(10):740-745.
56. Brissot R, Lassalle A, Vincendeau S, et al: Treatment of heterotopic ossification by extracorporeal shock wave: 26 patients. *Ann Readapt Med Phys* 2005;48(8):581-589.
57. Buschbacher R, McKinley W, Buschbacher L, Devaney CW, Coplin B: Warfarin in prevention of heterotopic ossification. *Am J Phys Med Rehabil* 1992;71(2):86-91.
58. Cassar-Pullicino VN, McClelland M, Badwan DA, McCall IW, Pringle RG, el Masry W: Sonographic diagnosis of heterotopic bone formation in spinal injury patients. *Paraplegia* 1993;31(1):40-50.
59. Cope R: Heterotopic ossification. *South Med J* 1990;83(9):1058-1064.
60. Fuller DA, Mark A, Keenan MA: Excision of heterotopic ossification from the knee: A functional outcome study. *Clin Orthop Relat Res* 2005;438: 197-203.
61. Garland DE, Blum CE, Waters RL: Periarticular heterotopic ossification in head-injured adults: Incidence and location. *J Bone Joint Surg Am* 1980; 62(7):1143-1146.
62. Garland DE, Alday B, Venos KG, Vogt JC: Diphosphonate treatment for heterotopic ossification in spinal cord injury patients. *Clin Orthop Relat Res* 1983;176:197-200.
63. Garland DE, Orwin JF: Resection of heterotopic ossification in patients with spinal cord injuries. *Clin Orthop Relat Res* 1989;242:169-176.
64. Garland DE, Shimoyama ST, Lugo C, Barras D, Gilgoff I: Spinal cord insults and heterotopic ossification in the pediatric population. *Clin Orthop Relat Res* 1989;245:303-310.
65. Jensen LL, Halar E, Little JW, Brooke MM: Neurogenic heterotopic ossification. *Am J Phys Med* 1987;66(6):351-363.
66. Keenan MA: Management of the spastic upper extremity in the neurologically impaired adult. *Clin Orthop Relat Res* 1988;233:116-125.
67. Keenan MA: Upper extremity dysfunction after stroke or brain injury, in Green DP, ed: *Green's Operative Hand Surgery*, ed 5. Philadelphia, PA, Elsevier Chruchill Livingstone, 2005, pp 1235-1269.
68. Lal S, Hamilton BB, Heinemann A, Betts HB: Risk factors for heterotopic ossification in spinal cord injury. *Arch Phys Med Rehabil* 1989;70(5): 387-390.
69. McCarthy EF, Sundaram M: Heterotopic ossification: A review. *Skeletal Radiol* 2005;34(10): 609-619.
70. Pittenger DE: Heterotopic ossification. *Orthop Rev* 1991;20(1):33-39.
71. van Kuijk AA, Geurts AC, van Kuppevelt HJ: Neurogenic heterotopic ossification in spinal cord injury. *Spinal Cord* 2002;40(7):313-326.
72. van Ooij A, van Kollenburg JA, Pons C, Walenkamp GH: Surgical removal of debilitating neurogenic heterotopic ossifications of the hip. *Ned Tijdschr Geneeskd* 2005;149(1):37-41.
73. Mendelson L, Grosswasser Z, Najenson T, Sandbank U, Solzi P: Periarticular new bone formation in patients suffering from severe head injuries. *Scand J Rehabil Med* 1975;7(4):141-145.
74. Mielants H, Vanhove E, de Neels J, Veys E: Clinical survey of and pathogenic approach to para-articular ossifications in long-term coma. *Acta Orthop Scand* 1975;46(2):190-198.
75. Couvée LM: Heterotopic ossification and the surgical treatment of serious contractures. *Paraplegia* 1971;9(2):89-94.

76. Domanski M: Heterotopic ossification in paraplegia: A clinical study. *J Bone Joint Surg Br* 1961;43: 125-127.
77. Hsu JD, Sakimura I, Stauffer ES: Heterotopic ossification around the hip joint in spinal cord injured patients. *Clin Orthop Relat Res* 1975;112: 165-169.
78. Stover SL, Hataway CJ, Zieger HE: Heterotopic ossification in spinal cord-injured patients. *Arch Phys Med Rehabil* 1975;56(5):199-204.
79. Tibone J, Sakimura I, Nickel VL, Hsu JD: Heterotopic ossification around the hip in spinal cord-injured patients: A long-term follow-up study. *J Bone Joint Surg Am* 1978;60(6):769-775.
80. Wharton GW: Heterotopic ossification. *Clin Orthop Relat Res* 1975;112:142-149.
81. Wharton GW, Morgan TH: Ankylosis in the paralyzed patient. *J Bone Joint Surg Am* 1970;52(1): 105-112.
82. Furman R, Nicholas JJ, Jivoff L: Elevation of the serum alkaline phosphatase coincident with ectopic-bone formation in paraplegic patients. *J Bone Joint Surg Am* 1970;52(6):1131-1137.
83. Orzel JA, Rudd TG: Heterotopic bone formation: Clinical, laboratory, and imaging correlation. *J Nucl Med* 1985;26(2):125-132.
84. Spielman G, Gennarelli TA, Rogers CR: Disodium etidronate: Its role in preventing heterotopic ossification in severe head injury. *Arch Phys Med Rehabil* 1983;64(11):539-542.
85. Akeson WH, Amiel D, Woo SL: Immobility effects on synovial joints the pathomechanics of joint contracture. *Biorheology* 1980;17(1-2):95-110.
86. Akeson WH, Amiel D, Abel MF, Garfin SR, Woo SL: Effects of immobilization on joints. *Clin Orthop Relat Res* 1987;219:28-37.
87. Botte MJ, Nickel VL, Akeson WH: Spasticity and contracture: Physiologic aspects of formation. *Clin Orthop Relat Res* 1988;233:7-18.
88. Woo SL, Matthews JV, Akeson WH, Amiel D, Convery FR: Connective tissue response to immobility: Correlative study of biomechanical and biochemical measurements of normal and immobilized rabbit knees. *Arthritis Rheum* 1975;18(3): 257-264.
89. Woo SL, Gomez MA, Woo YK, Akeson WH: Mechanical properties of tendons and ligaments: II. The relationships of immobilization and exercise on tissue remodeling. *Biorheology* 1982;19(3): 397-408.
90. Adams MM, Hicks AL: Spasticity after spinal cord injury. *Spinal Cord* 2005;43(10):577-586.
91. Benz EN, Hornby TG, Bode RK, Scheidt RA, Schmit BD: A physiologically based clinical measure for spastic reflexes in spinal cord injury. *Arch Phys Med Rehabil* 2005;86(1):52-59.
92. Bohannon RW: Tilt table standing for reducing spasticity after spinal cord injury. *Arch Phys Med Rehabil* 1993;74(10):1121-1122.
93. Burchiel KJ, Hsu FP: Pain and spasticity after spinal cord injury: Mechanisms and treatment. *Spine (Phila Pa 1976)* 2001;26(24, Suppl):S146-S160.
94. Casale R, Glynn CJ, Buonocore M: Reduction of spastic hypertonia in patients with spinal cord injury: A double-blind comparison of intravenous orphenadrine citrate and placebo. *Arch Phys Med Rehabil* 1995;76(7):660-665.
95. Davis R: Spasticity following spinal cord injury. *Clin Orthop Relat Res* 1975;112:66-75.
96. Guttmann L: Spinal shock and reflex behaviour in man. *Paraplegia* 1970;8(2):100-116.
97. Little JW, Burns SP, James JJ, Stiens SA: Neurologic recovery and neurologic decline after spinal cord injury. *Phys Med Rehabil Clin N Am* 2000; 11(1):73-89.
98. Livshits A, Rappaport ZH, Livshits V, Gepstein R: Surgical treatment of painful spasticity after spinal cord injury. *Spinal Cord* 2002;40(4):161-166.
99. Mahoney JS, Engebretson JC, Cook DF, Hart KA, Robinson-Whelen S, Sherwood AF: Spasticity experience domains in persons with spinal cord injury. *Arch Phys Med Rehabil* 2007;88(3): 288-294.
100. Priebe MM, Sherwood AM, Thornby JI, Kharas NF, Markowski J: Clinical assessment of spasticity in spinal cord injury: A multidimensional problem. *Arch Phys Med Rehabil* 1996;77(7):713-716.
101. Sangwan SS, Chand S, Siwach RC, Gupta IS: Treatment of intractable spasticity in spinal cord injured patients. *Indian J Med Sci* 1992;46(6): 169-173.
102. Maynard FM, Karunas RS, Waring WP III: Epidemiology of spasticity following traumatic spinal cord injury. *Arch Phys Med Rehabil* 1990;71(8): 566-569.
103. Jordan C: Current status of functional lower extremity surgery in adult spastic patients. *Clin Orthop Relat Res* 1988;233:102-109.
104. Smyth MD, Peacock WJ: The surgical treatment of spasticity. *Muscle Nerve* 2000;23(2):153-163.
105. Marsolais EB, Kobetic R: Development of a practical electrical stimulation system for restoring gait in the paralyzed patient. *Clin Orthop Relat Res* 1988;233:64-74.
106. Chen CL, Yeung KT, Bih LI, Wang CH, Chen MI, Chien JC: The relationship between sitting stability and functional performance in patients with paraplegia. *Arch Phys Med Rehabil* 2003;84(9): 1276-1281.
107. Franzoi AC, Castro C, Cardone C: Isokinetic assessment of spasticity in subjects with traumatic

spinal cord injury (ASIA A). *Spinal Cord* 1999; 37(6):416-420.

108. Haas BM, Bergström E, Jamous A, Bennie A: The inter rater reliability of the original and of the modified Ashworth scale for the assessment of spasticity in patients with spinal cord injury. *Spinal Cord* 1996;34(9):560-564.
109. Kakebeeke TH, Lechner H, Baumberger M, et al: The importance of posture on the isokinetic assessment of spasticity. *Spinal Cord* 2002;40(5): 536-543.
110. Patrick JH: Case for gait analysis as part of the management of incomplete spinal cord injury. *Spinal Cord* 2003;41(9):479-482.
111. Perell K, Scremin A, Scremin O, Kunkel C: Quantifying muscle tone in spinal cord injury patients using isokinetic dynamometric techniques. *Paraplegia* 1996;34(1):46-53.
112. Seib TP, Price R, Reyes MR, Lehmann JF: The quantitative measurement of spasticity: Effect of cutaneous electrical stimulation. *Arch Phys Med Rehabil* 1994;75(7):746-750.
113. Sköld C, Levi R, Seiger A: Spasticity after traumatic spinal cord injury: Nature, severity, and location. *Arch Phys Med Rehabil* 1999;80(12): 1548-1557.
114. Sköld C, Harms-Ringdahl K, Seiger A: Movement-provoked muscle torque and EMG activity in longstanding motor complete spinal cord injured individuals. *J Rehabil Med* 2002;34(2):86-90.
115. Suzuki T, Sonoda S, Saitoh E, et al: Prediction of gait outcome with the knee-ankle-foot orthosis with medial hip joint in patients with spinal cord injuries: A study using recursive partitioning analysis. *Spinal Cord* 2007;45(1):57-63.
116. van der Salm A, Veltink PH, Hermens HJ, Ijzerman MJ, Nene AV: Development of a new method for objective assessment of spasticity using full range passive movements. *Arch Phys Med Rehabil* 2005;86(10):1991-1997.
117. Elovic E: Principles of pharmaceutical management of spastic hypertonia. *Phys Med Rehabil Clin N Am* 2001;12(4):793-816, vii.
118. Gracies JM, Nance P, Elovic E, McGuire J, Simpson DM: Traditional pharmacological treatments for spasticity: Part II. General and regional treatments. *Muscle Nerve Suppl* 1997;6:S92-S120.
119. Hayes KC, Potter PJ, Wolfe DL, Hsieh JT, Delaney GA, Blight AR: 4-Aminopyridine-sensitive neurologic deficits in patients with spinal cord injury. *J Neurotrauma* 1994;11(4):433-446.
120. Hinderer SR, Lehmann JF, Price R, White O, deLateur BJ, Deitz J: Spasticity in spinal cord injured persons: Quantitative effects of baclofen and placebo treatments. *Am J Phys Med Rehabil* 1990; 69(6):311-317.
121. Jamous A, Kennedy P, Psychol C, Grey N: Psychological and emotional effects of the use of oral baclofen: A preliminary study. *Paraplegia* 1994; 32(5):349-353.
122. Kogel RW, Johnson PB, Chintam R, Robinson CJ, Nemchausky BA: Treatment of spasticity in spinal cord injury with Dronabinol, a Tetrahydrocannabinol derivative. *Am J Ther* 1995;2(10):799-805.
123. Segatore M, Miller M: The pharmacotherapy of spinal spasticity: A decade of progress I. Theoretical aspects. *SCI Nurs* 1994;11(3):66-69.
124. Segatore M, Miller M: The pharmacotherapy of spinal spasticity: A decade of progress. II: Therapeutics. *SCI Nurs* 1995;12(1):2-7.
125. Broderick CP, Radnitz CL, Bauman WA: Diazepam usage in veterans with spinal cord injury. *J Spinal Cord Med* 1997;20(4):406-409.
126. Abel NA, Smith RA: Intrathecal baclofen for treatment of intractable spinal spasticity. *Arch Phys Med Rehabil* 1994;75(1):54-58.
127. Aisen ML, Dietz M, McDowell F, Kutt H: Baclofen toxicity in a patient with subclinical renal insufficiency. *Arch Phys Med Rehabil* 1994;75(1): 109-111.
128. Akman MN, Loubser PG, Fife CE, Donovan WH: Hyperbaric oxygen therapy: Implications for spinal cord injury patients with intrathecal baclofen infusion pumps. Case report. *Paraplegia* 1994; 32(4):281-284.
129. Korenkov AI, Niendorf WR, Darwish N, Glaeser E, Gaab MR: Continuous intrathecal infusion of baclofen in patients with spasticity caused by spinal cord injuries. *Neurosurg Rev* 2002;25(4): 228-230.
130. Kravitz HM, Corcos DM, Hansen G, Penn RD, Cartwright RD, Gianino J: Intrathecal baclofen: Effects on nocturnal leg muscle spasticity. *Am J Phys Med Rehabil* 1992;71(1):48-52.
131. Lewis KS, Mueller WM: Intrathecal baclofen for severe spasticity secondary to spinal cord injury. *Ann Pharmacother* 1993;27(6):767-774.
132. Loubser PG, Narayan RK, Sandin KJ, Donovan WH, Russell KD: Continuous infusion of intrathecal baclofen: Long-term effects on spasticity in spinal cord injury. *Paraplegia* 1991;29(1):48-64.
133. Loubser PG, Akman NM: Effects of intrathecal baclofen on chronic spinal cord injury pain. *J Pain Symptom Manage* 1996;12(4):241-247.
134. Macdonell RA, Talalla A, Swash M, Grundy D: Intrathecal baclofen and the H-reflex. *J Neurol Neurosurg Psychiatry* 1989;52(9):1110-1112.
135. Meythaler JM, Steers WD, Tuel SM, Cross LL, Haworth CS: Continuous intrathecal baclofen in spinal cord spasticity: A prospective study. *Am J Phys Med Rehabil* 1992;71(6):321-327.

136. Ochs G, Struppler A, Meyerson BA, et al: Intrathecal baclofen for long-term treatment of spasticity: A multi-centre study. *J Neurol Neurosurg Psychiatry* 1989;52(8):933-939.
137. Penn RD, Savoy SM, Corcos D, et al: Intrathecal baclofen for severe spinal spasticity. *N Engl J Med* 1989;320(23):1517-1521.
138. Brenner R, Hyman N, Knobler R, O'Brien M, Stephan T: An approach to switching patients from baclofen to tizanidine. *Hosp Med* 1998; 59(10):778-782.
139. Gruenthal M, Mueller M, Olson WL, Priebe MM, Sherwood AM, Olson WH: Gabapentin for the treatment of spasticity in patients with spinal cord injury. *Spinal Cord* 1997;35(10):686-689.
140. Nance PW, Shears AH, Nance DM: Reflex changes induced by clonidine in spinal cord injured patients. *Paraplegia* 1989;27(4):296-301.
141. Nance PW: A comparison of clonidine, cyproheptadine and baclofen in spastic spinal cord injured patients. *J Am Paraplegia Soc* 1994;17(3):150-156.
142. Nance PW, Bugaresti J, Shellenberger K, Sheremata W, Martinez-Arizala A, North American Tizanidine Study Group: Efficacy and safety of tizanidine in the treatment of spasticity in patients with spinal cord injury. *Neurology* 1994; 44(11, Suppl 9)S44-S52.
143. Potter PJ, Hayes KC, Segal JL, et al: Randomized double-blind crossover trial of fampridine-SR (sustained release 4-aminopyridine) in patients with incomplete spinal cord injury. *J Neurotrauma* 1998;15(10):837-849.
144. Potter PJ, Hayes KC, Hsieh JT, Delaney GA, Segal JL: Sustained improvements in neurological function in spinal cord injured patients treated with oral 4-aminopyridine: Three cases. *Spinal Cord* 1998;36(3):147-155.
145. Priebe MM, Sherwood AM, Graves DE, Mueller M, Olson WH: Effectiveness of gabapentin in controlling spasticity: A quantitative study. *Spinal Cord* 1997;35(3):171-175.
146. Ridgeway B, Wallace M, Gerayli A: Ziconotide for the treatment of severe spasticity after spinal cord injury. *Pain* 2000;85(1-2):287-289.
147. Segal JL, Pathak MS, Hernandez JP, Himber PL, Brunnemann SR, Charter RS: Safety and efficacy of 4-aminopyridine in humans with spinal cord injury: A long-term, controlled trial. *Pharmacotherapy* 1999;19(6):713-723.
148. Weingarden SI, Belen JG: Clonidine transdermal system for treatment of spasticity in spinal cord injury. *Arch Phys Med Rehabil* 1992;73(9): 876-877.
149. Yablon SA, Sipski ML: Effect of transdermal clonidine on spinal spasticity: A case series. *Am J Phys Med Rehabil* 1993;72(3):154-157.
150. Zachariah SB, Borges EF, Varghese R, Cruz AR, Ross GS: Positive response to oral divalproex sodium (Depakote) in patients with spasticity and pain. *Am J Med Sci* 1994;308(1):38-40.
151. Rémy-Néris O, Barbeau H, Daniel O, Boiteau F, Bussel B: Effects of intrathecal clonidine injection on spinal reflexes and human locomotion in incomplete paraplegic subjects. *Exp Brain Res* 1999; 129(3):433-440.
152. Rémy-Néris O, Denys P, Bussel B: Intrathecal clonidine for controlling spastic hypertonia. *Phys Med Rehabil Clin N Am* 2001;12(4):939-951, ix.
153. Chabal C, Jacobson L, Schwid HA: An objective comparison of intrathecal lidocaine versus fentanyl for the treatment of lower extremity spasticity. *Anesthesiology* 1991;74(4):643-646.
154. Middleton JW, Siddall PJ, Walker S, Molloy AR, Rutkowski SB: Intrathecal clonidine and baclofen in the management of spasticity and neuropathic pain following spinal cord injury: A case study. *Arch Phys Med Rehabil* 1996;77(8):824-826.
155. Azouvi P, Mane M, Thiebaut JB, Denys P, Remy-Neris O, Bussel B: Intrathecal baclofen administration for control of severe spinal spasticity: Functional improvement and long-term follow-up. *Arch Phys Med Rehabil* 1996;77(1):35-39.
156. Becker WJ, Harris CJ, Long ML, Ablett DP, Klein GM, DeForge DA: Long-term intrathecal baclofen therapy in patients with intractable spasticity. *Can J Neurol Sci* 1995;22(3):208-217.
157. Berg-Johnsen J, Røste GK, Solgaard T, Lundar T: Continuous intrathecal infusion of baclofen: A new therapeutic method for spasticity. *Tidsskr Nor Laegeforen* 1998;118(21):3256-3260.
158. Boviatsis EJ, Kouyialis AT, Korfias S, Sakas DE: Functional outcome of intrathecal baclofen administration for severe spasticity. *Clin Neurol Neurosurg* 2005;107(4):289-295.
159. Burns AS, Meythaler JM: Intrathecal baclofen in tetraplegia of spinal origin: Efficacy for upper extremity hypertonia. *Spinal Cord* 2001;39(8): 413-419.
160. Chartier-Kastler E, Azouvi P, Yakovleff A, Bussel B, Richard F, Denys P: Intrathecal catheter with subcutaneous port for clonidine test bolus injection: A new route and type of treatment for detrusor hyperreflexia in spinal cord-injured patients. *Eur Urol* 2000;37(1):14-17.
161. Coffey JR, Cahill D, Steers W, et al: Intrathecal baclofen for intractable spasticity of spinal origin: Results of a long-term multicenter study. *J Neurosurg* 1993;78(2):226-232.
162. Elovic E, Kirshblum SC: Managing spasticity in spinal cord injury: Safe administration of bridge boluses during intrathecal baclofen pump refills. *J Spinal Cord Med* 2003;26(1):2-4.

163. Ethans KD, Schryvers OI, Nance PW, Casey AR: Intrathecal drug therapy using the Codman Model 3000 Constant Flow Implantable Infusion Pumps: Experience with 17 cases. *Spinal Cord* 2005;43(4):214-218.

164. Gardner B, Jamous A, Teddy P, et al: Intrathecal baclofen—a multicentre clinical comparison of the Medtronics Programmable, Cordis Secor and Constant Infusion Infusaid drug delivery systems. *Paraplegia* 1995;33(10):551-554.

165. Gerszten PC, Labirght AL, Barry MJ: Effect on ambulation of continuous intrathecal baclofen infusion. *Pediatr Neruosurg* 1997;27(1):40-44.

166. Gianino JM, York MM, Paice JA, Shott S: Quality of life: Effect of reduced spasticity from intrathecal baclofen. *J Neurosci Nurs* 1998;30(1):47-54.

167. Herman RM, D'Luzansky SC, Ippolito R: Intrathecal baclofen suppresses central pain in patients with spinal lesions: A pilot study. *Clin J Pain* 1992;8(4):338-345.

168. Ivanhoe CB, Tilton AH, Francisco GE: Intrathecal baclofen therapy for spastic hypertonia. *Phys Med Rehabil Clin N Am* 2001;12(4):923-938.

169. Kamensek J: Continuous intrathecal baclofen infusions: An introduction and overview. *Axone* 1999;20(3):67-72.

170. Kamensek J: Continuous intrathecal baclofen infusions: An introduction and overview. *Axone* 1999;20(4):93-98.

171. Nance P, Schryvers O, Schmidt B, Dubo H, Loveridge B, Fewer D: Intrathecal baclofen therapy for adults with spinal spasticity: Therapeutic efficacy and effect on hospital admissions. *Can J Neurol Sci* 1995;22(1):22-29.

172. Plassat R, Perrouin Verbe B, Menei P, Menegalli D, Mathé JF, Richard I: Treatment of spasticity with intrathecal Baclofen administration: Long-term follow-up, review of 40 patients. *Spinal Cord* 2004;42(12):686-693.

173. Thompson E, Hicks F: Intrathecal baclofen and homeopathy for the treatment of painful muscle spasms associated with malignant spinal cord compression. *Palliat Med* 1998;12(2):119-121.

174. Dario A, Scamoni C, Picano M, Casagrande F, Tomei G: Pharmacological complications of the chronic baclofen infusion in the severe spinal spasticity: Personal experience and review of the literature. *J Neurosurg Sci* 2004;48(4):177-181.

175. Douglas AF, Weiner HL, Schwartz DR: Prolonged intrathecal baclofen withdrawal syndrome: Case report and discussion of current therapeutic management. *J Neurosurg* 2005;102(6):1133-1136.

176. Green LB, Nelson VS: Death after acute withdrawal of intrathecal baclofen: Case report and literature review. *Arch Phys Med Rehabil* 1999; 80(12):1600-1604.

177. Kofler M, Kronenberg MF, Rifici C, Saltuari L, Bauer G: Epileptic seizures associated with intrathecal baclofen application. *Neurology* 1994; 44(1):25-27.

178. Protopapas MG, Bundock E, Westmoreland S, Nero C, Graham WA, Nesathurai S: The complications of scar formation associated with intrathecal pump placement. *Arch Phys Med Rehabil* 2007; 88(3):389-390.

179. Rivas DA, Chancellor MB, Hill K, Freedman MK: Neurological manifestations of baclofen withdrawal. *J Urol* 1993;150(6):1903-1905.

180. Schurch B: Errors and limitations of the multimodality checking methods of defective spinal intrathecal pump systems: Case report. *Paraplegia* 1993;31(9):611-615.

181. Soni BM, Mani RM, Oo T, Vaidyanathan S: Treatment of spasticity in a spinal cord-injured patient with intrathecal morphine due to intrathecal baclofen tolerance—a case report and review of literature. *Spinal Cord* 2003;41(10):586-589.

182. Soni BM, Oo T, Vaidyanathan S, Hughes PL, Singh G: Complications of sacral anterior root stimulator implantation in a cervical spinal cord injury patient: Increased spasms requiring intrathecal baclofen therapy followed by delayed fracture of lumbar spine leading to intractable spasms compelling disuse of the sacral anterior root stimulator. *Spinal Cord* 2004;42(2):136-138.

183. Teddy P, Jamous A, Gardner B, Wang D, Silver J: Complications of intrathecal baclofen delivery. *Br J Neurosurg* 1992;6(2):115-118.

184. Rushton DN, Lloyd AC, Anderson PM: Cost-effectiveness comparison of tizanidine and baclofen in the management of spasticity. *Pharmacoeconomics* 2002;20(12):827-837.

185. Savoy SM, Gianino JM: Intrathecal baclofen infusion: an innovative approach for controlling spinal spasticity. *Rehabil Nurs* 1993;18(2):105-113.

186. Stempien L, Tsai T: Intrathecal baclofen pump use for spasticity: A clinical survey. *Am J Phys Med Rehabil* 2000;79(6):536-541.

187. Vogt T, Urban PP: Optimized therapy of spastic syndrome by combination intrathecal baclofen with botulinum toxin. *Nervenarzt* 2000;71(12): 1007-1011.

188. Zahavi A, Geertzen JH, Middel B, Staal M, Rietman JS: Long term effect (more than five years) of intrathecal baclofen on impairment, disability, and quality of life in patients with severe spasticity of spinal origin. *J Neurol Neurosurg Psychiatry* 2004;75(11):1553-1557.

189. Botte MJ, Keenan MA: Reconstructive surgery of the upper extremity in the patient with head trauma. *J Head Trauma Rehabil* 1987;2(2):34-45.

190. Botte MJ, Abrams RA, Bodine-Fowler SC: Treatment of acquired muscle spasticity using phenol peripheral nerve blocks. *Orthopedics* 1995;18(2): 151-159.
191. Braun RM, Hoffer MM, Mooney V, McKeever J, Roper B: Phenol nerve block in the treatment of acquired spastic hemiplegia in the upper limb. *J Bone Joint Surg Am* 1973;55(3):580-585.
192. Garland DE, Lilling M, Keenan MA: Percutaneous phenol blocks to motor points of spastic forearm muscles in head-injured adults. *Arch Phys Med Rehabil* 1984;65(5):243-245.
193. Kirshblum S: Treatment alternatives for spinal cord injury related spasticity. *J Spinal Cord Med* 1999;22(3):199-217.
194. Mooney V, Frykman G, McLamb J: Current status of intraneural phenol injections. *Clin Orthop Relat Res* 1969;63:122-131.
195. Moore TJ, Anderson RB: The use of open phenol blocks to the motor branches of the tibial nerve in adult acquired spasticity. *Foot Ankle* 1991; 11(4):219-221.
196. Bell KR, Williams F: Use of botulinum toxin type A and type B for spasticity in upper and lower limbs. *Phys Med Rehabil Clin N Am* 2003;14(4): 821-835.
197. Ben Smaïl D, Denys P, Bussel B: Botulinum toxin and spinal cord injury. *Ann Readapt Med Phys* 2003;46(6):296-298.
198. Fried GW, Fried KM: Spinal cord injury and use of botulinum toxin in reducing spasticity. *Phys Med Rehabil Clin N Am* 2003;14(4):901-910.
199. O'Brien CF: Treatment of spasticity with botulinum toxin. *Clin J Pain* 2002;18(6, Suppl): S182-S190.
200. Richardson D, Edwards S, Sheean GL, Greenwood RJ, Thompson AJ: The effect of botulinum toxin on hand function after incomplete spinal cord injury at the level of C5/6: A case report. *Clin Rehabil* 1997;11(4):288-292.
201. Richardson D, Sheean G, Werring D, et al: Evaluating the role of botulinum toxin in the management of focal hypertonia in adults. *J Neurol Neurosurg Psychiatry* 2000;69(4):499-506.
202. Aydin G, Tomruk S, Keleş I, Demir SO, Orkun S: Transcutaneous electrical nerve stimulation versus baclofen in spasticity: Clinical and electrophysiologic comparison. *Am J Phys Med Rehabil* 2005; 84(8):584-592.
203. Barolat G, Singh-Sahni K, Staas WE Jr, Shatin D, Ketcik B, Allen K: Epidural spinal cord stimulation in the management of spasms in spinal cord injury: A prospective study. *Stereotact Funct Neurosurg* 1995;64(3):153-164.
204. Goulet C, Arsenault AB, Bourbonnais D, Laramée MT, Lepage Y: Effects of transcutaneous electrical nerve stimulation on H-reflex and spinal spasticity. *Scand J Rehabil Med* 1996;28(3):169-176.
205. Midha M, Schmitt JK: Epidural spinal cord stimulation for the control of spasticity in spinal cord injury patients lacks long-term efficacy and is not cost-effective. *Spinal Cord* 1998;36(3):190-192.
206. Ragnarsson KT: Physiologic effects of functional electrical stimulation-induced exercises in spinal cord-injured individuals. *Clin Orthop Relat Res* 1988;233:53-63.
207. Sadowsky CL: Electrical stimulation in spinal cord injury. *NeuroRehabilitation* 2001;16(3):165-169.
208. van der Salm A, Veltink PH, Ijzerman MJ, Groothuis-Oudshoorn KC, Nene AV, Hermens HJ: Comparison of electric stimulation methods for reduction of triceps surae spasticity in spinal cord injury. *Arch Phys Med Rehabil* 2006;87(2): 222-228.
209. Krause P, Straube A: Reduction of spastic tone increase induced by peripheral repetitive magnetic stimulation is frequency-independent. *NeuroRehabilitation* 2005;20(1):63-65.
210. Dalyan M, Sherman A, Cardenas DD: Factors associated with contractures in acute spinal cord injury. *Spinal Cord* 1998;36(6):405-408.
211. Braun RM, West F, Mooney V, Nickel VL, Roper B, Caldwell C: Surgical treatment of the painful shoulder contracture in the stroke patient. *J Bone Joint Surg Am* 1971;53(7):1307-1312.
212. Keenan MA, Abrams RA, Garland DE, Waters RL: Results of fractional lengthening of the finger flexors in adults with upper extremity spasticity. *J Hand Surg Am* 1987;12(4):575-581.
213. Botte MJ: Neuromuscular disorders, in Thordarson DB, ed: *Orthopaedic Surgery Essentials: Foot and Ankle*. Philadelphia, PA, Lippincott, Williams and Wilkins, 2004 pp 41-78.
214. Keenan MA, Ure K, Smith CM, Jordan C: Hamstring release for knee flexion contracture in spastic adults. *Clin Orthop Rel Res* 1988;236:221-226.
215. Botte MJ, Bruffey JD, Copp SN, Colwell CW: Surgical reconstruction of acquired spastic foot and ankle deformity. *Foot Ankle Clin* 2000;5(2): 381-416.
216. Botte MJ: Management of lower extremity deformity in acquired spasticity, in Myerson MS, ed: *Foot and Ankle Disorder*. Philadelphia, PA, WB Saunders, 2000, pp 900-918.
217. Botte MJ: Equinovarus deformity, in Nunley JA, Pfeffer GB, Sanders RW, Trepman E, eds: *Advanced Reconstruction: Foot and Ankle*. Rosemont, IL, American Academy of Orthopaedic Surgeons, 2004, pp 487-492.
218. Waters RL, Garland DE: Acquired neurologic disorders of the adult foot, in Mann RA, ed: *Surgery*

of the Foot. St. Louis, MO, CV Mosby, 1986, pp 332-341.

219. Moberg E, ed: *The Upper Limb in Tetraplegia: A New Approach to Surgical Rehabilitation*. Stuttgart, Germany, George Thieme Verlag, 1978.
220. Moberg EA, Lamb DW: Surgical rehabilitation of the upper limb in tetraplegia. *Hand* 1980;12(2): 209-213.
221. Moberg EA: Upper limb surgical rehabilitation in tetraplegia, in Evarts CM, ed: *Surgery of the Musculoskeletal System*. New York, NY, Churchill Livingstone, 1983.
222. Ejeskar A: Reconstruction of grip function in tetraplegia, in Fridén J, ed: *Tendon Transfers in Reconstructive Hand Surgery*. Federation of the European Societies for Surgery of the Hand. Boca Raton, FL, Taylor and Francis, 2005, pp 103-119.
223. Freehafer AA, Vonhaam E, Allen V: Tendon transfers to improve grasp after injuries of the cervical spinal cord. *J Bone Joint Surg Am* 1974;56(5): 951-959.
224. Freehafer AA: Tendon transfers in patients with cervical spinal cord injury. *J Hand Surg Am* 1991; 16(5):804-809.
225. Fridén J, Ejeskär A, Dahlgren A, Lieber RL: Protection of the deltoid to triceps tendon transfer repair sites. *J Hand Surg Am* 2000;25(1):144-149.
226. Fridén J, Lieber RL: Quantitative evaluation of the posterior deltoid to triceps tendon transfer based on muscle architectural properties. *J Hand Surg Am* 2001;26(1):147-155.
227. Fridén J: Reconstructive hand surgery improves hand function in tetraplegia: Basic research and clinical studies paved the way for this development. *Lakartidningen* 2003;100(24):2133-2139.
228. Fridén J: Reconstruction of elbow extension in tetraplegia, in Fridén J, ed: *Tendon Transfers in Reconstructive Hand Surgery*. Federation of the European Societies for Surgery of the Hand. Boca Raton, FL, Taylor and Francis, 2005.
229. Fridén J, ed: *Tendon Transfers in Reconstructive Hand Surgery*. Federation of the European Societies for Surgery of the Hand. Boca Raton, FL, Taylor and Francis, 2005.
230. Fridén J: New concepts in reconstruction of arm and hand function in tetraplegia—basic research and clinical application. *Handchir Mikrochir Plast Chir* 2005;37(4):223-229.
231. Hentz VR, Brown M, Keoshian LA: Upper limb reconstruction in quadriplegia: Functional assessment and proposed treatment modifications. *J Hand Surg Am* 1983;8(2):119-131.
232. Hentz VR, Hamlin C, Keoshian LA: Surgical reconstruction in tetraplegia. *Hand Clin* 1988;4(4): 601-607.
233. House JH, Gwathmey FW, Lundsgaard DK: Restoration of strong grasp and lateral pinch in tetraplegia due to cervical spinal cord injury. *J Hand Surg Am* 1976;1(2):152-159.
234. House JH, Shannon MA: Restoration of strong grasp and lateral pinch in tetraplegia: A comparison of two methods of thumb control in each patient. *J Hand Surg Am* 1985;10(1):22-29.
235. House JH: Reconstruction of the thumb in tetraplegia following spinal cord injury. *Clin Orthop Relat Res* 1985;195:117-128.
236. Kelly CM, Freehafer AA, Peckham PH, Stroh K: Postoperative results of opponensplasty and flexor tendon transfer in patients with spinal cord injuries. *J Hand Surg Am* 1985;10(6 Pt 1):890-894.
237. Lacey SH, Wilber RG, Peckham PH, Freehafer AA: The posterior deltoid to triceps transfer: A clinical and biomechanical assessment. *J Hand Surg Am* 1986;11(4):542-547.
238. Lamb DW, Chan KM: Surgical reconstruction of the upper limb in traumatic tetraplegia: A review of 41 patients. *J Bone Joint Surg Br* 1983;65(3): 291-298.
239. Landi A, Mulcahey MJ, Caserta G, Della Rosa N: Tetraplegia: Update on assessment. *Hand Clin* 2002;18(3):377-389.
240. Lieber RL, Fridén J, Hobbs T, Rothwell AG: Analysis of posterior deltoid function one year after surgical restoration of elbow extension. *J Hand Surg Am* 2003;28(2):288-293.
241. McDowell CL: Tetraplegia, in Green DP, ed: *Operative Hand Surgery*, ed 2. New York, NY, Churchill Livingstone, 1988, pp 1597-1618.
242. McDowell CL, Moberg EA, Smith AG: International conference on surgical rehabilitation of the upper limb in tetraplegia. *J Hand Surg Am* 1979; 4(4):387-390.
243. McDowell CL, Moberg EA, House JH: The second international conference on surgical rehabilitation of the upper limb in tetraplegia (quadriplegia). *J Hand Surg Am* 1986;11:604-608.
244. Moberg E: Surgical rehabilitation of the upper limb in tetraplegia. *Paraplegia* 1990;28(5): 330-334.
245. Mohammed KD, Rothwell AG, Sinclair SW, et al: Early complications with the Dacron deltoid to triceps prosthesis: Is Dacron any good? Presented at the *8th International Conference on Upper Limb Surgery for Tetraplegia*. Christchurch, New Zealand, 2004.
246. Mohammed KD, Rothwell AG, Sinclair SW, Willems SM, Bean AR: Upper-limb surgery for tetraplegia. *J Bone Joint Surg Br* 1992;74(6):873-879.
247. Revol M, Briand E, Servant JM: Biceps-to-triceps transfer in tetraplegia: The medial route. *J Hand Surg Br* 1999;24(2):235-237.

248. Smith AG: Early complications of key grip hand surgery for tetraplegia. *Paraplegia* 1981;19(2): 123-126.

249. Van Heest A: Tetraplegia, in Green DP, ed: *Green's Operative Hand Surgery*, ed 5. Philadelphia, PA, Elsevier Chruchill Livingstone, 2005, pp 1271-1295.

250. Waters RL, Moore KR, Graboff SR, Paris K: Brachioradialis to flexor pollicis longus tendon transfer for active lateral pinch in the tetraplegic. *J Hand Surg Am* 1985;10(3):385-391.

251. Zancolli EA: Midcervical tetraplegia with strong wrist extension: A two-stage synergistic reconstruction of the hand. *Hand Clin* 2002;18(3): 481-495.

252. McCarthy CK, House JH, Van Heest A, Kawiecki JA, Dahl A, Hanson D: Intrinsic balancing in reconstruction of the tetraplegic hand. *J Hand Surg Am* 1997;22(4):596-604.

253. Zancolli E: Surgery for the quadriplegic hand with active, strong wrist extension preserved: A study of 97 cases. *Clin Orthop Relat Res* 1975;112: 101-113.

254. Zancolli El: *Structural and Dynamic Basis of Hand Surgery*. Philadelphia, PA, JB Lippincott Co, 1979, p 231.

255. Botte MJ, Pacelli LL: Historical aspects of tendon transfers, in Fridén J, ed: *Tendon Transfers in Reconstructive Hand Surgery*. Federation of the European Societies for Surgery of the Hand. Boca Raton, FL, Taylor and Francis, 2005, pp 21-27.

256. Botte MJ, Pacelli LL: Basic principles in tendon transfer surgery, in Fridén J, ed: *Tendon Transfers in Reconstructive Hand Surgery*. Federation of the European Societies for Surgery of the Hand. Boca Raton, FL, Taylor and Francis, 2005, pp 29-49.

257. Johnson DL, Gellman H, Waters RL, Tognella M: Brachioradialis transfer for wrist extension in tetraplegic patients who have fifth-cervical-level neurological function. *J Bone Joint Surg Am* 1996; 78(7):1063-1067.

258. Lieber RL: Muscle architectural and biomechanical considerations in tendon transfer, in Fridén J, ed: *Tendon Transfers in Reconstructive Hand Surgery*. Federation of the European Societies for Surgery of the Hand. Boca Raton, FL, Taylor and Francis, 2005, pp 1-19.

259. Mulcahey MJ, Lutz C, Kozin SH, Betz RR: Prospective evaluation of biceps to triceps and deltoid to triceps for elbow extension in tetraplegia. *J Hand Surg Am* 2003;28(6):964-971.

260. Nickel VL, Perry J, Garrett AL: Development of useful function in the severely paralyzed hand. *J Bone Joint Surg Am* 1963;45:933-952.

261. Brand PW: *Clinical Mechanics of the Hand*. St. Louis, MO, CV Mosby, 1985.

262. Hiersche DL, Waters RL: Interphalangeal fixation of the thumb in Moberg's key grip procedure. *J Hand Surg Am* 1985;10(1):30-32.

263. Bajd T, Kralj A, Turk R, Benko H, Sega J: Use of functional electrical stimulation in the rehabilitation of patients with incomplete spinal cord injuries. *J Biomed Eng* 1989;11(2):96-102.

264. Bajd T, Karlj A, Stafanic M, Lavrac N: Use of functional electrical stimulation in the lower extremities of incomplete spinal cord injured patients. *Artif Orgnans* 1999;23(5):403-409.

265. Bajd T, Munih M, Kralj A: Problems associated with FES-standing in paraplegia. *Technol Health Care* 1999;7(4):301-308.

266. Bobet J: Can muscle models improve FES-assisted walking after spinal cord injury? *J Electromyogr Kinesiol* 1998;8(2):125-132.

267. Daly JJ, Marsolais EB, Mendell LM, et al: Therapeutic neural effects of electrical stimulation. *IEEE Trans Rehabil Eng* 1996;4(4):218-230.

268. Davis JA Jr, Triolo RJ, Uhlir J, et al: Preliminary performance of a surgically implanted neuroprosthesis for standing and transfers—where do we stand? *J Rehabil Res Dev* 2001;38(6):609-617.

269. Graupe D, Kohn KH: Transcutaneous functional neuromuscular stimulation of certain traumatic complete thoracic paraplegics for independent short-distance ambulation. *Neurol Res* 1997;19(3): 323-333.

270. Keith MW, Peckham PH, Thrope GB, Buckett JR, Stroh KC, Menger V: Functional neuromuscular stimulation neuroprostheses for the tetraplegic hand. *Clin Orthop Relat Res* 1988;233:25-33.

271. Kralj A, Bajd T, Turk R: Enhancement of gait restoration in spinal injured patients by functional electrical stimulation. *Clin Orthop Relat Res* 1988; 233:34-43.

272. Prochazka A, Mushahwar VK, McCreery DB: Neural prostheses. *J Physiol* 2001;533(Pt 1):99-109.

273. Peckham PH, Keith MW, Freehafer AA: Restoration of functional control by electrical stimulation in the upper extremity of the quadriplegic patient. *J Bone Joint Surg Am* 1988;70(1):144-148.

274. Waters RL, Campbell JM, Nakai R: Therapeutic electrical stimulation of the lower limb by epimysial electrodes. *Clin Orthop Relat Res* 1988;233: 44-52.

275. Peckham PH: Functional electrical stimulation: Current status and future prospects of applications to the neuromuscular system in spinal cord injury. *Paraplegia* 1987;25(3):279-288.

276. Popović D, Stein RB, Oğuztöreli N, Lebiedowska M, Jonić S: Optimal control of walking with functional electrical stimulation: A computer simulation study. *IEEE Trans Rehabil Eng* 1999;7(1): 69-79.

277. Aljure J, Eltorai I, Bradley WE, Lin JE, Johnson B: Carpal tunnel syndrome in paraplegic patients. *Paraplegia* 1985;23(3):182-186.

278. Bayley JC, Cochran TP, Sledge CB: The weight-bearing shoulder: The impingement syndrome in paraplegics. *J Bone Joint Surg Am* 1987;69(5): 676-678.

279. Blankstein A, Shmueli R, Weingarten I, Engel J, Ohry A: Hand problems due to prolonged use of crutches and wheelchairs. *Orthop Rev* 1985;14: 29-34.

280. Gellman H, Sie I, Waters RL: Late complications of the weight-bearing upper extremity in the paraplegic patient. *Clin Orthop Relat Res* 1988; 233:132-135.

281. Nichols PJ, Norman PA, Ennis JR: Wheelchair user's shoulder? Shoulder pain in patients with spinal cord lesions. *Scand J Rehabil Med* 1979; 11(1):29-32.

282. Nicholson BD: Evaluation and treatment of central pain syndromes. *Neurology* 2004; 62(5, Suppl 2):S30-S36.

283. Stefaniwsky L, Bilowit DS, Prasad SS: Reduced motor conduction velocity of the ulnar nerve in spinal cord injured patients. *Paraplegia* 1980; 18(1):21-24.

284. Ohry A, Brooks ME, Steinbach TV, Rozin R: Shoulder complications as a cause of delay in rehabilitation of spinal cord injured patients: (Case reports and review of the literature). *Paraplegia* 1978;16(3):310-316.

285. Silfverskiold J, Waters RL: Shoulder pain and functional disability in spinal cord injury patients. *Clin Orthop Relat Res* 1991;272:141-145.

286. Gellman H, Chandler DR, Petrasek J, Sie I, Adkins R, Waters RL: Carpal tunnel syndrome in paraplegic patients. *J Bone Joint Surg Am* 1988; 70(4):517-519.

287. Andrews LG, Armitage KJ: Sudeck's atrophy in traumatic quadriplegia. *Paraplegia* 1971;9(3): 159-165.

288. Gellman H, Eckert RR, Botte MJ, Sakimura I, Waters RL: Reflex sympathetic dystrophy in cervical spinal cord injury patients. *Clin Orthop Relat Res* 1988;233:126-131.

289. Sjölund BH: Pain and rehabilitation after spinal cord injury: The case of sensory spasticity? *Brain Res Brain Res Rev* 2002;40(1-3):250-256.

290. Wainapel SF, Freed MM: Reflex sympathetic dystrophy in quadriplegia: Case report. *Arch Phys Med Rehabil* 1984;65(1):35-36.

291. Little JW, Micklesen P, Umlauf R, Britell C: Lower extremity manifestations of spasticity in chronic spinal cord injury. *Am J Phys Med Rehabil* 1989; 68(1):32-36.

292. Benito-Ruiz J, Baena-Montilla P, Mena-Yago A, Miguel I, Montanana-Vizcaino J: A complicated trochanteric pressure sore: What is the best surgical management? Case report. *Paraplegia* 1993; 31(2):119-124.

293. Bielecki M, Skowroński R, Skowroński J: Sacral pressure sores and their treatment. *Chir Narzadow Ruchu Ortop Pol* 2006;71(1):51-56.

294. Stamate T, Budurcă AR: The treatment of the sacral pressure sores in patients with spinal lesions. *Acta Neurochir Suppl* 2005;93:183-187.

295. Krause JS, Vines CL, Farley TL, Sniezek J, Coker J: An exploratory study of pressure ulcers after spinal cord injury: Relationship to protective behaviors and risk factors. *Arch Phys Med Rehabil* 2001;82(1):107-113.

Index

A

B

C

D

E

F

G

H

J

K

L

M

N

O

P

Q

R

S

T

U

V

W

Z